AUTOIMMUNE DISEASES AND TREATMENT

Organ-Specific and Systemic Disorders

ANNALS OF THE NEW YORK ACADEMY OF SCIENCES

Volume 1051

AUTOIMMUNE DISEASES AND TREATMENT

Organ-Specific and Systemic Disorders

Edited by Yehuda Shoenfeld and M. Eric Gershwin

The New York Academy of Sciences
New York, New York
2005

⊗ *The paper used in this publication meets the minimum requirements of the American National Standard for Information Sciences—Permanence of Paper for Printed Library Materials, ANSI Z39.48-1984.*

Library of Congress Cataloging-in-Publication Data

International Conference on Autoimmunity (4th : 2004 : Budapest, Hungary)
Autoimmune diseases and treatment : organ-specific and systemic disorders / edited by Yehuda Shoenfeld and M. Eric Gershwin.
p. ; cm. — (Annals of the New York Academy of Sciences ; v. 1051)
Includes bibliographical references and index.
ISBN 1-57331-612-1 (cloth : alk. paper) — ISBN 1-57331-613-X (pbk. : alk. paper)
1. Autoimmune diseases—Congresses. I. Shoenfeld, Yehuda. II. Gershwin, M. Eric, 1946- . III. Title. IV. Series.
[DNLM: 1. Autoimmune Diseases—immunology—Congresses. 2. Autoimmune Diseases—therapy—Congresses. 3. Autoimmunity—Congresses. W1 AN626YL v.1051 2005 / WD 305 I603a 2005]
Q11.N5 vol. 1051
[RC600]
500 s—dc22
[616.97′8]

2005014243

GYAT / PCP

Printed in the United States of America
ISBN 1-57331-612-1 (cloth)
ISBN 1-57331-613-X (paper)
ISSN 0077-8923

ANNALS OF THE NEW YORK ACADEMY OF SCIENCES

Volume 1051
June 2005

AUTOIMMUNE DISEASES AND TREATMENT

Organ-Specific and Systemic Disorders

Editors
YEHUDA SHOENFELD AND M. ERIC GERSHWIN

This volume comprises part of the proceedings of the **Fourth International Congress on Autoimmunity**, which was supported by the American Autoimmune Related Diseases Association (AARDA) and the Associazione Patologie Autoimmuni Internazionale (APAI), and held November 3–7, 2004, in Budapest, Hungary.

CONTENTS

Part II. Systematic Autoimmune Diseases

Part III. Treatment

Foreword

As rheumatologists, we are keenly aware of the difficulties, including toxicity, in treating patients with autoimmune disease. Indeed, both of the editors have been practicing clinical rheumatologists for more than 30 years, and it is amazing to us that drugs commonly used in the 1970s remain standard fare today. For example, cyclophosphamide, a nitrogen mustard derivative first synthesized in 1958, is still widely used and is, in fact, carried as a stock item in most pharmacies. Cyclophosphamide has been widely used in rheumatology since at least 1974, and immunosuppressive agents have been used throughout the past 30 years in a variety of non-neoplastic settings—rheumatoid arthritis, systemic lupus erythematosus, Wegener's granulomatosis, polymyositis, scleroderma, glomerulonephritis, uveitis, inflammatory bowel disease, myasthenia gravis, idiopathic thrombocytopenic purpura, cryoglobulinemia, and bullous pemphigoid—with variable results.

Only within the past five years or so have we seen more specific therapy introduced. The highlight of these has been the introduction of anti-TNF agents in the treatment of rheumatoid arthritis, and we have witnessed dramatic improvements in the condition of our patients. On the other hand, we are also acutely aware of the case reports of multifocal leukoencephalopathy in patients receiving anti-TNF, and the long-term safety of these agents is clearly an issue. Other more specific monoclonal therapies have likewise been gaining favor, including anti-CD20, antibodies to the IL-6 receptor, and a host of others. We can only hope that specific therapies, coined the "magic bullet" by Paul Ehrlich, will some day be realized.

On the other hand, we are also aware of the plight of the young mother with rheumatoid arthritis who is unable to dress her children for school and is still unresponsive to the therapies available. In this volume (<http://www.nyas.org/annals/detail.asp?annalID=848>), the second in the series highlighting papers presented at the Fourth International Congress on Autoimmunity (<http://www.kenes.com/autoim2004/>), we present the latest and best science, which we hope will lead to new therapies. [The companion monograph, Volume 1050 (<http://www.nyas.org/annals/detail.asp?annalID=809>), deals with the concepts that underlie autoimmune disease in general.]

The present volume divides the diseases into organ-specific and organ-nonspecific diseases, and one section focuses entirely on treatment. We emphasize the cytokines, the chemokines, the cognate receptors, genetic interactions, the increasing use of intravenous immunoglobulins, and the more appropriate use of both monoclonal as well as immunosuppressive agents. A significant void remains, however, in the management of autoimmunity, a void too often filled with false hope and pharmacologic toxicity. We are reminded of a line from *Hamlet*: "Diseases desperate grown/By desperate appliance are relieved,/Or not at all."

We hope some day that the treatment of autoimmune disease will not be by "desperate appliance," but rather by specific manipulation to correct an underlying

Ann. N.Y. Acad. Sci. 1051: xiii–xiv (2005). © 2005 New York Academy of Sciences.
doi: 10.1196/annals.1361.200

immunological defect. We hope that we will no longer see young mothers unable to dress their children for school. We conclude, however, that although the papers presented in this meeting add a significant intellectual contribution to the underlying science of autoimmunity, the therapeutic void, regrettably, still remains.

—YEHUDA SHOENFELD
—M. ERIC GERSHWIN

Activation, Apoptosis, and Clearance of Neutrophils in Wegener's Granulomatosis

ANDRÉ P. VAN ROSSUM, PIETER C. LIMBURG, AND CEES G. M. KALLENBERG

Department of Internal Medicine, University Medical Center Groningen, 9713 GZ Groningen, the Netherlands

ABSTRACT: Wegener's granulomatosis (WG) is strongly associated with the presence of antineutrophil cytoplasmic autoantibodies (ANCAs). Within WG these ANCAs are usually (80–90%) directed against the azurophilic enzyme proteinase 3, the so called PR3-ANCA. A pathophysiological role for these autoantibodies, supported by numerous *in vitro* and *in vivo* studies, is specifically based on their capacity to bind and activate neutrophils and potentially may damage vessels. In this review, the pathogenic potential of different developmental stages of the neutrophil in the pathogenesis of WG is discussed. After release from the bone marrow into the circulation, neutrophils can be primed by TNFα and become attached to locally activated endothelium. Once attached to the endothelium, ANCAs can fully activate these primed neutrophils. In this activation process, the degree of activation after stimulation with PR3-ANCAs associates with the level of PR3 expression on the membrane of the neutrophil. Following activation, infiltrated neutrophils become apoptotic with further membrane expression of PR3. In WG patients, clearance of apoptotic neutrophils can be disturbed due to the opsonization of PR3-expressing apoptotic neutrophils with PR3-ANCAs, thereby perpetuating inflammation by the release of proinflammory cytokines during clearance; or it may favor autoimmunity by PR3 presentation in an inflammatory environment. Furthermore, the presence of ANCAs and the release of the vessel-related pentraxin PTX3 may lead to the persistence of late apoptotic neutrophils in tissues, thereby inducing leukocytoclastic lesions that are characteristic in patients with WG. All together, alive neutrophils as well as apoptotic neutrophils play a key role in different inflammatory phenomena seen in patients suffering from WG.

KEYWORDS: Wegener's granulomatosis (WG); antineutrophil cytoplasmic autoantibody (ANCA); T lymphocytes; B lymphocytes; inflammation

ANCA-ASSOCIATED VASCULITIS

The antineutrophil cytoplasmic autoantibody (ANCA)-associated vasculitides (AAV) are a group of autoimmune diseases characterized by necrotizing inflammation of arterioles, venules, and capillaries, although larger vessels may be involved as well.[1] These autoantibodies are in most cases directed against the azurophilic

Address for correspondence: Prof. Dr. C. G. M. Kallenberg, Department of Internal Medicine, University Medical Center Groningen, Hanzeplein 1, 9713 GZ Groningen, the Netherlands. Voice: +31-50-3612945; fax: +31-50-3619069.
c.g.m.kallenberg@int.azg.nl

**Ann. N.Y. Acad. Sci. 1051: 1–11 (2005). © 2005 New York Academy of Sciences.
doi: 10.1196/annals.1361.041**

granule proteins proteinase 3 (PR3) or myeloperoxidase (MPO) of the neutrophil designated as PR3-ANCA and MPO-ANCA, respectively. Based on histopathological and clinical manifestations, the Chapel Hill International Consensus Conference defined three major categories of AAV: Wegener's granulomatosis (WG), microscopic polyangiitis (MPA), and Churg–Strauss syndrome (CSS). PR3-ANCAs are found in 80–90% of WG patients and to a lesser extent in patients with MPA; they are found only incidentally in cases of CSS.[2,3] In patients with MPA and CSS, MPO-ANCAs are the dominant autoantibodies, but they occur in a minority of WG patients as well.[2,3]

These ANCAs are supposed to play an important role in the pathogenesis of AAV. Their pathophysiological role is supported by clinical data, animal experimental models, and *in vitro* data, all of which has been reviewed in various papers.[2,4–6] Clinically, ANCA titers have been shown to correlate, although not uniformly, with disease activity: specifically, an increase in ANCA titer frequently precedes a relapse, whereas a decline in titer is seen when remission is induced. In animal models, the pathophysiological role of ANCA has been supported by demonstrating that the transfer of splenocytes from MPO-deficient mice immunized with MPO to Rag2-deficient mice, which lack functional B and T lymphocytes, led to the development of severe necrotizing and crescentic glomerulonephritis.[7] Additionally, direct intravenous injection of anti-MPO antibodies, derived from MPO-immunized MPO-deficient mice, into wild-type or Rag2-deficient mice, resulted in focal necrotizing glomerulonephritis. Finally, *in vitro* studies have shown that ANCAs are capable of activating neutrophils leading to a respiratory burst and degranulation of noxious proteolytic enzymes that may induce endothelial injury.[8–10]

ACTIVATED NEUTROPHILS WITHIN ANCA-ASSOCIATED VASCULITIS

The hypothetical model of how these ANCAs activate neutrophils and harm the endothelium could be formulated as follows: first, neutrophils need to be primed with a low dose of tumor necrosis factor-α (TNFα) to upregulate surface expression of the autoantigens PR3 and MPO in order to allow ANCA binding. More importantly, next to surface expression of autoantigens, priming facilitates the clustering of FcγRIIa and β2 integrins and the formation of the NADPH oxidase complex. Second, neutrophils need to a have an adhesive state as reflected by CD11b/CD18 expression. Finally, when neutrophils are primed and firmly adhere to TNFα-activated endothelium, ANCAs can fully activate neutrophils resulting in degranulation and reactive oxygen species (ROS) production, eventually leading to injury of the vessels. In this activation process, $F(ab')_2$ fragments of ANCAs bind to their autoantigen, PR3 or MPO, whereas the Fc parts of ANCAs interact with neutrophil Fcγ-receptors resulting in full activation; $F(ab')_2$ fragments of ANCAs, as well, have been shown to induce minor activation.[11]

In biopsies from WG patients it has been shown that neutrophils are present and activated at sites of injury. These histological studies from the upper airways of Wegener's patients demonstrated large numbers of activated, apoptotic, and necrotic neutrophils in the early development of vasculitis.[12] Furthermore, in renal infiltrates, neutrophils are present next to monocytes.[13,14] In addition, the activated state of neutrophils and the extracellular localization of lysosomal enzymes was demonstrated in renal biopsies from patients with WG, and numbers of activated neutrophils present in renal biopsies correlated with renal tissue damage.[13]

So, neutrophils seem to play an important role in the pathogenesis of ANCA-associated vasculitis. Therefore, the key role of neutrophils during their cycle of activation, apoptosis, and clearance will be discussed in this review. The focus will be on neutrophils in PR3-ANCA-associated vasculitis.

PR3 EXPRESSION AND ACTIVATION

PR3 is a serine protease mainly stored in the azurophilic granules of neutrophils, but it can also be found in the specific and secretory vesicles as well.[15] Moreover, PR3 can be constitutively present on resting neutrophils. The priming of neutrophils with a low dose of TNFα facilitates the fusion of secretory vesicles and specific granules resulting in a two- to threefold upregulation of PR3 expression on the membrane of the neutrophil.[17] PR3 can be expressed on the membrane (mPR3) of the total population or on a subset of neutrophils (FIG. 1).[15–18] Individuals can be categorized according to their pattern of mPR3 expression on their resting neutrophils into those in whom all neutrophils express none to only minor levels of mPR3 ($mPR3^-$ individuals), individuals in whom all neutrophils express substantial levels of mPR3 ($mPR3^+$ individuals), and so-called bimodal individuals in whom two subsets are present: that is, a subset of neutrophils expressing none to minor levels of mPR3 and a subset expressing substantial levels of mPR3 ($mPR3^{-/+}$). This pattern seems to be genetically determined.[19] Interestingly, bimodal expression is not seen for elastase or other neutrophil markers. The clinical significance of this differential mPR3 expression on neutrophils has been studied by various groups.[18–20] Patients with PR3-ANCA–associated vasculitis have an inreased expression of mPR3 on their resting neutrophils as compared to healthy individuals. Furthermore, Rarok *et al.* demonstrated that an increased expression of mPR3 in vasculitis was associated with an increased incidence and rate of relapse.[18] In further *in vitro* studies, the functional

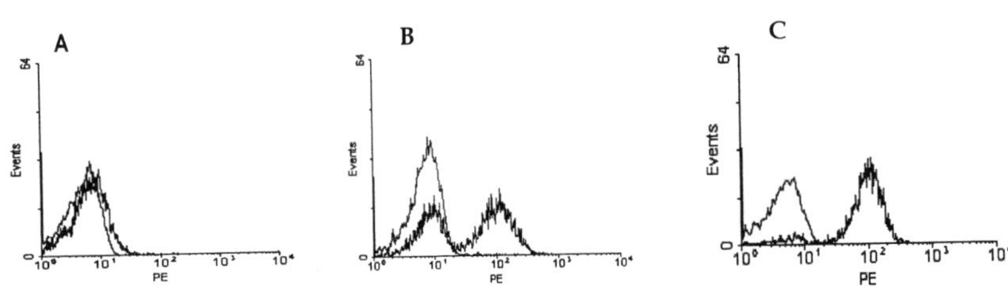

FIGURE 1. Patterns of PR3 surface expression on resting neutrophils: **(A)** $mPR3^-$ donor; **(B)** $mPR3^{-/+}$ or bimodal donor; **(C)** $mPR3^+$ donor. *Bold line* represents cells staining with anti-PR3 antibody; *thin line* respresents nonspecific binding.

significance of mPR3 expression for neutrophil activation after stimulation with anti-PR3 antibodies was analyzed.[17,21] We studied healthy individuals with different patterns of mPR3 expression and measured actin polymerization in neutrophils as an early event in neutrophil activation after stimulation with anti-PR3 antibodies.[17] This proved that even unprimed neutrophils can be activated by anti-PR3 antibodies, as measured by their F-actin polymerization. More importantly, levels of mPR3 expression were associated with the degree of F-actin polymerization after stimulation with anti-PR3 antibodies, further supporting the relation between mPR3 expression and susceptibility for relapses in patients with WG.[17] Thus, increased mPR3 expression on neutrophils in WG is a risk factor for relapse, probably due to increased sensitivity to activation by PR3-ANCAs.

EFFECTS OF APOPTOSIS ON PR3 EXPRESSION OF NEUTROPHILS

The fate of neutrophils after activation is apoptosis. Apoptosis is a genetically programmed cell suicide, characterized by the condensation of cytoplasm and intracellular organelles, cleavage of nuclear chromatin, and formation of apoptotic bodies with or without nuclear remnants.[22] During the induction of apoptosis, several genes encoding proinflammatory factors, signal transduction mediators, adhesion molecules, and other inflammation-related proteins are downregulated.[23] Therefore, several groups have studied changes in the expression of the autoantigens PR3 and MPO on neutrophils and basophilic cells during apoptosis.[24–29] The upregulation of PR3 and MPO during apoptosis could provide an alternative mechanism for ANCAs to interact with neutrophils. Gilligan *et al.* were the first to show that, in the absence of priming, aging neutrophils can translocate PR3 or MPO to the membrane during the apoptotic process, as assessed by increased ANCA binding.[26] Using electron microscopy, translocation to the membrane of cytoplasmic granules (containing PR3) was demonstrated, suggesting that the upregulation of the autoantigen was due to translocation of these granules. Four years later, Yang *et al.* observed that incubation of neutrophils *per se* is already sufficient to translocate ANCA antigens. In that study, unstimulated neutrophils showed increased ANCA antigen expression on the membrane after 4-h incubation; the same cells did not show signs of apotosis.[29] In addition, aging of neutrophils for 24 h, by which 30% became apoptotic, resulted in an increased expression of ANCA antigens. However, no significant difference in autoantigen expression could be found between apoptotic and nonapoptotic cells, implying that the upregulation of these autoantigens was merely a result of priming by minor trauma resulting from *in vitro* incubation. In another study,[27] apoptosis in neutrophils was accelerated by a low dose of TNFα (10 ng/mL) in combination with the protein synthesis inhibitor cycloheximide. By this method, the proapoptotic effect of TNFα is pronounced, whereas the antiapoptotic effects exerted via the NF-κB pathway are blocked by cycloheximide. TNFα-accelerated apoptotic neutrophils showed increased PR3 and MPO expression compared to TNFα-primed live neutrophils.[27] However, an increase of PR3 and MPO expression was only seen in a small proportion of apopotic neutrophils, probably leaky neutrophils, whereas most apoptotic neutrophils showed no increase in cell surface expression. We may conclude from these studies that PR3 and MPO remain on the membrane of neutrophils during apoptosis and are accessible for ANCAs. However, it is not conclusive whether apoptosis intrinsically upregulates expression of these autoantigens on the cell membrane of neutrophils.

APOPTOTIC NEUTROPHILS IN VASCULITIS

In ANCA-associated vasculitis, neutrophils from the peripheral blood show increased apoptosis after incubation *in vitro*.[31] In fact, these neutrophils are more primed, as assessed by increased ANCA-induced superoxide production, and they have increased expression of PR3 on their membrane in comparison to neutrophils of healthy controls. Aging of neutrophils up to 24 h results in their decreased ability to produce superoxides upon stimulation with ANCAs as well as with other potent stimuli.[31] Accelerating apoptosis by TNFα results in further abrogation of ANCA-mediated oxidative burst in neutrophils, which appears to be caspase-3-dependent.[27] Also, ANCAs themselves have been shown to accelerate apoptosis of neutrophils. In a study by Harper *et al.* TNFα-primed neutrophils incubated with IgG purified from ANCA-containing sera showed accelerated apoptosis when compared to control IgG, a process that was dependent on oxygen radical generation.[32] Interestingly, neutrophils in which accelerated apoptosis was induced by ANCAs showed typical features of apoptosis such as shrunken nuclei and internucleasomal cleavage of DNA but no increased externalization of phosphatidylserine. Thus, ANCAs induce increased apoptosis of neutrophils in AAV. These apoptotic neutrophils show upregulated surface expression of PR3 and are, as such, accessible by ANCAs, but they cannot be stimulated to superoxide production by ANCAs.

CLEARANCE OF NEUTROPHILS IN AN INFLAMMATORY CONTEXT

Apoptotic neutrophils are recognized by phagocytic cells, which results in their clearance by phagocytes. Clearance is a process of engulfment and digestion of apoptotic cells and is mainly executed by macrophages in tissues. Apoptotic cells are recognized by their expression of certain surface membrane molecules, mostly altered carbohydrates or phospholipids. A crucial phospholipid in the recognition of apoptotic cells is phosphatidylserine.[33,34]

Normally, the uptake of apoptotic cells by macrophages coincides with the suppression of proinflammatory cytokines such as TNFα and the enhanced production of anti-inflammatory cytokines such as TGF-β, PGE2, and PAF through autocrine and paracrine mechanisms.[35] In this way, clearance is safe and inflammation prevented. However, during ANCA-associated vasculitis, autoantibodies can opsonize apoptotic neutrophils that express PR3 or MPO, leading to an enhanced uptake and production of such proinflammotory cytokines as IL-1, IL-8, and TNFα.[28,31] As a result, clearance is unsafe and the inflammation perpetuated. Another potentially harmful mechanism associated with opsonization by autoantibodies in an inflammatory context is the potential breakdown of tolerance, resulting in autoimmunity. Whether tolerance or immunity is established depends on the maturity state of the dendritic cells (DCs). Immature DCs that internalize necrotic or apoptotic cells need maturation signals to mature. Maturation signals include lipopolysaccharide, interferon-α, and TNFα. Basically, T cell tolerance is induced when apoptotic cells are engulfed in the absence of maturation signals. In contrast, T cell activation and immunity may result when DCs ingest necrotic or apoptotic cells (for instance during a viral infection) leading to a release of maturation signals that induce the upregulation of MHC class II, and subsequently presentation of (auto)antigenic peptides in a MHC class II-restricted manner to T cells. Interestingly, the opsonization of apoptotic cells with anti-β2-glycoprotein I (GPI) autoantibodies facilitated MHC class II-antigen presentation by DCs.[36] In addition, DCs that were challenged with anti-β2-GPI-opsonized apoptotic cells secreted interleukin-1β (IL-1β), TNFα, and IL-10, as such increasing immunogenicity of these apoptotic cells.

Clayton *et al.* studied the effects of apoptotic and necrotic neutrophils on the phenotype of dendritic cells and their ability to stimulate allogeneic T cell proliferation.[37] They showed that the internalization of apoptotic and necrotic neutrophils by immature dendritic cells results in the upregulation of CD83 and MHC class II; whereas CD40, CD80, and CD86 were downregulated, resulting in a decreased ability to stimulate T cell proliferation. However, in the presence of TNFα, downregulation of these maturation markers after engulfment of apoptotic neutrophils was overcome to some extent, suggesting that apoptotic neutrophils in combination with cytokines at sites of inflammation may favor the development of autoimmunity. That apoptotic neutrophils under inflammatory conditions can be autoimmunogenic has been shown by a study by Patry *et al.*[38] They showed that the injection of syngeneic apoptotic neutrophils into Brown Norway rats resulted in the development of ANCAs, although the rats did not develope disease. Thus, clearance of apoptotic neutrophils opsonized by ANCAs will result in an inflammatory reaction that promotes autoantigen presentation and, as such, augments the autoimmune response.

DISTURBANCES IN THE CLEARANCE OF NEUTROPHILS

In WG, 40–50% of the patients have cutaneous manifestations which are, in most cases, histopathologically defined as leukocytoclastic vasculitis (FIG. 2).[39,40] Leukocytoclastic vasculitis is characterized by infiltration and accumulation of unscavenged apoptotic or necrotic neutrophils or fragmented nuclei of neutrophils in the tissues around the vessels (leukocytoclasia), and by the swelling of endothelial cells accompanied by fibrinoid necrosis of vessel walls.[41] Leukocytoclastic lesions are primarily found in the skin, but other organs may be involved as well. Recent studies on the nature of the neutrophilic infiltrate showed a strong positive staining with *in situ* nick end labeling techniques, thereby demonstrating DNA breakdown in the infiltrating neutrophils. In these lesions, only a minor part is typically apoptotic, whereas the majority of neutrophils shows breakdown of DNA with disintegrated cytoplasmic organelles and plasma membrane.[42,43] The phenomenon of leukocytoclasia is interesting since normally dying cells are quickly engulfed by phagocytes, particularly at sites of inflammation. Furthermore, the accumulation of dying cells and the presence of nuclear debris in these lesions suggest that the removal of apoptotic or necrotic cells is incomplete. Pentraxins have been shown to be involved in the removal of dying cells.[44] Classical pentraxins such as serum amyloid P (SAP) and C-reactive protein (CRP) bind to apoptotic cells in a calcium-dependent man-

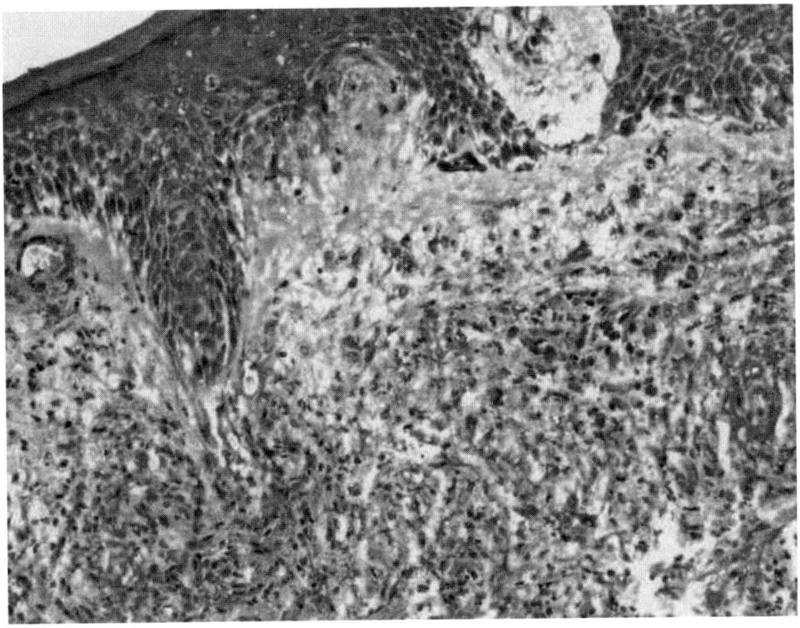

FIGURE 2. Histological specimen of leukocytoclastic vasculitis in the skin with infiltrating neutrophils, nuclear dust, and fibrinoid necrosis of the vessel (hematoxylin-eosin stain; original magnification: ×100). [Figure reduced to 50%.]

ner.[45,46] Subsequently, opsonization with CRP or SAP results in increased binding of the complement component C1q, thereby faciliating uptake.[47,48] In addition, Bijl *et al.* showed that SAP binds specifically to late apoptotic cells and regulates their clearance by macrophages.[49] In contrast, another pentraxin, PTX3, seems to inhibit, rather than facilitate, the uptake of apoptotic cells.[50,51] In view of the persistence of apoptotic neutrophils in leukocytoclastic vasculitis, the role of PTX3 in this phenomenon was further explored.

PTX3 IN VASCULITIS

In vasculitic patients, PTX3 levels correlate, independently from CRP, with disease activity.[52] PTX3 is produced locally at sites of inflammation under the control of proinflammatory signals, usually by endothelial cells or fibroblasts but also by cells of the monocytic lineage.[53,54] PTX3 specifically binds to dying cells, either necrotic or apoptotic,[50] although the binding of PTX3 to necrotic cells is less intense than to chemically or spontaneously induced apoptotic cells. Interestingly, human dendritic cells failed to phagocytose apoptotic cells in the presence of PTX3.[50] In the same study, Rovere *et al.* showed that PTX3 can bind to apoptotic neutrophils as well; however, this happens only in the case of late apoptotic neutrophils and not to vital or early apoptotic neutrophils. Subsequently, we showed that phagocytosis of late apoptotic neutrophils by macrophages was dose-dependently inhibited in the presence of PTX3, whereas SAP facilitated phagocytosis.[51] The inhibitory capacity of PTX3 on the clearance of late apoptotic neutrophils may explain the persistence of apoptotic and necrotic cells at sites of leukocytoclastic lesions. However, PTX3 only inhibits the clearance of late apoptotic neutrophils. In other words, early apoptotic neutrophils should be normally engulfed by phagocytes, particularly in inflammatory tissue. So, where do these late apoptotic or secondary necrotic neutrophils come from? A possible explanation comes from a study by Harper *et al.* in which TNFα-primed neutrophils incubated with IgG purified from ANCA-containing sera showed accelerated apoptosis compared to neutrophils incubated with control IgG.[32] The former neutrophils showed such typical features of apoptosis as shrunken nuclei and internucleosomal cleavage of DNA, but they showed no increased externalization of phosphatidylserine. Furthermore, these neutrophils were less well phagocytosed compared to apoptotic neutrophils incubated with control IgG, possibly due to defective phosphatidylserine expression.

Taken together, ANCAs and PTX3 both seem to be able to disturb the normal clearance of apoptotic neutrophils by macrophages, and, therefore, are candidate factors in the development of leukocytoclastic phenomena in vasculitis.

CONCLUSIONS

Neutrophils are key players in the pathogenesis of WG. Neutrophils are present at sites of injury and their numbers correlate with damage. PR3-ANCAs can activate these cells and, possibly, induce tissue damage. However, this is not their only function. The pathological potential of neutrophils continues after their death. Apoptotic neutrophils, expressing PR3 on their membrane, can be opsonized by PR3-ANCA, resulting in unsafe, proinflammotory clearance by macrophages and the presentation of PR3 or MPO by dendritic cells. In addition, in cases of WG, clearance of apoptotic neutrophils is sometimes incomplete, as shown by the persistence of apoptotic neutrophils (leukocytoclasia). In this phenomenon, ANCAs and a novel, vessel-related pentraxin (PTX3) are supposed to play a role. In conclusion, the pathogenic potential of neutrophils may be exerted in WG during two stages of their lifetime: in their vital and in their apoptotic state. Interaction of ANCAs with vital neutrophils results in the activation of these cells and tissue damage, whereas interaction with apoptotic neutrophils results in inflammatory clearance and the boosting of the PR3- or MPO-specific autoimmune response.

ACKNOWLEDGMENTS

This work was supported by the Dutch Kidney Foundation (Grant No. PC97).

REFERENCES

1. JENNETTE, J., R. FALK, K. ANDRASSY, *et al.* 1994. Nomenclature of systemic vasculitides: proposal of an international consensus conference. Arthritis Rheum. **37:** 187–192.

2. KALLENBERG, C.G., E. BROUWER, J.J. WEENING & J.W. TERVAERT. 1994. Anti-neutrophil cytoplasmic antibodies: current diagnostic and pathophysiological potential. Kidney Int. **46:** 1–15.
3. HOFFMAN, G.S. & U. SPECKS. 1998. Antineutrophil cytoplasmic antibodies. Arthritis Rheum. **41:** 1521–1537.
4. FALK, R.J. & J.C. JENNETTE. 2002. ANCAs are pathogenic—oh yes they are! J. Am. Soc. Nephrol. **13:** 1977–1979.
5. SAVAGE, C.O., L. HARPER & M. HOLLAND. 2002. New findings in the pathogenesis of antineutrophil cytoplasm antibody-associated vasculitis. Curr. Opin. Rheumatol. **14:** 15–22.
6. HUUGEN, D., J.W. TERVAERT & P. HEERINGA. 2004. Antineutrophil cytoplasmic autoantibodies and pathophysiology: new insights from animal models. Curr. Opin. Rheumatol. **16:** 4–8.
7. XIAO, H., P. HEERINGA, P. HU, *et al.* 2002. Antineutrophil cytoplasmic autoantibodies specific for myeloperoxidase cause glomerulonephritis and vasculitis in mice. J. Clin. Invest. **110:** 955–963.
8. CHARLES, L.A., M.L. CALDAS, R.J. FALK, *et al.* 1991. Antibodies against granule proteins activate neutrophils *in vitro*. J. Leukocyte Biol. **50:** 539–546.
9. FALK, R.J., R.S. TERRELL, L.A. CHARLES & J.C. JENNETTE. 1990. Antineutrophil cytoplasmic autoantibodies induce neutrophils to degranulate and produce oxygen radicals *in vitro*. Proc. Natl. Acad. Sci. USA **87:** 4115–4119.
10. MULDER, A.H., P. HEERINGA, E. BROUWER, *et al.* 1994. Activation of granulocytes by antineutrophil cytoplasmic antibodies (ANCAs): a Fc gamma RII-dependent process. Clin. Exp. Immunol. **98:** 270–278.
11. KETTRITZ, R., J.C. JENNETTE & R.J. FALK. 1997. Crosslinking of ANCA-antigens stimulates superoxide release by human neutrophils J. Am. Soc. Nephrol. **8:** 386–394.
12. TRAVIS, W.D., G.S. HOFFMAN, R.Y. LEAVITT, *et al.* 1991. Surgical pathology of the lung in Wegener's granulomatosis: review of 87 open lung biopsies from 67 patients. Am. J. Surg. Pathol. **15:** 315–333.
13. ROUWER, E., M.G. HUITEMA, A.H. MULDER, *et al.* 1994. Neutrophil activation *in vitro* and *in vivo* in Wegener's granulomatosis. Kidney Int. **45:** 1120–1131.
14. WEIDNER, S., M. CARL, R. RIESS & H.D. RUPPRECHT. 2004. Histologic analysis of renal leukocyte infiltration in antineutrophil cytoplasmic antibody-associated vasculitis: importance of monocyte and neutrophil infiltration in tissue damage. Arthritis Rheum. **50:** 3651–3657.
15. WITKO-SARSAT, V., E.M. CRAMER, C. HIEBLOT, *et al.* 1999. Presence of proteinase 3 in secretory vesicles: evidence of a novel, highly mobilizable intracellular pool distinct from azurophil granules. Blood **94:** 2487–2496.
16. HALBWACHS-MECARELLI, L., G. BESSOU, P. LESAVRE, *et al.* 1995. Bimodal distribution of proteinase 3 (PR3) surface expression reflects a constitutive heterogeneneity in the polymorphonuclear pool. FEBS Lett. **374:** 29–33.
17. VAN ROSSUM, A.P., A.A. RAROK, M.G. HUITEMA, *et al.* 2004. Constitutive membrane expression of proteinase 3 (PR3) and neutrophil activation by anti-PR3 antibodies. J. Leukocyte Biol. **76:** 1162–1170.
18. RAROK, A.A., C.A. STEGEMAN, P.C. LIMBURG & C.G. KALLENBERG. 2002. Neutrophil membrane expression of proteinase 3 (PR3) is related to relapse in PR3-ANCA-associated vasculitis. J. Am. Soc. Nephrol. **13:** 2232–2238.
19. SCHREIBER, A., A. BUSJAHN, F.C. LUFT & R. KETTRITZ. 2003. Membrane expression of proteinase 3 is genetically determined. J. Am. Soc. Nephrol. **14:** 68–75.
20. WITKO-SARSAT, V., P. LESAVRE, S. LOPEZ, *et al.* 1999. A large subset of neutrophils expressing membrane proteinase 3 is a risk factor for vasculitis and rheumatoid arthritis. J. Am. Soc. Nephrol. **10:** 1224–1233.
21. SCHREIBER, A., F.C. LUFT & R. KETTRITZ. 2004. Membrane proteinase 3 expression and ANCA-induced neutrophil activation. Kidney Int. **65:** 2172–2183.
22. MAIANSKI, N.A., A.N. MAIANSKI, T.W. KUIJPERS & D. ROOS. 2004. Apoptosis of neutrophils. Acta Haematol. **111:** 56–66.
23. KOBAYASHI, S.D., J.M. VOYICH, K.R. BRAUGHTON & F.R. DELEO. 2003. Down-regulation of proinflammatory capacity during apoptosis in human polymorphonuclear leukocytes. J. Immunol. **170:** 3357–3368.

24. DURANT, S., M. PEDERZOLI, Y. LEPELLETIER, *et al.* 2004. Apoptosis-induced proteinase 3 membrane expression is independent from degranulation. J. Leukocyte Biol. **75:** 87–98.
25. ESNAULT, V.L. 2002. Apoptosis: the central actor in the three hits that trigger antineutrophil cytoplasmic antibody-related systemic vasculitis. Nephrol. Dial. Transplant. **17:** 1725–1728.
26. GILLIGAN, H.M., B. BREDY, H.R. BRADY, *et al.* 1996. Antineutrophil cytoplasmic autoantibodies interact with primary granule constituents on the surface of apoptotic neutrophils in the absence of neutrophil priming. J. Exp. Med. **184:** 2231–2241.
27. KETTRITZ, R., J. SCHEUMANN, Y. XU, *et al.* 2002. TNF-alpha–accelerated apoptosis abrogates ANCA-mediated neutrophil respiratory burst by a caspase-dependent mechanism. Kidney Int. **61:** 502–515.
28. MOOSIG, F., E. CSERNOK, G. KUMANOVICS & W.L. GROSS. 2000. Opsonization of apoptotic neutrophils by antineutrophil cytoplasmic antibodies (ANCAs) leads to enhanced uptake by macrophages and increased release of tumor necrosis factor-alpha (TNF-alpha). Clin. Exp. Immunol. **122:** 499–503.
29. YANG, J.J., R.H. TUTTLE, S.L. HOGAN, *et al.* 2000. Target antigens for antineutrophil cytoplasmic autoantibodies (ANCAs) are on the surface of primed and apoptotic but not unstimulated neutrophils. Clin. Exp. Immunol. **121:** 165–172.
30. KETTRITZ, R., J. SCHEUMANN, Y. XU, *et al.* 2002. TNF-alpha-accelerated apoptosis abrogates ANCA-mediated neutrophil respiratory burst by a caspase-dependent mechanism. Kidney Int. **61:** 502–515.
31. HARPER, L., P. COCKWELL, D. ADU & C.O. SAVAGE. 2001. Neutrophil priming and apoptosis in antineutrophil cytoplasmic autoantibody-associated vasculitis. Kidney Int. **59:** 1729–1738.
32. HARPER, L., Y. REN, J. SAVILL, *et al.* 2000. Antineutrophil cytoplasmic antibodies induce reactive oxygen-dependent dysregulation of primed neutrophil apoptosis and clearance by macrophages. Am. J. Pathol. **157:** 211–220.
33. FADOK, V.A., D.L. BRATTON & P.M. HENSON. 2001. Phagocyte receptors for apoptotic cells: recognition, uptake, and consequences. J. Clin. Invest. **108:** 957–962.
34. HENSON, P.M., D.L. BRATTON & V.A. FADOK. 2001. The phosphatidylserine receptor: a crucial molecular switch? Nat. Rev. Mol. Cell Biol. **2:** 627–633.
35. FADOK, V.A., D.L. BRATTON, A. KONOWAL, *et al.* 1998. Macrophages that have ingested apoptotic cells *in vitro* inhibit proinflammatory cytokine production through autocrine/paracrine mechanisms involving TGF-beta, PGE2, and PAF. J. Clin. Invest. **101:** 890–898.
36. ROVERE, P., M.G. SABBADINI, C. VALLINOTO, *et al.* 1999. Dendritic cell presentation of antigens from apoptotic cells in a proinflammatory context: role of opsonizing antibeta2-glycoprotein I antibodies. Arthritis Rheum. **42:** 1412–1420.
37. CLAYTON, A.R., R.L. PRUE, L. HARPER, *et al.* 2003. Dendritic cell uptake of human apoptotic and necrotic neutrophils inhibits CD40, CD80, and CD86 expression and reduces allogeneic T cell responses: relevance to systemic vasculitis. Arthritis Rheum. **48:** 2362–2374.
38. PATRY, Y.C., D.C. TREWICK, M. GREGOIRE, *et al.* 2001. Rats injected with syngenic rat apoptotic neutrophils develop antineutrophil cytoplasmic antibodies. J. Am. Soc. Nephrol. **12:** 1764–1768.
39. BARKSDALE, S.K., C. W.HALLAHAN, G.S. KERR, *et al.* 1995. Cutaneous pathology in Wegener's granulomatosis: a clinicopathologic study of 75 biopsies in 46 patients. Am. J. Surg. Pathol. **19:** 161–172.
40. DAOUD, M.S., L.E. GIBSON, R.A. DEREMEE, *et al.* 1994. Cutaneous Wegener's granulomatosis: clinical, histopathologic, and immunopathologic features of thirty patients J. Am. Acad. Dermatol. **31:** 605–612.
41. LOTTI, T., I. GHERSETICH, C. COMACCHI & J.L. JORIZZO. 1998. Cutaneous small-vessel vasculitis. J. Am. Acad. Dermatol. **39:** 667–687.
42. BARDUAGNI, S., A. FREZZOLINI, G. FERRANTI, *et al.* 1998. *In situ* labeling of fragmented DNA in cutaneous necrotizing vasculitis. J. Dermatol. Sci. **17:** 160–164.
43. YAMAMOTO, T., Y. KABURAGI, S. IZAKI, *et al.* 2000. Leukocytoclasis: ultrastructural in situ nick end labeling study in anaphylactoid purpura. J. Dermatol. Sci. **24:** 158–165.

44. NAUTA, A.J., M.R. DAHA, C. VAN KOOTEN & A. ROOS. 2003. Recognition and clearance of apoptotic cells: a role for complements and pentraxins. Trends Immunol. **24:** 148–154.
45. FAMILIAN, A., B. ZWART, H.G. HUISMAN, *et al.* 2001. Chromatin-independent binding of serum amyloid P component to apoptotic cells. J. Immunol. **167:** 647–654.
46. GERSHOV, D., S. KIM, N. BROT & K.B. ELKON. 2000. C-Reactive protein binds to apoptotic cells, protects the cells from assembly of the terminal complement components, and sustains an antiinflammatory innate immune response: implications for systemic autoimmunity. J. Exp. Med. **192:** 1353–1364.
47. BHARADWAJ, D., M.P. STEIN, M. VOLZER, *et al.* 1999. The major receptor for C-reactive protein on leukocytes is Fc gamma receptor II. J. Exp. Med. **190:** 585–590.
48. BHARADWAJ, D., C. MOLD, E. MARKHAM & T.W. DU CLOS. 2001. Serum amyloid P component binds to Fc gamma receptors and opsonizes particles for phagocytosis. J. Immunol. **166:** 6735–6741.
49. BIJL, M., G. HORST, J. BIJZET, *et al.* 2003. Serum amyloid P component binds to late apoptotic cells and mediates their uptake by monocyte-derived macrophages. Arthritis Rheum. **48:** 248–254.
50. ROVERE, P., G. PERI, F. FAZZINI, *et al.* 2000. The long pentraxin PTX3 binds to apoptotic cells and regulates their clearance by antigen-presenting dendritic cells. Blood **96:** 4300–4306.
51. VAN ROSSUM, A.P., F. FAZZINI, P.C. LIMBURG, *et al.* 2004. The prototypic tissue pentraxin PTX3, in contrast to the short pentraxin serum amyloid P, inhibits phagocytosis of late apoptotic neutrophils by macrophages. Arthritis Rheum. **50:** 2667–2674.
52. FAZZINI, F., G. PERI, A. DONI, *et al.* 2001. PTX3 in small-vessel vasculitides: an independent indicator of disease activity produced at sites of inflammation. Arthritis Rheum. **44:** 2841–2850.
53. GOODMAN, A.R., T. CARDOZO, R. ABAGYAN, *et al.* 1996. Long pentraxins: an emerging group of proteins with diverse functions. Cytokine Growth Factor Rev. **7:** 191–202.
54. ALLES, V.V., B. BOTTAZZI, G. PERI, *et al.* 1994. Inducible expression of PTX3, a new member of the pentraxin family, in human mononuclear phagocytes. Blood **84:** 3483–3493.

Is PR3-ANCA Formation Initiated in Wegener's Granulomatosis Lesions?

Granulomas as Potential Lymphoid Tissue Maintaining Autoantibody Production

J. VOSWINKEL, A. MÜLLER, AND P. LAMPRECHT

Department of Rheumatology, University of Lübeck, Lübeck, Germany, and Rheumaklinik Bad Bramstedt, 24576 Bad Bramstedt, Germany

ABSTRACT: In Wegener's granulomatosis (WG), antiproteinase 3 (PR3) autoantibodies (PR3-ANCA) are crucial in the development of generalized vasculitis. Wegener's pathognomonic lesion, a granulomatous inflammation of the upper and lower respiratory tract, contains abundant lymphocytes and macrophages. Lymphocyte clusters in germinal center-like formation within the granulomatous lesion are frequently observed, which suggests antigen-driven B cell maturation. Wegener's autoantigen PR3, the target for autoreactive B and T cells, is expressed in granulomatous lesions. Disease progression in WG is accompanied by a profound generalized alteration of T cell differentiation with an increase of effector memory T cells ($CD4^+CD28^-$). The cytokine profile suggests an aberrant Th1-type response either to an environmental trigger and/or the autoantigen PR3 itself. *Staphylococcus aureus*, a risk factor for disease exacerbation, is widely present in the upper airways in WG. The Ig gene repertoire from WG lesions indicates a predominance of VH3+ B cells with affinity to PR3 as well as to the *S. aureus* B cell superantigen SPA. Hence, within the WG lesion, *S. aureus* might support the maturation of PR3-affinity B cells that enter a germinal center reaction in contact with PR3 and T cells and expand, leading to PR3-ANCA production. Thus, granulomatous lesions could represent a potential lymphoid tissue–maintaining autoantibody production rather than a simple, random leukocyte accumulation in WG.

KEYWORDS: Wegener's granulomatosis (WG); granuloma; lymphoid tissue; T lymphocytes; B lymphocytes

ALTERATION OF T CELL PHENOTYPE AND FUNCTION

T cells play a crucial role in upregulating or downregulating immune responses. Chronic inflammation and autoimmune disease, both of which are hallmarks of Wegener's granulomatosis (WG), might be consequences of a failure to adequately control T cell activity. There is substantial evidence that T cells are involved in the pathogenesis of WG. Vasculitic and granulomatous lesions contain abundant T cells,

Address for correspondence: Jan Voswinkel, M.D., Rheumaklinik Bad Bramstedt, Oskar Alexander Strasse 26, 24576 Bad Bramstedt, Germany. Voice: +49-41-92-902762; fax: +49-41-92-902389.

voswinkel@rheuma-zentrum.de

Ann. N.Y. Acad. Sci. 1051: 12–19 (2005).
doi: 10.1196/annals.1361.042

B cells, and macrophages in WG.[1] Soluble IL2-R and other markers are elevated, indicating T cell activation.[2,3] Activation markers such as CD25 and HLA-DR are upregulated on circulating T cells even during remission of the disease and in spite of treatment.[4,5] Oligoclonality and shortened telomeres suggest clonal expansion and replicative senescence of T cells in WG.[6,7] Premature senescence of T cells might be attributed to cytokine's effects, or they might be genetically determined or due to an antigen-driven process. There is evidence that T cell senescence might be antigen-driven in WG. Predominance of IgG1 and IgG3 PR3-ANCA suggests an antigen-driven T cell–dependent immune response.[8] T cells proliferate in response to "Wegener's autoantigen" PR3.[9] Moreover, treatments directed against T cells induce remission in WG.[10,11] Thus, therapeutic intervention disrupting T/B cell collaboration either by targeting T cells or B cells interferes with the disease processes important for the maintenance of WG activity.[10–12]

Whereas naïve T cells are critically dependent on co-stimulation through CD28, a member of the immunoglobulin superfamily, T cell activity of effector and memory T cells is differently regulated through a complex interplay of many receptors. Based on the analysis of cell surface markers and functional studies, it has been shown that CD28 expression is absent in so-called late-differentiated or effector memory T cells.[13,14] The fraction of circulating $CD28^-$ T cells is expanded in WG.[15–17] Organ involvement in WG correlates with the expansion of $CD28^-$ T cells.[17] Expansion of $CD28^-$ T cells in WG is independent of age and treatment. Similar to findings in cases of rheumatoid arthritis, not every patient is affected by this expansion, but the majority of patients are affected.[18,19] The expansion of $CD28^-$ T cells starts early in the disease process and is already evident in localized WG, such as early WG restricted to the respiratory tract. With disease progression to generalized WG, further expansion of $CD28^-$ T cells is seen.[20] In spite of the lack of co-stimulatory CD28 expression, CD28 T cells are not inert or apoptotic. Instead, they display potent effector functions. $CD28^-$ T cells are enriched in bronchoalveolar fluid and abundantly present in granulomatous lesions in WG.[18] Peripheral blood $CD4^+CD28^-$ T cells and $CD4^+CD28^-$ T cells found in granulomatous lesions are a major source of Th1-type cytokine secretion. Cytokine production of circulating $CD4^+CD28^-$ Th1-type cells and $CD4^+CD28^-$ Th1-type cells from granulomatous lesions is mainly restricted to TNF-α and IFN-γ.[19] $CD4^+CD28^-$ T cells display phenotypic markers typical of late-differentiated T cells. They express CD57 (differentiation marker), CD18 (activation marker and adhesion molecule β_2-integrin), and the Th1-type CC-chemokine receptor CCR5 (activation marker and adhesion molecule). A fraction of $CD4^+CD28^-$ T cells show intracytoplasmic perforin expression, indicating their cytotoxic potential.[19,20] Cytotoxic $CD4^+$ T cells have been recognized as a further $CD4^+$ T cell subset, but their role in inflammatory processes has still to be defined.[14]

Skewing of the T cell phenotype affects both $CD4^+$ T cells and $CD8^+$ T cells in WG.[19,21] Analysis of CMV-specific $CD8^+$ T cells shows that the phenotype of CMV-specific T cells is also altered and further skewed towards an effector phenotype. Thus, the alteration of T cell phenotype and function also seems to affect antigen-specific responses and might reflect a profound generalized alteration in T cell differentiation.[21] Although the cause of the expansion of $CD28^-$ T cells in WG is unknown, there is increasing evidence that the escape of prematurely senescent T cells from regulatory control contributes to the maintenance of chronic inflammation and facilitates autoreactivity.[22] Expansion of late differentiated CD28$^-$ Th1-type effector memory T cells on one side could be associated with a decrease of regulatory T cells on the other side. Recently, a reduction of potentially regulatory Th2-type Vα24$^+$Vβ11$^+$ NKT cells has been shown in WG.[23]

CYTOKINE PRODUCTION OF CIRCULATING T CELLS AND T CELLS FROM GRANULOMATOUS LESIONS

Circulating T cells, T cell lines and clones from peripheral blood and bronchoalveolar lavage, and granulomatous lesions from nasal biopsies all exhibit strong Th1-type cytokine responses upon unspecific stimulation in WG.[24,25] The number of CD3$^+$ T cells in granulomatous lesions ranges from 50–70%, whereas 30% of the cells are CD14$^+$ monocytes and macrophages. In localized WG, such as early WG still restricted to the respiratory tract, abundant IFN-γ and CD26 (optional Th1-type marker) expression is seen in the immunohistochemical staining of granulomatous lesions from nasal biopsies. IFN-γ and CD26 expression is less prominent in later stages of generalized WG.[26] Although these studies indicate a predispostion towards an exaggerated Th1-type response in WG,[27] the cytokine response becomes more complex with disease progression. Expression of Th1-type CC-chemokine receptor CCR5 and Th2-type CCR3 on CD4$^+$ and CD8$^+$ T cells is upregulated in localized and generalized WG, suggestive of activation and migratory capacity of T cells. In localized WG, Th1-type CCR5 expression is stronger on circulating T cells as well as in granulomatous lesions compared to generalized WG.[20,28] The CCR5- and CCR3-ligand RANTES (regulated on activation normal T cell expressed and secreted/CCL5) are expressed in granulomatous lesions from the respiratory tract in WG.[29] Predominance of CCR5 expression on T cells in early, localized WG might favor a stronger recruitment of Th1-type cytokine-secreting cells into granulomatous lesions in localized WG as compared to later stages of generalized WG.[20]

The importance of cytokines for the progress of disease activity in WG is underscored by an anecdotal report. A patient with localized WG was treated with IFN-α for acute hepatitis C virus (HCV) infection. IFN-α treatment resulted in reducing HCV to undetectable levels, while WG activity was exacerbated with IFN-α treatment.[30] Taken together, these data suggest that an aberrant Th1-type response to environmental triggers and/or the autoantigen PR3 itself might play an important role in the initiating of WG.[27] Disease progression is associated with a “switch” or further complexity of the collective T cell response. There is evidence of another subset of CCR3$^+$ Th2-type cells and a less prominent Th1-type cytokine production in granulomatous lesions of the upper respiratory tract in generalized WG. This “switch” or increasing complexity of the cytokine profile might be a consequence of further B cell expansion and T cell–dependent PR3-ANCA production during disease progression.[20,21,25,26,31]

PR3-SPECIFIC T CELLS

In WG, T cells proliferate in response to crude granular extraction of neutrophils, inactivated PR3, and single or overlapping linear PR3-derived peptides. However, similar proliferative responses to PR3 are also detected in healthy controls.[9,32–38] Although some studies report a preferential T cell reaction to certain PR3-derived peptide sequences, no immunodominant epitopes have been consistently reported for ANCA-associated vasculitides so far.[9,36,37] The frequency of peripheral blood PR3-specific CD4$^+$TNF-α^+ ($0.64 \pm 0.09\%$, mean $\pm$ SEM) and CD8$^+$TNF-α^+ T cells ($0.65 \pm 0.18\%$) has recently been determined by cytokine flow cytometry. This study used previously reported as well as newly generated HLA-DR and HLA-A and HLA-B binding PR3-derived peptide sequences. Similar to the aforementioned proliferation assays, there was no significant difference in the frequencies of PR3-specific T cells between WG and healthy controls.[39] High IL-10- but low IFN-γ secretion, and IL-4 secretion has been detected after stimulation with PR3 by ELISA.[38,40] Differences in methods and time kinetics with respect to the plasticity of the T cell cytokine response to PR3 may account for the discrepancies in cytokine responses to PR3 reported so far.[41] Thus, in spite of T cell dependent ANCA-production and evidence of T/B cell collaboration,[8,42] differences in the PR3-specific peripheral blood T cells responses have not consistently been detected between WG and healthy controls *in vitro*. However, the *in vivo* situation might be different. WG is characterized by granuloma formation predominantly affecting the respiratory tract. As mentioned above, granulomatous lesions contain abundant T cells, B cells, and macrophages, and may provide a place where such cells might collaborate to evoke autoreactivity.[1]

PR3-SPECIFIC B CELLS

Our group has presented preliminary evidence of lymphoid-like structures and potential maturation of autoreactive PR3-ANCA–producing B cells in granulomatous lesions in WG.[45] Granulomatous tissue specimens from different biopsy-proven localized and generalized WG disease stages were stained for B cells (FIG. 1). DNA from B cell clusters was characterized for rearranged immunoglobulin (Ig) genes. Gene analyzes revealed autoreactive B cells with potential affinity to PR3 in all samples in localized as well as in generalized WG. The mutational pattern of these B cells showed that aggressive courses of disease led to increased selective pressure, whereas the smouldering disease as well as effective immunosuppressive treatment led to Ig genes similar to the healthy repertoire.

ARE GRANULOMATOUS LESIONS A LYMPHOID TISSUE-LIKE STRUCTURE?

T cells are selected on self-peptide/self-MHC complexes in the thymus. Naïve T cells survive through recognition of the same or similar self-peptide/self-MHC complexes in the periphery. There is also some evidence that B cell maturation is also dependent on recognition of self-antigens.[43] After maturation naïve T cells with low affinity for self-antigens and T cells specific for self-antigens that do not access the thymus (such as CNS antigens) are generally ignored.[44] Currently favored mechanisms of a break of tolerance such as molecular mimicry, failure of negative feedback stimulation, impaired regulatory cytokine networks, and decrease in regulatory

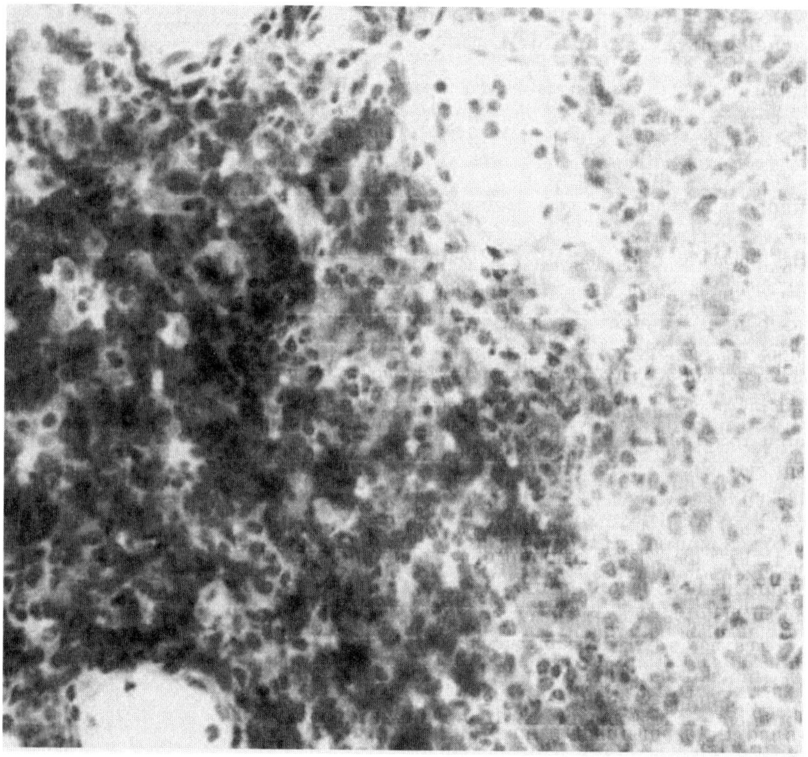

FIGURE 1. CD20 staining of a WG endonasal lesion. A frozen tissue section (8 μm) of an endonasal biopsy specimen from case 2 stained positive for B lymphocytes by anti-CD20 APAAP (red) and was counterstained by hematoxylin (blue). In proximity to an ill-defined Wegener's granuloma (*right*), there is a follicular infiltrate with a B lymphocyte content of more than 30% (original magnification: ×100; reduced to 67%). [Illustration in color online.]

T cells should favor autoimmunity against a random set of self-antigens rather than against particular groups of self-antigens or sole autoantigens as seen in human autoimmune diseases. Therefore, to recognize an autoantigen, break tolerance, and maintain autoimmune disease against a particular self-antigen such as PR3 T and B cells requires particular triggers and lymphoid structures for autoantigen presentation in predisposed individuals.

Neutrophil granulocytes are found more frequently in granulomatous lesions compared to other granulomatous diseases and PR3 is expressed in inflammatory lesions in WG.[46] Since chronic nasal carriage of *Staphylococcus aureus* is a risk factor for exacerbation of WG,[47] there is a possibiltity that such infections might trigger granuloma formation resembling tertiary lymphoid tissue in which faulty autoantigen presentation takes place in individuals predisposed to WG. The Ig gene repertoire from WG lesions indicates a predominance of VH3+ B cells with affinity to PR3 as well as to the *S. aureus* B cell superantigen SPA.[48] Thus, within the WG lesion, *S. aureus* might trigger PR3-affinity B cells that consecutively enter a germinal center reaction in contact with PR3 and T cells and expand, leading to PR3-ANCA production. The inactivation and processing of PR3 from apoptotic neutrophils via antigen-presenting cells such as dendritic cells is aberrant in patients with ANCA-associated vasculitis.[49] T cells could further drive granuloma formation—as suggested by *in vitro* and *in vivo* studies.[50] Alteration of the T cell response and anomalous autoantigen presentation in lymphoid structures could facilitate development of PR3-targeting autoimmune disease in WG.

Rather than being a consequence of random leukocyte recruitment subsequent to PR3-induced vasculitis, granuloma formation in WG could represent a lymphoid structure giving rise to autoantibody production. Induction of subsequent inflammatory lesions through ANCA-induced vasculitis would result in further lymphoid tisssue-like structure formation and induce further autoantibodies; if proven correct one day, this theory would present us with a *perpetuum mobile* of self-maintained inflammation.

REFERENCES

1. GEPHARDT, G.N., M. AHMAD & R.R. TUBBS. 1983. Pulmonary vasculitis (Wegener's granulomatosis): immunohistochemical study of T and B cell markers. Am. J. Med. **74:** 700–704.
2. SCHMITT, W.H., C. HEESEN, E. CSERNOK, *et al.* 1992. Elevated serum levels of soluble interleukin-2 recepetor in patients with Wegener's granulomatosis: association with disease activity. Arthritis Rheum. **35:** 1088–1096.
3. STEGEMAN, C.A., J.W. COHEN-TERVAERT, M.G. HUITEMA, *et al.* 1993. Serum markers of T cell activation in relapses of Wegener's granulomatosis. Clin. Exp. Immunol. **91:** 415–420.
4. POPA, E.R., C.A. STEGEMAN, N.A. BOS, *et al.* 1999. Differential B and T cell activation in Wegener's granulomatosis. J. Allergy Clin. Immunol. **103:** 885–894.
5. CHRISTENSSON, M., E. PETTERSSON, K.G. SUNDQVIST, *et al.* 2000. T cell activation in patients with ANCA-associated vasculitis: inefficient immune suppression by therapy. Clin. Nephrol. **54:** 435–442.
6. VOGT, S., C. IKING-KONERT, F. HUG, *et al.* 2003. Shortening of telomeres: evidence for replicative senescence of T cells derived from patients with Wegener's granulomatosis. Kidney Int. **63:** 2144–2151.
7. GISCOMBE, R., J. GRUNEWALD, S. NITYANAND, *et al.* 1995. T cell receptor (TCR) V gene usage in patients with systemic necrotizing vasculitis. Clin. Exp. Immunol. **101:** 213–219.
8. BROUWER, E., J.W. COHEN-TERVAERT, G. HORST, *et al.* 1991. Predominance of IgG1 and IgG4 subclasses of antineutrophil cytoplasmic antibodies (ANCA) in patients with Wegener's granulomatosi and clinically related disorders. Clin. Exp. Immunol. **83:** 379–386.
9. BALLIEUX, B.E., S.H. VAN DER BURG, E.C. HAGEN, *et al.* 1995. Cell-mediated autoimmunity in patients with Wegener's granulomatosis (WG). Clin. Exp. Immunol. **100:** 186–193.
10. LOCKWOOD, C.M., S. THIRU, J.D. ISAACS, *et al.* 1993. Long-term remission of intractable systemic vasculitis with monoclonal antibody therapy. Lancet **341:** 1620–1622.
11. SCHMITT, W.H., E.C. HAGEN, I. NEUMANN, *et al.* 2004. Treatment of refractory Wegener's granulomatosis with antithymocyte globulin (ATG): an open study in 15 patients. Kidney Int. **65:** 1440–1448.
12. KEOGH, K.A., M.E. WYLAM, J.H. STONE, *et al.* 2005. Induction of remission by B lymphocyte depletion in eleven patients with refractory antineutrophil cytoplasmic antibody-associated vasculitis. Arthritis Rheum. **52:** 262–268.

13. TOMIYAMA, H., T. MATSUDA & M. TAKIGUCHI. 2002. Differentiation of human CD8+ T cells from a memory to memory/effector phenotype. J. Immunol. **168:** 5538–5550.
14. APPAY, V. 2004. The physiological role of cytotoxic CD4(+) T cells: the holy grail. Clin. Exp. Immunol. **138:** 10–13.
15. SCHLESIER, M., T. KASPAR, J. GUTFLEISCH, *et al.* 1995. Activated CD4+ and CD8+ T cell subsets in Wegener's granulomatosis. Rheumatol. Int. **14:** 213–219.
16. GISCOMBE, R., S. NITYANAND, N. LEWIN, *et al.* 1998. Expanded T cell populations in patients with Wegener's granulomatosis: characteristics and correlates with disease activity. J. Clin. Immunol. **18:** 404–413.
17. MOOSIG, F., E. CSERNOK, G. WANG, *et al.* 1998. Costimulatory molecules in Wegener's granulomatosis (WG): lack of expression of CD28 and preferential up-regulation of its ligands B7-1 (CD80) and B7-2 (CD86) on T cells. Clin. Exp. Immunol. **114:** 113–118.
18. LAMPRECHT, P., F. MOOSIG, E. CSERNOK, *et al.* 2001. CD28 negative T cells are enriched in granulomatous lesions of the respiratory tract in Wegener's granulomatosis. Thorax **56:** 751–757.
19. KOMOCSI, A., P. LAMPRECHT, E. CSERNOK, *et al.* 2002. Peripheral blood and granuloma $CD4^+CD28^-$ T cells are a major source of IFN-γ and TNF-α in Wegerner's granulomatosis. Am. J. Pathol. **160:** 1717–1724.
20. LAMPRECHT, P., H. BRUHL, A. ERDMANN, *et al.* 2003. Differences in CCR5 expression on peripheral blood $CD4^+CD28^-$ T cells and in granulomatous lesions between localized and generalized Wegener's granulomatosis. Clin. Immunol. **108:** 1–7.
21. LAMPRECHT, P., A.L. VARGAS-CUERO, A. MULLER, *et al.* 2003. Alterations in the phenotype of CMV-specific and total CD8+ T cell populations in Wegener's granulomatosis. Cell Immunol. 2003 **224:**1–7.
22. VALLEJO, A.N., C.M. WEYAND & J.J. GORONZY. 2004. T cell senescence: a culprit of immune abnormalities in chronic inflammation and persistent infection. Trends Mol. Med. **10:** 119–124.
23. TAKAGI, D., K. IWABUCHI, C. IWABUCHI, *et al.* 2004. Immunoregulatory defects of V alpha 24V+ beta 11+ NKT cells in development of Wegener's granulomatosis and relapsing polychondritis. Clin. Exp. Immunol. **136:** 591–600.
24. LUDVIKSSON, B.R., M.C. SNELLER, K.S. CHUA, *et al.* 1998. Active Wegener's granulomatosis is associated with HLA-DR+ CD4+ T cells exhibiting an unbalanced Th1-type T cell cytokine pattern: reversal with IL-10. J. Immunol. **160:** 3602–3609.
25. CSERNOK, E., A. TRABANDT, A. MULLER, *et al.* 1999. Cytokine profiles in Wegener's granulomatosis: predominance of type 1 (Th1) in the granulomatous inflammation. Arthritis Rheum. **42:** 742–570.
26. MULLER, A., A. TRABANDT, K. GLOECKNER-HOFMANN, *et al.* 2000. Localized Wegener's granulomatosis: predominance of CD26 and IFN-gamma expression. J. Pathol. **192:** 113–120.
27. SNELLER, M.C. 2002. Granuloma formation, implications for pathogenesis of vasculitis. Cleveland Clin. J. Med. **69:** SII40–43.
28. LAMPRECHT, P., A. ERDMANN, A. MULLER, *et al.* 2003. Heterogeneity of CD4+ and CD8+ memory T cells in localized and generalized Wegener's granulomatosis. Arthritis Res. Ther. **5:** R25–31.
29. COULOMB-L'HERMINE, A., F. CAPRON, W. ZOU, *et al.* 2001. Expression of the chemokine RANTES in pulmonary Wegener's granulomatosis. Hum. Pathol. **32:** 320–326.
30. REINHOLD-KELLER, E., P. LAMPRECHT, A.C. FELLER & W.L. GROSS. 2001. Polyarthritis following interferon alpha treatment in a patient with localized Wegener's granulomatosis. Clin. Exp. Rheumatol. **19:** 227–228.
31. SANDERS, J.S., C.A. STEGEMAN & C.G. KALLENBERG. 2003. The Th1 and Th2 paradigm in ANCA-associated vasculitis. Kidney Blood Press Res. **26:** 215–220.
32. GRIFFITH, M.E., A. COULTHARD & C.D. PUSEY. 1996. T cell responses to myeloperoxidase (MPO) and proteinase 3 (PR3) in patients with systemic vasculitis. Clin. Exp. Immunol. **103:** 253–258.
33. MATHIESON, P.W., C.M. LOCKWOOD & D.B. OLIVEIRA. 1992. T and B cell responses to neutrophil cytoplasmic antigens in systemic vasculitis. Clin. Immunol. Immunopathol. **63:** 135–141.

34. RASMUSSEN N & J. PETERSEN. 1993. Cellular immune responses and pathogenesis in C-ANCA positive vasculitides. J. Autoimmun. **6:** 227–236.
35. BROUWER, E., C.A. STEGEMAN, M.G. HUITEMA, *et al.* 1994. T cell reactivity to proteinase 3 and myeloperoxidase in patients with Wegener's granulomatosis (WG). Clin. Exp. Immunol. **98:** 448–453.
36. KING, W.J., C.J. BROOKS, R. HOLDER, *et al.* 1998. T lymphocyte responses to antineutrophil cytoplasmic autoantibody (ANCA) antigens are present in patients with ANCA-associated systemic vasculitis and persist during disease remission. Clin. Exp. Immunol. **112:** 539–546.
37. VAN DER GELD, Y.M., M.G. HUITEMA, C.F. FRANSSEN, *et al.* 2000. *In vitro* T lymphocyte responses to proteinase 3 (PR3) and linear peptides of PR3 in patients with Wegener's granulomatosis (WG). Clin. Exp. Immunol. **122:** 504–513.
38. POPA, E.R., C.F. FRANSSEN, P.C. LIMBURG, *et al.* 2002. *In vitro* cytokine production and proliferation of T cells from patients with antiproteinase 3- and antimyeloperoxidase-associated vasculitis, in response to proteinase 3 and myeloperoxidase. Arthritis Rheum. **46:** 1894–1904.
39. WINEK, J., A. MUELLER, E. CSERNOK, *et al.* 2004. Frequency of proteinase 3 (PR3)-specific autoreactive T cells determined by cytokine flow cytometry in Wegener's granulomatosis. J. Autoimmun. **22:** 79–85.
40. MAYET, W.J., E. MARKER-HERMANN, J. SCHLAAK, *et al.* 1999. Irregular cytokine pattern of $CD4^+$ T lymphocytes in response to *Staphylococcus aureus* in patients with Wegener`s granulomatosis. Scand. J. Immunol. **49:** 585–594.
41. ASSENMACHER, M., M. LÖHNING, A. SCHEFFOLD, *et al.* 1998. Sequential production of IL-2, IFN-γ, and IL-10 by individual staphylococcal enterotoxin B-activated T helper lymphocytes. Eur. J. Immunol. **28:** 1534–1543.
42. CLAYTON, A.R. & C.O. SAVAGE. 2003. Production of antineutrophil cytoplasm antibodies derived from circulating B cells in patients with systemic vasculitis. Clin. Exp. Immunol. **132:** 174–179.
43. JANEWAY, C.A., JR. 2001. How the immune system works to protect the host from infection: a personal view. Proc. Natl. Acad. Sci. USA **98:** 7461–7468.
44. ZINKERNAGEL, R.M. & H. HENGARTNER. 1999. Regulation of the immune response by antigen. Science **293:** 251–253.
45. VOSWINKEL, J., A. MULLER, P. LAMPRECHT, *et al.* 2002. Does ANCA formation result from an antigen-triggered immune response in Wegener's endonasal inflamed tissue? Cleveland Clin. J. Med. **69**(suppl. 2)**:** SII-159.
46. BRAUN, M.G., E. CSERNOK, W.L. GROSS, *et al.* 1991. Proteinase 3, the target antigen of anticytoplasmic antibodies circulating in Wegener's granulomatosis: immunolocalization in normal and pathologic tissues. Am. J. Pathol. **139:** 831–838.
47. POPA, E.R., C.A. STEGEMAN, C.G.M. KALLENBERG, *et al.* 2002. *Staphylococcus aureus* and Wegener's granulomatosis. Arthritis Res. **4:** 77–79.
48. VOSWINKEL, J., J. KRAEMER, A. MUELLER, *et al.* 2004. B lymphocytes infiltrating Wegener's granuloma: the immunoglobulin VH gene repertoire from granulomatous tissues displays an antigen-driven maturation and suggests a microbial trigger. Arthritis Res. **6:** S24.
49. MOOSIG, F., E. CSERNOK, G. KUMANOVICS, *et al.* 2000. Opsonization of apoptotic neutrophils by antineutrophil cytoplasmic antibodies (ANCA) leads to enhanced uptake by macrophages and increased release of tumor necrosis factor-alpha (TNF-α). Clin. Exp. Immunol. **122:** 499–503.
50. EHLERS, S., J. BENINI, H.D. HELD, *et al.* 2001. αβ TCR+ cells and IFNγ, but not iNOS, are critical for granuloma necrosis in a mouse model for mycobacteria-induced pulmonary immunopathology. J. Exp. Med. **194:** 1847–1859.

Clinical Relevance of Antiphospholipid Antibodies in Primary Biliary Cirrhosis

PHILIPP VON LANDENBERG,[a] MICHAEL BAUMGARTNER,[b] JUERGEN SCHOELMERICH,[b] KARL J. LACKNER,[a] AND REINHILD KLEIN[c]

[a]*Institute of Clinical Chemistry and Laboratory Medicine, Johannes Gutenberg University, Mainz, Germany*

[b]*Department of Internal Medicine I, University of Regensburg, Regensburg, Germany*

[c]*Department of Internal Medicine II, University of Tübingen, Tübingen, Germany*

ABSTRACT: Primary biliary cirrhosis (PBC) is a cholestatic liver disease characterized by the presence of antimitochondrial autoantibodies (AMAs), but also with reactivities to other autoantigens. Recent studies showed that antibodies to phospholipids (APAs) represent an important group of autoantibodies identified in patients with PBC. In this study different types of APAs were identified in the sera of patients with PBC and autoimmune hepatitis (AIH) and control subjects. Sera from patients with PBC and AIH were tested for the presence of antibodies directed against cardiolipin (CL), phosphatidylserine (PS), and to β_2-glycoprotein I (β_2-GPI). Furthermore, an in-house test for antithromboplastin antibodies was performed. Antinuclear antibodies (ANAs) and antimitochondrial antibodies (AMAs) were tested with standard tests. IgM anti-PS antibodies were found in 75% of the 51 PBC patients, but only in 4% of the 48 AIH patients ($P < 0.0001$). IgM anti-CL antibodies were more frequently detected in AIH than in PBC (75% vs. 89%; $P = 0.045$). IgM anti-β_2-GPI antibodies were observed more frequently in patients with AIH (83%) than with PBC (59%; $P = 0.007$). The APAs of the IgG type did not differ significantly between the groups of patients. Considering the clinical/laboratory parameters, the levels of alkaline phosphatase ($P = 0.017$), glutamate pyruvate transaminase ($P = 0.035$), and glutamate oxalacetate transaminase ($P = 0.034$) were significantly higher in PBC patients who were positive for IgM anti-PS antibodies than in the anti-PS antibody–negative patients. In conclusion, APAs are present in PBC patients with a higher level of the disease or more intense liver damage than in patients without APAs. Thus IgM anti-PS antibodies represent a new marker of activity in PBC patients.

KEYWORDS: primary biliary cirrhosis (PBC); autoimmune hepatitis (AIH); antiphospholipid antibodies (APAs)

Address for correspondence: Prof. Dr. P. von Landenberg, Institute of Clinical Chemistry and Laboratory Medicine, Johannes Gutenberg University, Langenbeck Strasse 1, 55131 Mainz. Voice: +49-6131-17-5104; fax: +49-6131-17-6627.
landenberg@zentrallabor.klinik.uni-mainz.de

Ann. N.Y. Acad. Sci. 1051: 20–28 (2005). © 2005 New York Academy of Sciences.
doi: 10.1196/annals.1361.043

INTRODUCTION

Primary biliary cirrhosis (PBC) is a cholestatic liver disease characterized by autoreactive B and T cell responses directed against mitochondrial but also a variety of other autoantigens. The antimitochondrial antibodies (AMAs/anti-M2) react with the 2-oxoacid dehydrogenase complex of the inner mitochondrial membrane.[1–3] However, besides these diagnostically relevant AMAs, other autoantibodies can occur, such as antibodies to nuclear dots or nuclear membranes.[4,5] There is evidence from recent studies that antiphospholipid antibodies (APAs) may also be present.[6] These antibodies have been primarily described in systemic lupus erythematosus (SLE) and the antiphospholipid syndrome.[7–9] They are associated with clinical manifestations of thromboembolic events such as thrombocytopenia and habitual abortion, but also with other symptoms of vasculopathy such as amaurosis fugax, Raynaud's syndrome, sensorineural hearing loss or tinnitus, and others.[10] In this respect, their occurrence in PBC is of interest since some kind of vasculopathy of the small vessels surrounding bile ducts has been postulated to play a role in its pathogenesis.[11–13] However, APAs are a rather heterogeneous group of antibodies consisting of antibodies to negatively charged phospholipids such as cardiolipin, to aminoglycerophospholipids like phosphatidylserine and phosphatidylethanolamine, or to the phospholipid-binding protein β_2-glycoprotein.[14,15] Cardiolipin has long been recognized as the mitochondrial antigen M1 first described in secondary syphilis, and anti-M1 antibodies are the result of true molecular mimicry between bacterial (*Treponema pallidum*) and mitochondrial membranes.[16] Interestingly, phosphatidylserine and phosphatidylethanolamine are also present in relevant amounts in the mitochondrial membrane.[17]

In the present study we analyzed the subspecificity of APAs in patients with PBC as compared to AIH to see whether it might correlate with any clinical or laboratory parameters.

METHODS AND MATERIALS

Patients

Sera from 51 patients with clinically and serologically proven PBC were analyzed. All of the patients had a typical cholestatic constellation with increased alkaline phosphatase and gamma-glutamyltransferase as well as increased serum IgM levels and anti-M2 antibodies reacting with at least one component of the 2-oxoacid dehydrogenase complex of the inner mitochondrial membrane. Liver biopsy had been performed in 25 of the patients and was compatible with the diagnosis of PBC in all instances.

Furthermore, sera from 48 patients with autoimmune hepatitis (AIH) were included. All of these patients were in the active stage (first relapse of the disease), and none of them was undergoing immunosuppressive therapy at the time of serum analysis. All patients had increased transaminases and IgG levels (>20 g/L) and histologic studies performed on 20 of them revealed chronic active hepatitis. Thirty-five of the patients had antibodies to nuclei or actin (AIH I); one to liver/kidney microsomes (LKM); and twelve to the soluble liver/liver-pancreas antigen (SLA/LP).

Sera and clinical data from patients with autoimmune liver disease were kindly provided by colleagues from different hospitals in Germany. Control sera from 24 healthy blood donors were (kindly provided by Professor Dorothee Wernet, Department of Blood Transfusion, University of Tübingen. All sera was stored at –20°C.

Informed consent was obtained from each patient included in the study, and the study protocol (blood withdrawal) conforms to the ethical guidelines of the 1975 Declaration of Helsinki, as reflected in *a priori* approval by the institutions' Human Research Committee.

Demonstration of Antiphospholipid Antibodies

Antibodies to cardiolipin (CL), β_2-glycoprotein (β_2-GPI,) and phosphatidylserine (PS) of the IgG and IgM-type were tested by commercially available test kits (Fa. Aesku Diagnostics, Wendelsheim, Germany). The phospholipid antigens, CL and PS, were coated together with β_2-glycoprotein I. The ELISAs were performed according to the manufacturer's instructions. Levels below 8 U/mL were considered normal for all types of antibodies.

Furthermore, sera were tested against thromboplastin from rabbit brain by an in-house ELISA, as recently described. In brief, microtiter plates (Maxisorp, Nunc, Wiesbaden, Germany) were coated with thromboplastin (Sigma, St. Louis) at a concentration of 50 µg/mL. Patient's sera were diluted 1:800 for the detection of IgG and IgM antibodies. Monovalent peroxidase conjugated antihuman IgG and IgM antibodies from goat (DIANOVA, Hamburg, Germany) were diluted 1:2000, as substrate *o*-phenylendiamine was used. Optimal antigen and serum dilutions had been determined by serial dilutions.

Antibodies to mitochondria, nuclei, smooth muscle antigens/actin and liver-kidney microsomes (LKM) were analyzed by an immunofluorescence test (IFT) using cryostat sections from rat liver, kidney, stomach, and heart. Anti-M2 antibodies were determined by ELISA as previously described;[18] anti-liver-pancreas/soluble liver antibodies (SLA/LP) were detected by a complement fixation test and Western blotting using a purified antigen fraction from rat liver as previously described.[19] Anti-LKM antibodies in the IFT were verified by ELISA using recombinant CYP2D6 and the immunodominant epitopes.[20]

Laboratory Parameters

Alkaline phosphatase (AP), gamma glutamyltransferase (γ-GT), glutamate pyruvate transaminase (GPT) and glutamate oxalacetate transaminase (GOT), and bilirubin (BILI) were determined by standard laboratory methods. Serum IgG-, IgM-, and IgA levels were measured using nephelometry (Dade Behring, Marburg, Germany).

Statistical Analysis

Statistical analysis was performed employing the SPSS 10.0 program. Conventional Chi-square test and Fisher's exact test were used to analyze qualitative differences in univariate analysis. *P* values less than 0.05 were taken to indicate statistical significance.

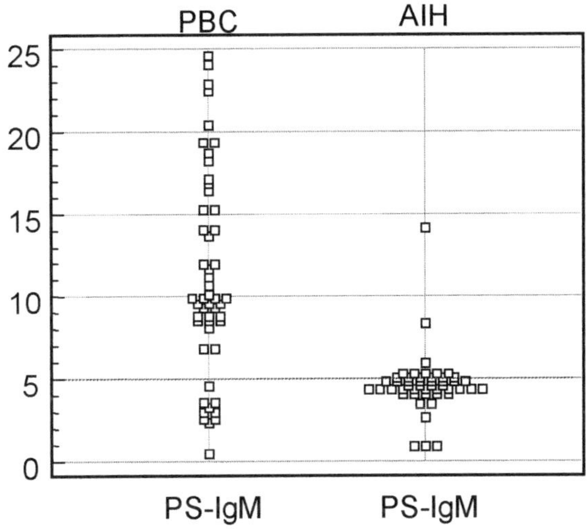

FIGURE 1. PBC versus AIH in PS IgM. Distribution of anti-PS IgM between PBC and AIH patients. Anti-PS IgM antibodies were measured using commercially available tests (Aesku Diagnostics, Wendelsheim, Germany). Cut-off level for considering positives was 8 U/mL.

RESULTS

Incidence of Antibodies to Phospholipids in Patients with PBC as Compared to Patients with AIH and Healthy Controls

Antibodies to phosphatidylserine of the IgM type were present in 38 of the 51 PBC patients (74.5%) but in only two (4.2%, $P < 0.0001$) of the AIH patients (FIG. 1). The test used revealed a sensitivity of 80.4% and a specificity of 95.8% for differentiation of these two entities. IgG antibodies to phosphatidylserine were observed only with a low incidence in the three groups of patients.

Antibodies to cardiolipin of the IgM type were more often present in patients with AIH (43 [89%] of the 48 patients), while only 38 (75%) of the patients with PBC and one of the controls had this antibody type (TABLE 1). Antibodies to cardiolipin of the IgG-type were rarely observed in patients with PBC. Thus, of the 51 patients, 8 (16%) were positive; similarly, only 5 (10%) of the 48 AIH patients and one of the healthy controls had this antibody type.

Antibodies to β_2-GPI of the IgG-type were hardly detected in any of the three groups, while anti-β_2-GPI-antibodies of the IgM-type were found in 30 of the 51 PBC (58.8%) and 40 of the 48 (83.3%) AIH-patients (TABLE 1).

Testing the patients' sera against thromboplastin, again, IgG antibodies were hardly detected. IgM antibodies were seen in 12 (23.5%) of the PBC patients, in 5 (10%) patients with AIH and in one control.

TABLE 1. Presence of antiphospholipid antibodies in patients and controls

Groups of Patients	Number of Patients Analyzed	IgM Antibodies to: Cardiolipin	β_2-Glycoprotein	Phosphatidyl-serine	Thromboplastin
		Number (%) Positive			
PBC	51	38 (75)	30 (59)	38 (75)	12 (23)
AIH	48	43 (89)	40 (83)	2 (4)	5 (10)
Controls	24	1 (4)	1 (4)	1 (4)	1 (4)
*P**		0.045	0.007	0.0001	NS

*Significance level comparing patients with PBC and AIH.

TABLE 2. Liver function parameters[a]

	Anti-PS IgM	N	Mean (U/L)	Significance level
AP	positive	38	208.74	$P = 0.017$
	negative	11	89.45	
γ–GT	positive	38	251.84	NS
	negative	11	276.00	
GOT	positive	38	26.21	$P = 0.034$
	negative	11	10.36	
GPT	positive	38	53.84	$P = 0.035$
	negative	11	11.45	

[a]Mean levels of liver enzymes and levels of significance in patients with and without anti-PS IgM antibodies.

Correlation of Anti-PS Antibodies with Laboratory Parameters

Considering the high incidence of anti-PS antibodies of the IgM type in PBC compared to AIH, we wanted to see whether they may correlate with clinical/laboratory parameters. Interestingly, levels of AP, GPT, and GOT were significantly higher in PBC patients, being positive for anti-PS antibodies of the IgM type, than in the anti-PS antibody–negative patients (FIG. 2), indicating an increased inflammatory activity in the former group. For the γ-GT and BILI levels no significant differences could be detected (TABLE 2). IgG and IgM serum levels did not differ significantly between PBC patients with or without anti-PS antibodies (data not shown).

Correlation between Antiphospholipid Antibodies of the IgM Type and Serum IgM Levels

Considering the fact that elevation of IgM globulins is a typical feature of PBC, we wondered whether this might be related to the high incidence of anti-PS antibodies of the IgM type in this disease. Therefore, we divided the patients into two groups: a group with pathologic IgM levels (>230 mg/L) and a group with normal

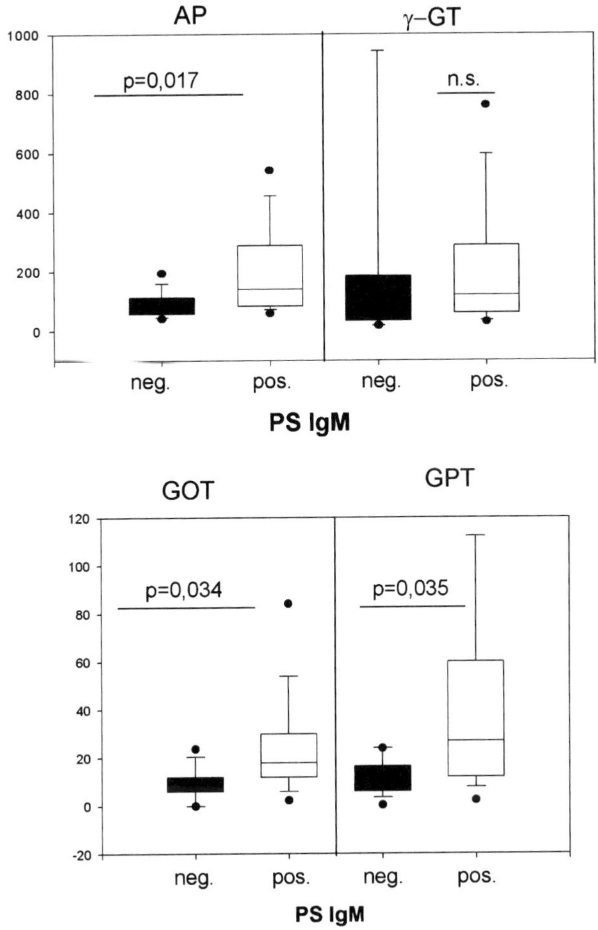

FIGURE 2. Liver enzymes associated with PS IgM antibodies in PBC patients. Mean levels of AP, γ-GT, GOT, and GPT in patients with anti-PS IgM. The liver enzymes were measured with standard routine tests. Comparison of bilirubin levels in the different groups showed no significant differences (data not shown).

IgM-levels. There was no significant difference between the two groups; anti-PS antibodies of the IgM type occurred independently whether IgM levels were increased or normal.

DISCUSSION

There are several reports showing that antiphospholipid antibodies may occur in autoimmune liver diseases. In the present study we observed that there is a significant difference between PBC and AIH, especially with respect to antibodies to phosphatidylserine and cardiolipin of the IgM-type. Thus, IgM anti-PS antibodies were found in 75% of the 51 PBC patients but only in 4% of the 48 AIH patients ($P < 0.0001$). In contrast, antibodies to cardiolipin of the IgM type were more frequently detected in AIH than in PBC, but—although statistically significant—this difference was not as obvious (75% vs. 89%; $P<0.045$) as for the anti-PS antibodies. Also, anti-β2-GPI-antibodies of the IgM-type were observed more frequently in patients with AIH (83%) than with PBC (59%; $P = 0.007$). In the case of the IgG subtype, the incidence of the different APAs did not differ significantly between the groups of patients.

The presence of IgM anti-PS antibodies in PBC patients was closely related to increased levels of laboratory markers indicating liver damage (transaminases, alkaline phosphatase). Interpretation of these results may assess the presence of APAs in PBC as a marker of disease activity or poor prognosis.

APAs have recently been described in another liver disease of unknown etiology, namely nodular regenerative hyperplasia (NRH) of the liver, and in this disease antibodies to cardiolipin were present in especially high numbers.[6] Vasculopathy may play an important role in the pathogenesis of NRH because it has been reported to occur in patients with systemic vasculitis or collagen disorders; it also occurs in patients with antiphospholipid syndrome. In this respect, the high incidence of antibodies to PS and cardiolipin in PBC is of interest considering the fact that in this cholestatic liver disease histologically hyperplastic regenerative nodules as well as vascular alterations can be observed.[11–13]

The mode of action of antibodies to PS in PBC remains unknown. From patients with antiphospholipid antibodies in nonliver diseases it is known that there is a good correlation between antibodies to cardiolipin, the lupus anticoagulants, and severe clinical symptoms such as thrombosis/embolism, infarction, or recurrent fetal loss. In contrast, in patients with moderate or rather "diffuse" symptoms of antiphospholipid syndrome such as Raynaud's syndrome, amaurosis fugax, sudden hearing loss, and tinnitus, antibodies to β_2-GPI seem to predominate (our own unpublished observation). Nevertheless, the induction of vascular inflammatory processes by these antibodies or interaction with coagulation factors leading to microthrombotic events have to be taken into consideration as a pathogenetic mechanism of these antiphospholipid antibodies in liver diseases of unknown etiology.

Furthermore, it has been shown that during the apoptosis of cells, expression of phosphatidylserine on cell membranes is enhanced, so that it is not unlikely that the antibodies to PS in PBC are not primarily present but rather induced in the course of the inflammatory process, leading to the destruction and apoptosis of epithelial cells.[21,22] This process may activate naturally occurring antibodies (including those to PS) with the aim of eliminating those apoptotic cells.[23,24] The fact that these antibodies are mainly of the IgM type would fit into this concept, as naturally occurring antibodies belong primarily to the IgM class.[25,26] A nonspecific stimulation of these antibodies as a result of elevated IgM globulins in PBC can, with certainty, be excluded, as we did not observe any correlation between the presence of these antibodies and serum IgM levels.

The relationship between anti-PS antibodies of the IgM type and a heightened inflammatory process as indicated by elevated AP, GPT, and GOT levels is in agreement with the suggestion of increased apoptosis in more active PBC. However, it has to be pointed out that the determination of antibodies to phospholipids in general and particularly to PS has several pitfalls and that the results obtained with commercially available test kits may vary to a large extent, despite the fact that all refer to international standards (our own unpublished observation).

Determination of antibodies to thromboplastin, a mixture of phospholipid and lipoproteins, also allowed a differentiation between PBC and AIH because they were nearly exclusively found in the PBC group. However, in the present study they have been detected in a lower incidence in PBC than previously reported.

In conclusion, we have shown that APAs occur frequently in autoimmune liver diseases. Of even greater relevance, we have also shown that antibodies to PS may serve as a prognostic marker because their presence correlated significantly with a heightened inflammatory process.

REFERENCES

1. Gershwin, M.E., I.R. Mackay, A. Sturgess & R.L. Coppel. 1987. Identification and specificity of a cDNA encoding the 70 kD mitochondrial antigen recognized in primary biliary cirrhosis. J. Immunol. **138:** 3525–3531.
2. Yeaman, S.J., D.J. Danner, D.J. Mutimer, *et al.* 1988. Primary biliary cirrhosis: identification of two major M2 mitochondrial autoantigens. Lancet **1:** 1067–1070.
3. Berg, P.A. & R. Klein. 1988. Molecular determination of the primary biliary cirrhosis-specific M2 antigen. Hepatology **8:** 200–202.
4. Lozano, F., A. Parés, L. Borche, *et al.* 1988. Autoantibodies against nuclear envelope-associated proteins in primary biliary cirrhosis. Hepatology **8:** 930–938.
5. Szostecki, C., H. Will, H.J. Netter & H.H. Guldner. 1984. Autoantibodies to the nuclear Sp 100 protein in primary biliary cirrhosis and chronic active hepatitis. Clin. Exp. Immunol. **55:** 553–560.
6. Klein, R., S. Goller & L. Bianchi. 2003. Nodular regenerative hyperplasia (NRH) of the liver—a manifestation of "organ-specific antiphospholipid syndrome"? Immunobiology **207:** 51–57.
7. Hughes, G.R. 1985. The anticardiolipin syndrome. Clin. Exp. Rheumatol. **3:** 285–286.
8. Harris, E.N., A.E. Gharavi, M.L. Boey, *et al.* 1983. Anticardiolipin antibodies: detection by radioimmunoassay and association with thrombosis in systemic lupus erythematosus. Lancet **2:** 1211–1214.
9. Wilson, W.A., A.E. Gharavi, T. Koike, *et al.* 1999. International consensus statement on preliminary classification criteria for definite antiphospholipid syndrome: report of an international workshop. Arthritis Rheum. **42:** 1309–1311.
10. Cervera, R., J.C. Piette, J. Font, *et al.* 2002. Antiphospholipid syndrome: clinical and immunologic manifestations and patterns of disease expression in a cohort of 1000 patients. Arthritis Rheum. **46:** 1019–1027.
11. Colina, F., F. Pinedo, J.A. Solis, *et al.* 1992. Nodular regenerative hyperplasia of the liver in early histological stages of primary biliary cirrhosis. Gastroenterology **102:** 1319–1324.
12. Buffet, C., M. Sinico, G. Adda, *et al.* 1991. Nodular regenerative hyperplasia and primary biliary cirrhosis. Gastroenterol. Clin. Biol. **15:** 856–858.
13. Abe, M., T. Masumoto, T. Ninomiya, *et al.* 2000. Hyperplastic liver nodules associated with early-stage primary biliary cirrhosis mimicking hepatocellular carcinoma. Dig. Dis. Sci. **45:** 1563–1567.
14. von Landenberg, P., J. Scholmerich, J. von Kempis & K.J. Lackner. 2003. The combination of different antiphospholipid antibody subgroups in the sera of patients with autoimmune diseases is a strong predictor for thrombosis: a retrospective study from a single center. Immunobiology **207:** 65–71.
15. Shoenfeld, Y., I. Krause, F. Kvapil, *et al.* 2003. Prevalence and clinical correlations of antibodies against six beta2-glycoprotein-I-related peptides in the antiphospholipid syndrome. J. Clin. Immunol. **23:** 377–383.

16. BERG, P.A. & R. KLEIN. 1986. Mitochondrial antigens and autoantibodies: from anti-M1 to anti-M9. Klin. Wochenschr. **64:** 897–909.
17. BIRNER, R. & G. DAUM. 2003. Biogenesis and cellular dynamics of aminoglycerophospholipids. Int. Rev. Cytol. **225:** 273–323.
18. KLEIN, R., H. POINTNER, W. ZILLY, *et al.* 1997. Antimitochondrial antibody profiles in primary biliary cirrhosis distinguish at early stages between a benign and a progressive course: a prospective study on 200 patients followed for 10 years. Liver **17:** 119–128.
19. STECHEMESSER, E., R. KLEIN & P.A. BERG. 1993. Characterization and clinical relevance of antiliver pancreas antibodies (anti-LP) in autoimmune hepatitis. Hepatology **18:** 1–8.
20. KLEIN, R., U.M. ZANGER, T. BERG, *et al.* 1999. Overlapping but distinct specificities of antiliver-kidney microsome antibodies in autoimmune hepatitis type II and hepatitis C revealed by recombinant native CYP2D6 and novel peptide epitopes. Clin. Exp. Immunol. **118:** 290–297.
21. FADOK, V.A. & P.M. HENSON. 2003. Apoptosis: giving phosphatidylserine recognition an assist—with a twist. Curr. Biol. **13:** R655–657.
22. SCHULTZ, D.R. & W.J. HARRINGTON, JR. 2003. Apoptosis: programmed cell death at a molecular level. Semin. Arthritis Rheum. **32:** 345–369.
23. KIM, S.J., D. GERSHOV, X. MA, *et al.* 2002. I-PLA(2) activation during apoptosis promotes the exposure of membrane lysophosphatidylcholine leading to binding by natural immunoglobulin M antibodies and complement activation. J. Exp. Med. **196:** 655–665.
24. PITTONI, V. & G. VALESINI. 2002. The clearance of apoptotic cells: implications for autoimmunity. Autoimmun. Rev. **1:** 154–161.
25. MOUTHON, L., S. LACROIX-DESMAZES, A. NOBREGA, *et al.* 1996. The self-reactive antibody repertoire of normal human serum IgM is acquired in early childhood and remains conserved throughout life. Scand. J. Immunol. **44:** 243–251.
26. COUTINHO, A., M.D. KAZATCHKINE & S. AVRAMEAS. 1995. Natural autoantibodies. Curr. Opin. Immunol. **7:** 812–818.

IL-10 and the Cytokine Network in the Pathogenesis of Human Autoimmune Hemolytic Anemia

CATERINA TORIANI-TERENZI AND ENZO FAGIOLO

Laboratory of Immunohematology, Catholic University "Sacro Cuore," Rome, Italy

ABSTRACT: In animal and human autoimmune hemolytic anemia (AIHA) immunologic tolerance loss against RBC self-antigens could be originated by several mechanisms: ignored self-antigens' epitopes, polyclonal lymphocyte activation, molecular mimicry between self- and foreign antigens, central or peripheral tolerance errors, or immunoregulatory disturbances including the alteration of a cytokine network. To identify the immunologic factors contributing to autoimmune onset and maintenance, several murine strains (such as NZB and NZB/NZW) that spontaneously develop a complex autoimmune syndrome, including AIHA, have been extensively studied. In human AIHA, the respective roles of IL-2, IL-4, IFN-γ, IL-10, and IL-12 were investigated by examining the spontaneous and mitogen-induced (OKT3 or LPS) production of these cytokines. ELISA methods were used in PBMCs to evaluate whether the manipulation of IL-10/IL-12 balance can have an effect on the incidence of autoimmune diseases and whether this might be useful for the control of AIHA. Results affirmed that AIHA is a disease that exhibits an increased basal synthesis of IL-4 and decreased levels of IFN-γ by AIHA PBMCs compared with controls and that there is a basal increase of Th2 cytokines. Th1-type cytokine decrease in the basal state occurred in parallel with an increase of constitutive IL-10 production and an IL-12 decrease. In conclusion, decreased production of Th1-type cytokines and the production of autoantibodies in AIHA may be secondary to the imbalance between IL-10 and IL-12, and the neutralization of IL-10 may be efficacious in diminishing the clinical pathology associated with Th2 subset prevalence. In the same way, the treatment with IL-12 could offer a second and independent level of blockade against the consequences of the overstimulation of B cells associated with AIHA.

KEYWORDS: **immunologic tolerance loss; cytokine network; AIHA**

INTRODUCTION

Autoimmune hemolytic anemia (AIHA) is the first recognized organ-specific autoimmune disease (AD) in humans; it is an antibody-mediated autoimmune disease caused by autoantibodies (autoAbs) against red blood cell (RBC) self-antigens. AIHA could be expressed in several species both in a spontaneous way and after induction by immune system manipulation. Anti-RBC autoAbs are detectable on patients' own erythrocytes by direct antiglobulin test (Coombs' test) or in their serum and/or eluate. AIHA patients could produce "warm" autoAbs (IgG or IgA),

Address for correspondence: Dr. Caterina Toriani-Terenzi, Viale dei Promontori, 438, 00122 Rome Italy. Voice/fax: +39-06-5665400.
cttoriani@tiscali.it

Ann. N.Y. Acad. Sci. 1051: 29–44 (2005). © 2005 New York Academy of Sciences.
doi: 10.1196/annals.1361.044

which best react at body temperature (T), or "cold" autoAbs (IgM or IgG), which have their maximal activity at lower T (<30°C), especially at 4°C. autoAbs have a clearly defined antigenic specificity and cause RBC destruction by macrophagic erythrophagocytosis (extravascular hemolysis) and/or direct lysis by complement activation (intravascular hemolysis), respectively. Most RBC "warm" autoAbs react against Rh proteins but, recently, in some AIHA cases, have been shown to be specific to Band 3, RBC anion channel protein, too. IgM "cold" agglutinins (CAs) are identified as anti-I, anti-i, anti-Pr, or anti-Gd autoAbs, while IgG "biphasic" autoAbs, in paroxysmal cold hemoglobinuria, are anti-P. The two last AIHA forms' antigenic epitopes are characterized by a carbohydrate structure found both in RBCs and in several tissues, leukocytes, and bacteria. In current studies on mechanisms of autoimmune response against RBCs, the identification of RBC antigenic epitopes, autoAbs' target, has been of decisive importance. But, in spite of serological and pathological evidence, the mechanism that produces a breakdown of immunologic tolerance versus RBC self-antigens is still unknown.

It is known that AIHA is one of the potential complications of a wide range of underlying diseases, including malignant lymphoproliferative disorders, other ADs, congenital immunodeficiencies, and viral infections. These associated conditions, which are characterized by complex modifications of immune response, make it difficult to investigate the etiology of AIHA. To identify the immunologic factors contributing to autoimmune onset and maintenance, several murine strains that spontaneously develop a complex autoimmune syndrome (such as NZB and NZB/NZW) have been extensively studied.[1] In fact, these murine strains share many features with human AIHA, including a susceptibility to neoplasia and/or other ADs. Functional abnormalities of B and T cells have been investigated, particularly lymphocyte activation, cytokine production, and their role in autoimmune onset. It is important to remember, however, that human AIHA differs from that in NZB mice or other human ADs because associated inflammatory events are not present.

Recently, in order to investigate the mechanisms of central and/or peripheral tolerance breakdown against RBC self-antigens, a transgenic (Tg) mouse model of AIHA has been produced,[2] and several theories have been proposed to explain the etiology of autoimmunity.[3] Some of these theories purport that autoimmunity is the consequence of immunoregulatory disorders or defects in peripheral or central tolerance; whereas, according to others, autoimmunity derives from a classic immune response against self- or cross-reactive antigens towards which, usually, tolerance need not be established. Different types of AIHA might be explained by experimental or human studies according to each of the following postulated mechanisms: (1) ignored self-antigens' epitopes; (2) polyclonal lymphocyte activation; (3) molecular mimicry between self- and foreign antigens; (4) errors in central or peripheral tolerance; and (5) disorders of immunoregulation.

Immunologic data that support these pathogenetic theories on autoimmunity derive from studies on animal models and human AIHA, as summarized in TABLE 1.

IGNORED SELF-ANTIGEN EPITOPES

Experimental data support the hypothesis of "self-ignorance" in human AIHA. Synthetic peptides corresponding to Rh polipeptide sequence, the most frequent

TABLE 1. Mice and human AIHA data supporting each postulated mechanism of autoimmunity

Ignored or cryptic self-epitopes

In NZB mice

Peptides of band 3 stimulate *in vitro* $CD4^+$ cells in MHC-II restricted manner

In humans

Rh or band 3 cryptic self-epitopes activate immunologically "ignorant" T cells

Rh-like proteins activate PMBCs only in patients with AIHA

Polyclonal B cell activation

In NZB mice

Accelerated proliferation of T and B cells ($CD5^+$) early in life.

In humans

High number of $PCA1^+$ cells in patients with AIHA

In chronic GVHD, activation of host B cells by donor T cells induces AIHA

Antigenic mimicry

In mice

Injection of rat erythrocytes in mice induces AIHA

Bacterial lipopolysaccharide activates B1 cells and induces AIHA in NZB mice

In humans

AIHA in patients with mycoplasma infection

Errors in central or peripheral tolerance

In mice

Neonatal thymectomy induces AIHA

Cortical atrophy of thymus and impaired ability to generate common lymphoid precursor in NZB mice

Killing of erythocyte autoantibody in transgenic mouse sequestered B1 cells improves AIHA in NZB mice.

Mice lacking IL2R chain develop lymphoproliferation and AIHA

Increased number of $TCR^+CD4^-CD8^-$ cells in peripheral blood of *lpr* and *gld* mice

In humans

Genetic defects of Fas/FasL apoptosis system induce lymphoproliferation and AIHA

Disorders of immunoregulation

In NZB mice

Th1/Th2 cytokine imbalance

IL-10 administration accelerates but anti-IL-10 delays the onset of autoimmune syndrome

Administration of IL-10 and IL-5 activates peritoneal B1 cells and induces AIHA

In the transgenic mouse, IL-5 and IL-10 activates peritoneal B1 cells and induces AIHA

TABLE 1. (*continued*) Mice and human AIHA data supporting each postulated mechanism of autoimmunity

In humans
Reduced number of peripheral $CD4^+$ and of $CD25^+$ cells in PHA-stimulated PMBC cultures
Increased *in vitro* basal proliferative response of T cells in nonstimulated PBMC cultures
Increased *in vitro* basal production of IL-10 and IL-4 in nonstimulated PMBC cultures
Basal *in vitro* reduction of INF- and IL-12 in anti-CD3-stimulated PMBC cultures
Increased serum levels of IL-4, TNF, IL-2, and soluble IL-2R
High serum levels of IL-10 in lymphoproliferative syndrome
IL-10 increases production of erythrocyte autoantibodies by PBMCs from AIHA patients

proteic target for the autoAbs in human "warm" type AIHA, were tested *in vitro* for their ability to stimulate normal T cells. Several peptides cause T cell activation and their proliferation can be blocked by anti-HLA-DR Ab. Most likely, autoreactive T cells ($CD45RA^+$) have not been deleted, but are anergic to autologous Rh polipeptides and therefore immunologically ignorant against cryptic self-antigens.[4] Subsequent studies show that synthetic peptides, corresponding to 30-KD Rh protein sequence associated with expression of D and Cc/Ee antigens, were able to stimulate the *in vitro* proliferation of mononuclear cells from the peripheral blood or spleen of AIHA patients. In the case of the greater number of patients, including all cases with Rh-specific autoAbs, two or more peptides stimulated proliferation, whereas cells in several cases of other kinds of anemia or healthy donors failed to respond to the peptides.[5] In several AIHA cases, autoAb production seems to be caused by the activation of class-II–restricted helper T cells specific for cryptic Rh epitopes. These autoreactive T cells seem to escape the clonal deletion and anergy during the induction of self-tolerance and remain quiescent even if the autoantigens they recognize are present.

POLYCLONAL LYMPHOCYTE ACTIVATION

Polyclonal T and/or B cell activation has been considered a starting mechanism of the autoimmune process, although B cell clone activation could also be the second step in the development of autoimmunity. Polyclonal B cell stimulators, as well as bacterial or viral molecules, can induce autoAb production from nondeleted and/or anergized self-reactive B cells.

Excessive B cell proliferation, particularly in early life, along with high amounts of IgM-secreting cells, have been described in NZB/W mice.[1] After intracerebral inoculation of lymphocytic choriomeningitis (LCM) virus, the CH3cB/FeJ mouse develops AIHA and hypergammaglobulinemia. A hemolysis reduction has been observed after the treatment with anti-CD4 monoclonal Abs.[6] An increased number of circulating cells express PCA1, a marker of B cells differentiation into plasma cells, and has been shown in all studied cases of human AIHA, confirming a state of B cell activation.[7]

Cold agglutinins, usually present at low levels, are increased during viral or mycoplasma infections due to AIHA. Newborn RBCs show mostly "i" structure; whereas, after the first months of life when branching transferases are expressed, "I" structure is formed. Therefore, only an incomplete tolerance has been established toward the "I" antigen which allows a nonhemolytic low CAs autoAb levels. The I/i carbohydrate structure is present both on RBCs and also on leukocytes, macrophages, platelets, and bacteria such as *Listeria monocytogenes* and *Streptococcus pneumoniae*. The I/i antigens sialylated form (Sia Ib), carried by glicolipides expressed on RBC surface, act as *Mycoplasma pneumoniae* receptors. It was suggested that the increased levels of CAs, induced by mycoplasma infection, are due to the presence of common antigenic epitopes on RBCs and mycoplasma;[8] otherwise the binding of mycoplasma to its receptor could be indirectly responsible for the activation of CA-producing B cell clones.[9] In Tg mouse expressing two Ig chain genes of a human anti-Sia-Ib IgM autoAbs, tolerance partially avoided CA expression by the peripheral deletion of autoreactive B cells, although a small number of B cells expressing human IgM are present in the peritoneal cavity.[10] In Tg mice expressing a human CA specific for sialylated carbohydrates, *Mycoplasma pulmonis* infection, which is similar in its pathologic features to human infection, high CA levels have been observed. Whereas in Tg-normal mice, only a small percentage of CA-expressing B cells could be detected and, in infected mice, most circulating B lymphocytes express the Tg Ig. These studies suggest that mycoplasma infection partly produces a breakdown of immune tolerance against specific activation of CA-expressing B cell clones.[11]

A clear example of T-dependent polyclonal B cell activation is the complex autoimmune syndrome associated with chronic graft-versus-host disease (GVHD), seen after bone marrow transplantation. In experimental and human chronic GVHD, alloreactive donor T cells that recognize the host histocompatibility antigens cause, by direct T–B interaction,[12] a selective stimulation of host self-reactive B cell clones, which produce a wide spectrum of autoAbs, including those against RBCs that give rise AIHA. In normal conditions these B cell clones still stay quiescent since their own tolerant T cells do not stimulate them.

MOLECULAR MIMICRY

Theories of self-ignorance or polyclonal T and/or B activation may be compatible with molecular mimicry hypothesis. Injected mice with rat RBCs produce autoAbs and then a hemolytic syndrome like warm-type AIHA in humans. It has been reported that mice have B cell clones able to identify rat RBC antigenic epitopes that are like RBC autoantigens. B cell clones usually do not react against self-antigens because they need a stimulus from autoreactive T cells that have been deleted or energized. Mice T cell clones could be able to react against foreign epitopes presented to the host in association with similar autologous epitopes.[13] Otherwise most cases of AIHA are associated with various bacterial or virus infections, probably due to the presence of common antigenic epitopes on RBC proteins or carbohydrates. It has been suggested that foreign, cross-reactive antigens could prevent clonal deletion and induce T-independent activation of self-reactive B cell clones.[14]

ERRORS IN CENTRAL OR PERIPHERAL TOLERANCE

T Cell Tolerance

In different animal models, including NZB and NZB/W mice, neonatal thymectomy induces or accelerates the immunopathological features, and severe cortical atrophy can be found in all of the studied models of murine lupus.[15] Several mechanisms have been proposed to explain post-thymectomy ADs: the reduction of T suppressor cells that produce cytokines able to avoid the autoreactive T cell clonal expansion;[16] self-tolerance breakage due to disequilibrium between Th1 and Th2 lymphocytes, as characterized by the reduction of Th1 activity;[17] and $CD4^+CD25^+$ immunoregulatory T cell depletion. Depletion of $CD4^+$ subpopulations, which co-express IL-2 receptor α-chain by thymectomy in most murine strains, results in the development of organ-specific ADs such as thyroiditis, gastritis, and insulin-dependent diabetes mellitus.[18] Mice lacking IL-2 receptor β-chain develop lymphadenopathy, a complex autoimmune syndrome that includes AIHA and an increase of $CD4^+CD69^+$ T cells spontaneously activated; this secretes greater amounts of both INF-γ and IL-4.[19] T cells seem to have an active role in promoting an autoAb response to self-RBCs in NZB mice. In fact, anti-$CD4^+$ Ab injection in these strains strongly reduce autoAb levels, both in young mice with negative antiglobulin test and in old mice, although, in most old mice, antiglobulin tests became positive 11 weeks after the last anti-$CD4^+$ Ab injection.[20] AIHA development in NZB mice seems to be associated with a predominant autoimmune response: T cell cultures from NZB mice stimulated with Band 3 proteins produce INF-γ and IL-4 prevalently, and IL-5 and IL-10 at low levels.[21] Th1 cytokines could produce a better presentation of cryptic RBC antigens by increasing MCH-II molecule expression on autoreactive T cells that escape to tolerance induction and remain quiescent (immunologically ignorant) in the peripheral lymphoid tissues. The larger part of responding T cells are $CD4^+$ and the response is MCH-II restricted.[22,23] Recently, one case of human AIHA with IgA autoAb Band 3 specificity has been reported: serum and eluate Ab reaction to normal RBCs was inhibited by RBC incubation with monoclonal Abs against the third extracellular loop of Band 3.[24]

The role of immunoregulatory T cells in maintaining immunologic tolerance has been supported. AD in NZB/W mice is prevented by stem cell transplants that restore $CD4^+CD25^+$ cells to normal count.[25] Experimental observations show that the reduced ability of NZB bone marrow cells to repopulate thymus seems to derive from an impaired ability of stem cells to generate common lymphoid precursors.[26] The $CD4^+CD25^+CD45RO$ regulatory/suppressor T cells are believed to maintain the immunologic self-tolerance, but their true regulatory mechanism has yet to be defined. These cells, which are in an anergic state, after *in vitro* stimulation by allogenic mature dendritic cells or anti-CD3, release IL-10 but not IL-2, IL-4, or INF-γ.[27]

In most patients affected by AIHA, idiopathic or associated diseases, excluding malignant lymphoproliferative disorders, a strong reduction in number of $CD4^+$ cells in peripheral blood and of percentage in CD25$^+$ cells in PHA-stimulated peripheral blood mononuclear cell (PBMC) cultures have been shown.[7]

B Cell Tolerance

The RBC autoAb Tg murine model provided important information about B cell autoreactivity and tolerance in AIHA. Mice expressing a transgene with IgM autoAb activity against murine RBCs were obtained from a hybridoma derived from NZB strain. In this model, B cells expressing Tg autoAbs were deleted in bone marrow and lymphoid organs; B1 CD5$^+$ trangene-expressing cells were found in the peritoneal cavity, too. This sequestered subpopulation, never before exposed to the antigen or escaped to tolerance, seems to be responsible for tolerance breakdown and then for the development of self-renewing AIHA. In fact, intraperitoneal injection of RBCs induced the apoptotic death of B1 cells and turned out the recovery of IIb and the decrease of autoAb levels and autoreactive B cells. Moreover, the hypotonic shock of killing peritoneal B cells produced consistent improvement in the AIHA patient. In fact, when crossed with the X-linked immune deficiency mutation *xid* (in which B1 cells are absent) the B cells did not show AIHA.[28] But the presence of B1 cells seems to be insufficient for the induction of autoimmunity; there is a need for additional factors. Mice bred in pathogen-free conditions did not suffer from AIHA, although they showed a a similar number of peritoneal B1 cells when compared with mice bred in normal conditions. However, the administration of gram-negative bacteria lipopolysaccharide activates B1 cells and induces AIHA.[29]

AIHA and Defects of Lymphocyte Apoptosis

Some forms of T cell tolerance and T-dependent forms of B cell tolerance could be caused by malfunctions such as an inefficient Fas/FasL apoptosis system, which is an important mechanism of programmed cell death in the maintenance of lymphocyte homeostasis and in establishment of self-tolerance, as shown by the genetic defects of Fas and FasL in both mice and human autoimmunity. In mice, genetic defects in the TFNRSF6-encoding Fas gene and TNFSF6-encoding FasL genes cause the *lpm* and *ged* phenotypes, respectively, which shows lymphoproliferation, autoAb production associated with autoimmune syndromes, and increased double-negative CD4$^-$ CD8$^-$ α/β^+ T cells.[30] A similar human form exists called "autoimmune lymphoproliferative syndrome" (ALPS), which is characterized by nonmalignant diffuse lymphadenopathy, IgG "warm" autoAb AIHA, thrombocytopenia, neutropenia, and an increase of double-negative T cells. Most patients have inherited heterozygous mutations in the *TNFRSF6* gene, which encodes Fas. ALPS patients without this mutation have other types of mutations, such as the TNFSF6 gene, which encodes FasL, or the CASP10 gene, which encodes caspase 10.[31]

DISORDERS OF IMMUNOREGULATION

The hypothesis about autoimmunity as a consequence of imunoregulatory disorders could be discussed together with the previous mechanism, which postulates the existence of errors in the establishement and/or maintenance of immunologic self-tolerance.

Immunoregulatory disorders have been considered as a primary cause of autoimmunity as well as being suggested by the high frequency of AIHA in patients with neoplasias or primary immunodeficiencies. In animals, ADs can be prevented or primed by the manipulation of certain T cell subpopulations. As mentioned above, ADs in rodents can be induced by eliminating $CD4^{+}CD25^{+}$ immunoregulatory T cells. Th1/Th2 cell cytokine imbalance may lead to similar pathologic effects. In fact, autoimmunity may be induced or improved by cytokines or anticytokine Ab administration. Studies of *in vitro* activation and cytokine production by lymphocytes and accessory cells seem to be one of the most promising attempts to explain AIHA pathogenesis.

Animal Models

A complex cytokine network dysregulation has been demonstrated in several animal ADs; yet, Th1, Th2, or accessory cell cytokines' respective contribution to the pathogenesis of ADs is still a matter of debate. Furthermore, several cytokines (for instance, IL-4, IL-6, and IL-10) are known to promote Ab production. It has been suggested that Th2 cells might play a role in the development of various autoAb-mediated diseases such as systemic lupus erythematosus (SLE) and AIHA.[32–34] IL-12, mostly produced by activated monocytes, promotes the development of Th1 cells *in vitro* and *in vivo* and may inhibit IL-4-induced Ab production.[35] INF-γ amplifies the IL-12 activation of Th1 cells and inhibits Th2 cell expansion. IL-4 and IL-10 inhibit the development of Th1 cell clones through downregulation of IL-12 production by the monocytes. In a recent effort to evaluate the role of IL-10 it has been observed that the continuous administration of anti-IL-10 Abs delays the onset of autoimmunity in NZB/W mice, owing to increases in TNF-α, whereas IL-10 administration accelerates the onset of the autoimmune syndrome.[36]

Administration of IL-5 and IL-10 activated peritoneal B1 cells and induced AIHA in Tg mice. IL-10-induced differentiation of B1 cells into Ab producing cells is strongly impaired in IL-5R-deficient Tg mice, suggesting that IL-5 is required for the activation and differentiation of B cells. In fact, when IL-5R is expressed in most peritoneal B1 cells, IL-5 Tg mice show a remarkable increase in the number of peritoneal B1 cells and in the level of RBC autoAbs.[37,38] Interestingly, in NZB mice, IL-10 seems to play a role in inducing B cell malignant lymphoproliferation. In fact, NZB mice B1 cells produce higher IL-10 mRNA levels than do normal ones and a strong correlation has been found between enhanced IL-10 mRNA levels and the development of malignant B1 clones.[39]

An involvement of Th1 cells has been suggested in NZB/W mice. In fact INF-γ, a Th1 cytokine, promotes B cell maturation and pathologic Ab generation, and its administration accelerates SLE, whereas administration of TNFα has the opposite effect.[40] Furthermore, in congenic MLR/lpm carrying one or both copies of the INF-γ gene inactivated, INF-γ enhancement is required for antinuclear Ab response, development of glomerulonephritis, and early mortality.[41]

Human AIHA

Since several Th2 cytokines, such as IL-4, IL-6, and IL-10, are known to promote Ab production by B cells, it has been suggested that Th2 cells might play a role in the development of autoAb-mediated diseases such as SLE and AIHA.

Some studies evaluate PBMC cultures' proliferative response and IL-10, IL-12, IL-IL-2, IL-4, and IFN-g production, respectively, by ^{3}H-thymidine incorporation and ELISA under basal conditions and after mitogen stimulation (LPS, PHA, and OKT3).[34,42,43] In untreated AIHA, patients have shown, in basal conditions, a proliferative response greater than that of controls, suggesting a basal state of hyperactivation. On the other hand, after mitogen stimulation, both by PHA and by OKT3, the Stimulation Index value is statistically lower in AIHA patients than in controls ($P<0.0001$), indicating that the patients' lymphocytes could be in a exhaustive condition due to their basal activation.[43]

In AIHA and human SLE, an increased IL-10 secretion has been observed. In fact, PBMCs obtained from AIHA patients show a constitutively increase of IL-10 production *in vitro* ($P<0.003$) compared to the controls. This significant difference is not maintained following LPS stimulation. Stimulation of PBMCs by LPS increased IL-10 production similarly in both AIHA patients ($P<0.03$) and controls ($P<0.0001$) compared to basal levels (FIG. 1).[42,43]

In AIHA, unstimulated cultures of IL-12 production were higher in 55% of cases compared to controls and the remaining values were similar to controls. On the other hand, cytokine production in LPS-stimulated AIHA PBMC cultures was lower when compared to controls. There was no statistically significant increase in IL-12 levels in LPS-stimulated vs. RPMI media–unstimulated AIHA PBMC cultures ($P = 0.40$), whereas a significant increase in control IL-12 levels after LPS stimulation ($P<0.0002$) was observed. Constitutional IL-12 levels were higher in patients' PBMCs compared to controls, but this was not statistically significant ($P = 0.10$). Finally, the level of LPS-driven cytokine production after stimulation were significally different among AIHA patients vs. controls ($P<0.04$) (FIG. 1).[43]

IL-2 production is slightly enhanced both in the absence of exogenous stimuli and in the presence of mitogens. IL-2 is a key cytokine, as it regulates the growth, differentiation, and function of lymphocytes; its high levels in AIHA patients, both in the absence of OKT3 and after OKT3 stimulation, justify the high basal proliferation/activation of T lymphocytes. Moreover, a basal decrease of IFN-γ, a Th1-type cytokine, has been noticed, but after mitogenic stimulation IFN-γ levels are similar both in AIHA patients and in controls. On the other hand IL-4, a Th2-type cytokine, increased basal production in AIHA patients ($P<0.01$), but after stimulation IL-4 levels are not statistically significant.

In absence of mitogenic stimuli there is a definite activation of AIHA T lymphocytes toward Th2 phenotype and consequent immunoglobulin production. It is important to notice that the increase of IL-4 and IFN-γ levels after mitogenic stimulation leads to similar levels both in patients and in controls—in fact, both could be activated but patients' T lymphocytes have a limited percentage of activation.[43]

In previous studies there was clear evidence of lymphocyte activation during the testing of the peripheral blood of AIHA patients showed by the enhancement of B PCA1+ lymphocytes, IL-2, soluble IL-2Rc high levels, and IL-1α high levels in all cases—and a reduced lymphocyte proliferative response to PHA, B lymphocyte response to PWM, and CD25$^+$ lymphocyte number after PHA stimulation in all cases. In summary, the data about the respective role of five cytokines in AIHA patients—at first diagnosis and before any transfusional or pharmacological treatment—was investigated by examining the spontaneous and mitogen-induced production of these

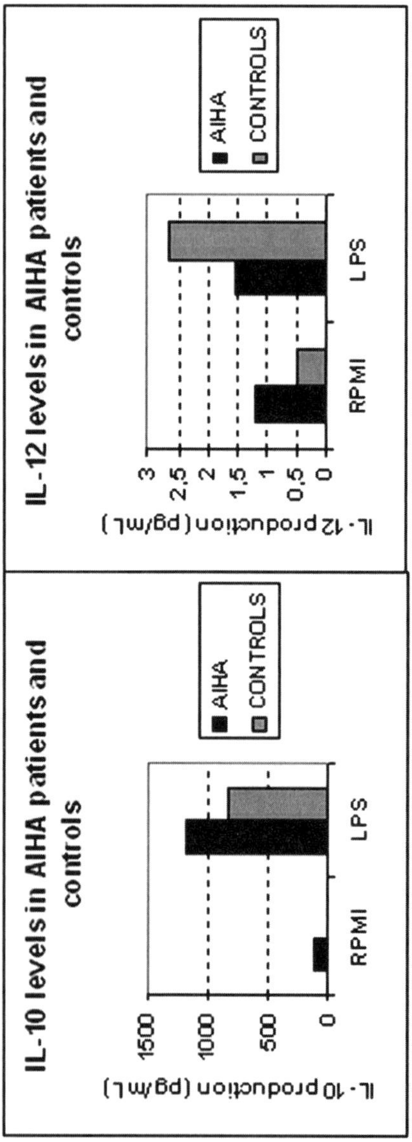

FIGURE 1. IL-10 and IL-12 levels in AIHA.

cytokines by ELISA methods. These show that AIHA is a disease with the following characterisitics:

1. IL-10 production is always higher in patients than in controls both in the basal state and after stimulation.
2. IL-12 levels in basal state are higher in patients than in controls; on the other hand, there is a statistically significant increase of IL-12 levels in controls but not in patients after stimulation, which could be explained as the consequence of an IL-10 inhibitory effect.
3. IL-2 production was slightly enhanced, in both the absence and presence of exogenous stimuli; this observation could justify the high basal activation of lymphocytes (both T and B cells).
4. There were constant but not significantly higher IL-4 and lower IFN-γ levels in AIHA patients as compared with healthy controls that experienced a prevalence of the Th2 pattern.

IL-10 AND CYTOKINE NETWORK DYSREGULATION

Studies on animal and human AIHA mentioned above suggest that loss of immunologic tolerance against RBC self-antigens could be primed by several mechanisms: self-antigens' ignorance, molecular mimicry between self and non-self-antigens, or polyclonal T and B cell activation (including the allogenic effect after bone marrow transplantation, central or peripheral tolerance errors, genetic defects in lymphocyte apoptosis, or immunoregulatory disturbances). The last mechanism, in human AIHA, focused on the central role of IL-10 in cytokine immunoregulatory network dysregulation. In fact, an increased IL-10 production by mononuclear blood cells is a common feature in several different AIHA models.

We have found several immunologic abnormalities in AIHA patients: decreased number of $CD4^+$ cells in peripheral blood, basal B and T cell hyperactivation, and high modifications of several cytokine production by PBMCs. All of these seem to be the consequence of increased production of IL-10. Interestingly, AIHA patients' PBMCs are able to produce high IL-10 levels in culture if stimulated by Rh(D) proteins, that are more often chosen as targets by RBC autoAbs.[44]

High IL-1α, IL-2, IL-4, and IL-2R serum levels have been found in AIHA patients— both idiophatic and those associated with other diseases or α-methyldopa therapy.[42] In addition, *in vitro* activation and cytokine production by PBMCs show that, in basal conditions, T cell proliferative response increased more than twofold that in controls, suggesting a state of hyperactivation, whereas, after stimulation with anti-CD3 Ab, T lymphocyte response was strongly decreased, indicating a probable cell exhaustive state that seems to be due to high IL-10 culture production. In fact, IL-10 production was high in patients' nonstimulated cultures when compared to controls; the same was true of IL-4 levels, though in a less evident manner. On the other hand, IL-12 basal production was higher in about 55% of cases, but in LPS-stimulated cultures IL-12 levels were lower in AIHA patients than in controls (FIG. 1), which could be ascribed to the cells' basal high activation state and their inability to react after stimulation, probably owing to IL-10's suppressive effect on IL-12 producer cells. It is easy to hypothesize that a disease-active state could be caused by decreased levels of IL-12 in AIHA as well as in SLE, because of its potent inhibitor role in loss of autoAb production. IL-2 slightly enhanced production, both in the absence of exogenous stimuli and after anti-CD3 stimulation; there is a basal low IFN-γ production in AIHA patients that became similar to that of controls after mitogenic stimulation. IL-2 increased levels in culture supernatant and in sera from AIHA patients and justified the high basal state of T cell activation and of autoreactive B cell clone activation. IL-4 basal production was increased in AIHA patients, while TNF-α was strongly increased in stimulated cultures and both cytokines together with IL-2 and IL-2R have also been found in high numbers in the sera of AIHA patients.[7,43]

Despite the evidence of the prevalence of Th2 cells during activation in animal and human AIHA, the above mentioned studies indicate that Th1 cell activation plays a decisive role in inducing loss of tolerance against self-RBCs. An immune response modulation through soluble mediators seems to induce a switch to Th2 response rather than to Th1, although experimental evidence from the Tg immunoglobulin mouse model suggest that self-imicking of foreign antigens rescues B cells from peripheral tolerance in a T-independent manner: tolerance loss may result from specific B cell receptor engagement.[45] High serum IL-10 levels have been found also in almost all patients affected by ALPS.[46] It has been suggested that Th2 prevalence in ADs is due to both an elevated IL-10 and a decreased IL-12 production. IL-12 inhibition by IL-10 produces a direct T cell differentiation toward Th2 activation.[47] In addition, increased IL-10 production inhibits B lymphocyte apoptosis by induction of Bcl-2, an anti-apoptotic protein.[48] Then, IL-10 overexpression could lead to the survival of autoreactive cell clones.

Immunologic abnormalities observed in human AIHA indicate a basal decrease of Th1 cytokine production and an increase of Th2 cytokines. IL-12 production in stimulated cultures from healthy controls (but not in AIHA patients) suggests that increased levels of IL-10 could cause a secondary decrease of IFN-γ basal production. These data support the hypothesis that IL-10 promotes autoimmunity and maintains ADs by continuous autoAb production, and that IL-10 and IL-12 together make an immunoregulatory circuit which can regulate the development and maintenance of ADs. Likewise, in AIHA and SLE PBMCs produce high levels of IL-10 *in vitro* but lower levels of IL-12 and other Th1 cytokines.[49] Recombinant IL-10 strongly inhibited IL-12 production *in vitro* both in SLE and in normal PBMC cultures; IL-10 reversed the IL-12 deficiency of SLE PBMCs.[50] These data suggest that a deficiency in IL-12 production may be the effect of excessive IL-10 production. IL-10 production was significantly downregulated in SLE PBMC cultures stimulated by IL-12; this effect was attributed to IFN-γ upregulation by IL-12. Moreover, it is possible that low IL-12 levels in AIHA, as well as in SLE, may contribute to produce the active state of the disease because this cytokine is a potent inhibitor of autoAb production.[51] It follows that decreased production of Th1 cytokines and tolerance loss in AIHA might be somehow connected to the imbalance between IL-10 and IL-12 and therefore to the alteration in IL-10/IL-12 immunoregulatory circuit (FIG. 2).

Some studies showed that IL-10 neutralization with anti-IL-10 Ab may produce some desirable consequences in NZB/W F1 mice, such as the reduction of autoAb production and delayed onset of autoimmune syndrome.[36] Administration of anti-IL-10 murine monoclonal Ab ameliorated cutaneous lesions and joint symptoms in patients with active and steroid-dependent SLE, independently of circulating anti-DNA Abs,[52] although it was found that anti-IL-10 strongly reduces *in vitro* synthesis

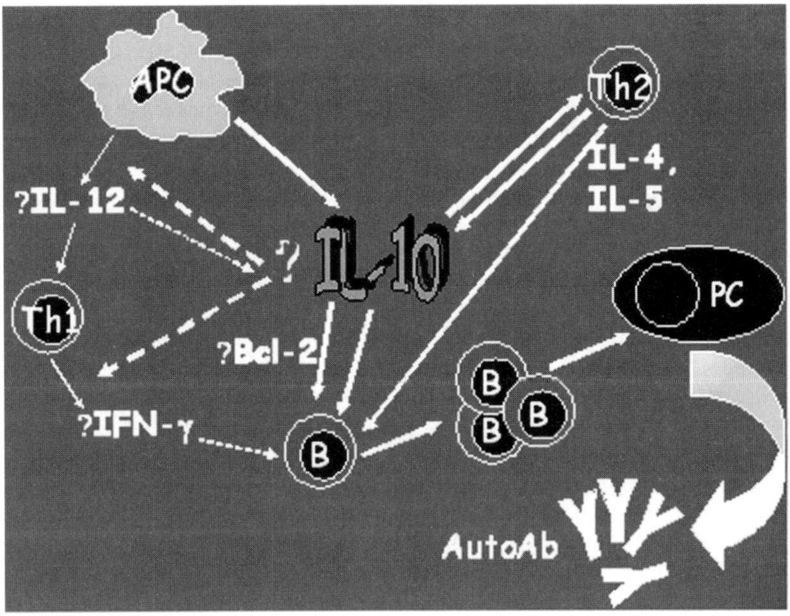

FIGURE 2. Increased production of IL-10 by Th2 cells and monocytes induce marked proliferation, differentiation of autoreactive B cell clones, and a reduced production of IL-12, which allows uncontrolled B cell clone expansion, inhibition of Th1 cell activation, IFN-γ production (which normally suppresses Th2 activation), and the induction of Bcl2 anti-apoptotic protein.

of IgM and IgG.[53] Moreover, IL-10, rather than IL-4 and IL-6, increases *in vitro* production of RBC autoAbs by AIHA patients' stimulated PBMCs.[54] Furthermore, *in vitro* studies indicated that the reduction of excessive autoAb production in SLE could be achieved by IL-12, independently of IFN-γ and IL-2 modulation. Then the treatment with IL-12 could offer a second and independent level of blockade against the consequences of the B cell overactivation associated with ADs like AIHA.[55]

Immunogenetic studies suggest a possible link between IL-10 promoter haplotypes and susceptibility to ADs. Single nucleotide polymorphism haplotypes in distal promoter that segregate with differences in quantitative IL-10 production are significantly associated with SLE and might define one component of the genetic susceptibility to disease.[56] On the basis of this evidence, it is also possible to hypothesize a genetic predisposition in AIHA.

REFERENCES

1. Theophilopoulos, A.N. & F.J. Dixon. 1985. Murine models of systemic lupus erythematosus. Adv. Immunol. **37:** 269–273.
2. Nisitani, S. *et al.* 1997. Anti-red blood cell immunoglobulin transgenic mice: an experimental model of autoimmune hemolytic anemia. Ann. N.Y. Acad. Sci. **815:** 245–252.

3. Theophilopoulos, A.N. 1995. The basis of autoimmunity: Part I. Mechanism of aberrant self-recognition. Immunol. Today **6:** 90–97.
4. Barker, R.N. & C.J. Elson. 1994. Multiple self epitopes on the rhesus polypeptide stimulate immunologically ignorant human T cells. Eur. J. Immunol. **24:** 1578–1582.
5. Barker, R.N. *et al.* 1997. Identification of T cell epitopes on the Rhesus polypeptides in autoimmune hemolytic anemia. Blood **90:** 2701–2715.
6. Coutelier, J.P. *et al.* 1994. Involvement of CD4+ cells in lymphocytic choriomeningitis virus-induced autoimmune anemia. J. Autoimm. **7:** 589–99.
7. Fagiolo, E. & L. Abenante. 1996. Lymphocyte activation and cytokine production in autoimmune hemolytic anemia (AIHA). Autoimmunity **24:** 147–156.
8. Yanney, F.A. *et al.* 1978. Cold agglutinating cross-reactivity with *Mycoplasma pneumoniae*. Infect. Immunol. **22:** 29–33.
9. Loomes, L.M. *et al.* 1984. Erythrocyte receptors for *Mycoplasma pneumoniae* are sialy lated oligosaccarides of type II antigens. Nature **307:** 560–563.
10. Havouis, S. *et al.* 2000. Negative regulation of autoreactive B cells in transgenic mice expressing a human pathogenic cold agglutinin. Eur. J. Immunol. **30:** 2290–2299.
11. Havouis, S. *et al.* 2002. Transgenic B lymphocytes expressing a human cold agglutinin escape tolerance following experimental infection of mice by *Mycoplasma pulmonis*. Eur. J. Immunol. **32:** 1147–1156.
12. Morris, S.C. *et al.* 1990. Autoantibodies in chronic graft versus host results from cognate T–B interactions. J. Exp. Med. **172:** 503–517.
13. Cox, K.O. & A. Howless. 1981. Induction and regulation of autoimmune hemolytic anemia in mice. Immnol. Rev. **55:** 90–97.
14. Gallart, T. *et al.* 1997. Anti-Sialb (anti-Gd) cold agglutinins bind the domain: neuNAcα 2-3 Gal in sialyl Lewis and related carbohydrates on nucleated cells in soluble cancer-associated mucins. Blood **90:** 1576–1587.
15. Sherer, Y. & Y. Shoenfeld. 1997. Thymectomy and autoimmune diseases. Sem. Clin. Immunol. **1:** 5–11.
16. Lo, D. *et al.* 1995. Regulation of CD4+ cells reactivity to self and nonself. Int. Rev. Immunol. **13:** 147–160.
17. Romagnani, S. 1997. The Th1 and Th2 paradigm. Immunol. Today **18:** 263–266.
18. Sakaguchi, S. *et al.* 1995. Immunologic tolerance mantained by activated T cells expressing IL2 receptor chain CD25: breakdown of a single mechanism of self tolerance causes various autoimmune diseases. J. Immunol. **155:** 1151–1164.
19. Suzuki, H. *et al.* 1995. Deregulated T cell activation and autoimmunity in mice lacking interleukin-2 receptor ‰ . Science **268:** 1472–1476.
20. Oliveira, G.G. *et al.* 1994. Production of erythrocyte autoantibodies in NZB mice is inhibited by CD4 antibodies. Clin. Exp. Immunol. **96:** 297–302.
21. Schen, C.R. *et al.* 1996. T-helper dominated responses to erythrocyte Band 3 in NZB mice. Immunology **89:**195–199.
22. Schen, C.R. *et al.* 2002. Characterization of the dominant autoreactive T-cell epitope in spontaneous autoimmune haemolytic anemia of the NZB mouse. J. Autoimmunity **18:** 149–157.
23. Schen, C.R. *et al.* 1999. Splenic but not thymic autoreactive T cells from New Zealand black mice respond to adominant Band 3 peptide. Immunology **96:** 595–599.
24. Janvier, D. *et al.* 2002. Severe autoimmune hemolytic anemia caused by a warm IgA autoantibody directed against the third loop of band 3. Transfusion **42:** 1547–1552.
25. Sardina, E.E. *et al.*1991. Transplantation of wheat germ agglutinin positive hematopoietic cells to cells to prevent or induce systemic lupus erythematosus. Proc. Natl. Acad. Sci. **88:** 1318–1323.
26. Hashimoto, Y. *et al.* 2002. Impaired development of T lymphoid precursors from pluripotent hematopoietic stem cells in New Zealand black mice. J. Immunol. **168:** 81–86.
27. Thornton, A.M. & E.M. Shevac. 1998. CD4+CD25+ immunoregulatory T cells suppress policlonal T cells activation *in vitro* by inhibiting IL2 production. J. Exp. Med. **188:** 287–296.
28. Murakami, M. & T. Honio. 1997. Transgenic mouse models for B dominant autoimmune diseases. Curr. Opin. Immunol. **9:** 846–850.

29. MURAKAMI, M. *et al.* 1994. Oral administration of lipopolysaccarides activates B1 cells in the peritoneal cavity and lamina propria of the gut an induces autoimmune symptoms in an autoantibody transgenic mice. J. Exp. Med. **180:** 111–121.
30. WATANABE-FUGUNAKA, R. *et al.* 1992. Lymphoproliferation disorder in mice explained by defects in Fas antigen that mediate apoptosis. Nature **356:** 314–317.
31. STRAUS, S.E. 1999. An inherited disorder of lymphocyte apoptosis the autoimmune lymphoproliferative syndrome. Ann. Int. Med. **130:** 591–601.
32. VIOLLARD, J.F. *et al.* 1999. Th1 and Th2 cytokine production by peripheral blood mononuclear cells from patients with systemic lupus erytematosus. Clin. Exp. Immunol. **115:** 189–195.
33. HORWITZ, D.A. *et al.* 1998. Decreased production of IL12 and other Th1 type cytokine in patients with recent onset systemic lupus erythematosus. Arthritis Rheum. **41:** 838–844.
34. FAGIOLO, E. & C. TORIANI-TERENZI. 1999. Enhanced IL10 production *in vitro* by monocytes in autoimmune hemolytic anemia. Immunol. Invest. **28:** 347–352.
35. ADORINI, L. 2000. The pathogenic role of IL12 in TH1-mediated autoimmune diseases. Immunol. Immunopharm. **20:** 29–35.
36. ISHIDA, H. *et al.* 1994. Continous administration of anti-IL10 antibodies delay onset of autoimmunity in NZB/W F1 mice. J. Exp. Med. **179:** 305–310.
37. NISITANI, S. *et al.* 1995. Administration of IL5 or IL10 activates peritoneal B1 cells and induces autoimmune hemolytic anaemia in anti-erythrocyte autoantibody transgenic mice. Eur. J. Immunol. **25:** 3047–3052.
38. SAKIYAMA, T. *et al.* 1999. Requirement of IL5 for induction of autoimmune hemolytic anemia in anti-red blood cell autoantibody transgenic mice. Int. Immunol. **11:** 995–1000.
39. RAMACANDRA, S. *et al.* 1996. Requirement IL10 of B1 lymphoproliferation disease in a murine model of CCL. J. Clin. Invest. **98:** 1788–1793.
40. JACOB, C.O. *et al.* 1987. *In vivo* treatement of (NZB x NZW) F1 lupus–like nephritis with monoclonal antibody to γ-interferon. J. Exp. Med. **166:** 798–803.
41. BALOMENOS, D. *et al.* 1998. Interferon-ã is required for lupus-like disease and lymphoaccumulation in MRL-lpr mice. J. Clin. Invest. **101:** 364–371.
42. FAGIOLO, E. *et al.* 1994. High cytokine serum levels in patients with autoimmune hemolytic anemia. Immunol. Inv. **23:** 449–456.
43. FAGIOLO, E. & C. TORIANI-TERENZI. 2002. Th1 and Th2 cytokine modulation by IL10/IL12 imbalance in autoimmune hemolytic anaemia. Autoimmunity **35:** 39–44.
44. HALL, A.M. *et al.* 2002. Interleukin-10 mediated regulatory T-cell responses to epitopes on a human red blood cell autoantigen. Blood **100:** 4529–4536.
45. KOUSCKOFF, V. *et al.* 2000. T cell-independent rescue of B lymphocytes from peripheral immune tolerance. Science **287:** 2501–2503.
46. FUSS, I.J. *et al.* 1997. Characteristic T helper-2 cell cytokine abnormalities in autoimmune lymphoproliferative syndrome. J. Immunol. **158:** 1912–1918.
47. SEGAL, B.M. *et al.* 1998. An IL10/IL12 immunoregulatory circuit controls susceptibility to autoimmune diseases. J. Exp. Med. **187:** 537–546.
48. LEVY Y. & J.C. BROUET. 1994. Interleukin-10 prevents spontaneous death of germinal center B cells by induction of the Bcl-2 protein. J. Clin. Invest. **93:** 424–428.
49. LORENTE, L. *et al.* 1993. Spontaneous production of interleukin-10 by lymphocytes and monocytes in systemic lupus erythematosus. Eur. Cytokine Net. **4:** 4221–4230.
50. LIU T.F. & B.M. JONES. 1998. Impaired production of IL12 in systemic lupus erythematosus: excessive production of IL10 suppress production of IL12. Cytokine **10:** 140–144.
51. HOUSSIAU, F.A. *et al.* 1997. IL12 inhibits *in vitro* immunoglobulin production by lupus PMBC. Clin. Exp. Immunol. **108:** 375–380.
52. LLORENTE, L. *et al.* 2000. Clinical and biologic effects of anti-interleukin-10 monoclonal antibody administration in systemic lupus erythematosus. Arthr. Rheum. **43:** 1790–1800.
53. AL-JANADI, M. *et al.* 1996. Interleukin-10 secretion in systemic lupus erythematosus and rheumatoid arthritis: IL-10 dependent CD4+CD45RO+ T cell–B antibody synthesis. J. Clin. Immunol. **16:** 198–207.

54. BARCELLINI, W. *et al.* 2000. *In vitro* quantification of anti-red blood cell antibody production in idiophatic autoimmune hemolytic anemia: effect of mitogen and cytokine stimulation. Br. J. Haematol. **111:** 452–460.
55. TORIANI-TERENZI, C. *et al.* 2002. Cytokine network in autoimmune hemolytic anemia: new probable targets for therapy. Cancer Prev. Det. **26:** 292–298.
56. GIBSON, A.E. *et al.* 2001. Novel single nucleotide polymorphism in the distal IL10 promoter affect IL10 production and enhance the risk of systemic lupus erythematosus. J. Immunol. **166:** 315–322.

Crohn's Disease Is Associated with Polymorphism of CARD15/NOD2 Gene in a Hungarian Population

ZSUZSANNA NAGY,[a] OSZKÁR KARÁDI,[a] GYÖRGY RUMI,[b] GYÖRGY RUMI, JR.,[a] ALAJOS PÁR,[a] GYULA MÓZSIK,[a] LÁSZLÓ CZIRJÁK,[c] AND GÁBOR SÜTŐ[c]

[a]*First Department of Medicine, Medical Faculty, University of Pécs, Pécs, Hungary*

[b]*Department of Medicine, Hospital Kaposi Mór, Kaposvár, Hungary*

[c]*Department of Immunology and Rheumatology, Medical Faculty, University of Pécs, Pécs, Hungary*

ABSTRACT: Crohn's disease (CD) is commonly classified as an immune-mediated disorder, but genetic and environmental factors seem to be important in its pathogenesis. Mutations within the CARD15/NOD2 gene have been associated with CD in the Caucasian population. The aim of our work was to investigate the allele frequency and clinical impact of the three common mutations in Hungarian CD patients and healthy controls. Seventy-four CD patients and 107 controls were examined. The genotyping of the three common CARD15/NOD2 mutations (Arg702Trp, Gly908Arg, and Leu1007fsinsC) was carried out by restriction fragment length polymorphism (RFLP) and amplification refractory mutation system (ARMS) techniques. The demographic and clinical parameters were correlated with χ^2 analysis. The overall prevalence of CARD15/NOD2 mutations in the Hungarian CD patients (33.78%) was significantly higher than in healthy control individuals (16.23%) ($P < 0.025$). The allele frequency of the Gly908Arg mutation did not differ, but the Arg702Trp and Leu1007fsinsC mutation were more common in CD patients than in controls. The onset of CD occurs about three years earlier in CARD15/NOD2 carriers. Carriage of the Arg702Trp and Leu1007fsinsC allele within the CARD15/NOD2 gene is associated with CD. These data are in line with similar findings showing a role of the CARD15/NOD2 protein in the etiopathogenesis of CD. The genotyping of these mutations might be used to identify high-risk patients.

KEYWORDS: Crohn's disease; CARD15/NOD2 mutation

INTRODUCTION

Crohn's disease (CD) is a chronic inflammatory disease that may involve any part of the gastrointestinal tract, but most frequently the terminal ileum and colon. Bowel inflammation is transmural and discontinuous and may contain granulomas. The

Address for correspondence: Gábor Sütő, M.D., Ph.D., Department of Immunology and Rheumatology, Medical Faculty, University of Pécs, Irgalmasok utcája 1, 7621 Pécs, Hungary. Voice: +36-72-507300; fax: +36-72-507339.
gabor.suto@aok.pte.hu

Ann. N.Y. Acad. Sci. 1051: 45–51 (2005). © 2005 New York Academy of Sciences.
doi: 10.1196/annals.1361.045

prevalence of the disease is approximately 100–200 of every 100,000 people in Western countries, but only about 53 of every 100,000 people in Hungary. However, the incidence of the disease in the Hungarian population has increased rapidly in the last decade.[1–3]

Many facts suggest that the basic etiology of IBD is a dysregulated immune response to microbial organisms in the gastrointestinal epithelial barrier. Specifically, the Th1-predominant proinflammatory mucosal immune response (for example, interleukin-2, interferon-γ, and tumor necrosis factor-α) is involved. The prevalence of inflammatory bowel disease is increased in individuals with other immune-mediated diseases, particularly ankylosing spondylitis, psoriasis, and sclerosing cholangitis.

The complexity of the genetic susceptibility in CD is supported by genome-wide scanning; eight major susceptibility loci suggested evidence of linkage.[4–9] Among the identified susceptibility loci the pericentromeric region on chromosome 16 (IBD1) was susceptible to CD only.[4] The importance of this locus has been confirmed by various groups, including the International IBD Genetics Consortium.[10]

The positional cloning and candidate gene analysis leads to the IBD1 locus,[11,12] which encodes the caspase recruitment domain gene protein (CARD15, previously known as NOD2), a member of the nucleotide-binding, oligomerization domain (NOD) family of inflammation and apoptosis regulators.[13] CARD15/NOD2 is expressed intracellularly in the monocytes and macrophages, where it appears to function as a sensor for bacterial products such as lipopolysaccharides (LPS) and peptidoglycanes (PGs) through the leucine-rich repeat (LRR) domain located in the C-terminal region of the gene. CARD15/NOD2 encodes a protein composed of two NH2-terminal caspase recruitment domains (CARDs), a nucleotide-binding domain (NBD), and 10 COOH-terminal leucine-rich repeats (LRR).[14] The response of the Crohn's disease–associated LRR mutant CARD15/NOD2 variants is impaired by the bacterial components, which indicates that the deficit of sensing bacteria might trigger the diffuse activation of nuclear factor-κB (NF-κB), and secondarily the inflammation and apoptosis through CARD15/NOD2-independent mechanisms.[15]

The frameshift mutation caused by a cytosine insertion (Leu1007fsinsC) results in a premature stop codon; the two missense mutations (Arg702Trp, Gly908Arg) in CARD15/NOD2 are associated with a susceptibility to CD. The presence of one copy of mutated alleles increases the risk by 2- to 4-fold, whereas it increases the relative risk for CD by 20- to 40-fold.[11,12] Twenty-seven rare additional mutations of the CARD15/NOD2 gene were reported; 93% of these were located in the distal third—the LRR part—of the gene. Patients with homozygosity or compound heterozygosity were characterized by an earlier onset (by two years) of the disease, a more frequent stricturing phenotype, and a less frequent colonic involvement.[16] We examined the genotype–phenotype correlation to elucidate the importance of the CARD15/NOD2 mutations and to collect data from central Europe. We investigated the three common mutations in 74 CD patients and compared the results with those of the 107 healthy controls.

PATIENTS AND METHODS

The study protocol conforms to the ethical guidelines of the Helsinki Declaration of 1975. Informed consent was obtained from all participants.

Patients

Patients were recruited from two southwestern Hungarian medical centers: the First Department of Medicine, Medical Faculty, University of Pécs in Pécs and the Medical Depatment of the Kaposi Mór Hospital in Kaposvár. We included 74 consecutive patients in the study. All of the patients had a diagnosis of CD, as supported by clinical, radiologic, endoscopic, and histologic findings.

We investigated the following data of patients: age, gender, age at diagnosis, disease behavior, extraintestinal manifestations (arthralgia, uveitis, skin affection).

One hundred and seven healthy subjects were collected for the control group. All patients and control participants were Caucasians.

Methods

Genomic DNA was extracted from EDTA anticoagulated peripheral blood by a salting out method.[17] Patients and control subjects were investigated for the three most common mutations (Arg702Trp, Gly908Arg, Leu1007fsinsC). The Arg702Trp mutation was genotyped using the amplification refractory mutation system (ARMS) with primers 5′-ATCTGAGAAGGCCCTGCTCC-3′ (wild-type, forward), 5′-ATCTGAGAAGGCCCTGCTCT-3′ (mutated, forward), and 5′-CCACACTTAGCCTTGATG-3′ (reverse). The Gly908Arg mutation creates a restriction site for *Hha*I and was genotyped by an restricition length polymorphism(RFLP)-PCR technique (5′-CCCAGCTCCTCCCTCTTC-3′ and 5′-AAGTCTGTAATGTAAAGCCAC-3′). The presence of a wild-type allele results in an intact 380-bp band, whereas the profile of the Gly908Arg variant is characterized by two bands of 138 bp and 242 bp on 2% agarose gel.[18] The ARMS technique, as described by Ogura *et al.*,[11] was used to genotype the Leu1007fsinsC with four primers: 5′-CTGAGCCTTTGTTGATGAGC-3′ (forward), 5′-TCTTCAACCACATCCCCATT-3′ (reverse), 5′-CAGAAGCCCTCCTGCAGGCCCT-3′ (forward, wild-type), and 5′-CGCGTGTCATTCCTTTCATGGGGC-3′ (mutated, reverse). The demographic and clinical parameters were correlated with χ^2 analysis.

RESULTS

We genotyped all the patients and healthy control participants for the three common CARD15/NOD2 variants. The mutational analysis of the CARD15/NOD2 showed that 33.7% of patients with CD carried at least one potential disease-causing mutation. We observed that the overall prevalence of CARD15 mutations in the Hungarian CD patients was significantly higher than in healthy control individuals (16.23%; 19/117) ($P < 0.025$). The percentage of CD patients with a double mutation was 8.1%; none of the controls had a double mutation. Of the three common mutations, two (Arg702Trp, Leu1007fsinsC) were confirmed to be intermittently associated with a susceptibility to Crohn's disease (TABLE 1). Of the 74 patients, three were homozygotes (two for the Arg702Trp mutation, one for the Leu1007fsinsC mutation), and three patients were compound heterozygotes.

The localization of the disease manifestation was recovered from the files of 25 patients. Both the colonic and the ileal occurrences were much more frequent in patients carrying the CARD15/NOD2 mutations.

TABLE 1. Allele frequencies for Arg702Trp, Gly908Arg, and Leu1007fsinsC in both populations

Mutation	Patients with CD (n = 74)	Control participants (n = 107)	χ^2
Arg702Trp	10.3%	4.7%	4.11 (P < 0.05)
Gly908Arg	2.7%	1.4%	0.81 (NS)
Leu1007fsins	8.9%	2.4%	6.36 (P < 0.025)
Overall	22.9%	8.5%	8.56 (P < 0.01)

NOTE: For the significance at the 0.05 level, χ^2 should be greater than or equal to 3.84; NS, nonsignificant.

TABLE 2. Baseline clinical characteristics of the 74 CD patients and the relationship between CARD15/NOD2 mutations and disease phenotypes

	No. (%) of CD patients	
Characteristic	CARD15 carrier	CARD15 noncarrier
Number	25 (34%)	49 (66%)
Age (yr)	36	38
Age at diagnosis (yr)	30	33
Gender (M/F)	11/14 (44%/56%)	20/29 (41%/59%)
History of smoking		
Never	15 (60%)	22 (45%)
Current	9 (36%)	19 (39%)
Ex-smoker	1 (4%)	8 (16%)
Duodenal involvement	2/7 (29%)	1/18 (6%)
Ileal involvement	7/7 (100%)	14/18 (78%)
Colonic involvement	5/7 (71%)	6/18 (33%)
Peripheral arthralgia	4 (16%)	18 (37%)

CD appears about three years earlier in CARD15/NOD2 carriers. There was no sexual difference between the CARD15/NOD2 carrier and noncarrier groups. The peripheral arthralgia was not different for any of the CARD15/NOD2 genotypes (TABLE 2).

DISCUSSION

Evidence for genetic heterogeneity in CD is known from varying results of genetic linkage studies.[4–9] This heterogeneity clearly exists at the CARD15/NOD2 gene locus, as only some patients have the CD-associated mutations of these gene. Data from other studies demonstrate that only 20–30% of the patients in the Caucasian population carried the three common susceptibility mutations, but none of these mutations were found in Japanese patients.[19] We found that CARD15/NOD2 mutations

TABLE 3. Comparison of allele frequencies of CARD15/NOD2-risk alleles in Hungarian CD patients to patients and controls (C) in previously published studies

	Arg702Trp		Gly908Arg		Leu1007fsinsC		Cumulative association	
	CD	C	CD	C	CD	C	CD	C
France[12]	11%		6%		12%		29%	
Germany[20]	7.2%	3.6%	4.2%	2.1%	12.2%	2.1%	23.6%	7.8%
USA[21]	10.7%	4%	4.3%	1.6%	8.4%	3.8%	23.4%	9.4%
Australia[22]	11%	5%	2%	1%	7%	1%	20%	9%
Japan[19]	0	0	0	0	0	0		
Hungary	10.3%	4.7%	2.7%	1.4%	8.9%	2.4%	22.9%	8.5%

are as frequent (22.9%) in Hungarian CD patients and healthy controls (8.5%) as in other reported Caucasian populations (TABLE 3).[12,19,20–22] As in other studies, Arg702Trp and Leu1007fsinsC mutations were the most common type found in CD patients, as in controls. The analysis of the demographic data suggested that CD appears about three years earlier in CARD15/NOD2 carriers. Similar findings were reported from other studies (TABLE 2).[16,20] It is well established that the ileal localization of CD is associated with frequent CARD15/NOD2 mutations. We found a similar result when we examined the localization of the disease and the mutation carriage.[16,20]

The exact molecular mechanism of CARD15/NOD2 in the immune response is unclear, but it is known that it plays an important role in inflammatory disorders. The mutations of the CARD15/NOD2 gene play a role in different pathologic processes: Blau syndrome (skin rash, cranial neuropathia, granulomatosus arthritis, uveitis),[23] Crohn's disease, psoriatic arthritis,[24] and allogenic stem cell transplantation–related mortality. The CARD15/NOD2 protein is expressed mainly in monocytes and is involved in the apoptosis, NF-κB activation; it is also a negative regulator of Toll-like receptor 2 (TLR-2)-mediated T helper 1 (Th1) responses.[25,26] If the CARD15/NOD2 gene is mutated, this negative regulation will be defective and the response to pathogenic and to the body's own bacteria will be bigger. CD is a immune-mediated disorder that may involve any part of the gastrointestinal tract and includes extra-intestinal inflammation of the skin, eyes, or joints. Because some mutations of the CARD15/NOD2 protein are related to the previously mentioned disorders with arthritis, we found the prevalence of the peripheral arthralgia in CARD15/NOD2 carriers and noncarriers to be an important question. The frequency of mutation carriers did not differ in the group with peripherial arthralgia (22.1%) nor in the group without arthralgia (35.5%). Among our CD patients, more than a quarter (28.5%) reported peripheral arthralgia, but the clinical evidence of arthritis was rare. From the extraintestinal manifestations in CD the phenotype arthralgia seems to not be related to the CARD15/NOD2 carriage. Because the prevalence of skin and eye involvement was uncommon among our patients, such a correlation was not investigated in this study.

Smoking, among other potentially relevant environmental factors of CD, has been shown to have an adverse effect on the clinical course of the disease.[27] We did not, however, find an association between CARD15/NOD2 risk alleles and tobacco exposure; nor did the frequency of smoking differ between CARD15/NOD2 carriers and noncarriers. Tobacco use and CARD15/NOD2 carriage seem to be independent risk factors in CD.

Our data suggested that carriage of the Arg702Trp and Leu1007fsinsC alleles within the CARD15/NOD2 gene is associated with CD. The genotyping of the CARD15/NOD2 mutations could also have clinical relevance because it is associated with severe involvement of the ileal region and with ileocecal resection.[20] A younger age at diagnosis is also related to the CARD15/NOD2 mutant alleles. The genotyping of these mutations might be used to identify high-risk patients.

ACKNOWLEDGMENTS

The CARD15/NOD2 mutations were analyzed with the assistance of Ágnes Bodrog. We are grateful to Tamás Szelestei, M.D., for the technical assistance. The study was supported by grants from the National Research Fund (OTKA), Budapest (Nos. F042912, F037639, T046437, and T034343) and from the Hungarian Ministry of Health (ETT 098/2001 and ETT 573/2003).

REFERENCES

1. Loftus, E.V., Jr., M.D. Silverstein, W.J. Sandborn, *et al.* 1998. Crohn's disease in Olmsted County, Minnesota, 1940–1993: incidence, prevalence, and survival. Gastroenterology **114:** 1161–1168.
2. Bernstein, C.N., J.F. Blanchard, P. Rawsthorne, *et al.* 1999. Epidemiology of Crohn's disease and ulcerative colitis in a central Canadian province: a population-based study. Am. J. Epidemiol. **149:** 916–924.
3. Lakatos, L., T. Pandur, G. David, *et al.* 2003. Association of extraintestinal manifestations of inflammatory bowel disease in a province of western Hungary with a disease phenotype: results of a 25-year follow-up study. World J. Gastroenterol. **9:** 2300–2307.
4. Hugot, J.P., P. Laurent-Puig, C. Gower-Rousseau, *et al.* 1996. Mapping of a susceptibility locus for Crohn's disease on chromosome 16. Nature **379:** 821–823.
5. Hampe, J., S. Schreiber, S.H. Shaw, *et al.* 1999. A genomewide analysis provides evidence for novel linkages in inflammatory bowel disease in a large European cohort. Am. J. Hum. Genet. **64:** 808–816.
6. Rioux, J.D., M.S. Silverberg, M.J. Daly, *et al.* 2000. Genomewide search in Canadian families with inflammatory bowel disease reveals two novel susceptibility loci. Am. J. Hum. Genet. **66:** 1863–1870.
7. Ma, Y., J.D. Ohmen, Z. Li, *et al.* 1999. A genome-wide search identifies potential new susceptibility loci for Crohn's disease. Inflamm. Bowel Dis. **5:** 271–278.
8. Cho, J.H., D.L. Nicolae, L.H. Gold, *et al.* 1998. Identification of novel susceptibility loci for inflammatory bowel disease on chromosomes 1p, 3q, and 4q: evidence for epistasis between 1p and IBD1. Proc. Natl. Acad. Sci. USA **95:** 7502–7507.
9. Satsangi, J., M. Parkes, E. Louis, *et al.* 1996. Two-stage, genome-wide search in inflammatory bowel disease provides evidence for susceptibility loci on chromosomes 3, 7, and 12. Nat. Genet. **14:** 199–202.
10. IBD International Genetics Consortium. 2001. International collaboration provides convincing linkage replication in complex disease through analysis of a large pooled data set: Crohn disease and chromosome 16. Am. J. Hum. Genet. **68:** 1165–1171.
11. Ogura, Y., D.K. Bonen, N. Inohara, *et al.* 2001. A frameshift mutation in NOD2 associated with susceptibility to Crohn's disease. Nature **411:** 603–606.

12. HUGOT, J.P., M. CHAMAILLARD, H. ZOUALI, *et al.* 2001. Association of NOD2 leucine-rich repeat variants with susceptibility to Crohn's disease. Nature **411:** 599–603.
13. INOHARA, N. & G. NUNEZ. 2003. NODs: intracellular proteins involved in inflammation and apoptosis. Nat. Rev. Immun. **3:** 371–382.
14. OGURA, Y., N. INOHARA, A. BENITO, *et al.* 2001. Nod2, a Nod1/Apaf-1 family member that is restricted to monocytes and activates NF-kB. J. Biol. Chem. **276:** 4812–4818.
15. INOHARA, N., Y. OGURA, F.F. CHEN, *et al.* 2001. Human Nod1 confers responsiveness to bacterial lipopolysaccharides. J. Biol. Chem. **276:** 2551–2554.
16. LESAGE, S., H. ZOUALI, J.P. CEZARD, *et al.* 2002. CARD15/CARD15 mutational analysis and genotype-phenotype correlation in 612 patients with inflammatory bowel disease. Am. J. Hum. Genet. **70:** 845–857.
17. MILLER, S., D. DYKES & H. POLESKY. 1988. A simple salting out procedure for extracting DNA from human nucleated cells. Nucl. Acids Res. **16:** 1215–1223.
18. VERMEIRE, S., G. WILD, K. KOCHER, *et al.* 2002. CARD15 genetic variation in a Quebec population: prevalence, genotype-phenotype relationship, and haplotype structure. Am. J. Hum. Genet. **71:** 74–83.
19. YAMAZAKI, K., M. TAKAZOE, T. TANAKA, *et al.* 2002. Absence of mutation in the NOD2/CARD15 gene among 483 Japanese patients with Crohn's disease. J. Hum. Genet. **47:** 469–472.
20. BÜNIG, C., J. GENSCHEL, S. BÜHNER, *et al.* 2004. Mutations in the NOD2/CARD15 gene in Crohn's disease are associated with ileocecal resection and are a risk factor for reoperation. Aliment. Pharmacol. Ther. **19:** 1073–1078.
21. BONEN, D.K., Y. OGURA, D.L. NICOLAE, *et al.* 2003. Crohn's disease-associated NOD2 variants share a signaling defect in response to lipopolysaccharide and peptidoglycan. Gastroenterology **124:** 140–146.
22. CAVANAUGH, J.A., K.E. ADAMS, E.J. QUAK, *et al.* 2003. CARD15/NOD2risk alleles in the development of Crohn's disease in Australian population. Ann. Hum. Genet. **67:** 531–541.
23. MICELI-RICHARD, C., S. LESAGE, M. RYBOJAD, *et al.* 2001. CARD15 mutations in Blau syndrome. Nat. Genet. **29:** 19–20.
24. RAHMAN, P., S. BARTLETT, F. SIANNIS, *et al.* 2003. CARD15: a pleiotropic autoimmune gene that confers susceptibility to psoriatic arthritis. Am. J. Hum. Genet. **73:** 677–681.
25. STAROS, E.B. 2003. Molecular discoveries alter our view of inflammatory bowel disease. Am. J. Clin. Pathol. **119:** 524–539.
26. BOUMA, G. & W. STROBER. 2003. The immunological and genetic basis of inflammatory bowel disease. Nat. Rev. Immun. **3:** 521–533.
27. CALKINS, B.M. 1989. A meta-analysis of the role of smoking in inflammatory bowel disease. Dig. Dis. Sci. **34:** 1841–1854.

Apoptosis in Human Skin

Role in Pathogenesis of Various Diseases and Relevance for Therapy

ESTHER REEFMAN, PIETER C. LIMBURG, CEES G. M. KALLENBERG, AND MARC BIJL

Departments of Rheumatology and Clinical Immunology, University Hospital, 9700 RB Groningen, the Netherlands

ABSTRACT: Cell death by apoptosis is a physiological process that enables the elimination of cells without causing an inflammatory response. In self-renewing tissue like the epidermal layers of the skin, cell numbers are tightly regulated by a delicate balance between proliferation, differentiation, and cell death. Besides cell death by terminal differentiation in normal skin, cell death can also be induced by exposure to sunlight. This paper will review the different forms of cell death in the skin and discuss the role of apoptosis in diseases like skin cancer, psoriasis, and systemic lupus erythematosus.

KEYWORDS: apoptosis; skin; UVB; cancer; SLE

INTRODUCTION

Apoptosis is a form of programmed cell death that plays a crucial role in the development and homeostasis of the human body. Especially in continuously renewing tissues like the skin, cell growth and cell death have to be tightly regulated to ensure correct tissue function and to prevent inappropriate excessive growth.

The skin is composed of three distinct layers. The deepest layer is the subcutaneous fat which is covered by the dermis. The dermis contains blood vessels, nerves, hair follicles, and sweat glands. The top layer is called the epidermis, a continuously renewing multilayered epithelium with a high turnover rate. The epidermis is composed of three cell types: Langerhans cells (LCs), melanocytes, and keratinocytes. Keratinocytes are the cells that form the largest part of the epidermis. Basal and suprabasal keratinocytes together contitute the rapidly proliferating compartment known as the stratum basale. Terminal keratinocyte differentiation is initiated upon detachment from the underlying basement membrane into the stratum spinosum.[1] Keratinocytes move upwards through the stratum spinosum into the stratum granulosum, where cells lose their nucleus. The end product is a mechanically rigid, cross-

Address for correspondence: Esther Reefman, M.Sc., Departments of Rheumatology and Clinical Immunology, University Hospital Groningen, P.O. Box 30.001, 9700 RB Groningen, the Netherlands. Voice: +31-50-363851; fax: +31-50-3619069.
e.reefman@med.rug.nl

Ann. N.Y. Acad. Sci. 1051: 52–63 (2005). © 2005 New York Academy of Sciences.
doi: 10.1196/annals.1361.046

linked, keratinous envelope in the stratum corneum and is shed as an enucleate corneocyte. Langerhans cells are the residential dendritic cells of the epidermis. Melanocytes produce pigment largely composed of melanin and are located in the basal layer of the epidermis.

Regulation of cell death is very important in the homeostasis of the epidermis. The turnover rate of keratinocytes is very high, and basal and suprabasal keratinocytes are constantly dividing and finally dying after terminal differentiation in the stratum granulosum. Furthermore, skin is continuously exposed to external factors such as chemicals and sunlight, which can damage keratinocytes. Cell death ensures that critically damaged keratinocytes are removed to prevent dysfunction of these cells.

ROLE OF APOPTOSIS IN TERMINAL DIFFERENTIATION

During the process of terminal differentiation keratinocytes eventually die. There is some controversy over whether terminal differentiation of keratinocytes is a variant of apoptosis. Some histological features of terminally differentiating keratinocytes resemble cellular changes associated with apoptosis: for example, pyknosis and fragmentation into nucleosome-sized pieces.[2] Both processes also share the activation of endonucleases,[3] caspase-3 activity,[4] and degradation of DNA. However, several reports also point out the differences between terminal differentiation and apoptosis. DNA fragmentation is hardly seen in terminally differentiated keratinocytes.[3] We could not detect the active form of caspase-3 in the skin of healthy controls.[5] Furthermore, Gandarillas *et al.* showed that keratinocytes undergo terminal differentiation *in vitro* without going into apoptosis.[6] Finally, in diseases characterized by defects in growth, differentiation, or adhesion, no increase of apoptotic nuclei were detected in affected epidermis as compared to normal skin. In combination, these data strongly suggest that in keratinocytes terminal differentiation and apoptosis are distinct cellular events.

SUNLIGHT-INDUCED APOPTOSIS IN SKIN

Apoptosis in the skin can be induced by chemicals and ionizing radiation; however, most relevant is the exposure of the skin to sunlight. Ultraviolet radiation (UVR) is a strong inducer of apoptosis in the skin. Apoptotic epidermal keratinocytes, known as sunburn cells (SBCs), were originally described by their distinctive appearance: pyknotic nuclei and a shrunken, eosinophilic cytoplasm.[7] These features make SBCs easily recognizable in hematoxylin-eosin (H&E)–stained sections. SBCs can be detected as early as 8 hours after UVR exposure with maximal numbers at 24–48 hours and disappearance by 60–72 hours.[8,9] *In vitro*, apoptosis will finally result in permeabilization of the plasma membrane, known as secondary necrosis, which may lead to inflammation. However, it is believed that this will not occur under physiological circumstances *in vivo* owing to the rapid clearance of apoptotic cells.[10] In the skin, loss of desmosomes on apoptotic keratinocytes [11] will result in more a rapid migration towards the stratum corneum. Subsequently, shedding will clear a large part of the SBCs from the skin. In addition, infiltrating macrophages,[12] Langerhans cells,[13] and keratinocytes[14] internalize SBCs before they reach the stratum corneum.

UV light (200–400 nm) is subdivided according to its wavelength in UVA (315–400 nm), UVB (280–315 nm), and UVC (200–280 nm) light. UVC is absorbed by the stratospheric ozone layer; therefore sunlight usually contains only UVA and UVB. UVA penetrates through epidermal and dermal layers of the skin, and is weakly absorbed by biomolecules. In contrast, UVB does not penetrate much further than the epidermal layer and is strongly absorbed by DNA and protein. UVB is therefore the most effective inducer of SBCs in the skin.[15,16] UVB-induced apoptosis has been recognized as a complex mechanism in which a variety of signaling pathways are involved: (1) apoptosis induced by direct DNA-damage; (2) death receptor–mediated

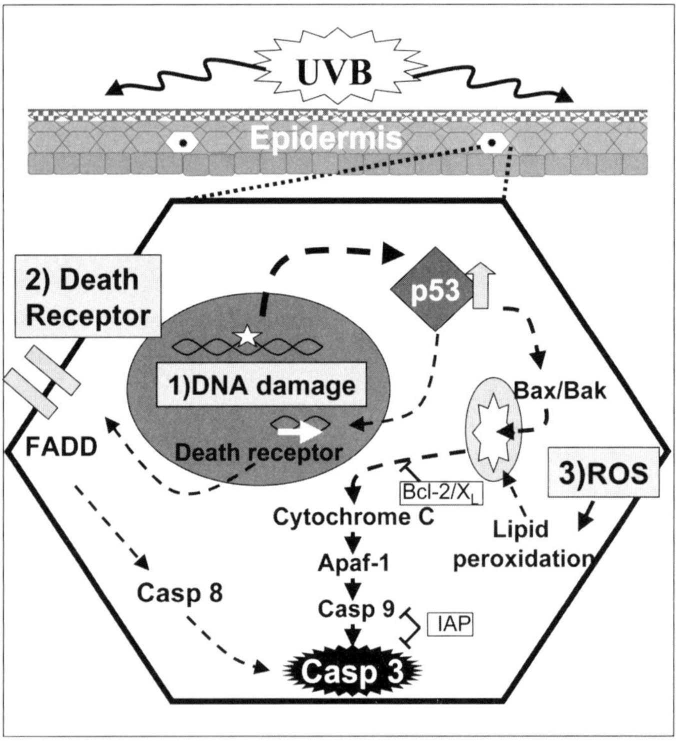

FIGURE 1. Schematic representation of the three signaling pathways involved in UVB-induced apoptosis. **(1)** Direct DNA-damage upregulates the expression and function of p53, which activates Bax/Bak, resulting in cytochrome *c* release from the mitochondria, subsequently leading to apoptotic protease-activating factor (Apaf-1), caspase-9, and caspase-3 activation, and the execution of apoptosis. P53 can also act as a transcription factor that is able to induce the transcription and expression of death receptors. **(2)** Death receptor clustering leads to recruitment and activation of FADD, which activates caspase-8, which in turn activates caspase-3. **(3)** Direct formation of reactive oxygen species (ROS) results in lipid peroxidation of the mitochondrial membrane and the subsequent release of cytochrome *c*, eventually leading to caspase-3 activation. Bcl-2 and Bcl-$X_L$can inhibit cytochrome *c* release, while inhibitors of apoptosis (IAPs) can inhibit activation of caspases.

apoptosis; and (3) apoptosis via the formation of reactive oxygen species (ROS). These pathways are discussed IN FIGURE 1.

1. Apoptosis Induced by Direct DNA Damage

UVB-induced DNA damage has long been proposed to be the only mediator of UVB-induced cell death. Absorbance of UVB energy by DNA results in two main types of lesions, known as cyclobutane pyrimidine dimers (CPDs) and 6-4 photoproducts. CPDs comprise 70–80% of all UV photoproducts. The majority of DNA lesions are removed by nucleotide excision repair (NER), which excises short single-stranded DNA nucleotide stretches (24–32 bases) around the damaged site and subsequently replaces the excised DNA lesion.[17] Increased numbers of SBCs are found in patients suffering form xeroderma pigmentosum, a disease in which genetic defects disable the nucleotide excision repair process.[18] The crucial role of DNA damage in UVB-induced apoptosis has been confirmed by *in vivo* studies in humans showing that the enhancement of DNA repair by the topical application of repair enzymes reduces the formation of SBCs.[19]

Cells with sustained DNA damage show a dramatic rise in the level of tumor suppressor gene p53 within minutes.[20] This upregulation was found to be proportional to the amount of CPD introduced into genomic DNA by UVB. P53 acts as a transcription factor, inducing transcription of a number of genes whose products trigger cell-cycle arrest during G1 phase. This allows the cell to repair DNA prior to DNA synthesis, thus reducing the DNA mutation rate.[8] In mice lacking functional p53, lower amounts of SBCs are induced.[8] When DNA damage is not sufficiently repaired, apoptosis is induced by the induction of pro-apoptotic factors like Bax or Bak, resulting in the release of cytochrome *c* from mitochondia. An apoptosome is formed by the binding of cytochrome *c* to apoptotic protease activating factor 1 (Apaf-1) and subsequently procaspase-9. This critical event leads to the initiation of the apoptotic cascade by the activation of caspase-9 and caspase-3 through cleavage.[21] Activation of these executer caspases in turn leads to cleavage of critical cellular substrates and DNA fragmentation. This mitochondrial pathway can be regulated by the anti-apoptotic Bcl-2 family of proteins (Bcl-2, Bcl-X_L), which prevent the release of cytochrome *c* from mitochondria,[22] and inhibitors of apoptosis (IAPs), which prevent caspase cleavage.[23] UV exposure leads to the downregulation of Bcl-2 in human skin, and promotes apoptosis.[24] Overexpression of Bcl-X_L and Bcl-X_S in the epidermis of transgenic mice contributes to cell survival after UV irradiation.[25] UV-induced DNA damage has also been shown to enhance the export and transcriptional activation of death receptors and their ligands mainly through p53-dependent pathways.[26,27]

2. Death Receptor–Mediated UV-Induced Apoptosis

Death receptors are members of the tumor necrosis factor (TNF) receptor superfamily, which includes the TNF receptor-1, the TNF-α-related apoptosis–inducing ligand (TRAIL) receptors, and Fas (CD95). Although all of these receptors have been linked to UV-induced apoptosis,[27–29] Fas-mediated cell death seems to play the most prominent role.[30]

Normal skin keratinocytes express Fas.[31] Expression is upregulated in chronically sun-exposed keratinocytes[32] but also after a single dose of UVB radiation,[33] demonstrating its involvement in sun-induced damage. CD95 mediates apoptosis via binding of its ligand, FasL (CD95L), which may be present in soluble form or expressed on the membrane of cells. FasL is also constitutively expressed by keratinocytes, and its expression is upregulated after UV exposure.[28,34] With respect to UVB-induced apoptosis, Aragene *et al.* demonstrated a direct and ligand-independent activation of Fas by the clustering of Fas at the cell membrane.[35] Clustering of Fas, ligand-dependent or -independent, leads to the activation of the intracellular death domains, which, in turn, can bind Fas-associated protein (FADD), thus triggering a cascade of proteases, starting with caspase-8. FADD has also recently been shown to be upregulated by UV irradiation.[36] Caspase-8 will cleave the executer caspase-3, which drives the apoptotic events described above.

3. Cell Stress Induced by UVB Irradiation

Reducing DNA damage and blocking death receptor signaling does not block apoptosis completely, indicating that at least a third independent signaling pathway is involved.[30] UVB is known to be a potent inducer of reactive oxygen species (ROS) in the cytoplasm. ROS have been shown to initiate cellular damage and apoptosis.[37–40] ROS can have multiple effects on a cell: it can damage DNA by inducing strand breaks, alter bases such as 8-hydroxyguanine, modify transcriptional binding sites on the DNA,[41] and cause lipid peroxidation. The cytotoxic potential of ROS lies in the latter effect. Lipid peroxidation changes the structure of plasma membranes[42] and damages the inner mitochondrial membrane, leading to cytochrome *c* release and subsequently resulting in apoptosis.[37] Mitochondria are not only a target for ROS but may also function as a source for ROS. In the late phase of UV-induced apoptosis, mitochondrial dysfunction leads to the enrichment of ROS in the cytoplasm.[43] Radical scavengers are able to partially inhibit UVB-induced apoptosis, although direct DNA damage induction and CD95 signaling are not affected by these scavengers.[30] Therefore, ROS contributes independently to UVB-mediated cell death.

ROLE OF UV-INDUCED APOPTOSIS IN PATHOGENESIS AND TREATMENT OF DISEASE

UV-induced apoptosis in the skin is known to be involved in the pathogenesis of multiple diseases. Defects in apoptosis may lead to hyperproliferation or even development of malignant cells. However, apoptotic cells themselves may also be involved in generating pathology. Next, we will discuss the three major diseases associated with UV induced apoptosis. A schemiatic representation is given in FIGURE 2.

Cancer Induction

Skin cancer is a very common form of cancer among Caucasians. Chronic repeated exposures to sunlight are epidemiologically shown to be the main cause of skin

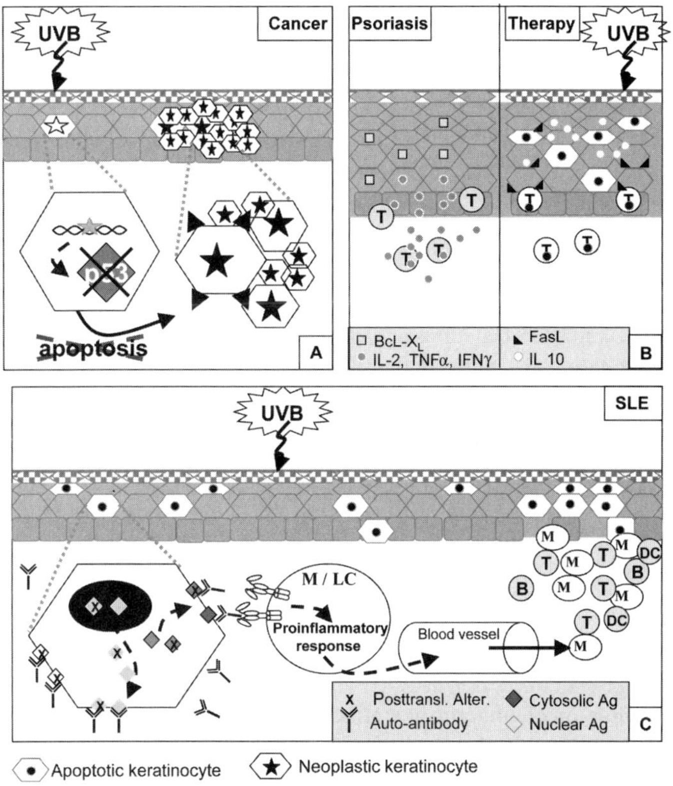

FIGURE 2. Schematic representation of the role of UVB-induced apoptosis in pathogenesis and treatment of disease. **(A) Cancer:** UVB induces damage to DNA that can lead to the formation of mutations in the tumor suppressor gene, p53. Loss of p53 function can result in a decrease of apoptotic signals, leading to the formation of a neoplastic keratinocyte. **(B) Psoriasis:** In the pathogenesis of psoriasis, keratinocytes are hyperproliferative and/or defective in terminal differentiation. Increased Bcl-X_L expression is involved in inhibition of apoptosis in psoriatic skin. Furthermore, infiltrating T cells producing proinflammatory cytokines (IL-2, TNFα, IFNγ) are also involved in the pathogenesis of psoriasis. Phototherapy, used for psoriatic lesions, induces apoptosis in keratinocytes and T cells directly and by upregulation of FasL on keratinocytes. IL-10 produced after irradiation also induces immunosuppression. Combining these effects will resolve psoriatic lesions. **(C) SLE:** Apoptotic keratinocytes induced by UVB express nuclear and cytosolic antigens (with or without posttranslational alteration induced by apoptosis) on their cell membrane. Autoantibodies present in SLE recognize these antigens. Inflammatory cells like residential Langerhans cells (LC), or macrophages (Mϕ) are recruited in the initial phase after irradiation and respond in a proinflammatory manner due to the interaction of Fc-gamma receptors and autoantibodies. This might lead to further recruitment of more inflammatory cells from the blood to the site where apoptotic cells reside, and thus inflammatory lesions develop.

cancer.[44] Skin malignancies are broadly divided into melanoma and nonmelanoma skin cancers. Nonmelanoma skin cancer (NMSC) occurs in sun-exposed sites and include basal cell and squamous cell carcinomas; they are derived from keratinocytes. Melanomas are derived from melanocytes and arise from naevi in both sun-exposed as well as nonexposed skin.

UVB in sunlight acts as a skin carcinogenic inducer, as well as a promoter, through the induction of DNA damage. Unrepaired photoproducts can lead to the incorporation of base mismatches. Mutations occur most commonly when a photoproduct contains a cytosine. Among CPDs, thymine-cytosine (T-C) and cytosine-cytosine (C-C) are shown to be the most mutagenic, while thymine–thymine dimers (T-T) are poorly mutagenic. The 6-4 photoproducts are very efficiently repaired within three hours after formation and are therefore less mutagenic.[45] As mentioned earlier, UV radiation can generate reactive oxygen species (ROS), which can cause oxidative damage to the DNA bases, forming 8-hydroxy-guanine that will result in G-to-T transversions.[46] Deletions and chromosomal aberrations can also be induced by UVB irradiation in mammalian cells.[47,48] The tumor suppressor gene p53 is commonly mutated after chronic UV exposure.[49,50] As discussed above, this protein plays a central role in induction of apoptosis via direct DNA damage and ROS formation. The mutations can result in loss of p53 function, leading to defective repair of UV-induced DNA damage[51] and a decreased apoptotic response.[52] Mutations that result in decreased apoptosis are associated with clonal expansion of these cells leading to tumor formation. Additionally, UV exposure causes transient immune suppression, which may also facilitate the growth of mutant cells without elimination.[53,54]

Psoriasis

Psoriasis is a common skin disorder characterized by hyperplasia and the incomplete differentiation of epidermal keratinocytes.[55] Aberrant expression of many regulatory molecules involved in proliferation might play a role in the pathogenesis of psoriasis. Bcl-X_L has been shown to be overexpressed in all layers of the psoriatic epidermis.[56] Furthermore, *in vitro* studies demonstrate that human keratinocytes derived from psoriatic plaques are resistant to induced apoptosis when compared to keratinocytes derived from normal skin.[57] However, several groups have reported that most keratinocytes in psoriatic epidermis have double-strand breaks in their DNA; this might reflect an apoptotic process.[56,58] Kwashima *et al.* recently showed that the increase in numbers of DNA double-strand breaks in psoriatic lesions was not the result of apoptotic processes but, rather, caused by active DNA replication.[59] Together, these reports show that defects in apoptosis might play an important role in the pathogenesis of psoriasis. Psoriasis is also accompanied by the infiltration of activated T lymphocytes in the dermis and epidermis, which in turn produce multiple inflammatory cytokines like IFN-γ, IL-2, and TNF-α. Whether the defects in apoptosis and differentiation are secondary to this influx is still unclear. UVB phototherapy is one of the most common treatments for extensive psoriasis and can induce long-lived clinical remissions. The main therapeutic effect of UVB irradiation seems to result from the depletion of T cells in lesions from epidermis and dermis. Apoptosis seems to be the primary mechanism involved in this depletion.[60] Although UVB can induce apoptosis in T lymphocytes and keratinocytes, at the doses used for treatment, mainly T lymphocytes are targeted.[61] Apoptosis of T cells can be induced directly by UVB or indirectly via upregulation of FasL in keratinocytes.[28] Besides the induction of apoptosis in immune-competent cells, UVB can also modulate immune responses, especially by the release of mediators from keratinocytes—IL-10 in particular.[62] IL-10 is normally decreased in psoriatic skin, and, upon the systemic administration of IL-10, antipsoriatic effects are seen.[63] Beneficial effects of UVB phototherapy can therefore be the result of the elimination of either T cells or keratinocytes by apoptosis, or immune modulation by IL-10.

Systemic Lupus Erythematosus

Systemic lupus erythematosus (SLE) is a systemic autoimmune disease characterized by the presence of autoantibodies to nuclear and cytoplasmic antigens in conjunction with a wide range of clinical manifestations. Photosensitivity is one of the characteristics of SLE; it affects 10–50% of patients.[64] Most, but not all, cutaneous lupus lesions occur in light-exposed areas and can be triggered by exposure to sunlight, which can even induce systemic disease activity. The processes inducing cutaneous and systemic inflammatory lesions have not been elucidated, but in recent years it has been suggested that apoptotic cells are one of the major factors involved. The accumulation of apoptotic cells due to an increased rate of apoptosis, decreased elimination of apoptotic cells, or a combination of both has been hypothesized to be an important factor in the development of inflammatory lesions, as seen in the skin.[65,66] During the apoptotic process, intracellular constituents are excessively presented to the immune systemowing to cell surface expression of intracellular constituents and/or posttranslational alteration of cellular proteins during apoptosis.[67–70] In SLE, autoantibodies are present that are specific for these antigens and binding to the apoptotic cell may change its clearance. In the skin of SLE patients deposition of IgG is often found at the dermal–epidermal junction, the so-called lupus band, or in the epidermal layer.[71] Increased numbers of apoptotic cells have been detected in LE skin lesions.[72] Keratinocytes from SLE patients have been shown to be more vulnerable to UV light *in vitro*.[73] Additionally, Baima *et al.* demonstrated an increase in Fas expression in keratinocytes in LE lesions, while Bcl-2 expression was decreased.[72] We have recently investigated the induction of apoptosis *in vivo* in SLE skin after UVB irradiation. Although SLE patients were more sensitive to UVB, similar numbers of apoptotic cells were induced in SLE patients and controls. However, the infiltrate seen after exposure was more extensive in 25% of the patients, and even persisted after ten days—while hardly any infiltrate was seen in the other patients and controls. After three days, in some patients, inflammatory lesions could be detected in the vicinity of apoptotic cells. We are currently characterizing the nature of this infiltrate to elucidate the mechanisms involved. However, these data indicate a more proinflammatory reaction after irradiation with UVB that is associated with apoptotic cells. We speculate that this might be caused by the opsonization of apoptotic keratinocytes by autoantibodies and subsequently alter clearance by macrophages and/or other phagocytes.

CONCLUSION

Because of daily exposure to sunlight, apoptosis in the skin is a daily event. In this way we are protected from cancer cell formation. However, when apoptotic mechanisms fail due to defects or mutations in key apoptotic proteins, pathological processes take over, as in skin cancer and psoriasis. Apoptotic cells themselves can also be the source from which the pathology develops. This might be the case in SLE, where binding of autoantibodies to apoptotic cells may lead to an altered recognition and clearance of these cells, thus leading to inflammation. Understanding these processes can result in an improvement in current therapies.

REFERENCES

1. GREEN, H. 1977. Terminal differentiation of cultured human epidermal cells. Cell **11:** 405–416.
2. MARUOKA, Y., H. HARADA, T. MITSUYASU, *et al.* 1997. Keratinocytes become terminally differentiated in a process involving programmed cell death. Biochem. Biophys. Res. Commun. **238:** 886–890.
3. MCCALL, C.A. & J.J. COHEN. 1991. Programmed cell death in terminally differentiating keratinocytes: role of endogenous endonuclease. J. Invest. Dermatol. **97:** 111–114.
4. ALLOMBERT-BLAISE, C., S. TAMIJI, L. MORTIER, *et al.* 2003. Terminal differentiation of human epidermal keratinocytes involves mitochondria- and caspase-dependent cell death pathways. Cell Death Differ. **10:** 850–852.
5. REEFMAN, E., H. KUIPER, M. JONKMAN, *et al.* 2004. Irradiation of systemic lupus erythematosus skin: sensitivity, apoptosis induction, and inflammation [abstract]. Autoimmun. Rev. **3**: 43.
6. GANDARILLAS, A., L.A. GOLDSMITH, S.G. SCHMEISSNER, *et al.* 1999. Evidence that apoptosis and terminal differentiation of epidermal keratinocytes are distinct processes. Exp. Dermatol. **8:** 71–79.
7. DANIELS, F., JR., D. BROPHY & W.C. LOBITZ, JR. 1961. Histochemical responses of human skin following ultraviolet irradiation. J. Invest. Dermatol. **37:** 351–357.
8. MURPHY, G., A.R. YOUNG, H.C. WULF, *et al.* 2001. The molecular determinants of sunburn cell formation. Exp. Dermatol. **10:** 155–160.
9. WOODCOCK, A. & I.A. MAGNUS. 1976. The sunburn cell in mouse skin: preliminary quantitative studies on its production. Br. J. Dermatol. **95:** 459–468.
10. PROSKURYAKOV, S.Y., A.G. KONOPLYANNIKOV & V.L. GABAI. 2003. Necrosis: a specific form of programmed cell death? Exp. Cell Res. **283:** 1–16.
11. WEISKE, J., T. SCHONEBERG, W. SCHRODER, *et al.* 2001. The fate of desmosomal proteins in apoptotic cells. J. Biol. Chem. **276:** 41175–41181.
12. COOPER, K.D., N. DURAISWAMY, C. HAMMERBERG, *et al.* 1993. Neutrophils, differentiated macrophages, and monocyte/macrophage antigen–presenting cells infiltrate murine epidermis after UV injury. J. Invest. Dermatol. **101:** 155–163.
13. REIS, C., E. SOUSA, P.D. STAHL & J.M. AUSTYN. 1993. Phagocytosis of antigens by Langerhans cells *in vitro*. J. Exp. Med. **178:** 509–519.
14. SHARLOW, E.R., C.S. PAINE, L. BABIARZ, *et al.* 2000. The protease-activated receptor-2 upregulates keratinocyte phagocytosis. J. Cell Sci. **113:** 3093–3101.
15. KUMAKIRI, M., K. HASHIMOTO & I. WILLIS. 1977. Biologic changes due to long-wave ultraviolet irradiation on human skin: ultrastructural study. J. Invest. Dermatol. **69:** 392–400.
16. YOUNG, A.R. 1987. The sunburn cell. Photodermatology **4:** 127–134.
17. DE LAAT, W.L., N.G. JASPERS & J.H. HOEIJMAKERS. 1999. Molecular mechanism of nucleotide excision repair. Genes Dev. **13:** 768–785.
18. PETIT-FRERE, C., E. CAPULAS, J.E. LOWE, *et al.* 2000. Ultraviolet B–induced apoptosis and cytokine release in xeroderma pigmentosum keratinocytes. J. Invest. Dermatol. **115:** 687–693.
19. STEGE, H., L. ROZA, A.A. VINK, *et al.* 2000. Enzyme-plus-light therapy to repair DNA damage in ultraviolet B–irradiated human skin. Proc. Natl. Acad. Sci. USA **97:** 1790–1795.

20. KASTAN, M.B., O. ONYEKWERE, D. SIDRANSKY, *et al.* 1991. Participation of p53 protein in the cellular response to DNA damage. Cancer Res. **51:** 6304–6311.
21. SITAILO, L.A., S.S. TIBUDAN & M.F. DENNING. 2002. Activation of caspase-9 is required for UV-induced apoptosis of human keratinocytes. J. Biol. Chem. **277:** 19346–19352.
22. HOCKENBERY, D., G. NUNEZ, C. MILLIMAN, *et al.* 1990. Bcl-2 is an inner mitochondrial membrane protein that blocks programmed cell death Nature **348:** 334–336.
23. DEVERAUX, Q.L., R. TAKAHASHI, G.S. SALVESEN & J.C. REED. 1997. X-linked IAP is a direct inhibitor of cell-death proteases. Nature **388:** 300–304.
24. WASHIO, F., M. UEDA, A. ITO & M. ICHIHASHI. 1999. Higher susceptibility to apoptosis following ultraviolet B irradiation of xeroderma pigmentosum fibroblasts is accompanied by upregulation of p53 and downregulation of bcl-2. Br. J. Dermatol. **140:** 1031–1037.
25. PENA, J.C., E. FUCHS & C.B. THOMPSON. 1997. Bcl-x expression influences keratinocyte cell survival but not terminal differentiation. Cell Growth Differ. **8:** 619–629.
26. BENNETT, M., K. MACDONALD, S.W. CHAN, *et al.* 1998. Cell surface trafficking of Fas: a rapid mechanism of p53-mediated apoptosis. Science **282:** 290–293.
27. KIBITEL, J., V. HEJMADI, L. ALAS, *et al.* 1998. UV-DNA damage in mouse and human cells induces the expression of tumor necrosis factor alpha. Photochem. Photobiol. **67:** 541–546.
28. LEVERKUS, M., M. YAAR & B.A. GILCHREST. 1997. Fas/Fas ligand interaction contributes to UV-induced apoptosis in human keratinocytes. Exp. Cell Res. **232:** 255–262.
29. QIN, J.Z., P. BACON, J. PANELLA, *et al.* 2004. Low-dose UV radiation sensitizes keratinocytes to TRAIL-induced apoptosis. J. Cell Physiol. **200:** 155–166.
30. KULMS, D., E. ZEISE, B. POPPELMANN & T. SCHWARZ. 2002. DNA damage, death receptor activation, and reactive oxygen species contribute to ultraviolet radiation–induced apoptosis in an essential and independent way. Oncogene **21:** 5844–5851.
31. OISHI, M., K. MAEDA & S. SUGIYAMA. 1994. Distribution of apoptosis-mediating Fas antigen in human skin and effects of anti-Fas monoclonal antibody on human epidermal keratinocyte and squamous cell carcinoma cell lines. Arch. Dermatol. Res. **286:** 396–407.
32. FILIPOWICZ, E., P. ADEGBOYEGA, R.L. SANCHEZ & Z. GATALICA. 2002. Expression of CD95 (Fas) in sun-exposed human skin and cutaneous carcinomas. Cancer **94:** 814–819.
33. BANG, B., J. RYGAARD, O. BAADSGAARD & L. SKOV. 2002. Increased expression of Fas on human epidermal cells after *in vivo* exposure to single-dose ultraviolet (UV) B or long-wave UVA radiation. Br. J. Dermatol. **147:** 1199–1206.
34. OUHTIT, A., A. GORNY, H.K. MULLER, *et al.* 2000. Loss of Fas-ligand expression in mouse keratinocytes during UV carcinogenesis. Am. J. Pathol. **157:** 1975–1981.
35. ARAGANE, Y., D. KULMS, D. METZE, *et al.* 1998. Ultraviolet light induces apoptosis via direct activation of CD95 (Fas/APO-1) independently of its ligand CD95L J. Cell Biol. **140:** 171–182.
36. KIM, P.K., R. WELLER, Y. HUA & T.R. BILLIAR. 2003. Ultraviolet irradiation increases FADD protein in apoptotic human keratinocytes. Biochem. Biophys. Res. Commun. **302:** 290–295.
37. FARBER, J.L. 1994. Mechanisms of cell injury by activated oxygen species. Environ. Health Perspect. **102:** 17–24.
38. MASAKI, H., T. ATSUMI & H. SAKURAI. 1995. Detection of hydrogen peroxide and hydroxyl radicals in murine skin fibroblasts under UVB irradiation. Biochem. Biophys. Res. Commun. **206:** 474–479.
39. PEUS, D., R.A. VASA, A. BEYERLE, *et al.* 1999. UVB activates ERK1/2 and p38 signaling pathways via reactive oxygen species in cultured keratinocytes. J. Invest. Dermatol. **112:** 751–756.
40. TYRRELL, R.M. 1995. Ultraviolet radiation and free radical damage to skin. Biochem. Soc. Symp. **61:** 47–53.
41. FLOYD, R.A. 1990. Role of oxygen free radicals in carcinogenesis and brain ischemia. FASEB J. **4:** 2587–2597.
42. DE KOK, T.M., F. TEN VAARWERK, I. ZWINGMAN, *et al.* 1994. Peroxidation of linoleic, arachidonic, and oleic acid in relation to the induction of oxidative DNA damage and cytogenetic effects. Carcinogenesis **15:** 1399–1404.

43. CADENAS, E. & K.J. DAVIES. 2000. Mitochondrial free radical generation, oxidative stress, and aging. Free Radic. Biol. Med. **29:** 222–230.
44. WOODHEAD, A.D., R.B. SETLOW & M. TANAKA. 1999. Environmental factors in nonmelanoma and melanoma skin cancer. J. Epidemiol. **9:** S102–114.
45. BRASH, D.E. & W.A. HASELTINE. 1982. UV-induced mutation hotspots occur at DNA damage hotspots. Nature **298:** 189–192.
46. SHIBUTANI, S., M. TAKESHITA & A.P. GROLLMAN. 1991. Insertion of specific bases during DNA synthesis past the oxidation-damaged base 8-oxodG. Nature **349:** 431–434.
47. EMRI, G., E. WENCZL, P. VAN ERP, *et al.* 2000. Low doses of UVB or UVA induce chromosomal aberrations in cultured human skin cells. J. Invest. Dermatol. **115:** 435–440.
48. HORIGUCHI, M., K.I. MASUMURA, H. IKEHATA, *et al.* 2001. Molecular nature of ultraviolet B light-induced deletions in the murine epidermis. Cancer Res. **61:** 3913–3918.
49. BRASH, D.E., J.A. RUDOLPH, J.A. SIMON, *et al.* 1991. A role for sunlight in skin cancer: UV-induced p53 mutations in squamous cell carcinoma. Proc. Natl. Acad. Sci. USA **88:** 10124–10128.
50. ZIEGLER, A., D.J. LEFFELL, S. KUNALA, *et al.* 1993. Mutation hotspots due to sunlight in the p53 gene of nonmelanoma skin cancers. Proc. Natl. Acad. Sci. USA **90:** 4216–4220.
51. SMITH, M.L., I.T. CHEN, Q. ZHAN, *et al.* 1995. Involvement of the p53 tumor suppressor in repair of UV-type DNA damage. Oncogene **10:** 1053–1059.
52. HILL, L.L., A. OUHTIT, S.M. LOUGHLIN, *et al.* 1999. Fas ligand: a sensor for DNA damage critical in skin cancer etiology. Science **285:** 898–900.
53. GUZMAN, E., J.L. LANGOWSKI & L. OWEN-SCHAUB. 2003. Mad dogs, Englishmen, and apoptosis: the role of cell death in UV-induced skin cancer. Apoptosis **8:** 315–325.
54. FISHER, M.S. & M.L. KRIPKE. 1977. Systemic alteration induced in mice by ultraviolet light irradiation and its relationship to ultraviolet carcinogenesis. Proc. Natl. Acad. Sci. USA **74:** 1688–1692.
55. MCKAY, I.A. & I.M. LEIGH. 1995. Altered keratinocyte growth and differentiation in psoriasis. Clin. Dermatol. **13:** 105–114.
56. WRONE-SMITH, T., T. JOHNSON, B. NELSON, *et al.* 1995. Discordant expression of Bcl-x and Bcl-2 by keratinocytes *in vitro* and psoriatic keratinocytes *in vivo*. Am. J. Pathol. **146:** 1079–1088.
57. WRONE-SMITH, T., R.S. MITRA, C.B. THOMPSON, *et al.* 1997. Keratinocytes derived from psoriatic plaques are resistant to apoptosis compared with normal skin. Am. J. Pathol. **151:** 1321–1329.
58. LAPORTE, M., P. GALAND, D. FOKAN, *et al.* 2000. Apoptosis in established and healing psoriasis. Dermatology **200:** 314–316.
59. KAWASHIMA, K., H. DOI, Y. ITO, *et al.* 2004. Evaluation of cell death and proliferation in psoriatic epidermis. J. Dermatol. Sci. **35:** 207–214.
60. OZAWA, M., K. FERENCZI, T. KIKUCHI, *et al.* 1999. 312-nanometer ultraviolet B light (narrow-band UVB) induces apoptosis of T cells within psoriatic lesions. J. Exp. Med. **189:** 711–718.
61. KRUEGER, J.G., J.T. WOLFE, R.T. NABEYA, *et al.* 1995. Successful ultraviolet B treatment of psoriasis is accompanied by a reversal of keratinocyte pathology and by selective depletion of intraepidermal T cells. J. Exp. Med. **182:** 2057–2068.
62. NISHIGORI, C., D.B. YAROSH, S.E. ULLRICH, *et al.* 1996. Evidence that DNA damage triggers interleukin 10 cytokine production in UV-irradiated murine keratinocytes. Proc. Natl. Acad. Sci. USA **93:** 10354–10359.
63. ASADULLAH, K., W. STERRY, K. STEPHANEK, *et al.* 1998. IL-10 is a key cytokine in psoriasis. Proof of principle by IL-10 therapy: a new therapeutic approach. J. Clin. Invest. **101:** 783–794.
64. PROVOST, T.T. & J.A. FLYNN. 2001. Cutaneous medicine. *In* Lupus Erythematosus. :41–81. Elsevier Science. London.
65. BIJL, M., P.C. LIMBURG & C.G. KALLENBERG. 2001. New insights into the pathogenesis of systemic lupus erythematosus (SLE): the role of apoptosis. Neth. J. Med. **59:** 66–75.
66. REEFMAN, E., H.M. DIJSTELBLOEM, P.C. LIMBURG, *et al.* 2003. Fc gamma receptors in the initiation and progression of systemic lupus erythematosus. Immunol. Cell Biol. **81:** 382–389.

67. Casciola-Rosen, L.A., G. Anhalt & A. Rosen. 1994. Autoantigens targeted in systemic lupus erythematosus are clustered in two populations of surface structures on apoptotic keratinocytes. J. Exp. Med. **179:** 1317–1330.
68. Saegusa, J., S. Kawano, M. Koshiba, *et al.* 2002. Oxidative stress mediates cell surface expression of SS-A/Ro antigen on keratinocytes. Free Radic. Biol. Med. **32:** 1006–1016.
69. Utz, P.J., M. Hottelet, P.H. Schur & P. Anderson. 1997. Proteins phosphorylated during stress-induced apoptosis are common targets for autoantibody production in patients with systemic lupus erythematosus. J. Exp. Med. **185:** 843–854.
70. Utz, P.J. & P. Anderson. 1998. Posttranslational protein modifications, apoptosis, and the bypass of tolerance to autoantigens. Arthritis Rheum. **41:** 1152–1160.
71. Halberg, P., S. Ullman & F. Jorgensen. 1982. The lupus band test as a measure of disease activity in systemic lupus erythematosus. Arch. Dermatol. **118:** 572–576.
72. Baima, B. & M. Sticherling. 2001. Apoptosis in different cutaneous manifestations of lupus erythematosus. Br. J. Dermatol. **144:** 958–966.
73. Furukawa, F., T. Itoh, H. Wakita, *et al.* 1999. Keratinocytes from patients with lupus erythematosus show enhanced cytotoxicity to ultraviolet radiation and to antibody-mediated cytotoxicity. Clin. Exp. Immunol. **118:** 164–170.

Cancer-Associated Myositis

Clinical Features and Prognostic Signs

ANDREA PONYI,[a,b] TAMÁS CONSTANTIN,[b] MIKLÓS GARAMI,[b] CSILLA ANDRÁS,[c] BÉLA TÁLLAI,[d] ANDREA VÁNCSA,[a] LAJOS GERGELY,[a] AND KATALIN DANKÓ[a]

[a]*Division of Clinical Immunology, Third Department of Internal Medicine,* [c]*Department of Oncology,* [d]*Department of Urology, Medical and Health Science Center, University of Debrecen, Debrecen, Hungary*

[b]*Second Department of Pediatrics, Faculty of Medicine, Semmelweis University, Budapest, Hungary*

ABSTRACT: Idiopathic inflammatory myositis is characterized by progressive weakness of the proximal muscles. There is a higher risk of malignancy than in the normal population. The aim of this study was to evaluate the frequency of malignancy among 251 myositis patients. We also compared clinical and immunological characteristics of cancer-associated myositis with primary myositis. There were no malignancies among polymyositis, overlap, or juvenile myositis patients. Twenty-two of ninety dermatomyositis patients also had a malignant disease. Patients with cancer-associated dermatomyositis were significantly older than primary myositis patients and had more severe cutaneous and muscle symptoms. Dysphagia and diaphragmatic involvement were more frequent among cancer-associated patients, while extramuscular features were less frequent. After successful treatment of the malignancy, we were able to manage myositis symptoms. One-year survival rate was significantly better in primary dermatomyositis patients. The subset of cancer-associated myositis differs from primary myositis in many aspects of its clinical and immunological features. Prognosis and life expectancy in cancer-associated myositis patients is determined by the underlying malignant disease. Therefore, age- and sex-specific examinations for detection of an underlying malignancy are important in the management of patients with dermatomyositis.

KEYWORDS: dermatomyositis; cancer; clinical features; prognostic signs; survival

INTRODUCTION

The heterogeneous group of idiopathic inflammatory myositis (IIM) consists of rare systemic autoimmune diseases. The hallmark of these disorders is a progressive weakness of the proximal muscles mediated by an autoimmune process. It has been

Address for correspondence: Andrea Ponyi, M.D., Third Department of Internal Medicine, Medical and Health Science Center, University of Debrecen, Moricz Zs Krt 22, 4004 Debrecen, Hungary. Voice/fax: +36-52-414-969.
ponyi@gyer2.sote.hu

Ann. N.Y. Acad. Sci. 1051: 64–71 (2005). © 2005 New York Academy of Sciences.
doi: 10.1196/annals.1361.047

well known for decades that IIM, mainly dermatomyositis (DM), can be associated with malignant diseases. The frequency in such case reports ranged widely from 3 to 60%. In recent years, it has been established in population-based cohort studies that the risk of malignancy is definitely higher than in the normal population and not only for dermatomyositis but for other forms of myositis as well. A great variety of tumors can accompany myositis. The nature of the temporal association between malignancy and myositis varies. Malignancy may occur before the diagnosis of myositis, or concurrently with it, or it may develop after the myositis. The etiology or the exact pathomechanism of the association of myositis with tumors has remained unclear. The most popular hypothesis is that myositis has a paraneoplastic nature in cancer-associated cases. It is assumed that compromised immune function or common environmental factors, such as Epstein-Barr virus, may also play a role in the development of cancer-associated myositis. On the contrary, if the malignancy occurs years after the myositis, the role of cytotoxic agents in the treatment of myositis may be supposed.

In the present work, the aim was to evaluate the relationship between malignancy and myositis among our patients. The clinical and immunological characteristics of patients with cancer-associated myositis (CAM) and primary myositis were compared.

PATIENTS AND METHODS

Two hundred fifty-one patients with different forms of IIM, who were studied from 1985 to 2003 by the Third Department of Internal Medicine, University of Debrecen, Hungary, were enrolled from our myositis database. Diagnosis of IIM was based upon the Bohan and Peter criteria in all cases.[1] Patients were classified into clinicopathological subsets: (1) polymyositis (PM); (2) DM; (3) overlap myositis (OM) or myositis in association with clinical and immunological features of another systemic autoimmune disease; (4) juvenile myositis; (5) CAM; and (6) other, uncommon forms of myositis.

Concerning the comparison of CAM and primary myositis, we analyzed retrospectively the following data: age, sex, muscle symptoms, skin and systemic symptoms (Raynaud's phenomenon, arthritis, dysphagia, dysphonia), diaphragmatic involvement, interstitial lung disease (ILD), cardiac involvement, laboratory data including creatinine kinase (CK), lactate dehydrogenase (LDH) serum activity, presence of autoantibodies (antinuclear factor [ANF], antibodies to extractable nuclear antigens (ENA), and the anti-Jo-1 antibody), treatment (glucocorticoid alone or with additional immunomodulatory agents including methotrexate, cyclosporine, azathioprine, cyclophosphamide, or intravenous immunoglobulin), and the date of death or the end of follow-up.

All data were analyzed using the SPSS for Windows 10.0 statistics software (SPSS Inc., Chicago, IL, USA). Student's t test or Fisher's exact test was applied to verify the statistical significance between patient groups. The survival curves were drawn using the Kaplan-Meier method. The log rank test was used to determine the statistical significance of the observed difference in survival rates between patient groups. P values less than 0.05 were considered significant.

RESULTS

In our cohort of IIM patients, we did not find cancer-associated myositis in the group of PM, OM, juvenile, or inclusion body myositis patients. Among patients with dermatomyositis, 24 had a malignancy at some point in their life. Considering the temporal connection between myositis and malignancy, there were 12 patients whose malignant disease occurred within one year of the myositis diagnosis. Six patients had a malignancy one year or more after the development of DM, and three patients had had a malignant disease one year or more before DM arose. One of our DM patients had multiple malignomas and recurrent episodes of myositis independently from her malignant diseases (endometrial carcinoma for 16 years and kidney tumor for 2 years before DM; then she had colon cancer, followed by a stomach cancer, 9 and 11 years later, respectively). Currently, this patient's myositis and malignant diseases are all in remission. The exact time limit of the association of a malignant disease with myositis is controversial. Therefore, we evaluated our patients as having CAM based upon evidence coming from the population-based cohort studies.[2] Patients with a malignancy that occurred more than two years before or more than five years after the diagnosis of myositis were discharged from further evaluation.

Among CAM patients, a broad range of malignant diseases was observed. The cancer site and histological types were as follows: breast cancer in four cases, gastric cancer in three cases, epipharyngeal cancer in two cases, colon cancer in two cases, lung cancer in two patients, urinary bladder cancer in one patient, ovarian cancer in one patient, and melanoma in one patient.

The summary of clinical and laboratory findings of patients with CAM and primary DM is presented in TABLE 1. CAM patients were significantly older than primary myositis patients at the time of myositis diagnosis ($P = 0.005$). A larger female-to-male ratio, which is characteristic of DM, was not observed among CAM patients. The distribution of cutaneous symptoms characteristic to DM (heliotropic rash, facial erythema, Gottron's papules, and Gottron's sign) was observed to a similar extent in both the groups. One striking feature of CAM patients is that they had more severe skin manifestations, which were often refractory to conventional therapy. In the area of muscle symptoms, the CAM group had more patients who seemed to have not only proximal, but also distal muscle weakness ($P = 0.007$). These patients had more severe muscle weakness, and a higher proportion became bedridden ($P = 0.021$). Classical features of systemic autoimmune diseases, arthritis, and Raynaud's phenomenon were more frequent in patients with primary DM ($P = 0.031$ and $P = 0.038$). Dysphagia, oropharyngeal dysfunction, and diaphragmatic involvement were more frequent in CAM patients, although in the case of dysphagia the difference was not significant. ILD were less frequent in CAM patients ($P = 0.043$), and we did not observed cardiac involvement among them.

Regarding the laboratory data, elevation of serum CK and LDH activity were observed in both groups. Nevertheless, primary DM patients seemed to have higher CK elevation than CAM patients ($P = 0.039$ and $P = 0.047$, respectively). Immunoserological alterations were less frequent among patients with CAM. All of ANF, ENA, and anti-Jo-1 testing showed positive results in a significantly higher proportion in DM patients. Tumor markers were also assessed in some patients. However, with the exception of CA 15-3, these markers did not serve as a clue to an underlying malignancy.

TABLE 1. Clinical and laboratory features of cancer-associated and primary dermatomyositis patients

	Cancer-associated Dermatomyositis	Primary Dermatomyositis
Number of patients	16	68
Mean age at myositis onset, yrs ± SD	56.0 ± 11.0[a]	46.2 ± 12.3
Male to female ratio	1.0:1.0	1.0:2.4
Cutaneous symptoms		
Heliotropic rash	13 (81%)	61 (89%)
Facial erythema	14 (87%)	59 (91%)
V-sign	11 (69%)	52 (76%)
Gottron's papules	14 (88%)	44 (65%)
Gottron's sign	10 (63%)	35 (52%)
Ulceration	7 (44%)[a]	9 (13%)
Symptoms		
Distal muscle weakness	8 (50%)[a]	4 (6%)
Became bedridden	7 (44%)[a]	8 (12%)
Fever	0 (0%)[a]	20 (29%)
Arthritis	3 (25%)[a]	34 (51%)
Raynaud's phenomenon	2 (17%)[a]	17 (26%)
Dysphagia	8 (50%)	24 (35%)
Oropharyngeal dysfunction	6 (38%)	8 (13%)
Diaphragmatic involvement	5 (31%)[a]	12 (17%)
Cardiac involvement	0 (0%)[a]	5 (7%)
Interstitial lung disease	3 (19%)[a]	17 (25%)
Laboratory features		
Mean CK activity, U/L	945 ± 654[a]	3612 ± 1450
Mean LDH activity, U/L	777 ± 206	1039 ± 966
ANF positivity	3 (19%)[a]	26 (39%)
ENA positivity	0 (0%)[a]	28 (41%)
Anti–Jo-1 positivity	0/12 (0%)[a]	10/59 (16%)
Tumor markers		
CEA	2/8 (25%)	2/29 (9%)
AFP	0/6 (0%)	0/34 (0%)
CA 72-4	0/6 (0%)	1/24 (4%)
CA 19-9	2/8 (25%)	2/27 (7%)
CA 15-3	1/7 (14%)[a]	2/27 (7%)
CA 125	3/6 (50%)	2/24 (8%)
Second-line immunosuppressive treatment required	9 (56%)[a]	29 (42%)

[a]$P < 0.05$ versus primary dermatomyositis patients.

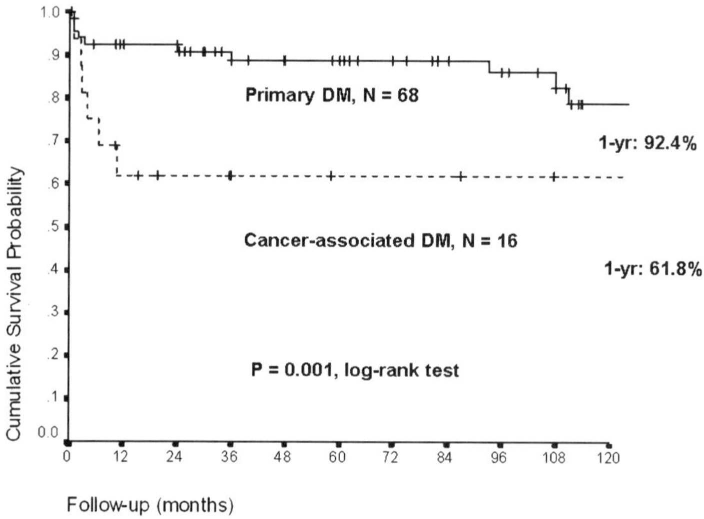

FIGURE 1. Survival of patients with primary and cancer-associated dermatomyositis.

In the management of CAM patients, more aggressive therapeutic protocols were required; second-line immunosuppressive agents were used in addition to high-dose glucocorticoids. After the appropriate treatment of the underlying malignancy, severe skin and muscle symptoms became manageable. The survival of CAM patients was determined by the underlying malignant disease; therefore that subgroup had significantly worse survival probability than patients with primary DM, as shown in FIGURE 1.

DISCUSSION

There has been much debate about a higher risk of malignant diseases in patients with IIMs, based on case series and previous case-control reports. In recent years, all of the large population-based studies found a remarkable association, mainly with DM, but to a modest extent with PM as well (TABLE 2). It should be mentioned that the diagnosis of myositis in some of the patients involved in these studies was not based on histological criteria.[2–4] The risk of cancer was found to be moderately higher in patients with inclusion body myositis.[5] Regarding the rarity of the disease, there are no other population-based studies to investigate the relationship between juvenile or overlap myositis and cancer.

Although a very great variety of types of cancer can occur, the most frequent are ovarian, lung, gastric, colorectal tumors and lymphomas in DM and lung, urinary bladder cancers, and lymphomas in PM.[2] Furthermore, in juvenile patients hematological malignancies are observed with greater frequency.[6] In Asian populations, nasopharyngeal and lung cancers are the most common types.[7,8]

In the majority of patients, CAM appears to have a paraneoplastic feature. In these cases, there is a strong correlation between the clinical course of myositis and

TABLE 2. Frequency of cancer-associated myositis in the literature

Author and Reference	Location	Patients		DM	PM
Hill[2]	Sweden, Finland, Denmark	1532, PM/DM	SIR	3.0	1.3
Stockton[3]	Scotland	708, PM/DM	SIR	7.7	2.1
Buchbinder[5]	Australia	537, PM/DM/IBM	RR	6.2	2.0
Zantos[4]	USA	1078, PM/DM	RR	4.4	2.1

ABBREVIATIONS: DM, dermatomyositis; PM, polymyositis; IBM, inclusion body myositis; SIR, standardized incidence ratio; RR, relative risk.

the malignant disease, as a relapse of the malignant diseases is accompanied by the reappearance of myositis. Another characteristic feature is the normal or slightly elevated CK.[9] Furthermore, these patients seldom have myositis-specific or myositis-associated autoantibodies. The successful treatment of the malignancy helps to relieve myositis symptoms. In turn, there are no specific antibodies that have been identified in CAM, and there is no specific association with a certain cancer type; these facts go against the theory of the paraneoplastic nature of myositis.

In the current study, we found remarkable differences between CAM and primary DM patients in respect to clinical and laboratory features. However, it should be mentioned that the small sample size allows for a limited interpretation of results. Similar to the data in the literature, our CAM patients were significantly older. Nevertheless, it should be kept in mind that there is evidence for a higher risk of malignancies in younger patients with DM compared to the normal population.[2,3] In contrast with the literature, there was no female predominance among patients with CAM. In view of the clinical manifestations, CAM patients had more extensive and severe skin symptoms than did primary DM patients. These skin symptoms were often exacerbated. We did not observe the presence of vasculitis among our CAM patients; vasculitis has traditionally been considered a sign of malignancy in DM patients.[10] Classic systemic features of myositis such as fever, arthritis, Raynaud's phenomenon, ILD, and cardiac involvement were less frequent. Given the severity of the disease, it was not surprising that dysphagia and diaphragmatic involvement were frequent among CAM patients. Immunoserologic alterations were less frequent in CAM patients. We also investigated the role of tumor markers, which seemed to be useless in detecting CAM patients. A limitation of these tests is that patients with systemic autoimmune diseases may have elevated serum levels of tumor markers.[11] The effective treatment of skin and severe muscle symptoms was a great challenge in our CAM patients. A cornerstone of management was the appropriate therapy for the malignant disease. While the survival of primary IIM patients has progressively improved worldwide,[12–15] CAM currently has the worse prognosis and survival rate among IIMs. On the other hand, our CAM patients had a 61.8% probability of survival at five years, which is a more positive number than the 10% value found in a recent study of Japanese patients.[16]

In conclusion, the recognition of particular risk factors that initiate a search for an underlying malignancy is very important in the management of myositis patients.[17] On the basis of our findings and the available literature, these are severe, exacerbated, or atypical cutaneous symptoms refractory to treatment in older patients, rapidly progressing severe muscle weakness, persistently elevated erythrocyte sedimentation rate, and the absence of immunoserologic alterations.[18–21] Therefore, an individually tailored screening is recommended, which should be based on the clinicopathological subgroup of myositis, age, and gender, and this awareness should extend through the follow-up as well.

ACKNOWLEDGMENTS

This work was supported by a Grant (T: 046931) from the Hungarian Scientific Research Fund.

REFERENCES

1. Bohan, A. & B.J. Peter. 1975. Polymyositis and dermatomyositis. Parts 1 and 2. N. Engl. J. Med. **292:** 344–347, 403–407.
2. Hill, C.L. *et al.* 2001. Frequency of specific cancer types in dermatomyositis and polymyositis: a population-based study. Lancet **357:** 96–100.
3. Stockton, D. *et al.* 2001. Risk of cancer in patients with dermatomyositis or polymyositis, and follow-up implications: a Scottish population-based cohort study. Br. J. Cancer. **85:** 41–45.
4. Zantos, D. *et al.* 1994. The overall and temporal association of cancer with polymyositis and dermatomyositis. J. Rheumatol. **21:** 1855–1859.
5. Buchbinder, R. *et al.* 2001. Incidence of malignant disease in biopsy-proven inflammatory myopathy: a population-based cohort study. Ann. Intern. Med. **134:** 1087–1095.
6. Rider, L.G. & F.W. Miller. 2000. Inflammatory muscle disease: clinical aspects. Baillière's Clin. Rheumatol. **14:** 37–54.
7. Ang, P. *et al.* 2000. Classical and amyopathic dermatomyositis seen at the National Skin Centre of Singapore: a three-year retrospective review of their clinical characteristics and association with malignancy. Ann. Acad. Med. Singapore **29:** 219–223.
8. Fujita, J. *et al.* 2001. Primary lung cancer associated with polymyositis/dermatomyositis, with a review of the literature. Rheumatol. Int. **20:** 81–84.
9. Fudman, E.J. & T.J. Schnitzer. 1986. Dermatomyositis without creatine kinase elevation: poor prognostic sign. Am. J. Med. **80:** 329–332.
10. Hunger, R.E. *et al.* 2001. Cutaneous leukocytoclastic vasculitis in dermatomyositis suggests malignancy. Dermatology **202:** 123–126.
11. Naschitz, J.E. *et al.* 1999. Rheumatic syndromes: clues to occult neoplasia. Semin. Arthritis Rheum. **29:** 43–55.
12. Marie, I. *et al.* 2001. Polymyositis and dermatomyositis: short term and long term outcome, and predictive factors of prognosis. J. Rheumatol. **28:** 2230–2237.
13. Danko K. *et al.* 2004. Long-term survival of patients with idiopathic inflammatory myopathies according to clinical features. A longitudinal study of 162 cases. Medicine (Baltimore) **83:** 35–42.
14. Maugars, Y.M. *et al.* 1996. Long-term prognosis of 69 patients with dermatomyositis or polymyositis. Clin. Exp. Rheumatol. **14:** 263–274.
15. Sultan, S.M. *et al.* 2002. Outcome in patients with idiopathic inflammatory myositis: morbidity and mortality. Rheumatology **41:** 22–26.
16. Wakata, N. *et al.* 2002. Polymyositis and dermatomyositis associated with malignancy: a 30-year retrospective study. Int. J. Dermatol. **41:** 729–734.
17. Sparsa, A. *et al.* 2002. Routine vs. extensive malignancy search for adult dermatomyositis and polymyositis: a study of 40 patients. Arch. Dermatol. **138:** 885–890.

18. AMENO, P. *et al.* 2002. Usefulness of erythrocyte sedimentation rate as tumor marker in cancer associated myositis. Eur. J. Dermatol. **12:** 165–169.
19. BASSET-SEGUIN, N. *et al.* 1990. Prognostic factors and predictive signs of malignancy in adult dermatomyositis. A study of 32 cases. Arch. Dermatol. **126:** 633–637.
20. GALLAIS, V. *et al.* 1996. Prognostic factors and predictive signs of malignancy in adult dermatomyositis. Ann. Dermatol. Venereol. **123:** 722–726.
21. CHEN, Y.J. *et al.* 2001. Predicting factors of malignancy in dermatomyositis and polymyositis: a case-control study. Br. J. Dermatol. **144:** 825–831.

Control of Type 1 Autoimmune Diabetes by Naturally Occurring $CD4^+CD25^+$ Regulatory T Lymphocytes in Neonatal NOD Mice

C. A. PICCIRILLO, M. TRITT, E. SGOUROUDIS, A. ALBANESE, M. PYZIK, AND V. HAY

Departments of Microbiology and Immunology, McGill University, Montreal, QC, Canada, H3A 2B4

ABSTRACT: **Nonobese diabetic (NOD) mice serve as a model of spontaneous type 1 diabetes (T1D), a T cell–mediated autoimmune disease leading to the destruction of pancreatic insulin-producing beta islet cells. A possible deficiency in regulatory T (T_{reg}) cell development or function may promote the activation, expansion, and recruitment of autoreactive T cells and the onset of T1D. Naturally occurring $CD4^+CD25^+$ T_{reg} (nT_{reg}) cells, which typically display potent inhibitory effects on T cell functions *in vitro* and *in vivo*, may be defective at controlling autoimmunity in T1D. We have examined the relative contribution of $CD4^+CD25^+$ nT_{reg} cells in the immune regulation of T1D in the NOD mouse model. $CD4^+CD25^+$ T cells represent 5–10% of $CD4^+$ thymocytes or peripheral T cells from prediabetic neonatal NOD mice, are anergic to TCR signals, and potently suppress activated T cells in a contact-dependent and cytokine-independent fashion *in vitro*. Unlike total $CD4^+$ T cells, prediabetic $CD25^+$-depleted $CD4^+$ T cells are potently diabetogenic when transferred in immunodeficient NOD mice. Co-transfer of $CD4^+CD25^+$ T cells from thymocytes or peripheral lymphoid tissues of neonatal NOD mice dramatically halts disease development and beta-islet cell lymphocytic infiltration, even when T1D is induced by $CD4^+$ T cells from BDC2.5 transgenic or diabetic NOD mice. Finally, we show that $CD4^+CD25^+$ T_{reg} preferentially accumulate in inflamed pancreatic environments, where they potently inhibit the antigen-specific expansion and cytokine effector functions of diabetogenic T cells. Thus, $CD4^+CD25^+$ T cell–mediated regulation is operative in the prediabetic neonatal T cell repertoire and can suppress the diabetogenic process and control the onset of T1D.**

KEYWORDS: **$CD4^+CD25^+$ regulatory T cells; diabetes; tolerance**

INTRODUCTION

Self/non-self discrimination requires a finely controlled balance between maintaining peripheral tolerance to autoantigens while maintaining the ability to mount

Address for correspondence: Dr. Ciriaco A. Piccirillo, Departments of Microbiology and Immunology & Center for the Study of Host Resistance, McGill University, 3775 University Street, Room 408, Lyman Duff Medical Building, Montreal, QC, Canada, H3A 2B4. Voice: 514-398-2872; fax: 514-398-7052.

Ciro.piccirillo@mcgill.ca

Ann. N.Y. Acad. Sci. 1051: 72–87 (2005). © 2005 New York Academy of Sciences.
doi: 10.1196/annals.1361.048

protective immune responses against invading pathogens.[1,2] In order to fine-tune and diversify its ability to control adaptive immune responses, a network of $CD4^+$ regulatory T cells (T_{reg}) cells exists to maintain this immunologic balance at various times, tissue locations, and inflammatory settings.[1–3]

The development of autoimmune diseases like type 1 diabetes (T1D) involves a breakdown in self-tolerance.[1,2] While autoreactive T cells are normally present in all individuals, clinical disease only affects a minority of the population, suggesting that mechanisms for peripheral self-tolerance must exist to completely control potentially pathogenic T cells.[3,4] Naturally occurring $CD4^+CD25^+$ T_{reg} cells (nT_{reg}) have emerged as a dominant peripheral mechanism of immune suppression of self-reactive T cells and a master-switch factor controlling the balance between tolerance and immunity.[5,6] This chapter briefly describes the tolerogenic functions of $CD4^+CD25^+$ nT_{reg} cells in a neonatal, nonobese diabetic (NOD) model of T1D.

T CELL–MEDIATED REGULATION OF ADAPTIVE IMMUNE RESPONSES

In an attempt to diversify its ability to control adaptive immune responses, the immune system has evolved numerous mechanisms, including T_{reg} cells, to downregulate immune responses. To this end, a network of T_{reg} cells exists to assure timely and efficient T cell immunoregulation at multiple levels, depending on the inflammatory status and anatomic location.[5,6] $CD4^+$ T cells endowed with the capacity to control the activation and function of other T cells exist in two general categories: induced and naturally occurring (FIG. 1).[5,6] Under unique activation conditions *in vivo* or *ex vivo,* non-regulatory $CD4^+$ T cell precursors (nT_{reg}-depleted $CD4^+$ T cells without intrinsic regulatory potential) can acquire CD25/Foxp3 expression and suppressive activity, and thus differentiate into induced $CD4^+CD25^+$ T_{reg} (iT_{reg}) cells.[6] Indeed, a variety of phenotypically and functionally distinct iT_{reg} cells have been described and include IL-4-producing Th2,[7] TGF-β1-producing Th3,[8] and IL-10 producing-Tr1 cells.[9]

In recent years, studies have indicated that normal $CD4^+$ T cells constitutively expressing the IL-2Rα chain (CD25) and the *Foxp3* transcription factor in the naïve T cell repertoire are potent regulators of T cell–mediated immune responses *in vitro* and *in vivo*.[1–6,10] Indeed, $CD4^+CD25^+$ T_{reg} cells, termed naturally occurring, have emerged as a dominant T cell population mediating peripheral tolerance to autoantigens. $CD4^+$ nT_{reg} cells develop during the normal process of T cell maturation in the thymus, survive in the periphery poised for normal surveillance of self-antigens, and prevent potential autoimmune responses. Most recent studies indicate that CD25 appears to be the most specific cell surface marker for nT_{reg} responsible for peripheral self-tolerance present in the normal T cell repertoire.[6] In recent years, $CD4^+CD25^+$ nT_{reg} cells have emerged as a dominant T cell population governing peripheral tolerance to self and non-self-directed immune responses, consist of 5–10% of peripheral $CD4^+$ T cells in mice and man,[4,11] and constitutively express CD25 and CTLA4 in the quiescent state in normal, unmanipulated, disease-free animals. Conventional $CD4^+$ T cells readily upregulate CD25 and CTLA-4 transiently after TCR activation and thus become unreliable markers after T cell activation.[2] Removal or abrogation of nT_{reg} cells from peripheral immune systems increases immunity to tu-

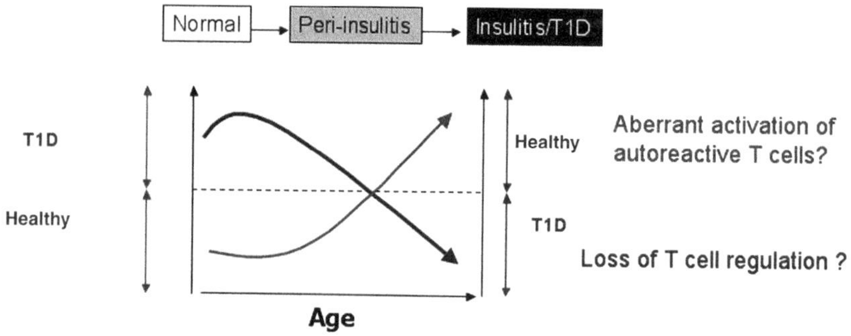

FIGURE 1. Pathogenesis of autoimmunity in T1D.

mors and allografts, and results in the development of multi-organ-specific autoimmune diseases, including autoimmune gastritis (AIG), T1D, inflammatory bowel disease (IBD), and thyroiditis.[12,13] $CD4^+CD25^+$ nT_{reg} cells are also able to prevent the development of autoimmune disease that occurs after a thymectomy[14] or following the transfer of autoreactive T cell clones,[15] as well as diseases induced by CD25-depleted $CD4^+$ T cells.[15] $CD4^+CD25^+$ T_{reg} cells have a diverse, polyclonal TCR repertoire allowing them to control immunity to bacterial, fungal, protozoal, nematodal, and viral pathogen–derived antigens.[16–19] $CD4^+CD25^+$ T_{reg} cells are anergic to *in vitro* antigenic stimulation but can actively expand and mediate antigen-specific suppression after antigen presentation by dendritic cells (DCs) *in vivo*.[4,20] $CD4^+CD25^+$ nT_{reg} cells require a TCR signal to activate their suppressor function *in vitro*, and suppress $CD4^+$ and $CD8^+$ T cell responses in an antigen-nonspecific manner, and contact-dependent fashion not requiring the action of immunosuppressive cytokines *in vitro*.[20–23] Recently, FoxP3 has been directly linked to the $CD4^+CD25^+$ T_{reg} cells, since FoxP3-deficient mice (Scurfy) and humans (IPEX syndrome) have a distinct inability to produce T_{reg} cells, and both succumb to a multi-organ autoimmune disease that includes T1D in the human newborn.[5,6,10] Treatment of $FoxP3^{-/-}$ mice with syngeneic T_{reg} cells from wild-type donors can protect against autoimmune disease, and retrovirally mediated transduction of naive $CD4^+$ cells with FoxP3 can induce T_{reg} cells.[10]

THE NOD MOUSE MODEL OF AUTOIMMUNE DISEASE

T1D is a chronic, organ-specific autoimmune disease that results in the destruction of the endocrine, insulin-producing beta (β) cells of the pancreatic islets of Langerhans.[1] The destruction of β cells results in an insulin deficiency that consequently leads to plasma glucose dysregulation, persistent hyperglycemia, and long-term complications. NOD mice represent a prototypic model of immune dysregulation since they spontaneously develop several autoimmune diseases such as thyroiditis, sialadenitis, and T1D (a disorder that shares many features with human T1D) and as such are an excellent experimental system with which to study the mechanisms controlling the initiation and termination of autoimmune responses.[24,25] Studies in normal NOD or NOD/BDC2.5 mice transgenic (Tg) for a diabetogenic TCR suggest that T1D development is influenced by genetic and environmental factors and comprises several stages.[24–26] Until the mice are 3 to 4 weeks of age, all the islets are free from lymphocytic infiltration, suggesting that the autoreactive T cells are silent during this period. An initial, nonpathogenic infiltration of the peri-islet regions then appears, indicating that activation and proliferation of self-reactive T cells is initiated (checkpoint 1).[24,25,27] Peri-insulitic lesions contain heterogeneous cellular infiltrates, including dendritic cells, macrophages, and T and B cells.[28] This stage is then followed by a breakdown of self-tolerance and a gradual T cell–dependent infiltration and destruction of β islet cells occurring around 12 weeks of age (checkpoint 2).[27,29] Although insulitis occurs in all NOD mice, in female mice the disease is clinically silent for many weeks with a higher T1D incidence.[25]

Studies in NOD mice demonstrate that β islet cell destruction and T1D pathogenesis is T lymphocyte-dependent, and that spontaneous disease generally requires the combined contributions of $CD4^+$ and $CD8^+$ T cells.[30,31] T cells from spontaneously diabetic NOD mice can adoptively transfer T1D to neonatal NOD and immunodeficient NOD-*scid* mice.[32] Coincident with the shift from nondestructive to destructive insulitis, there is also an imbalance between regulatory and proinflammatory cytokine production, which contributes to the development of disease.[33] Prior to β cell damage a relatively long period of Th2-dominated insulitis is observed followed by a destructive phase during which proinflammatory cytokines produced by Th1 cells and activated dendritic cells, namely IFNγ, IL-12, and TNF-α, play an important role in the development of these lesions.[33,34] Diabetes is transferable from NOD mice by Th1 cells, while treatments with Th2 cytokines such as IL-4 or IL-10 have generally been shown to be protective; however, no protection was observed in either NOD-IL-$4^{-/-}$ or NOD mice with Tg expression of IL-10 in β cells.[28,35,36] The role of TGF-β1 in altering the response of islet reactive $CD4^+$ T cells has also been suggested, as TGF-β1 Tg NOD mice exhibit a reduced incidence of diabetes.[37]

TOLEROGENIC FUNCTIONS OF CD4$^+$ REGULATORY T CELLS IN NOD MICE

NOD mice possess multiple immunoregulatory defects, which collectively contribute to spontaneous autoimmunity. In addition to expressing a disease-prone MHC II I-Ag7 haplotype, which may be responsible for poor negative selection in the $CD4^+$ T cell compartment,[38] numerous peripheral immune abnormalities occur in NOD mice by 3 to 4 weeks of age, coincident with the onset of insulitis.[39] These include reduced T cell proliferation and IL-2 and IL-4 cytokine production following TCR engagement,[39] a skewing towards pathogenic Th1 cell activation and effector functions,[24,25] and a functional deficiency in IL-4-producing CD-1-restricted, $NK1^+$ T cells.[40] More importantly, a disequilibrium between T effector (T_{eff}) and T_{reg} cells—which subsequently leads to excessive activation of islet antigen-specific Th1 cells, insulitis establishment, and diabetes progression—is believed to occur in NOD mice.[1,34] Thus, T_{reg} function represents a central control point in tolerance induction in T1D.

The time lag between the establishment of insulitis and the onset of overt diabetes suggests that the peripheral regulatory mechanisms that suppress immune reactivity to self-antigens and control disease progression are present in prediabetic NOD mice.[1,30] Studies in the NOD model have identified several functionally and phenotypically distinct protective T cell subsets, and numerous lines of evidence suggest that conventional αβ TCR^+CD4^+ T cells contain substantial regulatory functions in prediabetic NOD mice that are capable of either delaying or preventing diabetes. These include the prevention of adoptive transfer of diabetes by $CD4^+$ splenocytes from prediabetic NOD mice.[32,41] Onset of diabetes is accelerated by neonatal thymectomy,[42] cyclophosphamide,[43] CTLA-4-Ig,[44] or sublethal irradiation treatment[45]—all effects prevented by $CD4^+$ T cell infusion.[46] Futhermore, there is a striking difference in kinetics and severity of diabetes between conventional NOD/BDC2.5 and NOD/BDC2.5 *scid* mice, as the latter develop T1D more rapidly and more severely, suggesting that conventional BDC2.5/NOD mice potentially harbor a T_{reg} population.[10,12] Many attempts to define these T_{reg} cells in T1D have provided evidence that the suppressor cells are functionally and phenotypically heterogeneous in nature, and there is no consensus on the nature and phenotype of the predominant regulatory population operative in the NOD mouse. In fact, cell surface markers such as CD45Rb, CD62L, CD45RB, and DX5 have been used to define these $CD4^+$ T_{reg} cells and all appeared to partition with varying degrees of suppressor function.[46] The exact relationships between the above-described protective T cell subsets in an autoimmune setting are not well understood, and evidence supports the presence of multiple regulatory cell types that can potentially control autoreactive T cells via various mechanisms and in context-dependent fashions. In this regard, a recent study has shown that the depletion of distinct regulatory T cell subsets based on the markers CD4, CD25, CD62L, and $CD45RB^{low}$ in an adoptive transfer system led to the differential control of autoimmunity, such that $CD4^+CD62L^+$ cells controlled T1D, $CD4^+CD25^+$ T cells controlled AIG and TID, and $CD4^+CD45RB^{low}$ cells controlled IBD.[47] The reasons behind this tissue-specific mode of T cell regulation are unknown, but the data suggests that target organs confer unique regulatory pressures on infiltrating T_{eff} cells.

FUNCTIONAL $CD4^+CD25^+$ REGULATORY T CELLS IN NEONATAL NOD MICE

As discussed above, $CD4^+CD25^+$ nT_{reg} cells play a central, master-switch role in dampening peripheral self-reactive T cell responses and maintaining tolerance in several models of autoimmunity.[3,48] A central question is whether the onset of spontaneous autoimmune disease in NOD mice results from a decline in T cell regulation or from the overriding of such regulation by an uncontrollable activation, expansion, and differentiation of diabetogenic T cells (FIG. 2). The incidence of spontaneous T1D in NOD mice may in fact reflect developmental or functional deficiencies in $CD4^+CD25^+$ nT_{reg} cells, such that the balance between autoreactive and T_{reg} cells is altered and consequently tips the balance towards the activation, expansion, and recruitment of diabetogenic T cells, proinflammatory Th1 cytokine production and clinical T1D. Because the precise mechanism by which $CD4^+CD25^+$ nT_{reg} cells control autoimmune responses is still unknown, our laboratory examines specific questions regarding the tolerogenic functions of $CD4^+CD25^+$ nT_{reg} cells in the T cell repertoire of neonatal NOD mice.

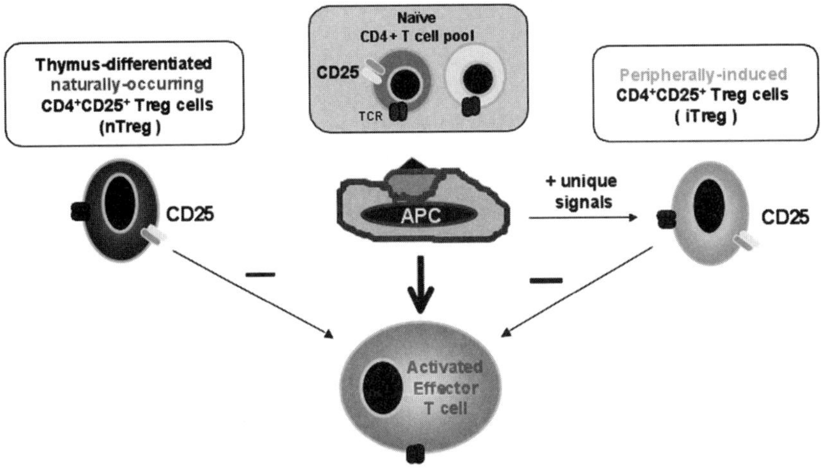

FIGURE 2. Naturally occurring and induced CD4$^+$ regulatory T cells.

CD4$^+$CD25$^+$ T$_{reg}$ cells have been implicated in T1D disease prevention in studies where immunodeficient NOD-*scid* recipient mice into which were transferred CD25-depleted splenocytes from prediabetic adult NOD mice (8–12 weeks old) succumbed to diabetes more rapidly than did those receiving unfractionated splenocytes.[49] These data are also consistent with the observation made in B7$^{-/-}$ and CD28$^{-/-}$ NOD mice, which notably lack CD4$^+$CD25$^+$ nT$_{reg}$ cells from birth. These mice show accelerated disease onset, and infusion of wild-type CD4$^+$CD25$^+$ T cells back into CD28$^{-/-}$ NOD recipient mice prevents disease.[49] Disruption of the B7/CD28 pathway in NOD mice causes T$_{reg}$ depletion by affecting both their thymic development and peripheral homeostasis, which leads to an accelerated diabetic phenotype.[50] Thus, effective CD28 co-stimulation is critical for the generation and maintenance of the CD4$^+$CD25$^+$ regulatory population. Recent studies have also reported a significant expansion of CD25-expressing CD4$^+$ T cells with apparent regulatory activity, sometimes correlating with the expression of a latent, membrane-bound form of TGF-β1 in inflamed pancreatic lymph nodes (pLN) of aged, diabetes-free mice.[51,52] Although T$_{reg}$ cell function was examined in the lymphoid tissues of adult, prediabetic, and, most likely, insulitic NOD mice, it remains unclear from the above-mentioned studies whether the CD4$^+$CD25$^+$ T cells are induced during pancreatic inflammation from CD4$^+$CD25$^-$ progenitors, or whether they emerge from the thymus-derived nT$_{reg}$ pool. While these studies illustrate the central role the CD4$^+$ T$_{reg}$ cells play in tolerance induction, a detailed analysis of the functional contibution made by CD4$^+$CD25$^+$ T$_{reg}$ cells of the naturally occurring lineage in the control of autoimmunity is lacking.

It is commonly stated that NOD mice have a defective CD4$^+$CD25$^+$ nT$_{reg}$ mechanism and that potentiation of these cells shifts the disease process towards tolerance to pancreatic antigens and T1D protection. In fact, we observed that CD4$^+$CD25$^+$ nT$_{reg}$ cells represent approximately 3–10% of total CD4$^+$ T cells from peripheral blood, thymocytes, lymph nodes (LNs), or spleen of prediabetic, wild-type or

BDC2.5 neonatal NOD mice (7–21 days of age). This proportion is comparable to T1D-resistant animal strains and refutes the view that NOD mice may have a generalized defect in their ability to generate sufficient numbers of nT_{reg} cells.[53] Neonatal nT_{reg} cells are phenotypically similar to $CD4^+CD25^+$ T_{reg} cells from T1D-resistant C57BL/6 mice, displaying a similar expression profile for various activation markers, including CD25 and CD62L, suggesting that the $CD4^+CD25^+$ T cell subset in neonatal mice does not emerge from the pre-activated T_{eff} cell pool.[53] This is in contrast to $CD4^+CD25^+$ T cells analyzed from prediabetic, adult NOD mice (8–12 weeks), a timepoint at which insulitis and β-islet immune responses are well engaged and as such display a higher proportion of $CD4^+$ T cells with an activated/memory phenotype ($CD4^+CD25^+CD62L^{low}$).[53] Although CD25 is a specific marker for resting $CD4^+CD25^+$ nT_{reg} in neonatal lymphoid environments, it becomes unreliable as conventional NOD $CD4^+$ T cells upregulate CD25 in adult, albeit prediabetic mice, thus precluding its use as a tracking biomarker of nT_{reg} cells in adult NOD mice whose autoimmune response is well initiated. Thus, neonatal $CD4^+CD25^+$ nT_{reg} cells, in contrast to their adult counterparts, display a surface phenotype like conventional nT_{reg} cells isolated from non-autoimmune-prone mice.[53] Lastly, neonatal $CD4^+CD25^+$ nT_{reg} cells from thymocytes and peripheral lymphoid tissues preferentially express FoxP3 in contrast to their $CD4^+CD25-$ T cell counterparts, further identifying them as classic nT_{reg} cells.[10,54]

Neonatal $CD4^+CD25^-$ nT_{reg} cells also display the function characteristics of normal nT_{reg} cells from non-autoimmune-prone animal strains.[53] They are anergic to TCR stimulation, and their responsiveness is restored in the presence of exogenous sources of IL-2.[20,55] Their anergic phenotype is further confirmed by the observation that, once stimulated via their TCR, neonatal nT_{reg} cells from NOD mice fail to transcribe the IL-2 gene.[55] Finally, $CD4^+CD25^+$ nT_{reg} cells isolated from either thymus or peripheral lymphoid tissues of neonatal NOD mice can potently suppress the *in vitro* proliferation of anti-CD3–activated T cells in a cytokine-independent fashion, since neutralization of IL-4, IL-10, or TGF-β1 failed to reverse suppression independently of antibody concentration or TCR signal strength.[53] Suppression mediated by nT_{reg} cells is also contact-dependent since suppression was abrogated in Transwell chambers.[53]

In order to monitor nT_{reg} activity *in vivo*, we have made use of an adoptive T cell transfer system whereby T1D is induced in immunodeficient NOD-*scid* recipient mice by the transfer of $CD4^+CD25^-$ T_{eff} cells from prediabetic NOD or BDC2.5 mice, and suppressed by the co-transfer of either $CD4^+CD25^+$ nT_{reg} cells from neonatal, prediabetic NOD or BDC2.5 mice.[53] Interestingly, $CD4^+CD25^-$ T cells from prediabetic NOD mice are potently diabetogenic when transferred alone in NOD-*scid* mice, as compared to unfractionated prediabetic $CD4^+$ T cells that never induce disease.[53] Similarly, $CD4^+CD25^+$ nTreg cells from neonatal BDC2.5 mice can also potently suppress the diabetogenic potential of BDC2.5 effector $CD4^+$ T cells. This suggests that nT_{reg} cells within the CD25-expressing fraction control β-islet cell reactivity in the normal repertoire. Our data also show that there is a time-dependent change in the ability of $CD4^+CD25^-$ T_{eff} to induce T1D *in vivo*, possibly indicating variable levels of priming in the diabetogenic donor T cell population.[53] However, when $CD4^+CD25^+$ nT_{reg} cells isolated from prediabetic neonatal NOD mice were transferred to NOD-*scid* recipient mice, even at T_{eff}/T_{reg} ratios > 1, T1D incidence and severity were dramatically reduced, while showing normal blood glucose levels, marked preservation insulin-producing β islet cells, and a significantly reduced insulitis grade.[53] We have also found that $CD4^+CD25^+$ T cells can suppress the induction of diabetes mediated by $CD4^+$ T cells isolated from overtly diabetic NOD mice or BDC2.5 Tg $CD4^+$ T cells, although greater numbers of nT_{reg} cells are generally required.[53] To further validate the involvement of $CD4^+CD25^+$ nT_{reg} cells in disease protection in NOD, we have also shown that $CD4^+CD25^+$ thymocytes confer a similar protective effect as nT_{reg} cells isolated from peripheral lymphoid tissues, suggesting that "virgin" nT_{reg} cells, which are not likely to come from a potentially activated peripheral compartment, are indeed a protective thymic-derived T cell subset operative in the NOD; this finding is consistent with other models of autoimmunity.[14,53,55] This is also consistent with studies showing that thymectomy in the NOD mouse leads to an acceleration of T1D onset.[42] In addition, recipients of $CD4^+CD25^-$ T_{eff} cells express significant levels of IFN-γ mRNA in the pancreas, consistent with the Th1 cell–mediated nature of T1D. Moreover, transfer of $CD4^+CD25^+$ T_{reg} cells significantly suppressed pancreatic IFN-γ mRNA expression, further confirming the protective role of nT_{reg} cells *in vivo*.[53] Subsequent studies have also shown the highest regulatory activity partitioned with the $CD4^+CD25^+$ cells expressing high levels of $CD62L^{high}$ cells *in vivo*, although both $CD62L^{low}$ and $CD62L^{high}$ subsets can potently suppress proliferative T cell responses to polyclonal stimuli *in vitro*.[47,53,56]

FUNCTIONAL DYNAMICS OF $CD4^+CD25^+$ nT_{reg} CELLS IN INFLAMED PANCREATIC ENVIRONMENTS

A major unresolved question about nT_{reg} cell–mediated suppression concerns the location at which tolerance induction occurs *in vivo*.[6] The differential ability of $CD4^+CD25^-$ and $CD4^+CD25^+$ T cells to resolve diabetes may indicate the different homing properties of each subset. The unreliable nature of CD25 as a specific marker for $CD4^+CD25^+$ nT_{reg} in inflammatory settings precludes its use as a marker of nT_{reg} cells in prediabetic or diabetic, adult NOD mice. In order to monitor nT_{reg} activity *in vivo*, we have made use of an adoptive T cell transfer system whereby T1D is induced in immunodeficient NOD-*scid* recipient mice by the transfer of $CD4^+CD25^-$ T_{eff} cells from prediabetic $Thy1.2^+$ mice, and suppressed by the cotransfer of $CD4^+CD25^+$ nT_{reg} cells from neonatal, prediabetic congenic $Thy1.1^+$ donor mice. This adoptive T cell transfer approach is an efficient way to track the functional dynamics of T_{eff} and T_{reg} cells independently in the context of an autoimmune response in the pancreatic environment. Following an initial recruitment/expansion of $CD4^+CD25-$ T_{eff} cells in pLN and pancreas, $CD4^+CD25^+$ nT_{reg} cells undergo a time-dependent migration/expansion in these environments, where, consequently, they actively suppress the expansion of T_{eff} cells.[53] The preferential accumulation of $CD4^+CD25^+$ T_{reg} in inflamed pLN and islets of T1D-protected mice possibly indicates that T_{reg} are activated or mediate their suppressor function once inflammation has been initiated by diabetogenic T cells in these sites. Similarly, a recent study using the BDC2.5 TCR Tg system suggests that the majority of T_{reg} cells present in NOD/BDC 2.5 mice are actively suppressing in the pancreas, rather than the pLN, where the initial priming of the autoreactive T cell response is presumably occurring.[51] This finding is also corroborated by Mottet *et al.*, who demonstrated in a model of murine IBD that CD4$^+$CD25$^+$ nT_{reg} cells actively proliferate in mesenteric LN and colon, where they suppress colitogenic CD4$^+$CD45Rb^{high} T_{eff} cells.[57]

The functional fate of autoreactive T cells that are targets of CD4$^+$CD25$^+$ nT_{reg} cell regulation is ill-defined. The protective effect observed in the above-described results indicates that CD4$^+$CD25$^+$ nT_{reg} cells may block the anti-islet CD4$^+$ T cell responses at multiple levels: (1) the priming of autoreactive T cells; (2) the expansion phase; (3) their differentiation into pathogenic Th1 effector cells; or (4) their homing in lymphoid and nonlymphoid tissues. Since nT_{reg} cells appear to home to or expand preferentially in pLN and pancreas, these tissues provide appropriate environments for regulating the priming, expansion, differentiation, and effector functions of antigen-specific, diabetogenic CD4$^+$ T cells.[58] In our system, the priming of T_{eff} cells did not seem to be affected in the presence of nT_{reg} cells, as determined by CD69, CD44, and CD62L activation marker expression on T_{eff} cells, suggesting that antigen presentation and initial TCR signals are not inhibited by nT_{reg} cells in an inflammatory setting.[53] Our studies also show that CD4$^+$CD25$^+$ T_{reg} cells proliferate in sites of inflammation. The precise relationship between inflammation, T_{reg} proliferation, and function is unclear, and it is conceivable that inflammation-derived mediators modulate autoimmune responses. Furthermore, these experiments are done in lymphopenic environments, and the relative contribution of homeostatic proliferation on the induction of T_{eff} and T_{reg} cell responses is unclear. However, it is known that they are anergic *in vitro*, can certainly expand homeostatically, and can preserve their anergic and suppressive phenotype in immunodeficient mice.[59] Adoptive transfer experiments in normal NOD mice have yielded similar results (unpublished observation). Thus, CD4$^+$CD25$^+$ nT_{reg} cells may lead to diminished differentiation and expansion of islet-infiltrating CD4$^+$ T cells into Th1 effectors in pLN, suppressed effector functions, or altered T_{eff} cell trafficking to the pancreas. This is consistent with our observation that nT_{reg} cells suppress disease transfer mediated by primed T cells from diabetic mice, which likely traffic directly to nonlymphoid tissues (islets), and circumventing priming in the pLN.[53] It remains to be seen whether nTreg cells employ diverse mechanisms to suppress in pLN or pancreas, or whether different subsets of nT_{reg} cells exist within the greater nTreg cell pool to inhibit immune responses in lymphoid or nonlymphoid tissues (FIG. 3).

Chemokine Basis for nT_{reg} Cell Recruitment into the Inflamed Pancreatic Environment

Lymphocyte trafficking to inflamed lymphoid and nonlymphoid tissues is largely dictated by a sequence of events involving the action of chemokines, which provide directional cues for the migration and recruitment of T cells into sites of inflammation.[60] The differential ability of CD4$^+$CD25$^-$ and CD4$^+$CD25$^+$ T cell subsets to resolve T1D may reflect differences in their homing *in vivo*. Our data strongly suggest that there may be an inflammation-related signal, which either triggers the recruitment or expansion of nT_{reg} cells in pancreas and pLN. Currently, the chemokine basis of nT_{reg} cell trafficking to sites of inflammation is not clearly understood. Some reports indicate that murine CD4$^+$CD25$^+$ T cells express CCR5 and that they may be attracted by macrophage inflammatory protein 1α or β (MIP-1α and MIP-1β), or RANTES.[61] These CCR5-chemokines are produced at high levels by activated antigen-presenting cells (APCs) and T cells, suggesting that CD4$^+$CD25$^+$ T cells may be

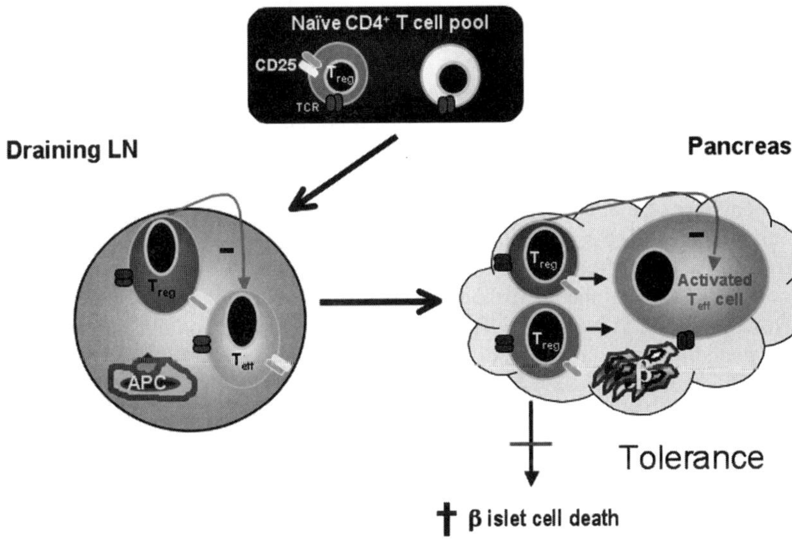

FIGURE 3. Naturally occurring CD4$^+$ CD25$^+$ T_{reg} cells and control T cell responses in T1D.

attracted to inflamed tissues to regulate or prevent autoimmune disease.[61] *In vitro* studies have also shown that CD4$^+$CD25$^+$ T cells from human peripheral blood selectively express CCR4 and CCR8 and show a strong chemotactic response to ligands for CCR4, namely macrophage-derived chemokine (MDC/CCL22) and thymus- and activation-regulated chemokine (TARC/CCL17), and I-309/CCL1, all of which are produced by activated T cells and professional APCs such as DCs and macrophages.[62] One recent study showed that nT_{reg} cells in prediabetic NOD mice are strongly restricted to the CD4$^+$CD25$^+$CD62L$^+$ subset expressing high levels of CCR7, and thus potentially migrating toward the lymphoid chemokines CCL19 and CCL21.[56] However, another study indicated that both CD62L$^+$ and CD62L$^-$ subsets could prevent the development of autoimmune gastritis and colitis in *scid* mice.[63] Thus, it remains to be seen whether chemokine receptors such as CCR4, CCR5, and CCR8 may endow T_{reg} cells with a competitive advantage over other T cells to respond to inflammatory signals by entering more efficiently in pLNs where they can potentially inhibit the activation of T_{eff} cell–mediated responses.

Role of Suppressor Cytokines in CD4$^+$CD25$^+$ T_{reg} Cell Effector Function in Vivo

In vitro, the consensus view is that CD4$^+$CD25$^+$ T cell–mediated suppression is contact-dependent and cytokine-independent:[2,20] nT_{reg} cells fail to suppress target T cells in Transwell experiments, neutralization of various suppressor cytokines does not block suppression, and IL-4$^{-/-}$, TGF-β1$^{-/-}$, or IL-10$^{-/-}$ T_{reg} cells remain functional *in vitro*.[20,23] The mechanisms by which CD4$^+$CD25$^+$ T cells regulate autoimmune diseases *in vivo* are far more complex, and several suppressor cytokines such as IL-4, IL-10, and TGF-β1 have been implicated in T_{reg} effector functions.[3] IL-$4^{-/-}$ $CD4^+CD25^+$ T cells have been shown to be suppressive in autoimmune gastritis (AIG).[64] While capable of suppressing AIG, IL-$10^{-/-}$ $CD4^+CD25^+$ T cells are incapable of suppressing inflammatory bowel disease (IBD) in the same mouse.[64,65] The role for TGF-β1 is controversial and has been reported to play a role in IBD protection mediated by nT_{reg} cells.[65] However, the sources of TGF-β1 are diverse and could be the $CD4^+CD25^+$ T cells, other T cell populations, or nonlymphoid cells such as epithelium that are part of the process of healing.[5] Thus, there appears to be a context-dependent requirement for some T_{reg}-derived suppressor cytokines. There is a possibility that different subsets of nT_{reg} cells exist such that some inhibit by a cell-contact-dependent mechanism, and others by the secretion of different suppressor cytokines. Alternatively, the inflammatory milieu in some contexts might dictate the mechanism by regulating the differentiation of nT_{reg} cells.[6]

IL-4, IL-10, and TGF-β1 have been shown to correlate with protection in T1D.[66] Although our data shows that $CD4^+CD25^+$ nT_{reg} from neonatal NOD mice can suppress T cell proliferation in the absence of IL-4, IL-10, or TGF-β1 *in vitro*, the cytokine-dependency of these cells *in vivo* is currently not known.[53] In our system, the presence of neutralizing monoclonal antibodies against IL-4, IL-10, and TGF-β1 had no effect on the ability of $CD4^+CD25^+$ nT_{reg} cells to suppress the diabetogenic potential of $CD4^+CD25^-$ T_{eff} cells.[53] Experiments are currently in progress to directly evaluate the contribution of these cytokines by comparing the regulatory potential of $CD4^+CD25^+$ nT_{reg} cells from wild-type, IL-$4^{-/-}$, IL-$10^{-/-}$, or IL-4/IL-10 double-deficient NOD mice. The direct analysis of TGF-$β1^{-/-}$ mice on a NOD genetic background is currently not possible, although we have recently shown that TGF-$β1^{-/-}$ nT_{reg} cells from neonatal mice remain fully capable of suppressing T cell–induced bacterial-driven mucosal inflammation *in vivo*.[67] Nonetheless, a recent study showed that a transient pulse of the cytokine TGF-β, when delivered in the islets, was able to induce the expansion of FoxP3-expressing $CD4^+CD25^+$ T_{reg} cells and correlated with the ability to suppress diabetes.[68] Thus, certain cytokines may help drive the induction/expansion of T_{reg} and may represent a potential target of immunotherapy.

Antigen Specificity and Effector Potential of $CD4^+CD25^+$ nT_{reg} Cells

A major unresolved question pertains to the antigen specificity of $CD4^+CD25^+$ T cells and its importance in T_{reg} development and function. Are they specific for the same antigens or epitopes as recognized by T_{eff} cells, or do they have a totally unrelated specificity for self-peptides that are expressed by the same or different APCs?[4,46] $CD4^+CD25^+$ nT_{reg} cells possess a polyclonal TCR repertoire, based on diverse gene expression of various TCR elements, and could conceivably recognize a wide array of self-antigens with high affinity.[3–6] Similarly, $CD4^+CD25^+$ T_{reg} cells isolated from thymus or peripheral lymphoid tissues of neonatal NOD mice display a diverse, polyclonal TCR repertoire as determined by immunoscope analysis of TCR repertoires (CDR3 spectra typing).[53] While there is some indication of antigen specificity *in vivo*, the evidence is still indirect. Evidence from a rat model of thyroiditis suggests that prenatal thyroid ablation leads to a state of thyroid hyper-reactivity postnatally, suggesting that the lack of exposure of immature T cells to the thyroid prevents T_{reg} differentiation.[69]

In T1D, several autoantigens to which tolerance is broken have been identified.[70,71] The relative contribution of these antigens in disease initiation, maintenance, and suppression is not fully understood. Although the induction of $CD4^+CD25^+$ T_{reg} suppressor activity depends on TCR engagement, the effector phase of nT_{reg} cells is MHC-unrestricted and antigen-nonspecific *in vitro*.[20,21] The current view is that self-antigen presentation in the thymus can induce the development of T_{reg} cells, which suggests that they may preferentially arise from self-antigen selection events in the thymus. Once exported to the periphery, they appear to continuously respond to autoantigen exposure, as supported by several studies: (1) $CD4^+CD25^+$ T_{reg} cells require sustained self-antigen MHC class II interactions, CD28/B7 engagement, and IL-2R signaling to be maintained in the periphery;[50,53] (2) adoptive transfer experiments involving the transfer of CSFE-labeled T_{reg} cells have demonstrated that these cells cycle continuously in the periphery in response to self-antigens in target organs.[50,53] The identification of the antigenic specificity of endogenous nT_{reg} cells has been difficult owing to their anergic phenotype, polyclonal reactivity, and their relatively low precursor frequency.[6] Recent studies have demonstrated that antigen-specific BDC2.5 T cells could be expanded *ex vivo* to induce a T_{reg} population, which, when co-transferred with diabetogenic T cells, could actively suppress any new onset and establish T1D at remarkably low cell numbers.[72,73] In one study, wild-type T_{reg} cells from NOD mice were less potent than their BDC2.5 T_{reg} cell counterparts *in vivo*, implying that antigen specificity plays an important role in the effectiveness of suppression.[72]

CONCLUSION

There are multiple immune tolerance pathways that regulate disease onset and progression in NOD mice. Amongst these, $CD4^+CD25^+$ T_{reg} cells represent a master switch of peripheral T cell tolerance induction to β-islet antigens, as abrogation of nT_{reg} function can break T cell tolerance to β-islet antigens and the onset of T1D (FIG. 3). The onset of spontaneous autoimmunity in NOD mice may result from a functional deficiency or waning of nTreg cells over time, such that diabetogenic T cells may preferentially activate, expand, and differentiate into pathogenic effector cells. Our results clearly show that $CD4^+CD25^+$ nT_{reg} cells from the prediabetic, T cell repertoire of newborn NOD mice are functionally capable of suppressing the diabetogenic potential of autoreactive $CD4^+$ T cells *in vitro*, and can control the onset and severity of T1D *in vivo*. In our model, nT_{reg} cells selectively home to, and expand in, inflamed pLNs and pancreas, where they may potentially suppress the development of diabetogenic $CD4^+$ T_{eff} cells by controlling their expansion, differentiation, trafficking, or effector function in order to limit histopathology. However, despite nT_{reg} cells actively suppressing the anti-islet T_{eff} cell responses in the neonatal immune system, this suppression is ultimately insufficient to maintain tolerance to pancreatic antigens since autoimmunity ultimately ensues in these mice. Functional analysis of T_{reg} and T_{eff} cells *in vivo* is critically important to fully elucidate the dynamics of $CD4^+CD25^+$ regulatory lymphocytes in inflamed lymphoid and nonlymphoid environments during tolerance induction. These studies may also provide insights into the cellular basis of T1D susceptibility, and may lead to the development of novel approaches to potentiate T_{reg} activity in T1D-prone hosts.

Furthermore, functional studies of $CD4^+CD25^+$ nT_{reg} cell activity in the control of TID will undeniably shed light on the central role of $CD4^+CD25^+$ T_{reg} in other autoimmune diseases.

ACKNOWLEDGMENTS

We would like to thank the McGill University Flow Cytometry Facility and McGill Animal Center for excellent technical assistance. We acknowledge the Canadian Institutes for Health Research (CIHR MOP 67211) and Canadian Foundation for Innovation for their financial support. C.A.P is a recipient of a Canada Research Chair.

REFERENCES

1. Anderson, M.S. *et al.* 2005. The NOD mouse: a model of immune dysregulation. Annu. Rev. Immunol. **23:** 447–485.
2. Piccirillo, C.A. *et al.* 2004. Naturally occurring $CD4^+CD25^+$ immunoregulatory T cells: central players in the arena of peripheral tolerance. Semin. Immunol. **16:** 81–88.
3. Shevach, E. *et al.* 2000. Regulatory T cells in autoimmmunity. Annu. Rev. Immunol. **18:** 423–449.
4. Sakaguchi, S. 2004. Naturally arising $CD4^+$ regulatory T cells for immunologic self-tolerance and negative control of immune responses. Annu. Rev. Immunol. **22:** 531–562.
5. Shevach E.M. 2002. $CD4^+CD25^+$ Suppressor T cells: more questions than answers. Nature Rev. Immunol. **2:** 389–400.
6. Piccirillo, C.A. *et al.* 2004. Cornerstone of peripheral tolerance: naturally occurring $CD4^+CD25^+$ regulatory T cells. Trends Immunol. **25:** 374–380.
7. Weiner, H.L. *et al.* 2001. Oral tolerance: immune mechanisms and the generation of Th3-type TGF-beta-secreting regulatory cells. Microbes Infect. **3:** 947–954.
8. Chen, Y. *et al.* 1994. Regulatory T cell clones induced by oral tolerance: suppression of autoimmune encephalomyelitis. Science **265:** 1237–1240.
9. Groux, H. *et al.* 1997. Generation of a novel regulatory $CD4^+$ T cell population which inhibits antigen-specific T cell responses. Nature **389:** 737–742.
10. Hori, S. *et al.* 2003. Control of regulatory T cell development by the transcription factor Foxp3. Science **299:** 1057–1061.
11. Levings, M.K. *et al.* 2001. Human $CD25^+CD4^+$ T regulatory cells suppress naive and memory T cell proliferation and can be expanded *in vitro* without loss of function. J. Exp. Med. **193:** 1295–1302.
12. Asano, M. *et al.* 1996. Autoimmune disease as a consequence of developmental abnormality of a T cell subpopulation. J. Exp. Med. **184:** 387–396.
13. Shimizu, J. *et al.* 1999. Induction of tumor immunity by removing $CD25^+CD4^+$ T cells: a common basis between tumor immunity and autoimmunity. J. Immunol. **163:** 5211–5218.
14. Sakaguchi, S. *et al.* 2001. Immunologic tolerance maintained by $CD25^+CD4^+$ regulatory T cells: their common role in controlling autoimmunity, tumor immunity, and transplantation tolerance. Immunol. Rev. **182:** 18–32.
15. Suri-Payer, E. *et al.* 1998. $CD4^+CD25^+$ T cells inhibit both the induction and effector function of autoreactive T cells and represent a unique lineage of immunoregulatory cells. J. Immunol. **160:** 1212–1218.
16. Hori, S. *et al.* 2002. $CD25^+CD4^+$ regulatory T cells suppress $CD4^+$ T cell-mediated pulmonary hyperinflammation driven by *Pneumocystis carinii* in immunodeficient mice. Eur. J. Immunol. **35:** 1282–1291.

17. BELKAID, Y. *et al.* 2002. $CD4^+CD25^+$ regulatory T cells control *Leishmania major* persistence and immunity. Nature **420:** 502–507.
18. HESSE, M. *et al.* 2004. $CD4^+CD25^+$ regulatory T cells are the major source of host-protective IL-10 in murine schistosomiasis. J. Immunol. **172:** 3157–3166.
19. SUVAS, S. *et al.* 2003. $CD4^+CD25^+$ T cells regulate virus-specific primary and memory $CD8^+$ T cell responses. J.Exp. Med. **198:** 889–901.
20. THORNTON, A.M. *et al.* 1998. $CD4^+CD25^+$ immunoregulatory T cells suppress polyclonal T cell activation *in vitro* by inhibiting interleukin 2 production. J. Exp. Med. **188:** 287–296.
21. THORNTON, A.M. *et al.* 2000. Suppressor effector function of $CD4^+CD25^+$ immunoregulatory cells is antigen nonspecific. J. Immunol. **164:** 183–190.
22. PICCIRILLO, C.A. *et al.* 2001. Control of $CD8^+$ T cell activation by $CD4^+CD25^+$ immunoregulatory cells. J. Immunol. **167:** 1137–1140.
23. PICCIRILLO, C.A. *et al.* 2002. $CD4^+CD25^+$ regulatory T cells can mediate suppressor function in the absence of transforming growth factor beta1 production and responsiveness. J. Exp. Med. **196:** 237–246.
24. SERREZE, D.V. *et al.* 2003. Genes and cellular requirements for autoimmune diabetes susceptibility in nonobese diabetic mice. Curr. Dir. Autoimmun. **4:** 31–67.
25. DELOVITCH, T.L. *et al.* 1997. The nonobese diabetic mouse as a model of autoimmune diabetes: immune dysregulation gets the NOD. Immunity **6:** 727–738.
26. GOTTLIEB, P.A. *et al.* 2002. Insulin-specific tolerance in diabetes. Clin. Immunol. **102:** 2–11.
27. SURI, A. *et al.* 1999. Dissecting the role of $CD4^+$ T cells in autoimmune diabetes through the use of TCR transgenic mice. Immunol. Rev. **169:** 55–65.
28. KING, C. *et al.* 1997. Organ-specific autoimmunity. Curr. Opin. Immunol. **9:** 863–871.
29. KATZ, J.D. *et al.* 1993. Following a diabetogenic T cell from genesis through pathogenesis. Cell **6:** 1089–1100.
30. ADORINI, L. *et al.* 2002. Understanding autoimmune diabetes: insights from mouse models. Trends Mol. Med. **8:** 31–38.
31. DILTS, S.M. *et al.* 1999. The role of CD4 and CD8 T cells in the development of autoimmune diabetes. J. Autoimmun. **3:** 285–290.
32. WICKER, L.S. *et al.* 1986. Transfer of autoimmune diabetes mellitus with splenocytes from nonobese diabetic (NOD) mice. Diabetes **8:** 855–860.
33. SUAREZ-PINZON, W.L. 2001. Approaches to type 1 diabetes prevention by intervention in cytokine immunoregulatory circuits. Int. J. Exp. Diabetes Res. **2:** 3–17.
34. BACH, J.F. 2001 Immunotherapy to insulin-dependent diabetes mellitus. Curr. Opin. Immunol. **13:** 601–605.
35. WANG, B. *et al.* 1998. Interleukin-4 deficiency does not exacerbate disease in NOD mice. Diabetes **8:** 1207–1211.
36. PENNLINE, K. *et al.* 1994. Recombinant human IL-10 prevents the onset of diabetes in the nonobese diabetic mouse. Clin. Immunol. Immunopathol. **71:** 169–175.
37. GREWAL, I.S. *et al.* 2002. Expression of transgene encoded TGF-beta in islets prevents autoimmune diabetes in NOD mice by a local mechanism. J. Autoimmun. **1–2:** 9–22.
38. KISHIMOTO, H. *et al.* 2001. A defect in central tolerance in NOD mice. Nat. Immunol. **11:** 1025–1031.
39. SALOJIN., K.V. *et al.* 1998. T cell anergy and altered T cell receptor signaling: effects on autoimmune disease. Immunol. Today **10:** 468–473.
40. SHARIF, S. *et al.* 2002. Regulation of autoimmune disease by natural killer T cells. J. Mol. Med. **8:** 290–300.
41. HASKINS, K. *et al.* 1989. Pancreatic islet-specific T cell clones from nonobese diabetic mice. Proc. Natl. Acad. Sci. USA **86:** 8000–8004.
42. DARDENNE, M. *et al.* 1989. Acceleration of the onset of diabetes in NOD mice by thymectomy at weaning. Eur. J. Immunol. **5:** 889–895.
43. CHARLTON, B. *et al.* 1989. Cyclophosphamide-induced diabetes in NOD/WEHI mice. Evidence for suppression in spontaneous autoimmune diabetes mellitus. Diabetes **4:** 441–447.
44. GREEN, J.M. *et al.* 1994. Absence of B7-dependent responses in CD28-deficient mice. Immunity **6:** 501–508.

45. MATHIEU, C. *et al.* 1993. Protection against autoimmune diabetes by induction of mixed bone marrow chimerism. Transplant Proc. **1:** 1266–1267.
46. BACH, J.F. *et al.* 2003. Regulatory T cells under scrutiny. Nat. Rev. Immunol. **3:** 189–198.
47. ALYANAKIAN, M.A. *et al.* 2003. Diversity of regulatory $CD4^+$ T cells controlling distinct organ-specific autoimmune diseases. Proc. Natl. Acad. Sci. USA **100:** 15806–15811.
48. SINGH, B. *et al.* 2001. Control of intestinal inflammation by regulatory T cells. Immunol. Rev. **182:** 1900–2001.
49. SALOMON, B. *et al.* 2000. B7/CD28 costimulation is essential for the homeostasis of the $CD4^+CD25^+$ immunoregulatory T cells that control autoimmune diabetes. Immunity **12:** 431–440.
50. TANG, Q. *et al.* 2003. CD28 controls peripheral homeostasis of $CD4^+CD25^+$ regulatory T cells. J. Immunol. **171:** 3348–3352.
51. HERMAN, A.E. *et al.* 2004. $CD4^+CD25^+$ T regulatory cells dependent on ICOS promote regulation of effector cells in the prediabetic lesion. J. Exp. Med. **199:** 1479–1489.
52. GREEN, E.A. *et al.* 2003. $CD4^+CD25^+$ T regulatory cells control anti-islet $CD8^+$ T cells through TGF-beta-TGF-beta receptor interactions in type 1 diabetes. Proc. Natl. Acad. Sci. **100:** 10878–10883.
53. TRITT, M. *et al.* 2004. Control of type 1 autoimmune diabetes by naturally occurring $CD4^+CD25^+$ regulatory T lymphocytes. Collected abstracts of the 4th International Autoimmunity Congress (Budapest, Hungary). No. A104.
54. MCHUGH, R.S. *et al.* 2002. $CD4^+CD25^+$ immunoregulatory T cells: gene expression analysis reveals a functional role for the glucocorticoid-induced TNF receptor. Immunity **16:** 311–323.
55. THORNTON, A. *et al.* 2004. IL-2 is critically required for activation of the suppressor function of $CD4^+CD25^+$ T cells *in vitro*. J. Immunol **172:** 6519–6523.
56. SZANYA, V. *et al.* 2002. The subpopulation of $CD4^+CD25^+$ splenocytes that delays adoptive transfer of diabetes expresses L-selectin and high levels of CCR7. J. Immunol. **169:** 2461–2465.
57. MOTTET, C. *et al.* 2003. Cure of colitis by $CD4^+CD25^+$ regulatory T cells. J. Immunol. **170:** 3939–3943.
58. GAGNERAULT, M.C. *et al.* 2002. Pancreatic lymph nodes are required for priming of cell reactive T cells in NOD mice. **196:** 369–377.
59. GAVIN, M.A. *et al.* 2001. Homeostasis and anergy of $CD4^+CD25^+$ suppressor T cells *in vivo*. Nat. Immunol. **3:** 33–41.
60. MOSER, B. *et al.* 2004. Chemokines: multiple levels of leukocyte migration control. Trends Immunol. **25:** 75–84.
61. BYSTRY, R.S. *et al.* 2001. B cells and professional APCs recruit regulatory T cells via CCL4. Nat. Immunol. **2:** 1126–1132.
62. IELLEM, A. *et al.* 2002. Unique chemotactic response profile and specific expression of chemokine receptors CCR4 and CCR8 by $CD4^+CD25^+$ regulatory T cells. J. Exp. Med. **194:** 847–853.
63. FU, S. *et al.* 2004. TGF-beta induces Foxp3+ T-regulatory cells from CD4+CD25- precursors. Am. J. Transplant. **4:** 1614–1627.
64. SURI-PAYER, E. *et al.* 2001. Differential cytokine requirements for regulation of autoimmune gastritis and colitis by $CD4^+CD25^+$ T cells. J. Autoimmun. **16:** 115–123.
65. THOMPSON, C. & F. POWRIE. 2004. Curr. Opin. Pharmacol. **4:** 408–414.
66. GOTTLIEB, P.A. *et al.* 2002. Cytokine and immunosuppressive therapies of type 1 diabetes mellitus. Endocrinol. Metab. Clin. North Am. **31:** 477–495.
67. KULLBERG, M.C. *et al.* TGF-β production by $CD4^+$ $CD25^+$ regulatory T cells is not essential for suppression of intestinal inflammation. Submitted for publication.
68. PENG, Y. *et al.* 2004 TGF-beta regulates in vivo expansion of Foxp3-expressing $CD4^+CD25^+$ regulatory T cells responsible for protection against diabetes. Proc. Natl. Acad. Sci. USA **101:** 4572–4577.
69. SEDDON, B. & D. MASON. 1999. Peripheral autoantigen induces regulatory T cells that prevent autoimmunity. J. Exp. Med. **189:** 877–881.

70. KASH, S.F. *et al.* 1999 Glutamate decarboxylase and GABA in pancreatic islets: lessons from knockout mice. Hormone Metab. Res. **31:** 340–344
71. WEGMANN, D.R. *et al.* 1994. Insulin-specific T-cells are a predominant component of islet infiltrates in pre-diabetic NOD mice. Eur. J. Immunol. **24:** 1853–1857.
72. TANG, Q. *et al.* 2004. *In vitro*-expanded antigen-specific regulatory T cells suppress autoimmune diabetes. J. Exp. Med. **199:** 1455–1465.
73. TARBELL, K.V. *et al.* 2004. CD25+ CD4+ T cells, expanded with dendritic cells presenting a single autoantigenic peptide, suppress autoimmune diabetes. J. Exp. Med. **199:** 1467–1477.

The Role of Methallothioneins in Experimental Autoimmune Encephalomyelitis and Multiple Sclerosis

CARMEN ESPEJO[a] AND EVA M. MARTÍNEZ-CÁCERES[b]

[a]*Unitat de Neuroimmunologia Clínica, Hospital Universitari Vall d'Hebron, Barcelona, Spain*

[b]*Laboratori d'Immunobiologia per a la Recerca i Aplicacions Diagnòstiques (LIRAD), Centre de Tranfusió i Banc de Teixits (CTBT), Institut d'Investigació en Ciències de la Salut Germans Trias i Pujol, Badalona, Barcelona, Spain*

ABSTRACT: Multiple sclerosis is a chronic inflammatory and demyelinating disease of the central nervous system (CNS) in which oxidative stress plays a pathogenic role. Metallothioneins are antioxidant proteins induced in the CNS under conditions where oxidative stress has taken place, such as tissue injury, stress, and some neurodegenerative diseases, which have been postulated to play a neuroprotective role. In this review we summarize recent progress in understanding the regulation and function of methallothioneins during experimental autoimmune encephalomyelitis and multiple sclerosis.

KEYWORDS: metallothionein; experimental autoimmune encephalomyelitis; multiple sclerosis; oxidative stress; antioxidant

INTRODUCTION

Multiple sclerosis (MS) is a chronic demyelinating disease of the central nervous system (CNS). It is the most frequent cause of nontraumatic neurological dysfunction in young adults. The mechanims involved in disease development have been extensively studied, and most of the available data support a model of lesion development mediated by Thelper 1 (Th1) $CD4^+$ lymphocytes secreting proinflammatory cytokines such as interferon-γ (IFN-γ) or tumor necrosis factor-α (TNF-α). Inflammatory CNS infiltrates are made up mostly of lymphocytes, macrophages, and various degrees of demyelination and axonal loss.[1,2] Experimental autoimmune encephalomyelitis (EAE) is an animal model for MS, with clinical signs and CNS lesions resembling those observed in MS.[3]

Address for correspondence: Eva M. Martínez-Cáceres, Laboratori d'Immunobiologia per a la Recerca i Aplicacions Diagnòstiques (LIRAD)—Centre de Tranfusió i Banc de Teixits (CTBT), Institut d'Investigació en Ciències de la Salut Germans Trias i Pujol, Badalona, Barcelona, Spain. Voice: +34-93-497-8892; fax: +34-93-497-8978.

evammc@ns.hugtip.scs.es

Ann. N.Y. Acad. Sci. 1051: 88–96 (2005). © 2005 New York Academy of Sciences.
doi: 10.1196/annals.1361.049

Although the actual pathogenic mechanisms involved in EAE/MS are not well understood, some literature points to the role of reactive oxigen species (ROS) in the ongoing inflammation and CNS damage.[4–7] In both EAE and MS, inflammatory cells produce nitric oxide (NO) and its oxidizing congeners such as peroxynitrite. Peroxynitrite and other reactive nitrogen species (RNS) exert a toxic effect on neurons, axons, and glial cells enhancing apoptosis. In addition, ROS and RNS increase blood–brain barrier (BBB) permeability and can therefore promote invasion of more inflammatory cells into the CNS. Brain cells protect themselves from oxidative stress by producing antioxidant enzymes, free radical scavengers, and proteins that bind transition metals like iron and copper.[8,9] Little is known about the role of antioxidants in MS. Antioxidants might prevent free radical–mediated tissue destruction and inhibit some of the early proinflammatory events, such as T cell activation and trafficking into the CNS, that result in inflammation and tissue damage. Indeed, several experimental studies support the hypothesis that antioxidants prevent or reduce the progression of EAE. Uric acid—a strong peroxynitrite scavenger—has been succesfully used in treating EAE.[10] Another potent antioxidant, bilirrubin, suppresses EAE,[11] whereas treatment with thymoquinone, an oxidative stress inhibitor,[12] or caffeic acid phenethyl ester,[13] alleviates the course of the disease in rats. On the other hand, it has been shown that MS patients have significantly lower levels of serum uric acid,[10] plasma vitamin E, plasma ubiquinone, lymphocyte ubiquinone, and erythrocyte glutathione peroxidase than controls.[14]

METALLOTHIONEINS

Metallothioneins (MTs) are a family of low molecular weight (6–7 kDa), heavy metal–binding, cystein-rich proteins. These proteins are found in the nucleus and cytoplasm of eukaryotic cells, sharing sequence and structural homology along the filogenetic scale. In mammals, MTs are polypeptides of 61–62 amino acids with 20 conserved Cys residues.[15] Seventeen different genes coding MT proteins have been described in humans in chromosome 16, from which at least 10 are functional.[16] In mice, MT genes are in chromosome 8, following an expression pattern similar to that of humans.

In mice and humans, the main classes of MTs found within the CNS are MT isoforms -I, -II, and -III. MT-I and -II are expressed coordinately in CNS and other tissues;[17] they are induced by inflammatory stimuli, glucocorticoids, and heavy metals. MT-I and –II isoforms are mainly expressed by astrocytes and activated microglia. In contrast, the MT-III isoform is mainly expressed by neurons, although it may be induced in astrocytes under some conditions.[18,19] In contrast to MT-I and-II, MT-III is relatively unresponsive to cytokines, hormones, and metals.

MT-I and -II are induced under conditions where oxidative stress has occurred,[20] such as in response to CNS injury; this includes freeze injury, focal ischemia, or spinal cord injury.[21] MT-I and -II expression is also elevated in neurodegenerative diseases such as Alzheimer's disease (even in the earliest stages),[22] Pick's disease, amyotrophic lateral sclerosis, alcoholism, and others;[23] in all of these diseases oxidative stress has been involved as a significant factor contributing to tissue injury.

Although the precise physiological role of MT-I and -II in the CNS remains unclear, it has been suggested that these proteins may protect cells from oxidative damage.[23] In relation to the mechanisms underlying their protective effect, it seems that the zinc-binding property of MTs (seven zinc ions per protein molecule) and their ability to scavenge free radicals, may play an important role. Moreover, MT-I and -II could also participate directly, reducing the inflammatory response associated with CNS injury. The function of MT-III, expressed mainly in neurons, is less well known, but it is different from that of MT-I and -II.[24]

METALLOTHIONEINS AND EAE

The different data on the role of MT-I and -II in the CNS suggest that these antioxidant proteins could also protect against the myelin and neuronal damage that occurs during EAE/MS. To investigate this hypothesis, we first analyzed MT-I and -II induction during EAE.[25] Twelve 129/Sv, H-2^b mice of either sex, at 8–14 weeks of age, were immunized with a subcutaneous injection of rat myelin oligodendrocyte glycoprotein peptide 40–55 (MOG_{40-55}) emulsified in Freund's adjuvant containing 4 mg/mL *Mycobacterium tuberculosis*. Control animals were immunized in the same way but without the MOG_{40-55} peptide. All animals were weighed and examined daily for neurological signs following the criteria described by Brocke *et al.*:[26] score 0 = no clinical signs; 0.5 = partial loss of tail tonus for two consecutive days; 1 = paralysis of whole tail; 2 = mild paraparesis of one or both hind limbs; 3 = paraplegia; 4 = tetraparesis; 5 = tetraplegia; 6 = death. Mice were sacrificed 28 days after immunization, and their brains and spinal cords were resected. MT-I and MT-III expression was evaluated by *in situ* hybridization. MT-II was not analyzed, given that MT-I and -II genes are expressed coordinately.[17] All animals with clinical signs of the disease showed inflammatory infiltrates with demyelination and astrogliosis in comparison with animals without EAE. We observed a strong induction of MT-I (and MT–II) in 129/Sv mice with clinical signs of EAE compared to animals that did not develop the disease, whose levels did not differ those of from nonimmunized control animals.[25] Furthermore, the level of expression was related to the severity of the disease, supporting the theory that induction of these antioxidant proteins may be part of a defense mechanism triggered during EAE induction.

To better understand the functions of MTs in the CNS, it is essential to characterize factors that control their expression. Interferons, inducers of the acute-phase response, and metallo-regulatory proteins have been shown to induce them.[27] Given that proinflammatory cytokines play an important role in the induction of EAE and are, at the same time, able to induce MTs, we analyzed MT induction in two different strains of IFN-γ receptor knockout mice. We observed that in both strains of knockout mice, EAE was more severe than in wild-type animals. When MT-I induction was analyzed, it also correlated with the severity of the clinical signs. These results demonstrate that, at least in our experimental model, IFN-γ is not necessary for the induction of MT-I and -II.[25]

In contrast to MT-I and -II, MT-III induction occurred differently. High levels of MT-III were constitutively expressed in the CNS of mice at basal levels (either wild-type or IFN-γ receptor knockout mice), but no significant induction of MT-III was observed adjacent to the inflammatory infiltrates in mice with EAE. The different expression patterns between MT-I (and -II) and MT-III, either basal or post-EAE induction, support a different function of these proteins in the CNS.

To further understand the role of MT-I and -II during EAE, we analyzed the expression profiles of the following group of markers:

(*a*) inflammation (IL-1b, IL-6, and TNF-α);
(*b*) demyelination (examined by detecting MBP immunoreactivity and its disappearance during EAE);
(*c*) axonal loss (detected by SMI-32 immunostaining, which marks axonal degeneration and transection due to demyelination, and amyloid precursor protein (APP), which is an early and sensitive marker for axonal pathology);
(*d*) oxidative stress (determined by using NITT and MDA immunoreactivity); and
(*e*) apoptotic cell death (judged by TUNEL)

Other markers were studied, such as those of tissue repair (studied by using immunostainings for PDGFa-receptor and NG2), which stain oligodendrocyte progenitor cells and detect oligodendroglial regeneration; and antibodies against GAP-43 and P-40, markers of neuroglial regeneration, sprouting, and regrowth. Similarly, anti-inflammatory cytokines like IL-10, TGF-α, and the growth factors bFGF and NGF were also analyzed. All these markers were compared with the expression of MT-I and -II during the exacerbation of EAE, with the aim of establishing the time relationship of these pathogenic processes.[28] Sixty SJL/J mice were immunized with a subcutaneous injection of proteolipid-protein peptide 139–151 ($PLP_{139-151}$), as described.[28] We chose this EAE model (SJL mice immunized with $PLP_{139-151}$) because these mice suffer from a relapsing–remitting course with inflammation and demyelination. Groups of five mice were sacrificed at different score points: score 0 (day 7 postimmunization (pi)), score 1 (day 13 pi), score 2 (days 15–19 pi), score 3–4 (days 22–24 pi), score 2, during clinical recovery (days 26–29 pi), and score 0, upon full recovery (days 34–37 pi). Tissue samples from nonimmunized (control group 1), and PBS-immunized (control group 2) mice were also obtained on day 7 pi. Overall, we could differentiate two different profiles of marker expression (FIG. 1): In the first profile (pattern 1), markers were expressed early after the induction of the disease, peaked at the highest clinical score, and decreased drastically at the beginning of clinical recovery. In the second profile (pattern 2), marker expression increased at a later point during relapse, peaked at highest clinical score, and remained elevated during recovery (FIG. 1F). Markers implicated in EAE-clinical ongoing as proinflammatory cytokines (FIG. 1A), oxidative stress (FIG. 1B), demyelination (not shown), axonal damage, and apoptosis (FIG. 1C) were found in the first profile while the second profile (pattern 2) included markers related to EAE-clinical recovery as anti-inflammatory cytokines, growth factors (FIG. 1D), oligodendroglial progenitor (FIG. 1E), and neuroglial regeneration markers (not shown). Interestingly, the expression of MTs were related to the second profile. The kinetics of the different molecules might be explained, at least in part, by their interaction with each other, supporting a beneficial role of MTs in the resolution of the relapse.

These results are also in agreement with those found in 129/sv MT-I + -II knockout mice, which suffer from a more severe EAE than control animals. Pathological analysis of those mice showed increased demyelination and axonal damage. Also, oligodendroglial regeneration, growth cone formation, and tissue repair including expression of trophic factors was significantly reduced in MT knockout mice during EAE.[29,30]

In summary, we think that the MT-I and -II proteins might have a role in the pathogenesis of EAE by mediating neuroregeneration, either by downmodulating neurodegenerative processes (such as inflammation, oxidative stress, demyelination, and axonal injury) or by upmodulating tissue repair processes (including the induction of growth factor expression), supporting the idea that the neuroprotective role previously described for MT-I and -II in other neuropathologic conditions such as

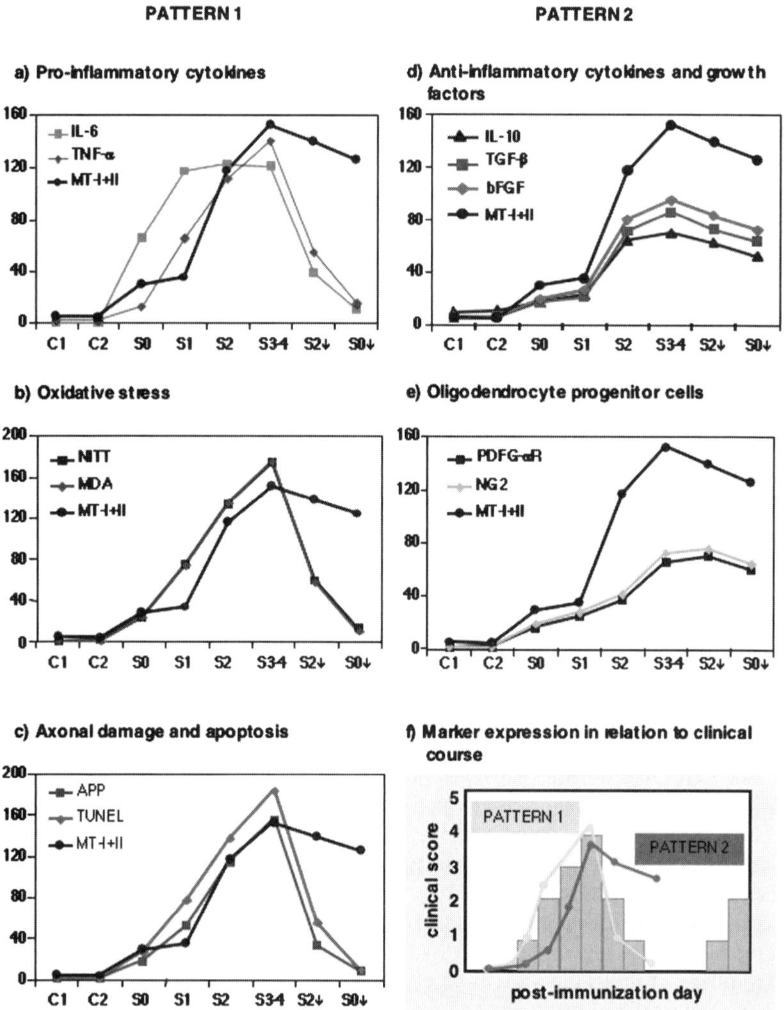

FIGURE 1. MT-I and -II expression in relation to CNS inflammatory, neurodegenerative tissue repair markers during EAE. **X axis: C1:** nonimmunized mice; **C2:** PBS immunized mice; **S0:** score 0 at day 7 postimmunization (pi); **S1:** score 1 at day 13 pi; **S2:** score 2 at days 15–19 pi; **S3–4:** score 3 at 4 days 22–24 pi; **S2↓:** score 2 during clinical recovery at days 26–29 pi; **S0↓:** score 0 upon full recovery-days 34–37 pi. Counts were carried out in n=5 mice per group. **Y axis:** number of positive cells/0.5 mm^2.

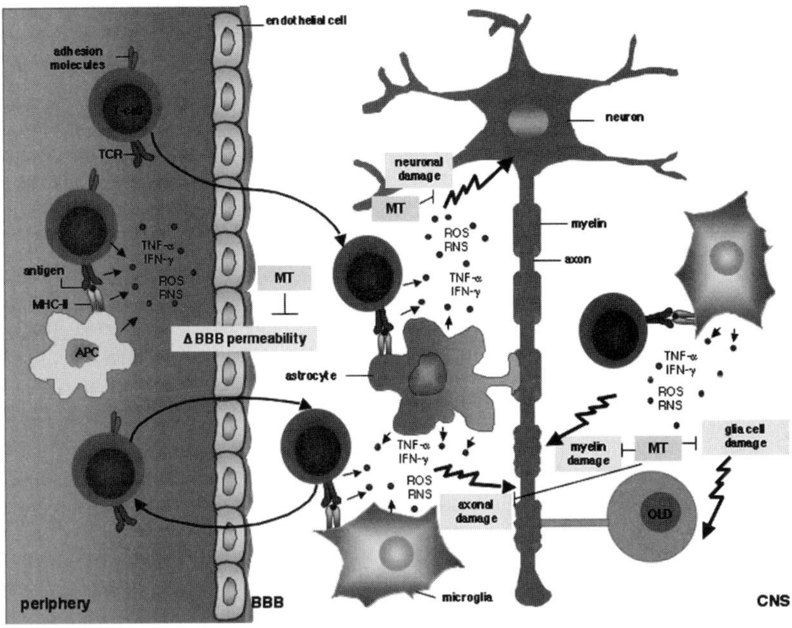

FIGURE 2. Role of MT-I and -II in the pathogenesis of EAE/MS during EAE/MS. Activated lymphocytes cross the blood–brain barrier (BBB) and enter into the CNS where, after a second activation induced by interaction with resident antigen presenting cells (APC), they secrete proinflammatory cytokines and reactive oxigen and nitrogen species, inducing neuronal and oligodendroglial damage, as well as direct injury to myelin and axons. The current literature on MI-I and -II suggest that MTs, induced by proinflammatory cytokines and oxidative stress, might act by downmodulating processes involved in neurodegeneration (such as inflammation, increase of the BBB permeability, oxidative stress, demyelination, neuronal damage, and axonal injury), at the same time that it would induce tissue repair processes (including the induction of growth factor expression).

trauma, ischemia, epilepsy, and neuroglial degeneration[31–34] may also be relevant in EAE/MS (FIG. 2).

METALLOTHIONEINS AND MS

In contrast to the increasing amount of data analyzing the role of MT-I and -II in EAE, little is known about the actual role of these proteins in MS. In our first approach, using immunohistochemistry, we analyzed MT induction in active and inactive lesions of brains from three deceased MS patients and two controls.[35] We found that in all MS cellular infiltrates, MT-I and -II increased significantly. The pattern of MT expression was similar to that found in the EAE model. Interestingly, MT levels were slightly increased in the inactive MS lesions in comparison with the active ones, suggesting that MTs could be related to disease remission. Lock *et al.*,[36] performing gene-microarray analysis of 4 MS lesions, found an increase in MT gene expression in all samples analyzed (acute, chronic active, and chronic silent lesions), which is in agreement with our findings at the protein level.

COULD MTs BE CONSIDERED A TREATMENT FOR MS?

Once synthesized, MTs may remain within the cell, where they may serve to sequester heavy metals, act as an antioxidant, or regulate gene activity by direct interactions with transcription factors like NF-κB.[37] MTs can also be released from cells and function as a soluble factor. This extracellular pool of MTs can interact with the surface of cells and modify their functions. In this regard, the existence of MT receptors has been reported on astrocytes.[38] Several reports describe altered serum MT levels in patients with autoimmune diseases, although the data are contradictory among authors.

In vitro experiments of Lynes *et al.* in mice have shown that soluble MTs can affect cell proliferation, macrophage, and cytotoxic T lymphocyte function, as well as humoral immunity to T-dependent antigens.[39] These authors have developed the hypothesis that extracellular MTs may act as negative regulators of the immune response and might play a role in suppressing the autoimmune attack by serving to limit the severity of the disease. This would point to a putative role of soluble MTs in the treatment of autoimmune diseases, including MS. In this context, it has been found that treatment with Zn-MT-II improves EAE,[40] and that MT-I+II treatment can block the disease process in experimental rheumatoid arthritis.[41]

Preliminary *in vitro* experiments from our laboratory in human peripheral blood mononuclear cells (PBMCs) show that soluble MTs inhibit IL-6 and IL-12 production (C. Espejo, unpublished results) in line with the results of Lynes *et al.* in mice.[39] More experiments are necessary to understand the interactions of MTs with the human immune system and their role in the autoimmune response; although, at this point, with the support of *in vitro* experiments and the studies in animal models, it is tempting to speculate that these antioxidant proteins might be potential therapeutic candidates in multiple sclerosis.

ACKNOWLEDGMENTS

We are very grateful to all our collaborators: Milena Penkowa, Irene Sáez-Torres, Javier Carrasco, Arancha Ortega, María Demestre, Joseph Graells, Tina Garcia, Juan Hidalgo, and especially to Xavier Montalban, Head of the Unitat de Neuroimmunologia Clínica, Hospital Vall d'Hebron.

REFERENCES

1. LASSMANN, H. 1999. The pathology of multiple sclerosis and its evolution. Philos. Trans. R. Soc. Lond. B. Biol. Sci. **354:** 1635–1640.
2. FERGUSON, B., M.K. MATYSZAK, M.M. ESIRI & V.H. PERRY. 1997. Axonal damage in acute multiple sclerosis lesion. Brain **120:** 393–399.

3. MARTIN, R., H.F. MCFARLAND & D.E. MCFARLIN. 1992. Immunological aspects of demyelinating diseases. Annu. Rev. Immunol. **10:** 153–187.
4. DE GROOT, C.J., S.R. RUULS, J.W. THEEUWES, *et al.* 1997. Immunocytochemical characterization of the expression of inducible and constitutive isoforms of nitric oxide synthase in demyelinating multiple sclerosis lesions. J. Neuropathol. Exp. Neurol. **56:** 10–20.
5. CROSS, A.H., P.T. MANNING, R.M. KEELING, *et al.* 1998. Peroxynitrite formation within the central nervous system in active multiple sclerosis. J. Neuroimmunol. **88:** 45–56.
6. VLADIMIROVA, O., J. O'CONNOR, A. CAHILL, *et al.* 1998. Oxidative damage to DNA in plaques of MS brains. Mult. Scler. **4:** 413–418.
7. GILGUN-SHERKI, Y., E. MELAMED & D. OFFEN. 2004. The role of oxidative stress in the pathogenesis of multiple sclerosis: the need for effective antioxidant therapy. J. Neurol. **251:** 261–268.
8. HALLIWELL, B. 1992. Reactive oxygen species and the central nervous system. J. Neurochem. **59:** 1609–1623.
9. PENTREATH V.W. & N.D. SLAMON. 2000. Astrocyte phenotype and prevention against oxidative damage in neurotoxicity. Hum. Exp. Toxicol. **19:** 641–649.
10. HOOPER, D.C., S. SPITSIN, R.B. KEAN, *et al.* 1998. Uric acid, a natural scavenger of peroxynitrite, in experimental allergic encephalomyelitis and multiple slerosis. Proc. Natl. Acad. Sci. USA **94:** 2528–2533.
11. LIU, Y., B. ZHU, X. WANG, *et al.* 2003. Bilirubin as a potent antioxidant suppresses experimental autoimmune encephalomyelitis: implications for the role of oxidative stress in the development of multiple sclerosis. J. Neuroimmunol. **139:** 27–35.
12. MOHAMED, A., A. SHOKER, F. BENDJELLOUL, *et al.* 2003. Improvement of EAE by thymoquinone, an oxidative stress inhibitor. Biomed. Sci. Instrum. **39:** 440–445.
13. ILHAN, A., O. AKYOL, A. GUREL, *et al.* 2004. Protective effects of caffeic acid phenethyl ester against experimental allergic encephalomyelitis-induced oxidative stress in rats. Free Radic. Biol. Med. **37:** 386–394.
14. SYBURRA, C. & S. PASSI. 1999. Oxidative stress in patients with multiple sclerosis. Ukr. Biokhim. Zh. **71:** 112–115.
15. BINZ, P.A. & J.H.R. KAGI. 1999. Metallothionein: molecular evolution and classification. *In* Metallothionein IV. C. D. Klaasen, Ed.: 7–13. Birkhauser Verlag. Basel.
16. SAMSON, S.L. & L. GEDAMU. 1998. Molecular analyses of metallothionein gene regulation. Prog. Nucleic Acid Res. Mol. Biol. **59:** 257–288.
17. YAGLE, M.K. & R.D. PALMITER. 1985. Coordinate regulation of mouse metallothionein I and II genes by heavy metals and glucocorticoids. Mol. Cell Biol. **5:** 291–294.
18. UCHIDA, Y., K. TAKIO, K. TITANI, *et al.* 1991. The growth inhibitory factor that is deficient in the Alzheimer´s disease brain is a 68 amino acid metallothionein-like protein. Neuron **7:** 337–347.
19. PALMITER, R.D., S.D FINDLEY, T.E. WHITMORE & D.M. DURNAM. 1992. MTs-III, a brain-specific member of the metallothionein gene family. Proc. Natl. Acad. Sci. USA **89:** 6333–6337.
20. SHIRAGA, H., R.F. PFEIFFER & M. EBADI. 1993. The effects of 6-hydroxydopamine and oxidative stress on the level of brain metallothionein. Neurochem. Int. **23:** 561–566.
21. HIDALGO J., M. ASCHNER, P. ZATTA & M. VASAK. 2001. Roles of the metallothionein family of proteins in the central nervous system. Brain Res. Bull. **55:** 133–145.
22. ADLARD P.A., A.K. WEST & J.C. VICKERS. 1998. Increased density of metallothionein I/II-immunopositive cortical glial cells in the early stages of Alzheimer's disease. Neurobiol. Dis. **5:** 349–356.
23. EBADI, M., P.L. IVERSEN, R. HAO, *et al.* 1995. Expression and regulation of brain metallothionein. Neurochem. Int. **27:** 1–22.
24. SOGAWA C.A., M. ASANUMA, N. SOGAWA, *et al.* 2001. Localization, regulation, and function of metallothionein-III/Growth inhibitory factor in the brain. Acta Med. Okayama **55:** 1–9.
25. ESPEJO, C., J. CARRASCO, J. HIDALGO, *et al.* 2001. Differential expression of metallothioneins in the CNS of mice with experimental autoimmune encephalomyelitis. Neuroscience **105:** 1055–1065.

26. BROCKE, S., K. GIJBELS & L. STEINMAN. 1994. Autoimmune Disease Models: A Guidebook. I. R Cohen & A. Miller, Eds.: 1–14. Academic Press. San Diego, CA.
27. HIDALGO J., B. CASTELLANO & I.L. CAMPBELL. 1997. Regulation of brain metallothioneins. Curr. Top. Neurochem. **1:** 1–26.
28. ESPEJO, C., M. PENKOWA, M. DEMESTRE, *et al.* 2005. Time course expression of CNS-inflammatory, neurodegenerative, tissue repair markers, and metallothioneins during experimental autoimmune encephalomyelitis. Neuroscience **132:** 1135–1149.
29. PENKOWA, M., C. ESPEJO, E.M. MARTÍNEZ-CÁCERES, *et al.* 2001. Altered inflammatory response and increased neurodegeneration in metallothionein I+II deficient mice during experimental autoimmune encephalomyelitis. J. Neuroimmunol. **119:** 248–260.
30. PENKOWA, M., C. ESPEJO, E.M. MARTÍNEZ-CÁCERES, *et al.* 2003. Increased demyelination and axonal damage in metallothionein I+II deficient mice during experimental autoimmune encephalomyelitis. Cell. Mol. Life Sci. **60:** 185–197.
31. VAN LOOKEREN-CAMPAGNE, M., H. THIBODEAUX, N. VAN BRUGGEN, *et al.* 1999. Evidence for a protective role of metallothionein-1 in focal cerebral ischemia. Proc. Natl. Acad. Sci. USA **96:** 12870–12875.
32. TRENDELENBURG, G., K. PRASS, J. PRILLER, *et al.* 2002. Serial analysis of gene expression identifies metallothionein-II as major neuroprotective gene in mouse focal cerebral ischemia. J. Neurosci. **22:** 5879–5888.
33. PENKOWA, M., J. CARRASCO, M. GIRALT, *et al.* 1999. CNS wound healing is severely depressed in metallothionein I- and II-deficient mice. J. Neurosci. **19:** 2535–2545.
34. PENKOWA, M., J. CARRASCO, M. GIRALT, *et al.* 2000. Altered central nervous system cytokine-growth factor expression profiles and angiogenesis in metallothionein-I+II deficient mice. J. Cereb. Blood Flow Metab. **20:** 1174–1189.
35. PENKOWA M., C. ESPEJO, A. ORTEGA-AZNAR, *et al.* 2003. Metallothionein expression in the central nervous system of multiple sclerosis patients. Cell. Mol. Life Sci. **60:** 1258–1266.
36. LOCK, C., G. HERMANS, R. PEDOTTI, *et al.* 2002. Gene-microarray analysis of multiple sclerosis lesions yields new targets validated in autoimmune encephalomyelitis. Nat. Med. **8:** 500–508.
37. SAKURAI, A., S. HARA, N. OKANO, *et al.* 1999. Regulatory role of metallothionein in NF-kappaB activation. FEBS Lett. **455:** 55–58.
38. EL REFAEY, H., M. EBADI, C.A. KUSZYNSKI, *et al.* 1997. Identification of metallothionein receptors in human astrocytes. Neurosci. Lett. **231:** 131–134.
39. CANPOLAT, E. & M.A. LYNES. 2001. *In vivo* manipulation of endogenous metallothionein with a monoclonal antibody enhances a T-dependent humoral immune response. Toxicol. Sci. **62:** 61–70.
40. PENKOWA, M. & J. HIDALGO. 2003. Treatment with metallothionein prevents demyelination and axonal damage and increases olygodendrocyte precursors and tissue repair during experimental autoimmune encephalomyelitis. J. Neurosci. Res. **72:** 574–586.
41. YOUN J., S.H. HWANG, Z.Y. RYOO, *et al.* 2002. Metallothionein suppresses collagen-induced arthritis via induction of TGF-beta and downregulation of proinflammatory mediators. Clin. Exp. Immunol. **129:** 232–239.

Oxidized Low-Density Lipoprotein/ β_2-Glycoprotein I Complexes and Autoantibodies in Patients with Type 2 Diabetes Mellitus

LUIS R. LOPEZ,[a] BETH L. HURLEY,[a] DANIEL F. SIMPSON,[a] AND EIJI MATSUURA[b]

[a]*Corgenix Inc., Westminster, Colorado 80234, USA*

[b]*Okayama University Graduate School of Medicine and Dentistry, Okayama 700-8558, Japan*

ABSTRACT: **Diabetes mellitus (DM) is associated with a high incidence of atherosclerotic cardiovascular complications that result from chronic metabolic abnormalities such as hyperglycemia-induced oxidative stress. The oxidative-modification of low-density lipoproteins (oxLDL) and oxLDL/β_2-GPI complex formation have been reported in patients with autoimmune disorders. OxLDL/ β_2-GPI complexes and autoantibodies to these complexes were measured by ELISA in serum samples from 50 type 2 DM patients and 50 age/sex–matched healthy controls. Mean OD for oxLDL/β_2-GPI complexes in DM was 0.099±0.065 with 50% of patients reacting above the assay cutoff (P<0.001 vs. controls). Mean OD for controls was 0.037±0.015 with 2% positives. Thirty-six (72%) DM patients were taking cholesterol-lowering statins and had a significantly lower mean OD complex level (0.092±0.071, P=0.05) compared to patients not taking statins (0.112±0.05). Mean OD for IgG anti-oxLDL/β_2-GPI antibodies in DM was 0.157±0.112, similar to the controls (0.146±0.098, P=0.328). Increased serum levels of oxLDL/β_2-GPI complexes may be a consequence of oxidative stress and LDL modification in DM. Lower levels of oxLDL/β_2GPI complexes in DM patients taking statins are in agreement with the antioxidant and antithrombotic properties of these drugs. No significant IgG autoantibody production was observed in this group of DM patients. The interaction of oxLDL with β_2-GPI in circulation suggests the intriguing possibility that oxLDL/β_2-GPI complexes may also play a role in the development of atherosclerosis and/or cardiovascular complications in DM.**

KEYWORDS: **atherosclerosis; low-density lipoprotein; β_2-glycoprotein I; oxidative stress**

INTRODUCTION

The metabolic abnormalities of diabetes mellitus (DM) predispose the development of micro- and macrovascular complications associated with significant

Address for correspondence: Luis R. Lopez, M.D., Corgenix Inc., 12061 Tejon Street, Westminster, Colorado 80234, USA. Voice: 303-457-4345; fax: 303-457-4519.
llopez@corgenix.com

Ann. N.Y. Acad. Sci. 1051: 97–103 (2005). © 2005 New York Academy of Sciences.
doi: 10.1196/annals.1361.050

morbidity and mortality. The arterial involvement is characterized by the development of accelerated (or premature) atherosclerosis, which leads to either coronary artery disease, cerobrovascular accidents, or peripheral vascular disease.[1] Chronic hyperglycemia and oxidative stress are risk factors for the development of atherothrombotic vascular disease by two main mechanisms: (1) the modification of platelet glycoproteins and production of platelet-active isoprostanes derived from arachidonic acid peroxidation, both stimulating *in vivo* platelet activation and aggregation; and (2) lipid peroxidation and vascular endothelium activation, producing increased adhesion, receptor expression, and proinflammatory/prothrombotic changes. Hyperglycemia-induced oxidative stress modifies the proatherogenic low-density lipoprotein (LDL) into an oxidized LDL form (oxLDL).[2,3] Patients with DM exhibit a decreased plasma antioxidant activity as well as increased levels of lipid hydroperoxides and F_2-isoprotanes. The latter two are recognized *in vivo* markers of ongoing oxidative stress.[4] Oxidative stress in DM may also depress plasma levels of anticoagulant proteins, further tilting the balance toward a proatherothrombotic state.[5] Decreased plasma activity of the HDL-associated antioxidant enzyme paraoxonase (PON) has been reported in patients with DM and has been proposed to be a contributor in the development of vascular complications.[6]

The accelerated (or premature) occurrence of atherosclerosis in patients with systemic lupus erythematosus (SLE) could not be fully explained by classic atherosclerosis risk factors and/or disease treatment.[7] Immunostaining of human atherosclerotic plaques has shown the presence of oxLDL, β_2-GPI, and CD4/CD8 immunoreactive cells,[8] indicating the participation of autoimmune mechanisms in atherogenesis. Oxidative stress, decreased PON activity, lipoprotein abnormalities, and prothrombotic states have been shown to occur frequently in patients with systemic autoimmune diseases (SLE) and antiphospholipid syndrome (APS).[9] We have previously shown that oxLDL binds β_2-GPI *in vitro* to form stable or nondissociable oxLDL/β_2-GPI complexes[10] and have demonstrated its presence in the serum of patients with autoimmune disease with vascular complications (SLE, APS). These findings suggest a pathogenic role of oxLDL/β_2-GPI complexes as atherogenic autoantigens.[11] Unlike SLE and APS patients that have both circulating oxLDL/β_2-GPI complexes and autoantibodies to these complexes,[12] nonautoimmune patients such as type 2 DM seem to have mainly circulating oxLDL/β_2-GPI complexes. These results open the intriguing possibility that oxLDL/β_2-GPI complexes may also play a role in the development of atherosclerosis and/or cardiovascular complications in DM.

MATERIAL AND METHODS

Subjects

Serum samples obtained from subjects enrolled in a diabetes patient registry (50 type 2 DM patients and 50 age and sex–matched healthy controls) were studied. Demographics and clinical characteristics of the patients and controls are summarized in TABLE 1.

TABLE 1. Demographics and clinical charateristics of type 2 DM patients and controls

	Patients with Diabetes	Control Subjects
Subjects (*n*)	50	50
Age in years (range)	70.4 (37–87)	71.8 (50–86)
Sex (M/F)	32/18	32/18
Glucose (mg/dL)	123	—
Hgb A1c (%)	6.7	—
T. Cholesterol (mg/dL)	177	—
HDL cholesterol (mg/dL)	46	—
LDL cholesterol (mg/dL)	95	—
Triglycerides (mg/dL)	157	—
Cardiovascular disease (*n*)	20	—
Statins (*n*)	34	—

ELISA for oxLDL/β_2-GPI Complexes

Murine IgG monoclonal antibody against human β_2-GPI (WB-CAL-1) was coated onto Nunc MaxiSorp 96-microwell plates (Nunc, Denmark). WB-CAL-1 monoclonal antibody used in this assay binds only oxLDL/β_2-GPI complexes, not free β_2-GPI.[10] Prediluted patients' serum in sample diluent containing 10mM $MgCl_2$ was added to the coated microwells and incubated for one hour at room temperature. $MgCl_2$ dissociates intermediate or electrostatically bound oxLDL/β_2-GPI complexes, allowing the specific detection of nondissociable or covalently bound complexes, if present.[10] Horseradish peroxidase (HRP)-conjugated antihuman Apo B100 murine monoclonal antibody was added to the microwells and incubated for an additional hour. Color was developed with tetramethylbenzydine (TMB)/H2O2, and the reaction stopped with 0.36N sulfuric acid. Optical density was read at a wavelength of 450 nm (650 nm reference). Reactivity of the assay was controlled with a curve built with oxLDL/β_2-GPI complex solution. The complexes were prepared in advance by incubating equal amounts of Cu^{2+}-oxidized LDL and purified human β_2-GPI. A normal cutoff value for the assay was established by testing serum samples from healthy blood donors (mean + three standard deviations).

ELISA for IgG Anti-oxLDL/β_2-GPI Antibodies

OxLDL/β_2-GPI complexes prepared by incubating equal amounts of Cu^{2+}-oxidized LDL with purified human β_2-GPI were coated onto Immunlon 1B™ 96-microwell plates (Dynex Technologies Inc., Virginia). These oxLDL/β_2-GPI complexes served as antigenic substrates to capture patients' antibodies. Diluted serum samples were added to the microwells and incubated for one hour at room temperature. HRP-conjugated antihuman IgG antibody was added to the microwells and incubated for one hour. Color was developed with TMB/H_2O_2, and the reaction stopped with 0.36N sulfuric acid. Optical density was read at a wavelength of 450 nm (650 nm reference). Reactivity of the assay was controlled with a curve built with serial dilution of selected positive sera for IgG anti-oxLDL/β_2-GPI antibodies. A normal cutoff value for the assay was established by testing serum samples from healthy blood donors (mean + three standard deviations).

RESULTS

oxLDL/β_2-GPI Complexes in Type 2 DM

The mean OD value for oxLDL/β_2-GPI complexes in type 2 DM patients was 0.099 ±0.065, which was significantly higher than the mean OD of the healthy control group (0.037 ± 0.015, P<0.001). With a cutoff value established at OD of 0.08 (mean + three SD of controls), 50% of DM patients and only one healthy control subject (2%) had elevated serum levels of oxLDL/β_2-GPI complexes. The control subject had a borderline elevated level (FIG. 1). No age or sex difference with respect to oxLDL/β_2-GPI complex levels was observed in this group of DM patients. Only LDL cholesterol levels showed a positive correlation with oxLDL/β_2-GPI complexes (r = 0.261), but this association did not reach statistical significance (P = 0.08). No correlation was found between oxLDL/β_2-GPI complex levels and fasting blood sugar, total cholesterol, HDL cholesterol, or triglycerides. The mean OD value of oxLDL/β_2-GPI complexes of 34 DM patients taking cholesterol-lowering statins was 0.092 ± 0.071, significantly lower than the mean of 16 patients not taking these drugs (0.112 ± 0.05, P = 0.05) (FIG. 2). However, the mean OD for oxLDL/β_2-GPI complexes in DM patients with overt clinical cardiovascular disease (0.096) was similar to that of patients without it (0.101).

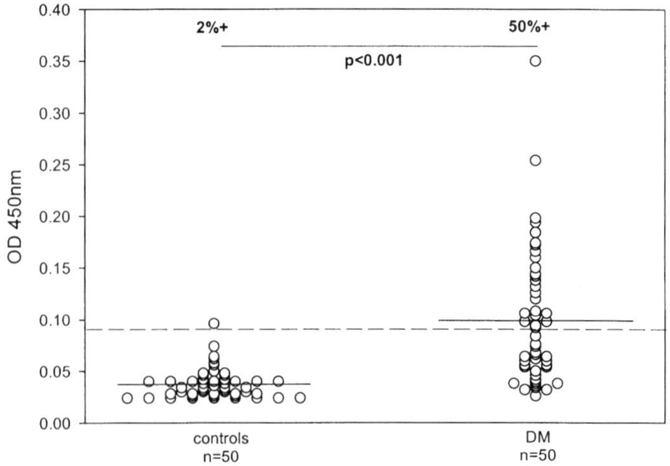

FIGURE 1. Serum levels of oxLDL/β_2GPI complexes measured by ELISA in 50 type 2 diabetes mellitus patients and 50 age/sex–matched healthy controls. Horizontal broken line represents the cutoff OD value of the assay (mean + three SD of 100 healthy controls). Solid lines represent the mean OD of each group. P value (Mann–Whitney rank test) significant if <0.05.

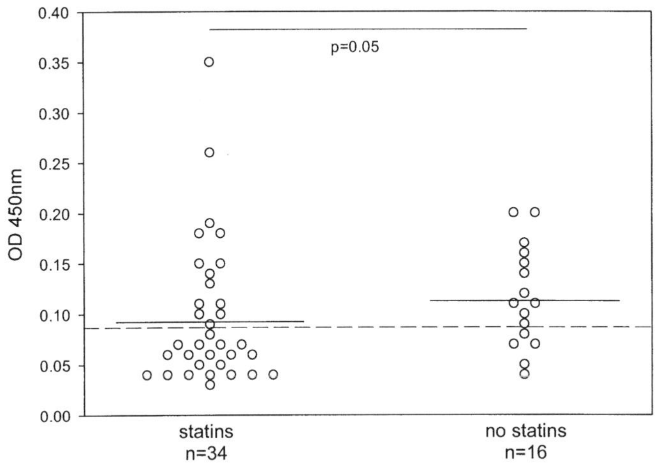

FIGURE 2. Serum levels of oxLDL/β_2GPI complexes measured by ELISA in 34 type 2 diabetes mellitus patients taking statins and 16 patients not taking statins. Horizontal broken line represents the cutoff OD value of the assay (mean + three SD of 100 healthy controls). Solid lines represent the mean OD of each group. *P* value (Mann–Whitney rank test) significant if <0.05.

IgG Anti-oxLDL/β_2GPI Antibodies in Type 2 DM

The mean OD for IgG anti-oxLDL/β_2-GPI antibodies in type 2 DM patients was 0.157 ± 0.112, similar to the mean OD of healthy controls (0.146 ± 0.098, $P = 0.328$).

DISCUSSION

These results demonstrate the presence of significantly higher serum levels of circulating oxLDL/β_2-GPI complexes in patients with type 2 DM compared to age- and sex-matched healthy controls. We have previously shown that high serum levels of oxLDL/β_2-GPI complexes are frequently found in autoimmune patients with vascular complications such as SLE and APS[13] and have proposed that these complexes play a pathogenic role in autoimmune-mediated thrombosis and atherosclerosis. In systemic autoimmune diseases, a generalized vascular inflammation frequently associated with decreased PON activity[9] may contribute to the initiation and progression of oxidative stress. These events may lead to the modification of LDL (oxLDL) and oxLDL/β_2-GPI complex formation. In patients with DM, low PON activity,[6] hyperglycemia-induced inflammation, and oxidative stress may also modify LDL, resulting in oxLDL/β_2-GPI complex formation.

In DM, chronic hyperglycemia seems to be an important cause of oxidative stress that produces thrombotic and atherosclerotic vascular complications.[2] The enzyme paraoxonase (PON) is normally associated with HDL cholesterol and protects LDL cholesterol from oxidative damage.[9] As in SLE, decreased PON activity has also been recently reported in DM patients.[6] Whether the decreased PON activity is the result or the consequence of chronic oxidative stress is not known. Nonetheless, the oxidative stress of DM modifies oxLDL and produces oxLDL/β_2-GPI complexes. Interestingly, DM patients taking cholesterol-lowering statins showed lower serum levels of oxLDL/β_2-GPI complexes. These results are in agreement with the antioxidant/antithrombotic effects of statins.[15] We found no difference in oxLDL/β_2-GPI complex levels between DM patients with and without cardiovascular disease. DM patients without cardiovascular disease may be asymptomatic with complexes and early arterial pathology that have not reached an end-stage point as in DM patients with clinical cardiovascular disease.

OxLDL/β_2-GPI complexes may function as atherogenic antigens because autoantibodies to this complex have been demonstrated in patients with SLE and APS.[14] IgG anti-oxLDL/β_2-GPI antibodies were present in SLE patients with active disease and with secondary APS.[13] Furthermore, these antibodies were strongly associated with arterial thrombosis in APS patients.[12] In contrast to patients with autoimmune disease, DM seem to produce no significant anti-oxLDL/β_2-GPI antibody response. In DM, serum levels of the proatherogenic IgG antibodies were similar to those of healthy controls.

A possible mechanism for atherosclerotic plaque formation in autoimmune disease involves the macrophage uptake of immune complexes (such as oxLDL/β_2-GPI/IgG). The *in vitro* macrophage uptake of oxLDL/β_2-GPI complexes was enhanced in the presence of anti-β_2-GPI antibodies, suggesting the participation of an efficient Fcγ macrophage receptor.[16] We also tested for IgG-containing oxLDL/β_2-GPI immune complexes by ELISA and found similar results to IgG anti-oxLDL/β_2-GPI antibodies. In the absence of antibodies and immune complexes in DM, oxLDL/β_2-GPI complexes are most likely taken up by macrophages via scavenger receptors, leading to the development of foam (fat-containing) cells in atherosclerotic plaques.

It is possible that other mechanisms than those described above, such as oxLDL forming complexes with other inflammatory molecules such as CRP, contribute to the development of accelerated atherosclerosis in DM. It is also possible that antibodies to other antigenic complexes may also participate. In addition, the metabolic or inflammatory abnormalities of DM may have an additive or even a synergistic effect in the development of vascular complications through platelet and endothelial activation (or dysfunction). Although preliminary, these results suggest that oxLDL/β_2-GPI complexes may play a pathogenic role in DM, and that they may be used as a serologic marker to assess the patient's risk for vascular complications. They also provide a rationale with which to develop vascular disease–preventive programs and/or more targeted therapeutic intervention.

COMPETING INTEREST: Luis R. Lopez is CEO of Corgenix, Inc., a manufacturer of ELISA test kits.

REFERENCES

1. HURST, R.T. & R.W. LEE. 2003. Increased incidence of coronary atherosclerosis in type 2 diabetes mellitus: mechanisms and management. Ann. Intern. Med. **139:** 824–834.
2. LAAKSO, M. 1999. Hyperglycemia and cardiovascular disease in type 2 diabetes. Diabetes **48:** 937–942.
3. EVANS, J.L., I.D. GOLDFINE, B.A. MADDUX & G.M. GRODSKY. 2002. Oxidative stress and stress-activated signaling pathways: a unifying hypothesis of type 2 diabetes. Endocr. Rev. **23:** 599–622.

4. TSAI, E.C., I.B. HIRSCH, J.D. BRUNZELL & A. CHAIT. 1994. Reduced plasma peroxyl radical trapping capacity and increased susceptibility of LDL to oxidation in poorly controlled IDDM. Diabetes **43:** 1010–1014.
5. DE CRISTOFARO, R., B. ROCCA, E. VITACOLONNA, *et al.* 2003. Lipid and protein oxidation contribute to a prothrombotic state in patients with type 2 diabetes mellitus. J. Thromb. Haemost. **1:** 250–256.
6. TSUZURA, S., Y. IKEDA, T. SUEHIRO, *et al.* 2004. Correlation of plasma oxidized low-density lipoprotein levels to vascular complications and human serum paraoxonase in patients with type 2 diabetes. Metabolism **53:** 297–302.
7. ESDAILE, J.M., M. ABRAHAMOWICZ, T. GRODZICKY, *et al.* 2001. Traditional Framingham risk factors fail to fully account for accelerated atherosclerosis in systemic lupus erythematosus. Arthritis Rheum. **44:** 2331–2337.
8. GEORGE, J., D. HARATS, B. GILBURD, *et al.* 1999. Immunolocalization of β_2-glycoprotein I (apolipoprotein H) to human atherosclerotic plaques. Circulation **99:** 2227–2230.
9. DELGADO ALVES, J., P.R.J. AMES, S. DONOHUE, *et al.* 2002. Antibodies to high-density lipoprotein and β_2-glycoprotein I are inversely correlated with paraoxonase activity in systemic lupus erythematosus and primary antiphospholipid syndrome. Arthritis Rheum. **46:** 2686–2694.
10. KOBAYASHI, K., M. KISHI, T ATSUMI, *et al.* 2003. Circulating oxidized LDL forms complexes with β2-glycoprotein I: implication as an atherogenic autoantigen. J. Lipid Res. **44:** 716–726.
11. MATSUURA, E. & L.R. LOPEZ. 2004. Are oxidized LDL/β_2-glycoprotein I complexes pathogenic antigens in autoimmune-mediated atherosclerosis? Clin. Dev. Immunol. **11:** 103–111.
12. LOPEZ, D., K. KOBAYASHI, J.T. MERRILL, *et al.* 2003. IgG autoantibodies against β_2-glycoprotein I complexed with a lipid ligand derived from oxidized low-density lipoprotein are associated with arterial thrombosis in antiphospholipid syndrome. Clin. Dev. Immunol. **10:** 203–211.
13. LOPEZ, D., I. GARCIA-VALLADARES, C.A. PALAFOX-SANCHEZ, *et al.* 2004. Oxidized low-density lipoprotein/β2-glycoprotein I complexes and autoantibodies to oxLig-1/β_2-glycoprotein I in patients with systemic lupus erythematosus and antiphopsholipid syndrome. Am. J. Clin. Pathol. **121:** 426–436.
14. MATSUURA, E., K. KOBAYASHI, T. KOIKE, *et al.* 2003. Atherogenic autoantigen: oxidized LDL complexes with β_2-glycoprotein I. Immunobiol. **207:** 17–22.
15. ROSENSON, R.S. 2004. Statins in atherosclerosis: lipid-lowering agents with antioxidant capabilities. Atherosclerosis **173:** 1–12.
16. LIU, Q., K. KOBAYASHI, J. FURUKAWA, *et al.* 2002. ω-Carboxyl variants of 7-ketocholesteryl esters are ligands for β_2-glycoprotein I and mediate antibody-dependent uptake of oxidized LDL by macrophages. J. Lipid Res. **43:** 1486–1495.

Autoantibodies to Human α6 Integrin in Patients with Bullous Pemphigoid

MÁRIA KISS,[a] ÁDÁM PERÉNYI,[a] ILONA MARCZINOVITS,[b] JÁNOS MOLNÁR,[b] ATTILA DOBOZY,[a,c] LAJOS KEMÉNY,[a,c] AND SÁNDOR HUSZ[a]

[a]*Department of Dermatology and Allergology, University of Szeged, Szeged, Hungary*

[b]*Department of Physiology, University of Szeged, Szeged, Hungary*

[c]*Dermatological Research Group of the Hungarian Academy of Sciences, Szeged, Hungary*

ABSTRACT: Bullous pemphigoid (BP) is characterized immunologically by tissue-bound and circulating autoantibodies targeting the hemidesmosomal proteins BP230 and BP180. Recent evidence suggests a pathophysiological role for autoantibodies against α6 integrin in the subepidermal blister formation of oral pemphigoid. The objective of our study was to investigate the presence of anti-α6 integrin antibodies in patients with classical BP. The autoantibody profiles of 30 patients with BP, 10 patients with pemphigus vulgaris, and 20 healthy persons were identified. With the use of PeptideStructure and PlotStructure software, four different antigenic epitopes for α6 integrin were predicted, and their fusion recombinant constructs were prepared in an *E. coli* expression system. Sera were tested for α6 integrin autoantibodies by an ELISA technique. Altogether, 52% of the patients with BP displayed circulating antibodies against at least one recombinant protein. Our findings provide the first evidence for the presence of anti-α6 integrin antibodies in patients with classical BP.

KEYWORDS: bullous pemphigoid; anti-α6 integrin antibodies; basement membrane; autoimmunity

INTRODUCTION

Pemphigoid is a heterogeneous group of autoimmune blistering diseases. When the disease predominantly involves the skin, it is called bullous pemphigoid (BP). BP is an IgG-mediated autoimmune blistering skin disease that is seen predominantly in elderly people. The disease is characterized immunologically by tissue-bound and circulating autoantibodies targeting the hemidesmosomal cytoplasmic plaque protein BP230 and the type II transmembrane protein BP180 (also known as collagen XVII).[1–3] Immunodominant and pathogenic epitopes of BP180 associated with BP have been mapped to the NC16A domain, a membrane-proximal noncollagenous stretch of the extracellular portion.[4] Autoantibodies to BP180 associated with BP

Address for correspondence: Mária Kiss, Ph.D., Department of Dermatology and Allergology, University of Szeged, H-6720 Szeged, Korányi fasor 6, Hungary. Voice: +36-62-545278; fax: +36-62-545954.

km@mail.derma.szote.u-szeged.hu

Ann. N.Y. Acad. Sci. 1051: 104–110 (2005). © 2005 New York Academy of Sciences.

doi: 10.1196/annals.1361.051

can release IL-6 and IL-8 from cultured human keratinocytes[5] and can induce dermal-epidermal separation in cryosections of human skin.[6] The pathogenic relevance of BP180 autoantibodies has been established by using experimental mouse model systems.[7] Immunodominant epitopes of BP230 have also been characterized, but the pathogenic role of anti-BP230 antibodies remains open to question.[8,9]

Integrins are cell surface receptors that are involved in cell-matrix adhesion and signaling. α6 integrin, a laminin receptor, contains 1050 amino acids present as a heavy (110 kDa) and a light chain (30 kDa) linked by a disulfide bond. The α6β4 integrin heterodimer, together with other members of the epidermal integrin family, is expressed by epidermal keratinocytes. This expression is restricted to the basal and suprabasal proliferative cell layers, both in the epidermis and in cultures of keratinocytes.[10] α6β4 integrin is localized at the basal pole of the basal cells and coordinates a structural linkage between intracellular filaments and the extracellular matrix of the basement membrane. The α6β4 integrin plays a crucial role in the assembly of hemidesmosomes,[11] and antibodies directed against α6β4 integrin induce a dermal-epidermal dissociation *in vitro*.[12] α6 integrin null-mutant mice die at birth, with severe blistering of the skin and other epithelia.[13]

It was demonstrated earlier that α6 integrin is a BP180 binding partner in the hemidesmosomal multimolecular complex and that this connection is essential for the functioning of hemidesmosomes. The protein associations of BP180 were mapped by Hopkinson *et al.*, who found that the 36 N-terminal residues of BP180 are essential for the polarization of the molecule to the basal surface, whereas the 27 extracellular residues immediately following the membrane-spanning domain of BP180 appear to mediate BP180 interactions with other hemidesmosomal proteins. Intriguingly, the same region contains the epitopes of pathogenic BP autoantibodies. Using a yeast two-hybrid assay, BP180 peptides, and *in vitro* assays of protein binding, Hopkinson *et al.* showed that specific domains of BP180 and α6 integrin can interact directly, and that the sequence containing the pathogenic autoantibody epitope in BP180 is most probably involved in this interaction.[14,15]

Recent evidence suggests a pathophysiological role for autoantibodies against α6 integrin in the subepidermal blister formation of oral pemphigoid, a subset of mucous membrane pemphigoid (MMP).[16] The objective of our study was to investigate the presence of anti-α6 integrin antibodies in patients with classical BP.

MATERIALS AND METHODS

Patients

Serum was studied from 30 BP patients (16 males and 14 females, mean age at onset 76 years, range 35 to 90 years) proven to have BP by clinical, histological, and immunohistological criteria. Sera from 20 healthy blood donors and 10 patients with pemphigus vulgaris served as controls. All the BP patients exhibited the specific clinical symptoms and histological picture. Direct immunofluorescence investigations demonstrated that all the patients had deposits of IgG and C3 along the basement membrane zone. Circulating autoantibodies in sera from the BP patients labeled the epidermal roof of the salt-split skin preparation, and all the BP patients

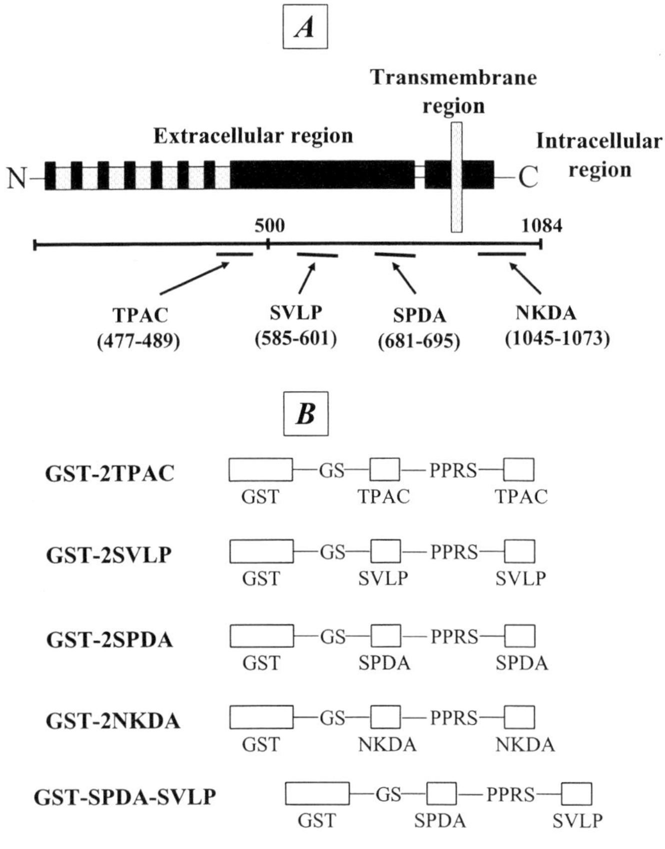

FIGURE 1. **(A)** Structural representation of human α6 integrin.[17] It contains seven weak sequence repeats (*dotted rectangles*) in the N-terminal region. The heavy and light chains of the molecule are linked by a disulfide bond. The antigenic epitopes of human α6 integrin were predicted via the programs PeptidStructure and PlotStructure. The localizations of the chosen four epitopes are demonstrated as *short lines* along the molecule. **(B)** Schematic diagrams of the recombinant products containing antigenic peptide epitopes of human α6 integrin. All recombinant fusion products are composed of GST at the -NH_2 terminal end, followed by the antigenic epitopes at the -COOH terminus. A dipeptide GS was inserted between GST and the particular epitope sequence. In the homologous and heterologous dimers, the peptides are linked through a tetrapeptide PPRS.

displayed autoantibodies against the BP230 and/or BP180 autoantigens detected by Western blotting.

Structures of the Chosen Antigenic Peptides of Human α6 Integrin

The sequence of human α6 integrin was from the Swiss-Prot and TrEMBL databanks; it was analyzed with the Wisconsin Package, Version 8 (Genetic Computer Group, Madison, WI) by means of the programs PeptideStructure and PlotStructure. The chosen epitopic fragments were as follows:

NKDA: NKKDHYDATYHKAEIHAQPSDKERLTSDA (NP_000201; 1045–1073) *intracellular*

TPAC: TPNRIDLRQKTAC (NP_000201; 477–489) *extracellular*

SVLP: SVEIQEPSSRRRVNSLP (NP_000201; 585–601) *extracellular*

SPDA: SPSNPRNPTKDGDDA (NP_000201; 681–695) *extracellular*

Schematic diagrams of human α6 integrin[17] and the chosen antigenic epitopes are presented in FIGURE 1.

Preparation of Recombinant Constructs Used for Autoantibody Detection

Nucleotide sequences coding for peptides NKDA, TPAC, SVLP, and SPDA were chemically synthesized *in vitro.* These synthetic DNA sequences were inserted through the *Bam*HI site to the glutathione-S transferase (GST) gene of the fusion-expression plasmid pGEX-4T-2 (Pharmacia, Sweden) in-frame. As a result of the cloning strategy, a dipeptide GS (one-letter code) was inserted between GST and the particular epitope sequence. In the homologous (GST-2NKDA, GST-2TPAC, GST-2SPDA, and GST-2SVLP) and heterologous (GST-SPDA-2SVLP) dimer constructs, DNA blocks encoding the peptides without stop codon were linked to one another by *Bam*HI and *Bgl*II restriction sites in-frame through a sequence coding for a tetrapeptide PPRS. The identities of the inserted DNA blocks and the flanking plasmid regions were controlled by sequencing. Recombinant plasmids were expressed in *E. coli* DH5a as described earlier.[18] The fusion protein was purified over a glutathione-Sepharose affinity matrix (Pharmacia, Sweden) from the soluble fraction of *E. coli* lysate and dialyzed against phosphate-buffered saline (PBS; pH 7.4) before being used for ELISA.

ELISA Investigations for Detection of Antibody against Human α6 Integrin

ELISA investigations were performed as previously described.[19] Briefly, recombinant proteins were dissolved and diluted in PBS, pH 7.4, at the optimal concentration of 1 μg/100 μL and allowed to coat overnight at 4°C. Control and patient serum samples were diluted 1:200. For the detection of the immune reactivity of the sera, peroxidase-conjugated anti-human IgG (Sigma-Aldrich, St. Louis, MO) was used. Optical density (OD) was measured at 492 nm. The optimal cutoff value was estimated carefully. Our earlier studies[19] indicated that the OD $> x + 2$ SD (x = mean OD of control subjects; SD = standard deviation of control OD) cutoff is the most

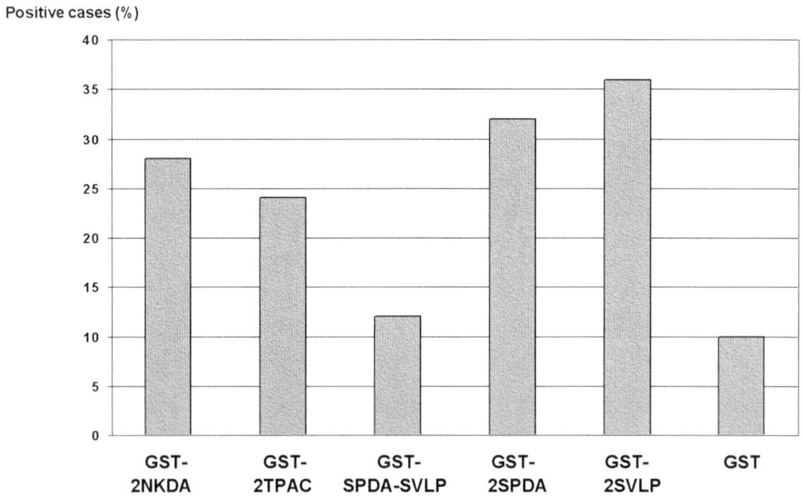

FIGURE 2. Immune reactivity in patients with classical BP against human α6 integrin represented by different recombinant fusion proteins. The structures of the recombinant proteins are depicted in FIGURE 1.

sensitive limit for the establishment of a screening procedure. We always used at least 18 healthy control samples per microplate, and each cutoff value was calculated for each microplate.

RESULTS

Sera were tested for α6 integrin autoantibodies using the fusion recombinant proteins in an ELISA system. Twenty-eight percent of the BP sera reacted with the construct containing the intracellular epitope, but positive reactions were demonstrated more frequently (32% and 36%) against the recombinant proteins containing the extracellular antigenic peptides of α6 integrin, which are close to the transmembrane region (FIG. 2). Altogether, 52% of the patients with BP displayed circulating antibodies against at least one recombinant protein. The healthy blood donors and the patients with pemphigus vulgaris did not exhibit immune reactivity with any of the recombinant constructs. Ten percent of the BP patients gave a slight borderline reaction with GST protein only.

DISCUSSION

MMP is a group of autoimmune, chronic inflammatory subepithelial blistering diseases predominantly affecting the mucous membranes. Autoantibodies against various epithelial basement membrane components (e.g., BP230, BP180, laminin 5, laminin 6, β4 integrin) probably play roles in the pathogenesis of this group of diseases.[20] Oral pemphigoid is a subset of MMP with disease limited to the oral cavity, without involvement of any other mucosa or skin. Bhol *et al.* identified the target antigen(s) recognized by sera from 20 untreated patients with oral pemphigoid.[16] They ascertained that patient sera selectively and specifically bound to human α6 integrin. In organ culture, they demonstrated the direct pathogenic role of anti-α6 integrin antibodies in subepidermal blister formation.[16] It has also been established that the titers of anti-α6 integrin antibodies correlate with disease activity, and clinical and serological remission has been achieved in patients using intravenous human immunoglobulin.[21]

The aim of our study was to investigate the occurrence of anti-α6 integrin antibodies in patients with classical BP, where skin symptoms predominate. The recombinant proteins we used for the detection of anti-α6 integrin antibodies were linear duplicates coupled to GST. In previous investigations, we demonstrated that tandem repetitions of antigenic epitopes increased the ligand affinity and the immune reactivity with the sera of BP patients.[19] We have observed that GST fusion forms with the antigenic epitopes to exhibit an increasing contribution of a-helix conformation in the dimer or multimer form, thereby enhancing the immunogenicity of the construct.[22]

Our findings provide the first evidence for the presence of anti-α6 integrin antibodies in patients with classical BP. As the BP patients with autoantibodies against α6 integrin did not reveal signs of mucosal involvement of their disease, the presence of α6 integrin autoantibodies might be a secondary autoimmune event. It suggests that antibodies directed against the transmembrane protein BP180 represent the pathogenic antibodies as a result of their accessibility for autoantibody induction, whereas antibodies directed against α6 integrin may represent an epiphenomenon. It has been speculated that patients first develop autoantibodies directed against BP180 and that, after these antibodies have bound to and damaged the epidermal cells, α6 integrin is made accessible and antibodies against it are formed as a consequence of intermolecular epitope spreading. Epitope spreading describes an immune phenomenon whereby an autoimmune disease process causes tissue damage in such a way that certain antigens originally "hidden" from the autoreactive T or B cells become exposed and evoke a secondary autoimmune response.[23,24] However, a direct pathogenic role of anti-α6 integrin autoantibodies in subepidermal blister formation in classical BP cannot be excluded. Further investigations are necessary to clarify this.

ACKNOWLEDGMENTS

This work was supported by the Hungarian Scientific Research Fund (OTKA Grants T 032 495, T 034 964, and TS 0443 826) and the Hungarian Ministry of Health (ETT 413/2003).

REFERENCES

1. Stanley, J.R. 1999. Bullous pemphigoid. *In* Fitzpatrick's Dermatology in General Medicine, pp. 666–671. McGraw-Hill. New York..
2. Labib, R.S., G.J. Anhalt, H.P. Patel, *et al.* 1986. Molecular heterogeneity of the bullous pemphigoid antigens as detected by immunoblotting. J. Immunol. **136:** 1231–1235.

3. YANCEY, K.B. & C.A. EGAN. 2000. Pemphigoid: clinical, histologic, immunopathologic, and therapeutic considerations. JAMA **284:** 350–356.
4. ZILLIKENS, D., P.A. ROSE, S.D. BALDING, *et al.* 1997. Tight clustering of extracellular BP180 epitopes recognized by bullous pemphigoid autoantibodies. J. Invest. Dermatol. **109:** 573–579.
5. SCHMIDT, E., S. REIMER, N. KRUSE, *et al.* 2000. Autoantibodies to BP180 associated with bullous pemphigoid release interleukin-6 and interleukin-8 from cultured human keratinocytes. J. Invest. Dermatol. **115:** 842–848.
6. SITARU, C., E. SCHMIDT, S. PETERMANN, *et al.* 2002. Autoantibodies to bullous pemphigoid antigen 180 induce dermal-epidermal separation in cryosections of human skin. J. Invest. Dermatol. **118:** 664–671.
7. LIU, Z. 2004. Bullous pemphigoid: using animal models to study the immunopathology. J. Investig. Dermatol. Symp. Proc. **9:** 41–46.
8. SKARIA, M., F. JAUNIN, T. HUNZIKER, *et al.* 2000. IgG antibodies from bullous pemphigoid patients recognize multiple antigenic reactive sites located predominantly within the B and C subdomains of the COOH-terminus of BP230. J. Invest. Dermatol. **114:** 998–1004.
9. KISS, M., S. HUSZ, T. JÁNOSSY, *et al.* 2005. Experimental bullous pemphigoid generated in mice with an antigenic epitope of the human hemidesmosomal protein BP230. J. Autoimmun. **24:** 1–10.
10. HERTLE, M.D., J.C. ADAMS & F.M. WATT. 1991. Integrin expression during human epidermal development in vivo and in vitro. Development **112:** 193–206.
11. GHOHESTANI, R.F., K. LI, P. ROUSSELLE & J. UITTO. 2001. Molecular organization of the cutaneous basement membrane zone. Clin. Dermatol. **19:** 551–562.
12. COLON, J.E., K.C. BHOL, M.S. RAZZAQUE & A.R. AHMED. 2001. *In vitro* organ culture model for mucous membrane pemphigoid. Clin. Immunol. **98:** 229–234.
13. GEORGES-LABOUESSE, E., N. MESSADDEQ, G. YEHIA, *et al.* 1996. Absence of integrin alpha 6 leads to epidermolysis bullosa and neonatal death in mice. Nat. Genet. **13:** 370–373.
14. HOPKINSON, S.B., S.E. BARKER & J.C. JONES. 1995. Molecular genetic studies of a human epidermal autoantigen (the 180-kD bullous pemphigoid antigen/BP180): identification of functionally important sequences within the BP180 molecule and evidence for an interaction between BP180 and α6 integrin. J. Cell Biol. **130:** 117–125.
15. HOPKINSON, S.B., K. FINDLAY, G.W. DE HART & J.C. JONES. 1998. Interaction of BP180 (type XVII collagen) and alpha 6 integrin is necessary for stabilization of hemidesmosome structure. J. Invest. Dermatol. **111:** 1015–1022.
16. BHOL, K.C., L. GOSS, S. KUMARI, *et al.* 2001. Autoantibodies to human alpha6 integrin in patients with oral pemphigoid. J. Dent. Res. **80:** 1711–1715.
17. DAVIS, T.L., I. RABINOVITZ, B.W. FUTSCHER, *et al.* 2001. Identification of a novel structural variant of the α6 integrin. J. Biol. Chem. **276:** 26099–26106.
18. MARCZINOVITS, I., C. SOMOGYI, A. PATTHY, *et al.* 1997. An alternative purification protocol producing hepatitis B virus X antigen on a preparative scale in *Eschericha coli.* J. Biotechnol. **56:** 81–88.
19. HUSZ, S., M. KISS, K. MOLNÁR, *et al.* 2000. Development of a system for detection of circulating antibodies against hemidesmosomal proteins in patients with bullous pemphigoid. Arch. Dermatol. Res. **292:** 217–224.
20. CHAN, L.S., A.R. AHMED, G.J. ANHALT, *et al.* 2002. The first international consensus on mucous membrane pemphigoid: definition, diagnostic criteria, pathogenic factors, medical treatment, and prognostic indicators. Arch. Dermatol. **138:** 370–379.
21. SAMI, N., K.C. BHOL & A.R. AHMED. 2002. Treatment of oral pemphigoid with intravenous immunoglobulin as monotherapy. Long-term follow-up: influence of treatment on antibody titres to human α6 integrin. Clin. Exp. Immunol. **129:** 533–540.
22. LACZKÓ, I., E. VASS, G.K. TÓTH, *et al.* 2000. Conformational consequences of coupling bullous pemphigoid antigenic peptides to glutathione-S-transferase and their diagnostic significance. J. Pept. Sci. **6:** 378–386.
23. VANDERLUGT, C.J. & S.D. MILLER. 1996. Epitope spreading. Curr. Opin. Immunol. **8:** 831–836.
24. CHAN, L.S., C.J. VANDERLUGT, T. HASHIMOTO, *et al.* 1998. Epitope spreading: lessons from autoimmune skin diseases. J. Invest. Dermatol. **110:** 103–109.

Soluble HLA Class I and Class II Molecules in Relapsing-Remitting Multiple Sclerosis

Acute Response to Interferon-β1a Treatment and Their Use as Markers of Disease Activity

ALIREZA MINAGAR,[a] IRENA ADAMASHVILLI,[a] STEPHEN L. JAFFE,[a] MICHAEL F. GLABUS,[b] EDUARDO GONZALEZ-TOLEDO,[c] AND ROGER E. KELLEY[a]

Departments of [a]Neurology, [b]Psychiatry, and [c]Radiology, Louisiana State University School of Medicine–Shreveport, Shreveport, Louisiana 71130, USA

ABSTRACT: During relapses in relapsing-remitting multiple sclerosis (RRMS), serum soluble HLA class I surface antigen (sHLA-I) levels are reported to either decrease or remain unchanged, whereas serum sHLA-II levels increase. Interferon-β1b therapy was recently reported to increase serum sHLA-I in RRMS. In the present prospective study, solid-phase enzyme-linked immunosorbent assay was used to measure sHLA-I and sHLA-II in the sera of 21 RRMS patients during a clinical exacerbation, and then six weeks after treatment with high-dose interferon-β1a (IFN-β1a). Pretreatment serum sHLA-I was significantly lower in patients than in normal controls ($P < 0.0005$). Pretreatment sHLA-II was also significantly lower than in normal controls ($P = .003$) unless enhancing MRI lesions (objectified relapse) were present; then sHLA-II levels were similar to normal controls (relative increase). Six weeks after initiation of IFN-β1a treatment, a significant increase in serum sHLA-I was observed in all 21 RRMS patients ($P < .0005$). Conversely, serum sHLA-II decreased significantly after treatment in the entire patient group ($P < .0005$). The acute effect of IFN-β1a on serum sHLA-I and sHLA-II was observed to be the opposite of that occurring during RRMS relapses. Monitoring of both sHLA-I and sHLA-II appears necessary if these molecules are to be developed as RRMS activity markers.

KEYWORDS: relapsing-remitting multiple sclerosis; soluble HLA I; soluble HLA II; interferon-β1a

INTRODUCTION

HLA cell surface class I and class II antigens, which are encoded by genes of the major histocompatibility complex (MHC), have been identified as probable mediators of autoimmune pathophysiology. HLA molecules are not only expressed on the

Address for correspondence: S. L. Jaffe, M.D., Magale Professor of Neurology, Department of Neurology, Louisiana State University Health Sciences Center, 1501 Kings Highway, Shreveport, LA 71130. Voice: 318-675-8394; fax: 318-675-6382.
sjaffe1@lsuhsc.edu

Ann. N.Y. Acad. Sci. 1051: 111–120 (2005). © 2005 New York Academy of Sciences.
doi: 10.1196/annals.1361.052

cell's surface, but can also be identified in a soluble (shed/secreted) form.[1–3] Such soluble class I (sHLA-I) and class II (sHLA-II) molecules may play a direct role in immunomodulation, or at least act as epiphenomenal markers.[4–6] Under stable conditions, the serum concentrations of soluble HLA antigens in each individual are relatively constant.[2,3] Increased levels of serum HLA-I and HLA-II have been reported with immune activation, both infectious and autoimmune.[7–9] sHLA-I also rises in the serum of patients treated with both interferon α and interferon γ.[10]

Multiple sclerosis (MS) is an immune-mediated disorder of the central nervous system that is characterized pathologically by loss of the myelin/oligodendrocyte complex and by axonal/neuronal degeneration. To date in relapsing-remitting MS (RRMS), there are no definitive *in vivo* markers of disease activity or markers of response to treatment with immunomodulators. Protection from or predisposition towards MS is clearly associated with certain MHC alleles.[11] In addition, $CD4^+$ T lymphocytes, which are present in acute plaques, only recognize antigen(s) in coordination with specific HLA gene products.[12] Moreover, sHLA-I and sHLA-II concentrations correlate quantitatively with specific HLA allotypes.[13] Therefore, soluble HLA molecules may be involved in the pathogenesis of MS, and recent findings (discussed below) further support more intensive investigation of these molecules in relation to RRMS.

Although a few studies have demonstrated alterations in sHLA-I and sHLA-II levels in the CSF of patients with MS,[14–17] the expression patterns of serum sHLA are not as well defined. In MS patients without distinction as to type or disease activity, serum sHLA-I has been found to be increased and sHLA-II decreased when compared with normal controls.[14–18] During RRMS exacerbations, serum sHLA-I has been reported to either decrease or remain unchanged, and sHLA-II to increase, although steroid treatment blocked this increase.[16,18,19] Beyond the ambiguities raised by these relapse correlational reports, the response of sHLA to β-interferon therapy in RRMS has only recently been reported (after the initiation of this study), and only the sHLA-I response to interferon-β1b treatment has been evaluated.[18] A significant sHLA-I increase from pretreatment levels was demonstrated after three months, with levels falling to baseline and slightly below during the next year; at 18 months, levels were only modestly above baseline. However, these levels were significantly higher in clinical responders versus nonresponders, suggesting a role for sHLA-I as a positive response marker to interferon-β1b therapy. In the present preliminary feasibility study, we investigated whether serial measurements of serum concentrations of both sHLA-I and sHLA-II might better serve as markers of disease activity in RRMS, as well as whether high-dose interferon-β1a (IFN-β1a) treatment initiated at the time of an RRMS relapse acutely affects the serum concentrations of sHLA-I and sHLA-II.

PATIENTS AND METHODS

Patient Population, Sampling, and Treatment

We prospectively studied 21 patients who were relapsing at study entry and who met the diagnostic criteria for RRMS as defined by McDonald.[20] At the time of study entry, all patients underwent neurological examination and brain MRI. None had received any immunomodulatory treatments for at least six months prior to study entry. As controls, we tested 82 racially and age-matched healthy individuals for sHLA-I levels, and 55 for sHLA-II.

After obtaining informed consent (IRB-approved), peripheral blood was drawn, clotted for 2 h, centrifuged, and stored at –20°C until analyzed. Patients were then treated with IFN-β1a, 44 mcg subcutaneously (Rebif), three times weekly. A second peripheral blood specimen was obtained six weeks after initiation of treatment and at least 24 h after the last interferon dose. No patient was on corticosteroid therapy at the time of sampling.

MRI Protocol

Brain MRI was performed on all patients using a 1.5 T machine with a standard head coil. The imaging protocol included sagittal T1-, axial T1-, T2-weighted, and FLAIR images. All MRI scans were performed before and after (Gd-DTPA) infusion. Axial T2-weighted and postcontrast T1-weighted images were used for assessment of MS plaques. The images were independently interpreted by a neuroradiologist, blinded as to patient status, using visual inspection and computer-assisted techniques.

Measurement of Soluble HLA Class I and Class II

Monoclonal antibodies: Hybridoma cell lines W6/32 (anti–HLA-A, B, C), L368 (anti-human β_2-microglobulin), Ab2.06, L203, and IVA-12 (anti–HLA-DR) were obtained from the American Type Culture Collection (Rockville, MD). These lines were expanded and the monoclonal antibodies (mAbs) were produced in BALB/c mice as described previously.[21] Anti–class I HLA monoclonal antibody W6/32 detects a common determinant on the α-chain of all HLA class I molecules. Monoclonal antibody L368 detects β_2-microglobulin, which is a constituent of all HLA class I molecules. Anti–class II HLA monoclonal antibodies AB2.06 and L203 react with noncompeting epitopes in the constant domain of HLA-DR molecules.

Solid-Phase Enzyme-Linked Immunosorbent Assay (ELISA)

The solid-phase ELISA for sHLA-I has been described previously.[2,9] The levels of sHLA-II were determined using a previously described assay, with minor modifications.[21] In brief: test samples were added to appropriate wells containing an anti–class I (W6/32) or an anti–class II (Ab2.06) mAb-coated bead. The reaction proceeded for 30 min for sHLA-I and 2 h for sHLA-II at 45°C. The beads were then washed three times with distilled water. Then, 200 µL of peroxidase-labeled anti–β_2-microglobulin mAb (L368) for sHLA-I or L2.03 mAb for sHLA-II was added to each bead and incubated for an additional hour at 45°C. After additional washes, the color reaction was initiated by adding the appropriate substrate. Absorbance was measured at 492 nm.

Standardization of sHLA-I and sHLA-II Assays

Each assay included a standard curve derived from negative controls. Negative controls consisted of 2% BSA and human serum, free of sHLA-I and sHLA-II. The sHLA-I positive control standard was prepared by chromatography, pooled serum being suffused over a CL-6B Sepharose mAb W6/32 gel column. The sHLA-I captured by the mAb column was eluted with glycine-HCl buffer (0.1 M glycine, pH 2.5). Fractions rich in sHLA-I were neutralized immediately with dibasic sodium phosphate, pooled, and dialyzed against saline. Total protein, which was assumed to be pure sHLA-I, was quantitatively analyzed with the Pierce BCA kit (Rockford, IL). With each assay, a standard curve was established by including in duplicate seven sHLA-I standards (1000, 750, 500, 250, 125, 62.5, and 0 ng/mL of pure sHLA-I protein). The test values were calculated from the curve described by these standards.

As regards sHLA-II values, the wide range of s-HLA-II concentrations reported from studies of sera from normal individuals seem likely to reflect either the use of multiple standards, or the different characteristics of the monoclonal antibodies used in the various described techniques.[3,21] Although initial standardization of the sHLA-II assay has been accomplished previously and reported,[21] due to the preliminary nature of this study, the amount of sHLA-II was inferred directly from the ELISA absorbance value (OD) of each sample of serum. The OD values of studied samples corresponding to sHLA-II values were compared with the OD values of 5% BSA used as the dilution factor and negative control within each procedure. To assess the specificity of the assay, parallel reactions were set up using preserved sera from previously tested individuals with known high or low levels of sHLA-II. The results for sHLA-II were expressed as units/mL, which represents the change in OD as compared with control. The lower limit of the test was about 0.030 units/mL. Any change in optical density less than that was considered negative.

Statistical Analysis

Data were analyzed with SPSS for Windows (v.11.0.1). All data sets were first evaluated using the Kolmogorov-Smirnov test to establish if they were normally distributed. Data that were not normally distributed were analyzed using nonparametric statistical tests. Values of $P < .05$ were considered statistically significant. The dependent variables were sHLA-1 and sHLA-2; they were measured pre- and post-treatment in patients, and at baseline only in healthy controls. Patients were then subgrouped according to the presence (P) or absence (M) of contrast-enhancing MRI lesions at the time of study inclusion, prior to treatment initiation. TABLE 1 summarizes the results of the statistical analyses. Means were tested using the appropriate paired and independent parametric and nonparametric tests. The General Linear Model was used to examine the first-order interaction effect between subjects, across groups.

RESULTS

Twenty-one patients with RRMS (female/male = 17/4) having a mean age of 35 years participated in this study. Serum sHLA-I and sHLA-II levels were measured during a clinical exacerbation prior to treatment with high-dose IFN-β1a, and six weeks after initiation of therapy. Those patients with enhancing MRI lesions at study entry were considered to have an objectively verified relapse.[11] TABLE 1 summarizes the mean values (SEM) for sHLA-I and sHLA-II for patients and controls.

Statistical analyses of these results are also presented in TABLE 1. Control sHLA-II levels, pre- and posttreatment sHLA-II levels of the entire patient group, and posttreatment sHLA-II levels in the nonenhancing (M) patient subgroup were not normally distributed.

TABLE 1. Mean sHLA-I and sHLA-II values for patient and control subjects with statistical analyses

	n	Mean (SEM)	Statistical analysis
sHLA I			
1. Control sHLA-I	82	240.8 (19.2)	1 vs. 2: $t = 4.9$; df = 101; $P < .0005$
2. Patient pretreatment sHLA-I	21	133.7 (10)	2 vs. 3: $t = 5.01$; df = 20; $P < .0005$
3. Patient posttreatment sHLA-I	21	337 (43.2)	
4. Patient pretreatment sHLA-I (P)	9	130.9 (12.6)	4 vs. 5: $t = 4.12$; df = 8; $P = .003$
5. Patient posttreatment sHLA-I (P)	9	348.3 (57.2)	1 vs. 4: $t = 1.88$; df = 89; $P < .0005$
6. Patient pretreatment sHLA-I (M)	12	137.5 (15.2)	6 vs. 7: $t = 3.2$; df = 11; $P = .009$
7. Patient posttreatment sHLA-I (M)	12	328.6 (64.3)	1 vs. 6: $t = 4.3$; df = 92; $P < .0005$
sHLA II			
8. Control sHLA-II*	55	0.262 (0.017)	8 vs. 9: $U = 326$; $P = .003$
9. Patient pretreatment sHLA-II*	21	0.259 (0.075)	9 vs. 10: $W = 4.02$; $P < .0005$
10. Patient posttreatment sHLA-II*	21	0.148 (0.044)	
11. Patient pretreatment sHLA-II (P)	9	0.261 (0.1)	11 vs. 12: $t = 2.24$; df = 8; $P = .04$
12. Patient posttreatment sHLA-II (P)	9	0.179 (0.09)	
13. Patient pretreatment sHLA-II (M)	12	0.258 (0.112)	13 vs. 14: $W = 3.01$; $P = .002$
14. Patient posttreatment sHLA-II (M)*	12	0.126 (0.044)	8 vs. 13: U = 170; $P = 0.006$

NOTE: P, contrast enhanced; M, no contrast enhancement; *t*, *t* value; *U*, Mann-Whitney U; *W*, Wilcoxon signed ranks; *not normally distributed.

Pretreatment sHLA-I and sHLA-II Levels

Pretreatment serum sHLA-I was significantly lower in patients than in controls ($P < .0005$) and a significant decrease was maintained when patients were divided into the two subgroups, one (9 patients) initially having enhancing MRI lesions (P) and the other (12 patients) not having enhancing MRI lesions (M). Moreover, serum sHLA-I was not significantly different between these two subgroups. Serum sHLA-II in the pretreatment patient group as a whole was significantly lower than in normal controls ($P = .003$), although when divided into the two subgroups (defined above), sHLA-II was significantly lower than in controls only in the nonenhancing patient subgroup (M) ($P = .006$). This suggests a relative sHLA-II increase at the time of an objectively verified exacerbation. However, sHLA-II concentrations were not significantly different between these MRI-defined patient subgroups, a significant variation demonstrated only in relation to controls.

Posttreatment sHLA-I and sHLA-II Levels

After six weeks of high-dose IFN-β1a treatment, mean serum sHLA-I increased significantly ($P < .0005$; TABLE 1 and FIG. 1) for the entire patient group as well as both MRI-defined subgroups (enhancing, $P = .016$; nonenhancing, $P = .009$). There was no significant difference between the two subgroups in terms of degree of sHLA-I concentration change over the six weeks of treatment.

The patient group as a whole had a significant decrease in sHLA-II after treatment with IFN-β1a ($P < .0005$; TABLE 1 and FIG. 2), and this decrease retained significance when the subjects were divided into the P and M subgroups (TABLE 1). First-order effects between subjects, across groups with respect to the degree of

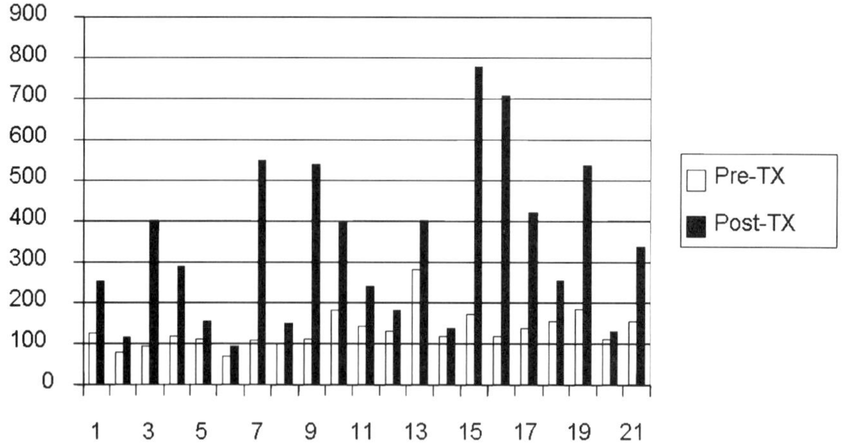

FIGURE 1. Comparison of patient serum concentrations of sHLA-I (ng/mL) pre- and six weeks posttreatment with high-dose interferon-β1a shows a significant increase. Enhancing MRI lesions at study entry were present in patients 1 to 9.

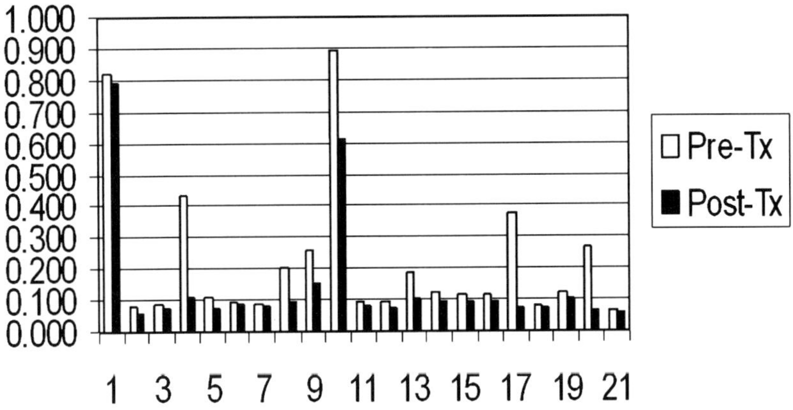

FIGURE 2. A comparison of patient serum concentrations of sHLA-II (units/mL) pre- and six weeks posttreatment with high-dose interferon-β1a demonstrated a significant decrease. Enhancing MRI lesions at study entry were present in patients 1 to 9.

patient sHLA-II decrease pre- to posttreatment between enhancing and nonenhancing subgroups, could not be performed because only levels in one subgroup distributed normally.

DISCUSSION

The purpose of this preliminary study was to evaluate the acute effects of high-dose IFN-β1a therapy on serum levels of sHLA-I and sHLA-II, and further evaluate the possibility of using these molecules in combination as markers of RRMS disease activity. sHLA-I levels in the entire patient group at baseline were found to be lower than in controls, and this reduction was significant in both subgroups, that is, those without and with MRI contrast–enhancing lesions, the latter representing an objective verification of RRMS relapse. After six weeks of IFN-β1a treatment, serum sHLA-I was significantly increased in the entire patient group and both subgroups. Our results with high-dose IFN-β1a mirror the findings of Fainardi *et al.*, who reported that IFN-β1b therapy also produces an early elevation of serum sHLA-I in RRMS.[18] Of particular note, these authors reported that those patients with a better clinical response to IFN-β1b had a higher serum sHLA-I at all sampling times over the 18 months of the study.

On the basis of the above observations, sHLA-I may exert an immunosuppressive effect in RRMS and accomplish this immunomodulation through multiple mechanisms. sHLA-I has been shown to induce antibody production in both allogeneic and xenogeneic combinations, to inhibit the activity of alloreactive cytotoxic T lymphocytes (CTLs), and to induce apoptosis in alloreactive and virus-specific CTLs as well as activated autologous and allogeneic CD8$^+$ T cells and CD8$^+$ NK cells.[22–25] The apoptotic effect of sHLA-I on CTLs is mediated by sHLA-TCR engagement.[26] The apparent mechanism for serum sHLA-I elevation induced by IFN-β1a is reported to be upregulation of MHC class I gene expression.[27,28]

Conversely, decreased sHLA-I during untreated relapses may allow proinflammatory Th1 cell proliferation and/or immune activation; and pathologically, acute MS lesions demonstrate decreased endothelial cell sHLA-I.[29] The degree of a patient's relapse/immune reactivity (i.e., using enhanced vs. nonenhanced MRI) had no impact upon the magnitude of posttreatment sHLA-I increase, implying that the effect was primarily IFN-β1a dependent. Additionally, there was no difference between the sHLA-I levels at exacerbation baseline of these two subgroups suggesting that sHLA-I levels cannot be considered specifically reflective of the degree of RRMS immunoreactivity, or perhaps MRI enhancement does not actually mirror efficiently the acute lesion load relapse severity.

Prior to exacerbation treatment, sHLA-II was found to be significantly decreased in the entire patient group compared with controls. But on further analysis, sHLA-II levels were relatively elevated in those patients with enhancing MRI lesions, that is, this group did not demonstrate a significant decrease versus controls, whereas the nonenhancing group did. This result corresponds to previous findings of elevated sHLA-II during relapse. Thus, an elevation of sHLA-II combined with an associated reduction in sHLA-I, when compared with the particular patient's remission levels, may have potential as a qualitative marker of RRMS relapse, as well as a quantitative marker for severity of relapse.

IFN-β1a treatment was associated with a decrease in sHLA-II across all patient groups, and this change may also be immunologically mechanistic. Class II HLA molecules appear to perform a crucial role in the pathogenesis of MS. HLA-II is not found in normal brain, but during RRMS exacerbations is expressed on approximately 10% of brain endothelial cells, although, interestingly, endothelial HLA-I expression (as discussed above, HLA-I/sHLA-I possibly being anti-inflammatory) is decreased.[29] This expression profile may allow circulating T cells adherence to, and passage through, brain capillary endothelium. Thus, HLA-II endothelial secretion/shedding directly into the circulation may account, at least in part, for serum sHLA-II elevation. Activated macrophages within acute MS brain lesions also express HLA-II, and these cells could also pass into the circulation during the relapse process, shedding/secreting sHLA-II. Therefore, increases in serum sHLA-II may reflect, and/or itself facilitate, the proinflammatory role of HLA-II in the pathogenesis of MS, whereas decreases in serum sHLA-II induced by IFN-β1a therapy may produce and/or mark an immunosuppressive, and, thus, salutory, effect on the course of RRMS. Because both corticosteroids and IFN-β1a appear to block sHLA-II increase during RRMS relapse, and, thus, likely HLA-II endothelial cell expression associated with blood-brain barrier destabilization, this blocking mechanism may explain relapse stabilization clinically, as well as the objective finding of decrease in MRI-enhancing lesion load.

Finally, the fact that sHLA-II levels were not always normally distributed suggests that quantitative expression of these molecules may be HLA allotype dependent, thus, perhaps, partially explaining the MS susceptibility of certain HLA genotypic individuals. Moreover, the variation of sHLA-I and sHLA-II concentrations among patients at the time of RRMS exacerbation (pretreatment, study entry) and the variable extent of change among patients posttreatment may well be, at least in part, HLA allotype dependent.[13]

We believe the positive results of this preliminary investigation of baseline sHLA-I and sHLA-II profiles in RRMS patients in relapse, as well as the short-term effects of IFN-β1a on sHLA-I and sHLA-II levels in these patients, justifies a better-controlled and more-detailed investigation of these phenomena over several years of RRMS treatment. Such a long-term study, which we have initiated, will be required to reliably define the role of soluble HLA molecules as markers of both disease activity and treatment response.

REFERENCES

1. Ivan Rood, J.J., A. van Leeuwen & M.C. van Santen. 1970. Anti HL-A2 inhibitor in normal human serum. Nature **226:** 366–367.
2. Gelder, F.B., J.C. McDonald, M.D. Landreneau, *et al.* 1991. Identification, characterization, and quantitation of soluble HLA antigens in the circulation and peritoneal dialysate of renal patients. Ann. Surg. **213:** 591–599.
3. Jendro, M., J.J. Goronzy & C.M. Weyand. 1991. Structural and functional characterization of HLA-DR molecules circulating in the serum. Autoimmunity **8:** 289–296.
4. Calne, R., R. Sells, J. Pena, *et al.* 1969. Induction of immunological tolerance by porcine liver allografts. Nature **223:** 472–476.
5. Davies, H., S. Pollard & R. Galne. 1989. Soluble HLA antigens in the circulation of liver graft recipients. Transplantation **49:** 659–660.
6. Nicolle, M., B. Nag, S. Sarma, *et al.* 1994. Specific tolerance to an acetylcholine receptor epitope induced in vitro in myasthenia gravis CD4+ lymphocytes by soluble major histocompatibility complex class II-peptide complexes. J. Clin. Invest. **93:** 1361–1369.
7. Ferreira, A., M.L. Villar, J.C. Alvarez-Cermeño, *et al.* 1988. Quantification of soluble serum HLA class I antigens in healthy volunteers and AIDS patients. Clin. Chim. Acta **174:** 207–211.
8. Inostroza, J., P. Munoz, R. Espinoza, *et al.* 1994. Quantitation of soluble HLA class I heterodimers and beta 2-microglobulin in patients with active pulmonary tuberculosis. Hum. Immunol. **40:** 179–182.
9. Adamashvili, I., R. McVie, F. Gelder, *et al.* 1997. Soluble HLA class I antigens in patients with type I diabetes and their family members. Hum. Immunol. **55:** 176–183.
10. Aulitzky, W.E., H. Grosse-Wilde, U. Westhoff, *et al.* 1991. Enhanced serum levels of soluble HLA class I molecules are induced by treatment with recombinant interferon-gamma (IFN-γ). Clin. Exp. Immunol. **86:** 236–239.
11. Noseworthy, J.H., C. Lucchinetti, M Rodriguez & B.G. Weinshenker. 2000. Multiple sclerosis. N. Engl. J. Med. **343:** 938–952.
12. Karandikar, N.J., M.P. Crawford, X. Yan, *et al.* 2002. Glatiramer acetate (Copaxone) therapy induces CD8(+) T cell responses in patients with multiple sclerosis. J. Clin. Invest. **109:** 641–649.
13. Adamashvili, I., P. Fraser & J. McDonald. 1996. Association of serum concentrations of soluble classI HLA with HLA allotypes. Transplantation **61:** 984–987.
14. Alvarez-Cermeño, J.C., L.M. Villar, M. Nocito, *et al.* 1992. Intrathecal synthesis of soluble class I antigens in multiple sclerosis. J. Neuroimmunol. **36:** 77–79.
15. Filaci, G., P. Contini, S. Brenci, *et al.* 1997. Soluble HLA class I and class II molecule levels in serum and cerebrospinal fluid of multiple sclerosis patients. Hum. Immunol. **54:** 54–62.
16. Fainardi, E., E. Granieri, M.R. Tola, *et al.* 2002. Clinical and MRI disease activity in multiple sclerosis are associated with reciprocal fluctuations in serum and cerebrospinal fluid levels of soluble HLA class I molecules. J. Neuroimmunol. **133:** 151–159.
17. Fainardi, E., R. Rizzo, L. Melchiorri, *et al.* 2003. Presence of detectable levels of soluble HLA-G molecules in CSF of relapsing-remitting multiple sclerosis: relationship with CSF soluble HLA-I and IL-10 concentrations and MRI findings. J. Neuroimmunol. **142:** 149–158.

18. FAINARDI, E., R. RIZZO, L. MELCHIORRI, *et al.* 2004. Beneficial effect of interferon-beta 1b treatment in patients with relapsing-remitting multiple sclerosis is associated with an increase in serum levels of soluble HLA-I molecules during the first 3 months of therapy. J. Neuroimmunol. **148:** 206–211.
19. OTT, M., C. SEIDL, U. WESTHOFF, *et al.* 1998. Soluble HLA class I and class II antigens in patients with multiple sclerosis. Tissue Antigens **51:** 301–304.
20. MCDONALD, W.I., A. COMPSTON, G. EDAN, *et al.* 2001. Recommended diagnostic criteria for multiple sclerosis: guidelines from the International Panel on the diagnosis of multiple sclerosis. Ann. Neurol. **50:** 121–127.
21. MCDONALD, J.C., I. ADAMASHVILI, J.M. HAYES, *et al.* 1994. Soluble HLA class II concentrations in normal individuals and transplant recipients: comparison with soluble HLA class I concentrations. Transplantation **58:** 1268–1272.
22. PUPPO, F., P. CONTINI, M. GHIO, *et al.* 2000. Soluble human MHC class I molecules induce soluble Fas ligand secretion and trigger apoptosis in activated CD8(+) Fas (CD95)(+) T lymphocytes. Int. Immunol. **12:** 195–203.
23. PUPPO, F., P. CONTINI, M. GHIO & F. INDIVERI, *et al.* 2002. Soluble HLA class I molecules/CD8 ligation trigger apoptosis of CD8+ cells by Fas/Fas-ligand interaction. Scientific WorldJournal **2:** 421–423.
24. SPAGGIARI, G.M., P. CONTINI, R. CAROSIO, *et al.* 2002. Soluble HLA class I molecules induce natural killer cell apoptosis through the engagement of CD8: evidence for a negative regulation exerted by members of the inhibitory receptor superfamily. Blood **99:** 1706–1714.
25. CONTINI, P., M. GHIO, A. POGGI, *et al.* 2003. Soluble HLA-A, -B, -C and -G molecules induce apoptosis in T and NK CD8+ cells and inhibit cytotoxic T cell activity through CD8 ligation. Eur. J. Immunol. **33:** 125–134.
26. SMITH, M.A., B. NAZIRUDDIN, N.J. POINDEXTER, *et al.* 2000. Liver transplant recipient sera derived soluble HLA mediates allele specific CTL apoptosis. Transplantation **69:** 157–162.
27. KUMAR, R. & L. KORUTLA. 1995. Induction of expression of interferon-stimulated gene factor-3 (ISGF-3) proteins by interferons. Exp. Cell Res. **216:** 143–148.
28. KIMURA, T., Y. KADOKAWA, H. HARADA, *et al.* 1996. Essential and non-redundant roles of p48 (ISGF3 gamma) and IRF-1 in both type I and type II interferon responses, as revealed by gene targeting studies. Genes Cells **1:** 115–124.
29. TRAUGOTT, U. 1987. Multiple sclerosis: relevance of class I and class II MHC-expressing cells to lesion development. J. Neuroimmunol. **16:** 283–302.

Proinflammatory Cytokines and Autoimmunity in Churg-Strauss Syndrome

B. HELLMICH, E. CSERNOK, AND W. L. GROSS

Poliklinik für Rheumatologie, Universitätsklinikum Schleswig-Holstein, Lübeck, Germany

ABSTRACT: **Churg-Strauss syndrome (CSS) belongs to the antineutrophil cytoplasmic antibody (ANCA)–associated vasculitides and is further characterized by severe eosinophilia and, often, granulomatous inflammation. The therapeutic efficacy of recombinant interferon-α (IFN-α) and tumor necrosis factor-α (TNF-α) blockade point toward a central role of cytokines in the pathogenesis of CSS. Recent data show that, in contrast to other primary systemic vasculitides, peripheral blood mononuclear cells (PBMCs) secrete not only large amounts of T helper type 1 (Th1) cytokines, particulary IFN-γ, but also release T helper type 2 (Th2) cytokines such as interleukin-4 (IL-4) and interleukin-13 (IL-13). Interleukin-5 is the most potent stimulator of eosinophil production and functional activation of mature eosinophils, the key effector cells in CSS. Data are presented showing that PBMCs from patients with CSS cultured with T cell–specific stimuli secrete significantly increased amounts of IL-5 compared with healthy controls, suggesting that IL-5 contributes substantially to the development of eosinophilia in CSS. As recombinant IFN-α downregulates IL-5 production of $CD4^+$ T cells *in vitro*, the increased secretion of IL-5 in patients with CSS may provide the clue for the therapeutic efficacy of recombinant IFN-α in the disease. Variations in the balance between Th1 and Th2 cytokines at different disease stages could contribute to the distinct clinical courses seen in patients with CSS, which can range from prominent Th1-mediated generalized vasculitis and granulomatous inflammation on one end of the spectrum to Th2-mediated systemic hypereosinophilia on the other. Although the association of ANCAs with CSS point toward an autoimmune origin of the disease, there is no direct evidence as yet for a direct pathogenic role of ANCAs in CSS.**

KEYWORDS: **Churg-Strauss syndrome; eosinophils; interleukin-5; cytokines**

INTRODUCTION

Churg-Strauss syndrome (CSS) is a rare necrotizing systemic vasculitis of small and medium-sized vessels. Two cardinal features distinguish CSS from other forms of primary systemic vasculitis: First, CSS is defined by blood eosinophilia of usually >10% and eosinophilic infiltration into affected tissues.[1–4] Second, with rare exceptions CSS occurs only in patients with bronchial asthma.[1–4] The idiopathic hyper-

Address for correspondence: Priv.-Doz. Dr. med. Bernhard Hellmich, Poliklinik für Rheumatologie, Universitätsklinikum Schleswig-Holstein, Campus Lübeck, Ratzeburger Allee 160, 23538 Lübeck, Germany.

gross@rheuma-zentrum.de

Ann. N.Y. Acad. Sci. 1051: 121–131 (2005).
doi: 10.1196/annals.1361.053

eosinophilic syndrome (HES) is another systemic disease associated with severe tissue and blood eosinophilia.[5] The etiopathogenesis of HES ("syndrome") varies broadly (see below); one variant may be the second phase of CSS, which usually starts with allergic manifestations in the upper (polyposis) and lower (asthma) respiratory tract.[6]

In contrast to CSS, asthma and vasculitis are *not* typical for idiopathic HES. However, besides eosinophilia, HES and CSS share many common clinical features, such as neuropathy, dyspnea, fatigue, fever, and skin rashes.[5] Furthermore, in both CSS and HES eosinophilic granulocytes are regarded as the primary effector cells.[5,7–9] This, along with the clinical similarities, may suggest a common etiology and pathogenesis for both entities, and raises the question whether CSS is simply the third disease stage of an HES in patients with asthma. On the other hand, the fact that two clinically distinctive features, asthma and systemic vasculitis, are always present in CSS, but are missing in HES could argue against a common etiology for both diseases. However, there are relapses of CSS restricted to other organs than the lung, that is, there are relapses without asthma.

The current literature regarding the etiology, epidemiology, and pathogenesis of CSS has been reviewed recently.[9] Therefore, this review will focus on the role of cytokines and immunoregulatory mechanisms operative in CSS. Data summarized in this review indicate that mechanisms stimulating eosinophilia as well as autoimmunity are involved in the pathogenesis of CSS, depending on the stage of the disease. Novel data are presented supporting a central role of interleukin-5 (IL-5) and other T helper type 2 (Th2) cytokines for the pathogenesis of CSS.

THREE CLINICALLY DISTINCT DISEASE STAGES CHARACTERIZE THE DEVELOPMENT OF CSS

In the majority of patients, disease progresses from bronchial asthma to full-blown CSS in three consecutive stages. The first stage is characterized by a severe, difficult-to-treat asthma, which is frequently accompanied by sinusitis.[2] Significant blood eosinophilia, an unusual finding in uncomplicated asthma,[10] may also be present at this early stage of disease. In the second disease stage, blood eosinophilia progresses and eosinophilic infiltration of tissues develops. Clinically, this stage is characterized by symptoms and findings related to tissue eosinophilia, such as pulmonary infiltrates.[11] Thus, the clinical picture at this disease stage is very similar to HES or other eosinophilic disorders, such as eosinophilic gastroenteritis or eosinophilic pneumonia. At this time, the presence of severe asthma may be the only indicator of CSS, which often renders differential diagnosis difficult in clinical practice. Vasculitis is still absent at this stage. According to current definitions, the term CSS may only be used in patients with vasculitis.[1–4] Thus, there is no general consensus for classifying patients with this nonvasculitic second stage of CSS. The third phase of disease is defined by the onset of systemic vasculitis and, sometimes, granulomatous disease, and usually develops several years after the onset of asthma.[11] As some manifestations of vasculitis—such as neuropathy—may be found in either CSS or HES, biopsies from sites of suspected vasculitis usually are necessary to confirm the diagnosis. Besides asthma and blood eosinophilia, the most common clinical manifestations at this stage are fleeting pulmonary infiltrates, peripheral neuropathy, purpura, and gastrointestinal and cardiac involvement.[1,2,9,12–14]

The point at which disease progresses from one stage to another varies considerably. In patients treated with systemic glucocorticoids for severe asthma, rapid tapering of the glucocorticoid dosage can result in rapid progression to systemic eosinophilia and vasculitis. Such latent cases of CSS that have been unmasked by reduction of systemic glucocorticoids have been termed *formes frustes* of CSS.[15] A similar mechanism has been proposed to explain the increased incidence of CSS in patients treated with leukotriene receptor antagonists (LRAs).[11,16,17] Improvement of asthmatic symptoms by treatment with LRAs often allows rapid reduction of systemic glucocorticoids, leading to unmasking of the underlying hypereosinophilic and vasculitic disease, as LRAs have no significant immunosuppressive properties.

ETIOLOGY AND PATHOGENESIS OF EARLY DISEASE STAGES OF CSS ARE UNKNOWN

In view of the above-mentioned differences in clinical presentations, it is rather likely that the three clinical stages of CSS are immunologically distinct. The first logical step in approaching the pathogenesis of CSS is to identify mechanisms that promote the development of esoinophilia (stage two) in patients with severe asthma (stage one). This, however, is a difficult task. To date, no valid prognostic factors have been identified that predict the development of CSS in patients with severe asthma. It seems, therefore, impossible to identify patients with CSS at their earliest disease stage. Given the low incidence of 1 to 3.4 new cases per 1 million inhabitants per year[18,19] and the absence of prognostic factors, it seems impossible to carry out systematic studies on the pathogenesis of early stages of CSS. In view of the above-mentioned difficulties in identifying patients at early disease stages, all published studies are based on patients with fully developed disease including both eosinophilia and vasculitis.

HES: A SYNDROME WITH PATHOGENETICALLY DISTINCT ENTITIES

As blood and tissue eosinophilia almost always precede the development of vasculitis, it seems crucial to understand the mechanisms leading to eosinophilia in CSS. Given the overlap of many clinical features in CSS and HES, similar pathogenetic mechanisms are not unlikely. In HES, several pathogenetically distinct variants with similar clinical presentations have been identified. One subtype of HES is suggestive of a myeloproliferative disease. In a recent study of 16 patients with HES, nine had an interstitial deletion on chromosome 4q12 resulting in the production of an abnormal constitutively activated tyrosine kinase (FIP1L1-PDGFRα).[7,20] These patients often are unresponsive to glucocorticoids, but frequently respond to imatinib mesilate, a tyrosine kinase inhibitor.[20] Whether chromosomal aberrations leading to constitutively activated tyrosine kinases represent a pathogenetic mechanism in CSS is unknown. The fact that progression of HES patients with such myeloproliferative variants of HES to CSS has not been reported argues against a central role of such mutations for the development of CSS. In addition, in a small number of patients studied we could not yet find an interstitial deletion on chromosome 4q12, and one patient receiving imatinib for treatment of CSS did not respond. Although clonal abnormalities in the eosinophils have been documented in some patients with HES,[5] such clonal expansion of eosinophils has not been reported in CSS.

A third subset of HES patients is characterized by the expansion of abnormal lymphocyte populations. Immunophenotyping demonstrated that these represent either double-negative immature T cells ($CD3^{+}CD4^{-}CD8^{-}$) or $CD3^{-}CD4^{+}$ cells.[21] In patients with T cell–mediated forms of HES, increased production of IL-5,[22] and in some cases also IL-4 and IL-13, has been documented,[7,21] suggesting that these T cells have a Th2 cytokine profile. There are presumably other subsets of HES, including the one that will ultimately transform into CSS.

INCREASED PRODUCTION OF IL-5, THE MOST POTENT STIMULATOR OF EOSINOPHILS, IN CSS

In view of the above-mentioned data in HES and many *in vitro* and *in vivo* data suggesting a key role of IL-5 for eosinophil production and activation, we performed a series of studies to elucidate the role of IL-5 in CSS. Previously reported results from these studies and recent novel data from our laboratory presented here indicate that IL-5 and other Th2 cytokines may in fact play an important role in the pathogenesis of CSS.

In an *in vitro* study, we analyzed the production of IL-5 and other cytokines in peripheral blood mononuclear cells (PBMCs) obtained from 15 patients with CSS and 14 healthy controls before and after stimulation with T cell–specific stimuli (anti-CD3 and anti-CD28) using cytometric bead arrays (CRA). Preliminary results from this study (B. Hellmich *et al.*, manuscript in preparation) are displayed in FIGURE 1

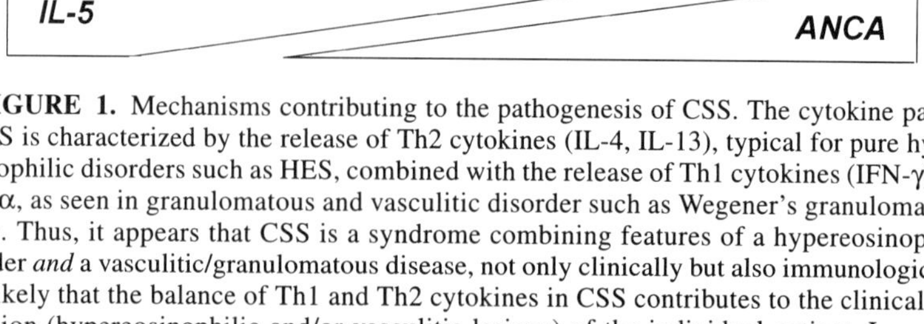

FIGURE 1. Mechanisms contributing to the pathogenesis of CSS. The cytokine pattern in CSS is characterized by the release of Th2 cytokines (IL-4, IL-13), typical for pure hypereosinophilic disorders such as HES, combined with the release of Th1 cytokines (IFN-γ) and TNF-α, as seen in granulomatous and vasculitic disorder such as Wegener's granulomatosis (WG). Thus, it appears that CSS is a syndrome combining features of a hypereosinophilic disorder *and* a vasculitic/granulomatous disease, not only clinically but also immunologically. It is likely that the balance of Th1 and Th2 cytokines in CSS contributes to the clinical presentation (hypereosinophilic and/or vasculitic lesions) of the individual patient. Increased release of IL-5 in subsets of patients with HES and CSS is a strong stimulus for eosinophil production and activation. The association with ANCAs in CSS is weaker compared with WG, and the pathogenic role of ANCAs in CSS is unclear at present.

and show that primed PBMCs from patients with CSS release significantly more IL-5 (85.0 pg/mL, interquartile range 48.50–226.3) compared with healthy controls (18.25 pg/mL, interquartile range 14.92–26.75; $P = .001$). However, IL-5 production in PBMCs cultured without T cell–specific stimuli (anti-CD3) and costimulatory signals (anti-CD28) was low in both CSS patients and controls (FIGURE 2), suggesting that PBMCs in CSS require T cell activation to secrete large amounts of IL-5. Cell surface and intracytoplasmatic staining for cytokines by flow cytometry demonstrated that the increased production of IL-5 *in vitro* is restricted to a small subset of activated monocytes (data not shown). In a previous study, we observed that IL-5 is also released by T cell clones obtained from patients with CSS after stimulation with phorbol myristate acetate (PMA) *in vitro*, but the amount of IL-5 released was not statistically different from healthy controls.[23] In another previous study, we analyzed the plasma levels of IL-5 in patients with CSS and other antineutrophil cytoplasmic antibody (ANCA)-associated vasculitides.[24] Although plasma IL-5 in healthy con trols and patients with Wegener's granulomatosis (WG) and microscopic polyangiitis (MPA) were low in both active disease as well as in remission, 30% of patients with CSS, especially those with active disease, had elevated plasma IL-5. In summary, data from the above-mentioned studies suggest that (i) the amount of circulating IL-5 is increased in patients with CSS in active disease; (ii) increased production of IL-5 by PBMCs is a likely source of elevated plasma IL-5 in CSS; and (iii) T cell activation is required for increased IL-5 release by PBMCs in CSS.

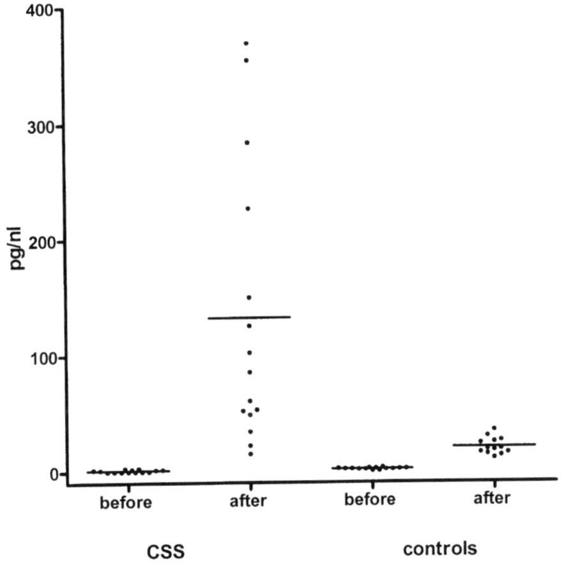

FIGURE 2. Significantly higher production of IL5 (P = .001) by PBMCs of patients with CSS cultured with T cell–specific stimuli compared with PBMCs from healthy controls. The production of IL-5 was analyzed using cytometric bead arrays before and after stimulation with anti-CD3 and anti-CD28-antibodies for 24 h. *Horizontal lines* represent medians.

IL-5 is the most potent cytokine to induce terminal differentiation of committed eosinophil precursors.[25] The fact that IL-5 not only stimulates eosinophil production, but also prolongs the survival of mature eosinophils in culture,[26] possibly via its ability to delay apoptosis,[27] makes IL-5 a likely candidate cytokine for hypereosinophilic disorders such as CSS or HES. In addition, IL-5 activates mature eosinophils and selectively induces degranulation and antibody-dependent cytotoxicity of eosinophils.[28,29]

Of particular interest with regard to the pathogenesis of CSS and vasculitis is the ability of IL-5 to promote the adhesion of eosinophils to vascular endothelium and CC chemokine receptor 3 (CCR3)–dependent migration of eosinophils from the vasculature.[8,30] Thus, the elevated production of IL-5 by PBMCs in CSS may be relevant pathogenetically not only for eosinophilia, but also for the development of vasculitis by promoting transvascular migration and functional activation of eosinophils. The fact that recombinant interferon-α (IFN-α) selectively inhibits the production of IL-5 by human $CD4^+$ T cells *in vitro*[31] may provide an explanation for the efficacy of therapeutic administration of IFN-α to patients with CSS.[32–34]

CSS IS CHARACTERIZED BY AN INCREASED PRODUCTION OF TH1 AND TH2 CYTOKINES

As mentioned above, T cell–mediated variants of HES are characterized by an increased release of Th2 cytokines, in particular IL-4, IL-5, and IL-13.[7] In contrast, T cell lines obtained from patients with CSS not only secrete large amounts of IL-4 and IL-13, but also secrete about 10 times more interferon-γ (IFN-γ) compared with T cell lines from healthy controls.[23] Recent data from our laboratory also show increased release of IFN-γ and IL-4 in PBMCs obtained from patients with CSS compared with healthy controls (B. Hellmich *et al.*, manuscript in preparation). We found that IFN-γ is released by unstimulated PBMCs from patients with CSS, whereas IL-4 release requires T cell activation and costimulatory signals (anti-CD28). Stratification of the T cell lines according to their IFN-γ to IL-4 ratio revealed that the majority of T cells belong to the Th0 type.[23] In contrast, WG is characterized by the predominance of a Th1 cytokine profile characterized by increased production of IFN-γ, but not IL-4.[23,35]

PROINFLAMMATORY CYTOKINES IN CSS: IMPLICATIONS FOR THE THERAPEUTIC EFFICACY OF TNF-α BLOCKADE AND THE DEVELOPMENT OF GRANULOMATOUS INFLAMMATION

Increased activity of other proinflammatory cytokines such as IL-1β and tumor necrosis factor-α (TNF-α) in patients with CSS has been reported.[36,37] Tsukadiara and coworkers documented increased serum TNF-α in 5 of 5 patients with CSS.[36] In a larger cohort of 33 patients with CSS, Grau *et al.* found elevated serum TNF-α in 18 cases.[37] As outlined above, PBMCs in CSS require T cell activation to secrete large amounts of IL-5 and other Th2 cytokines. Thus, elevated serum TNF-α may create the proinflammatory environment required for T cells to become activated and secrete IL-5 and other cytokines. The fact that therapeutic administration of TNF-α–

blocking agents to patients with refractory CSS can induce remission associated with decline of eosinophil counts[38] suggests that the above-mentioned hypothesis of TNF-α–mediated T cell activation resulting in the release of stimulators of eosinophil production and function may be operative *in vivo*.

Although data from autopsy studies suggest that granulomas are not found in every patient with CSS,[1,2,4] granulomatous inflammation is quite typical for the disease. In animal models of infection, neutralization of TNF-α and IFN-γ abrogates granuloma formation, suggesting that both cytokines are essential for granuloma formation and maintenance.[39–42] Therefore, the increased production of both TNF-α and IFN-γ in patients with CSS is likely to be relevant for the development of granulomatous inflammation in CSS. In animal models, blockade of TNF-α and IFN-γ shifts the cytokine pattern toward Th2, which then results in eosinophil infiltration and fibrotic degeneration.[39–42] Thus, variations in the balance between Th1 and Th2 cytokines at different disease stages may provide an explanation for distinct clinical courses in CSS, which may range from prominent Th1-mediated generalized vasculitis and granulomatous inflammation at one end of the spectrum to Th2-mediated systemic hypereosinophilia at the other.

In summary, the cytokine pattern in CSS is characterized by the release of Th2 cytokines, typical for pure hypereosinophilic disorders such as HES, combined with the release of Th1 cytokines, as seen in granulomatous and vasculitic disorder such as WG. Thus, it appears that CSS is a syndrome combining features of a hypereosinophilic disorder and a vasculitic/granulomatous disease not only clinically but also immunologically.

THE ROLE OF T CELLS IN CSS

As outlined above, T cells contribute to the pathogenesis of CSS by secretion of cytokines and chemokines, but need to be functionally activated to accomplish this. We earlier provided indirect evidence that T cells in patients with active CSS are in fact activated *in vivo*, by demonstrating increased levels of soluble interleukin-2 receptor (sIL-2R).[43] Although eosinophils activated by IL-3, IL-5, or GM-CSF *in vitro* express the IL-2R p55 subunit on their cell surface,[44] the majority of sIL2R is generated by activated T cells and, to a lesser degree, by B cells. We found that most of the *in vivo* activated T cells from patients with CSS are $CD4^+$.[23] This contrasts with findings in WG, where the T cell compartment consists mostly of $CD8^+$ cells. Clonal expansion of T cells in CSS has been reported.[23,45] In one series of eight CSS patients such clonal T cell expansion was associated with increased surface expression of CD95 and elevated serum levels of soluble CD95,[45] suggesting that this may delay apoptosis of CD95-positive T cells.

ANCA IN CSS: THE MISSING LINK BETWEEN HYPEREOSINOPHILIA AND AUTOIMMUNITY?

A prototype autoimmune disease is characterized at a minimum by the presence of autoantibodies against a defined and plausible autoantigen, and by proof that these antibodies are present in the vast majority of patients and cause the disease *in vivo*.

Convincing evidence that this definition of an autoimmune disease may be fulfilled in CSS is still lacking. Although antineutrophil cytoplasmic antibodies, most with a perinuclear pattern on indirect immunofluorescence (P-ANCA), are found in many patients with CSS,[12,46,47] the frequency of their detection ranges from 76% in patients with active disease[46] to less than 20% in other cohorts.[47] Myeloperoxidase (MPO), normally contained in the granules of polymorphonuclear neutrophils (PMNs), is the target antigen of P-ANCAs in most CSS patients that tested positive for P-ANCAs.[12,46,47] In a mouse model, anti-MPO-ANCA caused glomerulonephritis and vasculitic lesions, reassembling those found in MPA in humans,[48] suggesting that MPO-P-ANCAs are pathogenetically relevant in MPA.[49] As the pathology of CSS, including not only vasculitis, but also eosinophil-rich granulomatous inflammation, is quite different from that found in MPA, the results of this animal model are not directly transferable to CSS. An animal model for CSS has not yet been described.

If not directly pathogenic, it may be hypothesized that P-ANCAs in CSS may be a response to control the autoantigen. This raises the question, whether the autoantigens of ANCAs themselves may be relevant for the induction of the disease. In fact, preliminary data from our laboratory indicate that proteinase 3, the target antigen of "classic" ANCAs (C-ANCAs) in WG, can induce the activation of dendritic cells via protease activating receptor 2 (PAR-2).[50] It is as yet unknown whether dendritic cells play a role in the pathogenesis of CSS, as they do in animal models of giant cell arteritis.[51] However, activated eosinophils do play a role, as they express major histocompatibility complex II (MHC-II) and can process and present antigen.[8] Thus, eosinophil-like dendritic cells can function as antigen-presenting cells and stimulate T lymphocyte responses.[8] These eosinophil-mediated *in vivo* T cell proliferative responses are antigen-specific, CD80/CD86-dependent, and limited to $CD4^+$ cells.[8,52] Purified eosinophils from IL-5 transgenic mice are able to induce IL-4, IL-5, and IL-13 production in Th2 cells in an antigen-specific manner.[53] As eosinophils are activated in CSS *in vivo*,[36] and T cells in CSS are, in fact, mostly $CD4^+$ and secrete large amounts of IL-4, IL-5, and IL-13,[23] it may be hypothesized that eosinophils acting as antigen-presenting cells may participate in T cell activation in CSS. Further studies are needed to address this issue.

Preliminary data from our laboratory (in cooperation with G. Adamus, Oregon Health and Science University, Portland, OR) indicate that the prevalence of autoantibodies to the glycolytic enzyme α-enolase in patients with CSS is surprisingly high (82% in patients with active disease and 62% in patients in remission). Although α-enolase antibodies are not specific for CSS, their higher prevalence compared with other autoimmune diseases[54,55] warrants further investigation.

REFERENCES

1. Churg, J. & L. Strauss. 1951. Allergic granulomatosis, allergic angiitis, and periarteritis nodosa. Am. J. Pathol. **27:** 272–301.
2. Lanham, J., K. Elkon, C. Pusey & G. Hughes. 1984. Systemic vasculitis with asthma and eosinophilia: a clinical approach to the Churg-Strauss syndrome. Medicine **63:** 65–81.
3. Jennette, J.C., R. Falk, K. Andrassy, *et al.* 1994. Nomenclature of systemic vasculitides: proposal of an international consensus conference. Arthritis Rheum. **37:** 187–192.

4. Masi, A.T., G.G. Hunder, J.T. Lie, *et al.* 1990. The American College of Rheumatology 1990 criteria for the classification of Churg-Strauss syndrome (allergic granulomatosis and angiitis). Arthritis Rheum. **33:** 1094–1100.
5. Lin, D.A. & J.A. Boyce. 2003. The idiopathic hypereosinophilic syndrome. Allergy Asthma Proc. **24:** 417–420.
6. DeRemee, R.A., L.H. Weiland & T.J. McDonald. 1980. Respiratory vasculitis. Mayo Clin. Proc. **55:** 492–498.
7. Gotlib, J., J. Cools, J.M. Malone, 3rd, *et al.* 2004. The FIP1L1-PDGFRalpha fusion tyrosine kinase in hypereosinophilic syndrome and chronic eosinophilic leukemia: implications for diagnosis, classification, and management. Blood **103:** 2879–2891 [Epub: 2003. Nov. 20].
8. Shi, H.Z. 2004. Eosinophils function as antigen-presenting cells. J. Leukoc. Biol. **76:** 520–527 [Epub: 2004. June 24].
9. Hellmich, B., S. Ehlers, E. Csernok & W.L. Gross. 2003. Update on the pathogenesis of Churg-Strauss syndrome. Clin. Exp. Rheumatol. **21**(6)(suppl. 32)**:** S69–S77.
10. Loughlin, J., J. Cole, K. Rothman & E. Johnson. 2002. Prevalence of serious eosinophilia and incidence of Churg-Strauss syndrome in a cohort of asthma patients. Ann. Allergy Asthma Immunol. **88:** 319–325.
11. Lilly, C., A. Churg, M. Lazarovich, *et al.* 2002. Asthma therapies and Churg-Strauss syndrome. J. Allergy Clin. Immunol. **109:** S1–20.
12. Guillevin, L., P. Cohen, M. Gayraud, *et al.* 1999. Churg-Strauss syndrome: clinical study and long-term follow-up of 96 patients. Medicine **78:** 26–37.
13. Chumbley, L., E. Harrison & R. DeRemee. 1977. Allergic granulomatosis and angiitis (Churg-Strauss syndrome): report and analysis of 30 cases. Mayo Clin. Proc. **52:** 477–484.
14. Solans, R., J. Bosch, C. Perez-Bocanegra, *et al.* 2001. Churg-Strauss syndrome: outcome and long-term follow-up of 32 patients. Rheumatology **40:** 763–771.
15. Churg, A., M. Brallas, S. Cronin & J. Churg. 1995. Formes frustes of Churg-Strauss syndrome. Chest **108:** 320–323.
16. Wechsler, M., D. Finn, D. Gunawardena, *et al.* 2000. Churg-Strauss syndrome in patients receiving montelukast as treatment for asthma. Chest **117:** 708–713.
17. Hellmich, B. & W.L. Gross. 2003. Churg-Strauss Syndrom nach Behandlung mit Leukotrienrezeptorantagonisten: Demaskierung durch Steroidreduktion oder Nebenwirkung? Dtsch. Med. Wochenschr. **128:** 1469.
18. Reinhold-Keller, E., K. Herlyn, R. Wagner-Bastmeyer, *et al.* 2002. No difference in the incidences of vasculitides between north and south Germany: first results of the German vasculitis register. Rheumatology **41:** 540–549.
19. Watts, R., S. Lane, G. Bentham & D. Scott. 2000. Epidemiology of systemic vasculitis: a ten-year study in the United Kingdom. Arthritis Rheum. **43:** 414–419.
20. Cools, J., D.J. DeAngelo, J. Gotlib, *et al.* 2003. A tyrosine kinase created by fusion of the PDGFRA and FIP1L1 genes as a therapeutic target of imatinib in idiopathic hypereosinophilic syndrome. N. Engl. J. Med. **348:** 1201–1214.
21. Roufosse, F., L. Schandene, C. Sibille, *et al.* 1999. T-cell receptor-independent activation of clonal Th2 cells associated with chronic hypereosinophilia. Blood **94:** 994–1002.
22. Simon, H.U., S.G. Plotz, R. Dummer & K. Blaser. 1999. Abnormal clones of T cells producing interleukin-5 in idiopathic eosinophilia. N. Engl. J. Med. **341:** 1112–1120.
23. Kiene, M., E. Csernok, A. Mueller, *et al.* 2001. Elevated interleukin-4 and interleukin-13 production by T cell lines from patients with Churg-Strauss syndrome. Arthritis Rheum. **44:** 469–473.
24. Schonermarck, U., E. Csernok, A. Trabandt, *et al.* 2000. Circulating cytokines and soluble CD23, CD26, and CD30 in ANCA-associated vasculitides. Clin. Exp. Rheumatol. **18:** 457–463.
25. Clutterbuck, E.J., E.M. Hirst & C.J. Sanderson. 1989. Human interleukin-5 (IL-5) regulates the production of eosinophils in human bone marrow cultures: comparison and interaction with IL-1, IL-3, IL-6, and GMCSF. Blood **73:** 1504–1512.
26. Yamaguchi, Y., Y. Hayashi, Y. Sugama, *et al.* 1988. Highly purified murine interleukin 5 (IL-5) stimulates eosinophil function and prolongs *in vitro* survival. IL-5 as an eosinophil chemotactic factor. J. Exp. Med. **167:** 1737–1742.

27. Yamaguchi, Y., T. Suda, S. Ohta, *et al.* 1991. Analysis of the survival of mature human eosinophils: interleukin-5 prevents apoptosis in mature human eosinophils. Blood **78:** 2542–2547.
28. Lopez, A.F., C.J. Sanderson, J.R. Gamble, *et al.* 1988. Recombinant human interleukin 5 is a selective activator of human eosinophil function. J. Exp. Med. **167:** 219–224.
29. Fujisawa, T., R. Abu-Ghazaleh, H. Kita, *et al.* 1990. Regulatory effect of cytokines on eosinophil degranulation. J. Immunol. **144:** 642–646.
30. Shahabuddin, S., P. Ponath & R.P. Schleimer. 2000. Migration of eosinophils across endothelial cell monolayers: interactions among IL-5, endothelial-activating cytokines, and C-C chemokines. J. Immunol. **164:** 3847–3854.
31. Schandene, L., G.F. Del Prete, E. Cogan, *et al.* 1996. Recombinant interferon-alpha selectively inhibits the production of interleukin-5 by human $CD4^+$ T cells. J. Clin. Invest. **97:** 309–315.
32. Tatsis, E., A. Schnabel & W. Gross. 1998. Interferon-alpha treatment of four patients with the Churg-Strauss syndrome. Ann. Intern. Med. **129:** 370–374.
33. Termeer, C.C., J.C. Simon & E. Schopf. 2001. Low-dose interferon α-2b for the treatment of Churg-Strauss syndrome with prominent skin involvement. Arch. Dermatol. **137:** 136–138.
34. Hellmich, B. & W.L. Gross. 2004. Recent progress in the pharmacotherapy of Churg-Strauss syndrome. Expert Opin. Pharmacother. **5:** 25–35.
35. Csernok, E., A. Trabandt, A. Muller, *et al.* 1999. Cytokine profiles in Wegener's granulomatosis: predominance of type 1 (Th1) in the granulomatous inflammation. Arthritis Rheum. **42:** 742–750.
36. Tsukadiara, A., Y. Okubo, K. Kitano, *et al.* 1999. Eosinophil active cytokines and surface analysis of eosinophils in Churg-Strauss syndrome. Allergy Asthma Proc. **20:** 39–44.
37. Grau, G., P. Roux-Lombard, C. Gysler, *et al.* 1989. Serum cytokine changes in systemic vasculitis. Immunology **68:** 196–198.
38. Arbach, O., W. Gross & A. Gause. 2002. Treatment of refractory Churg-Strauss-syndrome (CSS) by TNF-alpha blockade. Immunobiology **206:** 496–501.
39. Amiria, P., R. Locksley, T. Parslow, *et al.* 1992. Tumour necrosis factor alpha restores granulomas and induced parasite egg-laying in schistosome-infected SCID mice. Nature **356:** 604–607.
40. Kindler, V., A. Sappino, G. Grau, *et al.* 1989. The inducing role of tumor necrosis factor in the development of bactericidal granulomas during BCG infection. Cell **56:** 731–740.
41. Joseph, A. & D. Boros. 1993. Tumor necrosis factor plays a role in Schistosoma mansoni egg-induced granulomatous inflammation. J. Immunol. **151:** 5461–5471.
42. Smith, D., H. Hansch, E. Bancroft & S. Ehlers. 1997. T-cell-independent granuloma formation in response to Mycobacterium avium: role of tumor necrosis factor-alpha and interferon-gamma. Immunology **92:** 413–421.
43. Schmitt, W., E. Csernok, K. Kobayashi, *et al.* 1998. Churg-Strauss syndrome: serum markers of lymphocyte activation and endothelial damage. Arthritis Rheum. **41:** 445–452.
44. Plumas, J., V. Guart & D. Aldebert. 1991. Human eosinophils from hypereosinophilic patients spontaneously express the p55 but not the p75 interleukin-2 receptor subunit. Eur. J. Immunol. **21:** 1265–1268.
45. Muschen, M., U. Warskulat, A. Perniok, *et al.* 1999. Involvement of soluble CD95 in Churg-Strauss syndrome. Am. J. Pathol. **155:** 915–925.
46. Keogh, K.A. & U. Specks. 2003. Churg-Strauss syndrome: clinical presentation, antineutrophil cytoplasmic antibodies, and leukotriene receptor antagonists. Am. J. Med. **115:** 284–290.
47. Arbach, O., E. Csernok, W. Gross & A. Gause. 2002. Is the Churg-Strauss syndrome an ANCA-associated vasculitis? Clevel. Clin. J. Med. **69:** 173–174.
48. Xiao, H., P. Heeringa, P. Hu, *et al.* 2002. Antineutrophil cytoplasmic autoantibodies specific for myeloperoxidase cause glomerulonephritis and vasculitis in mice. J. Clin. Invest. **110:** 955–963.

49. HELLMICH, B., E. CSERNOK & W. GROSS. 2003. Twenty years with ANCA (antineutrophil cytoplasmic antibodies): from seromarker to major pathogenic player in vasculitis. J. Leukoc. Biol. **74:** 1–2.
50. AI, M., P. JAGIELLO, J.T. EPPLEN, *et al.* 2004. Proteinase 3, Wegener's autoantigen, induces maturation of immunostimulatory dendritic cells via protease-activated receptor-2 [abstract]. Arthritis Rheum. **50** (Suppl.): S229.
51. MA-KRUPA, W., M.S. JEON, S. SPOERL, *et al.* 2004. Activation of arterial wall dendritic cells and breakdown of self-tolerance in giant cell arteritis. J. Exp. Med. **199:** 173–183.
52. SHI, H.Z., A. HUMBLES, C. GERARD, *et al.* 2000. Lymph node trafficking and antigen presentation by endobronchial lymphocytes. J. Clin. Invest. **105:** 945–953.
53. MACKENZIE, J.R., J. MATTES, L.A. DENT & P.S. FOSTER. 2001. Eosinophils promote allergic disease of the lung by regulating CD4(+) Th2 lymphocyte function. J. Immunol. **167:** 3146–3155.
54. LEE, K.H., H.S. CHUNG, H.S. KIM, *et al.* 2003. Human alpha-enolase from endothelial cells as a target antigen of anti-endothelial cell antibody in Behcet's disease. Arthritis Rheum. **48:** 2025–2035.
55. SAULOT, V., O. VITTECOQ, R. CHARLIONET, *et al.* 2002. Presence of autoantibodies to the glycolytic enzyme alpha-enolase in sera from patients with early rheumatoid arthritis. Arthritis Rheum. **46:** 1196–1201.

Rheumatic Fever

How *S. pyogenes*–Primed Peripheral T Cells Trigger Heart Valve Lesions

L. GUILHERME,[a,b] K. C. FAÉ,[a,b] S. E. OSHIRO,[a,b] A. C. TANAKA,[a] P. M. A. POMERANTZEFF,[a] AND J. KALIL[a,b,c]

[a]*Heart Institute (InCor), School of Medicine, University of São Paulo, São Paulo, Brazil*

[b]*Institute for Immunology Investigation, Millennium Institute, São Paulo, Brazil*

[c]*Clinical Immunology and Allergy, Department of Clinical Medicine, University of São Paulo, School of Medicine, São Paulo, Brazil*

ABSTRACT: The pathogenesis of rheumatic fever (RF) is related to autoimmune humoral and cellular responses against human tissues triggered by *Streptococcus pyogenes*. CD4$^+$ T cells are the ultimate effectors of chronic heart lesions in rheumatic heart disease (RHD). Heart-infiltrating CD4$^+$ T cell clones are able to recognize heart tissue and streptococcal antigens by molecular mimicry. The streptococcal M5(81–103) region, an immunodominant region, was recognized by both intralesional and peripheral T cell clones (62% and 38%, respectively). Peripheral T lymphocytes from Brazilian patients with severe RHD preferentially recognized the M5(81–96) peptide, in the context of HLA-DR7$^+$ and DR53$^+$ molecules. HLA-DR7 seems to be related to the development of multiple valvular lesions in RHD patients from different countries. In addition, the fact that peripheral and intralesional T cells recognized the M5(81–103) region points to this region as one of the streptococcal triggers of autoimmune reactions in RHD. T cell repertoire analysis from peripheral and intralesional T cell lines derived from RHD patients showed several oligoclonal expansions of BV families. Major expansions were found in the heart lesions, suggesting that such T cell populations preferentially migrate from the periphery to the heart. Some cross-reactive intralesional T cell clones displayed the same T cell receptor (TCR) BVBJ and CDR3 sequences, showing a degenerate pattern of antigen recognition. Heart tissue–infiltrating cells from myocardium and valvular tissue produced TNF-α, IFN-γ, IL-10, and IL-4, whereas few cells from valvular tissue produced IL-4, showing that the lack of regulation in the valves could be responsible for the permanent and progressive valvular lesions.

KEYWORDS: autoimmune disease; rheumatic fever; M protein; heart tissue proteins; molecular mimicry; T lymphocytes; T cell receptor; cytokines

Address for correspondence: Luiza Guilherme, Laboratório de Imunologia, Instituto do Coração (HC-FMUSP), Av. Dr. Eneas de Carvalho Aguiar, 44 – 9 andar., 05403-000 São Paulo, SP, Brazil. Voice: +55-11-3069-5901; fax: +55-11-3069-5953.
luizagui@usp.br

**Ann. N.Y. Acad. Sci. 1051: 132–140 (2005). © 2005 New York Academy of Sciences.
doi: 10.1196/annals.1361.054**

INTRODUCTION

The pathogenesis of rheumatic fever (RF) in susceptible individuals is related to autoimmune humoral and cellular responses directed towards human tissues, triggered by the response to *Streptococcus pyogenes.* Arthritis is one of the earliest and most common features of the disease, present in 60% to 80% of patients. It usually affects the peripheral large joints; knees, ankles, elbows, and wrists are most frequently affected. Small joints and the axial skeleton are rarely involved. The arthritis is usually migratory and very painful. Carditis, the most serious manifestation of the disease, affects 30% to 45% of RF patients and causes heart damage mainly in the valves, leading to rheumatic heart disease (RHD).

The *S. pyogenes* or group A streptococcus cell wall is composed primarily of carbohydrates such as *N*-acetyl β D-glucosamine, linked to a polymeric rhamnose backbone. Group A streptococci contain M, T, and R surface proteins and lipoteichoic acid (LTA), which are involved in bacterial adherence to pharyngeal epithelial cells. The M protein, which extends from the cell wall, is composed of two polypeptide chains with approximately 450 amino acid residues, in an alpha-helical coiled-coil conformation. The amino-terminal (N-terminal) portion presents antigenic variations—the first 11 amino acid residues define the different serotypes of the bacteria, of which 120 have been identified to date. The carboxy-terminal (C-terminal) half is conserved, and contains multiple repeat regions.[1] The M protein is the most important antigenic structure of the bacterium and shares structural homology with alpha-helical coiled-coil human proteins such as cardiac myosin, tropomyosin, keratin, laminin, vimentin (reviewed by Cunningham[2]), and several valvular proteins.[3]

The molecular mimicry mechanism is responsible for the cross-reactions between streptococcal antigens and human proteins, especially heart tissue proteins, in susceptible individuals. Humoral and cellular immune responses are involved in the development of RF autoimmune reactions, and it is now known that RHD lesions are mediated mainly by T cells.

GENETIC MARKERS

Genetic predisposition is one of the leading factors contributing to the development of autoimmunity in RF/RHD. Several HLA class II alleles have been associated with the development of disease in different countries.[4] HLA-DR7 is the allele most consistently associated with the disease. The association of HLA-DR7 with different DQ-B or DQ-A alleles seems to be associated with the development of multiple valvular lesions (MVL) or of mitral valve regurgitation (MVR) in RHD patients.[5,6]

PATHOGENIC MECHANISMS

T Cell Infiltration

RF/RHD is the most convincing example of postinfectious autoimmune disease mediated by a molecular mimicry mechanism in humans. As mentioned before, the disease is mediated by humoral and cellular immune responses. Although the humoral responses were described more than 50 years ago, their role in the development of RHD has not been completely understood. Recently, it was demonstrated that antibodies cross-reactive to M protein and heart tissue were able to bind to the endothelium, leading to inflammation, cellular infiltration, and valve scarring.[7,8]

The predominance of $CD4^+$ T cells in rheumatic heart lesions was the first evidence of the involvement of $CD4^+$ T cells in RHD lesions.[9,10]

Role of T Cells in Autoimmune Reactions

The functional role of these infiltrating T cells was first described by our group when we demonstrated T cell molecular mimicry as the mediator mechanism for heart tissue lesions in RHD. We have shown that heart-infiltrating T cells from RHD patients were able to recognize streptococcal M protein peptides as well as myocardium and valvular proteins.[3] Our results indicated three M5 regions (residues 1 to 25, 81 to 103, and 163 to 177) that cross-reacted with several heart protein fractions, mainly those derived from valvular tissue, with molecular masses of 95–150, 43, and 30–43 kDa.[3] By analyzing the reactivity of 90 heart tissue–derived T cell clones from several patients we were able to identify the M5(81–103) as an immunodominant region. This region comprises 22 amino acid residues, included in three overlapping peptides, M5(81–96), M5(83–103), and M5(91–103). Our results showed that 62% of M protein–reactive intralesional T cell clones recognized this region (FIG. 1). The same M5 epitopes were also preferentially recognized by peripheral T cell clones, also with a very high frequency (38%) (FIG. 1). These results suggest that peripheral M5-primed T cells preferentially migrate to the heart, and that this region could be one of the streptococcal triggers of autoimmune reactions in RHD. Interestingly, peripheral T lymphocytes preferentially recognized the M5(81–96) epitope in the context of HLA-$DR7^+$ and $DR53^+$ molecules in severe RHD patients.[11] As mentioned above, these two HLA class II alleles were shown to be genetic markers of susceptibility to RF/RHD in several populations, including Brazilian patients.

By employing a proteomics approach to the search for a putative cardiac tissue target autoantigen, we were able to characterize a number of mitral valve proteins, identified by molecular weight (MW) and isoelectric point (pI). Four valve-derived proteins with molecular masses ranging from 79 to 52 kDa and different pIs cross-reacted with the M5 immunodominant peptides and were recognized by intralesional T cell clones from severe RHD patients. Another mitral valve–derived protein, identified as 53 kDa, pI 5.12, showing 86% mass coverage with vimentin, was also recognized by B and peripheral and intralesional T lymphocytes from RHD patients (manuscript in preparation). Human light meromyosin peptides (LMM) were recognized with high frequency (63.2%) by heart-infiltrating T cell clones (manuscript submitted). Several LMM peptides presented cross-reactivity with M5 peptides and mitral valve–derived proteins, suggesting that cross-reactivity may occur first through mimicry and eventually through an epitope-spreading mechanism.[12] A high degree of sequence homology between streptococcal M5 and LMM peptides was observed, which corroborates the hypothesis of molecular mimicry during the autoimmune response.

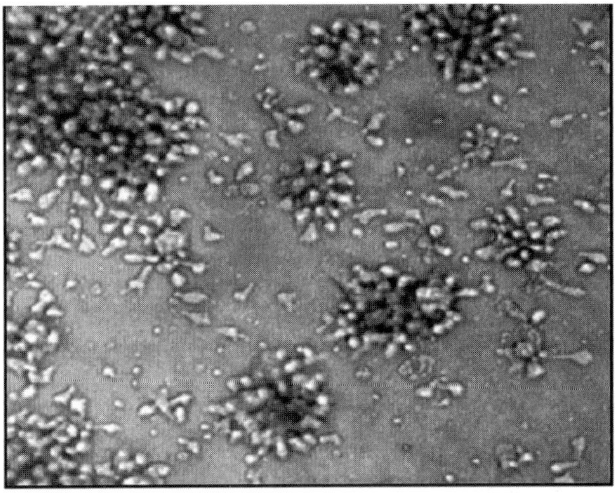

T cell clones	Total of positive T cell clones *	Streptococcal M5 immunodominant region			M5(81-103)⁺ / total ⁺
		M5(81-96)	M5(83-103)	M5(91-103)	
PBMC n = 13	**7** / 13	**2** / 13	**1** / 13	0 / 13	**3** / 7 (38 %)
Intralesional n = 90	**21** / 90	**6** / 90	**9** / 90	**2** / 90	**13** / 21** (62 %)

FIGURE 1. Reactivity of peripheral and heart tissue lesion-infiltrating T cell clones against the immunodominant streptococcal M5(81–103) region. Heart-infiltrating T cells are shown growing *in vitro*. In brief: heart tissue obtained from surgical fragments from RHD patients was minced finely using injection needles and small scissors and placed in flat-bottomed 96-well plates with Dulbecco's modified Eagle's medium supplemented with 2 mM L-glutamine, 10% pooled normal human serum, antibiotics, and 40 U/mL of human recombinant IL-2 on a HLA-DR–matched feeder layer of irradiated peripheral blood mononuclear cells as previously described.[3] (Photograph from Immunology Laboratory, Heart Institute; original magnification: ×200.) The reactivity against streptococcal M5 peptides by intralesional and peripheral T cell clones was measured by a proliferation assay. Positive proliferative responses had a stimulation index (SI) ≥ 2.5. Amino acid sequence of M5(81–103): DKLKQQRDTLSTQKETLEREVQN; M5(81–96), M5(83–103), and M5(91–103) are overlapping peptides.[11] *Reactivity against nine N-terminal streptococcal-M5–derived peptides; **some T cell clones recognized more than one peptide at the same time.

T Cell Repertoire

T cell recognition is mediated by the T cell receptor (TCR), which is composed of two molecules, the alpha and beta chains. The TCR α and β chains are produced by the assembly of variable (V), joining (J), and constant (C) gene segments, as well as of diversity (D) gene segments in the β chain only. Combinations between these genes generate around 1×10^{18} possible TCRs. Both chains have three regions termed complementarity-determining regions (CDR1, CDR2, and CDR3). CDR1 and CDR2 of the TCR interact with MHC molecules. The peptide side chains of the MHC-peptide complex on the surface of antigen-presenting cells (APCs) interact most closely with the CDR3 hypervariable region of the TCR, which is encoded by the V-D-J gene segments on the TCR β chain.

The TCR is one of the components of the trimolecular complex (MHC/peptide/TCR) involved in the activation of cellular immune responses. T cell activation and antigen recognition depend on the T cell repertoire. The 24 BV, 13 BJ, 31 AV, and 61 AJ families described vary in length and amino acid sequence. The analysis of these regions may detect antigen-driven T cell expansions involved in autoimmune responses.

Streptococcal M protein plays an important role in host anti-streptococcal immune responses and, for this reason, a putative superantigenic property was investigated by a number of researchers in the 1990s. Superantigens are proteins that polyclonally activate T cells through an MHC class II–dependent, but haplotype-unrestricted mechanism. Proliferative responses to superantigens are limited to T cells expressing a particular TCR-BV gene but are independent of antigen specificity.

A superantigenic effect of streptococcal M5 protein preparations (pepsin cleaved fragment, pepM5) for normal human T cells expressing TCR-BV2, BV4, and BV8 has been described.[13,14] However, the superantigenic effect was later dismissed by studies showing that the superantigenicity of pepM1 and pepM5 were actually due to contamination with pyrogenic exotoxins, which themselves have a potent superantigen effect on BV2-bearing human T cells.[15,16]

We analyzed the T cell repertoire in peripheral and intralesional T cell lines derived from RHD patients. Our results showed normal frequencies of the 24 BV families, excluding the superantigen effect of M protein. Several BVBJ oligoclonal expansions were observed in both myocardium and mitral valve tissue (TABLE 1A).[17] T cell clones cross-reactive to streptococcal and heart tissue proteins derived from these T cell lines showed some of the major BVBJ expansions detected in the intralesional T cell lines, giving support to the idea that streptococcus-primed T cells migrate from the periphery to the heart. As shown in TABLE 1B, BV13, BV3, BV5, and

TABLE 1A. T cell receptor BV families expressed in peripheral blood and in intralesional T cells

	BV oligoclonal T cell expansions	
Patients	PBMC	Intralesional T cell lines
1	3, **5**, **6**, 7, **8**, **9**, 12, **13**, **14**, **15**, **16**, 18, **21**, 22, **23**	1, 2, 3, 4, **5**, **6**, **8**, **9**, **13**, **14**, **15**, **16**, 17, **21**, **23**
2	**1**, **2**, **3**, 5, **7**, **8**, **16**, **17**, **20**, 22, 23	**1**, **2**, **3**, 4, **7**, **8**, 15, **16**, **17**, **20**, 21
3	**1**, 3, **4**, **5**, **7**, **8**, **13**, **15**, 16, **17**, **21**, 23	**1**, 2, **4**, **5**, 6, **7**, **8**, 9, **13**, 14, **15**, **17**, 18, 20, **21**
4	**7**, **8**, **9**, 12, **13**, **15**, **16**, **18**, **23**	1, 2, 3, 4, 5, 6, **7**, **8**, **9**, 11, **13**, 14, **15**, **16**, 17, **18**, 20, 21, 22, **23**, 24

NOTE: BV families in *bold type* represent oligoclonal T cell expansion shared by both peripheral blood and intralesional T cell repertoire.[17] RNA was extracted from PBMCs and intralesional T cell lines and amplified by RT-PCR using specific BV (22 families) and BJ (13 families) primers and an internal fluorescent BC primer. After running PCR products in a sequencing gel, results were analyzed using the Immunoscope software.[18]

TABLE 1B. TCR-BV BJ segments and CDR3 amino acid sequences from intralesional T cell clones obtained from patients 1 and 4

Patient no.	BV family	CDR3 amino acid sequence	BJ family	No. of cross-reactive T cell clones bearing BV family/total T cell clones analyzed
1	BV3	SFTGRLDNEQF	BJ2S1	2/10
	BV5	SPGSHEQY	BJ2S7	1/10
	BV5	SPGTEAPRTEAF	BJ1S1	1/10
	BV13	SGRQGRYEQY	BJ2S7	5/10
	BV14	STDSTSYEQY	BJ2S7	1/10
4	BV2	TWGSYGYT	BJ1S2	1/2
	BV3	SMVGYEQY	BJ2S7	1/2

NOTE: TCR-BV BJ families identified in the T cell clones from patients 1 and 4 were oligoclonally expanded in both peripheral and intralesional T cell lines. BV-BC PCR products were cloned into a vector and transfected into bacterial cells. Plasmids containing the inserts were purified by alkaline lysis, the DNA was amplified by PCR for BV-BC segments, and both strands were sequenced in an ABI377 automatic sequencer. Products were analyzed using Sequence Navigator software.[19]

BV14 were seen preferentially in the cross-reactive intralesional T cell clones from patient 1. Five cross-reactive T cell clones used the same BV13BJ2S7 and CDR3 sequence to recognize different antigens (data not shown), showing a degenerate pattern of reactivity. They expressed two alpha chains at the RNA level (data not shown) and recognized M5 epitopes or human cardiac beta chain synthetic myosin peptides or mitral valve–derived proteins.[19] In another patient, we found two cross-reactive T cell clones bearing two different BV families (BV2 and BV3) (TABLE 1B).

The fact that the same TCR defined by molecular analysis (BVBJ, AVAJ, and CDR3 sequence) was found in several T cell clones capable of recognizing different antigens suggests an intramolecular degenerate pattern of reactivity against streptococcal and human protein epitopes.

Cytokine Pattern

The evaluation of proinflammatory cytokine (TNF-α, IL-1) and IL-2 levels produced by peripheral blood mononuclear cells from RF/RHD patients without congestive heart failure after streptococcal antigen and pokeweed mitogen stimulation showed increased production of TNF-α, IL-1, and IL-2. Low levels of these cytokines were produced by tonsillar mononuclear cells from the same patients.[20] Increased production of IL-2 during acute rheumatic fever (ARF) and in patients with active RHD has also been reported.[21] These patients also showed high numbers of $CD4^+$ and $CD25^+$ T cells, suggesting an expansion of activated $CD4^+$ T cells in peripheral blood during the active phase of the disease.[21] Other authors have confirmed these findings, also showing increased plasma TNF-α in RF/RHD patients.[22–24]

Recently, we determined the cytokine pattern of heart tissue–infiltrating mononuclear cells from paired myocardium and valvular rheumatic heart lesions. Our

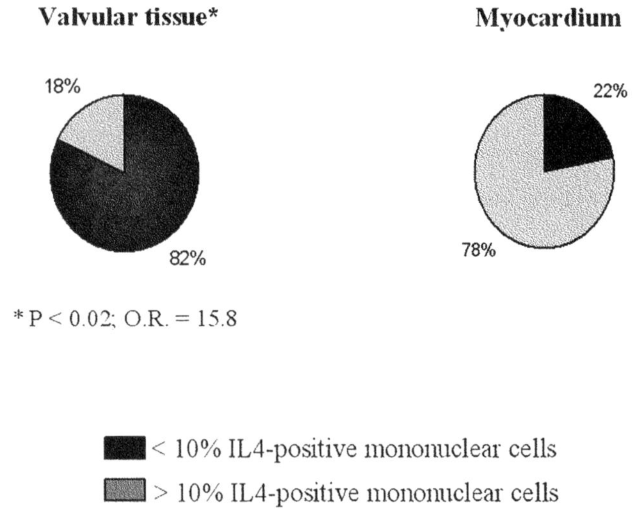

FIGURE 2. IL-4–producing mononuclear cells detected in valvular and myocardial paired tissues from RHD patients. Cytokine production was assessed by immunohistochemistry.[25] Valvular tissue fragments showed few IL-4–producing cells (<10%); myocardial tissue fragments showed several IL-4–producing cells (>10%). *$P < 0.02$, O.R. = 15.8 [number of valvular (82%) and myocardial (22%) tissue fragments with <10% IL-4–producing cells].

results showed a predominance of inflammatory cytokines TNF-α and IFN-γ, and scarce production of regulatory cytokines, such as IL-4, in the valvular tissue. We analyzed 20 heart tissue fragments, of which 11 were from valvular tissue and 9 from myocardial tissue. Eighty-two percent of valvular fragments (mitral and/or aortic valve) showed a low frequency (<10%) of IL-4–producing cells, whereas 78% of myocardial tissue fragments showed cells capable of producing IL-4 ($P < .02$, O.R. = 15.8) (FIG. 2). IL-10, a predominantly regulatory cytokine, was also secreted by a large number of cells in both valvular and myocardial tissue (FIG. 2).[25]

Consistent with the *in situ* results, stimulation of intralesional T cell lines with the immunodominant M5(81–96) peptide showed that most T cell lines were able to produce IFN-γ, suggesting a predominantly inflammatory response to this M5 epitope. IL-4 was not produced by mitral valve–derived T cell lines, and low amounts of IL-10 were produced by infiltrating T cell lines upon specific streptococcal stimulation.[25] Taken together, our data showed a mixed pattern of cytokines, suggesting the co-existence of intralesional inflammatory and regulatory T lymphocytes. However, regulatory cells are probably not efficient in neutralizing the aggressive autoreactive T cells and, consequently, in maintaining immunological self-tolerance.

CONCLUDING REMARKS

These results help us draw a new picture of the pathogenesis of RF/RHD. The role of the humoral immune response in the development of rheumatic heart disease lesions is in fact to trigger endothelial inflammation, leading to subsequent T cell infiltration. CD4$^+$ T cells are the major effectors of heart tissue lesions, and streptococcus-primed T cells are able to recognize heart proteins by molecular mimicry. These T cells show a degenerate pattern of antigen recognition (streptococcal antigens and autoantigens). The lack of IL-4, a regulatory cytokine, in the valvular tissue is involved in the progression and permanence of these lesions. In addition, the lack of IL-4 probably perpetuates and/or exacerbates the production of inflammatory cytokines (TNF-α and IFN-γ).

RF/RHD could be a prototype for the immunological events that may also be involved in other autoimmune diseases. In addition, these data will certainly open new possibilities for immunotherapy.

ACKNOWLEDGMENTS

This work was supported by grants from Fundação de Amparo a Pesquisa do Estado de São Paulo (FAPESP) Nos. 00/3402-2 and 99/035556-0, and by Conselho Nacional de Desenvolvimento Científico e Tecnológico (CNPq) No. 301775/83-4.

The authors declare that they have no competing financial interests.

REFERENCES

1. Fischetti, V. 1991. Streptococcal M protein. Sci. Am. **264:** 32–39.
2. Cunningham, M.W. 2000. Pathogenesis of group A streptococcal infections. Clin. Microbiol. Res. **13:** 470–511.
3. Guilherme, L., E. Cunha-Neto, V. Coelho, *et al.* 1995. Human heart-infiltrating T-cell clones from rheumatic heart disease patients recognized both streptococcal and cardiac proteins. Circulation **92:** 415–420.
4. Guilherme, L & J. Kalil. 2004. Rheumatic fever: how streptococcal throat infection triggers an autoimmune disease. *In* Infection and Autoimmunity. Y. Shoenfeld & N.R. Rose, Eds: 321–330. Elsevier. Amsterdam.
5. Stanevicha, V., J. Eglite, A. Sochevs, *et al.* 2003. HLA class II associations with rheumatic heart disease among clinically homogeneous patients in children in Latvia. Arthritis Res. Ther. **5:** 340–346.
6. Guédez, Y., A. Kotby, M. El-Demellaway, *et al.* 1999. HLA class II associations with rheumatic heart disease are more evident and consistent among clinically homogeneous patients. Circulation **99:** 2784–2790.
7. Galvin, J.E., M.E. Hemric, K. Ward & M.W. Cunningham. 2000. Cytotoxic mAb from rheumatic carditis recognizes heart valves and laminin. J. Clin. Invest. **106:** 217–224.
8. Roberts, S., S. Kosanke, D.S. Terrence, *et al.* 2001. Pathogenic mechanisms in rheumatic carditis: focus on valvular endothelium. J. Infect. Dis. **183:** 507–511.
9. Raizada, V., R.C. Williams, Jr., P. Chopra, *et al.* 1983. Tissue distribution of lymphocytes in rheumatic heart valves as defined by monoclonal anti-T cell antibodies. Am. J. Med. **74:** 90–96.
10. Kemeny, E., T. Grieve, R. Marcus, *et al.* 1989. Identification of mononuclear cells and T cell subsets in rheumatic valvulitis. Clin. Immunol. Immunopathol. **52:** 225–237.
11. Guilherme, L., S.E. Oshiro, K.C. Fae, *et al.* 2001. T-cell reactivity against streptococcal antigens in the periphery mirrors reactivity of heart-infiltrating T lymphocytes in rheumatic heart disease patients. Infect. Immun. **69:** 5345–5351.
12. Lehmann, P.V., T. Forsthuber, A. Miller & E.E. Sercarz. 1992. Spreading of T-cell autoimmunity to cryptic determinants of an autoantigen. Nature **359:** 155–157.
13. Kotb, M., H.S. Courtney, J.B. Dale & E.H. Beachey. 1989. Cellular and biochemical responses of human T lymphocytes stimulated with streptococcal M proteins. J. Immunol. **142:** 966–970.

14. WATANABE-OHNISHI, R., J. AELION, L. LEGROS, *et al.* 1994. Characterization of unique human TCR V beta specificities for a family of streptococcal superantigens represented by rheumatogenic serotypes of M protein. J. Immunol. **152:** 2066–2073.
15. FLEISCHER, B., K.H. SCHMIDT, D. GERLACH & W. KOHLER. 1992. Separation of T-cell-stimulating activity from streptococcal M protein. Infect. Immun. **60:** 1767–1770.
16. DEGNAN, B., J. TAYLOR, C. HAWKES, *et al.* 1997. Streptococcus pyogenes type 5 M protein is an antigen, not a superantigen, for human T cells. Hum. Immunol. **53:** 206–215.
17. GUILHERME, L., N. DULPHY, C. DOUAY, *et al.* 2000. Molecular evidence for antigen-driven immune responses in cardiac lesions of rheumatic heart disease patients. Int. Immunol. **12:** 1063–1074.
18. PANNETIER C., J. EVEN, P. KOURILSKY. 1995. T-cell repertoire diversity and clonal expansions in normal and clinical samples. Immunol. Today **16:** 176–181.
19. FAÉ, K., J. KALIL, A. TOUBERT & L. GUILHERME. 2004. Heart infiltrating T cell clones from a rheumatic heart disease patient display a common TCR usage and a degenerate antigen recognition pattern. Mol. Immunol. **40:** 1129–1135.
20. MILLER, L.C., E.D. GRAY, M. MANSOUR, *et al.* 1989. Cytokines and immunoglobulin in rheumatic heart disease: production by blood and tonsillar mononuclear cells. J. Rheumatol. **16:** 1436–1442.
21. MORRIS, K., C. MOHAN, P.L. WAHI, *et al.* 1993. Enhancement of IL-1, IL-2 production and IL-2 receptor generation in patients with acute rheumatic fever and active rheumatic heart disease; a prospective study. Clin. Exp. Immunol. **91:** 429–436.
22. NARIN, N., N. KÜTÜKÇÜLER, R. ÖZYÜREK, *et al.* 1995. Lymphocyte subsets and plasma IL-1α, IL-2, and TNF-α concentrations in acute rheumatic fever and chronic rheumatic heart disease. Clin. Immunol. Immunopathol. **77:** 172–176.
23. SAMSONOV, M.Y., G.P. TILZ, V.P. PISKLAKOV, *et al.* 1995. Serum-soluble receptors for tumor necrosis factor-α and interleukin-2 and neopterin in acute rheumatic fever. Clin. Immunol. Immunopathol. **74:** 31–34.
24. YEGIN, O., M. COSKUN & H. ERTUG. 1997. Cytokines in acute rheumatic fever. Eur. J. Pediatr. **156:** 25–29.
25. GUILHERME, L., P. CURY, L.M. DEMARCHI, *et al.* 2004. Rheumatic heart disease: pro-inflammatory cytokines play a role in the progression and maintenance of valvular lesions. Am. J. Pathol. **165:** 1583–1591.

Avidity of Anti-β_2-Glycoprotein I and Thrombosis or Pregnancy Loss in Patients with Antiphospholipid Syndrome

S. ČUČNIK, B. BOŽIČ, T. KVEDER, M. TOMŠIČ, AND B. ROZMAN

Department of Rheumatology, Univer sity Medical Center, Ljubljana, Slovenia

ABSTRACT: We aimed to evaluate avidity of anti-β_2-glycoprotein I antibodies (anti-β_2-GPIs) in patients with antiphospholipid syndrome (APS) at the time of acute thrombotic events or pregnancy loss as compared with clinical event–free periods. To do so, 69 sera samples from 16 patients (6 with primary APS and 10 with APS secondary to systemic lupus erythematosus) were selected on the basis of anti-β_2-GPI positivity. Avidity of IgG anti-β_2-GPIs was determined by chaotropic enzyme-linked immunosorbent assay (ELISA), using increased NaCl concentration during antibody binding. High, heterogeneous, and low-avidity anti-β_2-GPIs were measured in APS patients, with no clear pattern regarding the time of thrombotic events or pregnancy failure. In general, anti-β_2-GPI avidity did not change substantially during disease course. We concluded that avidity of anti-β_2-GPIs appears to be a rather stable parameter in an individual APS patient. Considering the previously shown association of high-avidity anti-β_2-GPIs with venous thrombosis, avidity of anti-β_2-GPIs may be a better predictor of predisposition to thrombosis and unsuccessful pregnancy than levels of antiphospholipid antibodies, which may fluctuate over time owing to several factors.

KEYWORDS: anti-β_2-glycoprotein I antibodies (anti-β_2-GPIs); avidity; antiphospholipid syndrome; thrombosis

INTRODUCTION

There is enormous heterogeneity among antibodies against β_2-glycoprotein I (anti-β_2-GPIs), with substantial differences in epitopic specificity and other properties. Avidity of anti-β_2-GPIs may be an important laboratory feature, correlating with thrombotic tendency. Generally, anti-β_2-GPIs are believed to be of low avidity,[1–3] but some authors have reported high-avidity anti-β_2-GPIs as well.[4–7] Recently, we showed an association of high-avidity anti-β_2-GPIs with venous but not with arterial and microvascular thrombosis in patients with antiphospholipid syndrome (APS).[4] However, in pediatric APS we were not able to demonstrate a significant correlation between anti-β_2-GPI avidity and thrombotic events or other relevant clinical manifestations and therapeutic procedures (unpublished observation).

Address for correspondence: Sasa Cucnik, Ph.D., Department of Rheumatology, University Medical Center, Vodnikova 62, SI-1000 Ljubljana, Slovenia. Voice: +386-1-5225479; fax: +386-1-5195338.
sasa.cucnik@guest.arnes.si

**Ann. N.Y. Acad. Sci. 1051: 141–147 (2005). © 2005 New York Academy of Sciences.
doi: 10.1196/annals.1361.055**

The aim of this study was to evaluate the avidity of anti-β_2-GPIs in patients with APS at the time of thrombotic events or miscarriage, and to examine whether anti-β_2-GPI avidity changes during the acute clinical phase as compared with event-free periods.

PATIENTS AND METHODS

Patients

From our serum and data bank we selected sera from anti-β_2-GPI–positive patients with APS whose blood samples were taken within 5 days of (1) diagnosis of a macrothrombotic event, (2) biopsy showing fresh microthrombotic changes, or (3) during the last month of unsuccessful pregnancy (abortion in the first trimester or fetal death according to APS clinical criteria).[8,9] Sixteen patients (6 with primary APS and 10 with APS secondary to systemic lupus erythematosus, SLE) fulfilled the enrollment criteria: 5 patients had arterial thrombosis (3 cerebrovascular insult, 2 upper extremity thrombosis), 4 had venous thrombosis (deep vein thrombosis of leg), 3 had microthromboses detected on kidney biopsy (in 2 cases during fatal catastrophic APS), and 4 suffered from pregnancy loss (2 abortions and 2 fetal deaths). Avidity of anti-β_2-GPIs and levels of anti-β_2-GPIs and anti-cardiolipin antibodies (aCLs) were measured in 69 sera samples obtained from the 16 studied patients during the acute phase and at least twice in event-free periods.

Detection of aCLs

IgG aCLs were determined in sera by standard aCL enzyme-linked immunosorbent assay (ELISA).[10,11] In brief: polystyrene microtiter plates (Medium Binding, Costar, Cambridge, MA) were coated with cardiolipin, blocked with 10% fetal calf serum in phosphate-buffered saline (PBS), and incubated with sera diluted 1:100 in fetal calf serum/PBS. Alkaline phosphatase–conjugated goat anti-human IgG (ACSC, Westbury, NY) and *p*-nitrophenyl phosphate (Sigma, Taufkirchen, Germany) in diethanolamine buffer was used as the detection system.

Detection of Anti-β_2-GPIs

IgG anti-β_2-GPIs were measured by our in-house ELISA,[4,12] evaluated through the European Forum for Antiphospholipid Antibodies.[12] Briefly, polystyrene microtiter plates (High Binding, Costar, Cambridge, MA) were coated with β_2-GPI in PBS and incubated with sera diluted 1:100 in PBS containing 0.05% Tween (PBS-Tween). After four washes, 50 μL/well of alkaline phosphatase–conjugated goat anti-human IgG second antibody in PBS-Tween was added. After 30 min of incubation at room temperature and four washes, 100 μL/well of disodium *p*-nitrophenyl phosphate dissolved at 1 g/L in 1 M diethanolamine buffer (pH 9.8) was added. Following color development, optical density versus a reagent blank was measured at 405 nm by a Rainbow microtiter plate reader (Tecan, Grödig/Salzburg, Austria). The level of anti-β_2-GPIs was derived from a standard curve according to the defined dilutions of monoclonal antibodies.[13]

TABLE 1. Avidity of anti-β_2-GPI in sera samples from 16 patients collected at time of acute thrombotic event or pregnancy loss and during event-free period

	Thrombotic event		Event-free period	
Patient no.	Type	Anti-β_2-GPI avidity	No. of sera samples	Anti-β_2-GPI avidity
1	Microthrombosis	Low	5	Low (4) Heterogeneous (1)
2		High	2	High
3		Low	2	Low
4	Venous thrombosis	Heterogeneous	4	High (1) Heterogeneous (3)
5		Low	2	Low
6		High	2	High
7		Heterogeneous	2	Low (1) Heterogeneous (1)
8	Arterial thrombosis	High	2	Heterogeneous
9		High	4	High (2) Heterogeneous (2)
10		Low	7	Low
11		Heterogeneous	2	Heterogeneous
12		Heterogeneous	3	Low (1) Heterogeneous (2)
13	Unsuccessful pregnancy	Low	3	Low
14		Low	3	Low (2) Heterogeneous (1)
15		Low	3	Heterogeneous
		High	7	High

Avidity Determination of IgG Anti-β_2-GPIs by Chaotropic Assay

Avidity of IgG anti-β_2-GPIs was determined by chaotropic ELISA as described recently.[4] Basically, the same procedure was used as in the anti-β_2-GPI ELISA by applying chaotropic conditions during antibody binding. Samples were diluted in PBS-Tween containing increasing concentrations of NaCl: 0.15, 0.25, 0.5, 1, and 2 M. Discrimination between anti-β_2-GPIs with high or low avidity was made arbitrarily, comparing the initial binding at 0.15 M NaCl with binding at 0.5 M NaCl. High-avidity anti-β_2-GPIs were considered to be present when binding at 0.5 M NaCl remained higher than 70% of initial binding. Low-avidity anti-β_2-GPIs were considered to be present when binding at 0.5 M NaCl decreased to or below 25% of initial binding. Samples which did not fulfill either of the above criteria were considered to be of heterogeneous avidity.[4]

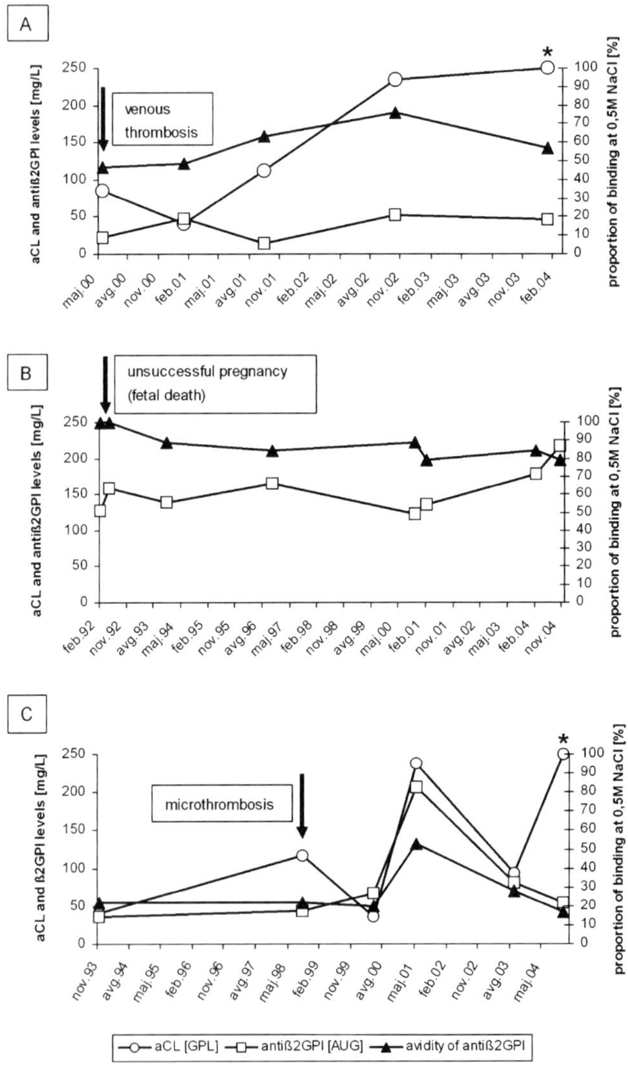

FIGURE 1. Dynamics of aCL and anti-β_2-GPI levels and avidity of anti-β_2-GPIs in patient follow-up. Anti-cardiolipin antibody: 1 mg/L aCL corresponds to 1 GPL unit;[22] example B: dynamics of aCL levels not shown because all values exceeded the measurement range of spectrophotometer; *values exceeded measurement range of spectrophotometer. Anti-β_2-GPI: 1 mg/L corresponds to activity of chimerical IgG monoclonal antibody (HCAL) in concentration of 1 mg/L.[13]

RESULTS

The presence of high, heterogeneous, and low-avidity anti-β_2-GPIs was detected in the APS patients, with no clear pattern regarding acute thrombotic events or pregnancy loss and event-free periods (TABLE 1).

Levels of aCLs and anti-β_2-GPIs, and anti-β_2-GPI avidity were monitored in all patients; three such cases are shown in FIGURE 1.

In the primary APS patient (FIG. 1A) a rather stable avidity of anti-β_2-GPIs (mostly heterogeneous) was demonstrated following iliofemoral thrombosis, for which he was first seen by us.

FIGURE 1B demonstrates the follow-up of an SLE patient with secondary APS, harboring persistent high-avidity anti-β_2-GPIs over a long disease course, regardless of several clinical remissions.

In another patient with APS secondary to SLE, the presence of low-avidity anti-β_2-GPIs at the time of fresh microthrombotic changes seen in a kidney biopsy specimen (along with old microthromboses) was followed by the presence of heterogeneous-avidity anti-β_2-GPIs, in parallel with higher anti-β_2-GPI levels, during the remission of SLE, with no clinical evidence of new thrombotic events or deterioration of renal function (FIG. 1C).

It should be noted that except in the patient in FIGURE 1C, showing clear parallelism of anti-β_2-GPI level and avidity, these two parameters generally behaved differently.

DISCUSSION

Anti-β_2-GPIs have generally been considered to be of low avidity, requiring bivalent binding to the antigen.[1–3] Recently, we showed an association of high-avidity anti-β_2-GPIs with venous but not with arterial or microvascular thrombosis, and with pregnancy complications in anti-β_2-GPI–positive APS patients, regardless of the time of the clinical event.[4] Our research was extended to a retrospective follow-up study of a group of APS patients with sera taken within 5 days of a thrombotic event or during the last month of unsuccessful pregnancy. In measuring anti-β_2-GPI avidity in individual patients before and after index events, we found that acute thromboses and miscarriages were not associated with substantial changes in anti-β_2-GPI avidity. Also, in classifying patients according to the type of thrombotic event (venous, arterial, microvascular) or unsuccessful pregnancy, we could not show any correlation between anti-β_2-GPI avidity and disease course.

Anti-cardiolipin antibodies may fluctuate during the time of a thrombotic event[14,15] or because of a number of other reasons. Anti-β_2-GPI level is known to be more strongly associated with thrombotic events than is aCL level.[16–18] However, Gomez-Pacheco *et al.* also observed a significant decrease in serum anti-β_2-GPI levels at the time of thrombosis as compared with serum levels before and after thrombosis.[19]

An interesting observation of this work is that anti-β_2-GPI avidity is a rather stable parameter in an individual patient. This suggests that avidity of anti-β_2-GPIs at a given point is a more reliable laboratory feature than antiphospholipid antibody level for assessing long-term thrombotic risk. There are several possible explanations for stability or minimal fluctuation in anti-β_2-GPI avidity in patients with APS. Persistence of an antigen has been suggested to be essential for long-term survival of memory B cells, and much clearer picture of affinity maturation in the course of long-lasting disease would be expected. After continuous stimulation of autoreactive B and T lymphocytes, antibody avidity would increase due to consequential somatic mutations. On the other hand, avidity would decrease after immunosuppressive therapy or immunodepletion, as a result of suppression/elimination of plasma cells and high-avidity antibodies. Thrombotic events with antibody consumption would add additional pressure to affinity maturation. Such situations were not very obvious in this study. Manz *et al.* reported long-lived plasma cell survival independent of an antigen in BALB/c mice after secondary immunization with ovalbumin.[20] Hoyer *et al.* recently showed that long-lived plasma cells, including autoreactive plasma cells, resistant to cyclophosphamide, constitute a major population in the spleen of NZB/W mice.[21] We speculate that overall avidity in the studied patients reflects cumulative binding of antibodies from short-lived plasma cells, with higher fluctuation in avidity, and long-lived plasma cells, with more stable antibody avidity.

In conclusion, the results of this study support our proposal that avidity of anti-β_2-GPIs is an important and stable laboratory parameter. Avidity of anti-β_2-GPIs should be taken into consideration when evaluating immune status in a patient with anitphospholipid syndrome.

ACKNOWLEDGMENTS

This work was supported in part by the Ministry of Higher Education, Science, and Technology of the Republic of Slovenia: Research Grant P3-314.

We express special thanks to Professor Takao Koike (Hokkaido University School of Medicine, Sapporo, Japan) for kindly providing HCAL monoclonal antibody.

REFERENCES

1. TINCANI, A., L. SPATOLA, E. PRATI, *et al.* 1996. The anti-beta2-glycoprotein I activity in human anti-phospholipid syndrome sera is due to monoreactive low-affinity autoantibodies directed to epitopes located on native beta2-glycoprotein I and preserved during species' evolution. J. Immunol. **157:** 5732–5788.
2. SHENG, Y., D.A. KANDIAH & S.A. KRILIS. 1998. Anti-beta 2-glycoprotein I autoantibodies from patients with the "antiphospholipid" syndrome bind to beta 2-glycoprotein I with low affinity: dimerization of beta 2-glycoprotein I induces a significant increase in anti-beta 2-glycoprotein I antibody affinity. J. Immunol. **161:** 2038–2043.
3. REGNAULT, V., E. DE MAISTRE, D. WAHL & T. LECOMPTE. 2000. Monovalent binding of autoantibodies to beta2-glycoprotein I, detected using surface plasmon resonance at low antigen density. Br. J. Haematol. **109:** 187–194.
4. CUCNIK, S., T. KVEDER, I. KRIZAJ, *et al.* 2004. High avidity anti-β2-glycoprotein I antibodies in patients with antiphospholipid syndrome. Ann. Rheum. Dis. **63:** 1478–1482.
5. ARVIEUX, J., Y. RENAUDINEAU, I. MANE, *et* al. 2002. Distinguishing features of anti-β2 glycoprotein I antibodies between patients with leprosy and the antiphospholipid syndrome. Thromb. Haemost. **87:** 599–605.
6. VLACHOYIANNOPOULOS, P.G., C. PETROVAS, M. TEKTONIDOU, *et al.* 1998. Antibodies to beta 2-glycoprotein-I: urea resistance, binding specificity, and association with thrombosis. J. Clin. Immunol. **18:** 380–391.

7. BLANK, M., A. WAISMAN, E. MOZES, *et al.* 1999. Characteristics and pathogenic role of anti-β2-glycoprotein I single-chain Fv domains: induction of experimental antiphospholipid syndrome. Int. Immunol. **11:** 1917–1926.
8. HOCHBERG, M.C. 1997. Updating the American College of Rheumatology revised criteria for the classification of systemic lupus erythematosus. Arthritis Rheum. **40:** 1725.
9. WILSON, W.A., A.E. GHARAVI, T. KOIKE, *et al.* 1999. International consensus statement on preliminary classification criteria for definite antiphospholipid syndrome: report of an international workshop. Arthritis Rheum. **42:** 1309–1311.
10. LOIZOU, S., J.D. MCCREA, J.C. RUDGE, *et al.* 1982 Measurement of anti-cardiolipin antibodies by an enzyme-linked immunosorbent assay (ELISA): standardization and quantitation of results. Clin. Exp. Immunol. **2:** 738–745.
11. BOZIC, B., M. STEGNAR, T. KVEDER, *et* al. 1997. Influence of degraded phosphatidylserine on binding of antiphospholipid antibodies. Int. Arch. Allerg. Immunol. **112:** 19–26.
12. CUCNIK, S., T. KVEDER, B. ROZMAN & B. BOZIC. 2004. Binding of high-avidity anti-β_2-glicoprotein I antibodies. Rheumatology **43:** 1353–1356.
13. CUCNIK, S., A. AMBROZIC, B. BOZIC, *et al.* 2000. Anti-β2-glycoprotein I ELISA: methodology, determination of cut-off values in 434 healthy Caucasians and evaluation of monoclonal antibodies as possible international standards. Clin. Chem. Lab. Med. **38:** 777–783.
14. DRENKARD, C., J. SANCHEZ-GUERRERO & D. ALARCON-SEGOVIA. 1989. Fall in antiphospholipid antibody at time of thromboocclusive episodes in systemic lupus erythematosus. J. Rheum. **16:** 614–617.
15. PRAPROTNIK, S. & B. BOZIC. 1996. A decrease in antiphospholipid antibodies before a thrombotic event. Clin. Rheumatol. **15:** 298–300.
16. CABIEDES, J., A.R. CABRAL & D. ALARCON-SEGOVIA. 1995. Clinical manifestations of the antiphospholipid syndrome in patients with systemic lupus erythematosus associate more strongly with anti-β_2-glycoprotein-I than with antiphospholipid antibodies. J. Rheumatol. **22:** 1899–1906.
17. TSUTSUMI, A., E. MATSUURA, K. ICHIKAWA, *et al.* 1996. Antibodies to β_2-glycoprotein I and clinical manifestations in patients with systemic lupus erythematosus. Arthritis Rheum. **39:** 1466–1474.
18. INANÇ, M., S. DONOHOE, C.T. RAVIRAJAN, *et al.* 1998. Anti-β_2-glycoprotein I, anti-prothrombin and anticardiolipin antibodies in a longitudinal study of patients with systemic lupus erythematosus and the antiphospholipid syndrome. Br. J. Rheumatol. **37:** 1089–1094.
19. GOMEZ-PACHECO, L., A.R. VILLA, C. DRENKARD, *et al.* 1999. Serum anti-β2-glycoprotein I and anticardiolipin antibodies during thrombosis in systemic lupus erythematosus patients. Am. J. Med. **106:** 417–423.
20. MANZ, R.A., M. LÖHNING, G. CASSESE, *et al.* 1998. Survival of long-lived plasma cells is independent of antigen. Int. Immunol. **10:** 1703–1711.
21. HOYER, B.F., K. MOSER, A.E. HAUSER, *et al.* 2004. Short-lived plasmablasts and long-lived plasma cells contribute to chronic humoral autoimmunity in NZB/W mice. J. Exp. Med. **199:** 1577–1584.
22. HARRIS, E.N. 1990. Special report: the Second International Anti-cardiolipin Standardization Workshop/the Kingston Anti-Phospholipid Antibody Study (KAPS) group. Am. J. Clin. Pathol. **94:** 476–484.

Neurological Complications of Celiac Disease and Autoimmune Mechanisms

Preliminary Data of a Prospective Study in Adult Patients

C. BRIANI,[a] G. ZARA,[a] E. TOFFANIN,[a] S. RUGGERO,[a] A. FERRARINI,[a] F. DE LAZZARI,[b] M. LUCA,[c] D. FAGGIAN,[d] F. GRASSIVARO,[a] M. ERMANI,[a] R. PEZZANI,[a] B. GIOMETTO,[e] AND A. D'ODORICO[b]

[a]*Department of Neurosciences, University of Padova, Padova, Italy*

[b]*Department of Surgical and Gastroenterological Science, University of Padova, Padova, Italy*

[c]*Department of Blood Transfusion Service Apheresis Unit, University of Padova, Padova, Italy*

[d]*Department of Laboratory Medicine, University of Padova, Padova, Italy*

[e]*Department of Neurology, General Hospital, Treviso, Italy*

ABSTRACT: **Antibodies to gangliosides and Purkinje cells have been reported in patients with celiac disease (CD) with neuropathy and ataxia, respectively. Whether these antibodies are pathogenic is not clear. The response of neurological symptoms and antibody titers to a gluten-free diet is still controversial. The objective of our study was to assess whether neurological manifestations in CD patients correlate with antibody titers and a gluten-free diet.Thirty-five CD patients (9 males, 26 females, mean age 37.1 ± 12.6 yrs) were followed prospectively. At initial evaluation, 23 were on a gluten-free diet, 12 were not. At recruitment and during follow-up, patients underwent neurological and electrophysiological evaluation. IgG, IgM, and IgA anti-ganglioside antibodies were assayed by ELISA; anti-neuronal antibodies were assessed by immunohistochemistry and Western blot. Four patients, all males, had electrophysiological evidence of neuropathy; three had been on a gluten-free diet for several months, and one was newly diagnosed. One had reduced tendon reflexes; another complained of distal paresthesias. With regard to anti-ganglioside antibodies, three patients had a moderate increase in antibodies without symptoms or signs of neuropathy. No patients had ataxia or cerebellar dysfunction, although in four patients reactivity to neuronal antigens was found. In 17 patients, an electrophysiological follow-up (mean duration of follow-up, 9 months) showed no changes. In conclusion, the preliminary results of this prospective study indicate that neuropathy, usually subclinical, may accompany CD. Antibody titers do not seem to correlate with neurological symptoms/signs**

Address for correspondence: Chiara Briani, M.D., Department of Neurosciences, University of Padova, Via Giustiniani, 5, 35128 Padova, Italy. Voice: +39-049-821-3600; fax: +39-049-875-1770.
chiara.briani@unipd.it

**Ann. N.Y. Acad. Sci. 1051: 148–155 (2005). © 2005 New York Academy of Sciences.
doi: 10.1196/annals.1361.056**

or diet. Ongoing follow-up will help confirm these data and clarify the role, if any, of antibodies in neurological involvement in CD.

KEYWORDS: celiac disease; autoantibodies; ganglioside; neuropathy; gluten; diet

INTRODUCTION

Celiac disease (CD) is an autoimmune disorder, affecting 0.3% to 1% of the population of the Western world. It is mediated by a T cell immune response against ingested gluten in genetically predisposed persons, with more than 95% of patients sharing the major histocompatibility complex class II human leukocyte antigen (HLA) DQ2 or DQ8 haplotype.[1] Tissue transglutaminase (TG) is the antigenic target recognized by anti-endomysial antibodies in CD, and serum anti-TG antibodies are a specific marker for the disease. Autoimmune disorders and organ-specific autoantibodies may be associated, especially type I diabetes mellitus and autoimmune thyroiditis.[1] Intestinal biopsy allows a definitive diagnosis, showing villous atrophy of the small intestinal mucosa, which improves after a gluten-free diet. Although the small bowel is often involved, approximately 50% of adult patients present with extraintestinal manifestations, mainly iron-deficiency anemia, but also osteoporosis, infertility, and neurological alterations. Among the latter, peripheral neuropathy and cerebellar ataxia are the most common.[2–4] The pathogenesis of neurological manifestations in CD is not clear. Moreover, the response of the neurological symptoms to a gluten-free diet is poor and still controversial. Emerging evidence points to humoral mechanisms for both ataxia and peripheral neuropathy in CD. Humoral response has been proposed in the pathogenesis of gluten ataxia, given the report of antibodies to Purkinje cells that cross-react with gliadin antigens in sera of celiac patients with ataxia.[5] These findings, however, have not been confirmed by other authors.[6,7] With regard to peripheral neuropathy, anti-ganglioside antibody reactivity has been reported in adult CD patients with neuropathy.[8,9] The antibodies are of IgG isotype, suggesting a T cell–mediated response to ganglioside antigens. A recent study from our group did not confirm these findings in a pediatric CD population, in which antibodies to gangliosides were found in two out of 42 celiac children with no symptoms or signs of neuropathy.[10] Moreover, the response of the antibodies to a gluten-free diet was controversial, with the antibody titer decreasing in one case and increasing in a second case after diet. Different biological and immunological characteristics in childhood and adulthood, however, make it difficult to compare our findings in CD children with those reported in adults. We therefore undertook a prospective study in an adult CD population to evaluate the incidence of neurological symptoms or signs, the presence of antibodies to peripheral nerve and neuronal antigens, and possible correlations with neurological manifestations and a gluten-free diet.

PATIENTS AND METHODS

Consecutively seen patients (>18 years of age) with histologically proven CD, recruited from the Department of Surgical and Gastroenterological Science of the University of Padova, were considered. Both patients with newly diagnosed (within one to three months) CD and patients already consuming a gluten-free diet were considered. Patients with associated diseases or conditions that were possible causes of neuropathy (diabetes, alcohol abuse, exposure to neurotoxic drugs) or ataxia (alcohol abuse, genetic disorders, syphilis, vitamin E or B_{12} deficiency) were excluded, so as to minimize possible confounding effects on neurological symptoms. All patients underwent neurological and electrophysiological evaluation at recruitment and at every follow-up visit. Blood samples were drawn for antibody determination. All investigations were performed under informed consent from each patient.

Neurological Evaluation

Standard neurological evaluation was performed. Strength was scored with the Medical Research Council (MRC) scale,[11] and deep tendon reflexes (biceps, triceps, knee, ankle) graded as follows: normal (2), diminished (1), absent (0) (16 maximum score). Symptoms were assessed with the Neurological Symptom Score (NSS)[12] (pathological >1).

Electrophysiological Study

Nerve conduction velocities (CV) were investigated by surface electrodes using standardized techniques. Compound muscle action potential (CMAP) amplitude and CV of median, ulnar, and peroneal nerves were recorded. CV and sensory nerve action potential (SNAP) amplitudes of the sural nerve were recorded bilaterally. The electrophysiological diagnosis of a baseline peripheral neuropathy was determined using laboratory reference values. Skin temperature was controlled and maintained above 32°C throughout the examination.

Follow-up Study

Follow-up was set at every six months for patients with a recent (within one to three months) diagnosis of CD, and who were to start a gluten-free diet, and every 12 months for patients with long-standing CD already on a gluten-free diet. At every follow-up evaluation, patients underwent neurological and electrophysiological evaluations, as well as antibody testing.

Anti-TG and Anti-gliadin Antibodies

Anti-TG antibodies were assessed using a quantitative ELISA with h-tTG2 (Inova Diagnostics, Inc.). IgG and IgA anti-gliadin antibodies were tested with a standardized ELISA (Inova Diagnostics, Inc.).

Anti-ganglioside Antibodies

The wells of ELISA microtiter plates were coated with 100 μL of methanol containing 0.5 μg of ganglioside (GM1, GM2, GD1a, GD1b) (Sigma Immunochemical, St. Louis, MO) antigens, and the methanol allowed to evaporate. After saturation with 1% bovine serum albumin (BSA) in PBS, increasing dilutions of patient sera were added in triplicate and incubated overnight at 4°C, followed by incubation with peroxidase-conjugated goat anti-human IgM, IgG, and IgA (0.8 mg/mL) (Jackson

Immunoresearch Laboratories, West Grove, PA), diluted 1:1000, for 2 h. Sera added to microwells coated with 1% BSA only served as the control for each dilution. After washing, 100 μL of developing solution containing 0.05 M Na_2HPO_4, 0.024 M sodium citrate, pH 5, 0.08 % *o*-phenylenediamine, and 0.008% H_2O_2 were added. Reaction products were measured spectrophotometrically at 450 nm in a Biotek EIA reader. The titer for each specimen was taken as the highest dilution at which the optical density reading was 0.1 units greater than in the corresponding BSA-coated wells.

Anti-neuronal Antibodies

Anti-neuronal antibodies were assessed by immunohistochemistry and Western blot.

Immunohistochemistry was performed on both paraformaldehyde-fixed frozen and paraffin-embedded sections from rat cerebellum. In brief: 8-μm-thick paraformaldehyde-fixed frozen and paraffin-embedded sections from rat cerebellum were used. After blocking nonspecific immunoglobulin binding with normal rabbit serum (diluted 1:20 in PBS) for 10 min at room temperature (RT), the sections were incubated with sera (diluted 1:100 and 1:500) for 1 h at RT or overnight at 4°C. After washing with PBS, sections were incubated with rabbit biotinylated anti-human IgG (1:200) in PBS for 1 h at RT (Dako, Denmark). After further washing, an avidin-peroxidase complex was applied for 30 min at RT (Dako, Denmark), and the reactions developed with 3,3'-diaminobenzidine tetrahydrochloride and 0.01% H_2O_2 in PBS. Human cerebellar tissue, formalin-fixed and paraffin-embedded, from patients without neurological disorders was used to confirm the reactivity on rat tissues, applying the same procedures as described above.

Western blot was performed on neuronal proteins extracted from rat brain homogenate, as previously described.[13] Electrophoresis was done in 10 cm × 8 cm minigels with a Tris-glycine buffer system. After separation, proteins were transferred electrophoretically to a nitrocellulose membrane, and the membrane was incubated for 1 h at RT with 2% nonfat milk in PBS. Patient sera diluted 1:500 in 0.1% nonfat milk in PBS were applied overnight at 4°C. After washing, horse radish peroxidase (HRP)-conjugated rabbit anti human immunoglobulins (1:1000; Dako, Denmark) were applied, and the reaction developed using ethylaminocarbazole-hydrogen peroxide.

Immunoblot with recombinant Yo, Hu, Ri, and amphiphysin proteins (Milenia Biotec GmbH, Germany) was done in positive cases.

RESULTS

Thirty-five CD patients (9 males, 26 females, mean age 37.1 ± 12.6 yrs) were enrolled and prospectively followed for a median of 9 months (range 6–18 months). Twenty-three patients were on a gluten-free diet at recruitment, with a median duration of diet of 37 months (range 18–61 months) and median duration of disease of 25 months. Adherence to the diet was assessed by testing anti-TG antibodies. Twelve patients were not on a gluten-free diet at first evaluation, and had a median time from

TABLE 1. Clinical data and electrophysiological findings in four CD patients with neuropathy

Patient	Sex	Age (yr)	Gluten-Free Diet Duration (mo)	MDL (msec)	Peroneal MCV (m/s)	Sural CV (m/s)	NSS	DTR
1	M	38	1	4.3	42.5	Normal	0	16
2	M	54	139	4.15	42.4	Normal	2	16
3	M	32	66	5.55	38.5	38.3	0	14
4	M	53	28	3.8	41.3	Normal	0	16

ABBREVIATIONS: MDL, motor distal latency; MCV, motor conduction velocity; CV, conduction velocity; NSS, neuropathy sensory score[12]; DTR, deep tendon reflexes.

Laboratory reference values: sural CV 42–53 m/sec; peroneal MCV, 45–55 m/sec; MDL, equal to or less than 5 msec.

diagnosis of 1.5 months. HLA was available for 20 of the 35 patients; all bore HLA DQ2 aplotype, none had DQ8.

At recruitment, four patients, all males, had electrophysiological evidence of mild neuropathy, which was motor in three (slowing of peroneal nerve CV, with normal CMAP amplitude), and sensory-motor in one (slowing of both peroneal and sural nerve CV, with normal CMAP and SNAP amplitude). One of the four patients had reduced deep tendon reflexes, another had symptoms of neuropathy (cramps and distal paresthesias in the lower limbs). Three of the four patients had been consuming a gluten-free diet for several months (28, 66, and 139 months, respectively), whereas one was newly diagnosed (one month). No known causes of neuropathy or other associated autoimmune diseases were present. Serum levels vitamin B_{12} and folate were within normal limits. The characteristics of the four patients are summarized in TABLE 1. With regard to antibodies to gangliosides, three patients, all females, had an increased titer of anti-ganglioside antibodies, without symptoms or signs of peripheral neuropathy. In two cases, the antibodies were of IgM isotype (titers 1:6,400 to GM1, 1:6,400 to GD1a), in one case IgG (1:1,600 to GD1b). One patient had an associated, medically treated, autoimmune hypothyroidism (Hashimoto's disease). All three had been consuming a gluten-free diet (for 17, 192, and 60 months, respectively).

No patients had ataxia or cerebellar dysfunction, although in four patients low reactivity to neuronal antigens was found by immunohistochemistry, with morphological staining limited to Purkinje cell cytoplasm and apical dendrites (FIG. 1). Western blot with neuronal extracts and immunoblot with recombinant onconeuronal antigens were negative.

A follow-up evaluation is available for 17 patients so far. The mean duration of follow-up is 9 months (range 6–18). None of the patients asymptomatic at enrollment have developed neurological symptoms or signs, or electrophysiological or antibody modifications at follow-up. The mild CV abnormalities present in four patients at recruitment have shown no changes at follow-up (last follow-up at months 15, 13, 9, and 9, for patients 1, 2, 3, and 4, respectively), including those in patient 1, who started a gluten-free diet soon after initial evaluation (TABLE 1).

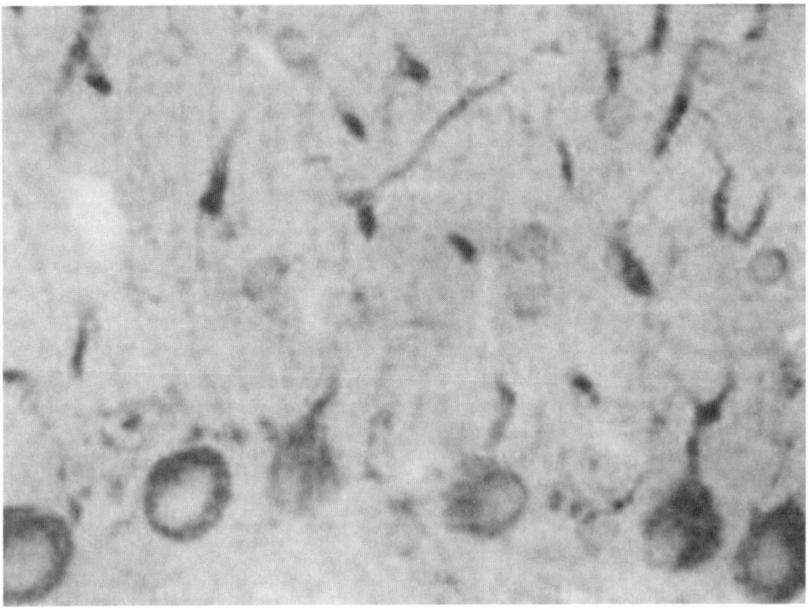

FIGURE 1. Granular staining of Purkinje cell cytoplasm and scattered apical dendrites of rat cerebellum (×250; reduced by 60%).

One of the three patients with increased anti-ganglioside antibody titer had a second antibody testing 12 months later; the antibody titer (anti-GD1a IgM, 1:6,400) showed no change.

DISCUSSION

The results of our study demonstrated the presence of electrophysiological abnormalities, often subclinical, in 4 of 35 (11%, CI 95%: 0.6%–21.3%) CD patients. The absence in these patients of other known causes of neuropathy points to a possible role of CD in the occurrence of neuropathy. The presence of neuropathy seems to be independent of a gluten-free diet. Three of the four patients with electrophysiological alterations, in fact, had been on a gluten-free diet since the establishment of the CD diagnosis, 139, 66, and 28 months before our first evaluation. Moreover, the patient whose subclinical neuropathy was detected only one month after the diagnosis of CD did not show any clinical or electrophysiological modification at follow-up evaluation 15 months after the initiation of a strict gluten-free diet. These preliminary results seem to question a direct neurotoxic effect of gluten exposure, and point to different mechanisms that might be responsible for, or contribute to, the development of peripheral neuropathy in CD patients. Our results are in agreement with those by Luostarinen *et al.* in patients with well-treated CD.[14]

Antibodies to ganglioside, when present in our population of CD patients, do not seem to correlate with clinical manifestations or gluten-free diet. In two cases, the antibodies were of IgM isotype, and in one case of IgG isotype. The different isotypes may reflect a different function of the antibodies, with IgM reflecting a more nonspecific autoimmune reactivity, and IgG a possible T cell–mediated pathogenic role. Consistently, CD adults with neuropathy have been found to have IgG antibodies to gangliosides.[8,9] The absence of symptoms or signs of peripheral nerve involvement in our patients, however, suggest that the antibodies might be unrelated to, or not sufficient to, induce nerve damage, unless other, as yet unidentified, factors are involved.

On the other hand, anti-ganglioside antibodies were not present in the four patients with electrophysiological evidence of neuropathy. It is possible that severe nerve damage is required before anti-ganglioside antibodies are generated as a secondary response.

Also, antibodies to neuronal antigens do not seem to correlate with neurological complications. In addition, the reactivity in immunohistochemistry was not suggestive of an onconeuronal antibody pattern, as confirmed by the negativity of the immunoblot with recombinant onconeuronal proteins.

In conclusion, the preliminary results of this prospective study indicate that neuropathy, including subclinical neuropathy, may complicate CD (11% of the cases in our study). Antibodies to gangliosides and to neuronal antigens do not seem to correlate with neurological symptoms or signs. The ongoing follow-up study will help to better address the relationship among CD, autoimmunity, and gluten-free diet, and to clarify whether antibodies, when present, might be predictive of neurological involvement in CD patients, as already shown for other antibodies to peripheral nerve antigens.[15]

REFERENCES

1. Farrell, R.J. & C.P. Kelly. 2002. Celiac sprue. N. Engl. J. Med. **346:** 180–188.
2. Cooke, W.T. & T.W. Smith. 1966. Neurological disorders associated with adult coeliac disease. Brain **89:** 683–722.
3. Burk, K., S. Bosch, C.A. Muller, *et al.* 2001. Sporadic cerebellar ataxia associated with gluten sensitivity. Brain **124:** 1013–1019.
4. Hadjivassiliou, M., R.A. Grunewald & G.A. Davies-Jones. 2002. Gluten sensitivity as a neurological illness. J. Neurol. Neurosurg. Psychiatry **72:** 560–563.
5. Hadjivassiliou, M., S. Boscolo, G.A. Davies-Jones, *et al.* 2002. The humoral response in the pathogenesis of gluten ataxia. Neurology **58:** 1221–1226.
6. Wiendl, H., M. Mehling, J. Dichgans, *et al.* 2003. The humoral response in the pathogenesis of gluten ataxia [comment]. Neurology **60:** 1397.
7. Wurster, U. 2003. The humoral response in the pathogenesis of gluten ataxia [comment]. Neurology **60**:1397.
8. Alaedini, A., P.H. Green, H.W. Sander, *et al.* 2002. Ganglioside reactive antibodies in the neuropathy associated with celiac disease. J. Neuroimmunol. **127:** 145–148.
9. Chin, R.L., H.W. Sander, T.H. Brannagan, *et al.* 2003. Celiac neuropathy. Neurology **60:** 1581–1585.
10. Briani, C., S. Ruggero, G. Zara, *et al.* 2004. Anti-ganglioside antibodies in children with coeliac disease: correlation with gluten-free diet and neurological complications. Aliment. Pharmacol. Ther. **20:** 231–235.
11. Medical Research Council. 1943. Aids to the investigation of peripheral nerve injuries, 2nd ed. (revised). War Memorandum Series, No. 7: 11–46. HMSO. London.

12. DYCK, P.J. 1988. Detection, characterization, and staging of polyneuropathy: assessed in diabetics. Muscle Nerve **11:** 21–32.
13. VIANELLO, M., R. VITALIANI, R. PEZZANI, *et al.* 2004. The spectrum of antineuronal autoantibodies in a series of neurological patients. J. Neurol. Sci. **220:** 29–36.
14. LUOSTARINEN, L., S.L. HIMANEN, M. LUOSTARINEN, *et al.* 2003. Neuromuscular and sensory disturbances in patients with well treated coeliac disease. J. Neurol. Neurosurg. Psychiatry **74:** 490–494.
15. MEUCCI, N., L. BALDINI, A. CAPPELLARI, *et al.* 1999. Anti-myelin-associated glycoprotein antibodies predict the development of neuropathy in asymptomatic patients with IgM monoclonal gammopathy. Ann. Neurol. **46:** 119–122.

E2F1$^{-/-}$ C57BL/6 Mice Overexpressing a Human Bcl-2 Transgene in B Cells Develop a Mild Autoimmune Syndrome

MARÍA J. MARÍN,[a] ITXASO GARCÍA,[b] MARTA PEÑA,[a] AINHOA BOLÍVAR,[a] ANA ZUBIAGA,[b] AND MARCOS LÓPEZ-HOYOS[a]

[a]*Inmunology Unit, Hospital Universitario Marqués de Valdecilla, Santander, Spain*

[b]*Department of Genetics, Physical Anthropology and Animal Physiology, Faculty of Science and Technology, University of the Basque Country, Bilbao, Spain*

ABSTRACT: Bcl-2, besides having an anti-apoptotic function, delays cell cycle progression at G1 to S. Overexpression of Bcl-2 in B cells induces an autoimmune syndrome (AIS) in pro-autoimmune genetic backgrounds. E2F1, a member of the E2F transcription factors, controls cell cycle, but it also induces cell death. E2F1$^{-/-}$ mice show an altered negative thymic selection but a conserved peripheral tolerance. As a consequence, these mice do not develop autoimmunity. Our aim was to evaluate whether deregulation of both apoptosis and cell cycle alters the mechanisms of tolerance and induces an AIS. C57BL/6 E2F1$^{-/-}$ mice were crossed with C57BL/6 mice overexpressing a human Bcl-2 transgene in B cells to obtain *E2F1$^{-/-}$ hbcl-2* Tg mice. These mice were followed for up to 15 months of age with bleedings every three months to obtain serum and whole blood. The production of an AIS was assessed by quantitation of serum anti-DNA antibodies, renal light microscopy, and direct immunofluorescence in search of immunoglobulin deposits. *E2F1$^{-/-}$ hbcl-2* Tg mice developed an AIS characterized by anti-DNA autoantibody production with renal damage observed after the 9th month of age. The lesions consisted mainly on cellular proliferation and mesangial deposits, compatible with a mesangial glomerulonephritis. The composition of deposits was predominantly of IgA, followed by IgM and IgG. Despite the development of renal damage, the AIS observed did not induce an accelerated mortality. The coexistence of an altered B cell apoptosis, together with the lack of E2F1, induces a mild AIS in the non-autoimmune background of C57BL/6 mice.

KEYWORDS: apoptosis; cell cycle; Bcl-2; E2F; mice; autoimmune syndrome

INTRODUCTION

In the past, cell death and cell proliferation seemed to be independent cellular processes that were regulated by different molecular pathways that never encountered each other. However, accumulating evidence suggests that both death and pro-

Address for correspondence: Marcos López-Hoyos, Servicio de Inmunología, Hospital Universitario Marqués de Valdecilla, Santander 39008, Spain. Voice and fax: 34-942203453. inmlhm@humv.es

Ann. N.Y. Acad. Sci. 1051: 156–165 (2005). © 2005 New York Academy of Sciences. doi: 10.1196/annals.1361.057

liferation are connected, and molecules thought to play a role only in one pathway have been found to regulate the other one.[1–3]

E2F1 is a member of a family of seven transcriptional factors essential for regulating the correct cell cycle progression through the transcription of genes necessary for the progression from the G1 to S phase of cell cycle.[4] This protein functions as a heterodimer with members of the DP family, although the specificity for the DNA binding is determined by the E2F subunit.[5,6] This heterodimer is associated with members of the retinoblastoma protein, which are unphosphorylated during G0 and early G1 stages of the cell cycle. This union inhibits E2F1 function. In the presence of mitogenic signals, several cyclin-dependent kinases phosphorylate the retinoblastoma protein, which, in turn, dissociates from E2F1. As a consequence, free E2F1 can activate the E2F-responsive genes, initiating the DNA replication.[5,6]

E2F1 not only regulates cell cycle progression, but also been reported to participate in the regulation of apoptotic pathways, both intrinsic and extrinsic.[7] E2F2 and E2F3, members of the same subfamily as E2F1, may also regulate the apoptotic pathways, although their role in this process remains controversial. The E2F1-DP heterodimer may directly induce the expression of some pro-apoptotic genes, such as Apaf-1, a component of the apoptosome complex, essential in the mitochondrial pathway of apoptosis.[8] E2F1 may also promote apoptosis through activation of p53 by three different mechanisms: (1) protection of p53 degradation through induction of $p19^{arf}$ expression; (2) induction of expression of the p53 kinase Atm; and (3) direct binding to the p53 and subsequent increase in p53-mediated transcriptional function.[9–11]

With regard to the consequences of the apoptotic control by E2F1, we have previously described the role of E2F1 in thymic apoptosis.[12] E2F1 protects thymocytes from *in vitro* apoptosis induced by anti-CD3 stimulation, but not from glucocorticoid treatment. Such an effect results in an increase in the number of thymocytes in E2F1 knockout mice. The protection from apoptosis is dependent on a decrease of the p53 levels of $CD4^+CD8^+$ thymocytes. In addition, E2F1 plays a role in the negative selection of double-positive thymocytes, since the lack of function of E2F impairs the deletion of autoreactive thymocytes after staphylococcus enterotoxin B injection. Furthermore, the thymocytes that do not undergo negative selection are functional and responsive to polyclonal stimuli.[12]

Bcl-2 is another example of connection between apoptotic and proliferative pathways. Bcl-2 was the first member described of an expanding family of proteins with both anti- and pro-apoptotic functions.[13] The main mechanism by which Bcl-2 protects from apoptosis is by inhibiting the formation of homodimers Bax-Bax at the outer membrane of the mitochondria, which facilitates the exit of cytochrome *c* to the cytosol to form the apoptosome.[13] In addition to its well-established role as an anti-apoptotic protein, Bcl-2 was shown to delay entry into the cell cycle through an unknown mechanism. In fact, a mutant Bcl-2 protein transfected into cell lines has been shown to inhibit both the ability to delay cell cycle as well as the anti-apoptotic function.[14] Vairo *et al.* proposed a mechanism for the cell cycle–inhibitory effect of Bcl-2.[15] When Bcl-2 levels are low, mitogenic stimulation provokes destruction of p130 and p27, facilitating cell cycle entry. However, when Bcl-2 is overexpressed, p27 expression increases and inhibits the cdk2 activity. As a consequence, p130 and p27 are not phosphorylated and the E2F4-p130 repressor complex remains stable, inducing cell cycle delay by repressing the E2F1 activity. It seems that Bcl-2-dependent cell cycle control is mediated by a region of the molecule different from the region involved in the anti-apoptotic regulation, specifically on a tyrosine at position28, near the N-terminal end.[15]

In our laboratory we have previously demonstrated how inhibition of B cell apoptosis through the overexpression of a human Bcl-2 transgene is able to induce an autoimmune syndrome, both in induced murine models or spontaneously.[16,17] However, Bcl-2 by itself is not able to induce such an effect. It requires additional factors, such as a polyclonal activation, similar to what has been described in a model of host-versus-graft disease.[16] Likewise, in the presence of a pro-autoimmune genetic background, such as that of the New Zealand white mice, Bcl-2 is able to induce autoimmunity.[17] In this latter case, the production of autoantibodies and the autoimmune syndrome is dependent on the presence of $CD4^+$ T cells, together with the genetic abnormalities of the New Zealand white mouse.

Taken together data from the E2F1 knockout mice and the Bcl-2 transgenic mice, and considering the molecular connections proposed between these two molecules, our objective is to evaluate whether deregulation of both apoptosis and cell cycle alters the mechanisms of tolerance and induces an autoimmune syndrome, by backcrossing Bcl-2 transgenic mice with E2F1 knock out mice.

MATERIAL AND METHODS

Mice

C57BL/6-SV40-Eμ-*hbcl-2* Tg mice[18] were purchased from the Jackson Laboratories (Bar Harbor, ME). B6-SV40-Eμ-*hbcl-2* Tg mice were crossed with $E2F1^{-/-}$ mice in our animal facilities. F1 hybrids (Bcl-$2^{+/-}$ E2F$1^{+/-}$) were intercrossed to obtain the $E2F1^{-/-}$ *hbcl-2* Tg mice. As control groups the $E2F1^{-/-}$ non-Tg mice and the $E2F1^{+/+}$ *hbcl-2* Tg mice were employed. Eight to nine mice from each group were followed up to 15 months of age.

The presence of the *hbcl-2* Tg in F1 mice was assessed in peripheral blood mononuclear cells by flow cytometry using a specific mAb against human Bcl-2 (clone 6C8; Pharmingen, San Diego, CA), as described previously.[16] The detection of the wild-type (170 bp) or mutant *E2F1* allele (230 bp) was made by a PCR reaction previously described.[12]

Mice were bled every three months from the retro-orbital plexus, and the resulting sera were stored at –20°C until use. In addition, a sample from each bleeding was used for flow cytometry studies.

Serologic Studies

The presence of IgG anti-DNA antibodies (Abs) was determined in sera by ELISA[16] and the results expressed in TU in reference to a standard curve obtained from a serum pool from 6–8-month old MRL *lpr/lpr* mice.

Flow Cytometry Studies

The number of the main blood lymphocyte subsets in the different groups of mice was evaluated by flow cytometry. Fifty μL of whole blood were stained with different combinations of fluorescein isothiocyanate- (FITC), phycoerythrin- (PE), peridinin chlorophyll protein- (PerCP) and allophycocianin (APC)-conjugated mAbs (Pharmingen) directed against surface T and B cell antigens: CD3, CD4, CD5, CD8, CD25, CD38, CD45, CD69, B220 and IgM. A total of 10^4 viable cells were analyzed in a FACS Calibur flow cytometer using Cell Quest Pro software (Becton Dickinson, Mountain View, CA).

Histopathologic Study

Samples of all major organs were obtained at autopsy. For light microscopy studies of the kidney, the organs were immersed in a fixative solution containing 10% formaldehyde in 0.12 M PBS (pH 7.4) for 24 hours at room temperature. After fixation, samples were embedded in paraffin, and 3-µm-thick sections were processed for hematoxylin–eosin staining.

Tissue-bound IgM, IgG and IgA antibodies were studied by immunofluorescence on kidney cryosections using fluoresceinated goat anti-mouse IgM and goat anti-mouse IgG antibodies (Jackson ImmunoResearch, West Grove, PA) or fluoresceinated goat anti-mouse IgA antibody (Cappel Laboratories, Cochranville, PA).

Statistical Analysis

Statistical analysis of differences between groups of mice was performed using the Mann–Whitney test. Probability values <0.05 were considered significant.

RESULTS

Production of Serum Anti-DNA Antibodies

We first looked at the production of anti-DNA antibodies as a serum marker of autoimmunity. *E2F1*$^{-/-}$ non-Tg mice showed no positive titers of anti-DNA Abs during all the study (FIG. 1). One and four mice from the *E2F1*$^{+/+}$ *hbcl-2* Tg group produced low positive levels of anti-DNA Abs at 3 and 6 months of age, respectively. The frequency of positive sera and the titers of anti-DNA Abs in this group increased after 9 months of age. When the overexpression of Bcl-2 and the lack of E2F1 were combined in the *E2F1*$^{-/-}$ *hbcl-2* Tg mice, the production of anti-DNA was increased, especially at 9 and 12 months of age.

Histopathologic Findings

The production of anti-DNA antibodies was followed by the production of kidney damage in *hbcl-2* Tg mice, either E2F1$^{-/-}$ or E2F1$^{+/+}$. However, all the *E2F1*$^{-/-}$ *hbcl-2* Tg mice demonstrated more severe lesions with mesangial proliferation and deposits. In some cases peritubular lymphoplasmacytic infiltrates were observed. In addition, one *E2F1*$^{-/-}$ *hbcl-2* Tg mouse had extracapillar proliferation. These lesions destroyed the glomerular structure in many cases. The *E2F1*$^{+/+}$ *hbcl-2* Tg mice showed only moderate mesangial proliferation. In both types of mice, abundant tubular casts could be observed (FIG. 2). None of the *E2F1*$^{-/-}$ non-Tg mice suffered any kidney damage. No pathologic findings were detected in any other tissue or organ (lungs, liver, brain, spleen and lymph nodes).

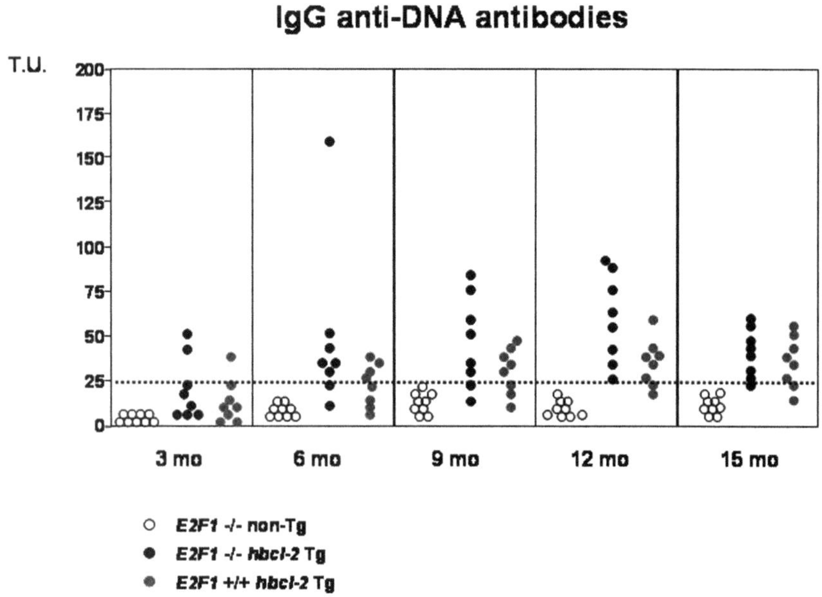

FIGURE 1. Serum levels of IgG anti-DNA in *E2F1*$^{-/-}$ non-Tg mice (*open circles*), *E2F1*$^{-/-}$ *hbcl-2* Tg mice (*solid circles*) and *E2F1*$^{+/+}$ *hbcl-2* Tg mice (*gray circles*). Values of individual mice are expressed in titration units (TU) for anti-DNA autoAbs. *Dashed horizontal line* represents the cutoff value obtained with sera from 15*E2F1*$^{+/+}$ non-Tg mice.

As observed for serologic and histologic data, direct immunofluorescence showed more intense deposits of immunoglobulins in the kidneys of *E2F1*$^{-/-}$ *hbcl-2* Tg mice than in those from *E2F1*$^{+/+}$ *hbcl-2* Tg mice. Such deposits were of both IgG and IgM. However, prominent granular IgA deposits localized primarily in the mesangium were observed in *E2F1*$^{-/-}$ *hbcl-2* Tg mice, but not in *E2F1*$^{+/+}$ *hbcl-2* Tg mice (FIG. 3). Altogether, these findings were compatible with the development of a mesangial nephropathy.

Despite the serologic and histologic findings, *E2F1*$^{-/-}$ non-Tg mice, *E2F1*$^{+/+}$ *hbcl-2* Tg mice, and *E2F1*$^{-/-}$ *hbcl-2* Tg mice did not show an increased mortality, all remaining alive at 15 months of age.

Lymphocyte Homeostasis

It is possible that the autoimmune phenomena observed in E2F1$^{-/-}$ hbcl-2 Tg mice are secondary to a disturbance in the lymphocyte homeostasis as a consequence of deregulation in both cell death and proliferation. Thus, flow cytometry analysis of peripheral blood cells after staining with specific mAbs was performed. The only major finding was a relative decrease of T cells, both CD4^{+} and CD8^{+}, in *E2F1*$^{+/+}$ *hbcl-2* Tg mice. Such decrease was dependent on almost two-fold increase in the frequency of B cells (B220^{+}IgM^{+}). The changes were observed from 3 months of age. This pattern was exactly the same in the *E2F1*$^{-/-}$ *hbcl-2* Tg mice (data not shown).

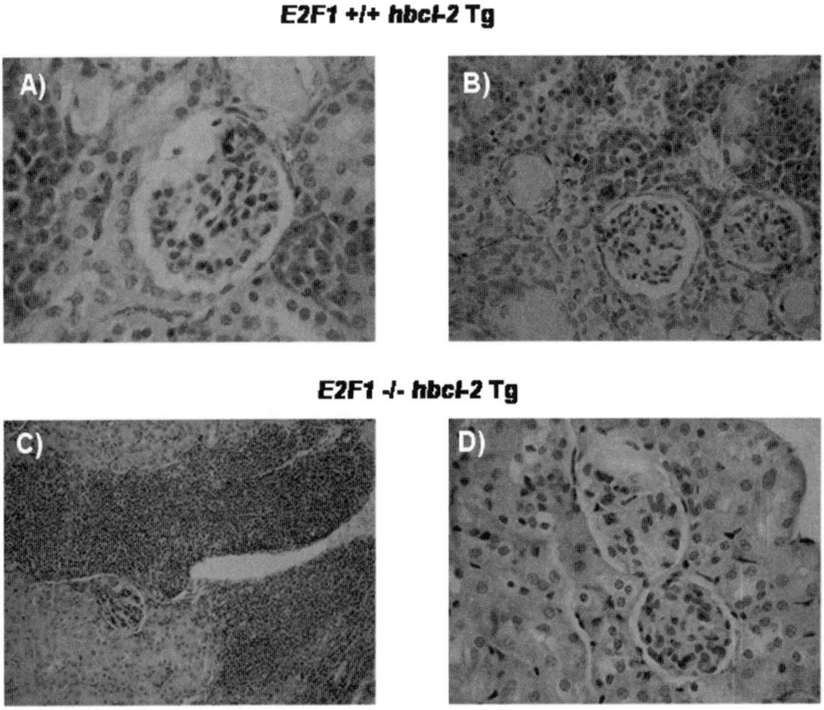

FIGURE 2. Histologic appearance of glomeruli from 10-month-old *E2F1*$^{+/+}$*hbcl-2* Tg mice (**A**,**B**) and *E2F1*$^{-/-}$ *hbcl-2* Tg mice (**C**,**D**). *E2F1*$^{+/+}$ *hbcl-2* Tg mice showed moderate mesangial cell proliferation (**A**) with cellular peritubular infiltrates and tubular casts (**B**). Lesions were more severe in *E2F1*$^{-/-}$ *hbcl-2* Tg mice, with important pericapillary lymphoplasmacytic infiltrates (**C**) and mesangial deposits and proliferation that disrupted the glomerular architecture (**D**).

Additional lymphocyte subsets were studied in peripheral blood, such as regulator T cells ($CD4^+$CD25high) or B-1 cells ($B220^+IgM^+CD5^+$). No significant differences in the frequency of these cells were found among the three groups of mice studied. In addition, there was no difference in the expression of activation markers, such as CD38 or CD69.

DISCUSSION

In the last years, the evidence for a link between pathways regulating cell death and those controlling cell cycle have been described at the molecular level.[1–3] Here, preliminary data show that in E2F1$^{-/-}$ *hbcl-2* Tg mice, defects in the regulation of B cell apoptosis, as a result of the overexpression of Bcl-2, together with the alteration in the cell cycle control, lead to the development of a mild autoimmune syndrome in C57BL/6 mice.

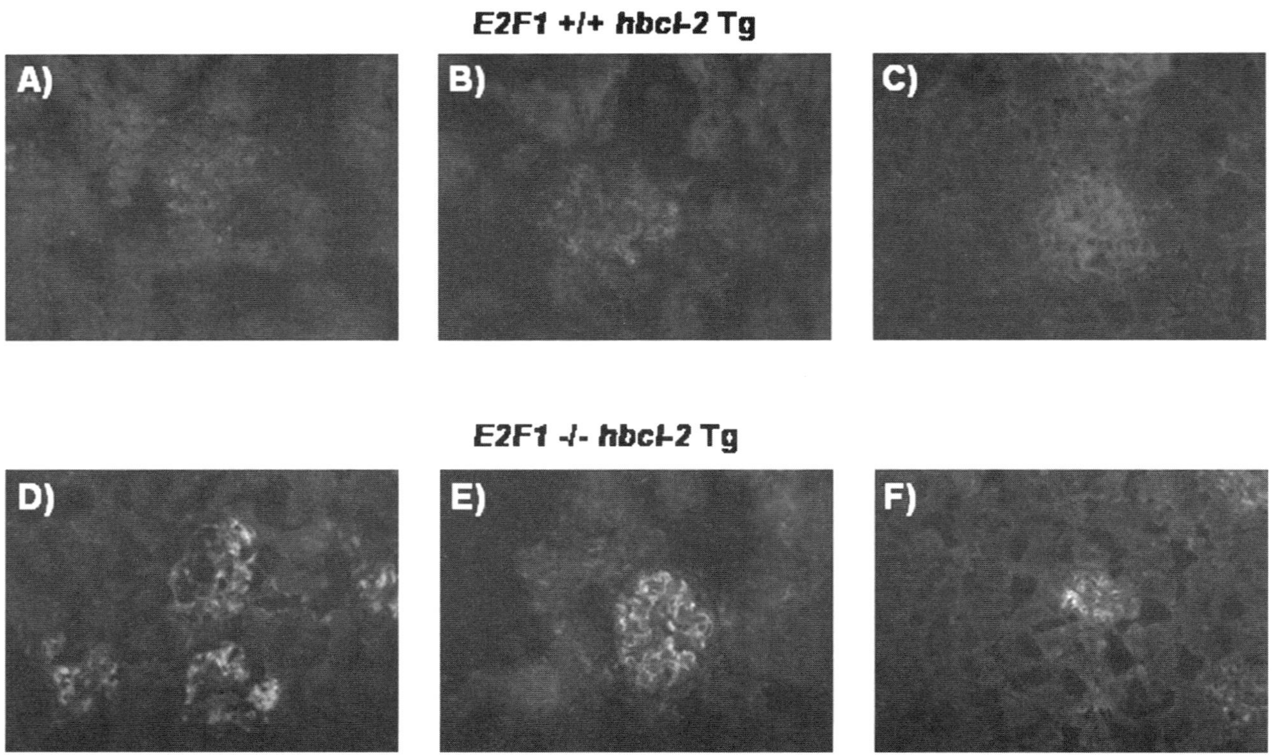

FIGURE 3. Presence of IgA (**A,D**), IgM (**B,E**), and IgG (**C,F**) deposits in the glomeruli of 10-month-old *E2F1*$^{+/+}$ *hbcl-2* Tg mice and *E2F1*$^{-/-}$ *hbcl-2* Tg mice (original magnification ×40; reduced by 44%).

Classical models of autoimmune disease have been described in so-called autoimmune-prone strains (i.e., MRL, NZW, NZB). It was suggested that the genetic background of these animals carried a number of predisposing genes for the induction of autoimmunity.[19] With the development of molecular methods and mapping studies, many loci have been associated with different autoimmune traits, especially in the NZW and NZB strains.[19] Our data indicate that two isolated genetic modifications in a non-lupus-prone background are sufficient to induce autoimmunity. Nonetheless, it is hard to explain the presence of autoimmune traits in *E2F1*$^{+/+}$*hbcl-2* Tg mice, which only carry the overexpression of the Bcl-2 transgene in B cells. Although these mice are in a non-autoimmune background, some lupus traits have been mapped to regions derived from C57BL/6 mice.[19]

We have previously demonstrated that inhibition of B cell apoptosis through the overexpression of Bcl-2 induce an autoimmune disease in experimental and spontaneous murine models.[16,17] However, in both cases, the presence of additional factors was necessary to develop a full syndrome. Among these factors, a T $CD4^+$ help is crucial since the deletion of this cell subset completely abrogates the syndrome.[17] This type of T–B interaction is also present in the *E2F1*$^{-/-}$ *hbcl-2* Tg mice. The additive effect of the deletion of E2F1$^{-/-}$ and the overexpression of Bcl-2 in our animals may be explained by a dysfunction in the mechanisms of tolerance at central and/or peripheral lymphoid tissues. E2F1 is necessary for the negative selection of thymocytes in TCR-transgenic mice by inducing overexpression of p53.[12] The lack of E2F1 does not protect thymocytes from passive death, but from activation-induced cell death, facilitating the escape of autoreactive thymocytes to the peripheral lymphoid organs. However, peripheral tolerance mechanisms seem to be E2F1-independent because E2F1$^{-/-}$ mice do not develop autoimmunity.[12] On the other hand, constitutive expression of Bcl-2 in B cells may promote the survival of autoantibody-producing B cells at the bone marrow and/or germinal centers.[20,21] These autoreactive B cells would interact with the autoreactive T cells that survive from the thymic negative selection in the E2F1$^{-/-}$ mice and, as a consequence, induce autoantibody production and development of an autoimmune syndrome.

Recently, E2F1 has been proposed to enable the mitochondrial pathway of apoptosis during activation-induced cell death (AICD).[2] AICD is essential to control those immune responses in which the antigen persists, such as self-antigens, to avoid the production of autoimmune diseases.[22] The MRL *lpr/lpr* mouse is the best demonstration that a failure in AICD induces an autoimmune disease.[23] The continuing proliferation of autoreactive T cells has been demonstrated to induce activation of E2F1 that may potentiate Bid-dependent apoptosis, which suggests that E2F1 may help in AICD.[2] In the *E2F1*$^{-/-}$ mice, the lack of E2F1 would result in defective connection with the mitochondrial pathway of apoptosis, leading to the survival of autoreactive T and B cells. In the case of B cells, such an effect would be additive, with the increased survival induced by the ove expression of Bcl-2 in B cell of the *E2F1*$^{-/-}$ *hbcl-2* Tg mice.

Finally, there may be additional immune factors that may help to the production of autoimmunity in the *E2F1*$^{-/-}$ *hbcl-2* Tg mice. Thl/Th2 imbalance has been proposed as a pathogenic mechanism in a number of autoimmune diseases, both in humans and mice.[24] We have previously demonstrated that E2F1$^{-/-}$ show an increased production of Th2 cytokines after polyclonal *in vitro* stimulation.[25] These data must be confirmed in the *E2F1*$^{-/-}$ *hbcl-2* Tg mice and could help us to understand the mild phenotype observed.

In conclusion, these preliminary data indicate that the molecular connections proposed at the molecular level between Bcl-2 and E2F1 may have some implications *in vivo*, causing an autoimmune disease. Nonetheless, it must be addressed whether this effect is a consequence of a breakdown of immune tolerance due to disturbances in cell death and/or cell proliferation, and how much Bcl-2 and E2F1 contribute to it.

ACKNOWLEDGMENTS

This work was supported by grants from the Fondo de Investigaciones Sanitarias (PI020417) and the Fundación Marqués Valdecilla (to M.L.H.) and by grants from Fondo de Investigaciones Sanitarias (PI021561) and from the Basque Government (Etortek-IE019) (to A.M.Z.). M.J.M. is a recipient of the Fundación Marqués Valdecilla fellowship for graduate studies. A.B. is a recipient of a grant from the Fondo de Investigaciones Sanitarias (RITC C3/03), and I.G. is a recipient of a Basque Government fellowship for graduate studies.

REFERENCES

1. Woo, M.J. *et al.* 2003. Caspase-3 regulates cell cycle in B cells: a consequence of substrate specificity. Nat. Immunol. **4:** 1016–1022.
2. Cao, Q. *et al.* 2004. The E2F-1 transcription factor promotes caspase-8 and Bid expression, and enhances Fas signaling in T cells. J. Immunol. **173:** 1111–1117.
3. Salmena, L. *et al.* 2003. Essential role for caspase-8 in T-cell homeostasis and T-cell-mediated immunity. Genes Dev. **17:** 883–895.
4. Kovesdi, I., R. Reichel & J.R. Nevins. 1987. Role of an adenovirus E2 promoter binding factor in E1A-mediated coordinate gene control. Proc. Natl. Acad. Sci. USA **84:** 2180–2184.
5. Dyson, N. 1998. The regulation of E2F by pRB-family proteins. Genes Dev. **12:** 2245–2262.
6. Helin, K. 1998. Regulation of cell proliferation by the E2F transcription factors. Curr. Opin. Genes Dev. **8:** 28–35.
7. Phillips, A.C. & K.H. Vousden. 2001. E2F-1 induced apoptosis. Apoptosis **63:** 173–182.
8. Moroni, M.C. *et al.* 2001. Apaf-1 is a transcriptional target for E2F and p53. Nat. Cell Biol. **3:** 552–558.
9. Lissy, N.A. *et al.* 2000. A common E2F-1 and p73 pathway mediates cell death induced by TCR activation. Nature **407:** 642–645.
10. Irwin, M. *et al.* 2000. Role for the p53 homologue p73 in E2F-1 induced apoptosis. Nature **407:** 645–648.
11. Zhu, J.W. *et al.* 1999. A role for E2F1 in the induction of ARF, p53, and apoptosis during thymic negative selection. Cell Growth Differ. **10:** 829–838.
12. Garcia, I. *et al.* 2000. A role for E2F1 in the induction of apoptosis during thymic negative selection. Cell Growth Differ. **11**: 91–98.
13. Chao, D.T. & S.J. Korsmeyer. 1998. Bcl-2 family: regulators of cell death. Annu. Rev. Immunol. **16:** 395–419.
14. O'Reilly, L.A., D.C.S. Huang & A. Strasser 1996. The cell death inhibitor Bcl-2 and its homologues influence control of cell cycle entry. EMBO J. **15:** 6979–6990.
15. Vairo, G. *et al.* 2000. Bcl-2 retards cell cycle entry through p27kip1, pRB relative p130, and altered E2F regulation. Moll. Cell. Biol. **20:** 4745–4753.

16. Lopez-Hoyos, M. *et al.* 1996. Constitutive expression of Bcl-2 in B cells causes a lethal form of lupuslike autoimmune disease after induction of neonatal tolerance to H-2b alloantigens. J. Exp. Med. **183:** 2523–2531.
17. Marquina, R. *et al.* 2004. Inhibition of B cell death causes the development of an IgA nephropathy in (New Zealand White x C57BL/6)F1-bcl-2 transgenic mice. J. Immunol. **172:** 7177–7185.
18. Strasser, A. *et al.* 1991. Enforced Bcl-2 expression in B-lymphoid cells prolongs antibody responses and elicits autoimmune disease. Proc. Natl. Acad. Sci. USA **88:** 8661–8665.
19. Kono, D.H., R. Baccala & A.N. Theofilopoulos. 2004. Genes and genetics of murine lupus. *In* Systemic Lupus Erythematosus. R.G. Lahita, Ed.: 225–263. Elsevier. London.
20. Lang, J. *et al.* 1997. Enforced Bcl-2 expression inhibits antigen-mediated elimination of peripheral B cells in an antigen dose-dependent manner and promotes receptor editing in autoreactive immature B cells. J. Exp. Med. **186:** 1513–1522.
21. Smith, K.G.C. *et al.* 2000. Bcl-2 transgene expression inhibits apoptosis in the germinal center and reveals differences in the selection of memory B cells and bone marrow antibody-forming cells. J. Exp. Med. **191:** 475–484.
22. Opferman, J.T. & S.J. Korsmeyer. 2003. Apoptosis in the development and maintenance of the immune system. Nat. Immunol. **4:** 410–415.
23. Van Parijs, L., A. Biuckians & A.K. Abbas. 1998. Functional roles of Fas and Bcl-2-regulated apoptosis of T lymphocytes. J. Immunol. **160:** 2065–2071.
24. Mosmann, T.R. & S. Sad. 1996. The expanding universe of T-cell subsets: Th1, Th2 and more. Immunol. Today **17:** 138–146.
25. Infante, A. *et al.* 2004. Altered Th1 and Th2 responses in E2F1- and E2F2-deficient mice. Presented at the 12th International Congress of Immunology. Montreal, July 21, 2004.

Systemic Thromboembolism in Inflammatory Bowel Disease

Mechanisms and Clinical Applications

GILAD TWIG, GISELE ZANDMAN-GODDARD, MARTINE SZYPER-KRAVITZ, AND YEHUDA SHOENFELD[a]

Department of Medicine B and Center for Autoimmune Diseases, Sheba Medical Center Tel-Hashomer, Sackler Faculty of Medicine, Tel-Aviv University, Israel

ABSTRACT: Systemic thromboembolism is an extraintestinal manifestation of inflammatory bowel disease (IBD), and an important cause of patient morbidity and mortality. The underlying basis for the hypercoagulable state in IBD is complex, and involves altered activity of all three components that govern hemostasis: platelets, fibrinolysis, and the coagulation cascade. Currently, there are no distinct guidelines for treating or preventing thromboembolic (TE) events in IBD patients compared with the general population. However, the prothrombotic state in IBD stems, at least in part, from several modifiable factors, such as hyperhomocysteinemia and an active inflammatory state. In this review we summarize the mechanisms that favor thrombosis in IBD, and the principles that need to be applied for the primary and secondary prevention of TE in this selected group of patients.

KEYWORDS: thrombosis; hypercoagulable state; inflammatory bowel disease; homocysteinemia

CLINICAL FEATURES OF THROMBOEMBOLISM IN INFLAMMATORY BOWEL DISEASE

Thromboembolic (TE) events in inflammatory bowel disease (IBD) patients were first described in 1936.[1] Ever since, a mounting body of evidence has accumulated suggesting an increased prevalence of TE events in IBD patients. Thrombosis is characterized by both focal microthrombi in the vasculature of the inflamed intestine[2] and systemic TE events,[3,4] leading to extensive morbidity[5,6] and mortality within two years of a TE event.[7]

Two large cohort studies have shown that the overall incidence of TE events is ~6.5% in both Crohn's disease and ulcerative colitis patients, with a three-fold increase in the risk of a systemic TE event compared with the general population.[3,4] However, the fact that in postmortem autopsies the incidence of systemic throm-

[a]Incumbent of the Laura Schwartz-Kipp Chair of Autoimmune Diseases.

Address for correspondence: Prof. Yehuda Shoenfeld, M.D., FRCP (Hon.), Laura Schwarz-Kipp Chair of Autoimmune Diseases, Department of Medicine B, Sheba Medical Center, Tel-Hashomer, 52621, Israel. Voice: 972-3-5302652; fax: 972-3-5352855.

shoenfel@post.tau.ac.il

Ann. N.Y. Acad. Sci. 1051: 166–173 (2005). © 2005 New York Academy of Sciences.
doi: 10.1196/annals.1361.058

TABLE 1. Clinical features of thrombosis in inflammatory bowel disease

	Inflammatory Bowel Disease	References
Overall incidence of thrombosis	6.2%	3, 4
Risk ratio for TE event	3.0–3.6	3, 4
Median time to occurrence of first TE event	~5 years	3, 7
Two-year mortality following a TE event	22–25%	5, 7
Evidence for bowel disease activity at the time of TE event	CD: 60–89% UC: 45–60%	3, 6
Prevalence of DVT or PE	79–87%	3, 7

ABBREVIATIONS: CD, Crohn's disease; DVT, deep vein thrombosis; IBD, inflammatory bowel disease; PE, pulmonary embolus; TE, thromboembolic; UC, ulcerative colitis.

boembolism is nearly six-fold higher than that seen in clinical studies[8] suggests that a large fraction of cases remains undiagnosed. These figures raise the possibility that thromboembolism is a more common extraintestinal manifestation than previously appreciated.

In IBD, systemic TE events occur mainly in the venous circulation,[3,5] but can also develop in the arterial circulation.[9] Deep vein thrombosis (DVT) and pulmonary embolus are the most common types of TE,[3,5] but thromboses are also reported in unusual sites such as cerebral, innominate, retinal, hepatic, and mesenteric veins.[5,6,10,11]

The degree of activity and the extent of inflammatory intestinal disease are generally considered to correlate well (but not invariantly) with the patient's risk for a TE event.[7,12,13] In two large cohort studies, about two-thirds of IBD patients that experienced a TE event had at least one clinical manifestation of active bowel disease.[3,5] In several series of IBD patients, the control of disease activity led to a partial normalization of disturbed coagulation factor profile and platelet activity,[14] and, in turn, anticoagulation therapy attenuated inflammation.[15] Yet at least two lines of evidence suggest that intestinal inflammation cannot account for the hypercoagulable state in IBD patients: (1) One-third of IBD patients experience TE events in the absence of active bowel disease,[3,5] or, in ulcerative colitis patients, even after undergoing proctocolectomy.[6,7] (2) The hypercoagulable state is not found in other autoimmune diseases such as celiac disease, which is also characterized by a substantial inflammatory component.[3] Thus, factors other than inflammation need to be considered for the prothrombotic state in IBD. The clinical features of IBD patients that experienced TE events are shown in TABLE 1.

THE CELLULAR BASIS FOR THE HYPERCOAGULABLE STATE IN INFLAMMATORY BOWEL DISEASE

The cellular basis that underlies the hypercoagulable state in IBD is complex and includes impaired function of all three components that govern hemostasis: platelets, coagulation, and fibrinolysis. These mechanisms are summarized in TABLE 2.

TABLE 2. Potential mechanisms underlying hypercoagulability in inflammatory bowel disease

Platelet/endothelial	Spontaneous platelet aggregation Hyperhomocysteinemia Elevated titers of autoantibodies: aCL, LAC, anti-β_2-GPI Increased levels of von Willebrand factor
Hypercoagulation	Elevated coagulation factors: I, prothrombin. thrombin-antithrombin, V, VII, VIII Decreased AT-III Decreased protein S Decreased protein C Decreased endothelial protein C receptor Elevated titers of autoantibodies: aCL, LAC, anti-β_2-GPI
Hypofibrinolysis	Decreased tPA Decreased PAI Increased TAFI

ABBREVIATIONS: aCL, anti-cardiolipin; AT III, antithrombin III; β_2-GPI, beta2 glycoprotein 1; IBD, inflammatory bowel disease; LAC, lupus anticoagulant; PAI, plasminogen activating inhibitor; TAFI, thrombin-activatable fibrinolysis inhibitor; tPA, tissue plasminogen activator.

Impaired Platelets and Platelet–Endothelial Interactions

Spontaneous platelet aggregation or platelet hypersensitivity to low concentrations of aggregating agents occurs in nearly 50% of IBD patients.[16] Although this feature of IBD platelets may be independent of the disease activity,[16,17] recent evidence suggests that platelet hyperactivation is, at least in part, mediated by the CD40–CD40 ligand (CD40L) pathway. This pathway is increasingly recognized to play a central role in the chronic inflammation that promotes atherosclerosis[18] and platelet activation. IBD platelets overexpress CD40L protein up to four times more frequently than normal platelets and release more soluble CD40L (sCD40L) to the plasma, leading to a ~15-fold increase in CD40L plasma levels.[19] As elevated levels of sCD40 are associated with an increased risk for developing a TE event,[20] the CD40-CD40L pathway may contribute to thrombosis in IBD.[19,21] At the mechanistic level, CD40L overexpression in IBD platelets is likely to originate from interaction with the activated endothelium of the microvasculature of the inflamed mucosa. Two findings support this suggestion: (1) normal platelets exposed to activated human intestinal microvascular endothelial cells (HIMECs) become activated and overexpress CD40L, and (2) platelet CD40L overexpression and increased plasma levels of sCD40L in IBD patients correlate with the extent of bowel disease.[19]

Hyperhomocysteinemia (hyper-Hcy) is a risk factor for arterial and venous thrombosis, having an incidence of about 5% in the general population.[22] Hyper-Hcy is approximately three times more frequent in IBD than in the normal population,[11] and can be secondary to medications (methotrexate, salazopyrine, corticosteroids) and nutritional causes. The latter include decreased levels of vitamin B6,[23] vitamin B12,[24] and folate.[25] Thus, the conversion of homocysteine by the remethylation cycle (folate- and B12-dependent) to methionine or by the trans-sulfuration pathway to cysteine (B6-dependent) are impaired. A comparison between the homocysteine levels of IBD patients with a TE event and those without such a history shows no significant difference in Hcy levels.[11] However, this lack of correlation likely reflects the multifactorial basis for hypercoagulability in IBD patients, and not a lack of contribution of hyper-Hcy to the prothrombotic state in IBD.[12] Therefore, folate and B vitamin supplementation are recommended for IBD patients, as they can successfully lower Hcy levels.[26]

Disturbed Coagulation

Several sites of the coagulation cascade are altered in IBD patients, including increased fibrinogen,[17] increased prothrombin fragments and thrombin-antithrombin complexes,[27] and increased factors V, VII, and VIII.[5,28] This increase in coagulation factors favors clot formation, and therefore predisposes to thrombosis.

The levels of proteins that regulate the coagulation cascade are also altered. The levels of antithrombin III (AT III), a potent endogenous thrombin inhibitor, are significantly lower in the plasma of IBD patients.[13,28] Under normal conditions, activated protein C with its cofactor protein S inhibit activated factors V and VIII, and thereby prevent uncontrolled thrombosis. Although reports on the levels of protein C and protein S in IBD patients are conflicting, a few reports show a deficiency of protein C[29,30] and of protein S[31–33] during active bowel disease. IBD patients also have significantly lower expression of endothelial protein C receptor and thrombomodulin,[34] which impair protein C activation and consequently lead to lower effective protein C activity.[34]

Several studies report that the prevalence of factor V Leiden mutation (activated protein C resistance), the most common inherited thrombophilia, is more frequent in IBD patients than in the general population. However, subsequent works found that the prevalence of this mutation in IBD is similar to that of the general population.[35] Two other common inherited thrombophilias (prothrombin G20210A mutation and C677T variant of the methylenetetrahydrofolate reductase, MTHFR) were as frequent in IBD patients as in the general population.[35] These findings suggest that genetic factors do not account for the hypercoagulable state in IBD.

Fibrinolysis

Impaired systemic fibrinolytic capacity is another potential contributor to the hypercoagulable state in IBD patients. The plasma levels of tissue plasminogen activator (tPA), the principal activator of the fibrinolytic system, are significantly lower in IBD patients than in the general population.[36] In addition, an increase in two proteins that inhibit fibrinolysis, plasminogen activator inhibitor[36] and thrombin-activatable fibrinolysis inhibitor,[37] have been reported. Thus, both decreased activation and increased inhibition of the fibrinolytic system can contribute to hypofibrinolysis in IBD patients.

Autoantibodies

Autoantibodies against several components of the coagulation system are present at a higher frequency in IBD patients and may predispose for thrombosis. Antiphospholipid antibodies that include anti-cardiolipin (aCL) antibodies and lupus anticoagulant (LAC) facilitate thrombosis by activating endothelial cells and platelets and by impairing the activity of anticoagulation proteins. The prevalence of aCL antibodies in IBD patients is higher than in controls, with an average incidence of ~20%, but with a reported incidence in excess of 30%.[38] Antibodies against β2-glycoprotein I (β2-GPI), the cofactor that mediates the binding of aCL antibodies to cardiolipin, is a more specific parameter for evaluating the risk for thrombosis.[39] The incidence of β2-GPI antibodies in IBD patients is ~9%, compared with none in healthy controls.[39] Reports on the association of LAC with IBD patients are more conflicting, as one report indicated a 19% incidence,[40] whereas others found no difference between IBD patients and healthy controls.[6]

Antibodies against protein S were described in ~8% of IBD patients, but they were independent of protein S level. However, elevated titers of protein S antibodies, LAC, and aCL and β2-GPI antibodies, were not shown to be significantly different in IBD patients with TE events compared with IBD patients without such a history.[33,39,40] Follow-up studies will be necessary to assess the predictive value of these autoantibodies on the subsequent development of TE events.

TREATMENT

Despite numerous studies on the link between IBD and thrombosis, there are currently no distinct guidelines for the management of a TE event in this selected group of patients. In this section we list the recommendations for minimizing the risk of thrombosis, based on recent published clinical work in the field (TABLE 3).

In an outpatient setting, minimizing modifiable risk factors is a critical step in patient treatment that cannot be overemphasized. Smoking, oral contraceptive therapy, and hormone replacement therapy (HRT) should be avoided.[41] Immobility is a principal risk factor for TE events in IBD patients[7] that needs to be avoided, together with other conditions that facilitate blood stasis, such as obesity. Vitamins B6 and B12 and folate supplements should be included in the diet of IBD patients to avoid hyperhomocysteinemia, especially in the case of extensive bowel disease. It is advisable to measure the plasma level of homocysteine to assess the response to these supplements. Attenuation of mucosal inflammation is an important step in minimizing the procoagulant state, as coagulation function is partially normalized during remission of bowel disease. In fact, one report even suggested venous thromboembolism to be an indication for surgical resection of the inflamed bowel,[5] but currently no further evidence supports this approach.

Screening for inherited thrombophilia, such as Factor V Leiden mutation, prothrombin G20210A mutation, and C677T variant of the MTHFR, as well as screening for protein C and protein S deficiency, AT III deficiency, aCL, LAC, and hyper-Hcy in IBD patients is a complex and controversial issue of great clinical significance. Currently, no special guidelines for IBD patients exist. Yet several factors such as (i) the degree of bowel disease activity, (ii) patient history of a TE event, or (iii) family history of TE event(s) may suggest a need for thrombophilia screening. Such screening in IBD patients, especially in the presence of a family history of thrombosis, is advisable, as a positive screening may change therapeutic management and necessitate primary prevention with heparin or low-molecular-weight he-

TABLE 3. Prevention of thromboembolic events in patients with IBD

Strategy	Treatment
Minimize modifiable risk factors	
Avoid procoagulant agents	Avoid smoking, HRT/OCT
Minimize blood stasis	Mobilization, support stockings, and avoiding obesity
Minimize vessel injury	Restricted use of central intravenous catheters
Reduce hyperhomocysteinemia	Nutrient supplements (vitamin B6, vitamin B12, folic acid) Follow-up of homocysteine level
Control bowel inflammation activity	Consider heparin treatment depending on: Degree of immobility History of thrombosis Bowel disease activity
Assess risk for thrombosis	Consider thrombophilia screening: Prior events of thrombosis Family history of thrombosis Concurrence with other risk factors Degree of bowel inflammation

ABBREVIATIONS: IBD, inflammatory bowel disease; HRT, hormone replacement therapy; OCT, oral contraception therapy; TE event, thromboembolic event.

parin. In IBD patients who have had a TE event, the concurrence of IBD activity and positive screening for thrombophilia justifies the inclusion of heparin in the patient's therapy, as it is a relative indication for lifelong anticoagulation.[7] Thus, the similar prevalence of inherited thrombophilia among IBD patients and among the general population does not mean that the indications for thrombophilia screening should also be similar.

On an inpatient basis, support stockings and early mobilization are recommended to minimize blood stasis, the leading prothrombotic risk factor in IBD patients.[7] Restricted use of central intravenous catheters is recommended to minimize vessel injury. Primary prevention with heparin or low-molecular-weight heparin in a patient with extensive and aggravated bowel disease that is steroid resistant is increasingly recognized as an acceptable treatment.[15,42–44] This is an intriguing and paradoxical effect of heparin, considering that aggravation of bowel disease is often accompanied by anemia and gastrointestinal bleeding. The emerging anti-inflammatory properties of heparin, *in vitro* and *in vivo*, provide the basis for this therapy.[45] Double-blind placebo-controlled studies are needed to define accurately the degree of bowel disease severity that justifies treatment with heparin.

To conclude, IBD patients have an approximately threefold greater risk for developing a TE event compared with the normal population. The risk for thrombosis correlates well with disease activity in Crohn's disease, and to lesser extent in ulcerative colitis. The cellular basis for hypercoagulability in these patients is not completely understood but is likely to be multifactorial, and, therefore, there is no single laboratory marker that reliably correlates with the occurrence of thrombosis. Modifiable risk factors should be minimized, early inpatient mobilization should be encouraged, and folate and vitamin B supplementation should be prescribed to control homocysteine levels. Heparin treatment may have a central role in the treatment of IBD patients with active bowel disease and/or increased risk for thrombosis, due to its dual anticoagulation and anti-inflammatory benefits. Further studies are needed to characterize the criteria for its use.

REFERENCES

1. BARGEN, J.A. & N.W. BARKER. 1936. Extensive arterial and venous thrombosis complicating ulcerative colitis. Arch. Intern. Med. **58:** 17–31.
2. WAKEFIELD, A.J. *et al.* 1989. Pathogenesis of Crohn's disease: multifocal gastrointestinal infarction. Lancet **334:** 1057–1062.
3. MIEHSLER, W. *et al.* 2004. Is inflammatory bowel disease an independent and disease specific risk factor for thromboembolism? Gut **53:** 542–548.
4. BERNSTEIN, C.N., J.F. BLANCHARD, D.F. HOUSTON & A. WAJDA. 2001. The incidence of deep venous thrombosis and pulmonary embolism among patients with inflammatory bowel disease: a population-based cohort study. Thromb. Haemost. **85:** 430–434.
5. TALBOT, R.W., J. HEPPELL, R.R. DOZOIS & R.W. BEART, JR. 1986. Vascular complications of inflammatory bowel disease. Mayo Clin. Proc. **61:** 140–145.
6. JACKSON, L.M. *et al.* 1997. Thrombosis in inflammatory bowel disease: clinical setting, procoagulant profile and factor V Leiden. QJM **90:** 183–188.
7. SOLEM, C.A., E.V. LOFTUS, W.J. TREMAINE & W.J. SANDBORN. 2004. Venous thromboembolism in inflammatory bowel disease. Am. J. Gastroenterol. **99:** 97–101.
8. GRAEF, V. *et al.* 1965. Venous thrombosis occurring in non-specific ulcerative colitis. Arch. Intern. Med. **117:** 377–382.
9. NOVACEK, G. *et al.* 2004. Aortic mural thrombi in patients with inflammatory bowel disease: report of two cases and review of the literature. Inflamm. Bowel Dis. **10:** 430–435.
10. MURATA, S. *et al.* 2004. Cerebral sinus thrombosis associated with severe active ulcerative colitis. Intern. Med. **43:** 400–403.
11. OLDENBURG, B. *et al.* 2000. Homocysteine in inflammatory bowel disease: a risk factor for thromboembolic complications? Am. J. Gastroenterol. **95:** 2825–2830.
12. SAIBENI, S., L. SPINA & M. VECCHI. 2004. Exploring the relationships between inflammatory response and coagulation cascade in inflammatory bowel disease. Eur. Rev. Med. Pharmacol. Sci. **8:** 205–208.
13. SOUTO, J.C. *et al.* 1995. Prothrombotic state and signs of endothelial lesion in plasma of patients with inflammatory bowel disease. Dig. Dis. Sci. **40:** 1883–1889.
14. HOMMES, D.W. *et al.* 1997. Beneficial effect of treatment with a monoclonal anti-tumor necrosis factor-alpha antibody on markers of coagulation and fibrinolysis in patients with active Crohn's disease. Haemostasis **27:** 269–277.
15. GAFFNEY, P.R. *et al.* 1995. Paradoxical response to heparin in 10 patients with ulcerative colitis. Am. J. Gastroenterol. **90:** 220–223.
16. WEBBERLEY, M.J., M.T. HART & V. MELIKIAN. 1993. Thromboembolism in inflammatory bowel disease: role of platelets. Gut **34:** 247–251.
17. CHIARANTINI, E. *et al.* 1996. Hemostatic abnormalities in inflammatory bowel disease. Thromb. Res. **82:** 137–146.
18. LIBBY, P. 2003. Vascular biology of atherosclerosis: overview and state of the art. Am. J. Cardiol. **91:** 3A–6A.
19. DANESE, S. *et al.* 2003. Activated platelets are the source of elevated levels of soluble CD40 ligand in the circulation of inflammatory bowel disease patients. Gut **52:** 1435–1441.
20. VARO, N. *et al.* 2003. Soluble CD40L: risk prediction after acute coronary syndromes. Circulation **108:** 1049–1052.
21. KOUTROUBAKIS, I.E. *et al.* 2004. Association between enhanced soluble CD40 ligand and prothrombotic state in inflammatory bowel disease. Eur. J. Gastroenterol. Hepatol. **16:** 1147–1152.

22. McCully, K.S. 1996. Homocysteine and vascular disease. Nat. Med. **2:** 386–389.
23. Saibeni, S. *et al.* 2003. Low vitamin B(6) plasma levels, a risk factor for thrombosis, in inflammatory bowel disease: role of inflammation and correlation with acute phase reactants. Am. J. Gastroenterol. **98:** 112–117.
24. Romagnuolo, J. *et al.* 2001. Hyperhomocysteinemia and inflammatory bowel disease: prevalence and predictors in a cross-sectional study. Am. J. Gastroenterol. **96**: 2143–2149.
25. Lashner, B.A. *et al.* 1989. Effect of folate supplementation on the incidence of dysplasia and cancer in chronic ulcerative colitis. A case-control study. Gastroenterology **97:** 255–259.
26. Cattaneo, M. *et al.* 1998. High prevalence of hyperhomocysteinemia in patients with inflammatory bowel disease: a pathogenic link with thromboembolic complications? Thromb. Haemost. **80:** 542–545.
27. Chamouard, P. *et al.* 1995. Prothrombin fragment 1 +,2 and thrombin-antithrombin III complex as markers of activation of blood coagulation in inflammatory bowel diseases. Eur. J. Gastroenterol. Hepatol. **7:** 1183–1188.
28. Lake, A.M., J.Q. Stauffer & M.J. Stuart. 1978. Hemostatic alterations in inflammatory bowel disease: response to therapy. Am. J. Dig. Dis. **23:** 897–902.
29. Jorens, P.G. *et al.* 1990. Acquired protein C and S deficiency, inflammatory bowel disease and cerebral arterial thrombosis. Blut **61:** 307–310.
30. Larsen, T.B. *et al.* 2002. Platelets and anticoagulant capacity in patients with inflammatory bowel disease. Pathophysiol. Haemost. Thromb. **32:** 92–96.
31. Wyshock, E., M. Caldwell & J.P. Crowley. 1988. Deep venous thrombosis, inflammatory bowel disease, and protein S deficiency. Am. J. Clin. Pathol. **90:** 633–635.
32. Koutroubakis, I.E. *et al.* 2000. Resistance to activated protein C and low levels of free protein S in Greek patients with inflammatory bowel disease. Am. J. Gastroenterol. **95:** 190–194.
33. Saibeni, S. *et al.* 2001. Reduced free protein S levels in patients with inflammatory bowel disease: prevalence, clinical relevance, and role of anti-protein S antibodies. Dig. Dis. Sci. **46:** 637–643.
34. Faioni, E.M. *et al.* 2004. Expression of endothelial protein C receptor and thrombomodulin in the intestinal tissue of patients with inflammatory bowel disease. Crit. Care Med. **32:** S266–270.
35. Papa, A. *et al.* 2003. Review article: inherited thrombophilia in inflammatory bowel disease. Am. J. Gastroenterol. **98:** 1247–1251.
36. Gris, J.C. *et al.* 1990. Impaired fibrinolytic capacity in patients with inflammatory bowel disease. Thromb. Haemost. **63:** 472–475.
37. Saibeni, S. *et al.* 2004. Assessment of thrombin-activatable fibrinolysis inhibitor (TAFI) plasma levels in inflammatory bowel diseases. Am. J. Gastroenterol. **99:** 1966–1970.
38. Koutroubakis, I.E. 2000. Role of thrombotic vascular risk factors in inflammatory bowel disease. Dig. Dis. **18:** 161–167.
39. Koutroubakis, I.E. *et al.* 1998. Anti-cardiolipin and anti-beta2-glycoprotein I antibodies in patients with inflammatory bowel disease. Dig. Dis. Sci. **43:** 2507–2512.
40. Heneghan, M.A. *et al.* 1998. Activated protein C resistance, thrombophilia, and inflammatory bowel disease. Dig. Dis. Sci. **43:** 1356–1361.
41. Wakefield, A.J. *et al.* 1991. Smoking, the oral contraceptive pill, and Crohn's disease. Dig. Dis. Sci. **36:** 1147–1150.
42. Vrij, A.A. *et al.* 2001. Low molecular weight heparin treatment in steroid refractory ulcerative colitis: clinical outcome and influence on mucosal capillary thrombi. Scand. J. Gastroenterol, Suppl. **234:** 41–47.
43. Kao, A. *et al.* 2002. Anticoagulation therapy in cerebral sinovenous thrombosis and ulcerative colitis in children. J. Child Neurol. **17:** 479–482.
44. Ageno, W. *et al.* 2002. Thrombosis prophylaxis in medical patients: a retrospective review of clinical practice patterns. Haematologica **87:** 746–750; discussion 250.
45. Tyrrell, D.J. *et al.* 1999. Heparin in inflammation: potential therapeutic applications beyond anticoagulation. Adv. Pharmacol. **46:** 151–208.

Pregnancy Loss and Endometriosis

Pathogenic Role of Anti-Laminin-1 Autoantibodies

JUNKO INAGAKI,[a] AKANE KONDO,[a,b] LUIS R. LOPEZ,[c] YEHUDA SHOENFELD,[d] AND EIJI MATSUURA[a]

[a]*Department of Cell Chemistry, Okayama University Graduate School of Medicine and Dentistry, Okayama, Japan*

[b]*Department of Obstetrics and Gynecology, Tokai University, Isehara, Japan*

[c]*Corgenix, Inc., Westminster, Colorado, USA*

[d]*Department of Medicine B and Center for Autoimmune Diseases, Sheba Medical Center, Tel-Hashomer, Israel*

ABSTRACT: Laminin-1 is a major multifunctional glycoprotein that forms an integral part of the scaffolding network of basement membranes, and is the earliest synthesized component during embryogenesis. This protein (α1β1γ1) plays an important role in basement membrane assembly and epiblast differentiation during embryonic development. Anti-laminin-1 autoantibodies are known to cause infertility and recurrent spontaneous abortion in animals. Recently, we reported that the presence of IgG anti-laminin-1 antibodies (Abs) in the blood is significantly associated with recurrent first-trimester miscarriages and subsequent negative pregnancy outcomes. Interestingly, these antibodies are also strongly associated with infertility, especially infertility caused by endometriosis. Laminin-α1, laminin-β1, and laminin-γ1 mRNAs were also detected in 90% of endometriotic lesions, and all laminin-α1, laminin-β1, and laminin-γ1 chains were localized to the basement membranes of glandular epithelium in endometriotic peritoneal lesions. ELISA showed specific reactivity of the autoantibodies to a particular region of the laminin-1 molecule, that is, the α1 chain G domain. IgM monoclonal anti-laminin-1 Abs, which we recently established, also recognized the G domain and cross-reacted with human α1 chain located in the basement membrane of the glandular epithelium of human endometrium. We also established an animal model that produced high titers of anti-laminin-1 Abs after immunization with mouse laminin-1. Anti-laminin-1 Abs from the immunized mice caused a higher fetal resorption rate with lower embryonic and placental weights. Thus, anti-laminin-1 Abs may be important in the development of autoimmune-mediated reproductive failures, and the assessment of the such antibodies may provide a novel means for noninvasive diagnosis of endometriosis.

KEYWORDS: anti-laminin-1 autoantibody; recurrent spontaneous abortion; infertility; endometriosis; adenomyosis

Address for correspondence: Eiji Matsuura, Ph.D., Associate Professor, Department of Cell Chemistry, Okayama University Graduate School of Medicine and Dentistry, 2-5-1 Shikata-cho, Okayama 700-8558, Japan. Voice: +81-86-235-7402; fax: +81-86-235-7404.
eijimatu@md.okayama-u.ac.jp

**Ann. N.Y. Acad. Sci. 1051: 174–184 (2005). © 2005 New York Academy of Sciences.
doi: 10.1196/annals.1361.059**

LAMININ ISOFORMS

Laminins are major scaffolding network–forming components of basement membranes (BMs) organized in thin layers of extracellular matrix found at the basal surface of many cell types. These proteins are cruciform heterotrimeric glycoproteins composed of α, β, and γ chains.[1] Five distinct α chains, three β chains, and three γ chains have been identified, and these subunits assemble into at least 15 laminin isoforms that display tissue-specific expression during different stages of development.[2,3]

Of the 15 laminin isoforms, laminin-1 (α1β1γ1) and laminin-10 (α5β1γ1) are expressed earliest during embryogenesis. In blastocysts or in the early implanting mouse embryo, laminin-1 is expressed in the inner cell mass and in trophectoderm basement membrane, whereas laminin-10 is expressed in the matrix between the cells of the inner cell mass and the polar trophectoderm basement membrane. As implantation proceeds, although laminin-1 and laminin-10 are found in both embryonic basement membrane and Reithert's membrane, laminin-1 is the predominant laminin in Reithert's membrane and laminin-10 is predominantly expressed in embryonic basement membrane.[4]

The laminin-β1 and laminin-γ1 chains are detected starting from the two-cell stage of the preimplantation mouse embryo, and are widely expressed in adult tissues. Laminin-α1 chain appears at the 8- to 16-cell stage, and its expression is decreased or absent at most sites during maturation.[2,5,6] Therefore, the distribution of laminin-1 is extremely limited in adult tissues.[7] Laminin-2 (α2β1γ1) and laminin-4 (α2β2γ1) are the most abundant isoforms in muscle and nerve tissues.[8–10] Laminin-5 (α3β3γ2) is an epidermis-specific isoform.[11] Laminin-10 (α5β1γ1) and laminin-11 (α5β2γ1) are widely expressed in both embryonic and adult tissues such as lung, heart, bone marrow, pancreas, and kidney.[2,12] Laminin-8 (α4β1γ1) is typically distributed in mesenchyme or mesenchyme-derived cells (adipocytes, muscle cells, bone marrow, and blood vessels), and is found in all vascular endothelial basement membranes of fetal and adult tissues.[2,13–15]

STRUCTURE AND BIOLOGICAL FUNCTIONS OF LAMININS

The carboxy (C)-terminal of the three laminin chains associate into a triple-stranded coiled-coil arrangement to form a cruciform structure with three short arms and one long arm. The amino (N)-terminal moieties of each chain form three short arms and join together to form the long arm ending in the carboxyl-terminal globular domain (G domain).[16] Although some chains exist as alternatively spliced forms, these chains have common structural features, such as the tandem distribution of globular, rod-like, and coiled-coil domains.[16–18] Laminins play significant roles in the adhesion, migration, proliferation, and differentiation of cells, and in the maintenance of tissue architecture.[19] These biological processes occur through signal transduction and cell-matrix interactions mediated by laminin-specific receptors and other matrix components.[20] In particular, the carboxyl-terminal G domain of the laminin-α chain has five tandemly arrayed subdomains, and contains the recognition sites of several integrin receptors and sites for heparin binding, thus playing a role in various biological activities.[19,21,22]

Laminin-1, first isolated from the mouse Engelbreth-Holm-Swarm tumor,[23] is the most extensively characterized isoform. Although this protein remains present as a major epithelial laminin in some adult tissues, its expression is extremely limited in adult tissues.[7] This protein appears very early during epithelial morphogenesis in the embryo and plays a critical role in embryonic development and placentation.[2,19,24] The absence of laminin-1 causes abnormal morphogenesis of embryonic BM and a lack of development of Reichert's membrane, leading to very early embryonic death.[24,25]

The multiple biological activities of laminin-1 have been dissected using proteolytic laminin fragments, recombinant proteins, and synthetic peptides. According to studies with synthesized peptides, the YIGSR sequence located on the β1 chain promotes cell adhesion and migration, and inhibits angiogenesis and tumor metastasis.[26–28] The IKVAV sequence located on the α1 chain promotes cell adhesion, neurite outgrowth, experimental metastasis, collagenase IV induction, angiogenesis, cell growth, and tumor growth.[29–32] In particular, the laminin-α1 chain carboxyl-terminal G domain has been identified as a site of multiple biological activities. Nineteen potentially active sequences, including five peptides (AG-10, AG-22, AG-32, AG-56, and AG-73) with cell attachment activities, have been identified in the domain.[22] These peptides promote heparin binding, cell adhesion, neurite outgrowth, and tumor growth and metastasis.

Furthermore, recent studies using laminin-γ1 or β1-integrin null mouse embryonic stem cells demonstrated that these cells were unable to synthesize laminin-1, form basement membranes, or undergo epiblast differentiation and cavitation. In each cell line, exogenous laminin-1 rescued basement membrane formation, epiblast differentiation, and cavitation.[33,34] These studies showed the critical role of laminin-α1 chain in basement membrane assembly and epiblast differentiation. Analysis using laminin-1 fragments or recombinant laminin-α1 domains demonstrated that embryonic basement membrane assembly and cellular differentiation required polymerization of laminin-1 through its three short arms, and interaction (anchorage) with the cells of the inner cell mass through a heparin-binding sequence in the laminin-α1 chain G domain. Of all identified laminin isoforms, laminin-1 appears to be essential in very early embryogenesis and the peri-implantation period.

AUTOANTIBODIES TO LAMININ-1 AND REPRODUCTIVE FAILURE

Reproductive failure, including recurrent spontaneous abortion and infertility, can result from multiple causes. More than 60% of spontaneous abortions are caused by fetal death due to chromosomal abnormalities, whereas the remainder are due to maternal causes, including infection, physical defects, hormonal factors, immune dysfunction, and systemic disease. Autoimmune dysfunction in clinically asymptomatic patients also may lead to recurrent spontaneous abortions.[35] Some recurrent aborters have, in fact, one or more types of abnormal autoantibodies (auto-Abs). Although autoimmune mechanisms in reproductive failure have not been clarified entirely, antiphospholipid Abs in particular, such as β2-glycoprotein I (β2GPI)-dependent anticardiolipin Abs and lupus anticoagulants, anti-DNA Abs, and antinuclear Abs, have been implicated in recurrent abortions. One mechanism in spontaneous abortion is thought to be thrombosis of the placental vasculature and placental infarction, caused by the reaction of auto-Abs against β2-glycoprotein I, prothrombin, and/or annexin V. Another possible cause is direct binding of auto-Abs to cytotrophoblast cells, impairing trophoblast invasion into maternal decidua and implantation by preventing differentiation to syncytiotrophoblast.[36] Many investigators have attempted to establish an association between specific auto-Abs and reproductive failure, yet the potential immunological causes of recurrent abortions are still only poorly understood. The presence of each auto-Ab alone or even the combination of at least two types of auto-Abs cannot satisfactorily predict miscarriages.[37] We have found that in some cases miscarriages recurred even with low-dose aspirin treatment, in spite of significantly reduced antiphospholipid Ab and/or antinuclear Ab titers. Therefore, it is necessary to identify other auto-Abs that potentially can serve as markers for miscarriage risk.

The presence of serum auto-Abs against laminin-1 was initially associated with recurrent miscarriages in monkeys.[38] These sera subsequently were found to cause abnormalities in cultured rat embryos.[39] Immunization with murine laminin-1 or laminin-1 peptides (i.e., YIGSR or RGD) of monkeys that previously had had multiple successful pregnancies caused embryotoxicity and infertility or spontaneous abortion.[40,41] Passive immunization with rabbit anti-laminin-1 Abs in pregnant mice also induced spontaneous abortion. These Abs were detected in Reichert's membrane and visceral yolk sac endoderm cells from the embryos.[42] These data suggested that anti-laminin-1 auto-Abs could be one cause of reproductive failure.

We also established an animal model that produced high titers of anti-laminin-1 Abs after immunization with mouse laminin-1. Anti-laminin-1 Abs from the immunized mice caused a higher fetal resorption rate with lower embryonic and placental weights.[43] Thus, anti-laminin-1 Abs may affect implantation and/or the fetal development in the mouse model.

CLINICAL SIGNIFICANCE OF IgG ANTI-LAMININ-1 ANTIBODIES

Recurrent Abortions

Our recent clinical study showed that serum IgG anti-laminin-1 Abs are significantly associated with recurrent first-trimester miscarriages in humans.[44]

A total of 177 recurrent aborters with a history of two or more consecutive first-trimester miscarriages were enrolled into a study and were tested for the presence of anti-laminin-1 Abs, β2GPI-dependent anticardiolipin Abs, lupus anticoagulants, anti-DNA Abs, and antinuclear Abs before they conceived again. These recurrent aborters were then followed-up during subsequent pregnancies, and the outcomes were evaluated relative to their blood test results prior to pregnancy. Fifty-five (31.1%) women out of 177 recurrent aborters were positive for IgG anti-laminin-1Abs. IgG anti-laminin-1 Ab levels (but not IgM Abs) in recurrent aborters were significantly higher than those of healthy pregnant women and healthy nonpregnant women ($P = .0043$ and $P = .0073$, respectively; FIG. 1). The live-birth rate of subsequent pregnancies of IgG anti-laminin-1 auto-Ab-positive recurrent aborters was significantly lower than that of IgG anti-laminin-1 auto-Abs-negative recurrent aborters ($P = .032$). There were no significant relationships observed between IgG anti-laminin-1 Abs and the other auto-Abs tested. This study demonstrated that IgG

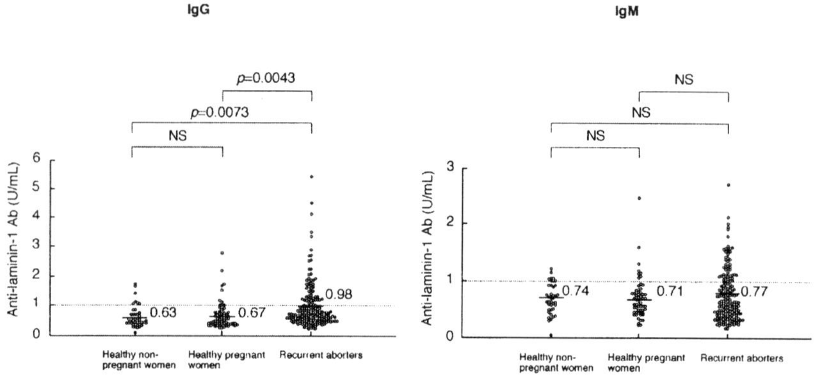

FIGURE 1. Levels of IgG or IgM anti-laminin-1 antibodies in recurrent spontaneous aborters. Anti-laminin-1 antibodies were detected by ELISA using a laminin-1-coated plate. *Dotted line* shows 1 U/mL (1 U/mL = OD, the mean + 3 SD of healthy nonpregnant women), as a cut-off value for the antibodies. *Solid lines* show mean values.[44]

anti laminin-1 auto-Abs are closely related to recurrent miscarriages and subsequent pregnancy outcomes of recurrent aborters. Our findings suggest that IgG anti-laminin-1 Abs may have a harmful effect on events during early stages of pregnancy, such as embryonic implantation, embryogenesis, placental vascularization, and/or placental nutrient transport.

Infertility Caused by Endometriosis

Our recent clinical study also showed that IgG anti-laminin-1 Abs are significantly associated with endometriosis in infertile patients.[45]

Sixty-eight infertile patients who underwent laparoscopy or laparotomy were tested for the presence of IgG anti-laminin-1 Abs. Twenty infertile patients (29%) were positive for anti-laminin-1 Abs. Antibody levels in these patients were significantly higher than those in healthy nonpregnant women (P = .0005; FIG. 2). The presence of auto-Abs correlated significantly with endometriosis in these patients (P = .0096). Seventeen of 42 infertile patients with endometriosis (40%) tested positive for anti-laminin-1 Abs. Other causes of infertility (tubal factor, hormonal abnormality, uterine anomaly, and unexplained) were not associated with these Abs. The values of anti-laminin-1 Abs were compared between infertile patients with and without endometriosis. Significantly elevated values of these Abs were observed in 42 infertile patients with endometriosis (mean value = 1.1 ± 1.2 U/mL) compared with those without endometriosis (0.46 ± 0.33 U/mL) (P = .015); FIG. 3).

In addition, ELISA showed specific auto-Ab reactivity to a particular region of the laminin-1 molecule, that is, the $\alpha 1$ chain G domain. Laminin-$\alpha 1$, laminin-$\beta 1$, and laminin-$\gamma 1$ mRNAs were also detected in 90% of endometriotic lesions. The mRNAs were detected in tissues at all four stages of endometriosis.

In this study, we demonstrate that infertile patients have significantly higher levels of anti-laminin-1 Abs. These results suggest that anti-laminin-1 Abs may be involved not only in recurrent first-trimester miscarriages, but also in infertility in humans. We

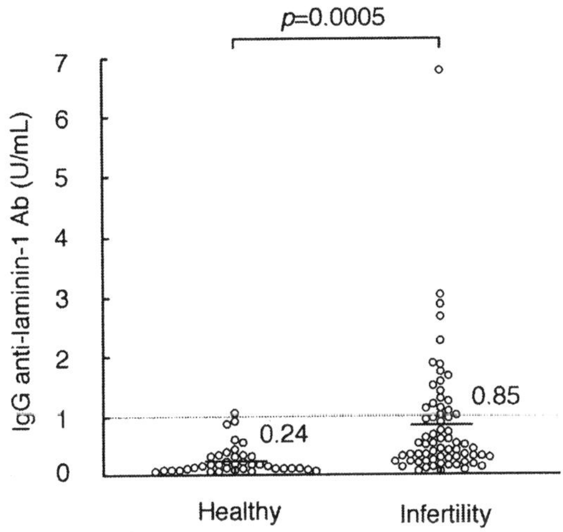

FIGURE 2. IgG values of anti-laminin-1 antibodies in 68 infertile patients who underwent laparoscopy or laparotomy. Anti-laminin-1 antibodies were detected by ELISA using a laminin-1-coated plate. *Dotted line* shows 1 U/mL (1 U/mL = OD, the mean + 3 SD of healthy nonpregnant women), as a cut-off value for the antibodies. *Solid lines* show mean values.[45]

also show that these Abs are strongly associated with infertility, and especially with endometriosis, a widely accepted cause of infertility. A number of studies indicate that infertile patients with endometriosis frequently have elevated levels of auto-Abs specific for endometrial, ovarian, nuclear, and other antigens.[46–48] Although the mechanism of infertility in this disease is poorly understood, it has been suggested that an aberrant immunological mechanism, including the production of auto-Abs, may be involved in infertility. The presence of anti-laminin-1 Abs in infertile patients with endometriosis, and the function of laminin-1 in embryogenesis, implantation, and placentation, suggest that anti-laminin-1 Abs may play a role in modulating very early reproductive processes, and may be responsible for endometriosis-associated infertility.

From our data, anti-laminin-1 Abs in infertile patients with endometriosis clearly recognize the G domain of the laminin-α1 chain. The G domain contains the recognition sites of several integrin receptors, playing a role in various biological activities.[19,21,22] It has been shown that the direct inhibition of laminin-1 binding to integrin receptors and to other basement membrane components by anti-laminin-1 Abs impairs normal basement membrane formation and epithelial morphogenesis.[49] Therefore, it is possible that these antibodies may also interfere directly with the function of laminin-1, disrupt early reproductive stages, and be involved in endometriosis-associated infertility.

Adenomyosis

Endometriosis and adenomyosis are benign estrogen-dependent diseases that are found in women of reproductive age. Although these diseases often result in similar symptoms and have many similarities pathophysiologically, they are considered dis-

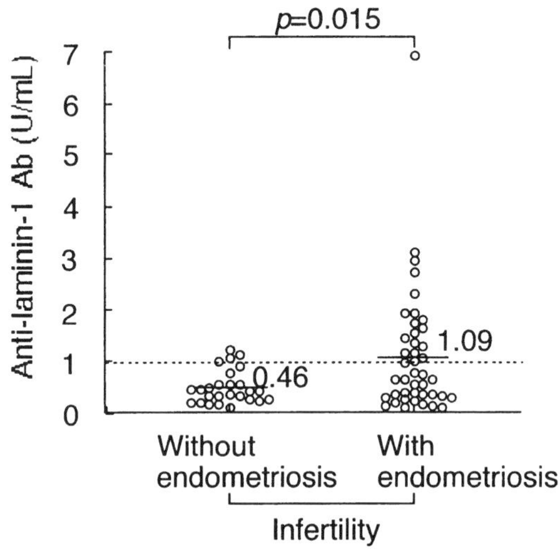

FIGURE 3. Comparison of IgG values of anti-laminin-1 antibodies between infertile patients with and without endometriosis. The *dotted* and *solid lines* show the cut-off and mean values for the antibodies, respectively.[45]

tinct entities. Endometriosis is defined as the presence of endometrial glands and stroma outside the uterine cavity, whereas adenomyosis is characterized by the penetration of endometrial glands and stroma into the myometrium. More recently, we examined the presence of IgG anti-laminin-1 auto-Abs in patients with adenomyosis to assess whether these Abs are associated with adenomyosis as well as endometriosis. IgG anti-laminin-1 Abs were significantly associated with endometriosis, but not with adenomyosis (manuscript in preparation).

LAMININ-1 EXPRESSION IN ENDOMETRIOTIC AND ADENOMYOTIC LESIONS

Immunohistochemical study with specific monoclonal Abs demonstrated that laminin-α1, laminin-β1, and laminin-γ1 chains are present in the basement membranes of ectopic glandular epithelium of both endometriotic and adenomyotic lesions. Laminin-α1 chain was detected only in the basement membranes of glandular epithelium, whereas laminin-β1 and laminin-γ1 chains were strongly expressed in the basement membranes of vascular endothelium and in connective tissue stroma, in addition to the basement membranes of glandular epithelium (manuscript in preparation). Anti-laminin-1 Abs were significantly associated with endometriosis but not with adenomyosis, despite the expression of laminin-1 in the basement membranes of the ectopic glandular epithelium of both endometriotic and adenomyotic lesions. Although the reason is not clear, this difference may be related to the location of endometriotic and adenomyotic foci, that is, in the peritoneal cavity versus myometrium, and to their etiologies.

SPECIFICITY OF ANTI-LAMININ-1 ANTIBODIES

Using Western blot analysis, we showed that anti-laminin-1 Abs from both recurrent aborters and infertile patients with endometriosis reacted with all laminin-1 chains, that is, laminin-α1, laminin-β1, and laminin-γ1. ELISA also confirmed that a target epitope for the Abs is present in a particular region of the laminin-1 molecule, that is, the carboxyl-terminal G domain of the α1 chain. It has been reported that many sites responsible for various biological activities, including promotion of heparin binding, cell attachment, and neurite outgrowth, are located in the G domain. Therefore, we examined the binding specificity of the Abs, using direct and inhibition ELISA with 113 systematically synthesized 12-mer peptides (AG peptides) that cover the entire amino acid sequence of the laminin-α1 chain G domain. Anti-laminin-1 Abs recognized several particular AG-peptide sequences from the G domain. A few of the AG peptide sequences recognized by the Abs included sites with activities involving cell adhesion and spreading. Interestingly, the anti-laminin-1 Abs bound most avidly to the peptide with the strongest cell attachment activity (manuscript in preparation). This peptide has an important role in multiple biological activities, such as cell adhesion and spreading, cell differentiation, neurite outgrowth, and basement membrane remodeling. Therefore, Abs that bind to this peptide sequence may interfere with important biological functions of laminin-1. Further, we recently have established a mouse IgM monoclonal Ab (mAb) against the laminin-α1 chain G domain from mice immunized with mouse laminin-1, and have characterized its specificity and the structure of its epitope.[50] Immunohistochemical analysis showed that this mAb specifically cross-reacts to basement membranes of endometrial glandular epithelium in both mouse and human. It has been suggested that this mAb may recognize a structure common to the G domain of the laminin-α1 chain of both mice and humans. In addition, the specificity of this mAb to peptides derived from the G domain was similar to that of anti-laminin-1 Abs from patients with endometriosis.[50] The epitope recognized by this mAb may be a site commonly recognized by human auto-Abs. Although human serum anti-laminin-1 auto-Abs are polyclonal, at least one of the major epitopes was also recognized by this mouse mAb.

As previously described, anti-laminin-1 Abs induced by active immunization with mouse laminin-1 affect fetal development in the immunized mice. Our greatest interest is in whether such anti-laminin-1 Abs associated with recurrent spontaneous abortions and endometriosis-associated infertility may prevent cell-cell interactions, impair the formation of normal basement membranes, and disrupt early reproductive stages, that is, whether such Abs are pathogenic, protective, or merely an epiphenomenon.

CONCLUSIONS

- Laminin α1 chain differs from other laminin chains. It is generally expressed during specific early stages of embryogenesis (8- to 16-cell stage); it is also found in some adult tissues, but its distribution is extremely limited.
- Laminin-1 appears to be essential for embryonic basement membrane assembly and epiblast differentiation during very early embryogenesis.
- IgG (but not IgM) anti-laminin-1 Abs are occasionally present in recurrent aborters.

- In animal models, active immunization with mouse laminin-1 causes abortions in the anti-laminin-1 Ab–positive group.
- The appearance of IgG anti-laminin-1 Abs is significantly related to infertility associated with endometriosis, but not with adenomyosis.
- Laminin-1 has been detected in the basement membranes of ectopic glandular epithelium of both endometriotic and adenomyotic lesions.
- Measurement of IgG anti-laminin-1 Abs may be a useful tool for diagnosing reproductive failure, such as recurrent abortion and infertility associated with endometriosis.

REFERENCES

1. BURGESON, R.E., M. CHIQUET, R. DEUTZMANN, *et al.* 1994. A new nomenclature for the laminins. Matrix Biol. **14:** 209–211.
2. MINER, J.H., B.L. PATTON, S.I. LENTZ, *et al.* 1997. The laminin a chains: expression, developmental transitions, and chromosomal locations of a1-5, identification of heterotrimeric laminins 8-11, and cloning of a novel a3 isoform. J. Cell Biol. **137:** 685–701.
3. LIBBY, R.T., M.F. CHAMPLIAUD, T. CLAUDEPIERRE, *et al.* 2000. Laminin expression in adult and developing retinae: evidence of two novel CNS laminins. J. Neurosci. **20:** 6517–6528.
4. KLAFFKY, E., R. WILLIAMS, C.C. YAO, *et al.* 2001. Trophoblast-specific expression and function of the integrin α7 subunit in the peri-implantation mouse embryo. Dev. Biol. **239:** 161–175.
5. COOPER, A.R. & H.A. MAC QUEEN. 1983. Subunits of laminin are differentially synthesized in mouse eggs and early embryos. Dev. Biol. **96:** 467–471.
6. DZIADEK, M. & R. TIMPL. 1985. Expression of nidogen and laminin in basement membranes during mouse embryogenesis and in teratocarcinoma cells. Dev. Biol. **111:** 372–382.
7. VIRTANEN, I., D. GULLBERG, J. RISSANEN, *et al.* 2000. Laminin α1-chain shows a restricted distribution in epithelial basement membranes of fetal and adult human tissues. Exp. Cell Res. **257:** 298–309.
8. SUNADA, Y., S.M. BERNIER, C.A. KOZAK, *et al.* 1994. Deficiency of merosin in dystrophic dy mice and genetic linkage of laminin M chain gene to dy locus. J. Biol. Chem. **269:** 13729–13732.
9. XU, H., P. CHRISTMAS, X.R. WU, *et al.* 1994. Defective muscle basement membrane and lack of M-laminin in the dystrophic dy/dy mouse. Proc. Natl. Acad. Sci. USA **91:** 5572–5576.
10. COLOGNATO, H., M. MACCARRICK, J.J. O'REAR & P.D. YURCHENCO. 1997. The laminin α2-chain short arm mediates cell adhesion through both the α1β1 and α2β1 integrins. J. Biol. Chem. **272:** 29330–29336.
11. HISAMATSU, Y., T. NISHIYAMA, S. AMANO, *et al.* 2003. Usefulness of immunoblotting using purified laminin 5 in the diagnosis of anti-laminin 5 cicatricial pemphigoid. J. Dermatol. Sci. **33:** 113–119.
12. MINER, J.H., R.M. LEWIS & J.R. SANES. 1995. Molecular cloning of a novel laminin chain, a5, and widespread expression in adult mouse tissues. J. Biol. Chem. **270:** 28523–28526.
13. IIVANAINEN, A., K. SAINIO, H. SARIOLA & K. TRYGGVASON. 1995. Primary structure and expression of a novel human laminin α4 chain. FEBS Lett. **365:** 183–188.
14. NIIMI, T., C. KUMAGAI, M. OKANO & Y. KITAGAWA. 1997. Differentiation-dependent expression of laminin-8 (α4β1γ1) mRNAs in mouse 3T3-L1 adipocytes. Matrix Biol. **16:** 223–230.
15. PETAJANIEMI, N., M. KORHONEN, J. KORTESMAA, *et al.* 2002. Localization of laminin α4-chain in developing and adult human tissues. J. Histochem. Cytochem. **50:** 1113–1130.

16. SASAKI, M., H.K. KLEINMAN, H. HUBER, *et al.* 1988. Laminin, a multidomain protein. The A chain has a unique globular domain and homology with the basement membrane proteoglycan and the laminin B chains. J. Biol. Chem. **263:** 16536–16544.
17. GALLIANO, M.F., D. ABERDAM, A. AGUZZI, *et al.* 1995. Cloning and complete primary structure of the mouse laminin α 3 chain. Distinct expression pattern of the laminin α 3A and α 3B chain isoforms. J. Biol. Chem. **270:** 21820–21826.
18. KALLUNKI, P., K. SAINIO, R. EDDY, *et al.* 1992. A truncated laminin chain homologous to the B2 chain: structure, spatial expression, and chromosomal assignment. J. Biol. Chem. **119:** 679–693.
19. COLOGNATO, H. & P.D. YURCHENCO. 2000. Form and function: the laminin family of heterotrimers. Dev. Dyn. **218:** 213–234.
20. BELKIN, A.M. & M.A. STEPP. 2000. Integrins as receptors for laminins. Microsc. Res. Tech. **51:** 280–301.
21. MERCURIO, A.M. 1995. Laminin receptors: achieving specificity through cooperation. Trends Cell Biol. **5:** 419–423.
22. NOMIZU, M., W.H. KIM, K. YAMAMURA, *et al.* 1995. Identification of cell binding sites in the laminin a 1 chain carboxyl-terminal globular domain by systematic screening of synthetic peptides. J. Biol. Chem. **270:** 20583-20590.
23. TIMPL, R., H. ROHDE, P.G. ROBEY, *et al.* 1979. Laminin—a glycoprotein from basement membranes. J. Biol. Chem. **254:** 9933–9937.
24. SMYTH, N., H.S. VATANSEVER, P. MURRAY, *et al.* 1999. Absence of basement membranes after targeting the LAMC1 gene results in embryonic lethality due to failure of endoderm differentiation. J. Cell Biol. **144:** 151–160.
25. MINER, J.H., C. LI, J.L. MUDD, *et al.* 2004. Compositional and structural requirements for laminin and basement membranes during mouse embryo implantation and gastrulation. Development **131:** 2247–2256.
26. GRAF, J., Y. IWAMOTO, M. SASAKI, *et al.* 1987. Identification of an amino acid sequence in laminin mediating cell attachment, chemotaxis, and receptor binding. Cell **48:** 989–996.
27. IWAMOTO, Y., F.A. ROBEY, J. GRAF, *et al.* 1987. YIGSR, a synthetic laminin pentapeptide, inhibits experimental metastasis formation. Science **238:** 1132–1134.
28. SAKAMOTO, N., M. IWAHANA, N.G. TANAKA & Y. OSADA. 1991. Inhibition of angiogenesis and tumor growth by a synthetic laminin peptide, CDPGYIGSR-NH2. Cancer Res. **51:** 903–906.
29. GRANT, D.S., K. TASHIRO, B. SEGUI-REAL, *et al.* 1989. Two different laminin domains mediate the differentiation of human endothelial cells into capillary-like structures in vitro. Cell **58:** 933–943.
30. TASHIRO, K., G.C. SEPHEL, B. WEEKS, *et al.* 1989. A synthetic peptide containing the IKVAV sequence from the A chain of laminin mediates cell attachment, migration, and neurite outgrowth. J. Biol. Chem. **264:** 16174–16182.
31. KANEMOTO, T., R. REICH, L. ROYCE, *et al.* 1990. Identification of an amino acid sequence from the laminin A chain that stimulates metastasis and collagenase IV production. Proc. Natl. Acad. Sci. USA **87:** 2279–2283.
32. NOMIZU, M., A. UTANI, N. SHIRAISHI, *et al.* 1992. The all-D-configuration segment containing the IKVAV sequence of laminin A chain has similar activities to the all-L-peptide in vitro and in vivo. J. Biol. Chem. **267:** 14118–14121.
33. MURRAY, P. & D. EDGAR. 2000. Regulation of programmed cell death by basement membranes in embryonic development. J. Cell. Biol. **150:** 1215–1221.
34. LI, S., D. HARRISON, S. CARBONETTO, *et al.* 2002. Matrix assembly, regulation, and survival functions of laminin and its receptors in embryonic stem cell differentiation. J. Cell. Biol. **157:** 1279–1290.
35. GLEICHER, N. & A. EL-ROEIY. 1988. The reproductive autoimmune failure syndrome. Am. J. Obstet. Gynecol. **159:** 223–227.
36. ROTE, N.S. 1996. Antiphospholipid antibodies and recurrent pregnancy loss. Am. J. Reprod. Immunol. **35:** 394–401.
37. INFANTE-RIVARD, C., M. DAVID, R. GAUTHEIR, *et al.* 1991. Lupus anticoagulants, anticardiolipin antibodies, and fetal loss. A case-control study. N. Engl. J. Med. **325:** 1063–1066.

38. WEEKS, B.S., N.W. KLEIN, H. KLEINMAN, *et al.* 1989. Laminin immunized monkeys develop sera toxic to cultured rat embryos and fail to reproduce. Teratology **40:** 47–57.
39. CAREY, S.W. & N.W. KLEIN. 1989. Autoantibodies to laminin and other basement membrane proteins in sera from monkeys with histories of reproductive failure identified by cultures of whole rat embryos. Fertil. Steril. **51:** 711–718.
40. WEEKS, B.S., M. NOMIZU, R.S. RAMCHANDRAN, *et al.* 1998. Laminin-1 and the RKRLQVQLSIRT laminin-1 α1 globular domain peptide stimulate matrix metalloproteinase secretion by PC12 cells. Exp. Cell Res. **243:** 375–382.
41. CHAMBERS, B.J., N.W. KLEIN, S.H. CONRAD, *et al.* 1995. Reproduction and sera embryotoxicity after immunization of monkeys with the laminin peptides YIGSR, RGD, and IKVAV. Proc. Natl. Acad. Sci. USA **92:** 6818–6822.
42. FOIDART, J.M., M. YAAR, A. FIGUEROA, *et al.* 1983. Abortion in mice induced by intravenous injections of antibodies to type IV collagen or laminin. Am. J. Pathol. **110:** 346–357.
43. MATALON, S.T., M. BLANK, E. MATSUURA, *et al.* 2003. Immunization of naive mice with mouse laminin-1 affected pregnancy outcome in a mouse model. Am. J. Reprod. Immunol. **50:** 159–165.
44. INAGAKI, J., E. MATSUURA, M. NOMIZU, *et al.* 2001. IgG anti-laminin-1 autoantibody and recurrent miscarriages. Am. J. Reprod. Immunol. **45:** 232–238.
45. INAGAKI, J., M. SUGIURA-OGASAWARA, M. NOMIZU, *et al.* 2003. An association of IgG anti-laminin-1 autoantibodies with endometriosis in infertile patients. Hum Reprod. **18:** 544–549.
46. MATHUR, S., M.R. PERESS, H.O. WILLIAMSON, *et al.* 1982. Autoimmunity to endometrium and ovary in endometriosis. Clin. Exp. Immunol. **50:** 259–266.
47. PILLAI, S.P., V.L. HOLT, J.H. LEE, *et al.* 1998. Levels of antibodies to transferrin and a2-HS glycoprotein in women with and without endometriosis. Am. J. Reprod. Immunol. **40:** 69–73.
48. MATHUR, S.P. 2000. Autoimmunity in endometriosis: relevance to infertility. Am. J. Reprod. Immunol. **44:** 89–95.
49. KADOYA, Y., K. KADOYA, M. DURBEEJ, *et al.* 1995. Antibodies against domain E3 of laminin-1 and integrin a6 subunit perturb branching epithelial morphogenesis of submandibular gland, but by different modes. J. Cell Biol. **129:** 521–534.
50. KONDO, A., J. INAGAKI, K. KOBAYASHI, *et al.* 2005. Characterization of a murine anti-laminin-1 monoclonal antibody (AK8) produced by immunization with mouse-derived laminin-1. Clin. Dev. Immunol. **12:** 67–73.

Primary Biliary Cirrhosis

Solving the Enigma

ALESSIA GIORGINI,[a] CARLO SELMI,[a,b] PIETRO INVERNIZZI,[a] MAURO PODDA,[a] MASSIMO ZUIN,[a] AND M. ERIC GERSHWIN[b]

[a]*Division of Internal Medicine, Department of Medicine, Surgery and Dentistry, San Paolo School of Medicine, University of Milan, Milan, Italy*

[b]*Division of Rheumatology, Allergy and Clinical Immunology, University of California at Davis, Davis, California, USA*

ABSTRACT: Primary biliary cirrhosis (PBC) is a chronic cholestatic liver disease, most commonly affecting female patients between 40 and 60 years of age. Patient sera present autoantibodies against mitochondrial antigens (AMA) and elevated serum IgM. Histologic studies demonstrate progressive destruction of small- and medium-sized intrahepatic bile ducts and, ultimately, liver cirrhosis. The precise mechanisms leading to selective destruction of such biliary epithelial cells are still unknown, although a number of immunomediated pathways have been proposed. Genetic background is critical in determining susceptibility to the disease, although no clear association with haplotypes of the major histocompatibility complex has been identified. Molecular mimicry by either infectious agents or xenobiotics has been proposed as a means of breaking tolerance in genetically predisposed individuals, thus leading to the onset of PBC. In this review, available data and current theories regarding the immunomediated pathogenesis of PBC will be described.

KEYWORDS: autoimmune cholangitis; immunology; autoantibodies; genetic susceptibility; environmental factors

INTRODUCTION

Primary biliary cirrhosis (PBC) is a chronic inflammatory cholestatic liver disease of unknown etiology in which autoimmunity seems to be the most likely pathogenic mechanism. Liver histology in PBC is characterized by mononuclear infiltration of portal tracts and progressive destruction of small intrahepatic bile ducts, followed by liver fibrosis and, ultimately, cirrhosis.[1] The precise mechanisms leading to selective destruction of biliary epithelial cells (BECs) lining only small- and medium-size intrahepatic bile ducts are still unknown, although a number of immunomediated pathways have been proposed. The importance of genetic suscepti-

Address for correspondence: M. Eric Gershwin, M.D., Division of Rheumatology, Allergy and Clinical Immunology, Genome and Biomedical Sciences Facility, University of California at Davis, 451 E. Health Sciences Drive, Suite 6510, Davis, California 95616. Voice: 530-752-2884; fax: 530-752-4669.
megershwin@ucdavis.edu

Ann. N.Y. Acad. Sci. 1051: 185–193 (2005).
doi: 10.1196/annals.1361.060

bility to PBC has recently been stressed by the high concordance among monozygotic twin sets,[2] and is critical to disease onset, whereas other mechanisms such as molecular mimicry by either microorganisms[3] or xenobiotics[4] have also been proposed. Thus, the resulting hypothesis is that environmental factors may initiate PBC in genetically predisposed individuals, with epidemiological observations supporting this view.

EPIDEMIOLOGY AND CLINICAL FEATURES OF PBC

Most of the reported epidemiological data used to determine the incidence and prevalence rates of PBC are descriptive, with some studies presenting methodological limitations such as non-uniform case definition. Currently, PBC is considered to be most prevalent in England, Scandinavia, and in specific areas of the United States, where prevalence rates have been reported to be as high as 402 cases per million.[5] PBC is also more frequent in relatives of affected individuals, with 1% to 6% of PBC cases presenting with at least one other family member with the disease.[6] Patients are typically middle-aged women, and present with elevated serum IgM and alkaline phosphatase in the vast majority of cases.[7] The diagnosis is based on the presence of two out of the three internationally accepted criteria: (1) detectable serum antimitochondrial autoantibodies (AMAs, titer >1:40), (2) increased alkaline phosphatase level for longer than six months, and (3) a compatible or diagnostic liver histology. Liver histology shows vanishing bile ducts with inflammatory infiltrates, with staging according to Ludwig and colleagues into four stages, from mild periportal inflammation (stage I) to frank cirrhosis (stage IV).[8] Currently, PBC is diagnosed in the absence of symptoms in the majority of cases; however, fatigue and pruritus are the most common symptoms at earlier stages of disease. Jaundice is a late symptom and is a marker of advanced or end-stage PBC, alongside signs and symptoms of liver cirrhosis. Comorbidities with other autoimmune diseases, particularly Sjögren's syndrome and scleroderma, is common at all stages of PBC.[9] Ursodeoxycholic acid (UDCA) at a dose of 13 to 20 mg/kg/d is the only approved treatment for PBC, and has been shown to improve symptoms and biochemical findings, and to slow the progression of the disease, thus increasing patient survival.[10] However, UDCA is not curative, whereas orthotopic liver transplantation (OLT) is considered the only and ultimate treatment for end-stage PBC.

PATHOGENESIS

Autoimmune Features

Several clinical and serological characteristics as well as experimental findings strongly imply an autoimmune pathogenesis for PBC, whereas others make PBC a peculiar entity among autoimmune diseases. The disease is characterized by the presence of detectable AMAs in approximately 90% of affected individuals,[11] although we note that patients lacking AMAs present a similar disease and progression compared with AMA-positive subjects,[12] seemingly arguing against a pathogenic role for these autoantibodies. Autoreactive T cells, both $CD4^+$ and $CD8^+$, have been identified in PBC regardless of the AMA status, and such lymphocytes and AMAs recognize overlapping epitopes within the mitochondrial autoantigens.[13] Other characteristics that indicate an autoimmune pathogenesis for PBC include the striking female predominance (9:1 female to male ratio)[14] and the increased incidence among family members of affected individuals, in both cases similar to findings in other autoimmune conditions.[6] Other characteristics make an autoimmune pathogenesis for PBC less likely. First, no direct proof has been provided for a direct pathogenic role of AMAs in bile duct injury and no convincing animal model has been described, although the induction of AMAs in experimental animals can be achieved by immunization with different mimics.[15] Further, it is well established that most autoimmune diseases are responsive to immunosuppressive therapy. In PBC, all immunosuppressive agents have proven relatively ineffective. Lastly, and again different from most autoimmune diseases, we note the lack of a clear association with human leukocyte antigen (HLA) haplotypes that suggests a unique genetic background.

Immunological Markers

AMA

In most cases, indirect immunofluorescence is used for the screening of AMAs in suspected cases, but this technique possesses limited sensitivity and, particularly at lower dilutions of sera, low specificity for PBC. When AMAs are tested with more recently developed techniques, based on the use of recombinant mitochondrial antigens (with immunoblotting), the sensitivity and specificity of the test are significantly higher, approaching 100%.[16] AMAs are directed against components of the 2-oxoacid dehydrogenase (2-OADC) family of enzymes located on the inner membrane of mitochondria.[17] Specifically, the main antigens recognized are the E2 and E3 binding protein (E3BP) components of the pyruvate dehydrogenase complex PDC (frequently presenting cross-reactivity), and the E2 components of the 2-oxoglutarate dehydrogenase (OGDC) and branched-chain 2-oxoacid dehydrogenase (BCOADC) complexes. AMAs recognize closely related conformational epitopes, including the inner lipoylated domain of PDC-E2, BCOADC-E2, and OGDC-E2.[17] Several studies have attempted to associate AMA patterns or titers with a number of variables, including disease severity, but have failed to clearly demonstrate any correlation.[15] Because of these data and the observation that a subgroup of patients with PBC lack detectable AMAs, as mentioned above, it is unclear whether these autoantibodies have a direct pathogenic role in bile duct destruction, or whether they should be considered mere epiphenomena of the disease.

Anti-nuclear Antibodies (ANAs)

Serum ANAs have been detected in a subset (in some cases approaching 50%) of patients with PBC. The two immunofluorescence patterns specific to PBC are "nuclear rim" and "multiple nuclear dots," based on the recognition by the autoantibodies of gp210 and nucleoporin 62 (within the nuclear pore complex) and nuclear body protein sp100 and PML, respectively.[18] Most recently, it has been proposed that small ubiquitin-like molecules (SUMO) might play a role in the cross-reactivity of Sp100-specific ANA with other self antigens.[19]

Autoreactive T Cells

A number of different mononuclear cells can be found in the area surrounding damaged bile ducts in PBC. T helper ($CD4^+$) TCR ab^+ and $CD8^+$ are the most common T cell phenotypes encountered,[13] perhaps secondary to IFN-γ as a chemotaxic stimulus.[20]

Autoreactive liver $CD4^+$ T cells in PBC specifically recognize PDC-E2.[21] Similar to what has been observed for AMAs, the PDC-E2 amino acid residues E, D, and K at positions 170, 172, and 173, respectively, are essential for the recognition of the epitope by HLA-restricted T cell clones. In addition, PDC-$E2_{163–176}$–specific $CD4^+$ T cell clones also recognize other mitochondrial autoantigens, including the E2 subunits of OGDC and BCOADC, as well as E3BP.[22,23]

Several findings suggest that CD8 T cells play a role in the immunopathogenesis of PBC.[13,24] Recent data indicate that the amino acid residues 159 to 167 of PDC-E2 constitute an HLA-restricted CD8 T cell epitope, and that autoreactive PDC-$E2_{159–167}$–specific cells are found in the peripheral blood of patients with PBC.[25] Moreover, the frequency of PDC-$E2_{159–167}$–specific CD8 T cells is 10-fold higher in PBC liver than in peripheral blood.[26]

Natural killer T (NKT) cells constitute a lymphoid lineage that is distinct from classical T, B, or natural killer (NK) cells; they can be studied specifically using a CD1d tetramer. The frequency of tetramer-restricted NKT cells is significantly higher in the liver than in the peripheral blood of patients with PBC, and such cells also represent a greater proportion of cells in both of these compartments in patients with PBC, compared with controls.[27]

Targeting of BECs

The highly selective destruction of BECs is one of the unique features of PBC. As all nucleated cells in the body contain at least some mitochondria, the target antigens are continually being presented in association with major histocompatibility complex (MHC) class I antigens in all tissues, whereas in PBC they are targeted only in BECs. An explanation for this comes from the observation that certain anti–PDC-E2 antisera react not only with PDC-E2 in mitochondria but also with additional material located at the apical end of the BEC in close apposition to the surface.[28] Further, this apical staining occurs very early in the natural history of PBC, even before the appearance of MHC class II antigens on BECs,[29] and it is not detected in other liver diseases, such as chronic active hepatitis or primary sclerosing cholangitis. Finally, this aberrant apical staining is detected in liver samples from patients with AMA-negative PBC.[29] However, the molecule aberrantly expressed may be a truncated product of PDC-E2 that is complexed with other molecules (perhaps xenobiotics) in a way that masks epitopes. The matter rests there at present, but the increasing sensitivity of proteomics methods may eventually provide a means to sequence or otherwise fingerprint the material. In the interim, it is only possible to speculate. If the material is derived from PDC-E2, perhaps there are sequence variants common to PBC patients that lead to an altered turnover of the molecule, thus leading to the accumulation of PDC-E2 only in specific BECs. Whatever its identity, it is noteworthy that the material is found in association with IgA and the polymeric immunoglobulin receptor[30,31] on the cell membranes of BECs.

The Role of Immunoglobulin A

IgA is the most common immunoglobulin isotype found on epithelial surfaces, including the biliary epithelium. It is therefore possible that the selective injury in PBC is mediated by AMA-IgA binding to the mitochondrial antigen, thus inducing cell dysfunction and death. Our group has demonstrated that IgA from PBC patients localizes with PDC-E2 (or cross-reactive material), both in the cell cytoplasm and on the apical membrane of BECs, whereas no co-localization could be observed with antibodies from healthy subjects.[31] The IgA that is found on the mucosal surface arrives there by uptake and trafficking across the BEC in association with the polymeric immunoglobulin receptor. It is possible that during this transport process, IgA with anti-mitochondrial specificity may contact its cognate antigen and that the complex may lead to apoptosis.[32]

GENETICS

The epidemiology of PBC indicates that family members of patients have an increased risk of being diagnosed with the disease, with concordance rates between monozygotic twins among the highest ever reported for an autoimmune disease. No family study of genetic linkage has been performed in PBC, possibly because of the rarity of the disease and the difficulty in obtaining DNA samples from a large number of representative families. All available studies to date have had a controlled, cross-sectional design but have been prone to multiple sampling errors and biases of incorrect estimations. Moreover, a multi-hit genetic model has been proposed for PBC, with different genetic variants conferring susceptibility (first hit) and others influencing disease progression (second hit).

Major Histocompatibility Complex Haplotypes

Based on results obtained in other autoimmune diseases, most association studies have concentrated on MHC haplotypes and their role in PBC. First, researchers from different sites examined the association of HLA class I molecules with PBC, with no consistent results.[6] Our group recently reported that PBC may be associated with various HLA-B alleles, although such associations were found only in a small proportion of the 138 patients typed, and the patients were from one geographical area.[33] Further, several studies have reported an association of HLA class II alleles and PBC in populations of Caucasian and Asian ethnicity. Among Caucasians, an association between PBC susceptibility and HLA-DR8 (DRB1*08) has been found most frequently,[6] whereas more recently it has been reported that the linkage of the DQA1*0401 allele and the DR8$^-$ DQB1*0402 haplotype may be associated with disease progression.[34] We note, however, that several European studies have failed to confirm an association with DR8, or report other associations, such as PBC with DR3 or DPB1*0301.[6] Our data suggest that the DRB1*11 allele has a protective effect against PBC in Italian subjects.[33] Within the MHC class III region, scrutinized genes in PBC include tumor necrosis factor alpha (TNF-α), again with conflicting results.[35] Consequently, we propose that the association of MHC haplotypes with susceptibility to PBC should be regarded as different according to different population groups or geographical areas, and is substantially weaker than that observed in other autoimmune diseases.[36]

Non-MHC Polymorphisms

Controversial findings were also reported from the study of the polymorphism of genetic variants of immunomodulatory molecules (such as chemokines, CTLA-4, IL-2, or IL-10, polymorphisms of the vitamin D receptor), enzymes producing vasoactive compounds, and bile acid transporters; no clear association with the onset or the severity of PBC has been found.[6]

Sex Chromosomes

Genes mapping on the X chromosome are critical to the maintenance of physiological sex hormone levels and, more important, of immune responsiveness.[14] Our group has recently reported an enhanced monosomy X (i.e.., a major defect of the X chromosome) in the peripheral white blood cells of women with PBC[37] at a case frequency of 5% compared with 2% for age-matched control females, with age dependency in both groups. Our findings suggest a polygenic model with an X-linked major locus of susceptibility in which genes that escape X chromosome inactivation are the major candidates for PBC susceptibility.

We also note that the role of microchimerism in PBC has been studied widely.[38] In particular, it has been suggested that the presence of fetal DNA in the liver of affected women years after pregnancy may predispose to PBC; independent studies, however, have not confirmed such a hypothesis.[6]

ENVIRONMENTAL FACTORS

The geographical pattern of PBC distribution, experimental data, and lack of strong genetic associations have suggested that environmental factors play a role in initiating PBC. Attention has focused mainly on infectious agents (bacteria and viruses) and chemicals (xenobiotics).

The ability of infectious agents, particularly bacteria, to induce autoimmune responses in experimental settings has been documented, and molecular mimicry is the most widely considered mechanism explaining these observations.[39] Briefly, this model suggests that microbes present peptides sharing different degrees of homology with self-proteins, thus leading to a promiscuous antibody and cell-mediated immune response capable of reacting with both microbial and self-epitopes. T cell activation produces cross-reacting T cells, leading to self-tissue destruction, thus perpetuating the autoimmune response, possibly through the degeneracy of the T cell receptor and cross-priming. Of the bacterial strains suggested to lead to PBC through molecular mimicry,[39] the most evidence has been reported for *Escherichia coli*, primarily based on reports of an increased prevalence of urinary tract infections in patients with PBC.[9] Recently, our group has provided serological data suggesting that a ubiquitous xenobiotic-metabolizing Gram-negative bacterium, *Novosphingobium aromaticivorans*, is the best candidate yet for the induction of PBC.[40] The reactivity against *N. aromaticivorans* was estimated to be 100- to 1000-fold higher than against *E. coli*.[40] For completeness, we also note that a novel human betaretrovirus has been suggested in the etiology of PBC[41]; however, our laboratory was unable to confirm such data.[42]

Xenobiotics are foreign compounds that may either alter or complex with defined self or non-self-proteins, inducing a change in the molecular structure of the native protein sufficient to induce an immune response. Such immune responses may then result in the cross-recognition of the self form, which could in turn perpetuate the immune response, thus leading to chronic autoimmunity. Experimental evidence showed that specific organic structures attached to the mitochondrial antigens were recognized by sera from PBC patients with a higher affinity than native forms of such antigens.[43] Similarly, one halogenated compound was capable of inducing AMA production in animal models[40] with no liver lesions.

CONCLUSIONS

Available evidence suggests that PBC should be considered as a unique yet representative autoimmune disease. Future research efforts will need to focus on several critical issues. First, to provide prevalence and incidence rates in different geographical areas, large epidemiological studies should be performed, and novel noninvasive, highly sensitive, and specific markers for diagnosis should be developed to overcome the limitations of serum AMA testing. Second, further studies are hampered by our current poor understanding of the interplay between genetic and environmental factors, the variability of disease progression, and the absence of informative animal models. To provide better diagnostic tools and therapeutic options in the future, researchers should dedicate their efforts to achieving a better knowledge of the pathogenetic mechanisms. The promising data obtained with xenobiotics or bacteria, if confirmed, together with large international familial studies of the genetic background of PBC, could provide important clues to unraveling the mystery of PBC.

REFERENCES

1. PARES, A. & J. RODES. 2003. Natural history of primary biliary cirrhosis. Clin. Liver Dis. **7:** 779–794.
2. SELMI, C. *et al.* 2004. Primary biliary cirrhosis in monozygotic and dizygotic twins: genetics, epigenetics, and environment. Gastroenterology **127:** 485–492.
3. SELMI, C. & M.E. GERSHWIN. 2004. Bacteria and human autoimmunity: the case of primary biliary cirrhosis. Curr. Opin. Rheumatol. **16:** 406–410.
4. LONG, S.A., J. VAN DE WATER & M.E. GERSHWIN. 2002. Antimitochondrial antibodies in primary biliary cirrhosis: the role of xenobiotics. Autoimmun. Rev. **1:** 37–42.
5. SELMI, C. *et al.* 2004. Epidemiology and pathogenesis of primary biliary cirrhosis. J. Clin. Gastroenterol. **38:** 264–271.
6. INVERNIZZI, P. *et al.* 2005. From bases to basis: linking genetics to causation in primary biliary cirrhosis. Clin. Gastroenterol. Hepatol. **3:** 401–410.
7. TALWALKAR, J.A. & K.D. LINDOR. 2003. Primary biliary cirrhosis. Lancet **362:** 53–61.
8. LUDWIG, J., E.R. DICKSON & G.S. MCDONALD. 1978. Staging of chronic nonsuppurative destructive cholangitis (syndrome of primary biliary cirrhosis). Virchows Arch. A Pathol. Anat. Histol. **379:** 103–112.
9. PARIKH-PATEL, A. *et al.* 2001. Risk factors for primary biliary cirrhosis in a cohort of patients from the United States. Hepatology **33:** 16–21.

10. GLUUD, C. & E. CHRISTENSEN. 2002. Ursodeoxycholic acid for primary biliary cirrhosis. Cochrane Database Syst. Rev. (1): CD000551.
11. MACKAY, I.R. *et al.* 2000. The peculiar autoimmunity of primary biliary cirrhosis. Immunol. Rev. **174:** 226–237.
12. INVERNIZZI, P. *et al.* 1997. Comparison of the clinical features and clinical course of antimitochondrial antibody-positive and -negative primary biliary cirrhosis. Hepatology **25:** 1090–1095.
13. ISHIBASHI, H., M. NAKAMURA, S. SHIMODA & M.E. GERSHWIN. 2003. T cell immunity and primary biliary cirrhosis. Autoimmun. Rev. **2:** 19–24.
14. SELMI, C. *et al.* 2004. Primary biliary cirrhosis: does X mark the spot? Autoimmun. Rev. **3:** 493–499.
15. BOGDANOS, D.P., H. BAUM & D. VERGANI. 2003. Antimitochondrial and other autoantibodies. Clin. Liver Dis. **7:** 759–777.
16. MIYAKAWA, H. *et al.* 2001. Detection of antimitochondrial autoantibodies in immunofluorescent AMA-negative patients with primary biliary cirrhosis using recombinant autoantigens. Hepatology **34:** 243–248.
17. GERSHWIN, M.E. *et al.* 2000. Primary biliary cirrhosis: an orchestrated immune response against epithelial cells. Immunol. Rev. **174:** 210–225.
18. WORMAN, H.J. & J.C. COURVALIN. 2003. Antinuclear antibodies specific for primary biliary cirrhosis. Autoimmun. Rev. **2:** 211–217.
19. JANKA, C. *et al.* 2005. Small ubiquitin-related modifiers: a novel and independent class of autoantigens in primary biliary cirrhosis. Hepatology **41:** 609–616.
20. KITA, H., I.R. MACKAY, J. VAN DE WATER & M.E. GERSHWIN. 2001. The lymphoid liver: considerations on pathways to autoimmune injury. Gastroenterology **120:** 1485–1501.
21. VAN DE WATER, J. *et al.* 1991. Evidence for the targeting by 2-oxo-dehydrogenase enzymes in the T cell response of primary biliary cirrhosis. J. Immunol. **146:** 89–94.
22. SHIMODA, S. *et al.* 1995. HLA DRB4 0101-restricted immunodominant T cell autoepitope of pyruvate dehydrogenase complex in primary biliary cirrhosis: evidence of molecular mimicry in human autoimmune diseases. J. Exp. Med. **181:** 1835–1845.
23. SHIMODA, S. *et al.* 1998. Identification and precursor frequency analysis of a common T cell epitope motif in mitochondrial autoantigens in primary biliary cirrhosis. J. Clin. Invest. **102:** 1831–1840.
24. MEUER, S.C. *et al.* 1988. Clonal analysis of human T lymphocytes infiltrating the liver in chronic active hepatitis B and primary biliary cirrhosis. Eur. J. Immunol. **18:** 1447–1452.
25. KITA, H. *et al.* 2002. Identification of HLA-A2-restricted CD8(+) cytotoxic T cell responses in primary biliary cirrhosis: T cell activation is augmented by immune complexes cross-presented by dendritic cells. J. Exp. Med. **195:** 113–123.
26. KITA, H. *et al.* 2002. Quantitative and functional analysis of PDC-E2-specific autoreactive cytotoxic T lymphocytes in primary biliary cirrhosis. J. Clin. Invest. **109:** 1231–1240.
27. KITA, H. *et al.* 2002. Quantitation and phenotypic analysis of natural killer T cells in primary biliary cirrhosis using a human CD1d tetramer. Gastroenterology **123:** 1031–1043.
28. VAN DE WATER, J. *et al.* 1993. Molecular mimicry in primary biliary cirrhosis. Evidence for biliary epithelial expression of a molecule cross-reactive with pyruvate dehydrogenase complex-E2. J. Clin. Invest. **91:** 2653–2664.
29. TSUNEYAMA, K. *et al.* 1995. Abnormal expression of the E2 component of the pyruvate dehydrogenase complex on the luminal surface of biliary epithelium occurs before major histocompatibility complex class II and BB1/B7 expression. Hepatology **21:** 1031–1037.
30. MIGLIACCIO, C. *et al.* 1998. Monoclonal antibodies to mitochondrial E2 components define autoepitopes in primary biliary cirrhosis. J. Immunol. **161:** 5157–5163.
31. FUKUSHIMA, N. *et al.* 2002. Characterization of recombinant monoclonal IgA anti-PDC-E2 autoantibodies derived from patients with PBC. Hepatology **36:** 1383–1392.

32. MATSUMURA, S. *et al.* 2004. Caspase induction by IgA antimitochondrial antibody: IgA-mediated biliary injury in primary biliary cirrhosis. Hepatology **39:** 1415–1422.
33. INVERNIZZI, P. *et al.* 2003. Peculiar HLA polymorphisms in Italian patients with primary biliary cirrhosis. J. Hepatol. **38:** 401–406.
34. DONALDSON, P. *et al.* 2001. HLA and interleukin 1 gene polymorphisms in primary biliary cirrhosis: associations with disease progression and disease susceptibility. Gut **48:** 397–402.
35. DONALDSON, P.T. 1999. TNF gene polymorphisms in primary biliary cirrhosis: a critical appraisal. J. Hepatol. **31:** 366–368.
36. SELDIN, M.F., C.I. AMOS, R. WARD & P.K. GREGERSEN. 1999. The genetics revolution and the assault on rheumatoid arthritis. Arthritis Rheum. **42:** 1071–1079.
37. INVERNIZZI, P. *et al.* 2004. Frequency of monosomy X in women with primary biliary cirrhosis. Lancet **363:** 533–535.
38. LAMBERT, N. & J.L. NELSON. 2003. Microchimerism in autoimmune disease: more questions than answers? Autoimmun. Rev. **2:** 133–139.
39. VAN DE WATER, J., H. ISHIBASHI, R.L. COPPEL & M.E. GERSHWIN. 2001. Molecular mimicry and primary biliary cirrhosis: premises not promises. Hepatology **33:** 771–775.
40. SELMI, C. *et al.* 2003. Patients with primary biliary cirrhosis react against a ubiquitous xenobiotic-metabolizing bacterium. Hepatology **38:** 1250–1257.
41. XU, L. *et al.* 2003. Does a betaretrovirus infection trigger primary biliary cirrhosis? Proc. Natl. Acad. Sci. USA **100:** 8454–8459.
42. SELMI, C. *et al.* 2004. Lack of immunological or molecular evidence for a role of mouse mammary tumor retrovirus in primary biliary cirrhosis. Gastroenterology **127:** 493–501.
43. LONG, S.A. *et al.* 2001. Immunoreactivity of organic mimeotopes of the E2 component of pyruvate dehydrogenase: connecting xenobiotics with primary biliary cirrhosis. J. Immunol. **167:** 2956–2963.

The Stages of Type 1A Diabetes

NARU BABAYA, MAKI NAKAYAMA, AND GEORGE S. EISENBARTH

Barbara Davis Center for Childhood Diabetes,
University of Colorado Health Sciences Center,
Aurora, Colorado 80010-1763, USA

ABSTRACT: We can now predict the development of type 1 diabetes in man because it is a chronic autoimmune disorder with defined stages of disease. We can also readily prevent the disorder in animal models. A major goal is safe prevention in man, and for this we will almost certainly need a better understanding of pathogenesis, coupled with rigorous clinical trials.

KEYWORDS: NOD mouse; prediction; genetic susceptibility; environmental factor; autoantibody; trial; transplantation; review

INTRODUCTION

It is now possible to predict the development of type 1A (immune-mediated) diabetes in man [1,2] and to prevent the disorder in animal models.[3,4] Furthermore, experimental therapies have been shown to delay loss of beta cell function in man.[5] The ability to predict the disease comes from the realization that type 1A diabetes is a chronic autoimmune disorder, from improvements in immunogenetic and anti-islet autoantibody assays, and from the development of relatively simple predictive paradigms, such as "combinatorial" autoantibody prediction.[2,4]

Despite these advances there are many gaps in our current knowledge of the pathogenesis of this common and extensively studied autoimmune disorder. We will emphasize recent conceptual advances in our understanding of the stages of type 1A diabetes (FIG. 1) and, in parallel, consider the disease in man and in the NOD mouse model.[6]

A major advantage of the NOD model is the ability to sample at will from the site of pathology, combined with the availability of multiple genetic and immunologic tools applicable to murine models. The major disadvantage of this model is that relatively small perturbations of the immune system can prevent progression to diabetes, though such therapies usually cannot prevent insulitis. The NOD mouse is inbred and usually raised in a "pathogen-free" environment, and only a portion of mice progress to diabetes, even given these restrictions. Thus, it is very likely that most of the therapies effective in NOD mice will have little utility in man, but it is nevertheless very likely that understanding the pieces of the puzzle that lead to spontaneous

Address for correspondence: George S. Eisenbarth, M.D., Ph.D., Barbara Davis Center for Childhood Diabetes, University of Colorado Health Sciences Center, 12801 East 17th Avenue, Aurora, CO 80010-1763, USA. Voice: 303-724-6847; fax: 303-724-6839.
george.eisenbarth@uchsc.edu

Ann. N.Y. Acad. Sci. 1051: 194–204 (2005). © 2005 New York Academy of Sciences.
doi: 10.1196/annals.1361.061

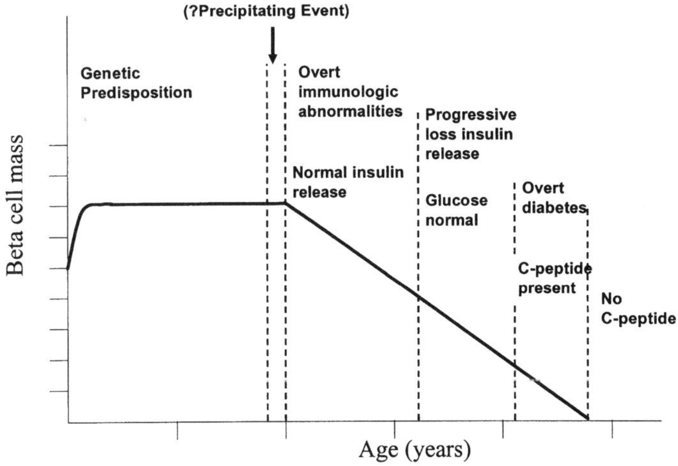

FIGURE 1. Stages in the development of type 1A diabetes. (From Eisenbarth.[82] Reproduced by permission.)

immune-mediated diabetes in the NOD mouse will inform the more difficult development of effective and safe therapies for man.

PATHOPHYSIOLOGY

To provide focus and to highlight gaps in our current knowledge we will emphasize the hypothesis that type 1A diabetes in the NOD mouse, and perhaps man, results predominantly from CD4 T cell–mediated pathogenic loss of tolerance to a single epitope of a primary islet autoantigen. For the NOD mouse this epitope may be the insulin B:9–23 peptide discovered by Wegmann and Daniel.[7] We have evidence that insulin is a primary autoantigen in NOD mice, and deletion of the insulin 2 gene accelerates disease, whereas deletion of the insulin 1 gene prevents development of diabetes.[8] It is likely that memory CD4 T lymphocytes reacting with the B:9–23 insulin peptide are present as a natural consequence of the lack of thymic deletion in both normal (e.g., BALB/c) and NOD mice of the appropriate MHC genotype. Specific activation of these memory T lymphocytes results in T cell expansion and homing to islets, with concomitant production of insulin autoantibodies,[9] collateral priming[10] with inter- and intramolecular epitope spreading, and islet beta cell destruction.[11–13] The destruction is beta cell–specific, owing to the presence of the beta cell–specific molecule insulin. The relatively slow and progressive time course of islet destruction is a result of asynchronous destruction of the beta cells of different islets.[14] Such asynchronous destruction probably is the result of the equivalent of a plaque assay, determined by the relatively uncommon event of an activated pathogenic T lymphocyte entering a specific islet through a fenestrated islet capillary, expanding, recruiting additional effector cells, and not being suppressed by regulatory T cells. In addition, it is likely that the frequency of the hypothesized plaquing CD4 T cell in the circulation is determined by a complex interplay of cells within the pancreatic lymph node, including an important role of regulatory T lymphocytes in the lymph node.[15–17] At present, we do not know with certainty which islet molecules are important targets and which are ancillary, how pathogenic T lymphocytes escape thymic deletion, where initial activation occurs, what their route to islets and dynamics within islets is, how autoantibodies and B lymphocytes contribute to disease, the importance of multiple additional cells in pathogenesis (e.g., NK cells),[18] and why some islets escape destruction and therefore some mice escape diabetes. As we develop a better understanding of each of the stages of type 1A diabetes we believe we will have more complete answers.

STAGE I: GENETIC SUSCEPTIBILITY

Diabetes in the NOD mouse is a polygenic disorder, and different combinations of susceptibility loci lead to different phenotypes (e.g., expression of insulin autoantibodies and insulitis but lack of diabetes).[19] Linkage analysis and congenic mapping have identified 21 loci (*Idd1-21*)[20,21] that contribute to the development of autoimmune type 1 diabetes in the NOD mouse. Among susceptibility genes, class II major histocompatibility complex (MHC) genes (e.g., specific amino acids of the I-A molecule (I-A^{g7}) and lack of I-E expression) are the most important determinants of diabetes.[22]

In humans, several genome-wide linkage studies[23,24] have been conducted to identify about 20 candidate regions that may contain unidentified diabetes susceptibility genes. Until recently, only two susceptibility regions had been reproducibly identified, namely HLA genes and the insulin gene VNTR (variable nucleotide tandem repeat).[25] However, a major advance in the genetics of type 1A diabetes is the discovery that the LYP (lymphocyte tyrosine phosphatase) gene contributes to diabetes risk.[26–28]

Bottini *et al.* initially described the LYP polymorphism (arginine to tryptophan at position 620 of the *PTPN22* gene) leading to increased susceptibility, and the association of the T variant with type 1A diabetes has been confirmed in a large study from Great Britain.[27,28] With an odds ratio of approximately 1.7 this is a relatively potent locus for type 1A diabetes susceptibility (on order of insulin[29] and much greater than cytotoxic T lymphocyte antigen 4, *CTLA4*).[26] The LYP molecule down modulates signaling through the T cell receptor, and the specific polymorphism associated with diabetes risk (arginine to tryptophan) blocks the binding of LYP to the signaling molecule Csk.[27,28] This specific tryptophan polymorphism is associated with a series of autoimmune disorders (e.g., rheumatoid arthritis, lupus erythematosus), probably by its influence on T cell signaling.[28,30,31]

A recent report by Wang and coworkers has implicated a gene termed *SUMO4* in type 1A diabetes in some but not all populations.[32] CTLA-4, by means of its ligand-binding domain, may compete with CD28 for the receptors (CD80 and CD86) that they share, and is a "counter-regulator" of CD28 T cell antigen receptor (TCR) activation of T cells.[33] In a very large study, linkage to type 1A diabetes was demonstrated for a polymorphism of *CTLA4* (*IDDM12*, 2q32.1-q33), but the relative risk was only 1.14.[26] In NOD mice, *Idd5.1* (insulin-dependent diabetes 5.1) has been defined to a 2.1-Mb region containing *Ctla4*, with *Cd28* located in the same genetic region.[21] In addition, there are two "single" gene mutations causing autoimmunity and type 1A diabetes: mutations of the AIRE gene, causing APS-I (autoimmune polyendocrine syndrome type 1), and mutations of the FOXP3 gene, resulting in the IPEX syndrome.[34–36] FOXP3 is a transcription factor, essential for the generation of $CD4^+CD25^+$ regulatory cells, and in its absence neonates die of overwhelming autoimmunity, including neonatal diabetes.

STAGE II: TRIGGERING/ ENVIRONMENTAL FACTORS

At present it is not known how or even where T cell autoimmunity directed at islet autoantigens first develops. In man, specific anti-islet autoantibodies react with glutamic acid decarboxylase, insulin, IA-2, and IA-2b.[13,37] In the NOD mouse, only specific anti-insulin antibodies have been confirmed,[3,38] whereas multiple T cell molecular targets are well known.[11] There are several hypotheses relative to the initiation of islet autoimmunity, including (1) molecular mimicry, (2) physiologic beta cell apoptosis, and (3) activation of the innate immune system in a genetically susceptible host.

Environmental factors are important to the development type 1A diabetes, and many potential candidates are under evaluation, among them dietary factors, such as cow's milk and cereals,[39–41] and viral infections.[42] Cow's milk–based infant formulas and cow's milk consumption in childhood have been suggested to trigger the development of type 1A diabetes mellitus. However, the issue is far from being resolved. In animal models, cow's milk proteins are modestly and variably diabetogenic, and when introduced at weaning trigger insulitis and diabetes,[43] perhaps through molecular mimicry.[44] In humans, several epidemiologic studies have not shown an association between early exposure to cow's milk and type 1A diabetes mellitus.[45–47] Recent reports by Norris *et al.*[39] and Ziegler *et al.*[40] found that timing of exposure to cereals is important in developing anti-islet autoantibodies.

Viral infections have been associated with the development of type 1A diabetes. Multiple reports suggest that molecular mimicry may lead to autoimmunity, and viral infections have been implicated as a trigger of autoimmune diabetes.[48,49] Polyinosinic-polycytidylic acid (PolyIC), a mimic of double-stranded viral RNA can, with the insulin B:9–23 peptide, induce insulitis and diabetes in modified $H\text{-}2^d$ mice (e.g., BALB/c)[9] and, with RT1-u, in multiple rat strains .[50] Other groups have reported that a viral epitope that mimics a self-antigen accelerates a previously established autoimmune process but does not initiate autoimmune diabetes.[51]

Mathis *et al.* hypothesized that antigen-presenting cells (APCs) in the pancreatic lymph nodes recognize their antigens because of physiological beta cell death (apoptosis), which takes place in islets of rodents, peaking at 14 to 17 days after birth.[52] Recently, the group reported that physiological apoptosis precipitates the availability of islet beta cell antigens carried to the pancreatic lymph node by dendritic cells.[53] The test system utilized was activation of BDC2.5 anti-islet CD4 T cells, but was only partially inhibited by the irreversible pancaspase inhibitor ZVAD or a knockout of caspase 12.

STAGE III: ACTIVE AUTOIMMUNITY

In an NOD mouse, insulin autoantibodies can be detected as early as three weeks of age, insulitis is histologically observed in almost all female NOD mice after five weeks of age, and lymphocytic infiltration gradually expands. The majority of the infiltration consists of T cells, although B cells, macrophages, and other immune cells are also likely to contribute to the initiation and expansion of autoimmunity against beta cells.[54,55] In humans, insulitis is observed in the pancreas of newly diagnosed diabetic patients.[56] These autoreactive T cells may kill insulin-producing beta cells by inducing apoptosis and necrosis mediated by perforin/granzymes,[57] Fas/FasL interaction,[58,59] and cytokine production. [60] Beta cell mass is thought to be reduced progressively, accompanied with increased beta cell proliferation in NOD animal models.[61]

One of the earliest indicators of anti-islet autoimmunity is the detection of autoantibodies to beta cell antigens. At present, we utilize three major types of antibodies for the diagnosis and prediction of type 1A diabetes (FIG. 2). These are antibodies to insulin (IAA), glutamic acid decarboxylase (GAD-AA), and the protein tyrosine phosphatase IA2 (IA2-AA). The prediction of type 1A diabetes in NOD mice has been evaluated prospectively, measuring the development of IAA (insulin autoantibodies). The expression of IAA at a younger age was strongly associated with early development of type 1A diabetes.[3] In man, type 1A diabetes is "predictable" among relatives, using a combination of the above three autoantibodies.[1,2] With a combination of immunogenetic, autoantibody, and metabolic parameters, it is possible to predict diabetes with an accuracy that allows trials of type 1A diabetes prevention, though some individuals express multiple autoantibodies for decades prior to developing overt diabetes, and the majority of individuals expressing a single autoantibody are unlikely to progress.

To improve diabetes prediction, T cell assays, rather than autoantibody assays, may be more important, because autoreactive T cells are believed to mediate beta cell destruction. The enzyme-linked immunospot assay for detection of cytokine-secreting cells (CK ELISpot) detects specific T cells through their cytokine secretion.[62] Tetramers and other multimers of MHC molecules (class I and class II) with

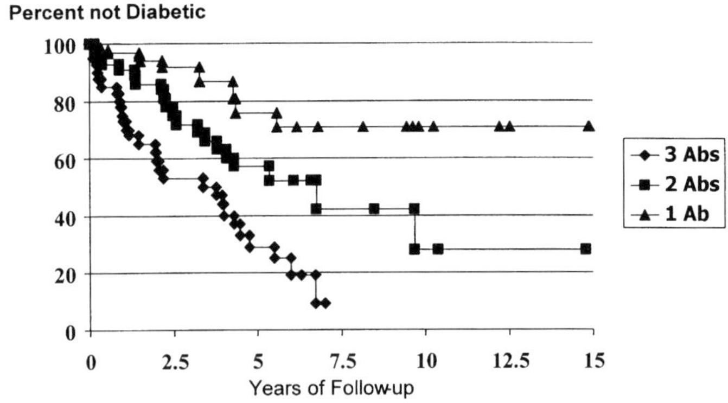

3 Abs	n =	41	17	8	1		
2 Abs	n =	44	27	15	4	2	1
1 Ab	n =	93	23	14	10	6	4

FIGURE 2. Progression of first-degree relatives to type 1A diabetes relative to the number of anti-islet autoantibodies expressed (of GAD65, IA-2 (ICA512), or insulin). (Modified from Verge *et al.*[1] Reprinted by permission.)

TABLE 1. Selected immunotherapy trials

Status/Trials	Reagents	Comment
	New-Onset Diabetes	
Anti-CD3[67]	ChAglCD3	Ongoing
Anti-CD3[5,68]	hOKT3γ1 Ala-Ala	Mitigates deterioration in insulin production
ATGAM[77]	Anti-thymocyte globin	No lasting effect
Heat-shock protein[78]	DiaPep277	One report of preservation of endogenous insulin production in adults
Cyclosporin A[79]	Cyclosporin A	Preservation of C-peptide only during administration
	Prediabetic (Antibody-Positive)	
DPT-1[80]	Subcutaneous insulin	No effect
DPT-1	Oral insulin	No effect overall; potential delay in pregression in those with high-level IAA
	Genetically Susceptible	
DIPP[81]	Nasal insulin	Ongoing

relevant peptide epitopes are also used to assess specific T cells. Trudeau *et al.* reported that diabetogenic $CD8^+$ T cells in the peripheral blood of NOD mice were detected using tetramers.[63]

STAGE IV: LOSS OF INSULIN SECRETION/LOSS OF BETA CELL MASS

Because beta cell mass decreases before development of clinically symptomatic diabetes, metabolic abnormalities can usually be demonstrated before diagnosis of diabetes. The first-phase insulin response following intravenous glucose load (FPIR) is often but not always an early abnormality, as is impaired glucose tolerance (e.g., glucose at 2 h 140 mg/dL and less than 200 mg/dL on an oral glucose tolerance test). Children carrying high-risk HLA-DQB1 with multiple islet autoantibodies have lower FPIR, and children with abnormal FPIR have a higher risk of developing overt diabetes.[64] Of note, there is heterogeneity in the timing of decreasing FPIR, and insulin resistance associated with puberty and obesity may affect the FPIR. However, the FPIR, in combination with islet autoantibodies, is a good predictive parameter of the approximate time to onset of type 1A diabetes.[65]

STAGE V: OVERT DIABETES

Once diabetes is diagnosed, significant beta cell loss is usually present, but significant numbers of beta cells still remain. The function of residual beta cells is usually assessed by measuring C-peptide.[66] One of the most promising therapies to slow bets cell loss at this stage is infusion of modified monoclonal (mAb) anti-CD3 antibodies. The original mouse anti-human CD3 mAb, OKT3, could not be used in patients with autoimmune disease because of its severe toxicity, ascribed to cytokine release. To eliminate this toxicity two different monoclonal antibodies, ChAglyCD3[67] and hOKT3g1 Ala-Ala,[16,68] were produced by different groups. Clinical trials of these anti-CD3 antibodies for the treatment of several autoimmune diseases are under way.[69] Preclinical studies in NOD mice, where anti-CD3 therapy is effective at the onset of diabetes but not before, implicates induction of TGFβ-secreting regulatory T cells.[70] In one clinical trial, one year after a single 14-day course of hOKT3g1 Ala-Ala treatment, a significant mitigation of the deterioration in insulin production and improvement in metabolic control was observed in treated patients compared with controls.[5] Monoclonal antibodies, not only anti-CD3 antibodies, but also antibodies targeting other T cell molecules, will be extensively evaluated for therapy of type 1A diabetes over this next decade.

STAGE VI: INSULIN-DEPENDENT DIABETES

In this last stage, almost all of the beta cells have been destroyed and patients require insulin therapy. Preventing the progression of chronic complications, microangiopathy (neuropathy, retinopathy, and nephropathy) and macroangiopathy (e.g., myocardial infarction, brain infarction) while avoiding severe hypoglycemia is difficult to achieve.

In patients with "brittle" diabetes with recurrent episodes of severe hypoglycemia, islet transplantation is a consideration. Prolonged insulin independence can be achieved after islet transplantation.[71–73] Despite significant success and cure of recurrent hypoglycemia, with time most patients again require some insulin therapy, and all patients must be on immunosuppression.[74] A major limitation is the inadequate supply of cadaveric pancreases as a source of islets. Potential sources of transplantable islets in the future may come through the expansion of beta cells, the harnessing of embryonic stem cells or adult stem cells, and the use of beta cell lines, as well as the use of xenogeneic islets.[75,76]

CONCLUSION

Our improved understanding of the pathogenesis of type 1A diabetes has led to the current implementation of clinical trials at multiple stages of the disease, from genetic susceptibility (e.g., dietary trials) to trials of islet transplantation. A major deficiency at present is the inability to directly measure the T cells destroying beta cells, but it is hoped that newer knowledge and approaches in this area will facilitate therapeutic trials leading to disease prevention.

ACKNOWLEDGMENTS

This work was supported by grants from the National Institutes of Health (DK32083, AI39213, DK55969, DK62718, DK32493), Diabetes Endocrine Research Center (P30 DK57516), Clinical Research Centers (MO1 RR00069, MO1 RR00051), Immune Tolerance Network (AI15416), Autoimmunity Prevention Center (AI50864), Autoimmunity Center of Excellence, the American Diabetes Association, the Juvenile Diabetes Foundation, and the Children's Diabetes Foundation.

REFERENCES

1. VERGE, C.F. *et al.* 1996. Prediction of type I diabetes in first-degree relatives using a combination of insulin, GAD, and ICA512bdc/IA-2 autoantibodies. Diabetes. **45:** 926–933.
2. BARKER, J.M. *et al.* 2004. Prediction of autoantibody positivity and progression to type 1 diabetes: Diabetes Autoimmunity Study in the Young (DAISY). J. Clin. Endocrinol. Metab. **89:** 3896–3902.
3. YU, L. *et al.* 2000. Early expression of antiinsulin autoantibodies of humans and the NOD mouse: evidence for early determination of subsequent diabetes. Proc. Natl. Acad. Sci. USA **97:** 1701–1706.
4. EISENBARTH, G.S. *et al.* 2002. Insulin autoimmunity: prediction/precipitation/prevention type 1A diabetes. Autoimmun. Rev. **1:** 139–145.
5. HEROLD, K.C. *et al.* 2002. Anti-CD3 monoclonal antibody in new-onset type 1 diabetes mellitus. N. Engl. J. Med. **346:** 1692–1698.
6. MAKINO, S. *et al.* 1980. Breeding of a non-obese, diabetic strain of mice. Jikken Dobutsu. **29:** 1–13.
7. DANIEL, D., R.G. GILL, N. SCHLOOT & D. WEGMANN. 1995. Epitope specificity, cytokine production profile and diabetogenic activity of insulin-specific T cell clones isolated from NOD mice. Eur. J. Immunol. **25:** 1056–1062.
8. MORIYAMA, H. *et al.* 2003. Evidence for a primary islet autoantigen (preproinsulin 1) for insulitis and diabetes in the nonobese diabetic mouse. Proc. Natl. Acad. Sci. USA **100:** 10376–10381.
9. MORIYAMA, H. *et al.* 2002. Induction and acceleration of insulitis/diabetes in mice with a viral mimic (polyinosinic-polycytidylic acid) and an insulin self-peptide. Proc. Natl. Acad. Sci. USA **99:** 5539–5544.
10. EISENBARTH, S.C. *et al.* 2004. IL-4-dependent Th2 collateral priming to inhaled antigens independent of Toll-like receptor 4 and myeloid differentiation factor 88. J. Immunol. **172:** 4527–4534.
11. PANAGIOTOPOULOS, C., J.D. TRUDEAU & R. TAN. 2004. T-cell epitopes in type 1 diabetes. Curr. Diab. Rep. **4:** 87–94.
12. ANDERSON, M.S. & J.A. BLUESTONE. 2004. The NOD mouse: a model of immune dysregulation. Annu. Rev. Immunol. Nov 29 (e-pub ahead of print).
13. WINTER, W.E., N. HARRIS & D. SCHATZ. 2002. Type 1 diabetes islet autoantibody markers. Diabetes Technol. Ther. **4:** 817–839.
14. KIKUTANI, H. & S. MAKINO. 1992. The murine autoimmune diabetes model: NOD and related strains. Adv. Immunol. **51:** 285–322.
15. HOGLUND, P. *et al.* 1999. Initiation of autoimmune diabetes by developmentally regulated presentation of islet cell antigens in the pancreatic lymph nodes. J. Exp. Med. **189:** 331–339.
16. BLUESTONE, J.A. & Q. TANG. 2004. Therapeutic vaccination using CD4+CD25+ antigen-specific regulatory T cells. Proc. Natl. Acad. Sci. USA **101** (Suppl. 2)**:** 14622–14626.
17. BOUR-JORDAN, H. *et al.* 2004. Costimulation controls diabetes by altering the balance of pathogenic and regulatory T cells. J. Clin. Invest. **114:** 979–987.
18. POIROT, L., C. BENOIST & D. MATHIS. 2004. Natural killer cells distinguish innocuous and destructive forms of pancreatic islet autoimmunity. Proc. Natl. Acad. Sci. USA **101:** 8102–8107.
19. WICKER, L.S., J.A. TODD & L.B. PETERSON. 1995. Genetic control of autoimmune diabetes in the NOD mouse. Annu. Rev. Immunol. **13:** 179–200.
20. HALL, R.J. *et al.* 2003. An autoimmune diabetes locus (Idd21) on mouse chromosome 18. Mamm. Genome **14:** 335–339.

21. WICKER, L.S. *et al.* 2004. Fine mapping, gene content, comparative sequencing, and expression analyses support Ctla4 and Nramp1 as candidates for Idd5.1 and Idd5.2 in the nonobese diabetic mouse. J. Immunol. **173:** 164–173.
22. HATTORI, M. *et al.* 1986. The NOD mouse: recessive diabetogenic gene in the major histocompatibility complex. Science **231:** 733–735.
23. DAVIES, J.L. *et al.* 1994. A genome-wide search for human type 1 diabetes susceptibility genes. Nature **371:** 130–136.
24. POCIOT, F. *et al.* 2004. Novel analytical methods applied to type 1 diabetes genome-scan data. Am. J. Hum. Genet. **74:** 647–660.
25. HORNUM, L. & H. MARKHOLST. 2004. New autoimmune genes and the pathogenesis of type 1 diabetes. Curr. Diab. Rep. **4:** 135–142.
26. UEDA, H. *et al.* 2003. Association of the T-cell regulatory gene CTLA4 with susceptibility to autoimmune disease. Nature **423:** 506–511.
27. BOTTINI, N. *et al.* 2004. A functional variant of lymphoid tyrosine phosphatase is associated with type I diabetes. Nat. Genet. **36:** 337–338.
28. SIMINOVITCH, K.A. 2004. PTPN22 and autoimmune disease. Nat. Genet. **36:** 1248–1249.
29. WALTER, M. *et al.* 2003. IDDM2/insulin VNTR modifies risk conferred by IDDM1/HLA for development of Type 1 diabetes and associated autoimmunity. Diabetologia **46:** 712–720.
30. BEGOVICH, A.B. *et al.* 2004. A missense single-nucleotide polymorphism in a gene encoding a protein tyrosine phosphatase (PTPN22) is associated with rheumatoid arthritis. Am. J. Hum. Genet. **75:** 330–337.
31. KYOGOKU, C. *et al.* 2004. Genetic association of the R620W polymorphism of protein tyrosine phosphatase PTPN22 with human SLE. Am. J. Hum. Genet. **75:** 504–507.
32. GUO, D. *et al.* 2004. A functional variant of SUMO4, a new I kappa B alpha modifier, is associated with type 1 diabetes. Nat. Genet. **36:** 837–841.
33. SHARPE, A.H. & G.J. FREEMAN. 2002. The B7-CD28 superfamily. Nat. Rev. Immunol. **2:** 116–126.
34. GAMBINERI, E., T.R. TORGERSON & H.D. OCHS. 2003. Immune dysregulation, polyendocrinopathy, enteropathy, and X-linked inheritance (IPEX), a syndrome of systemic autoimmunity caused by mutations of FOXP3, a critical regulator of T cell homeostasis. Curr. Opin. Rheumatol. **15:** 430–435.
35. RAMSDELL, F. 2003. Foxp3 and natural regulatory T cells: key to a cell lineage? Immunity **19:** 165–168.
36. ANDERSON, M.S. *et al.* 2002. Projection of an immunological self shadow within the thymus by the aire protein. Science **298:** 1395–1401.
37. YU, L. & G. EISENBARTH. 2002. Humoral autoimmunity. *In* Type 1 Diabetes: Cellular, Molecular and Clinical Immunology [published online <http://www.uchsc.edu/misc/diabetes/books.html>]. G. Eisenbarth & K. Lafferty, Eds. University of Colorado Health Sciences Center. Denver.
38. YU, L. *et al.* 2003. The second murine autoantibody workshop: remarkable interlaboratory concordance for radiobinding assays to identify insulin autoantibodies in nonobese diabetic mice. Ann. N.Y. Acad. Sci. **1005:** 1–12.
39. NORRIS, J.M. *et al.* 2003. Timing of initial cereal exposure in infancy and risk of islet autoimmunity. JAMA **290:** 1713–1720.
40. ZIEGLER, A.G. *et al.* 2003. Early infant feeding and risk of developing type 1 diabetes-associated autoantibodies. JAMA **290:** 1721–1728.
41. KNIP, M. 2003. Environmental triggers and determinants of beta-cell autoimmunity and type 1 diabetes. Rev. Endocr. Metab. Disord. **4:** 213–223.
42. WASMUTH, H.E. & H. KOLB. 2000. Cow's milk and immune-mediated diabetes. Proc. Nutr. Soc. **59:** 573–579.
43. ATKINSON, M.A. *et al.* 1988. Dietary protein restriction reduces the frequency and delays the onset of insulin dependent diabetes in BB rats. Autoimmunity **2:** 11–19.
44. Martin, J.M. *et al.* 1991. Milk proteins in the etiology of insulin-dependent diabetes mellitus (IDDM). Ann. Med. **23:** 447–452.
45. ATKINSON, M.A. *et al.* 1993. Lack of immune responsiveness to bovine serum albumin in insulin-dependent diabetes. N. Engl. J. Med. **329:** 1853–1858.

46. Norris, J.M. *et al.* 1996. Lack of association between early exposure to cow's milk protein and beta-cell autoimmunity: Diabetes Autoimmunity Study in the Young (DAISY). JAMA **276:** 609–614.
47. Couper, J.J. *et al.* 1999. Lack of association between duration of breast-feeding or introduction of cow's milk and development of islet autoimmunity. Diabetes **48:** 2145–2149.
48. Wen, L., J. Peng, Z. Li & F.S. Wong. 2004. The effect of innate immunity on autoimmune diabetes and the expression of Toll-like receptors on pancreatic islets. J. Immunol. **172:** 3173–3180.
49. Hiemstra, H.S. *et al.* 2001. Cytomegalovirus in autoimmunity: T cell crossreactivity to viral antigen and autoantigen glutamic acid decarboxylase. Proc. Natl. Acad. Sci. USA **98:** 3988–3991.
50. Ellerman, K.E. & A.A. Like. 2000. Susceptibility to diabetes is widely distributed in normal class IIu haplotype rats. Diabetologia **43:** 890–898.
51. Christen, U. *et al.* 2004. A viral epitope that mimics a self antigen can accelerate but not initiate autoimmune diabetes. J. Clin. Invest. **114:** 1290–1298.
52. Mathis, D., L. Vence & C. Benoist. 2001. beta-Cell death during progression to diabetes. Nature **414:** 792–798.
53. Turley, S. *et al.* 2003. Physiological beta cell death triggers priming of self-reactive T cells by dendritic cells in a type-1 diabetes model. J. Exp. Med. **198:** 1527–1537.
54. Jansen, A. *et al.* 1994. Immunohistochemical characterization of monocytes-macrophages and dendritic cells involved in the initiation of the insulitis and beta-cell destruction in NOD mice. Diabetes **43:** 667–675.
55. Serreze, D.V. *et al.* 1996. B lymphocytes are essential for the initiation of T cell-mediated autoimmune diabetes: analysis of a new "speed congenic" stock of NOD.Ig mu null mice. J. Exp. Med. **184:** 2049–2053.
56. Itoh, N. *et al.* 1993. Mononuclear cell infiltration and its relation to the expression of major histocompatibility complex antigens and adhesion molecules in pancreas biopsy specimens from newly diagnosed insulin-dependent diabetes mellitus patients. J. Clin. Invest. **92:** 2313–2322.
57. Kagi, D. *et al.* 1997. Reduced incidence and delayed onset of diabetes in perforin-deficient nonobese diabetic mice. J. Exp. Med. **186:** 989–997.
58. Moriwaki, M. *et al.* 1999. Fas and Fas ligand expression in inflamed islets in pancreas sections of patients with recent-onset Type I diabetes mellitus. Diabetologia **42:** 1332–1340.
59. Savinov, A.Y. *et al.* 2003. Contribution of Fas to diabetes development. Proc. Natl. Acad. Sci. USA **100:** 628–632.
60. Arnush, M. *et al.* 1998. IL-1 produced and released endogenously within human islets inhibits beta cell function. J. Clin. Invest. **102:** 516–526.
61. Sreenan, S. *et al.* 1999. Increased beta-cell proliferation and reduced mass before diabetes onset in the nonobese diabetic mouse. Diabetes **48:** 989–996.
62. Schloot, N.C. *et al.* 2003. Comparison of cytokine ELISpot assay formats for the detection of islet antigen autoreactive T cells. Report of the third immunology of diabetes society T-cell workshop. J. Autoimmun. **21:** 365–376.
63. Trudeau, J. D. *et al.* 2003. Prediction of spontaneous autoimmune diabetes in NOD mice by quantification of autoreactive T cells in peripheral blood. J. Clin. Invest. **111:** 217–223.
64. Keskinen, P. *et al.* 2002. First-phase insulin response in young healthy children at genetic and immunological risk for Type I diabetes. Diabetologia **45:** 1639–1648.
65. Bleich, D., R.A. Jackson, J.S. Soeldner & G.S. Eisenbarth. 1990. Analysis of metabolic progression to type I diabetes in ICA+ relatives of patients with type I diabetes. Diabetes Care **13:** 111–118.
66. Palmer, J.P. *et al.* 2004. C-peptide is the appropriate outcome measure for type 1 diabetes clinical trials to preserve beta-cell function: report of an ADA workshop, 21–22 October 2001. Diabetes **53:** 250–264.
67. Bolt, S. *et al.* 1993. The generation of a humanized, non-mitogenic CD3 monoclonal antibody which retains in vitro immunosuppressive properties. Eur. J. Immunol. **23:** 403–411.

68. ALEGRE, M.L. *et al.* 1994. A non-activating "humanized" anti-CD3 monoclonal antibody retains immunosuppressive properties in vivo. Transplantation **57:** 1537–1543.
69. CHATENOUD, L. 2004. Anti-CD3 antibodies: towards clinical antigen-specific immunomodulation. Curr. Opin. Pharmacol. **4:** 403–407.
70. BELGHITH, M. *et al.* 2003. TGF-beta-dependent mechanisms mediate restoration of self-tolerance induced by antibodies to CD3 in overt autoimmune diabetes. Nat. Med. **9:** 1202–1208.
71. SHAPIRO, A.M. *et al.* 2000. Islet transplantation in seven patients with type 1 diabetes mellitus using a glucocorticoid-free immunosuppressive regimen. N. Engl. J. Med. **343:** 230–238.
72. RYAN, E.A. *et al.* 2001. Clinical outcomes and insulin secretion after islet transplantation with the Edmonton protocol. Diabetes **50:** 710–719.
73. RYAN, E.A. *et al.* 2002. Successful islet transplantation: continued insulin reserve provides long-term glycemic control. Diabetes **51:** 2148–2157.
74. BERTUZZI, F., A. SECCHI & V. DI CARLO. 2004. Islet transplantation in type 1 diabetic patients. Transplant Proc. **36:** 603–604.
75. ITKIN-ANSARI, P. *et al.* 2003. Cell-based therapies for diabetes: progress towards a transplantable human beta cell line. Ann. N.Y. Acad. Sci. **1005:** 138–147.
76. ITKIN-ANSARI, P. & F. LEVINE. 2004. Sources of beta-cells for human cell-based therapies for diabetes. Cell Biochem. Biophys. **40:** 103–112.
77. EISENBARTH, G. S. *et al.* 1985. Anti-thymocyte globulin and prednisone immunotherapy of recent onset type 1 diabetes mellitus. Diabetes Res. **2:** 271–276.
78. RAZ, I. *et al.* 2001. Beta-cell function in new-onset type 1 diabetes and immunomodulation with a heat-shock protein peptide (DiaPep277): a randomised, double-blind, phase II trial. Lancet **358:** 1749–1753.
79. CAREL, J.C. *et al.* 1996. Cyclosporine delays but does not prevent clinical onset in glucose intolerant pre-type 1 diabetic children. J. Autoimmun. **9:** 739–745.
80. DIABETES PREVENTION TRIAL—TYPE I DIABETES STUDY GROUP. 2002. Effects of insulin in relatives of patients with type 1 diabetes mellitus. N. Engl. J. Med. **346**: 1685–1691.
81. KUPILA, A. *et al.* 2001. Feasibility of genetic and immunological prediction of type I diabetes in a population-based birth cohort. Diabetologia **44:** 290–297.
82. EISENBARTH, G. 2004. Prediction of type 1 diabetes: the natural history of the prediabetic Period (teaching slides). *In* Type 1 Diabetes: Cellular, Molecular and Clinical Immunology [published online <http://www.uchsc.edu/misc/diabetes/books.html>]. G. Eisenbarth & K. Lafferty, Eds. University of Colorado Health Sciences Center. Denver.

Soluble CD40L in Plasma of Patients with Primary Biliary Cirrhosis

SABINE OERTELT,[a,b] PIETRO INVERNIZZI,[b] CARLO SELMI,[a,b] MAURO PODDA,[b] AND M. ERIC GERSHWIN[a]

[a]*Division of Rheumatology, Allergy and Clinical Immunology, University of California at Davis, Davis, California 95616, USA*

[b]*Divison of Internal Medicine, Department of Medicine, Surgery and Dentistry, San Paolo School of Medicine, University of Milan, Milan, Italy*

ABSTRACT: CD40 ligand (CD40L) is expressed by activated T cells and interacts with the CD40 molecule present on B cells and endothelial cells, promoting immunoglobulin switching in the former and cytokine upregulation in the latter. CD40L exists in both a soluble (sCD40L) and a membrane-bound form. Because primary biliary cirrhosis (PBC) is characterized by targeting of small intrahepatic bile ducts by autoreactive T cells, plasma concentrations of sCD40L were investigated using enzyme-linked immunosorbent assay (ELISA) to measure plasma concentrations of sCD40L in 12 patients with PBC and 12 healthy controls. No difference could be detected between plasma concentrations of sCD40L in patients versus controls ($P = 0.977$). No correlation between age and plasma levels of sCD40L could be identified ($P = 0.24$). We concluded that PBC patients do not exhibit higher plasma concentrations of sCD40L than age-matched controls, a finding common to several autoimmune diseases. Further investigation of the CD40-CD40L system is strongly encouraged.

KEYWORDS: primary biliary cirrhosis (PBC); soluble CD40L; autoimmunity; biliary epithelial cells

INTRODUCTION

Primary biliary cirrhosis (PBC) is an autoimmune disease of the liver, characterized by the presence of circulating anti-mitochondrial antibodies (AMAs)[1] and infiltrating autoreactive T lymphocytes, leading to the progressive destruction of small intrahepatic bile ducts and, eventually, to cirrhosis and liver failure.[2] The high prevalence of circulating antibodies and the existence of a major immunogenic epitope shared between B and autoreactive T lymphocytes suggests a strong interaction among different branches of the immune system.[3]

Address for correspondence: M. Eric Gershwin, M.D., Division of Rheumatology, Allergy and Clinical Immunology, University of California at Davis School of Medicine, Genome and Biomedical Sciences Facility, 451 E. Health Sciences Drive, Suite 6510, Davis, CA 95616. Voice: 530-752-2884; fax: 530-752-4669.

megershwin@ucdavis.edu

Ann. N.Y. Acad. Sci. 1051: 205–210 (2005). © 2005 New York Academy of Sciences.

doi: 10.1196/annals.1361.062

The CD40–CD40 ligand system constitutes one of the fundamental accessory molecules in T–B cell activation. CD40 is expressed by B cells, as well as macrophages and epithelial cells;[4] CD40 ligand (CD40L) is upregulated upon activation of Th cells through TCR involvement. CD40L, a 39 kDa cellular membrane component, is a member of the tumor necrosis factor (TNF) ligand superfamily of receptors.[5] It stimulates B cell activation, immunoglobulin production, and class switching, as well as endothelial cell response, leading to production of inflammatory cytokines and upregulation of cell adhesion molecules.[6] Two different sources of soluble CD40L (sCD40L) have been identified: T cells, which release sCD40L by enzymatic cleavage at a metalloproteinase-sensitive site in the membrane-proximal region of the extracellular domain; and platelets, which release sCD40L from intracytoplasmic vesicles upon contact-activated degranulation.

In recent years many associations between the plasma concentration of soluble CD40L and disease activity and severity have been documented in several autoimmune diseases, especially those correlated with vascular inflammation, such as systemic lupus erythematosus,[7] diabetes type I,[8] and inflammatory bowel diseases.[9] We investigated the role of soluble CD40L in PBC because of the definite pathogenetic role of activated T cells in disease initiation and progression, and the potential role of CD40L in two of the typical findings of PBC—high IgM titers and a predisposition to certain types of infection, especially urinary tract infections.

Hyper-IgM syndrome (XHIM) is a disorder associated with a mutation of the X-linked CD40L gene;[10] patients characteristically exhibit a defect in immunoglobulin switching, with elevated blood IgM concentrations, immunodeficiency, and a high incidence of opportunistic infections. These findings resemble those detected in PBC, even if the clinical expression is much reduced. Moreover, biliary epithelial cells (BECs) express CD40 on their surface and undergo apoptosis after stimulation of CD40 with CD40L and subsequent Fas upregulation;[11] thus, these cells could represent both a potential trigger and a target source. Both the T cell–bound CD40L and its soluble form might interact with BEC CD40, stimulating the release of proinflammatory cytokines, resembling the findings in atherogenesis.[12,13]

In addition, a predictive molecular marker for T cell activation and disease severity in PBC is not available and would represent a valuable biochemical tool for prognosis. Indeed, the appropriate counseling and clinical management of the growing number of individuals with early PBC requires the accurate identification of patients with rapidly progressing disease. Unfortunately, current prognostic variables are based on data from patients with advanced disease, proving less appropriate for subjects with normal levels of most variables.[14]

MATERIALS AND METHODS

Patient Samples

After obtaining written consent, blood was drawn from 12 patients with PBC and 12 healthy controls. The diagnosis of PBC was made according to internationally accepted criteria.[2] Classification of histological features was determined by Ludwig's staging, no or little fibrosis corresponding to stage I-II, fibrosis or cirrhosis to stage III-IV.[15] Patients had a mean age of 54 years (range: 28 to 70); controls were matched to the PBC patients by age classes and sex ratio, the mean age being 51 years (range: 31 to 66). All patients were AMA-positive and on therapy with ursodeoxycholic acid (UDCA, 12 to 15 mg/kg/d). One patient was affected by CREST syndrome. The study protocol excluded patients and healthy subjects with known specific signs of inflammation, as this could interfere with T cell activation.

Whole blood was collected into EDTA tubes and immediately centrifuged at 100 × *g* for 10 min to obtain platelet-free plasma; an additional centrifugation at 100 × *g* for 10 min was performed to ensure elimination of all platelets. This technique was selected because of the variable findings related to collection method in previous studies.[16,17] Plasma was stored at –80° until analysis.

Determination of Soluble CD40L Concentration by ELISA

Commercial sCD40L ELISA kits were obtained (R&D Systems, Minneapolis, MN) and assays performed following the manufacturer's instructions. In brief: diluted samples of patient plasma were applied in duplication 96-well plates precoated with polyclonal anti-CD40L antibody and incubated for 2 h on a shaker. After washing four times, the plates were incubated for other 2 h with polyclonal enzyme-linked anti-CD40L antibody conjugated with horseradish peroxidase. The plates were washed an additional four times and substrate was added to determine the quantity of CD40L bound. The plates were then analyzed on a microplate reader (Wallac, Victor2, Wellesley, MA).

Statistical Analysis

Differences in the concentrations of soluble CD40L between patients and controls were determined by Mann-Whitney nonpaired nonparametric test, two-tailed probabilities were used for significance testing, and $P < .05$ was considered signifi-

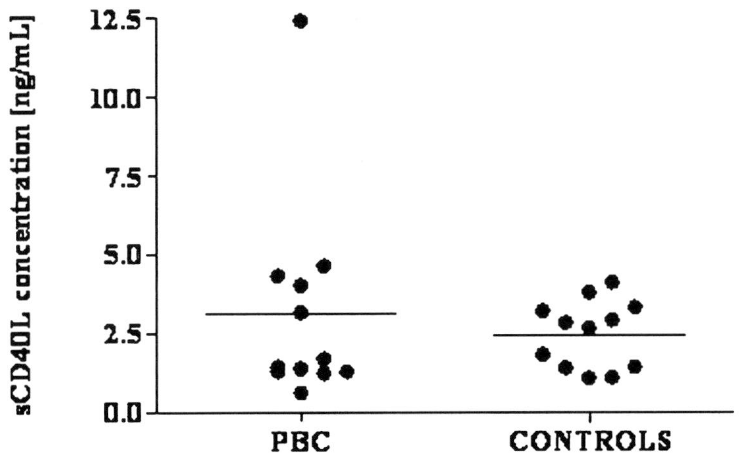

FIGURE 1. Distribution of plasma sCD40L values among PBC patients and controls.

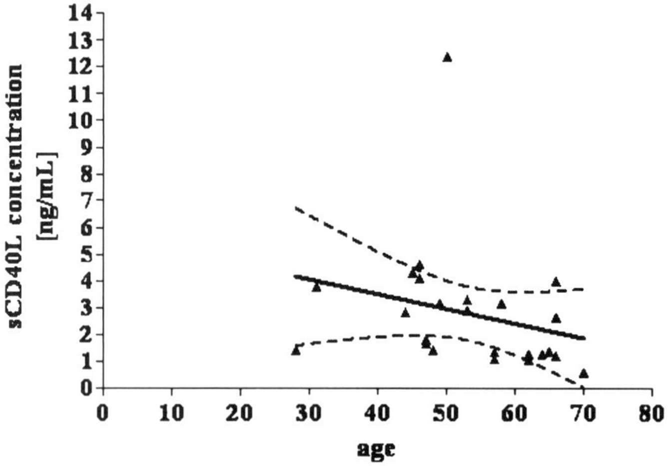

FIGURE 2. Correlation between sCD40L concentrations and age.

cant. All statistical analysis was performed using GraphPad Prism software, version 4.0 (GraphPad Software, Inc., San Diego, CA).

RESULTS

Twelve PBC patients and 12 healthy controls were enrolled for determination of soluble CD40L levels in plasma samples. Normal values for sCD40L in plasma are 0.03 to 3.98 ng/mL. Values can be modified by any condition involving T cell and platelet activation. Comparing the two groups, no significant difference could be identified ($P = .977$). The median concentration of sCD40L was 1.535 ng/mL in patients (range: 0.58–12.4) and 2.72 ng/mL in controls (range: 1.05–4.09). No difference could be detected between patients with more advanced disease and those staged I-II. Despite one male patient, affected also by CREST, who showed a particularly elevated titer of sCD40L (12.4 ng/mL) compared with the study population, no differences in the overall distribution could be detected between the two groups (FIG. 1). No correlation could be identified between plasma CD40L titer and age ($P = .24$; FIG. 2).

DISCUSSION

The absence of significant differences in the plasma concentrations of sCD40L among PBC patients versus healthy controls in this study may be related to several factors. The source of the systemic increase of sCD40L in other diseases, especially those with vascular involvement, has been identified as platelets activated through local stimulation.[18,19] Previous studies have been performed using serum instead of plasma, leading to potential platelet degranulation[20,21] and modified sCD40L gradients. T cells are known to be a source of sCD40L, but their role in the systemic increase of the factor has not been established. The localized inflammation in PBC, restricted to small intrahepatic bile ducts, might not be sufficient to trigger variation of plasma sCD40L concentration. Moreover, the absence of a systemic elevation of sCD40L cannot role out the presence of a localized increase exerting a paracrine effect. Furthermore, UDCA, the most commonly administered medication in PBC, has demonstrated immunomodulatory activity on disease progression[22] and adjuvant effect on engraftment, reducing the rejection rate.[23] The direct toxicological activity of UDCA is not known, but according to its effects, this agent could be cause a reduction in T cell activation and, consequently, a reduction of the circulating CD40L titer. All enrolled patients were taking UDCA therapy; an analysis of patients prior to therapy or after washout could thus give divergent results.

Thc negative result cannot exclude a potential role of CD40L in both its soluble and membrane-bound form in PBC. A high incidence of chronic cholangiopathies, cirrhosis, and malignancies have been seen in XHIM as a consequence of infection and persistent inflammation, most likely due to *Cryptosporidium*.[24,25] The involvement of bacterial infections as potential triggers of PBC is a commonly accepted theory, even if no causative agent has been identified thus far.[26] These findings, associated with the higher prevalence of X monosomy in PBC patients,[27] could point to a selective quantitative or functional defect of the CD40–CD40L interaction. It is not possible to rule out whether our findings are related to reduced T cell activation, insufficient concentrations of the molecule on a systemic basis, or molecular modifications. Higuchi and colleagues[28] investigated the presence of mutations in the CD40L gene in PBC patients by single-strand conformational polymorphism (SSCP), finding no differences between patients and controls. Nonetheless, both the absence of the same mutation conducing to hyper-IgM syndrome and the absence of an elevated sCD40L titer should be considered as preliminary data, acquired in small populations of patients and thus only indicative; further investigation of this intriguing molecule in the pathogenesis of PBC should be strongly encouraged.

REFERENCES

1. Gershwin, M.E., I.R. Mackay, A. Sturgess & R.L. Coppel. 1987. Identification and specificity of a cDNA encoding the 70 kd mitochondrial antigen recognized in primary biliary cirrhosis. J. Immunol. **138:** 3525–3531.
2. Kaplan, M.M. *et al.* 2005. Primary biliary cirrhosis. N. Engl. J. Med. In press.
3. Stout, R.D. & J. Suttles. 1996. The many roles of CD40 in cell-mediated inflammatory responses. Immunol. Today **17:** 487–492.
4. Durie, F.H. *et al.* 1994. The role of CD40 in the regulation of humoral and cell-mediated immunity. Immunol. Today **15:** 406–411.
5. Banchereau, J. *et al.* 1994. The CD40 antigen and its ligand. Annu. Rev. Immunol. **12:** 881–922.
6. Mach, F. *et al.* 1997. Functional CD40 ligand is expressed on human vascular endothelial cells, smooth muscle cells, and macrophages: implications for CD40-CD40 ligand signaling in atherosclerosis. Proc. Natl. Acad. Sci. USA **94:** 1931–1936.
7. Kato, K. *et al.* 1999. The soluble CD40 ligand sCD154 in systemic lupus erythematosus. J. Clin. Invest. **104:** 947–955.
8. Lim, H.S., A.D. Blann & G.Y. Lip. 2004. Soluble CD40 ligand, soluble P-selectin, interleukin-6, and tissue factor in diabetes mellitus: relationships to cardiovascular disease and risk factor intervention. Circulation **109:** 2524–2528.

9. DANESE, S., M. SANS & C. FIOCCHI. 2004. The CD40/CD40L costimulatory pathway in inflammatory bowel disease. Gut **53:** 1035–1043.
10. ETZIONI, A. & H.D. OCHS. 2004. The hyper IgM syndrome—an evolving story. Pediatr. Res. **56:** 519–525.
11. AFFORD, S.C. *et al.* 2001. CD40 activation-induced, Fas-dependent apoptosis and NF-kappaB/AP-1 signaling in human intrahepatic biliary epithelial cells. FASEB J. **15:** 2345–2354.
12. SCHONBECK, U. & P. LIBBY. 2001. CD40 signaling and plaque instability. Circ. Res. **89:** 1092–1103.
13. HOLLENBAUGH, D. *et al.* 1995. Expression of functional CD40 by vascular endothelial cells. J. Exp. Med. **182:** 33–40.
14. SPRINGER, J. *et al.* 1999. Asymptomatic primary biliary cirrhosis: a study of its natural history and prognosis. Am. J. Gastroenterol. **94:** 47–53.
15. LUDWIG, J. 1987. New concepts in biliary cirrhosis. Semin. Liver Dis. **7:** 293–301.
16. THOM, J. *et al.* 2004. Measurement of soluble P-selectin and soluble CD40 ligand in serum and plasma. J. Thromb. Haemost. **2:** 2067–2069.
17. AHN, E.R., *et al.* 2004. Differences of soluble CD40L in sera and plasma: implications on CD40L assay as a marker of thrombotic risk. Thromb. Res. **114:** 143–148.
18. DANESE, S. *et al.* 2003. Activated platelets are the source of elevated levels of soluble CD40 ligand in the circulation of inflammatory bowel disease patients. Gut **52:** 1435–1441.
19. HARDING, S.A. *et al.* 2004. Increased CD40 ligand and platelet-monocyte aggregates in patients with type 1 diabetes mellitus. Atherosclerosis **176:** 321–325.
20. VAKKALANKA, R.K. *et al.* 1999. Elevated levels and functional capacity of soluble CD40 ligand in systemic lupus erythematosus sera. Arthritis Rheum. **42:** 871–881.
21. KOMURA, K. *et al.* 2004. Elevated circulating CD40L concentrations in patients with systemic sclerosis. J. Rheumatol. **31:** 514–519.
22. KOULENTAKI, M. *et al.* 2004. Survival of anti-mitochondrial antibody-positive and -negative primary biliary cirrhosis patients on ursodeoxycholic acid treatment. Dig. Dis. Sci. **49:** 1190–1195.
23. FRIMAN, S. *et al.* 1992. Adjuvant treatment with ursodeoxycholic acid reduces acute rejection after liver transplantation. Transpl. Int. (Suppl. 1) **5:** S187–189.
24. HAYWARD, A.R. *et al.* 1997. Cholangiopathy and tumors of the pancreas, liver, and biliary tree in boys with X-linked immunodeficiency with hyper-IgM. J. Immunol. **158:** 977–983.
25. STEPHENS, J., M. COSYNS, M. JONES & A. HAYWARD. 1999. Liver and bile duct pathology following *Cryptosporidium parvum* infection of immunodeficient mice. Hepatology **30:** 27–35.
26. BAUM, H. 1995. Mitochondrial antigens, molecular mimicry and autoimmune disease. Biochim. Biophys. Acta. **1271:** 111–121.
27. INVERNIZZI, P. *et al.* 2004. Frequency of monosomy X in women with primary biliary cirrhosis. Lancet **363:** 533–535.
28. HIGUCHI, M. *et al.* 1998. Analysis of CD40 ligand gene mutations in patients with primary biliary cirrhosis. Scand. J. Clin. Lab. Invest. **58:** 429–432.

Decreased Serum Leptin Levels in Primary Biliary Cirrhosis

A Link between Metabolism and Autoimmunity?

ROMAN RIEGER,[a,c] SABINE OERTELT,[a,c] CARLO SELMI,[a,b]
PIETRO INVERNIZZI,[b] MAURO PODDA,[b] AND M. ERIC GERSHWIN[a]

[a]*Division of Rheumatology, Allergy and Clinical Immunology, University of California at Davis, Davis, California 95616, USA*

[b]*Division of Internal Medicine, San Paolo School of Medicine, University of Milan, Milan, Italy*

ABSTRACT: Primary biliary cirrhosis (PBC) is an autoimmune liver disease of unknown etiology resulting in the progressive destruction of the intrahepatic bile ducts and leading to chronic cholestasis and ultimately liver cirrhosis and failure. The immune response in PBC seems to be mediated by autoantibodies as well as autoreactive T lymphocytes directed against mitochondrial antigens in biliary epithelial cells, primarily PDC-E2. Experimental evidence suggests a role of the hormone/cytokine leptin in autoimmune diseases. Leptin is an adipocyte-derived molecule that acts as a hormone influencing food intake and energy metabolism as well as a cytokine with pro-inflammatory, immune-regulatory functions. To study serum leptin in PBC and its association with disease severity, we evaluated serum levels in 37 patients with PBC (27 with no signs of fibrosis or cirrhosis at histologic examination) and 37 age- and sex-matched healthy controls using a validated ELISA method. We found that patients with PBC had significantly lower leptin serum levels compared with healthy controls (13.6 ± 13.8 vs. 17.6 ± 11.6; $P < 0.05$). No correlation between disease severity and serum leptin levels was found. This study has demonstrated that leptin levels are decreased in the serum of patients with PBC but do not seem to be associated with disease severity. Data do not seem to indicate a direct role of leptin in the perpetuation of the autoimmune response in PBC. However, further studies are warranted to further characterize the functions of leptin during the natural history of autoimmunity.

KEYWORDS: primary biliary cirrhosis; leptin; autoimmune disease

INTRODUCTION

Initially discovered as a regulator of body weight through inhibition of food intake,[1] the mainly adipocyte-produced hormone leptin has been recently recognized

Address for correspondence: M. Eric Gershwin, M.D., Division of Rheumatology, Allergy and Clinical Immunology, University of California at Davis School of Medicine, GBSF Suite 6510, Davis, CA 95616. Voice: 530-752-2884; fax: 530-752-4669.
megershwin@ucdavis.edu
[c]These authors contributed equally to this work.

**Ann. N.Y. Acad. Sci. 1051: 211–217 (2005). © 2005 New York Academy of Sciences.
doi: 10.1196/annals.1361.124**

as an active modulator of the induction and plasticity of the immune system. In fact, leptin influences neutrophil chemotaxis, macrophage phagocytosis, and T cell apoptosis.[2–4] Moreover, it can contribute to the switch toward a T helper (Th) type I response in specific experimental conditions, through autocrine IFN-γ and TNF-α upregulation, as well as NK cell activation.[5,6] These particular functions of leptin have prompted an intense investigation of its potential effects as a trigger and severity marker in autoimmune diseases.[7] Nonetheless, despite the apparent univocal effect of leptin on disease susceptibility and progression observed in animal models, the association of the molecule with human autoimmunity remains controversial (TABLE 1). The apparently conflicting data might represent the necessity of other cytokines to elicit leptin functions[8] or the existence of more complex regulatory networks.

Primary biliary cirrhosis (PBC) is an autoimmune liver disease characterized by the presence of circulating antimitochondrial antibodies (AMA), chronic cholestasis, and progressive destruction of the intrahepatic bile ducts eventually leading to cirrhosis and liver failure.[9] The condition is associated with the presence of autoreactive liver-infiltrating T and NK cells that give rise to a local inflammatory response without a univocal Th response for the simultaneous presence of divergent cytokine subsets.[10] Two recent studies have investigated leptin levels in PBC with conflicting results.[11,12] In the following study we attempted to shed further light on the role of leptin in PBC by analyzing serum levels in a population of well-defined patients with PBC and matched healthy controls.

MATERIAL AND METHODS

Patient Samples

Serum samples were obtained from 37 female patients with PBC and 37 age-matched healthy control women after overnight fasting. The diagnosis of PBC was based on internationally accepted criteria, including detectable serum AMA, a cholestatic pattern of serum biochemical tests (elevated serum alkaline phosphatase) for at least 6 months, and/or compatible liver histology.[13] The median age of patients at enrollment was 67 years (range 41–89 years) (healthy controls: 66 years, range 36–89 years) with a median disease duration of 11 years (range 1–37 years). All patients had undergone liver biopsy within 18 months prior to enrollment and histologic staging was defined in accordance with Ludwig's criteria.[14] In our series, 27/37 patients presented histologic evidence of liver fibrosis or cirrhosis (i.e., stages I and II) and 10/37 had stages III and IV. Clinical parameters and therapy of the study population are represented in TABLE 2. Serum samples from patients and controls were collected at the San Paolo University Hospital, Milan and frozen at –20°C until used for the detection assay. The study protocol followed the ethical guidelines of the most recent Declaration of Helsinki (Edinburgh, 2000), and all subjects enrolled in the study provided written informed consent.

Determination of Serum Leptin Concentrations

Serum leptin concentrations were measured in duplicate samples using an enzyme-linked immunosorbent assay (ELISA) kit (Linco Research, St. Charles, MI) according to the instructions of the manufacturer.

Statistical Analysis

The Mann-Whitney non-parametric U-test was used to compare leptin levels between groups and P values < 0.05 were considered statistically significant. A Spearman correlation was used to determine correlation between leptin levels and clinical parameters. Statistical analyses were performed using Prism software (GraphPad Software, San Diego, CA). Continuous variables are expressed as mean ± standard deviation (SD) unless specified otherwise.

RESULTS

Sera from 37 female patients with PBC and 37 age-matched female healthy controls were studied for leptin levels. Results observed are represented in FIGURE 1. Serum leptin levels were significantly lower in PBC patients compared with healthy controls (8.7 ± 13.8 ng/mL vs. 15.6 ± 11.6 ng/mL; median ± SD, $P < 0.037$). Among patients with PBC, no significant difference in serum leptin levels was found between histologic stage I/II (8.7 ± 15.2 ng/mL) and stage III/IV patients (7.6 ± 9.0 ng/mL, median ± SD). No significant correlation between leptin levels and patient age or disease duration, as well as serum ALT, alkaline phosphatase, or albumin levels or prothrombin time ratio could be found (data not shown). Finally, ongoing treatment of PBC with ursodiol (UDCA) or other immunomodulatory treatment, did not influence leptin levels (data not shown).

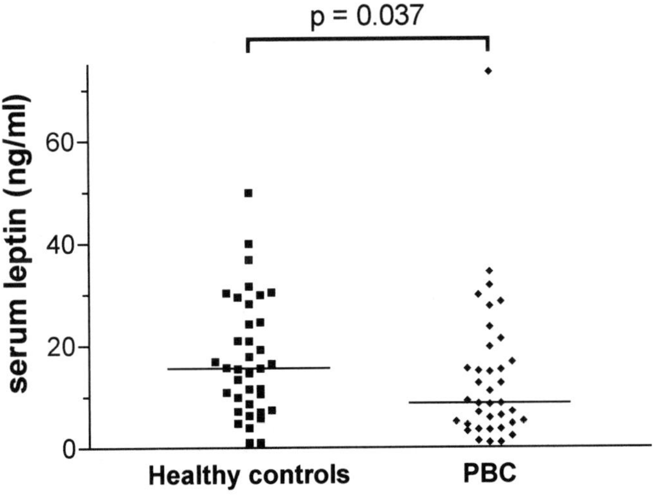

FIGURE 1. Serum leptin levels in patients with PBC and healthy controls.

TABLE 1. Available evidence for the role of leptin in human autoimmune disease

Circulating leptin levels	Reference
Inflammatory bowel disease	
Association among BMI and leptin, no correlation with disease severity	20
Higher levels associated with the disease, due to *in situ* production by epithelial cells	15
Graves' disease	
Thyroid hormones could increase serum leptin level during suppression of beta-adrenergic receptors in patients with Graves' disease	16
Thyroid function has no effect on leptin but has an effect on adiponectin and resistin	21
Type 1 diabetes	
Serum leptin levels are not altered in adolescents with diabetes mellitus	22
Leptin levels are higher in patients with DM I and correlate with disease duration and insulin therapy	17
Rheumatoid arthritis	
Plasma leptin was significantly increased; synovial fluid leptin levels were significantly lower	18
Correlation among BMI and leptin in patients with rheumatoid arthritis; no correlation with disease activity	23
Systemic lupus erythematosis	
Patients with SLE have higher levels of serum leptin, but these levels do not correlate with SLEDAI score, age, duration, or steroid therapy	19

DISCUSSION

In the present study, we investigated the serum concentration of leptin in patients with PBC and age-matched healthy controls. Recent studies have indicated an important function for leptin in innate and adaptive immunity and, as a result of that, also in autoimmune conditions. Indeed, leptin reportedly plays a role in autoimmune diseases such as inflammatory bowel disease (IBD), multiple sclerosis, type 1 diabetes, Graves' disease, systemic lupus erythematosus (SLE), and rheumatoid arthritis (RA). In particular, increased levels of leptin have been reported in all these conditions compared with controls[15–19] (TABLE 1). In these settings, we can hypothesize that leptin acts as a pro-inflammatory cytokine and promotes the typical Th1 cell differentiation and cytokine production during the autoimmune process. Interestingly, moreover, intestinal cells from patients with IBD have been demonstrated to secrete locally active leptin, thus contributing to the increase of the overall circulating pool.[15] However, other authors have reported that the observed serum leptin concentrations are within the physiological range in all of the above conditions except SLE,[20–23] thus questioning the function of leptin in autoimmunity.

TABLE 2. Clinical, histologic, and biochemical characteristics of patients with PBC

	Variable
Stage of disease	
Stage I–II	27
Stage III–IV	10
Age (years)	66 (41–89)
Duration of disease (years)	11.2 (1–7)
Bilirubin (mg/dL)	1.4 (0.4–12.8)
ALT (SGPT) (UI/L)	61.8 (11–354)
Alkaline phosphatase (UI/L)	450 (84–1526)
Albumin (g/dL)	3.97 (3.1–4.9)
PT (INR)	1.04 (0.97–1.5)
Therapy (no. of patients)	
No therapy	7
UDCA only	12
UDCA and other therapy	18

NOTE: Continuous variables are expressed as median (range).

The presence and function of leptin in PBC, an autoimmune disorder affecting the liver, is also controversial. In fact, data from two recent studies are conflicting. One study by Breidert *et al.* reported higher serum leptin in patients with PBC compared with controls, whereas serum levels of ghrelin, a leptin antagonist, were decreased.[11] On the other hand, a study from Spain indicated that PBC sera were characterized by lower leptin plasma levels and that such levels correlated with the histologic stage and severity of the disease.[19] In the present study, we observed lower serum leptin levels in patients with PBC compared with healthy controls, in line with the findings of Garcia-Gonzalez *et al.* However, we could not confirm the correlation between disease stage and serum levels of leptin. The presence of autoreactive T cell infiltrates in PBC livers suggests elevated serum levels of leptin compared with normal controls, assuming a function of leptin as a pro-inflammatory cytokine. However, similar to others,[19] we could not verify this hypothesis and report opposite findings. A possible explanation might be the occurrence of malabsorption associated with long-standing cholestasis in PBC[24] and the concurrent weight loss secondary to reduced assimilation of lipids.[25] This might in turn cause hypoplasia of the adipose tissue, thus resulting in an interference with leptin biosynthesis. These concomitant factors might exert a confounding effect in the correlation between leptin levels and the severity of PBC. The clinical significance and the question of whether leptin plays a role in the progression of PBC still remain to be elucidated. Moreover, it appears interesting that the presence of an enhanced metabolic rate has been postulated in patients with PBC.[26] Further, we note that the humoral and cellular autoimmune reactions in PBC are directed against enzymes such as pyruvate dehydrogenase that influence glucose levels, thus ultimately contributing to the metabolic requirements of the cell.[27] Finally, the effects of leptin as a pro-inflammatory cytokine in PBC also need to be elucidated.

In conclusion, our data obtained in a cross-sectional fashion demonstrate reduced serum levels of leptin in patients with PBC compared with healthy controls. Because leptin could play a role in the generation of clinical symptoms in PBC, longitudinal studies are necessary to investigate the changes in leptin levels over the natural history of the disease. In particular, it is currently unknown whether altered leptin levels are active determinants in the perpetuation of the immune-mediated tissue injury or else accompanying phenomena secondary to the injury itself. Moreover, it would be interesting to analyze the metabolic state of patients with PBC using methods for estimating the metabolic rates made available in the past decade.[28] Ultimately, only a multidisciplinary approach that requires expertise in biochemistry, metabolism, and immunology will allow a better definition of the role of leptin in the autoimmune pathogenesis of PBC.

ACKNOWLEDGMENTS

This work was supported by National Institutes of Health Grants DK39588 and DK037003

REFERENCES

1. Friedman, J.M. & J.L. Halaas. 1998. Leptin and the regulation of body weight in mammals. Nature **395:** 763–770.
2. Caldefie-Chezet, F., A. Poulin & M.P. Vasson. 2003. Leptin regulates functional capacities of polymorphonuclear neutrophils. Free Radic. Res. **37:** 809–814.
3. Mancuso, P. *et al.* 2002. Leptin-deficient mice exhibit impaired host defense in Gram-negative pneumonia. J. Immunol. **168:** 4018–4024.
4. Howard, J.K. *et al.* 1999. Leptin protects mice from starvation-induced lymphoid atrophy and increases thymic cellularity in ob/ob mice. J Clin Invest. **104:** 1051–1059.
5. Lord, G.M. *et al.* 1998. Leptin modulates the T-cell immune response and reverses starvation-induced immunosuppression. Nature. **394:** 897–901.
6. Tian, Z., *et al.* 2002. Impaired natural killer (NK) cell activity in leptin receptor deficient mice: leptin as a critical regulator in NK cell development and activation. Biochem. Biophys. Res. Commun. **298:** 297–302.
7. La Cava, A. & G. Matarese. 2004. The weight of leptin in immunity. Nat. Rev. Immunol. **4:** 371–379.
8. Zarkesh-Esfahani, H. *et al.* 2004. Leptin indirectly activates human neutrophils via induction of TNF-alpha. J. Immunol. **172:** 1809–1814.
9. Gershwin, M.E. *et al.* 2000. Primary biliary cirrhosis: an orchestrated immune response against epithelial cells. Immunol. Rev. **174:** 210–225.
10. Ishibashi, H. *et al.* 2003. T cell immunity and primary biliary cirrhosis. Autoimmun. Rev. **2:** 19–24.
11. Breidert, M. *et al.* 2004. Ghrelin/leptin-imbalance in patients with primary biliary cirrhosis. Exp. Clin. Endocrinol. Diabetes **112:** 123–126.
12. Garcia-Suarez, C. *et al.* 2004. [Plasma leptin levels in patients with primary biliary cirrhosis and their relationship with degree of fibrosis]. Gastroenterol. Hepatol. **27:** 47–50.
13. Kaplan, M.M. 1996. Primary biliary cirrhosis. N. Engl. J. Med. **335:** 1570–1580.
14. Ludwig, J., E.R. Dickson & G.S. McDonald. 1978. Staging of chronic nonsuppurative destructive cholangitis (syndrome of primary biliary cirrhosis). Virchows Arch. A. Pathol. Anat. Histol. **379:** 103–112.

15. SITARAMAN, S. *et al.* 2004. Colonic leptin: source of a novel proinflammatory cytokine involved in IBD. FASEB J. **18:** 696–698.
16. SERA, N. *et al.* 2000. Thyroid hormones influence serum leptin levels in patients with Graves' disease during suppression of beta-adrenergic receptors. Thyroid **10:** 641–646.
17. BIDECI, A., P. CINAZ & F. S. EZGU. 2002. Leptin levels in children with insulin dependent diabetes mellitus. Turk. J. Pediatr. **44:** 211–214.
18. BOKAREWA, M. *et al.* 2003. Leptin consumption in the inflamed joints of patients with rheumatoid arthritis. Ann. Rheum. Dis. **62:** 952–956.
19. GARCIA-GONZALEZ, A. *et al.* 2002. Serum leptin levels in women with systemic lupus erythematosus. Rheumatol. Int. **22:** 138–141.
20. HOPPIN, A.G. *et al.* 1998. Serum leptin in children and young adults with inflammatory bowel disease. J. Pediatr. Gastroenterol. Nutr. **26:** 500–505.
21. YATURU, S., S. PRADO & S.R. GRIMES. 2004. Changes in adipocyte hormones leptin, resistin, and adiponectin in thyroid dysfunction. J. Cell. Biochem. **93:** 491–496.
22. MYERS, S.E. *et al.* 2004. Pubertal changes in serum leptin levels in adolescents with type 1 diabetes mellitus: a controlled longitudinal study. J. Pediatr. Endocrinol. Metab. **17:** 1653–1662.
23. ANDERS, H.J. *et al.* 1999. Leptin serum levels are not correlated with disease activity in patients with rheumatoid arthritis. Metabolism.. **48**: 745–748.
24. DI LEO, V. *et al.* 2003. Gastroduodenal and intestinal permeability in primary biliary cirrhosis. Eur. J. Gastroenterol. Hepatol. **15:** 967–973.
25. LANSPA, S.J. *et al.* 1985. Pathogenesis of steatorrhea in primary biliary cirrhosis. Hepatology **5:** 837–842.
26. GREEN, J.H., P.N. BRAMLEY & M.S. LOSOWSKY. 1991. Are patients with primary biliary cirrhosis hypermetabolic? A comparison between patients before and after liver transplantation and controls. Hepatology **14**: 464–472.
27. SUGDEN, M.C. & M.J. HOLNESS. 2003. Recent advances in mechanisms regulating glucose oxidation at the level of the pyruvate dehydrogenase complex by PDKs. Am. J. Physiol. Endocrinol. Metab. **284:** E855–E862.
28. GIBNEY, E. *et al.* 1997. Total energy expenditure in patients with small-cell lung cancer: results of a validated study using the bicarbonate-urea method. Metabolism **46:** 1412–1417.

Analysis of the Foxp3/Scurfin Gene in Crohn's Disease

OGYI PARK,[a,b] IRINA GRISHINA,[a] PATRICK S. LEUNG,[b] M. ERIC GERSHWIN,[b] AND T. PRINDIVILLE[a]

[a]*Division of Gastroenterology and* [b]*Division of Rheumatology, Allergy and Clinical Immunology, Department of Internal Medicine, University of California at Davis, School of Medicine, Davis, California 95616, USA*

ABSTRACT: Crohn's disease (CD) is a chronic inflammatory bowel disease typified by transmural inflammation affecting any part of the gastrointestinal tract. CD4$^+$CD25$^+$ regulatory T cells (T_{reg} cells) play important roles in intestinal homeostasis. Adoptive transfer of regulatory T cells into mice with chronic colitis prevented inflammation and reappearance of normal intestinal architecture. The *Foxp3* gene encodes a protein that is a member of the forkhead/winged-helix family of transcriptional regulators and is involved in the regulation of T cell activation. Mutation of *Foxp3* gene may lead to development of autoimmune disease and inflammatory bowel disease. We investigated 10 single-nucleotide polymorphisms (SNPs) of the *Foxp3* gene in CD patients and assessed allele and genotype frequencies in 93 patients with Crohn's disease (61 female and 32 male), 82 patients with primary biliary cirrhosis (PBC) (all female), and 108 normal controls (51 female and 57 male). We found that 3 SNPs (−6054, –/ATT; −3279, A/C; −924, A/G) in the promoter region and 1 SNP (IVS9+459, T/C) in the intron 9 region existed in CD patients. No significant differences of allele and genotype frequencies of all four SNPs were observed between CD patients and controls (both female and male groups). However, there was a significance difference of the comparison between PBC patients and controls in the IVS9+459 SNP. These data indicate that SNPs of the Foxp3 gene are not significantly associated with CD but are associated with PBC.

KEYWORDS: Crohn's disease; primary biliary cirrhosis; single-nucleotide polymorphism; Foxp3; forkhead/winged helix box; T_{reg} cells; regulatory T cells

INTRODUCTION

Inflammatory bowel disease (IBD) is a complex polygenetic disease that phenotypically appears as two specific disorders: ulcerative colitis (UC) and Crohn's disease (CD). These diseases are typified by episodes of intense inflammation with periods of remission, a cycle that persists throughout the life of the patient, impli-

Address for correspondence: Thomas Prindiville, M.D., Division of Gastroenterology, University of California at Davis, School of Medicine, One Shields Avenue, Surge III, Davis, CA 96516. Voice: 530-752-3296.
tpprindiville@ucdavis.edu

**Ann. N.Y. Acad. Sci. 1051: 218–228 (2005). © 2005 New York Academy of Sciences.
doi: 10.1196/annals.1361.125**

cating significant immune dysregulation. The pathogenesis of IBD consists of three interacting elements: genetic background, priming by the enteric microflora, and immune-mediated tissue injury. These interactions lead to a cascade of events that result in the activation of inflammatory cells, the production of inflammatory cytokines and mediators, and tissue damage.[1,2] The genetic events responsible for these diseases highlight the complexity of the chronic inflammatory disease processes. Data from gene screening studies support the existence of a group of at least four susceptibility genes that predispose the host to the IBD phenotype of chronic inflammation. Superimposed on this susceptibility background is one of many specific diverse genetic abnormalities that result in the disease's subphenotypic expression. The additive effect of multiple susceptibility genes associated with one of at least five specific genes responsible for the CD subphenotype and one for the UC subphenotype complicate genomic scan studies.[3–5] Although the susceptibility genes are not completely delineated, several reside in the HLA, IBD5, and cytokine regions.[3,6–8]

The gastrointestinal tract is home to the largest number of leukocytes in the body as well as the site where these cells encounter abundant exogenous stimuli. In the gastrointestinal tract, regulation of the immune response is a balance between the need to mount protective immunity against pathogens, while not activating damaging inflammatory responses to the abundance of harmless antigens present, including those derived from resident bacteria.[9,10] To maintain intestinal homeostasis, the regulatory T cells (T_{reg} cells), a subset of $CD4^+$ T cells that express the marker CD25, are thought to perform the specialized role of peripheral regulation of both the adaptive and the innate immune system mediated by secretion of IL-10 and TGF-β.[11] T_{reg} cells also protect lymphopenic mice from induced inflammatory bowel disease, experimental autoimmune encephalomyelitis, diabetes, and allergy.[12–15]

$CD4^+CD25^+$ T cells, which constitute ~10 % of peripheral murine and human $CD4^+$ T cells, express CTLA-4, a glucocorticoid-induced TNFR family-related protein (GITR), and the forkhead/winged helix transcription factor Foxp3. Foxp3 has been shown to program the development and function of T_{reg} cells.[16–20]

Interestingly, the autoimmune response and inflammation produced by manipulating $CD25^+CD4^+$ T_{reg} cells and the genetic defects in *Foxp3* are quite similar. For example, $CD4^+$ T cell–mediated lymphoproliferative disease characterized by cachexia and multiorgan lymphocytic infiltrates has been shown to carry mutation in the *Foxp3* gene in the mouse strain scurfy.[21] Furthermore, the absence of the *Foxp3* gene in mice is associated with severe autoimmune disease that rapidly leads to the death of the host.[22] The human genetic disease immune dysregulation, polyendocrinopathy, enteropathy, X-linked syndrome (IPEX: also called X-linked autoimmunity–allergic dysregulation syndrome, XLAAD) is caused by mutations in the human homologue of *Foxp3*.[23–26] In contrast, overexpression of the gene in transgenic mice decreases T cell responsiveness and results in fewer peripheral T cells. $CD4^+CD25^-$ T cells transduced with *Foxp3* gene block the induction of IBD and gastritis in lymphopenic mice and inhibit the proliferation of naïve T cells *in vitro*.[20,27,28]

The *Foxp3* gene is located on chromosome Xp11.23 and encodes transcription factors possessing a forkhead/winged helix DNA binding domain.[23] Bassuny and colleagues studied microsatellite polymorphisms and single-nucleotide polymorphisms (SNPs) in human *Foxp3* gene. Their study showed that the functional polymorphism in the promoter/enhancer region of the *Foxp3* gene is associated with type

1 diabetes.[29] Antigen-specific *Foxp3*–transduced T cells have been shown to be effective in controlling established type 1 diabetes.[30]

It is believed that regulatory T cells play an important role in intestinal homeostasis and its dysregulation could lead to development of IBD. Recently, Malita *et al.* reported that $CD4^+CD25^+$ (bright) T cells residing in human intestinal lamina propria retained functional regulatory activity and are significantly increased in patients with IBD, suggesting that $CD4^+CD25^+$ (bright) T cells in the intestinal mucosa contribute to intestinal homeostasis.[31] However, the underlying mechanism is unknown. Here, we hypothesized that defects of *Foxp3* gene may be involved in Crohn's disease. In this study, we identified four SNPs (three in the promoter region and one in the intron 9 region) in CD patients, and assessed the association of genotype and allele frequencies between patients with Crohn's disease, patients with primary biliary cirrhosis, and normal controls.

MATERIAL AND METHODS

Study Subjects

The study populations consisted of 93 (61 females and 32 males) unrelated patients with Crohn's disease (CD), 82 female patients with primary biliary cirrhosis (PBC), and 108 (51 females and 57 males) normal healthy controls. The diagnosis of CD was based on conventional clinical, endoscopic, and pathologic criteria. Peripheral blood was collected from all patients after informed consent using University of California at Davis–approved Human Subjects protocols. Genomic DNA was extracted from peripheral whole blood using a QIAamp DNA Blood kit (Qiagen, Valencia, CA) according to the manufacturer's instruction.

Searching for Single-Nucleotide Polymorphisms in the Human FOXP3 Gene

To verify the existence of the SNPs, we performed PCR-direct sequencing for ten SNP candidates in the promoter and intron regions previously described.[29] PCR primers are shown in TABLE 1. PCR was performed in 25 μL volumes, containing 20 ng of genomic DNA (pooled DNA of 20 CD patients' samples), 10 pmol of each primer, 0.6 units of Taq DNA polymerase (Roche, Indianapolis, IN,), and 5 nmol of each dNTP under the following conditions; denaturation at 94°C for 5 min, followed by 40 cycles of 94°C for 30 sec, 60°C for 30 sec, and 72°C for 30 sec, with the final extension of 72°C for 10 min. PCR products were loaded on 2% agarose gels and extracted from the agarose gels. PCR products were then analyzed by direct sequencing using a fluorescent dideoxyterminator method by ABI PRISM 3100 Genetic Analyzer (Applied Biosystems, Foster City, CA).

Genotyping of Single-Nucleotide Polymorphism in the FOXP3 Gene by TaqMan Allelic Discrimination

Predeveloped TaqMan SNP Genotyping Assays were used for the genotyping of –3279 and –924 in the promoter region and IVS9+459 in the intron 9 region (C__22476877_10, C__15942641_10, and C__27476877_10, Applied Biosystems, Foster City, CA). TaqMan minor groove binder (MGB) probes and primers for –6054

TABLE 1. Primers used in the screening of SNPs in the promoter and intron regions of the FOXP3/Scurfin gene

Position	Forward primer	Reverse primer
SNPs in the promoter region		
–6054 ATT/- (rs590234)	5′-ATGGCAGGGAGGTAGGCAC-3′	5′-GAGATGAGAGAGATGCAGTTG-3′
–5906 T/A (rs2869211)	5′-GGTGAAGTACTTAATGCATGGG-3′	5-GAGATGAGAGAGATGCAGTTG-3′
–3499 A/G (rs3761547)	5′-CTCGCTCTTTGTGTGTGTCTCTT-3′	5′-AGGCGTGGAGTAGACAAGGG-3′
–3279 A/C (rs3761548)	5′-ACCGAAATGCAGCGGCAGAGTT-3′	5′-CCAACGTGTGAGAAGGCAGAA-3′
–2383 C/T (rs3761549)	5′-GTGGCCAGATGGACATCACC-3′	5′-GTCATGGCGGCCGGAT- GC-3′
–1383 C/T (rs2232364)	5′-AAGGAGCAACTGCTCCCCCA-3′	5′-CTTTCTTTAGGAAGTGTTTCCG-3′
–924 A/G (rs2232365)	5′-CCAGGCTTGAGGGCCAGAAA-3′	5′-GGGTCTGGATCTCAGGGCAA-3′
SNPs in the intron regions		
IVS1 +87 G/T (rs2232366)	5′-AGGCCCTGGGCCCAGGAT-3′	5′-GGGGATTTTCTTGGCCCTGC-3′
IVS5 –20 G/A (rs2232368)	5′-AGGAGAGAACTCCCAGAGGG-3′	5′-GTACCATCTCTCTCTGGAGGA-3′
IVS9 +459 A/G (rs2280883)	5′-CCTTCCCCAGCCTTTATGCC-3′	5′-AGAAGGCATTGGGGAGGCTG-3′

NOTE: The location of each SNP in the promoter and intron regions was determined regarding the translation start site.

were designed. Sequences of primers were forward primer; 5′-CTGCCCATGCAT-TAAGTACTTCAC-3 and reverse primer; 5′-CATTCCAGCCAGGTAA GGTCTT-TA-3′, and MGB probes were VIC-CCATTTATTCTATTATTATTTTTT-8NFQ and FAM-CCATTTATTCTATTATTTTTT-8NFQ (Assays-by-Design; Applied Biosystems, Foster City, CA).

Allelic discrimination reactions were carried out using 20 ng of DNA in a final volume of 15 μL using TaqMan Universal PCR Master Mix (Applied Biosystems, Foster City, CA). PCR conditions consisted of an initial incubation at 95°C for 10 min, followed by 40 cycles at 92°C for 15 sec and at 60°C for 1 min using the Thermocycler 9700 (Applied Biosystems, Foster City, CA). Allelic discrimination was performed using the 7900H SDS and genotype analysis was performed using the ABI Prism SDS v.1.9 software (Applied Biosystems, Foster City, CA).

Statistical Analysis

The observed frequencies of each polymorphism in CD, PBC, and normal controls were analyzed by standard χ^2 tests. Data were considered significant when *P* value was less than 0.05, and the risk associated with individual alleles or genotypes was calculated as the odds ratio with 95% confidence intervals (CI) using InStat program.

RESULTS

Identification of Single-Nucleotide Polymorphism of the FOXP3 Gene in Patients with Crohn's Disease

To identify the existence of SNPs of the *Foxp3* gene in CD patients, we performed PCR with 20 pooled DNA samples from CD patients with 10 different primer pairs according to the NCBI SNPs Database (TABLE 1) and directly sequenced the PCR products. We found that four SNPs existed in *Foxp3* gene of CD patients. Three of four were located in the promoter region, –6054 (deletion/ATT, rs5902434), –3279 (A/C, rs376158) and –924 (A/G, rs2232365), and one in the intron 9 region, IVS9+459 (T/C, re2280883).

Analysis of Allele and Genotypic Frequencies

The *P* values of each polymorphic site were analyzed with respect to the comparison of CD patients and the controls, and of PBC patients and controls (TABLES 2 and 3). No significant differences were observed between controls and CD, but genotypes in CD revealed a trend toward increasing homozygosity, –6054 (del/del, 25% vs. 34%), –3279 (A/A, 14% vs. 21%), –924 (G/G, 25% vs. 33%) and IVS9+459 (T/T, 16% vs. 25%), compared to controls. However, the comparison with control and PBC demonstrated significant difference of IVS9+450 SNP ($P = 0.003$ by χ^2 test) (TABLE 2). For the analysis of allele frequencies, CD patients and normal controls were divided into female and male groups because allele frequencies of *FOXP3* gene, located on X-chromosomes, are different from female and male. The observed allele frequency of the –6054 (deletion to ATT) and –924 (A to G) polymorphism was not significantly different between CD patients and controls as well as PBC

TABLE 2. Genotype analyses in polymorphisms of *Foxp3* gene among CD, PBC and normal controls

			Control vs. CD			Control vs. PBC		
Position[a]	Gender	Allele	Control *n* (%)	CD *n* (%)	*P* value[b]	Control *n* (%)	PBC *n* (%)	*P* value[b]
-6054	F	-/-[c]	13 (25)	21 (34)	0.544	13 (25)	27 (33)	0.422
		-/ATT	28 (55)	28 (46)		28 (55)	45 (55)	
		ATT/ATT	10 (20)	12 (20)		10 (20)	10 (12)	
-3279	F	A/A	7 (14)	13 (21)	0.284	7 (14)	16 (20)	0.436
		A/C	24 (47)	32 (52)		24 (47)	42 (51)	
		C/C	20 (39)	16 (26)		20 (39)	24 (29)	
-924	F	A/A	11 (22)	13 (21)	0.676	11 (22)	14 (17)	0.735
		A/G	27 (53)	28 (46)		27 (53)	43 (52)	
		G/G	13 (25)	20 (33)		13 (25)	25 (31)	
IVS9+459	F	T/T	8 (16)	15 (25)	0.205	8 (16)	31 (38)	0.003
		T/C	22 (43)	30 (49)		22 (43)	36 (44)	
		C/C	21 (41)	16 (26)		21 (41)	15 (18)	

[a]Calculated from the translation start site.
[b]Value was determined by χ^2 test from 2×3 contingency table.
[c]Deletion.

patients and controls in the female group. The −3279 SNP (A to C) was 52% in CD patients, 55% in PBC patients, and 63% in controls. The allele frequencies were not significantly different compared with disease groups and control, but the tendency of polymorphism was increased in CD and PBC patients. Furthermore, the comparison of allele frequencies of IVS9+459 SNP (T to C) revealed significant difference between PBC and controls ($P = 0.001$ by χ^2 test), whereas there was no significant difference between CD and controls (TABLE 3). No significant differences of all the SNPs were observed in male population between CD and controls. In addition, the comparison of allele frequencies and genotype analysis between CD and PBC revealed no differences observed (data not shown).

TABLE 3. Allele frequencies of SNPs of Foxp3 gene among patients with CD or PBC and normal controls

			Control vs. CD			Control vs. PBC		
Position[a]	Gender	Allele	Control n (%)	CD n (%)	P value[b]	Control n (%)	PBC n (%)	P value[b]
-6054	F	—[c]	54 (53)	70 (57)	0.281	54 (53)	99 (60)	0.287
		ATT	48 (47)	52 (43)		48 (47)	65 (40)	
	M	—	31 (53)	17 (53)	0.909	31 (53)	—	
		ATT	26 (46)	15 (47)		26 (46)	—	
-3279	F	A	38 (37)	58 (48)	0.157	38 (37)	74 (45)	0.256
		C	64 (63)	64 (52)		64 (63)	90 (55)	
	M	A	23 (40)	14 (44)	0.930	23 (40)	—	
		C	34 (60)	18 (56)		34 (60)	—	
-924	F	A	49 (48)	54 (44)	0.667	49 (48)	71 (43)	0.256
		G	53 (52)	68 (56)		53 (52)	93 (57)	
	M	A	24 (42)	14 (44)	0.880	24 (42)	—	
		G	33 (58)	18 (56)		33 (58)	—	
IVS9 +459	F	T	38 (37)	60 (49)	0.098	38 (37)	98 (60)	0.001
		C	64 (63)	62 (51)		64 (63)	66 (40)	
	M	T	21 (37)	15 (47)	0.484	21 (37)	—	
		C	36 (63)	17 (53)		36 (63)	—	

[a] Calculated from the translation start site.
[b] Value was determined by χ^2 test from 2×2 contingency table with Yates correction.
[c] Deletion.

DISCUSSION

IBD is a chronic inflammatory bowel disease typified by significant immune dysregulation. The pathogenesis in CD involves high-level production of proinflammatory cytokines and upregulated expression of costimulatory molecules.[32] The chronic mucosal inflammatory responses in patients with IBD are directed at or in response to the intraluminal commensal microbial populations. In the normal mucosa the individual is tolerant to commensal bacterial flora and food-derived antigens. In murine models, a fine balance has been shown to exist between stimulation and regulation in response to enterobacterial antigens. The $CD4^+CD25^+$ T_{reg} cells regulate the proliferative responses to enteroantigens and have controlled mucosal inflammation in experimental animal models of colitis.[33] A recent study demonstrated that $CD4^+CD25^+$ T_{reg} cells reside in normal and inflamed gastrointestinal lamina propria. A significantly increased number of $CD4^+CD25^+$ T_{reg} cells and activities in patients with inflammatory bowel disease exist.[31] These data support that $CD4^+CD25^+$ T_{reg} cells play key roles in regulation of immune response and maintain intestinal homeostasis mediated by secreting suppressor cytokines, such as IL-10 and tumor growth factor beta (TGF-β).[10,15] In patients with myasthenia gravis $CD4^+CD25^+$ T_{reg} cells are present in normal numbers, although severe functional regulatory defects exist that are correlated with the expression of Foxp3.[34] The expression of Foxp3 and T_{reg} function are IL-6–dependent.[35] In CACO2 cells, IL-6 has been identified as a inducer of nuclear factor kappa B (NF-κB) activation in intestinal epithelial cells and a putative target for therapy.[36] IBD is characterized by upregulation of TNF-α that subsequently induces increased production of IL- 6.[37]

The *Foxp3* gene, mainly expressed in $CD4^+CD25^+$ T_{reg} cells in physiological conditions, encodes a protein that is a member of the forkhead/winged-helix family of transcriptional regulators, and is involved in the regulation of T cell activation. The Foxp3 protein acts as a repressor of T cell transcription by downregulating cytokine production.[16,20] Deficiency of Foxp3 may lead to various autoimmune diseases, probably because of the lack of functional $CD4^+CD25^+$ T_{reg} cells.[25] On the other hand, transgenic mice with the *Foxp3* gene demonstrated that overproduction of Foxp3 in lymphoid tissues caused a decrease in the number of peripheral T cells and suppression of immune system, while cytolytic activity was relatively preserved.[27] Furthermore, transfer of $CD4^+CD25^+$ T cells into mice with colitis led to disappearance of the lymphocytic infiltration in the lamina propria and reappearance of normal architecture of the intestine.[38]

The Foxp3 protein consists of 431 amino acids in humans and 429 amino acids in mice with 86% identity.[22] In humans, 13 mutations in the *FOXP3* gene have been reported and linked to autoimmune disease, X-linked autoimmunity allergic dysregulation syndrome (XLAAD) or immune dysfunction, polyendocrinopathy, enteropathy, X-linked (IPEX).[23,24,26,39] Most of these mutations lie in the forkhead domain, possibly disrupting the DNA binding activity of the protein. These mutations may result in altering function of Foxp3 protein. The dysregulation of T cell resulting from the loss of protein function demonstrates that the critical role Foxp3 plays in the control of activation-induced T cell expansion and differentiation. The phenotype of patients with point mutations in the *FOXP3* gene is just as severe, suggesting that the amino acids affected by these mutations may be critical for normal protein function.[25] In transient assays, transfection of the human *FOXP*3 gene into Jurkat cells with a luciferase reporter, driven by a multimer NFAT site in IL-2 promoter, leads to decrease in activation-induced promoter activity, consistent with an inhibitory function.[20]

Bassuny and his colleagues studied polymorphism of microsatellite and SNP of human *FOXP3* gene in paatients with type 1diabetes. They found that the polymorphisms of microsatellite in the intron zero regions were transiently expressed in the cell lines. These polymorphisms expressed in the cell lines showed the significant difference in the enhancer activity and were associated with type 1 diabetes.[29]

In an animal model of induced intestinal autoreactivity T_{reg} cells inhibited the proliferative response.[40] Additionally, functional abnormalities of T_{reg} cells have been implicated in a number of other human diseases such as psoriasis, myasthenia gravis, schistosomiasis, juvenile idiopathic arthritis, Kawasaki's disease and graft-versus-host disease.[34,41–45] Foxp3 is just one of a number of forked-head transcription factors that have significant immunoregulatory functions and play important roles in lymphocyte function and development.[46] Dysregulation of any one of these transcription factors may play important roles in human diseases.

In this study, we investigated 10 SNPs of *FOXP3* gene and identified four SNPs (three in promoter region and one in intron 9) existing in CD patients. With these four SNPs, we analyzed allele and genotype frequencies in CD patients, PBC patients, and controls. The allele frequencies showed no significant differences in the comparison of the CD patient group and controls. However, the tendency for polymorphism was increased in CD patients. The sample size of each group used for this study consisted of 51 females in the CD group and 82 in the PBC group and therefore further studies would be required using a larger sample size. These data do not support immune dysregulation secondary to promoter heterogeneity in the *FOXP3* gene. They suggest other mechanisms for dysregulation such as cytokine inhibition of T_{reg} cell function. It is interesting, however, that PBC patients and controls revealed significant differences of allele frequencies ($P = 0.001$) in IVS9+459 SNP (TABLE 3). This might suggest that there are differences or inadequate T_{reg} function in PBC. The effects of IVS9+459 SNP and other possible SNPs like the *FOXP3* SNPs in PBC remain to be investigated. Primary biliary cirrhosis (PBC) is an organ-specific autoimmune disease characterized by presence of high titer of antimitochondrial antibody in the patient's serum, lymphocytic infiltrates in the liver, and bile duct destruction.[47] We speculate that patients having allele T might be more susceptible to dysregulation than patients with allele C. In conclusion, four SNPs of human *FOXP3* are not associated with Crohn's disease but are associated with the autoimmune disease PBC.

REFERENCES

1. PODOLSKY, D.K. 1991. Inflammatory bowel disease (1). N. Engl. J. Med. **325:** 928–937.
2. HAMILTON, S.R. 1987. The differential diagnosis of idiopathic inflammatory disease by colorectal biopsy. Int. J. Colorectal Dis. **2:** 113–117.
3. STOLL, M. *et al.* 2004. Genetic variation in DLG5 is associated with inflammatory bowel disease. Nat. Genet. **36:** 476–480.
4. HUGOT, J.P. *et al.* 2001. Association of NOD2 leucine-rich repeat variants with susceptibility to Crohn's disease. Nature **411:** 599–603.

5. OGURA, Y. *et al.* 2001. A frameshift mutation in NOD2 associated with susceptibility to Crohn's disease. Nature **411:** 603–606.
6. VAN HEEL, D.A. *et al.* 2004. Inflammatory bowel disease susceptibility loci defined by genome scan meta-analysis of 1952 affected relative pairs. Hum. Mol. Genet. **13:** 763–770.
7. HUGOT, J.P. 2004. Inflammatory bowel disease: a complex group of genetic disorders. Best Pract. Res. Clin. Gastroenterol. **18:** 451–462.
8. GIALLOURAKIS, C. *et al.* 2003. IBD5 is a general risk factor for inflammatory bowel disease: replication of association with Crohn disease and identification of a novel association with ulcerative colitis, in Am J Hum Genet. 2003. p. 205–121.
9. ASSEMAN, C., S. FOWLER & F. POWRIE. 2000. Control of experimental inflammatory bowel disease by regulatory T cells. Am. J. Respir. Crit. Care Med. **162:** S185–S189.
10. ANNACKER, O. & F. POWRIE 2002. Homeostasis of intestinal immune regulation. Microbes Infect. **4:** 67–74.
11. OCHS, H.D., S.F. ZIEGLER & T.R. TORGERSON. 2005. FOXP3 acts as a rheostat of the immune response. Immunol. Rev. **203:** 156–164.
12. FURTADO, G.C. *et al.* 2001. Regulatory T cells in spontaneous autoimmune encephalomyelitis. Immunol. Rev. **182:** 122–134.
13. CUROTTO DE LAFAILLE, M.A. & J.J. LAFAILLE. 2002. CD4(+) regulatory T cells in autoimmunity and allergy. Curr. Opin. Immunol. **14:** 771–778.
14. BLUMBERG, R.S., L.J. SAUBERMANN & W. STROBER. 1999. Animal models of mucosal inflammation and their relation to human inflammatory bowel disease. Curr. Opin. Immunol. **11:** 648–656.
15. SINGH, B. *et al.* 2001. Control of intestinal inflammation by regulatory T cells. Immunol. Rev. **182:** 190–200.
16. HORI, S., T. NOMURA & S. SAKAGUCHI. 2003. Control of regulatory T cell development by the transcription factor Foxp3. Science **299:** 1057–1061.
17. TAKAHASHI, T. *et al.* 2000. Immunologic self-tolerance maintained by CD25(+)CD4(+) regulatory T cells constitutively expressing cytotoxic T lymphocyte-associated antigen 4. J. Exp. Med. **192:** 303–310.
18. MCHUGH, R.S. *et al.* 2002. CD4(+)CD25(+) immunoregulatory T cells: gene expression analysis reveals a functional role for the glucocorticoid-induced TNF receptor. Immunity **16:** 311–323.
19. READ, S., V. MALMSTROM & F. POWRIE. 2000. Cytotoxic T lymphocyte-associated antigen 4 plays an essential role in the function of CD25(+)CD4(+) regulatory cells that control intestinal inflammation. J. Exp. Med. **192:** 295–302.
20. SCHUBERT, L.A. *et al.* 2001. Scurfin (FOXP3) acts as a repressor of transcription and regulates T cell activation. J. Biol. Chem. **276:** 37672–37679.
21. KASPROWICZ, D.J. *et al.* 2003. Scurfin (FoxP3) controls T-dependent immune responses in vivo through regulation of CD4+ T cell effector function. J. Immunol. **171:** 1216–1223.
22. BRUNKOW, M.E. *et al.* 2001. Disruption of a new forkhead/winged-helix protein, scurfin, results in the fatal lymphoproliferative disorder of the scurfy mouse. Nat. Genet. **27:** 68–73.
23. BENNETT, C.L. & H.D. OCHS. 2001. IPEX is a unique X-linked syndrome characterized by immune dysfunction, polyendocrinopathy, enteropathy, and a variety of autoimmune phenomena. Curr. Opin. Pediatr. **13:** 533–538.
24. CHATILA, T.A. *et al.* 2000. JM2, encoding a fork head-related protein, is mutated in X-linked autoimmunity-allergic disregulation syndrome. J. Clin. Invest. **106:** R75–81.
25. WILDIN, R.S. *et al.* 2001. X-linked neonatal diabetes mellitus, enteropathy and endocrinopathy syndrome is the human equivalent of mouse scurfy. Nat. Genet. **27:** 18–20.
26. GAMBINERI, E., T.R. TORGERSON & H.D. OCHS. 2003. Immune dysregulation, polyendocrinopathy, enteropathy, and X-linked inheritance (IPEX), a syndrome of systemic autoimmunity caused by mutations of FOXP3, a critical regulator of T-cell homeostasis. Curr. Opin. Rheumatol. **15:** 430–435.
27. KHATTRI, R. *et al.* 2001. The amount of scurfin protein determines peripheral T cell number and responsiveness. J. Immunol. **167:** 6312–6320.

28. Khattri, R. *et al.* 2003. An essential role for Scurfin in CD4+CD25+ T regulatory cells. Nat. Immunol. **4:** 337–342.
29. Bassuny, W.M. *et al.* 2003. A functional polymorphism in the promoter/enhancer region of the FOXP3/Scurfin gene associated with type 1 diabetes. Immunogenetics **55:** 149–156.
30. Jaeckel, E., H. von Boehmer & M.P. Manns. 2005. Antigen-specific FoxP3-transduced T cells can control established type 1 diabetes. Diabetes **54:** 306–310.
31. Makita, S. *et al.* 2004. CD4+CD25bright T cells in human intestinal lamina propria as regulatory cells. J. Immunol. **173:** 3119–3130.
32. James, S.P. & J.M. Klapproth. 1996. Major pathways of mucosal immunity and inflammation: cell activation, cytokine production and the role of bacterial factors. Aliment. Pharmacol. Ther. **10** (Suppl. 2): 1–9.
33. Powrie, F. 2004. Immune regulation in the intestine: a balancing act between effector and regulatory T cell responses. Ann. N.Y. Acad. Sci. **1029:** 132–141.
34. Balandina, A. *et al.* 2005. Functional defect of regulatory CD4(+)CD25+ T cells in the thymus of patients with autoimmune myasthenia gravis. Blood **105:** 735–741.
35. Doganci, A. *et al.* 2005. The IL-6R alpha chain controls lung CD4+CD25+ Treg development and function during allergic airway inflammation in vivo. J. Clin. Invest. **115:** 313–325.
36. Kitamura, K. *et al.* 2004. Pivotal roles of interleukin-6 in transmural inflammation in murine T cell transfer colitis. J. Leukoc. Biol. **76:** 1111–1117.
37. Heinrich, P.C. *et al.* 2003. Principles of interleukin (IL)-6-type cytokine signalling and its regulation. Biochem. J. **374:** 1–20.
38. Mottet, C., H.H. Uhlig & F. Powrie. 2003. Cutting edge: cure of colitis by CD4+CD25+ regulatory T cells. J. Immunol. **170:** 3939–3943.
39. Nieves, D.S. *et al.* 2004. Dermatologic and immunologic findings in the immune dysregulation, polyendocrinopathy, enteropathy, X-linked syndrome. Arch, Dermatol. **140:** 466–472.
40. Westendorf, A.M. *et al.* 2005. CD4+ T cell mediated intestinal immunity: chronic inflammation versus immune regulation. Gut **54:** 60–69.
41. Sugiyama, H. *et al.* 2005. Dysfunctional blood and target tissue CD4+CD25high regulatory T cells in psoriasis: mechanism underlying unrestrained pathogenic effector T cell proliferation. J. Immunol. **174:** 164–173.
42. Singh, K.P. *et al.* 2005. Retroviral Foxp3 gene transfer ameliorates liver granuloma pathology in *Schistosoma mansoni* infected mice. Immunology **114:** 410–417.
43. de Kleer, I.M. *et al.* 2004. CD4+CD25 bright regulatory T cells actively regulate inflammation in the joints of patients with the remitting form of juvenile idiopathic arthritis. J. Immunol. **172:** 6435–6443.
44. Miura, Y. *et al.* 2004. Association of Foxp3 regulatory gene expression with graft-versus-host disease. Blood **104:** 2187–2193.
45. Furuno, K. *et al.* 2004. CD25+CD4+ regulatory T cells in patients with Kawasaki disease. J. Pediatr. **145:** 385–390.
46. Jonsson, H. & S.L. Peng. 2005. Forkhead transcription factors in immunology. Cell Mol. Life Sci. **62:** 397–409.
47. Mackay, I.R. *et al.* 2000. The peculiar autoimmunity of primary biliary cirrhosis. Immunol. Rev. **174:** 226–237.

Juvenile Systemic Sclerosis

A Follow-up Study of Eight Patients

SZILVIA SZAMOSI,[a] LÁSZLÓ MARÓDI,[b] LÁSZLÓ CZIRJÁK,[c] ZOLTÁN ELLENES,[b] AND GABRIELLA SZÜCS[a,d]

[a]*Third Department of Medicine, Division of Rheumatology,* [b]*Department of Paediatric Immunology, University of Debrecen Medical Center, Debrecen, Hungary*

[c]*Department of Immunology and Rheumatology, University of Pécs, Pécs, Hungary*

[d]*Research Group of Autoimmune Diseases, Hungarian Academy of Sciences, Debrecen, Hungary*

ABSTRACT: Juvenile systemic sclerosis (jSSc) is a rare form of systemic sclerosis (also known as scleroderma). Fewer than 10% of SSc cases have their onset before age 20 and fewer than 2% before the age of 10. Few case reports and cohort studies on jSSc have been published. Our objective was to assess the clinical and laboratory characteristics of eight cases of juvenile-onset SSc followed up at our institution. Clinical manifestations of SSc were recorded, and immunologic laboratory tests including antinuclear antibodies (ANAs), anti-centromere antibodies (ACAs), and anti-Scl-70 antibodies were assessed. The female-to-male ratio was 7:1, and age at onset ranged from 3–17 years. At the time of analysis, 2 of 8 patients were still under 18 years of age, and 6 of 8 patients were adults. The mean follow-up period from the onset of disease was 19.1 years. Raynaud's phenomenon was present in all cases. Only 2 of 8 patients had diffuse SSc. During follow-up, pulmonary fibrosis developed in only 2 of 8 patients and cardiovascular manifestations in 3 of 8 patients. Secondary sicca syndrome was present in 2 of 8 cases. Regarding immunologic laboratory markers, 7 of 8 patients were ANA positive. However, none of these patients ever carried anti-Scl-70 antibodies, and only 2 of 8 patients had ever had ACA seropositivity. Our results suggest that in jSSc, Raynaud's phenomenon is more severe, whereas internal organ manifestations and the frequency of autoantibodies are far less pronounced than in adult-onset SSc. Also, the survival rate and final outcome of patients with jSSc appear to be better than those in patients with adult-onset SSc.

KEYWORDS: juvenile systemic sclerosis; scleroderma; Raynaud's phenomenon; fibrosis; connective tissue disease

Address for correspondence: Gabriella Szücs, M.D., Ph.D., Third Department of Medicine, Division of Rheumatology, University of Debrecen Medical Center, 22 Moricz Zs Street, Debrecen, H-4004, Hungary. Voice: +36-52-311-087; fax: +36-52-414-489.
szucsg@iiibel.dote.hu

**Ann. N.Y. Acad. Sci. 1051: 229–234 (2005). © 2005 New York Academy of Sciences.
doi: 10.1196/annals.1361.063**

INTRODUCTION

Systemic sclerosis (SSc) is an autoimmune connective tissue disease characterized by diffuse inflammation and subsequent fibrosis of the skin, accompanied by varying degrees of internal organ involvement. Internal organ manifestations indicate a poor prognosis, and death results primarily from pulmonary failure and cardiac events.[1,2]

Systemic sclerosis is a rare disease in adults and children. Of all patients with SSc, fewer than 10% developed evidence of the disease before the age of 20, and only about 1.5% developed signs of SSc before the age of 10. Although information on survival and prognostic factors for survival in adult SSc patients is increasing, our knowledge of the outcome of juvenile systemic sclerosis (jSSc) is still limited.[3–5] Therefore, to learn more about jSSc, we analyzed the clinical and laboratory characteristics of jSSc patients undergoing follow-up at the University of Debrecen.

PATIENTS AND METHODS

Eight cases of SSc of juvenile onset were included in the study. Patients had either the limited or the diffuse cutaneous form of SSc (lSSc and dSSc, respectively), as defined by LeRoy and colleagues,[1] and fulfilled the American College of Rheumatology (ACR) criteria for the classification of SSc.[2] Clinical symptoms, internal organ manifestations, and immunologic laboratory tests were analyzed. These tests included assessment of Raynaud's phenomenon (intermittent ischemia of the fingers or toes), pulmonary function testing, echocardiography, esophageal radiography, and determination of autoantibodies in serum samples.

RESULTS

Eight patients with juvenile-onset SSc (7 female and 1 male; mean age 30.1 years [range 13–47 years]) were enrolled in the study from a pool of 230 SSc patients undergoing regular follow-up at our institution. Duration of disease (calculated from the time of diagnosis of SSc) ranged from 3–37 years (mean 19.25 years). The mean age at disease onset was 10.87 years (range 3–17). At the time of analysis, 2 of 8 patients were still under 18 years or age, and 6 of 8 were adults.

TABLE 1 shows the patients' demographic data. Two patients were affected by dSSc and six by lSSc. Raynaud's phenomenon was present in all cases, but ulcers of the fingers developed in only two. Analysis of internal organ manifestations revealed that pulmonary fibrosis developed in only two patients during follow-up (alveolitis was found in only one case [patient 4] by high-resolution computed tomography [HRCT]). Forced vital capacity (FVC) and diffusing capacity of the lung for carbon monoxide (DLCO) tests showed no impairment of pulmonary function in any of the cases.

Three patients had cardiac manifestations with diastolic function abnormalities as assessed by echocardiography, and three patients had gastrointestinal manifestations, such as esophageal dysmotility revealed by esophageal barium swallow.

TABLE 1. Clinical and demographic characteristics and follow-up of eight patients with juvenile systemic sclerosis (jSSc)

Patient	Sex	Age	Age (yr) at onset of SSc	Subset	R/U	Lung	Heart	GI	Secondary Sjögren's syndrome
1	F	47	10	ldSSc	R/U	–	+	–	+
2	F	46	17	ldSSc	R/U	+	+	+	–
3	M	34	3	ldSSc	R	–	–	–	+
4	F	29	13	ldSSc	R	+	+	+	–
5	F	40	16	ldSSc	R	–	–	+	–
6	F	13	7	dcSSc	R	–	–	–	–
7	F	14	11	dcSSc	R	–	–	–	–
8	F	18	10	ldSSc	R	–	–	–	–

Abbreviations: dcSSc, diffuse cutaneous SSc; lcSSc, limited cutaneous SSc; GI, gastrointestinal; R/U = Raynaud's phenomenon/ulcers of the fingers; SSc, systemic sclerosis.

TABLE 2. Autoantibody profiles of eight patients with juvenile systemic sclerosis (jSSc)

Patient	ANA	ACA	TopoI Ab	Other auto-antibodies
1	+	–	–	RF, ENA, CL, B2GP, SSA
2	+	+	–	—
3	+	–	–	SSA, SSB, B2GP
4	+	–	–	B2GP
5	–	+	–	RF
6	+	–	–	dsDNA
7	+	–	–	—
8	+	–	–	dsDNA

Abbreviations: ACA, anticentromere antibody; ANA, antinuclear antibody; B2GP, beta-2-glycoprotein; CL, cardiolipin; dsDNA, double-stranded DNA; ENA, extractable nuclear antigen; RF, rheumatoid factor; topoI Ab, anti-topoisomerase I antibody.

Finally, secondary sicca (Sjögren's) syndrome was present in two of eight cases. No renal manifestations developed in any patient during follow-up.

Analysis of autoantibody profiles revealed that seven of eight patients showed antinuclear antibody (ANA) positivity, and one patient was ANA negative (TABLE 2). We found anticentromere-antibody (ACA) positivity in only two cases; however, neither of these patients had ever carried the anti-topoisomerase (anti-Scl70) autoantibody. Other autoantibodies were randomly present in serum samples of a few scattered cases, showing no clinical relevance whatsoever. These autoantibodies included anti-dsDNA, anti-ENA, anti-RNP, anti-SSA, anti-SSB, anti–beta-2-glycoprotein I (B2GPI, anticardiolipin (aCL), and rheumatoid factor.

Our jSSc patients' therapy included drugs to improve microcirculation, such as pentoxifyllin, calcium-channel blockers, and acetylcholinesterase (ACE) inhibitors.

Two patients received D-penicillamine at disease onset, whereas two patients were administered corticosteroids to control myositis and alveolitis, respectively.

DISCUSSION

Systemic sclerosis is a rare childhood disease. The largest series of cases of childhood onset reported features similar to those of adult-onset disease.[3–5] In 2001, consensus was reached by the First International Workshop on Juvenile Scleroderma in Italy to establish classification criteria for jSSc.[3] This classification system differs slightly from the ACR criteria[2] adapted for adult patients and currently being validated in pediatric rheumatology. At the same time, knowledge of the prognosis and survival of jSSc is limited,[3–5] even as classification criteria are being developed for jSSc and more information is available on survival and prognostic factors in adult SSc.

Systemic sclerosis is an uncommon systemic autoimmune disease characterized by diffuse inflammation and subsequent fibrosis of the skin together with varying degrees of internal organ involvement. Pulmonary, cardiac, and renal manifestations signal a poor prognosis and are the leading cause of death in SSc. Cardiac involvement includes myocardial inflammation and fibrosis, conduction-system abnormalities, arrhythmias, or pericardial disease. In addition, scleroderma renal crisis and pulmonary hypertension may lead to significant cardiac dysfunction. Lung manifestations include mild or severe pulmonary fibrosis, or fibrosing alveolitis.[6–9] In the adult SSc population, the presence of cardiac, pulmonary, or renal involvement is predictive of a poor outcome, as are the presence of the diffuse skin symptoms and skin hypo- and/or hyperpigmentation.[10]

Although systemic sclerosis confers a high risk of mortality, there is considerable heterogeneity across settings. Age at onset may be an important factor in the outcome, as jSSc and adult-onset SSc may have different organ manifestations and therefore different prognoses. Therefore, comparisons between jSSc and adult-onset SSc may have great clinical relevance for disease management and prognosis. Nonetheless, only a limited number of case reports and cohort studies on jSSc are available.[3] For example, some investigators have reported a correlation between anti-topoisomerase I antibody levels and skin sickness score, renovascular resistance, and decreasing vital capacity. Sato and colleagues[11] followed some patients (some under 18 years) in whom higher anti-topoisomerase I antibody levels correlated with increased disease activity.

Foeldvari and colleagues[12] collected data from 324 pediatric rheumatology centers and analyzed 135 jSSc patients in a multicenter international study. An improved five-year survival rate of 95% was found in jSSc in this study than in a previously presented adult study that included data from 1,863 SSc patients; in the latter, the five-year survival rate was only 78%.[13] Foeldvari and colleagues compared organ involvement in the jSSc patient group with fatal versus nonfatal outcomes. In the group with fatal outcomes (8/135), the authors noted a trend towards a greater number of patients with pulmonary and CNS involvement as well as a significant increase in cardiovascular and renal involvement. These results are similar to reports on adult patients.[14,15]

Goldenberg and colleagues described the clinical features and disease course of 11 jSSc patients whose prognosis was good. In this group, there were no deaths, and no patients suffered significant visceral organ damage.[4]

CONCLUSION

Summarizing the results of our present study, the female-to-male ratio was 7:1 among our jSSc patients. This ratio differs from that of other published reports, where the female-to-male ratio was 1:1 for patients with disease onset before 8 years of age and 3:1 among older patients. Our results resemble the female-to-male ratio found in adult-onset cases of SSc. None of the patients in the present study developed severe pulmonary, cardiac, or other internal organ manifestations during the follow-up period. In fact, these patients remain fully active in their daily lives. These results suggest that internal organ manifestations and the frequency of autoantibodies are far less pronounced in the jSSc than in the adult-onset SSc population; furthermore, these findings resemble those described by Foeldvari and colleagues[12] and Goldenberg and colleagues.[4]

In conclusion, our study accords with the reports of other researchers. It suggests that the survival rate and outcome of patients with jSSc is better than that of patients with adult-onset SSc. However, it is still not clear whether this difference reflects slower disease progression or a much weaker influence of comorbidity factors in the pediatric group. To collect more evidence to support this conclusion will require additional multicenter international studies.

REFERENCES

1. LeRoy, E.C., C. Black, R. Fleischmajer, *et al.* 1988. Scleroderma (systemic sclerosis): classification, subsets and pathogenesis. J. Rheumatol. **15:** 202–205.
2. Subcommittee for Scleroderma Criteria of the American Rheumatism Association Diagnostic and Therapeutic Criteria Committee. 1980. Preliminary criteria for the classification of systemic sclerosis(scleroderma). Arthritis Rheum. **23:** 581–590.
3. Cassidy, J.T. & R.E. Petty. 1995. The sclerodermas and related disorders. I. Textbook of Pediatric Rheumatology, 3d Ed.: 423–465. W.B. Saunders. Philadelphia.
4. Goldenberg, J., A. Pinto-Pessoa, M. Odete-Hilario, *et al.* 1993. Scleroderma in children. A report of eleven cases. Rev. Rheum. (Engl. Edn.). **60:** 131–136.
5. Cassidy, J.T., D.B. Sullivan, L. Dabich & R.E. Petty. 1977. Scleroderma in children. Arthritis Rheum. **20:** 351–354.
6. Geirsson, A.J., F.A. Wollheim & A. Akesson. 2001. Disease severity of 100 patients with systemic sclerosis over a period of 14 years: using a modified Medsger scale. Ann. Rheum. Dis. **60:** 592–598.
7. Ioannidis, J.P., P.G. Vlachoyiannopoulos, A.B. Haidich, *et al.* 2005. Mortality in systemic sclerosis: an international meta-analysis of individual patient data. Am. J. Med. **118:** 2–10.
8. Mukerjee, D., D. St. George, C. Knight, *et al.* 2004. Echocardiography and pulmonary function as screening tests for pulmonary arterial hypertension in systemic sclerosis. Rheumatology (Oxford). **43:** 461–466.
9. Steen, V. 2004. The heart in systemic sclerosis. Curr. Rheumatol. Rep. **6:** 137–140.
10. Czirják, L., Z. Nagy & G. Szegedi. 1993. Survival analysis of 118 patients with systemic sclerosis. J. Intern. Med. **234:** 335–337.

11. SATO, S., Y. HAMAGUCHI, M. HASEGAWA & K. TAKEHARA. 2001. Clinical significance of anti-topoisomerase I antibody levels determined by ELISA in systemic sclerosis. Rheumatology (Oxf.) **40:** 1135–1140.
12. FOELDVARI, I., M. ZHAVANIA, N. BIRDI, *et al.* 2000. Favourable outcome in 135 children with juvenile systemic sclerosis: results of a multi-national survey. Rheumatology (Oxf.) **39:** 556–559.
13. STEEN, V.D. & T.A. MEDSGER. 1997. Survival studies in systemic sclerosis: demographic features. Arthritis Rheum. **40:** S124.
14. CALLAHAN, L.F. & T. PINCUS. 1997. Mortality in the rheumatic diseases. Arthritis Care Res. **8:** 229–241.
15. ALTMAN, R.D., T.A. MEDSGER, JR., D.A. BLOCH & B.A. MICHEL. 1991. Predictors of survival in systemic sclerosis (scleroderma). Arthritis Rheum. **34:** 403–413.

Antifodrin Antibodies in Sjögren's Syndrome

A Review

TORSTEN WITTE

Abteilung Klinische Immunologie, Zentrum Innere Medizin der Medizinischen Hochschule Hannover, Hannover, Germany

ABSTRACT: Establishing the diagnosis of Sjögren's syndrome has been difficult in light of its nonspecific symptoms (dry eyes and mouth) and lack of both sensitive and specific laboratory markers. Recently, antibodies against alpha-fodrin have been characterized: first in animal models of Sjögren's syndrome, and later in humans. Antibodies against alpha-fodrin have been shown to be present in up to 98% of untreated patients. These antibodies are directed against an apoptotic cleavage product of alpha-fodrin. Anti-alpha-fodrin is clearly involved in the pathogenesis of murine models of Sjögren's syndrome. However, in humans, conflicting data have recently been generated with regard to the prevalence of antibodies against alpha-fodrin in the disease. These differences may be caused by interference of treatment with antibody concentrations, but may also reflect varying methods of patient selection. Further studies on untreated patients are needed to establish the diagnostic efficiency of antibodies against alpha-fodrin in Sjögren's syndrome, which may be a potential diagnostic marker in addition to antibodies against Ro. In this review, the potential of antifodrin antibodies as laboratory markers of Sjögren's syndrome is discussed.

KEYWORDS: Sjögren's syndrome; antifodrin antibodies; anti-Ro antibodies; IgA anti-alpha-fodrin; IgG anti-alpha-fodrin; disease classification criteria

INTRODUCTION

Sjögren's syndrome is an autoimmune disease characterized by lymphocytic infiltration of the salivary and lacrimal glands. It is a major cause of dry eyes (keratoconjunctivitis sicca) and dry mouth (xerostomia) and affects up to 0.5% of the population. Nevertheless, establishing the diagnosis of Sjögren's syndrome has been difficult for several reasons:

1. *Objective signs of dry eyes and mouth are frequent.* They may be iatrogenic (caused by radiation, tricyclic antidepressants, or beta blockers) or the result of infections (e.g., hepatitis C and HIV) or sarcoidosis and are often observed in the elderly.[1,2]

Address for correspondence: Torsten Witte, M.D. Abteilung Klinische Immunologie, Zentrum Innere Medizin der Medizinischen Hochschule Hannover, Carl-Neuberg-Strasse 1, 30625 Hannover, Germany. Voice: +49-511-5323014; fax: +49-511- 5325648.
witte.torsten@mh-hannover.de

Ann. N.Y. Acad. Sci. 1051: 235–239 (2005). © 2005 New York Academy of Sciences.
doi: 10.1196/annals.1361.064

2. *Symptoms of the disease are nonspecific.* In most studies, the association-between subjective symptoms and objective tests of reduced tear and saliva flow was weak.[2] Conversely, these symptoms are frequently observed in patients with depression or fibromyalgia, one of the most important differential diagnoses in clinical practice.

3. *No available laboratory markers are both sensitive and specific.* Antibodies against Ro (SSA) and La (SSB) are regarded as disease markers. Therefore, these antibodies are part of most sets of classification criteria. In some studies, the prevalence of antibodies against Ro in Sjögren's syndrome is 90%; in other studies, however, the prevalence of antibodies against Ro is only 20–40%.[3] Also, antibodies against Ro are not associated with symptoms of and objective tests for sicca syndrome in the general population.[1,2] Therefore, a search for better diagnostic markers for Sjögren's syndrome is under way. One result has been the recent discovery of autoantibodies against alpha-fodrin.

ANTIBODIES AGAINST ALPHA-FODRIN

As Markers of Sjögren's Syndrome

Alpha-fodrin is a 240-kDa protein forming a heterodimer with beta-fodrin, a 235-kDa molecule homologous to alpha-fodrin. The heterodimers are anchored to the plasma membrane, bind to actin, calmodulin, and microtubules,[4] and are present in most cells of the body. Alpha-fodrin appears to be involved in exocytosis and secretion, and antibodies against alpha-fodrin block secretion at least in chromaffin cells.[5]

In 1997, antibodies against alpha-fodrin were first described in NFS/sld mice thymectomized on day 3, a murine model of Sjögren's syndrome.[6] During apoptosis, alpha-fodrin is cleaved by caspase-3 into smaller fragments of 150 kDa and 120 kDa.[7]

In these mice, the development of antibodies against alpha-fodrin and Sjögren's syndrome could be prevented by treatment with caspase inhibitors as well as injection of alpha-fodrin before thymectomy.[8] Conversely, injecting apoptotic cleavage products of alpha-fodrin induced autoantibodies, T cell stimulation, and lymphocytic infiltration of the salivary glands in normal mice.[8] Thus, strong evidence points to a crucial role for antibodies against alpha-fodrin in murine models of Sjögren's syndrome.

Prevalence in Sjögren's Syndrome

In initial studies of patients with Sjögren's syndrome classified according to Japanese criteria, the prevalence of IgG antibodies against alpha-fodrin (detected by immunoblot analysis) was 67–95%.[6] Recent studies of the same group used larger fragments of alpha-fodrin, including the 150-kDa cleavage product, as antigens. In these studies, the prevalence of immunoglobulin A (IgA) and/or IgG antibodies against alpha-fodrin was 98% in patients classified according to the San Diego criteria.[9,12]

Our own observations using an enzyme-linked immunosorbent assay (ELISA) determined the prevalence of both IgG and IgA antibodies against alpha-fodrin in Sjögren's syndrome. The disease was classified according to the revised European-

Community Study Group (ESG) criteria,[10] the American-European Consensus Group criteria,[11] and the highly stringent San Diego criteria.[12]

IgA antibodies against alpha-fodrin were consistently more prevalent than IgG autoantibodies. IgA antibodies against alpha-fodrin were present in 88%, IgG antibodies in 64%, and IgA and/or IgG antibodies in 93% of a total of 85 patients classified according to San Diego criteria.[13] Prevalence was lower in patients classified according to both ESG and American-European Consensus Group criteria. In the latter group, IgA antibodies against alpha-fodrin were present in 64% and IgG antibodies against alpha-fodrin in 50% of the patients.[13]

Specificity for Sjögren's Syndrome

Because the neoantigen of alpha-fodrin is an apoptotic cleavage product, it is expected that antibodies against alpha-fodrin would be observed in a number of diseases characterized by chronic apoptosis. In fact, cleavage products of alpha-fodrin have been identified in plaques localized in the CNS of patients with multiple sclerosis (MS).[14] As these data led us to expect, we detected IgG antibodies against alpha-fodrin in approximately 10–20% of patients with MS, but also in 20% of patients with rheumatoid arthritis, even in the absence of secondary Sjögren's syndrome, and in 2% of blood donors. However, IgA antibodies against alpha-fodrin, produced locally in salivary glands, were more specific for Sjögren's syndrome. They were detected in only 2% of blood donors and in fewer than 10% of MS patients. It is difficult to distinguish between Sjögren's syndrome and CNS involvement from MS. A recent study has shown that one of six patients with primary-progressive MS also suffer from Sjögren's syndrome. These patients were better identified by antibodies against alpha-fodrin than by antibodies against Ro or La.[15]

Furthermore, in systemic lupus erythematosus (SLE), there is a highly significant association between IgA antibodies against alpha-fodrin and antibodies against Ro and La. IgA antibodies against alpha-fodrin were present in 36 of 135 (27%) SLE patients. Antibodies against Ro were observed in 72% of patients with IgA alpha-fodrin antibodies, but in only 37% of patients without them ($P = 0.0002$). Antibodies against La were observed in 44% of patients with IgA alpha-fodrin antibodies, but in only 12% of patients without them ($P = 0.0002$) (unpublished data).

As Activity Markers of Sjögren's Syndrome

A highly significant association has been made between the concentration of IgA- and IgG-antibodies against alpha-fodrin and the degree of lymphocytic infiltration in the salivary glands of patients classified according to San Diego criteria (unpublished data). Antibodies against alpha-fodrin were measured during follow-up of patients treated with antimalarials or low-dose glucocorticosteroids. In the majority of patients, the concentration of antibodies against alpha-fodrin normalized within three months. Therefore, antibodies against alpha-fodrin not only are markers of Sjögren's syndrome, but also reflect inflammatory disease activity.

Differing Views on Prevalence in Sjögren's Syndrome

Some authors have reported a lower prevalence of antibodies against alpha-fodrin in Sjögren's syndrome. Some of these studies are summarized in TABLE 1. In most

TABLE 1. Summary of representative studies for the prevalence of alpha-fodrin antibodies in Sjögren's syndrome

Author	Test system	Classification criteria	Patients (*n*)	Prevalence of IgA anti-alpha-fodrin	Prevalence of IgG anti-alpha-fodrin	Prevalence of IgA and/or IgG anti-alpha-fodrin
Haneji[6]	Immunoblot	Japanese	43	Not done	95%	Not done
Witte[16]	ELISA	ESG	85	64%	55%	79%
Witte[13]	ELISA	San Diego	85	88%	64%	93%
de Seze[17]	ELISA	ESG	84	Not shown	Not shown	70%
Ruffatti[18]	ELISA	ESG	80	32.5%	21.1%	40%
Maruyama[9]	ELISA	San Diego	60	Not done	Not done	98%
Szanto[19]	ELISA	ESG	67	37.3%	38.8.%	Not shown

ABBREVIATIONS: ELISA, enzyme-linked immunosorbent assay; ESG, European Community Study Group; Ig, immunoglobulin.

of the studies, the proportion of patients who were treated with medications that reduce the concentration of alpha-fodrin antibodies has not been mentioned. Therefore, a rigorous comparison of the prevalence of alpha-fodrin antibodies in different studies has been impossible so far. If the prevalence of alpha-fodrin antibodies differs even in untreated patients, then the patient selection method and the mode of establishing a diagnosis in Sjögren's syndrome are likely the reason.

CONCLUSIONS

Antibodies against alpha-fodrin are sensitive markers of Sjögren's syndrome. Their exact prevalence appears to be between 50% and 90%, but it needs to be studied further in untreated patients. Through ongoing attempts at epitope mapping, the sensitivity of antibodies against alpha-fodrin may be increased even further. Therefore, they may be used as markers for screening Sjögren's syndrome, in addition to antibodies against Ro.

Furthermore, antibodies against alpha-fodrin appear to be markers for disease activity in Sjögren's syndrome. Therefore, they may become relevant tools for identifying selected patients who have a high degree of inflammation for the appropriate therapeutic interventions.

REFERENCES

1. SCHEIN, O.D., M.C. HOCHBERG, B. MUNOZ, *et al.* 1999. Dry eye and dry mouth in the elderly: a population-based assessment. Arch. Intern. Med. **159:** 1359–1363.
2. HAY, E.M., E. THOMAS, B. PAL, *et al.* 1998. Weak association between subjective symptoms or and objective testing for dry eyes and dry mouth: results from a population based study. Ann. Rheum. Dis. **57:** 20–24.
3. DELALANDE, S., J. DE SEZE, A.L. FAUCHAIS, *et al.* 2004. Neurologic manifestations in primary Sjögren's syndrome: a study of 82 patients. Medicine **83:** 280–291.
4. NAKANO, M., S. NOGAMI, S. SATO, *et al.* 2001. Interaction of syntaxin with alpha-fodrin, a major component of the submembranous cytoskeleton. Biochem. Biophys. Res. Commun. **288:** 468–475.

5. PERRIN, D., O.K. LANGLEY & D. AUNIS. 1987. Anti-alpha-fodrin inhibits secretion from permeabilized chromaffin cells. Nature **326:** 498–501.
6. HANEJI, N., T. NAKAMURA, K. TAKIO, *et al.* 1997. Identification of alpha-fodrin as a candidate autoantigen in primary Sjögren's syndrome. Science **276:** 604–607.
7. JANICKE, R.U., P. NG, M.L. SPRENGART & A.G. PORTER. 1998. Caspase-3 is required for alpha-fodrin cleavage but dispensable for cleavage of other death substrates in apoptosis. J. Biol. Chem. **273:** 15540–15545.
8. SAEGUSA, K., N. ISHIMARU, K. YANAGI, *et al.* 2002. Prevention and induction of autoimmune exocrinopathy is dependent on pathogenic autoantigen cleavage in murine Sjögren's syndrome. J. Immunol. **169:** 1050–1057.
9. MARUYAMA, T., I. SAITO, Y. HAYASHI, *et al.* 2004. Molecular analysis of the human autoantibody response to alpha-fodrin in Sjögren's syndrome reveals novel apoptosis-induced specificity. Am. J. Pathol. **165:** 53–61.
10. VITALI, C., S. BOMBARDIERI, H.M. MOUTSOPOULOS, *et al.* 1996. Assessment of the European classification criteria for Sjögren's syndrome in a series of clinically defined cases: results of a prospective multicentre study. The European Study Group on Diagnostic Criteria for Sjögren's syndrome. Ann. Rheum. Dis. **55:** 116–121.
11. VITALI, C., S. BOMBARDIERI, R. JONSSON, *et al.* 2002. For the European Study Group on Classification criteria for Sjögren's syndrome. Classification criteria for Sjögren's syndrome: a revised version of the European criteria proposed by the American-European Consensus Group. Ann. Rheum. Dis. **61:** 554–558.
12. FOX, R.I., C.A. ROBINSON, J.G. CURD, *et al.* 1986. Sjögren's syndrome. Proposed criteria for classification. Arthritis Rheum. **29:** 577–585.
13. WITTE, T., T. MATTHIAS, M. OPPERMANN, *et al.* 2003. Prevalence of antibodies against alpha-fodrin in Sjögren's syndrome: comparison of two sets of classification criteria. J. Rheumatol. **30:** 2157–2159.
14. SHIELDS, D.C., K.E. SCHAECHER, T.C. SAIDO & N.L. BANIK. 1999. A putative mechanism of demyelination in multiple sclerosis by a proteolytic enzyme, calpain. Proc. Natl. Acad. Sci. USA. **96:** 11486–11491.
15. DE SEZE, J., S. DUBUCQUOI, A.L. FAUCHAIS, *et al.* 2003. Alpha-fodrin autoantibodies in the differential diagnosis of MS and Sjögren syndrome. Neurology **61:** 268–269.
16. WITTE, T., T. MATTHIAS, F.C. ARNETT, *et al.* 2000. IgA and IgG autoantibodies against alpha-fodrin as markers for Sjögren's syndrome. J. Rheumatol. **27:** 2617–2620.
17. DE SEZE, J., S. DUBUCQUOI, A.L. FAUCHAIS, *et al.* 2004. Autoantibodies against alpha-fodrin in Sjögren's syndrome with neurological manifestations. J. Rheumatol. **31:** 500–503.
18. RUFFATTI, A., P. OSTUNI, P. GRYPIOTIS, *et al.* 2004. Sensitivity and specificity for primary Sjögren's syndrome of IgA and IgG anti-alpha-fodrin antibodies detected by ELISA. J. Rheumatol. **31:** 504–507.
19. SZANTO, A., I. CSIPO & M. ZEHER. 2005. Sensitivity and specificity of anti-alpha-fodrin antibodies in primary Sjögren's syndrome. J. Rheumatol. **32:** 197–198.

Generation and Characterization of Three Monoclonal IgM Antiphospholipid Antibodies Recognizing Different Phospholipid Antigens

CATHARINA BUSCHMANN, CHRISTIAN FISCHER, VIOLA OCHSENHIRT, CAROLIN NEUKIRCH, KARL J. LACKNER, AND PHILIPP VON LANDENBERG

Institute of Clinical Chemistry and Laboratory Medicine, Johannes Gutenberg University of Mainz, Mainz, Germany

ABSTRACT: Antiphospholipid antibodies (APLs) might be involved in the pathogenesis of the antiphospholipid syndrome (APS). This study analyzes the structural characteristics of monoclonal APLs derived from patients with this disease. Patient-derived B cells were immortalized using Epstein-Barr virus transformation and subsequent fusion to the myeloma cell line CB-F7. APL-producing hybridomas were cloned to obtain cell lines producing monoclonal APL. DNA encoding the variable region of heavy and light chains of the antibodies was sequenced and analyzed regarding their usage within the V-gene family and the existence of somatic hypermutation. Binding patterns of APL to various phospholipids and beta-2-glycoprotein-I (β2-GPI) were determined using ELISA, with special regard to β2-GPI dependency. As a result, three APL-producing hybridoma cell lines from patients with APS were established: JGG9, HVA2, and HLC9. APLs were of the IgM isotype and showed different binding patterns toward phospholipids and β2-GPI. One of them, JGG9, showed extensive somatic hypermutations in both the CDR3 region and a framework region of the heavy chain. JGG9 bound to cardiolipin in the presence of the protein cofactor β2-GPI. In contrast, the antibodies HVA2 and HLC9 (which also showed somatic hypermutations in the CDR3 region) presented polyreactivity to several phospholipids—cardiolipin, phosphatidylserine, -ethanolamine, -inositol, -choline, and sphingomyelin—but not to β2-GPI. In conclusion, JGG9 presents a high degree of mutation in the CDR3 and framework region resulting from the deletions of nucleotides, and affects amino acid composition. Polyreactivity and the absence of cofactor dependency present HLC9- and HVA2-like natural antibodies that have no contact with any antigen. Nonetheless, these natural antibodies show somatic hypermutation of the heavy chain, indicating antigen-driven maturation. Regarding the possible role of APL in infection, HVA2 in particular may represent a pathogen-maturated antibody showing cross-reactivity between phospholipids and infectious agents. Further experiments are needed to reveal the functional activity of these antibodies.

KEYWORDS: antiphospholipid antibodies; monoclonal antibodies; somatic hypermutation; germline sequences; natural antibodies; antiphospholipid syndrome; infectious disease; immunoglobulin M; anticardiolipin syndrome

Address for correspondence: Prof. Dr. Philipp von Landenberg, Institute of Clinical Chemistry and Laboratory Medicine, Johannes Gutenberg University of Mainz, Langenbeckstrasse 1, 55131 Mainz, Germany. Voice: +49-6131-175104; fax: +49-6131-176627.
Landenberg@zentrallabor.klinik.uni-mainz.de

**Ann. N.Y. Acad. Sci. 1051: 240–254 (2005). © 2005 New York Academy of Sciences.
doi: 10.1196/annals.1361.065**

INTRODUCTION

Antiphospholipid antibodies (APLs) have long been known. Besides their well-recognized appearance in certain infectious diseases such as syphilis, they have been associated with antiphospholipid syndrome (APS; also known as anticardiolipin syndrome).[1,2] Typical manifestations of APS are recurrent arterial and venous thrombosis and recurrent spontaneous abortions. Numerous other clinical manifestations have been associated with APL.[3,4] While initially it was thought that APLs bind directly to phospholipids, the discovery that most APLs require protein cofactors to interact with their phospholipid antigen was an important step forward in the understanding of APLs' binding specificity. Researchers have since discovered antibodies binding proteins alone.[5–10] Additional evidence suggests that protein cofactor dependency might be related to the pathogenic potential of APLs.[10]

However, APLs are also known in the context of infectious diseases. So-called natural autoantibodies are present in healthy individuals and are often nonspecific with regard to peptides. These antibodies recognize antigens, like carbohydrates or lipids, mostly in a polyreactive way, so many APL might be natural autoantibodies.[11] In contrast to disease-related hypermutated immunoglobulin G (IgG) antibodies, natural autoantibodies are predominantly of the IgM type, encoded mostly by unmutated variable-region genes and independent of T-cell help for activation.[12] Although the function of these natural autoantibodies is not completely clear, they seem to play a role in innate immunity and first-line defense against pathogens.[13]

In APL research, analysis of monoclonal antibodies has been applied by several research groups in the past to gain insight into structural characteristics and potential functions of these antibodies.[14–18] Although the pathogenic potential of these monoclonals must always be demonstrated for each antibody, they are valuable tools for investigating APLs' mechanisms of action on the molecular level.

In this study, we characterized three monoclonal APLs derived from APS patients with regard to binding specificities, heavy- and light-chain composition, and DNA structure encoding the variable regions of the antibodies. Even though the monoclonal APLs are secreted by APS patients' B cells, further studies are needed to reveal whether they are relevant for the pathogenesis of APS and infectious disease or whether they are natural antibodies.

METHODS

Generation of APL-Producing Monoclonal Cell Lines

APL-producing cell clones were generated by Epstein-Barr virus (EBV) infection of patient-derived B cells, followed by fusion to the mouse-human heteromyeloma cell line CB-F7[19] by either pegylated (PEG) fusion or electrofusion. Shortly thereafter, mononuclear cells were isolated from 30 mL of heparinized blood of APS patients using Ficoll gradient centrifugation. Cells were washed twice with phosphate-buffered saline (PBS) and resuspended at a density of 3×10^6 cells/mL in RPMI 1640 medium supplemented with the following: 10% heat-inactivated fetal calf serum (FCS), 100 U/mL each of penicillin and streptomycin, and 2 mM L-glutamine. Monocytes were depleted by adhering them to the plastic surface of cell culture flasks. EBV infection was performed by adding 2 mL EBV-containing supernatant of the B95-8 cell line to 1 mL of the cell suspension, followed by incubation for 12 hours at 37°C in a humidified atmosphere containing 5% CO_2. Thereafter, cells were pelleted and resuspended in fresh RPMI medium (supplemented as described above) containing 2 μg/mL phytohemagglutinine and 1 μg/mL cyclosporin A, and seeded in 96-well plates at 10^5 cells/well.

After 2 to 3 weeks, supernatants of growing cell colonies were screened for APL production by phospholipid-8S enzyme-linked immunosorbent assay (ELISA; Aesku.Diagnostics, Wendelsheim, Germany). Cell populations with antiphospholipid activity were expanded and fused to histone acetyltransferase (HAT)-sensitive,ouabain-resistant, nonsecreting CB-F7 heteromyeloma cells.

PEG fusion was performed in a 3-to-1 ratio of B cells to CB-F7 cells using a minimum of 3×10^7 cells, as described.[19] After fusion, cells were seeded at 5×10^6 cells/mL in 96-well plates in RPMI 1640 medium supplemented with FCS, penicillin, streptomycin, and L-glutamine, as previously mentioned. After 24 hours of incubation, the medium was replaced by HAT-ouabain medium; the new medium comprised RPMI, supplemented as described above, with 5 mM hypoxanthin, 20 μM aminopterin, 800 μM thymidin, and 10 μM ouabain.

For electrofusion, 2.5×10^5 B cells and CB-F7 cells were mixed and pelleted by centrifugation (5 minutes, $160 \times g$). The pellet was washed twice with hypo-osmolar electrofusion buffer (Eppendorf, Hamburg, Germany) and centrifuged for 7 minutes and 70 g. After the last centrifugation step, cells were resuspended in 200 μL hypo-osmolar fusion buffer and poured into the fusion chamber of an Eppendorf Multiporator. Cells were fused using a standard protocol: 30 seconds, 5 V (alignment of cells); 3×30 μs, 30 V (fusion); and 30 seconds, 5 V (postfusion). After fusion, cells were distributed into four chambers of a cloning plate (Greiner BioOne, Frickenhausen, Germany) in a postfusion medium (RPMI 1640 without phenyl red, supplemented with 10% FCS and 2 mM L-glutamine). After 24 hours of incubation, HAT-sensitive ouabain medium was added.

Identification of Antibody Heavy and Light Chains

Antibody heavy and light chains were analyzed using western blot technology. Cell culture supernatants containing APLs were concentrated in Vivaspin 4 concentrators (Vivascience, Hannover, Germany) with a molecular weight cutoff of 50 kDa and separated by denaturing SDS-polyacrylamide gel electrophoresis (SDS-PAGE). Gels were blotted onto nitrocellulose membranes. Mu heavy chains were detected using donkey-anti-human IgM Fc5μ (Jackson ImmunoResearch, West Grove, PA).Mouse-anti-human kappa-chain or mouse-anti-human lambda-chain (both ICN Biomedicals, Ohio [new company name, MP Biomedicals, Irvine, CA]) were used to detect κ- or λ-chains, respectively. Alkaline phosphatase (AP)–conjugated secondary antibodies against rabbit-, donkey-, and mouse-IgG were used and visualized with 5-bromo-4-chloro-3-indoyl phosphate/nitro blue tetrazolium (BCIP/NBT) substrate.

ELISA Procedures

The binding of APLs to six different phospholipids (cardiolipin, phosphatidylserine, phosphatidylethanolamine, phosphatidylinositol, phosphatidylcholine, and sphingomyelin) and β2-GPI was tested using phospholipid-8-pro-ELISA (Aesku.Diagnostics) according to the manufacturer's instructions.

Amplification of V-Region cDNA of APL

The RNA of hybridoma cells was isolated using an RNeasy Kit (Qiagen, Hilden, Germany) according to the manufacturer's instructions. The OneStep RT-PCR Kit (Qiagen) was used for the reverse transcription of V-region mRNA and the subsequent amplification of cDNA. Four reactions were performed for four different possible heavy and light chains. We also employed a mixture of family-specific primers (each 20 μM), binding at the beginning of the V region, and a specific primer, binding in the constant region of the antibody mRNA, as follows.[20]

1. Primers for μ-chain:

Forward: VHL-1: 5′ TCACCATGGACTGCACCTGGA 3′
VHL-2: 5′ CCATGGACACACTTTGCTCCAC 3′
VHL-3: 5′ TCACCATGGAGTTTGGGCTGAGC 3′
VHL-4: 5′ AGAACATGAAACACCTGTGGTTCTT 3′
VHL-5: 5′ ATGGGGTCAACCGCCATCCT 3′
VHL-6: 5′ ACAATGTCTGTCTCCTTCCTCAT 3′
Backward: CμII: 5′ CAGGAGACGAGGGGGAAAAG 3′

2. Primers for γ-chain:

Forward: VHL-1: 5′ TCACCATGGACTGCACCTGGA 3′
VHL-2: 5′ CCATGGACACACTTTGCTCCAC 3′
VHL-3: 5′ TCACCATGGAGTTTGGGCTGAGC 3′
VHL-4: 5′ AGAACATGAAACACCTGTGGTTCTT 3′
VHL-5: 5′ ATGGGGTCAACCGCCATCCT 3′
VHL-6: 5′ ACAATGTCTGTCTCCTTCCTCAT 3′
Backward: CγII: 5′ GCCAGGGGGAAGACGGATG 3′

3. Primers for κ-chain:

Forward: V_{κ}L-1: 5′ GCTCAGCTCCTGGGGCTCCTG 3′
V_{κ}L-2: 5′ CTGGGGCTGCTAATGCTCTGG 3′
V_{κ}L-3: 5′ TTCCTCCTGCTACTCTGGCTC 3′
V_{κ}L-4: 5′ CAGACCCAGGTCTTCATTTCT 3′
Backward: CκII: 5′ TTTCAACTGCTCATCAGATGGCGG 3′

4. Primers for λ-chain:

Forward: V_{λ}L-1: 5′ CCTCTCCTCCTCACCCTCCT 3′
V_{λ}L-2: 5′ CTCCTCACTCAGGGCACA 3′
V_{λ}L-3: 5′ ATGGCCTGGACCCCTCTCC 3′
Backward: CλII: 5′ AGCTCCTCAGAGGAGGGCGG 3′

OneStep-RT-PCR was performed according to the manufacturer's instructions.

Family-Specific PCR of the APL Variable Region

cDNA mixtures from OneStep-RT-PCR, just described, were split and used for subsequent family-specific PCRs using single family-specific primers. For each reaction, the following were mixed: 3 μL of cDNA mixture, 5 μL of 10 × Pfu PCR buffer (Stratagene, La Jolla, CA), 1.25 μL of 10 mM deoxynucleotide mix, PCR grade (dNTP), 1 μL of 20 μM family-specific *forward*-primer, 1 μL of 20 μM constant-region *backward* primer, 1 μL (2.5 U) PfuTurbo DNA Polymerase (Stratagene), and 38 μL of water. PCR conditions were as follows: 45 seconds at 94°C, 45 seconds at 50°C, and 1 minute 45 seconds at 72°C, repeated for 30 cycles and followed by a 10-minute incubation time.

Determining cDNA Sequence Encoding the Variable Region of APL Light and Heavy Chains

PCR products of family-specific PCR were cleaned with Centri-Sep columns (Princeton Separations, Adelphia, NJ) and directly sequenced using a CEQ 8000 sequencer (Beckmann Coulter, Krefeld, Germany). Single family-specific and constant-region primers, just described, were used for sense and antisense sequencing. V-region sequences were analyzed and aligned to homologous germline genes by reference to either the VBase database (www.mrc-cpe.cam.ac.uk) [21] or the BLAST Ig database.

RESULTS

Three different monoclonal APLs—JGG9, HLC9, and HVA2—were obtained from different APS patients. JGG9 was derived from a 49-year-old female patient (JG) with secondary APS, and HLC9 and HVA2 were isolated from male patients (HL, a 51 year old, and HV, a 58 year old) with primary APS. All three antibodies were shown to be of the IgM type and to carry κ light chains, as determined by western blot analysis and sequence analysis. Our results are summarized in TABLE 1.

TABLE 1. Sequence analysis of the monoclonal APLs JGG9, HLC9, and HVA2

Antiphospholipid antibody		JGG9	HLC9	HVA2
V-gene family (heavy chain)		VH3	VH3	VH2
V-gene family (light chain)		VκII	VκIII	VκII
Sequence H	V		DP-49	VII-5
	D		D6-13	D3-3
	J	{JH3?}	JH4b	JH5
Sequence L	V	DPK13	DPK21	DPK22
	J	Jκ2	Jκ2	Jκ4
Homology H			DNA = 95.87% Protein = 90.7%	DNA = 96.44% Protein = 94.65%
Homology L		DNA = 98.75% Protein = 99.06%	DNA = 97.86% Protein = 95.41%	DNA = 99.69% Protein: 100%
Insertion H	V–D		Yes	Yes
	D–J		Yes	Yes
Insertion L	V–J	No	Yes	No (rather, deletion)

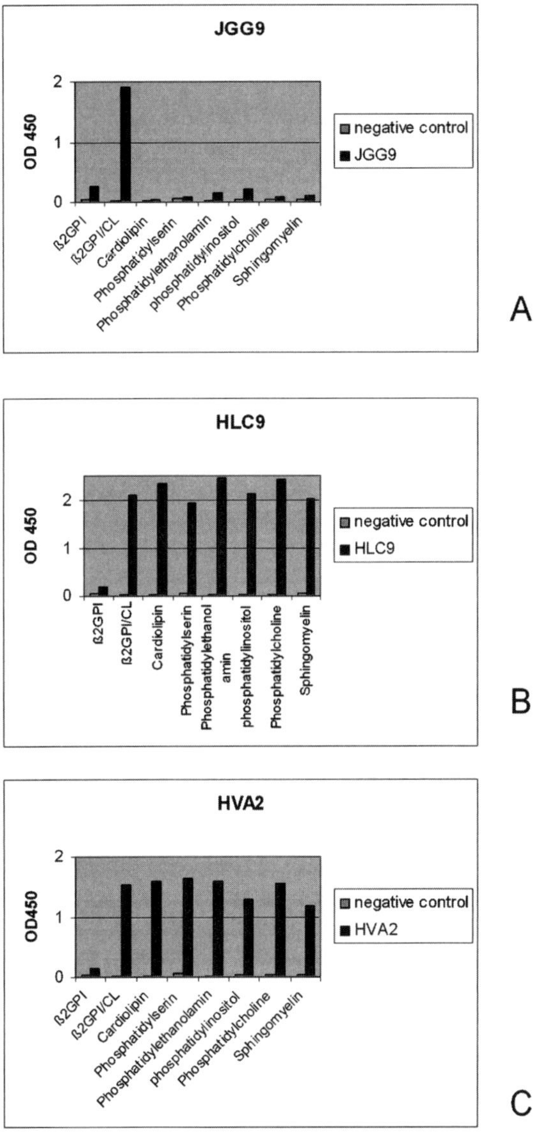

FIGURE 1. Binding profiles of the three antiphospholipid antibodies (APLs): JGG9 (**A**), HLC9 (**B**), and HVA2 (**C**). Binding to indicated phospholipid and protein antigens was tested with a microtiter-plate-based enzyme-linked immunosorbent assay (ELISA).

Analysis of binding of APL to cardiolipin, phosphatidylserine, phosphatidylethanolamine, phosphatidylinositol, phosphatidylcholine, sphingomyelin, and β2-GPI revealed different binding patterns for JGG9, HLC9, and HVA2, especially with regard to β2-GPI dependency of phospholipid binding. Whereas JGG9 binds to β2-GPI, and even better to the cardiolipin/β2-GPI complex, HLC9 and HVA2 bind to all displayed antigens, except for β2-GPI, and do not depend on the presence of β2-GPI (FIG. 1).

When the VH genes of JGG9, HLC9, and HVA2 were analyzed after amplification of the coding sequence of mRNA for IgM, it was shown that JGG9's heavy-chain variable region (FIG. 2A and B) belongs to the VH3 family. The closest germline V segment is DP-53. A homologous D segment was found by neither VBase nor

```
DP-53     GAGGTGCAGCTGGTGGAGTCCGGGGGAGGCTTAGTTCAGCCTGGGGGGTCCCTGAGACTC
JGG9 μ    GAGGTGCAGCTGGTGGAGTCCGGGGGAGGCTTAGTTCAGCCTGGGGGGTCCCTGAGACTC

          TCCTGTGCAGCCTCTGGATTCACCTTCAGTAGCTACTGGATGCACTGGGTCCGCCAAGCT
          TCCTGTGCAGCCTCTGGATTCACCTTCAGTAGTTACTGGATGCACTGGGTCCGCCAAGCT

          CCAGGGAAGGGGCTGGTGTGGGTCTCACGTATTAATAGTGATGGGAGTAGCACAAGCTAC
          CCAGGGAAGGGGCTGGTGTGGGTCTCACATATTAATAGTGATGGGAGTACCACAACCTAC

          GCGGACTCCGTGAAGGGCCGATTCACCATCTCCAGAGACAACGCCAAGAACACGCTGTAT
          GCGGACTCCGTGAAGGGCCGATTCACCATCTCCAGAGACAACGCCAAGTACACGCTGTAT

          -C-TGCA-AATG-AACAGTCTGAGAGCCGAGGACACGG-CTG-TGTATTACTGTGCAAGA
          GCGTGCGGAATGGAACAGTCTGAGAGCCGACGACACGGTCTGATGTATTACTGTGCAAGG

JH3                   GCTTTT-GATGT-C-TGGGGCCAAGGG-ACA-ATGGTCAC-CGT-CTC
          GAGCATACTGACGGTATGAGACGTACATGGGGCCAAGGGTACCTACGGTCACACGTACTC

          TT-CAG
          CTACAGGGA
```

FIGURE 2. (**A**) JGG9 heavy chain.

FIGURE 2. Alignment of APL variable-region sequences with antibody germline regions. Because the optimal alignments of DNA and protein for the heavy-chain region of JGG9 differed slightly, both are shown in panels **A** and **B**.

```
DP-53           GAG GTG CAG CTG GTG GAG TCC GGG GGC GGA TTA GTT CAG CCT GGG GGG TCC
JGG9 μ          GAG GTG CAG CTG GTG GAG TCC GGG GGC GGA TTA GTT CAG CCT GGG GGG TCC
                 E   V   Q   L   V   E   S   G   G   G   L   V   Q   P   G   G   S

                                                                 $
                CTG AGA CTC TCC TGT GCA GCC TCT GGA TTC ACC TTC AGT AGC TAC TGG ATG
                CTG AGA CTC TCC TGT GCA GCC TCT GGA TTC ACC TTC AGT AGT TAC TGG ATG
                 L   R   L   S   C   A   A   S   G   F   T   F   S   S   Y   W   M

                                                                     R
                CAC TGG GTC CGC CAA GCT CCA GGG AAG GGG CTG GTG TGG GTC TCA CGT ATT
                CAC TGG GTC CGC CAA GCT CCA GGG AAG GGG CTG GTG TGG GTC TCA CAT ATT
                 H   W   V   R   Q   A   P   G   K   G   L   V   W   V   S   H   I

                                     S
                AAT AGT GAT GGG AGT AGC ACA AGC TAC GCG GAC TCC GTG AAG GGC CGA TTC
                AAT AGT GAT GGG AGT ACC ACA ACC TAC GCG GAC TCC GTG AAG GGC CGA TTC
                 N   S   D   G   S   T   T   T   Y   A   D   S   V   K   G   R   F

                                                 N               -   L   Q       -
                ACC ATC TCC AGA GAC AAC GCC AAG AAC ACG CTG TAT --- CTG CAA ATG ---
                ACC ATC TCC AGA GAC AAC GCC AAG TAC ACG CTG TAT GCG TGC GGA ATG GAA
                 T   I   S   R   D   N   A   K   Y   T   L   Y   A   C   G   M   E

                 N       L   R   A   E   D   T   A   V
                AAC AGT CTG AGA GCC GAG GAC ACG GCT GTG TAT TAC TGT GCA AGA
                CAG TCT GAG AGC CGA CGA CAC GGT CTG ATG TAT TAC TGT GCA AGG GAG CAT
                 Q   S   E   S   R   R   H   G   L   M   Y   Y   C   A   R   E   H

                             A   F   D   V                   T   M   V   T   V   S
JH3                         GCT TTT GA  GTC                 ACA A G GTC ACC GT  TCT
                ACT GAC GGT ATG AGA CGT ACA TGG GGC CAA GGG TAC CTA CGG TCA CAC GTA
                 T   D   G   M   R   R   T   W   G   Q   G   Y   L   R   S   H   V

                 S   V
                TCA  G
                CTC CTA CAG GGA
                 L   L   Q   G
```

FIGURE 2 — *continued.* (**B**) JGG9 heavy chain.

BLAST Ig search. JH3 was determined to be the J segment with the greatest homology to the JGG9 heavy chain. Alignment with germline segments using Heidelberg Unix Sequence Analysis Resources (HUSAR) software showed several insertions of nucleotides into the JGG9 sequence, compared with the germline sequence. Whereas the homology was 92.3% on the DNA level, it was only 76.9% on the protein level owing to frame shifts. Strikingly, most amino acid exchanges occurred in framework regions, and only 6 of 28 replacements (21.4%) could be found in complementarity-determining regions (CDRs).

The JGG9 light-chain variable region (FIG. 2C) carried a V segment of the VκII family. It is most homologous to the DPK13 germline V gene. In addition, the J segment is nearly identical to the Jκ2 segment of the Jκ locus in germline configuration.

```
               D   I   V   M   T   G   T
DPK13          GAT ATT GTG ATG ACC CAG ACT CCA CTC TCC CTG CCC GTC ACC CCT GGA GAG
JGG9 κ                                   T CCA CTC TCC CTG CCC GTC ACC CCT GGA GAG
                                           P   L   S   L   P   V   T   P   G   E

               CCG GCC TCC ATC TCC TGC AGG TCT AGT CAG AGC CTC TTG GAT AGT GAT GAT
               CCG GCC TCC ATC TCC TGC AGG TCT AGT CAG AGC CTC TTG GAT AGT GAT GAT
                P   A   S   I   S   C   R   S   S   Q   S   L   L   D   S   D   D
                                                   CDR1
                                                $
               GGA AAC ACC TAT TTG GAC TGG TAC CTG CAG AAG CCA GGG CAG TCT CCA CAG
               GGA AAC ACC TAT TTG GAC TGG TAC CTC CAG AAG CCA GGG CAG TCT CCA CAG
                G   N   T   Y   L   D   W   Y   L   Q   K   P   G   Q   S   P   Q

                    $
               CTC CTG ATC TAT ACG CTT TCC TAT CGG GCC TCT GGA GTC CCA GAC AGG TTC
               CTC CTC ATC TAT ACG CTT TCC TAT CGG GCC TCT GGA GTC CCA GAC AGG TTC
                L   L   I   Y   T   L   S   Y   R   A   S   G   V   P   D   R   F

                                           CDR 2
               AGT GGC AGT GGG TCA GGC ACT GAT TTC ACA CTG AAA ATC AGC AGG GTG GAG
               AGT GGC AGT GGG TCA GGC ACT GAT TTC ACA CTG AAA ATC AGC AGG GTG GAG
                S   G   S   G   S   G   T   D   F   T   L   K   I   S   R   V   E

                                                                               Y
jκ2                                                                           TAC
               GCT GAG GAT GTT GGA GTT TAT TAC TGC ATG CAA CGT ATA GAG TTT CCT
               GCT GAG GAT GTT GGA GTT TAT TAC TGC ATG CAA CGT ATA GAG TTT CCT TGG
                A   E   D   V   G   V   Y   Y   C   M   Q   R   I   E   F   P   W

                                                                   CDR3
               ACT TTT GGC CAG GGG ACC AAG CTG GAG ATC AAA C

               ACT TTT GGC CAG GGG ACC AAG CTG GAG ATC AAA CGA ACT GTG GCT GCA C
                T   F   G   Q   G   T   K   L   E   I   K   R   T   V   A   A
```

FIGURE 2 — *continued.* (**C**) JGG9 light chain.

Compared with germline segments, the JGG9 light chain showed three mutations at the DNA level: two silent mutations in framework regions and one mutation in the CDR3 region resulting in a single amino-acid exchange (Y→W). No inserted P- or N-nucleotides could be detected at the junction between the V and J segments. These results indicate 98.8% homology of the JGG9 light chain to germline segments on the DNA level and 99% homology on the protein level.

HLC9-variable regions have VH3 family and VκIII family V segments, respectively. Heavy-chain variable region segments (FIG. 2D) were found to be most homologous to DP-49 (V segment), D6-13 (D segment), and JH4b (J segment). On the DNA level, 16 mutations were found, leading to a homology to germline segments of 95.9%. The mutations resulted in nine amino acid exchanges, so homology on the protein level was 90.7%. Of all amino acid exchanges, 75% occurred in CDR regions. At both the V-D and D-J junctions, insertions of bases could be observed, which also led to insertions of amino acids.

The V segment of the HLC9 light chain (FIG. 2E) is closely homologous to the DPK21 germline V segment; the J segment is closely related to the Jκ2 germline J segment. As a consequence of seven mutations on the DNA level, there are five mutations in amino acid composition, with 97.9% homology on the DNA level and

```
DP-49                                               CAG GTG CAG CTG GTG GAG TCT GGG
HLC9 μ        T GCT CTT TTA AGA GGT GTC CAG TGT CAG GTG CAG CTG GTG GAG TCT GGG
                 A   L   L   R   G   V   Q   C   Q   V   Q   L   V   E   S   G

                                                                 A
              GGA GGC GTG GTC CAG CCT GGG AGG TCC CTG AGA CTC TCC TGT GCA GCC TCT
              GGA GGC GTG GTC CAG CCT GGG AGG TCC CTG AGA CTC TCC TGT GTA GCC TCT
               G   G   V   V   Q   P   G   R   S   L   R   L   S   C   V   A   S

                                              M
              GGA TTC ACC TTC AGT AGC TAT GGC ATG CAC TGG GTC CGC CAG GCT CCA GGC
              GGA TTC ACC TTC AGT AGC TAT GGC ATA CAC TGG GTC CGC CAG GCT CCA GGC
               G   F   T   F   S   S   Y   G   I   H   W   V   R   Q   A   P   G
                                 CDR1
                                                       Y               N
              AAG GGG CTG GAG TGG GTG GCA GTT ATA TCA TAT GAT GGA AGT AAT AAA TAC
              AAG GGG CTG GAG TGG GTG GCA GTT ATA TCA TTT GAT GGA AGT AGT AAA TAC
               K   G   L   E   W   V   A   V   I   S   F   D   G   S   S   K   Y
                                                               CDR2
                   A
              TAT GCA GAC TCC GTG AAG GGC CGA TTC ACC ATC TCC AGA GAC AAT TCC AAG
              TAT ACA GAC TCC GTG AAG GGC CGA TTC ACC ATC TCC AGA GAC AAT TCC AAG
               Y   T   D   S   V   K   G   R   F   T   I   S   R   D   N   S   K

                           Y               N
              AAC ACG CTG TAT CTG CAA ATG AAC AGC CTG AGA GCT GAG GAC ACG GCT GTG
              AAC ACG CTG CAT CTG CAA ATG AGC AGC CTG AGA GCT GAG GAC ACG GCT GTG
               N   T   L   H   L   Q   M   S   S   L   R   A   E   D   T   A   V

                                                   G               S   W   Y
D6-13                                             GGG TAT AGC AGC AGC TGG TA
              TAT TAC TGT GCG AAA
              TAT TAC TGT GCG AAA TCG GTT CGA CTC TTG TAT AGC AGC AGA GAG ACC CCG
               Y   Y   C   A   K   S   V   R   L   L   Y   S   S   R   E   T   P
                                                           CDR3
                                  Y
JH4b                              TAC TTT GAC TAC TGG GGC CAG GGA ACC CTG GTC ACC GTC

              AGG GGG GAC GGC CCC TTT GAC TAC TGG GGC CAG GGA ACC CTG GTC ACC GTC
               R   G   D   G   P   F   D   Y   W   G   Q   G   T   L   V   T   V


              TCC TCA

              TCC TCA GGG AGT GCA TCC GCC CCA ACC C
               S   S   G   S   A   S   A   P   T
```

FIGURE 2 — *continued.* (**D**) HLC9 heavy chain.

95.4% homology on the protein level. Only 40% of amino acid exchanges took place in CDR regions (two exchanges). At the V-J junction, we found comparatively fewer insertions of nucleotides.

The HVA2 variable region of the heavy chain (FIG. 2F) shows a V segment most closely similar to the VII-5 gene of the germline V-gene locus. An analysis of D-segment usage yielded a less obvious result, though the germline D segment D3-3 was indicated as the most homologous. The JH5 germline J segment was used as such without any modifications. On the DNA level, 14 mutations were observed, many of them successive (that is, two or three base exchanges often occurring in one triplet). These mutations led to seven amino acid exchanges, mostly in the CDR3 region of the HVA2 μ-chain. Homology to the germline variable-region segment on the DNA

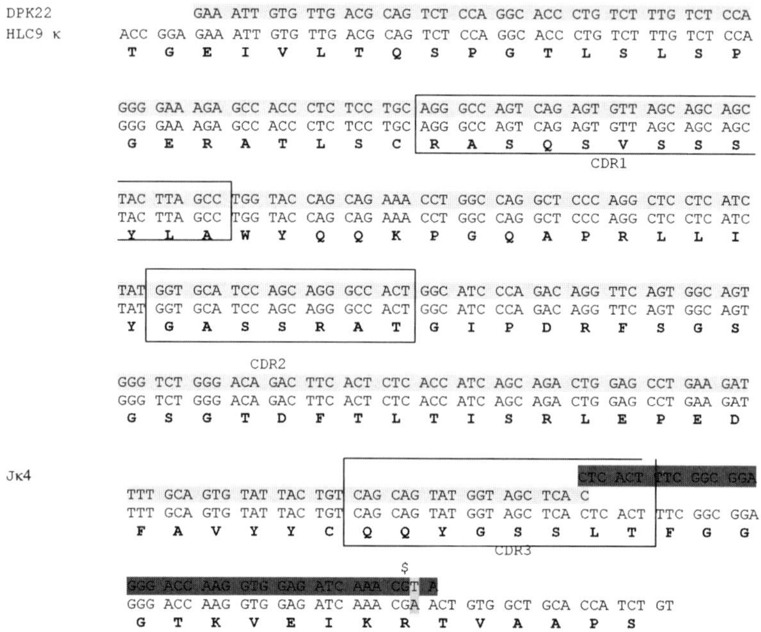

FIGURE 2 — *continued.* (E) HLC9 light chain.

level was 96.4%, and 94.7% on the protein level; 85.7% of all amino acid exchanges took place in CDR regions, 71.4% of them in CDR3. Inserted nucleotides between segments V and D and only one between segments D and J could be detected.

The HVA2 light-chain variable region (FIG. 2G) is composed of a V segment, being identical to the DPK22 germline segment, and a J segment, nearly identical to the Jκ4 gene. Only one conservative base-pair exchange in the framework region was observed. There was 99.7% homology on the DNA level and 100% homology on the protein level. There were no insertions at the V-J junction, but a minor overlap of the V and J segments was observed, indicating that at least one nucleotide had been deleted from the V or J segment.

DISCUSSION

This study generated human monoclonal antibodies to gain insight into structural characteristics of antibody molecules binding to phospholipids, with special regard to DNA organization. APLs are well recognized in the context of several diseases, mainly APS, infectious conditions, and as components of the natural autoantibody repertoire. Highly specific APL binding is described mainly as a feature of somatically mutated IgG, whereas more-specific IgM antibodies are thought to be encoded

```
VII-5                                          CAG ATC ACC TTG AAG GAG TCT
HVA2 µ     TG CTG ACC ATC CCT TCA TGG GTC TTG TCC CAG ATC ACC TTG AAG GAG TCT
              L   T   I   P   S   W   V   L   S   Q   I   T   L   K   E   S

           GGT CCT ACG CTG GTG AAA CCC ACA CAG ACC CTC ACG CTG ACC TGC ACC TTC
           GGT CCT ACG CTG GTG AAA CCC ACA CAG ACC CTC ACG CTG ACC TGC ACC TTC
            G   P   T   L   V   K   P   T   Q   T   L   T   L   T   C   T   F

           TCT GGG TTC TCA CTC AGC ACT AGT GGA GTG GGT GTG GGC TGG ATC CGT CAG
           TCT GGG TTC TCA CTC AGC ACT AGT GGA GTG GGT GTG GGC TGG ATC CGT CAG
            S   G   F   S   L   S   T   S   G   V   G   V   G   W   I   R   Q
                                            CDR1

                                                                N
           CCC CCA GGA AAG GCC CTG GAG TGG CTT GCA CTC ATT TAT TGG AAT GAT GAT
           CCC CCA GGA AAG GCC CTG GAG TGG CTT GCA CTC ATT TAT TGG GAT GAT GAT
            P   P   G   K   A   L   E   W   L   A   L   I   Y   W   D   D   D

                                                                  CDR2
           AAG CGC TAC AGC CCA TCT CTG AAG AGC AGG CTC ACC ATC ACC AAG GAC ACC
           AAG CGC TAC AGC CCA TCT CTG AAG AGC AGG CTC ACC ATC ACC AAG GAC ACC
            K   R   Y   S   P   S   L   K   S   R   L   T   I   T   K   D   T

                                            M
           TCC AAA AAC CAG GTG GTC CTT ACA ATG ACC AAC ATG GAC CCT GTG GAC ACA
           TCC AAA AAC CAG GTG GTC CTT ACA TTG ACC AAC ATG GAC CCT GTG GAC ACA
            S   K   N   Q   V   V   L   T   L   T   N   M   D   P   V   D   T

                                                        V
D3-3                                                   GTA TTA CGC TTT TTG GAG
           GCC ACA TAT TAC TGT GCA CAC AGA C
           GCC ACA TAT TAC TGT GCA CAC AGA CGG GCA CTT GGG TTA CGC TTT TTG GAG
            A   T   Y   Y   C   A   H   R   R   A   L   G   L   R   F   L   E

                L   L   Y   P
           TGG TTA TTA TAC C
JH5                           C AAC TGG TTC GAC CCC TGG GGC CAG GGA ACC CTG GTC
           TGG ACC AAA GGT GCC AAC TGG TTC GAC CCC TGG GGC CAG GGA ACC CTG GTC
            W   T   K   G   A   N   W   F   D   P   W   G   Q   G   T   L   V
                      CDR3

           ACC GTC TCC TCA G
           ACC GTC TCC TCA GGG AGT G
            T   V   S   S   G   S
```

FIGURE 2 — *continued.* (**F**) HVA2 heavy chain.

by germline sequences; however, both result in an accumulation of arginine, asparagine, and lysine residues that are responsible for phospholipid binding.[22] The APLs found in APS patients are believed to be predominantly IgG type and bind phospholipids in a cofactor-dependent manner,[23–26] whereas nonpathogenic APLs have been associated with infections and are thought to interact with phospholipids with low affinity and no cofactor dependency.[27] Antibodies of the natural autoantibody repertoire also bind to their antigens with low affinity. Furthermore, they display polyreactivity and use variable-region segments in germline configuration,[12] indicating that infection-associated APLs are of natural antibody origin and are upregulated as a consequence of defense against pathogens.

Regarding their binding specificity, HLC9 and HVA2 have properties ascribed to nonpathogenic, natural autoantibodies. That is, they show polyreactivity towards

```
DPK22             GAA ATT GTG TTG ACG CAG TCT CCA GGC ACC CTG TCT TTG TCT CCA
HVA2 κ    ACC GGA GAA ATT GTG TTG ACG CAG TCT CCA GGC ACC CTG TCT TTG TCT CCA
           T   G   E   I   V   L   T   Q   S   P   G   T   L   S   L   S   P

          GGG GAA AGA GCC ACC CTC TCC TGC|AGG GCC AGT CAG AGT GTT AGC AGC AGC
          GGG GAA AGA GCC ACC CTC TCC TGC|AGG GCC AGT CAG AGT GTT AGC AGC AGC
           G   E   R   A   T   L   S   C | R   A   S   Q   S   V   S   S   S
                                                         CDR1

          TAC TTA GCC|TGG TAC CAG CAG AAA CCT GGC CAG GCT CCC AGG CTC CTC ATC
          TAC TTA GCC|TGG TAC CAG CAG AAA CCT GGC CAG GCT CCC AGG CTC CTC ATC
           Y   L   A | W   Y   Q   Q   K   P   G   Q   A   P   R   L   L   I

          TAT|GGT GCA TCC AGC AGG GCC ACT|GGC ATC CCA GAC AGG TTC AGT GGC AGT
          TAT|GGT GCA TCC AGC AGG GCC ACT|GGC ATC CCA GAC AGG TTC AGT GGC AGT
           Y | G   A   S   S   R   A   T | G   I   P   D   R   F   S   G   S

                      CDR2
          GGG TCT GGG ACA GAC TTC ACT CTC ACC ATC AGC AGA CTG GAG CCT GAA GAT
          GGG TCT GGG ACA GAC TTC ACT CTC ACC ATC AGC AGA CTG GAG CCT GAA GAT
           G   S   G   T   D   F   T   L   T   I   S   R   L   E   P   E   D

Jκ4                                                   CTC ACT TTC GGC GGA
           TTT GCA GTG TAT TAC TGT|CAG CAG TAT GGT AGC TCA C
           TTT GCA GTG TAT TAC TGT|CAG CAG TAT GGT AGC TCA CTC ACT|TTC GGC GGA
            F   A   V   Y   Y   C | Q   Q   Y   G   S   S   L   T | F   G   G
                                                CDR3
                                       $
           GGG ACC AAG GTG GAG ATC AAA CGT A
           GGG ACC AAG GTG GAG ATC AAA CGA ACT GTG GCT GCA CCA TCT GT
            G   T   K   V   E   I   K   R   T   V   A   A   P   S
```

FIGURE 2 — *continued.* (**G**) HVA2 light chain.

different phospholipid antigens and no cofactor dependency, at least not to β2-GPI. JGG9 (although carrying a μ-chain as its heavy chain) shows characteristics of an APS-related antibody, as demonstrated by its clear dependency on β2-GPI. Drawing attention to its molecular structure, JGG9's heavy-chain region shows the highest degree of mutations in comparison with germline sequences; a homologous D segment was not found. This may have been the result of nucleotides deleted during the rearrangement process or of an extremely intensive process of mutation that changed the sequence of this segment completely. Surprisingly, most of the mutations led to changes of the amino acid composition of framework regions 3 and 4. Even insertions of amino acids could be detected. Because sides for antigen contact lie preferentially in CDR regions, mutations in the framework regions are not likely to result from antigen-driven processes. Nonetheless, a comparatively high number of mutations could also be found in the CDR3 region. Because no D segment could be aligned, conclusions about the actual state of mutations cannot be made.

Although HLC9 and HVA2 display polyreactivity, indicating that they could belong to the natural antibody repertoire, certain mutations can be detected even in their DNA and protein structure. Both have a limited number of mutations and amino acid exchanges, mainly in their CDR regions. Therefore, it cannot be ruled out that HLC9 and HVA2 have undergone a process of somatic hypermutation. This process would be compatible with antigen contact leading to affinity maturation, which would be unusual for a polyreactive "natural" antibody.

Strikingly, accumulations of amino acid exchanges to arginine, asparagine, or lysine were not found either in JGG9 or in HLC9 and HVA2 sequences.

To gain deeper insight into the nature of the antibodies and the possibility of affinity maturation as the cause for mutation, verification by statistical methods is planned.[28,29] Furthermore, functional analyses and animal experiments are needed to reveal whether JGG9, HLC9, and HVA2 are involved in the pathogenesis of APS or are more likely to play a role in natural antibody repertoire and pathogen defense.

REFERENCES

1. Hughes, G.R., N.N. Harris & A.E. Gharavi. 1986. The anticardiolipin syndrome. J. Rheumatol. **13:** 486–489.
2. Harris, E.N., A.E. Gharavi, M.L. Boey, *et al.* 1983. Anticardiolipin antibodies: detection by radioimmunoassay and association with thrombosis in systemic lupus erythematosus. Lancet. **2:** 1211–1214.
3. Shapiro, S.S. 1996. The lupus anticoagulant/antiphospholipid syndrome. Annu. Rev. Med. **47:** 533–553.
4. Alarcon-Segovia, D. 1992. Clinical manifestations of the antiphospholipid syndrome. J. Rheumatol. **19:** 1778–1781.
5. Galli, M., P. Comfurius, C. Maassen, *et al.* 1990. Anticardiolipin antibodies (ACA) directed not to cardiolipin but to a plasma protein cofactor. Lancet **335:** 1544–1547.
6. McNeil, H.P., R.J. Simpson, C.N. Chesterman & S.A. Krilis. 1990. Anti-phospholipid antibodies are directed against a complex antigen that includes a lipid-binding inhibitor of coagulation: beta 2-glycoprotein I (apolipoprotein H). Proc. Natl. Acad. Sci. USA. **87:** 4120–4124.
7. Bevers, E.M., M. Galli, T. Barbui, *et al.* 1991. Lupus anticoagulant IgG's (LA) are not directed to phospholipids only, but to a complex of lipid-bound human prothrombin. Thromb. Haemost. **66:** 629–632.
8. Sammaritano, L.R., A.E. Gharavi, C. Soberano, *et al.* 1992. Phospholipid binding of antiphospholipid antibodies and placental anticoagulant protein. J. Clin. Immunol. **12:** 27–35.
9. Matsuda, J., N. Saitoh, K. Gohchi, *et al.* 1994. Anti-annexin V antibody in systemic lupus erythematosus patients with lupus anticoagulant and/or anticardiolipin antibody. Am. J. Hematol. **47:** 56–58.
10. Roubey, R.A. 1994. Autoantibodies to phospholipid-binding plasma proteins: a new view of lupus anticoagulants and other "antiphospholipid" autoantibodies. Blood **84:** 2854–2867.
11. Lieby, P., A. Soley, A.M. Knapp, *et al.* 2003. Memory B cells producing somatically mutated antiphospholipid antibodies are present in normal healthy individuals. Blood **5**: 5.
12. Hayakawa, K., M. Asano, S.A. Shinton, *et al.* 1999. Positive selection of natural autoreactive B cells. Science. **285:** 113–116.
13. Hayakawa, K. & R.R. Hardy. 2000. Development and function of B-1 cells. Curr. Opin. Immunol. **12:** 346–353.
14. Lieby, P., A. Soley, H. Levallois, *et al.* 2001. The clonal analysis of anticardiolipin antibodies in a single patient with primary antiphospholipid syndrome reveals an extreme antibody heterogeneity. Blood. **97:** 3820–3828.
15. Olee, T., S.S. Pierangeli, H.H. Handley, *et al.* 1996. A monoclonal IgG anticardiolipin antibody from a patient with the antiphospholipid syndrome is thrombogenic in mice. Proc. Natl. Acad. Sci. USA. **93:** 8606–8611.
16. Pierangeli, S.S., X. Liu, R. Espinola, *et al.* 2000. Functional analyses of patient-derived IgG monoclonal anticardiolipin antibodies using in vivo thrombosis and in vivo microcirculation models. Thromb. Haemost. **84:** 388–395.

17. von Landenberg, C., K.J. Lackner, P. von Landenberg, *et al.* 1999. Isolation and characterization of two human monoclonal anti-phospholipid IgG from patients with autoimmune disease. J. Autoimmun. **13:** 215–223.
18. Zhu, M., T. Olee, D.T. Le, *et al.* 1999. Characterization of IgG monoclonal anti-cardiolipin/anti-beta2GP1 antibodies from two patients with antiphospholipid syndrome reveals three species of antibodies. Br. J. Haematol. **105:** 102–109.
19. Grunow, R., S. Jahn, T. Porstmann, *et al.* 1988. The high efficiency, human B cell immortalizing heteromyeloma CB-F7. Production of human monoclonal antibodies to human immunodeficiency virus. J. Immunol. Methods. **106:** 257–265.
20. Wang, X. & B.D. Stollar. 2000. Human immunoglobulin variable region gene analysis by single cell RT-PCR. J. Immunol. Methods. **244:** 217–225.
21. Tomlinson, I., S.C. Williams, S.J. Corbett, *et al.* 1996. VBASE sequence directory. http://www.mrc-cpe.cam.ac.uk/imt-doc/public/INTRO.html. MRC Centre for Protein Engineering, Cambridge, UK.
22. Giles, I.P., J.D. Haley, S. Nagl, *et al.* 2003. A systematic analysis of sequences of human antiphospholipid and anti-beta2-glycoprotein I antibodies: the importance of somatic mutations and certain sequence motifs. Semin. Arthritis Rheum. **32:** 246–265.
23. Alarcon-Segovia, D., M. Deleze, C.V. Oria, *et al.* 1989. Antiphospholipid antibodies and the antiphospholipid syndrome in systemic lupus erythematosus. A prospective analysis of 500 consecutive patients. Medicine (Baltimore) **68:** 353–365.
24. Lynch, A., R. Marlar, J. Murphy, *et al.* 1994. Antiphospholipid antibodies in predicting adverse pregnancy outcome. A prospective study. Ann. Intern. Med. **120:** 470–475.
25. Matsuura, E., Y. Igarashi, M. Fujimoto, *et al.* 1990. Anticardiolipin cofactor(s) and differential diagnosis of autoimmune disease. Lancet **336:** 177–178.
26. Ordi, J., A. Selva, F. Monegal, *et al.* 1993. Anticardiolipin antibodies and dependence of a serum cofactor. A mechanism of thrombosis. J. Rheumatol. **20:** 1321–1324.
27. Loizou, S., C.G. Mackworth-Young, C. Cofiner & M.J. Walport. 1990. Heterogeneity of binding reactivity to different phospholipids of antibodies from patients with systemic lupus erythematosus (SLE) and with syphilis. Clin. Exp. Immunol. **80:** 171–176.
28. Chang, B. & P. Casali. 1994. The CDR1 sequences of a major proportion of human germline Ig VH genes are inherently susceptible to amino acid replacement. Immunol. Today **15:** 367–373.
29. Lossos, I.S., R. Tibshirani, B. Narasimhan & R. Levy. 2000. The inference of antigen selection on Ig genes. J. Immunol. **165:** 5122–5126.

Premature Immunosenescence in Rheumatoid Arthritis and Multiple Sclerosis Patients

MARIELLE THEWISSEN, LOES LINSEN, VEERLE SOMERS, PIET GEUSENS, JEF RAUS, AND PIET STINISSEN

Biomedisch Onderzoeksinstituut, Limburgs Universitair Centrum and School of Life Sciences, Transnational University Limburg, Universitary Campus, Diepenbeek, Belgium

ABSTRACT: **Patients with T-cell-mediated autoimmune diseases show immune system abnormalities that resemble the typical characteristics of autoimmune dysfunction described in the elderly. In addition, the incidence of autoimmune disease increases with advancing age. To evaluate whether patients with rheumatoid arthritis (RA) and multiple sclerosis (MS) have premature immunosenescence, we measured two indicators of aging: the number of T-cell-receptor excision circles (TRECs) and the percentage of $CD4^+CD28^{null}$ T cells. We studied them in the peripheral blood mononuclear cells (PBMCs) of 60 RA patients, 32 MS patients, and 40 healthy controls (HCs). We found that TREC numbers were lower in RA and MS patients than in age-matched HCs, indicating premature thymic involution. Moreover, a subset of these patients contained age-inappropriate high frequencies of $CD4^+CD28^{null}$ T cells. This study provides evidence of premature immune system senescence in both RA and MS patients. Premature aging could be a risk factor for developing autoimmune disorders in genetically predisposed individuals in a susceptible environment.**

KEYWORDS: **premature aging; $CD4^+CD28^{null}$ T cells; T-cell homeostasis; immunosenescence; multiple sclerosis; thymic involution; T-cell-receptor excision circles; TREC number; rheumatoid arthritis**

INTRODUCTION

Autoimmune diseases (AIDs) often arise as age advances. Patients with T-cell-mediated AIDs show immune system abnormalities that resemble the typical characteristics of immune dysfunction described in the elderly. Several research groups have observed T-cell clonal expansions in the peripheral blood of rheumatoid arthritis (RA) patients.[1–4] Others have reported a population of T cells in RA patients with signs of replicative stress.[2–6] An important aspect of immunosenescence is thymic involution,[7] during which the epithelial space (where T-cell maturation and selection take place) is replaced by fatty tissue. This restructuring process causes a decline in

Address for correspondence: Dr. P. Stinissen, Biomedisch Onderzoeksinstituut, Limburgs Universitair Centrum, Universitary Campus, Building A, B-3590 Diepenbeek, Belgium. Voice: +32-11-26-92-04; fax: +32-11-26-92-09.
piet.stinissen@luc.ac.be

Ann. N.Y. Acad. Sci. 1051: 255–262 (2005).
doi: 10.1196/annals.1361.066

the output of new T cells from the thymus.[7] A space-filling autoproliferation mechanism, known as homeostatic proliferation, keeps peripheral T-cell numbers at a constant level throughout life and becomes particularly important with advancing age.[8] However, this mechanism induces replicative stress on peripheral T cells. Replicatively stressed cells have lost the expression of the major costimulatory molecule CD28, accompanied by phenotypic and functional changes.[9–12]

Premature aging, associated thymic involution, and compensatory autoproliferation could play an important role in the pathogenesis of autoimmunity. It has been shown in mice that severe T-cell depletion or the transfer of small numbers of T cells into T-cell–deficient hosts induces immunopathology and the development of AIDs.[13,14] Apparently, the control mechanisms that maintain a stable and diverse repertoire of naive and memory T cells in a healthy functional immune system are severely compromised in lymphopenic conditions.[15] In addition, lymphopenia-induced autoproliferation causes the accumulation of potential auto-aggressive T cells, whose functional capacities could confer an increased risk for developing autoimmunity.

To evaluate whether the immune systems of patients with RA or multiple sclerosis (MS) have undergone premature aging, we measured the number of T-cell–receptor excision circles (TRECs) and the percentage of $CD4^{+}CD28^{null}$ T cells in peripheral blood mononuclear cells (PBMCs). These parameters are important indicators of aging within the immune system.

MATERIAL AND METHODS

Patients and Controls

Peripheral blood samples were obtained from 40 healthy controls (HCs), 60 rheumatoid arthritis (RA) patients, and 32 clinically definite multiple sclerosis (MS) patients.[30] All RA patients fulfilled the 1988 American College of Rheumatology (ACR) criteria for RA. TABLE 1 summarizes characteristics of patients and controls enlisted in this study. In RA patients, disease activity was evaluated by clinical examination. Patients and controls were divided into three groups according to their age. The youngest age group (15–40 years) contained 16 HCs, 5 RA patients, and 17 MS patients; the middle age group (41–60 years) consisted of 14 HCs, 30 RA patients, and 14 MS patients; and the oldest group (61 years and older) contained 10 HCs and 24 RA patients.

Analysis of $CD4^{+}CD28^{null}$ T-Cell Frequencies

Peripheral blood mononuclear cells (PBMCs) were isolated by means of Ficoll-Hypaque density gradient centrifugation (Sigma-Aldrich, St. Louis, MO). Percentages of $CD4^{+}CD28^{null}$ T cells were determined by flow-cytometric analysis. PBMCs were stained with fluorescein isothiocyanate (FITC)-labeled anti-CD4 and phycoerytrin (PE)-labeled anti-CD28 antibodies (BD Biosciences, Erembodegem, Belgium). Cells were analyzed with a FACS Calibur (BD Biosciences). The percentage of $CD28^{null}$ T cells within the $CD4^{+}$ T-cell population was then calculated.

TABLE 1. Characteristics of rheumatoid arthritis patients, multiple sclerosis patients, and healthy controls

	Healthy controls ($n = 40$)	Rheumatoid arthritis patients ($n = 60$)	Multiple sclerosis patients ($n = 32$)
Age range (mean)	21–75 (45.0)	34–84 (56.7)	16–58 (39.4)
Gender (male/female)	16/24	20/40	12/20
Disease duration (yr)	—	6.9	6.5
RF status (positive/negative)	—	25/33	—
Disease status (active/stable)	—	26/34	—
Mean EDSS	—	—	3.9
MS subtype (RR/SP)	—	—	27/5

ABBREVIATIONS: EDSS, Expanded Disability Status Score; RF, rheumatoid factor; RR, relapsing-remitting; SP, secondary-progressive.

Quantification of TREC Numbers

Genomic DNA (gDNA) was isolated by incubating cells in lysis buffer (75 mM NaCl, 25 mM EDTA, 1% sodium dodecyl sulfate [SDS], and 50 μg/mL proteinase K) for 1 hour at 37°C, followed by chloroform:isoamylalcohol (24:1) extraction. TREC numbers in 100 ng of gDNA were measured with quantitative real-time PCR LightCycler technology (Roche Diagnostics GmbH, Mannheim, Germany). Each LightCycler run was reproduced at least once. Primers (5′-TCC CTT TCA ACC ATG CTG-3′ and 5′-GGC TTG GGA TAG CTG T-3′) were constructed to amplify a fragment including the δRecφ Jα signal joint. The TREC 5′-probe (5′-GGC CCT GTC TGC TCT TCA-3′-) was labeled at the 3′ end with fluorescein, whereas the TREC 3′ probe (5′-CAC CGT TCT CAC GAG TTGp-3′) was labeled at the 5′ end with LightCycler Red 640. For amplicon detection, the LightCycler FastStart DNA Master Hybridization Probes kit was used according to the manufacturer's instructions (Roche Diagnostics GmbH). In addition, reaction mixtures contained 100 ng gDNA, 3 mM $MgCl_2$, 0.5 pmol primers, and 0.2 pmol probes. The PCR program consisted of an initial 10 minutes at 95°C for FastStart Taq DNA polymerase activation followed by 43 cycles of repeated denaturation (3 seconds at 95°C), annealing (10 seconds at 59°C), and chain extension (15 seconds at 72°C). A serial dilution of TREC-containing plasmids was used as a standard for absolute quantification.

Statistical Analysis

Using SPSS software, one-way analysis of variance (ANOVA) was performed to compare TREC numbers and percentages of $CD4^{+}CD28^{null}$ T cells among RA patients, MS patients, and HCs. Tukey tests were performed as post-hoc tests. Student's *t* tests were used to compare different subgroups of patients and controls. A *P* value of less than 0.05 was considered statistically significant.

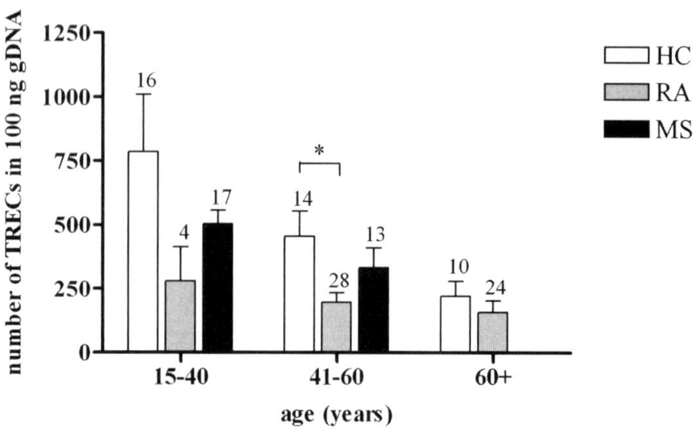

FIGURE 1. TREC numbers in rheumatoid arthritis (RA) patients, multiple sclerosis (MS) patients, and healthy controls (HCs). Patients and HCs were divided into three age groups. The average number of TRECs in 100 ng of gDNA was determined for all subgroups. *Error bars* illustrate SEM. Numbers on top of SEM indicate the number of patients or controls tested in the corresponding group. $*P < .05$. Abbreviations: gDNA, genomic DNA; SEM, standard error of the mean; TREC, T-cell–receptor excision circle.

RESULTS

Premature Thymic Involution in RA and MS Patients

Thymic output can be estimated by evaluating the TREC content of PBMCs. TRECs are generated as extrachromosomal by-products during the recombination of V(D)J gene segments of the T-cell receptor (TCR). TRECs are stable, do not replicate, and are therefore diluted with every cell division.[16] The δRec-φJα signal joint (sj) TREC was described to be a good measure for thymic output.[17] FIGURE 1 shows that TREC numbers declined progressively with age in the PBMCs of HCs, indicating an age-dependent decrease in thymic output. Remarkably, TREC numbers in the youngest RA patients (aged 15–40 years) were comparable to TREC numbers in the oldest HCs (61 years and older) and did not decline further with age. A statistically significant lower number of TRECs was observed in RA patients compared with HCs in the age group 41–60 years (FIG. 1). In addition, TREC numbers in MS patients were lower than those in age-matched healthy individuals, especially in the youngest MS patients. However, these differences were not statistically significant (FIG. 1). Apparently, during the first decades of life, thymic involution had progressed at a faster rate in RA and MS patients than in HCs.

Age-Independent High Frequencies of $CD4^{+}CD28^{null}$ T Cells in RA and MS Patients

Studies on human aging have identified the loss of CD28 expression on both $CD4^{+}$ and $CD8^{+}$ T cells as the best biologic indicator of aging in the immune system.[18] Surprisingly, in HCs, frequencies of $CD4^{+}CD28^{null}$ T cells did not increase

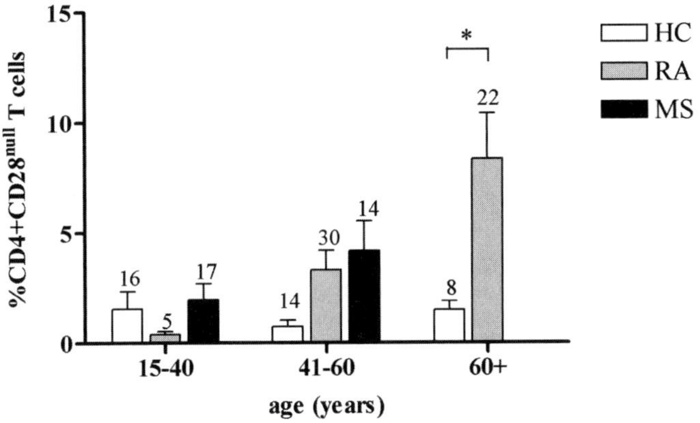

FIGURE 2. Percentages of $CD4^+CD28^{null}$ T cells in rheumatoid arthritis (RA) patients, multiple sclerosis (MS) patients, and healthy controls (HCs). The average percentage of $CD4^+CD28^{null}$ T cells was determined for all subgroups. *Error bars* illustrate SEM. Numbers on top of SEM indicate the number of patients or controls tested in the corresponding group. $^*P < .05$. SEM, standard error of the mean.

with advancing age (FIG. 2). In the youngest age groups, no difference in the percentage of $CD4^+CD28^{null}$ T cells among HCs, RA patients, and MS patients could be observed. However, percentages of $CD4^+CD28^{null}$ T cells did increase with advancing age in RA and MS patients. In the oldest age group, RA patients had significantly more $CD4^+CD28^{null}$ T cells than did age-matched HCs (FIG. 2). For RA patients, no correlation could be detected between the percentage of $CD4^+CD28^{null}$ T cells and gender, disease duration, rheumatoid factor (RF) status, and disease status. In addition, for MS patients, no relation was seen between the Expanded Disability Status Score (EDSS), gender, MS subtype, and the percentage of $CD4^+CD28^{null}$ T cells.

DISCUSSION

Several lines of evidence suggest that T cells play an important role in the pathogenesis of RA and MS. A skewed TCR repertoire was observed in RA patients, but none of the Vβ genes was found to be consistently overexpressed in all, or a subgroup, of RA patients.[2,4,19] Although several putative autoantigens have been implicated as candidate antigens in RA (collagen, proteoglycans, heat-shock proteins [HSPs]) and MS (myelin components), the "disease-triggering" antigen (or antigens) has not been identified.[20] These findings support the concept that autoimmune diseases are not caused by a single autoantigen, but rather result from a general dysfunction of peripheral immune system tolerance or homeostasis mechanisms.

CONCLUSION

This study examined TREC content and the percentage of $CD4^+CD28^{null}$ T cells as indicators of immunosenescence. Although group sizes were often too small to obtain significant differences, the observed age-inappropriate low TREC numbers indicate that both RA and MS patients had premature thymic involution. However, several biologic parameters could complicate the interpretation of TREC data.[21] TREC numbers can be diluted by peripheral T-cell proliferation. Chronic T-cell stimulation induces increased T-cell turnover in RA patients, as evidenced by age-inappropriate short T-cell telomere lengths in RA patients.[22] Decreased thymic output will induce compensatory autoproliferation, a process that contributes to TREC dilution. Age-inappropriate thymic involution and increased peripheral T-cell turnover will each contribute to the lower TREC numbers observed in RA patients. These findings are in agreement with the results of other reports that have described decreased TREC numbers in RA and MS patients.[3,22,23]

In addition, we observed age-inappropriate high percentages of $CD4^+CD28^{null}$ T cells in RA and MS patients. Although $CD4^+CD28^{null}$ T cells are devoid of a major costimulatory signal, they are neither anergic nor functionally paralyzed.[2] Instead, they have gained proinflammatory capacities and cytotoxic function and are resistant to apoptosis.[5,24] The presence of these cells early in disease, and the fact that they do not correlate with disease duration, suggests that $CD4^+CD28^{null}$ T cells not only are a marker for T-cell aging but may be actively involved in the pathogenesis of AIDs. Our data are in line with the findings of other research groups that have reported on increased percentages of $CD4^+CD28^{null}$ T cells in RA and MS patients.[2,5,6,24–26]

Besides thymic involution, several other mechanisms could have contributed to the age-inappropriate high frequencies of $CD4^+CD28^{null}$ T cells. For example, a viral infection can cause massive proliferation of peripheral T cells. Normally, most of these newly generated effector cells are deleted at the end of the response, thereby restoring total T-cell numbers to normal levels. However, defects in these deletion mechanisms can lead to several immune system abnormalities, including contracted TCR diversity and the accumulation of large numbers of clonally expanded T cells. These T cells can persist for many years and compromise immune competence. Several research groups have claimed that the $CD4^+CD28^{null}$ T cells that emerge in the elderly are indeed cytomegalovirus (CMV)-specific cells.[27,28] However, the TCR specificity of the $CD4^+CD28^{null}$ T cells in RA and MS patients has yet to be determined.

The decline in immunocompetence with age is accompanied by a steadily increasing incidence rate of autoimmune diseases.[29] Reduced thymic output induces compensatory autoproliferation of T cells, and this process can lead to premature T-cell senescence and contribute to the immune system abnormalities associated with autoimmunity and aging. Although the incidence of autoimmune diseases increases with advancing age, immunosenescence alone is clearly not sufficient to induce autoimmunity. This finding illustrates that autoimmunity is a complex, multifactorial disorder. Premature aging could be a risk factor for developing autoimmunity in genetically prone individuals in a susceptible environment.

REFERENCES

1. WAGNER, U.G., K. KOETZ, C.M. WEYAND & J.J. GORONZY. 1998. Perturbation of the T cell repertoire in rheumatoid arthritis. Proc. Natl. Acad. Sci. USA **95:** 14447–14452.

2. SCHMIDT, D., J.J. GORONZY & C.M. WEYAND. 1996. $CD4^+CD7^-CD28^-T$ cells are expanded in rheumatoid arthritis and are characterized by autoreactivity. J. Clin. Invest. **97:** 2027–2037.
3. PONCHEL, F., A.W. MORGAN, S.J. BINGHAM, *et al.* 2002. Dysregulated lymphocyte proliferation and differentiation in patients with rheumatoid arthritis. Blood **100:** 4550–4556.
4. BAKAKOS, P., C. PICKARD, W.M. WONG, *et al.* 2002. Simultaneous analysis of T cell clonality and cytokine production in rheumatoid arthritis using three-colour flow cytometry. Clin. Exp. Immunol. **129:** 370–378.
5. FASTH, A.E., D. CAO, R. VAN VOLLENHOVEN, *et al.* 2004. CD28nullCD4+ T cells—characterization of an effector memory T-cell population in patients with rheumatoid arthritis. Scand. J. Immunol. **60:** 199–208.
6. WAGNER, U., M. PIERER, S. KALTENHAUSER, *et al.* 2003. Clonally expanded CD4+CD28null T cells in rheumatoid arthritis use distinct combinations of T cell receptor BV and BJ elements. Eur. J. Immunol. **33:** 79–84.
7. LINTON, P.J. & K. DORSHKIND. 2004. Age-related changes in lymphocyte development and function. Nat. Immunol. **5:** 133–139.
8. GOLDRATH, A.W. 2002. Maintaining the status quo: T-cell homeostasis. Microbes Infect. **4:** 539–545.
9. WARRINGTON, K.J., S. TAKEMURA, J.J. GORONZY & C.M. WEYAND. 2001. CD4+,CD28– T cells in rheumatoid arthritis patients combine features of the innate and adaptive immune systems. Arthritis Rheum. **44:** 13–20.
10. GROH, V., A. BRUHL, H. EL-GABALAWY, *et al.* 2003. Stimulation of T cell autoreactivity by anomalous expression of NKG2D and its MIC ligands in rheumatoid arthritis. Proc. Natl. Acad. Sci. USA **100:** 9452–9457.
11. YEN, J.H., B.E. MOORE, T. NAKAJIMA, *et al.* 2001. Major histocompatibility complex class I: recognizing receptors are disease risk genes in rheumatoid arthritis. J. Exp. Med. **193:** 1159–1167.
12. SNYDER, M.R., L.O. MUEGGE, C. OFFORD, *et al.* 2002. Formation of the killer Ig-like receptor repertoire on CD4+CD28null T cells. J. Immunol. **168:** 3839–3846.
13. BELL, E.B., S.M. SPARSHOTT, M.T. DRAYSON & W.L. FORD. 1987. The stable and permanent expansion of functional T lymphocytes in athymic nude rats after a single injection of mature T cells. J. Immunol. **139:** 1379–1384.
14. GLEESON, P.A., B.H. TOH & I.R. VAN DRIEL. 1996. Organ-specific autoimmunity induced by lymphopenia. Immunol. Rev. **149:** 97–125.
15. BARTHLOTT, T., G. KASSIOTIS & B. STOCKINGER. 2003. T cell regulation as a side effect of homeostasis and competition. J. Exp. Med. **197:** 451–460.
16. DOUEK, D.C., R.D. MCFARLAND, P.H. KEISER, *et al.* 1998. Changes in thymic function with age and during the treatment of HIV infection. Nature **396:** 690–695.
17. HAZENBERG, M.D., M.C. VERSCHUREN, D. HAMANN, *et al.* 2001. T cell receptor excision circles as markers for recent thymic emigrants: basic aspects, technical approach, and guidelines for interpretation. J. Mol. Med. **79:** 631–640.
18. VALLEJO, A.N., C.M. WEYAND & J.J. GORONZY. 2004. T-cell senescence: a culprit of immune abnormalities in chronic inflammation and persistent infection. Trends Mol. Med. **10:** 119–124.
19. VANDERBORGHT, A., P. GEUSENS, C. VANDEVYVER, *et al.* 2000. Skewed T-cell receptor variable gene usage in the synovium of early and chronic rheumatoid arthritis patients and persistence of clonally expanded T cells in a chronic patient. Rheumatology (Oxford) **39:** 1189–1201.
20. FIRESTEIN, G.S. 2003. Evolving concepts of rheumatoid arthritis. Nature **423:** 356–361.
21. HAZENBERG, M.D., J.A. BORGHANS, R.J. DE BOER & F. MIEDEMA. 2003. Thymic output: a bad TREC record. Nat. Immunol. **4:** 97–99.
22. KOETZ, K., E. BRYL, K. SPICKSCHEN, *et al.* 2000. T cell homeostasis in patients with rheumatoid arthritis. Proc. Natl. Acad. Sci. USA **97:** 9203–9208.
23. HUG, A., M. KORPORAL, I. SCHRODER, *et al.* 2003. Thymic export function and T cell homeostasis in patients with relapsing remitting multiple sclerosis. J. Immunol. **171:** 432– 437.

24. MARKOVIC-PLESE, S., I. CORTESE, K.P. WANDINGER, *et al.* 2001. $CD4^{+}CD28$-costimulation-independent T cells in multiple sclerosis. J. Clin. Invest. **108:** 1185–1194.
25. GERLI, R., G. SCHILLACI, A. GIORDANO, *et al.* 2004. $CD4^{+}CD28^{-}$T lymphocytes contribute to early atherosclerotic damage in rheumatoid arthritis patients. Circulation. **109:** 2744 –2748.
26. PAWLIK, A., L. OSTANEK, I. BRZOSKO, *et al.* 2003. The expansion of $CD4^{+}CD28^{-}$T cells in patients with rheumatoid arthritis. Arthritis Res. Ther. **5:** R210–R213.
27. VAN LEEUWEN, E.M., E.B. REMMERSWAAL, M.T. VOSSEN, *et al.* 2004. Emergence of a CD4+CD28–granzyme B^{+}, cytomegalovirus-specific T cell subset after recovery of primary cytomegalovirus infection. J. Immunol. **173:** 1834–1841.
28. OUYANG, Q., W.M. WAGNER, W. ZHENG, *et al.* 2004. Dysfunctional CMV-specific CD8(+) T cells accumulate in the elderly. Exp. Gerontol. **39:** 607–613.
29. WEYAND, C.M., J.W. FULBRIGHT & J.J. GORONZY. 2003. Immunosenescence, autoimmunity, and rheumatoid arthritis. Exp. Gerontol. **38:** 833–841.
30. ARNETT, F.C., C. EDWORTHY, D.A. BLOCH, *et al.* 1988. The American Rheumatism Association 1987 revised criteria for the classification of rheumatoid arthritis. Arthritis Rheum. **31:** 315–324.

Association of Rheumatoid Arthritis with HLA-DR1 and HLA-DR4 in Hungary

ANIKÓ KAPITÁNY,[a] ERIKA ZILAHI,[a] SÁNDOR SZÁNTÓ,[b] GABRIELLA SZÜCS,[b] ZOLTÁN SZABÓ,[b] ANIKÓ VÉGVÁRI,[b] PÉTER RASS,[a] SÁNDOR SIPKA,[a] GYULA SZEGEDI,[c] AND ZOLTÁN SZEKANECZ[b,c]

[a]*Laboratory of Immunology,* [b]*Division of Rheumatology, Third Department of Medicine, University of Debrecen Medical Center, Debrecen, Hungary*

[c]*Research Group of Autoimmune Diseases, Hungarian Academy of Sciences, Debrecen, Hungary*

ABSTRACT: Susceptibility to and outcome for rheumatoid arthritis (RA) have been associated with particular HLA-DR alleles, but these alleles vary among ethnic groups and geographic areas. The frequency of HLA-DR1 (HLA-DRB1*0101, DRB1*0102) and HLA-DR4 (DRB1*0401, DRB1*0404) alleles is elevated among Caucasian patients with RA. We studied a northeastern Hungarian population of RA patients to determine the frequency of HLA-DR1 and HLA-DR4 phenotypes in this population and to compare it with healthy control subjects, as well as to investigate whether the presence of these alleles could be a marker for RA. We performed HLA-DRB1 genotyping (DRB1*01-DRB1*16) in 83 RA patients and 55 healthy controls using polymerase chain reaction with sequence-specific primers (PCR-SSP). In the case of HLA-DR1– or HLA-DR4–positive patients, the DR1 and DR4 subtypes were also determined. The frequency of HLA-DR4 alleles was significantly higher in RA patients than in controls (31.3 vs. 10.9%; P <.05). HLA-DR1, in particular, tended to be more frequent in patients than in controls (32.5 vs. 18.1%). Among the HLA-DR4 subtypes, DRB1*0401 and DRB1*0404 were the most common alleles found in both groups. However, no significant differences were seen in the frequency of HLA-DRB1*0401 and HLA-DRB1*0404 between RA patients and controls. In contrast, HLA-DRB1*0405 and HLA-DRB1*0408 were significantly more common in RA patients than in control subjects. Among HLA-DR1 subtypes, the DRB1*0101 allele was most commonly detected, but HLA-DRB1*0101 as well as DRB1*0102 and DRB1*0105 were similarly frequent in RA patients and controls. HLA-DR12 was more common among controls than in RA patients (18.1 vs. 0%; P <.05). Our results generally agree with the findings in other Caucasian populations. Nonetheless, we found differences in the frequency of HLA-DR1 and HLA-DR4 subtypes among Hungarian patients compared with reports from other geographic regions (e.g., Finland and Asia). Our data suggest that in northeastern Hungary, HLA-DR4 as well as its subtypes DRB1*0405 and DRB1*0408 may be involved in susceptibility to RA, but HLA-DR1 may not. In addition, the presence of HLA-DR12, at least in Hungary, may protect from this disease.

Address for correspondence: Zoltan Szekanecz, M.D., Ph.D., D.Sc., Third Department of Medicine, Rheumatology Division, University of Debrecen Medical Center, 22 Moricz Zs Street, Debrecen H-4004, Hungary. Voice: +36-52-311-087; fax: +36-52-414-489.
szekanecz@iiibel.dote.hu

**Ann. N.Y. Acad. Sci. 1051: 263–270 (2005). © 2005 New York Academy of Sciences.
doi: 10.1196/annals.1361.067**

KEYWORDS: **rheumatoid arthritis; shared epitope; HLA-DR alleles; Hungary**

INTRODUCTION

Rheumatoid arthritis (RA) is an autoimmune disease, leading to chronic synovitis and eventually bone and joint destruction. Its etiology is still unknown; however, both genetic and environmental factors play important roles in the onset of RA.[1–3] The major histocompatibility complex (MHC) is encoded in human leukocyte antigen (HLA) gene clusters on chromosome 6.[3] Among MHC class II molecules, various HLA-DR alleles have been associated with susceptibility to RA in several ethnic groups[2–20] (TABLE 1). In addition, some HLA-DRB1 alleles have been related to disease severity and outcome in RA[2,8,9] (TABLE 1).

These disease-associated HLA molecules share a common amino acid sequence in the third hypervariable region of the DRB chain, the so-called "shared epitope" (SE).[3,13] The SE is a sequence of five amino acids. Among SE variants, the QKRAA motif is found in DRB1*0401 and DRB1*0409; the QRRAA sequence has been described in DRB1*0101, DRB1*0102, DRB1*0404, DRB1*0405, DRB1*0408, DRB1*0410, DRB1*1402, and DRB1*1406 variants; and the RRRAA motif is specific for the DRB1*1001 subtype[2,3,13] (TABLE 1).

Significant ethnic and geographic differences are related to gene expression among RA patient populations. For example, in RA patients from Northern Europe, HLA-DRB1*04 is strongly associated with RA,[4,14] whereas Mediterranean RA patients carry the DRB1*01 and DRB1*10 alleles.[15] Furthermore, in North American natives, DRB1*14 is associated with susceptibility to RA.[16] One recent report on Hungarian RA patients showed a strong association of the HLA-DRB1*0404 subtype with RA.[10]

TABLE 1. HLA-DR association with rheumatoid arthritis in various ethnic groups

HLA-DRB1	Amino acid sequence (70-74 loci)	Association in ethnic groups	Susceptibility	Prognostic value
**0101*	QRRAA	Asian Indians, Caucasians, Japanese	+	–
**0102*	QRRAA	Ashkenazy Jews	+	–
**0401*	QKRAA	Caucasians, Koreans	+	+
**0404*	QRRAA	Caucasians, Southern Chinese	+	+
**0405*	QRRAA	Koreans, Japanese, Southern Chinese, Spanish	+	+
**0408*	QRRAA	Caucasians	–	+
**0410*	QRRAA	Japanese, Chinese	+	+
**1001*	RRRAA	Southern Africans, Spanish	+	–
**1402*	QRRAA	Yakima Indians (North America), Peruvians	+	–

In general, the HLA-DR4 allele is found in 75% of Caucasian RA patients as well as 30% of the healthy Caucasian population. Among the DRB1*04 alleles, DRB1*0401 and DRB1*0404 have been associated with increased susceptibility to RA among Caucasian patients with RA,[2,4,17] whereas the frequency of the DRB1*0405 allele is higher among Japanese[18] and Chinese[19] patients. Among HLA-DR1 subtypes, the association of the DRB1*0101 allele with RA has been reported in Ashkenazy Jews [20] and in various other Caucasians patient populations[2,4,8,10,12,14,15] (TABLE 1).

In this study, we determined the frequency of various HLA-DRB1*01 and DRB1*04 alleles in a northeastern Hungarian population of RA patients.

PATIENTS AND METHODS

Selection of Rheumatoid Arthritis Patients and Controls

Eighty-three Hungarian RA patients (70 females and 13 males, all Caucasian) were included in our study. All patients fulfilled the 1987 revised classification criteria of the American College of Rheumatology (ACR).[21] The mean age of the patients was 50 ± 15 years (range 17–82). The mean disease duration at the time of the study was 6 ± 4 years (range 0.5–22 years). Peripheral blood was drawn from each patient for DNA isolation.

Peripheral blood was also obtained from 55 healthy Caucasian controls (47 females and 8 males) with similar mean age (46 ± 13 years). These individuals were either hospital employees or visitors who were unrelated to the patients. Informed consent was obtained from each RA patient and control subject. For this study, we also obtained ethical committee approval.

Polymerase Chain Reaction with Sequence-Specific Primers

Genomic DNA was isolated from buffy coats of EDTA-anticoagulated blood using a QIAamp Blood Mini Kit (Qiagen) according to the instructions of the manufacturer.

Polymerase chain reaction (PCR)-based HLA-DRB genotyping (DRB1*01-DRB1*16) was performed with the help of sequence-specific primers (Olerup SSP, GenoVision, Oslo, Norway).[22] Then HLA-DR1– or HLA-DR4–positive samples were further analyzed for DR1 and DR4 subtypes (GenoVision). All samples were processed according to the instructions of the manufacturer using recombinant Taq DNA polymerase (Invitrogen, Carlsbad, CA). PCR amplification of DNA was performed using a PCR Express Thermal Cycler (Hybaid, Middlesex, UK). HLA genotypes were determined on the basis of the PCR product pattern obtained using 2% agarose gel electrophoresis. DNA bands were detected using an Alpha Imager Multi-Image Light Cabinet (Alpha Innotech, San Leandro, CA).

Statistical Analysis

HLA-DR allele frequencies in patients with RA were compared with those obtained from healthy subjects. Frequency comparisons for different antigens were performed by chi-square analysis with Yartes' correlation or by Fischer's exact test

TABLE 2. Distribution of various HLA-DR alleles among RA patients and controls

HLA-DR	RA n (%) (n = 83)	Control n (%) (n = 55)	Significance
DR1	27 (32.5)	10 (18.1)	NS (P = 0.06)
DR3	(18.1)	14 (25.4)	NS
DR4	26 (31.3)	6 (10.9)	S (P <.05)
DR7	17 (20.5)	12 (21.8)	NS
DR8	4 (4.8)	2 (3.6)	NS
DR9	3 (3.6)	2 (3.6)	NS
DR10	3 (3.6)	2 (3.6)	NS
DR11	23 (27.7)	19 (34.5)	NS
DR12	0 (0)	10 (18.1)	S (P <.05)
DR13	13 (15.7)	9 (16.4)	NS
DR14	3 (3.6)	3 (5.4)	NS
DR15	11 (13.2)	8 (14.5)	NS
DR16	8 (9.6)	9 (16.4)	NS

ABBREVIATIONS: *n*, number of subjects; S , significant; NS, nonsignificant.

using SPSS 11.0.0 statistical software. Differences between any two data groups were considered significant if the P value was less than 0.05.

RESULTS

Distribution of HLA-DRB1 Alleles

The distribution of HLA-DR antigens in our population is shown in TABLE 2. HLA-DR1 (HLA-DRB1*01) alleles were detected in 32.5% of RA patients compared with 18.1% of controls. However, this difference was not statistically significant ($P = 0.06$). HLA-DR4 (HLA-DRB1*04) alleles were expressed in significantly more RA patients (31.3%) than controls (10.9%) (P <.05). The frequency of HLA-DR12 (HLA-DRB1*12) was significantly lower among RA patients than controls (0 vs 18.1%, respectively) (P <.05). No differences were found between RA patients and controls with regard to HLA-DR3, DR7-11, and DR13-16 allele frequencies (TABLE 2).

Distribution of HLA-DR1 Subtypes

We also performed HLA-DR1 (HLA-DRB1*01) subtyping in HLA-DR1-positive RA patients ($n = 27$) and controls ($n = 10$). Results are shown in TABLE 3. Among RA patients, 92.6% expressed the DRB1*0101 allele, 3.7% expressed the DRB1*0102, and 3.7% the DRB1*0105. The distribution of these DRB1*01 subtypes was statistically equivalent in the control group (90%, 10%, and 0%, respectively).

TABLE 3. Distribution of HLA-DR1 subtypes among RA patients and controls

HLA-DR1 subtype	RA *n* (%) (*n* = 27)	Control *n* (%) (*n* = 10)	Significance
*DRB1*0101*	25 (92.6)	9 (90.0)	NS
*DRB1*0102*	1 (3.7)	1 (10.0)	NS
*DRB1*0105*	1 (3.7)	0 (0)	NS

ABBREVIATIONS: *n*, number of subjects; S, significant; NS, nonsignificant.

TABLE 4. Distribution of HLA-DR4 subtypes among RA patients and controls

HLA-DR4 subtype	RA n (%) (*n* = 26)	Control n (%) (*n* = 6)	Significance
*DRB1*0401*	16 (61.5)	4 (66.7)	NS
*DRB1*0402*	0 (0)	1 (16.7)	NS
*DRB1*0404*	5 (19.2)	1 (16.7)	NS
*DRB1*0405*	3 (11.5)	0 (0)	S (P <.05)
*DRB1*0406*	1 (3.8)	0 (0)	NS
*DRB1*0407*	1 (3.8)	0 (0)	NS
*DRB1*0408*	2 (7.7)	0 (0)	S (P <.05)

ABBREVIATIONS: *n*, number of subjects; S, significant; NS, nonsignificant.

Distribution of HLA-DR4 Subtypes

HLA-DR4 (HLA-DRB1*04) subtyping was performed in HLA-DR4–positive RA patients (n = 26) and controls (n = 6). Results are shown in TABLE 4. HLA-DRB1*0401 was the most frequently expressed allele in both RA patients (61%) and controls (66%). Interestingly, the DRB1*0404 subtype, which has been described as important among Caucasians, was similarly common among RA patients (19.2%) and controls (16.7%). No statistically significant differences were found between patients and controls with regard to DRB1*0401 and DRB1*0404 expression. In contrast, small but significant differences were seen among RA patients and controls regarding DRB1*0405 (11.5 versus 0%) and DRB1*0408 subtypes (7.7 versus 0%) (P <.05). Among other allele subtypes, DRB1*0402, DRB1*0406, and DRB1*0407 were each detected only in a single subject (TABLE 4).

Among HLA-DR4–positive RA patients, three were DRB1*0401 homozygotes, two were DRB1*0401/*0404 heterozygotes, and one was a DRB1*0401/*0407 heterozygote. Twenty patients carried only one copy of DRB1*04 alleles (data not shown).

DISCUSSION

The association between certain HLA-DR alleles and RA has been well established in many ethnic groups[2–20] (TABLE 1). HLA-DRB1 genes have also been associated with disease severity and outcome[2,8,9] (TABLE 1). It has been suggested that susceptibility to RA may be related to specific epitopes in the third hypervariable region of the first domain of the DRB1 chain, termed the *shared epitope*.[3,13] These specific sequences span amino acid residues 70 through 74; the most relevant sequences are QKRAA, QRRAA, and RRRAA. These motifs have been found in susceptible HLA-DR1 and HLA-DR4 subtypes, including HLA-DRB1*0101, DRB1*0401, DRB1*0404, DRB1*0405, as well as HLA-DRB1*1001 and DRB1*1402[3,13] (TABLE 1). Among Caucasians, HLA-DR1 (the HLA-DRB1*0101 allele) and HLA-DR4 (the HLA-DRB1*0401, DRB1*0404, and DRB1*0408 alleles) have been implicated primarily in susceptibility to and severity of disease in RA[2,3] (TABLE 1). Only one published report on Hungarian RA patients has reported the strongest association in RA to be the HLA-DRB1*0404 allele.[10]

In this study, we assessed HLA-DRB1 genotype frequencies in a northeastern Hungarian population of RA patients and compared these frequencies with those of healthy controls. HLA-DR4 was significantly more common in RA patients. In addition, HLA-DR1 showed a tendency to be more frequent in RA than in healthy controls. Great geographic differences pertain to this issue. Similar to our results, HLA-DR4 has been strongly associated with RA in Northern Europe, the United States, Germany, and Argentina.[4,6,8,9,14] In a single recent Hungarian study, HLA-DR4 as well as HLA-DR1 was associated with RA,[10] supporting our current findings. However, Mediterranean RA patients tend to carry HLA-DR1, as well as HLA-DR10, rather than HLA-DR4, [15] and Native North American Indians tend to carry HLA-DR14.[16] Thus, with regard to the association of HLA-DRB1 with RA, our Hungarian RA patient population seems to more closely resemble northern and western, rather than southern, European RA patients.

We also found diminished frequency of the HLA-DR12 allele among our RA patients compared with controls. A study from Finland similarly suggests that HLA-DR12 plays a protective role in RA.[4]

Regarding HLA-DR1 (HLA-DRB1*01) subtypes, DRB1*0101, DRB1*0102, and DRB1*0105 were the most frequent alleles expressed by our RA patients and controls. However, all three alleles were equally common in patients and healthy subjects. In addition to our results showing a slight increase in HLA-DR1 frequency among RA patients compared with controls, our data suggest that in northeastern Hungary, HLA-DR1 and its subtypes may not play an important role in RA. In contrast to our results, the role of HLA-DR1 in the pathogenesis of RA was addressed in Ashkenazy Jews[20] as well as in various other Caucasian populations.[2,4,6,8,12,14,15] Note, however, that the authors of the only related published Hungarian study did not perform HLA-DR1 subtyping.[10]

Among HLA-DR4 subtypes, DRB1*0401 and DRB1*0404 were the most common among our RA patients and controls. However, we did not find any differences among HLA-DR4 subtypes between the two subject groups. In other Caucasian populations, the DRB1*0401 and DRB1*0404 alleles have been associated with increased susceptibility to RA.[2,17]

In contrast, DRB1*0405 and DRB1*0408 were much less common, but the frequencies of these alleles were significantly higher in RA patients than in controls. The frequency of the DRB1*0405 allele is reportedly higher in Asian populations, such as Koreans,[5,13] Japanese,[18] and Chinese.[19] Also, HLA-DRB1*0408 has been associated with increased susceptibility to RA in Finland. [4] Thus, our results support a role for DRB1*0405 and DRB1*0408 in the pathogenesis of RA among northeastern Hungarian patients. In addition, with regard to HLA-DR4 allele subtypes, our Hungarian subpopulation may reflect genetic patterns found in Finland and Asia.

ACKNOWLEDGMENTS

This work was supported by Grants 60/2000 and 60/2001 from the Hungarian Medical Research Council (ETT) (Z.S.) and Grant 18/2000 from the Research and Development Fund for Highest Education (FKFP) (Z.S.).

REFERENCES

1. Harris, E.D., Jr. 1990. Rheumatoid arthritis: pathophysiology and implications for therapy. N. Engl. J. Med. **332:** 1277–1287.
2. Weyand, C.M., K.C. Hicok, D.L. Conn & J.J. Goronzy. 1992. The influence of HLA-DRB1 genes on disease severity in rheumatoid arthritis. Ann. Intern. Med. **117:** 801–806.
3. Gregersen, P.K., J. Silver & R.J. Winchester. 1987. The shared epitope hypothesis: an approach to understanding the molecular genetics of susceptibility to rheumatoid arthritis. Arthritis Rheum. **30:** 1205 –1213.
4. Laivoranta-Nyman, S., T. Mottonen, R. Hermann, *et al.* 2004. HLA-DR-DQ haplotypes and genotypes in Finnish patients with rheumatoid arthritis. Ann. Rheum. Dis. **63:** 1406–1412.
5. Lee, H.S., K.W. Lee , G.G. Song, *et al.* 2004. Increased susceptibility to rheumatoid arthritis in Koreans heterozygous for HLA-DRB1*0405 and *0901. Arthritis Rheum. **50:** 3468–3475.
6. Gorman, J.D., E. David-Vaudey, M. Pai, *et al.* 2004. Particular HLA-DRB1 shared epitope genotypes are strongly associated with rheumatoid arthritis. Arthritis Rheum. **50:** 3476–3484.
7. Agrawal, S., A. Agrawal, S. Dabadghao, *et al.* 1995. Compound heterozygosity of HLA-DR4 and DR1 antigens in Asian Indians increases the risk of extra-articular features in rheumatoid arthritis. Br. J. Rheumatol. **34:** 41 –44.
8. Seidl, C., U. Koch, T. Buhleier, *et al.* 1997. HLA-DRB1*04 subtypes are associated with increased inflammatory activity in early rheumatoid arthritis. Br. J. Rheumatol. **36:** 941–944.
9. Citera, G., L.A. Padulo, G. Fernandez, *et al.* 2001. Influence of HLA-DR alleles on rheumatoid arthritis: susceptibility and severity in Argentine patients. J. Rheumatol. **28:** 1486–1491 .
10. Varga, É., É. Palkonyai, P. Temesvári, *et al.* 2003. The role of HLA-DRB1*04 alleles and their association with HLA-DQB genes in genetic susceptibility to rheumatoid arthritis in Hungarian patients. Acta Microbiol. Immunol. Hung. **50:** 33–41.
11. Hameed, K., S. Bowman , E. Kondeatis , *et al.* 1997. The association of HLA-DRB genes and the shared epitope with rheumatoid arthritis in Pakistan. Br. J. Rheumatol. **36:** 1184–1188.
12. Van Jaarsveld, C.H.M., H.G. Otten, J.W.G. Jacobs, *et al.* 1998. Association of HLA-DR with susceptibility to and clinical expression of rheumatoid arthritis: re-evaluation by means of genomic tissue typing. Br. J. Rheumatol. **37:** 411–416 .
13. Hong, G.H., M.H. Park, F. Takeuchi, *et al.* 1996. Association of specific amino acid sequence of HLA-DR with rheumatoid arthritis in Koreans and its diagnostic value. J. Rheumatol. **23:** 1699–1703.
14. Stastny, P. 1978. Association of the B-cell alloantigen DRw4 with rheumatoid arthritis. N. Engl. J. Med. **298:** 869–871.
15. Boki, K.A., G.S. Panayi, R.W. Vaughan, *et al.* 1992. HLA class II sequence polymorphisms and susceptibility to rheumatoid arthritis in Greeks. The HLA-DR shared-epitope hypothesis accounts for the disease in only a minority of Greek patients. Arthritis Rheum. **35:** 749–755.

16. WILLKENS, R.F., G.T. NEPOM, C.R. MARKS, *et al.* 1991. Association of HLA-Dw16 with rheumatoid arthritis in Yakima Indians. Further evidence for the "shared epitope" hypothesis. Arthritis Rheum. **34:** 43–47.
17. WORDSWORTH, B.P., J.S. LANCHBURY, L.I. SAKKAS, *et al.* 1989. HLA-DR4 subtype frequencies in rheumatoid arthritis indicate that DRB1 is the major susceptibility locus within the HLA class II region. Proc. Natl. Acad. Sci. USA **86:** 10049–10053.
18. 18. WATANABE, Y., K. TOKUNAGA, K. MATSUKI, *et al.* 1989. Putative amino acid sequence of HLA-DRB chain contributing to rheumatoid arthritis susceptibility. J. Exp. Med. **169:** 2263–2268.
19. MOLKENTIN, J., P.K. GREGERSEN, X. LIN, *et al.* 1993. Molecular analysis of HLA-DR beta and DQ beta polymorphism in Chinese with rheumatoid arthritis. Ann. Rheum. Dis. **52:** 610–612.
20. DE VRIES, N., K.S. RONNINGEN, M.G. TILANUS, *et al.* 1993. HLA-DR1 and rheumatoid arthritis in Israeli Jews: sequencing reveals that DRB1*0102 is the predominant HLA-DR1 subtype. Tissue Antigens **41:** 26–30.
21. ARNETT, F.C., S.M. EDWORTHY, D.A. BLOCH, *et al.* 1988. The American Rheumatism Association 1987 revised criteria for the classification of rheumatoid arthritis. Arthritis Rheum. **31:** 315–324.
22. OLERUP, O. & H. ZETTERQUIST. 1992. HLA typing by PCR amplification with sequence-specific primers (PCR-SSP) in 2 hours: an alternative to serological DR typing in clinical practice including donor-recipient matching in cadaveric transplantation. Tissue Antigens **39:** 225–235.

Plasminogen Activator Inhibitor-1 Is Associated with Impaired Endothelial Function in Women with Systemic Lupus Erythematosus

EMILY C. SOMERS,[a,b] WENDY MARDER,[a] MARIANA J. KAPLAN,[a] ROBERT D. BROOK,[c] AND W. JOSEPH McCUNE[a]

[a]*University of Michigan,* [a]*Division of Rheumatology,* [c]*Division of Cardiology, Ann Arbor, Michigan 48109, USA*

[b]*London School of Hygiene & Tropical Medicine, Infectious Disease Epidemiology Unit, London WC1E 7HT, UK*

ABSTRACT: Endothelial function, measured noninvasively by brachial artery flow-mediated dilatation (FMD), has been shown to be impaired in patients with systemic lupus erythematosus (SLE). We hypothesized that depressed FMD in SLE patients is associated with increased levels of plasminogen activator inhibitor-1 (PAI-1), an inhibitor of fibrinolysis and regulator of vasoactivity. In this cross-sectional study of female SLE patients under the age of 55, putative markers of cardiovascular disease (CVD) such as PAI-1 were measured in addition to lupus-related disease activity (SLEDAI). The primary outcome, FMD, was measured using high-resolution ultrasound of the brachial artery gated to the R wave to determine endothelial-dependent vasomotion. Endothelial-independent vasomotion was measured in response to nitroglycerin (NMD). Seventy-six female SLE patients, mean age 38.3 ± 9.4 years, were included. All patients demonstrated normal NMD responses, indicating that depression of FMD was related to decreased endothelial nitric oxide production. Increased PAI-1 was related to depressed FMD by univariate regression ($P = 0.004$). In a multivariable regression model adjusting for t-PA (tissue plasminogen activator)/PAI-1 ratio, SLEDAI, age at visit, family history of cardiovascular disease, SLE disease duration and body mass index, every 1 ng/mL increase in PAI-1 was associated with a reduction of 0.07 units FMD ($P = 0.039$). PAI-1 was associated with impaired endothelial dysfunction, after controlling for several potential confounders. Given the high incidence of cardiovascular disease in SLE, further investigation of the role of subclinical markers of CVD is needed.

KEYWORDS: systemic lupus erythematosus (SLE); plasminogen activator inhibitor-1 (PAI-1); endothelium; flow-mediated dilatation

Address for correspondence: Emily C. Somers, University of Michigan Health System, Division of Rheumatology, 1150 W. Medical Center Dr., 5520 MSRB 1, Ann Arbor, MI 48109-0680. Voice: 734-936-1166; fax: 734-763-4151.
emsomers@umich.edu

**Ann. N.Y. Acad. Sci. 1051: 271–280 (2005). © 2005 New York Academy of Sciences.
doi: 10.1196/annals.1361.068**

BACKGROUND

Morbidity and mortality due to cardiovascular disease (CVD) was recognized in systemic lupus erythematosus (SLE) patients as early as 1939, when Soma Weiss wrote "In this disease myocardial failure of varying degrees is rather common ... the skin manifestations may be slight, preterminal, or even completely absent and the heart failure dominates the picture.... Histologic examination may reveal either no changes or interstitial edema, scarring, and at times thrombosis of the coronary arterioles."[1] More recently, a bimodal mortality pattern has been recognized in the SLE population, whereby a substantial number of late SLE deaths are related to CVD, in contrast to early deaths which are ascribed to active lupus and concomitant infections.[2] Estimates of the increased risk for development of CVD in lupus patients range from an overall 8- to 9-fold increase, to a 50-fold increase in young women.[3] Vascular insults characteristic of SLE are likely to underlie part of the excess risk of CVD in this population.

The plasminogen activation (PA) system constitutes a critical response mechanism to vascular injury. The central reaction of this system is the conversion of plasminogen to plasmin by tissue-type (t-PA) and urinary-type (u-PA) plasminogen activators. Plasminogen activator inhibitor 1 (PAI-1), a member of the serpin superfamily of protease inhibitors, plays a key role in regulating the PA system by serving as the primary inhibitor of t-PA and u-PA. PAI-1 also directly inhibits plasmin and appears to play a major role in determining the proliferative response to vascular injury by inhibiting the degradation of fibrin and several extracellular matrix proteins by plasmin. PAI-1 may also modulate vascular disease progression by plasmin-independent mechanisms.[4]

As reviewed by Lyon and Hsueh, clinical studies have reported that circulating PAI-1 levels are correlated with cardiovascular events, including those occurring among specific populations such as diabetes patients.[5] An epidemiologic study based in Sweden demonstrated that increased PAI-1 concentrations increased risk of future incident myocardial infarctions.[6] These relationships need to be confirmed in the lupus population. However, defects in the fibrinolytic system, such as decreased tissue-type plasminogen activator (t-PA) activity and elevated levels of PAI-1 in patients with SLE have been associated with an increased tendency to thrombosis.[7,8] In addition, autoantibodies to recombinant PAI-1 have been described in SLE and correlate with clinical parameters measured by the BILAG disease activity index including global clinical score. Further, autoantibodies to fibrin-bound t-PA have been proposed to play a role in the pathogenesis of vascular disease in some SLE patients.[9–11]

This study was undertaken to characterize endothelial function in SLE patients, and to examine whether PAI-1 is associated with impaired flow-mediated dilatation, a measure of endothelial dysfunction, in young to middle-aged women with SLE.

PATIENTS AND METHODS

Study Population

A cross-sectional study of women with SLE was performed to examine markers of cardiovascular disease. Patients were recruited from the Michigan Lupus Cohort and University of Michigan outpatient rheumatology clinics. SLE patients fulfilling at least four American College of Rheumatology criteria for SLE,[12,13] and aged less than 55 years, were invited to participate in the cardiovascular assessment. Patients were excluded if they were current smokers (within the previous 6 months), had a personal history of cardiovascular disease, thrombosis, or diabetes, were pregnant, or had a current infection. Acute infections may perturb endothelial function, and have been shown to be associated with a transient increase in risk of vascular events.[14] Patients taking more than one antihypertensive medication in addition to a diuretic were also excluded as a safety precaution, since study participants were asked to postpone all medications on the morning of the study until after the cardiovascular assessments were performed. This research was approved by the University of Michigan Institutional Review Board, and all study participants signed written, informed consent forms.

Study Procedures

Study visits were performed at the University of Michigan General Clinical Research Center, in a temperature- and light-controlled room. To control for circadian variations, all visits were performed during morning hours. Patients were asked to fast, refrain from physical activity, and postpone any medications the morning of the visit until all functional assessments had been performed. Patients underwent vascular function measurements prior to venipuncture for the procurement of blood samples.

Data collection: Patients had a medical history and physical examination conducted by a rheumatologist, which included assessment of SLE activity as measured by the Systemic Lupus Erythematosus Disease Activity Index (SLEDAI).[15] The Systemic Lupus International Collaborating Clinics/American College of Rheumatology (SLICC/ACR) Damage Index was used to evaluate accumulated damage (of at least 6 months' duration) owing to previous lupus activity, treatment, or intercurrent illness.[16] Height and weight were measured with stadiometers and calibrated scales. Body mass index (BMI) was calculated as weight (kg)/height squared (m^2). BMI was categorized in accordance with guidelines from the obesity task force of the National Heart, Lung and Blood Institute (NHLBI), as follows: underweight <18.5 kg/m^2, normal 18.5–24.9 kg/m^2, overweight 25–29.9 kg/m^2, obese I 30–34.9 kg/m^2, obese II 35–39.9 kg/m^2, obese III ≥ 40 kg/m^2.[17] Family history of cardiovascular disease was considered to be positive if a first-degree relative had experienced a cardiovascular event at age less than 55 or 65 years for male and female relatives, respectively.

Measurement of vascular function: Flow-mediated dilation (FMD) and nitroglycerin-mediated dilation (NMD) were measured noninvasively by ultrasound, with the study participant resting in the supine position. A 10-mHz linear array transducer and an HP Image Point ultrasound system (Hewlett Packard, Andover, MA) were used for image acquisition. Baseline measurements of the brachial artery diameter were taken. Subsequently, a blood pressure cuff was inflated to 50 mmHg above the participant's systolic blood pressure over the proximal portion of the right forearm for 4 minutes. FMD was determined 1 minute after release of the cuff. Brachial artery diameter was allowed to then return to baseline over a period of 15 minutes. To evaluate endothelium-independent nitric oxide responsiveness, 0.4 mg nitroglycerin was administered sublingually; brachial artery images were obtained 3 minutes later. Serial longitudinal images of the brachial artery were obtained with image acquisition gated to the R wave from the electrocardiogram (24 sequential frames). Measurements were performed by an individual who was unaware of the clinical status of the participants. Individual frames were assessed utilizing a standard program (Brachial Analyzer with DICOM, Medical Imaging Applications LLC, Iowa City, IA). Only frames in which the image clarity was sufficient to ensure an accurate measurement were included. The end point of measurement was the percentage of change in mean brachial diameter in response to reactive hyperemia (FMD) or to nitroglycerin (NMD). The reproducibility of this technique in our unit has been reported previously.[18,19]

Assays: PAI-1 plasma levels were measured by an ELISA sandwich procedure using a solid-phase monoclonal antibody and an enzyme-labeled goat second antiserum for detection (IMUBIND plasma PAI-1 ELISA, American Diagnostica, Greenwich, CT). Tissue-plasminogen activator (t-PA) was measured in plasma using a double antibody ELISA (IMUBIND t-PA ELISA, American Diagnostica, Greenwich, CT). The assay utilizes human single chain t-PA as a standard calibrated against an international standard (NIBSAC, Hertfordshire, England). Assays for fibrinolytic markers were performed at the Medical Research Laboratories (Highland Heights, KY). In previous quality-control assessments performed by members of our research team, the monthly interassay coefficients of variation were found to be 4–9% for PAI-1 and 3.8–8.7% for t-PA. Medical Research Laboratories has been certified by the National Heart Lung and Blood Institute, Centers for Disease Control Part III program.[20]

Statistical analysis: Baseline summary statistics were computed as mean ± standard deviation for continuous variables, or frequency and proportion for categorical variables. Variables were assessed for normality and log-transformed if appropriate. Pearson correlation coefficients were calculated to examine the strength and direction of associations between continuous variables. To estimate the effect of PAI-1 on vascular function, univariate linear regression was performed. Multivariable regression was performed to account for potential confounders. *P* values less than 0.05 were considered statistically significant. Data management and analysis were performed using Stata version 8 (StataCorp, College Station, TX).

RESULTS

Seventy-six female SLE patients participated in this research. In accordance with eligibility criteria, none of the study participants had previously experienced a cardiovascular event. Baseline characteristics of the population are presented in TABLE 1. Overall, lupus disease activity was relatively low among patients at the time of the study visit (mean SLEDAI score 3.6 ± 3.8). Although average disease duration was long (12 ± 7.2 years), accumulated damage was notably low (ACR/SLICC damage score 1.1 ± 1.8). The majority of patients (71%) had no family history of premature cardiovascular disease in a first-degree relative.

The primary outcome measure, FMD, was normally distributed with a mean of 4.0 ± 4.6 SD (range, 8.8 to 13.5%). All patients demonstrated normal NMD responses, suggesting that cases of FMD impairment were related to deficits in endothelial

TABLE 1. Baseline characteristics of the study population

	SLE Patients (n = 76)
Female	100%
Age at visit	38.3 ± 9.4
Race/ethnicity	
White	65 (86%)
Black	10 (13%)
Hispanic	1 (1%)
Body Mass Index (kg/m^2)	
Underweight (<18.5)	2 (2.6%)
Normal (18.5–24.9)	39 (51.3%)
Overweight (25–29.9)	21 (27.6%)
Obese I (30–34.9)	8 (10.5%)
Obese I (35–39.9)	2 (2.6%)
Obese III (≥40)	4 (5.3%)
Family history of CVD	
No	54 (71%)
Yes	19 (25%)
Unknown	3 (4%)
Duration of SLE (yr)	12 ± 7.2
SLICC damage score	1.1 ± 1.8
SLEDAI score	3.6 ± 3.8
FMD (%)	4.0 ± 4.6
PAI-1 (ng/mL)	20.2 ± 19
t-PA (ng/mL)	7.9 ± 9.1

NOTE: Data expressed as mean ± SD or frequency (%).

nitric oxide production rather than altered responses of arterial smooth muscle to nitric oxide. PAI-1 levels were negatively correlated with FMD ($r = -0.33$, $P = 0.004$). When PAI-1 was categorized according to quartile, mean FMD ranged from 5.3% for the lowest PAI-1 quartile to 2.7% for the highest PAI-1 quartile (FIG. 1). Increased PAI-1 was related to depressed FMD by univariate regression; for each 1 ng/mL increase in PAI-1 there was a corresponding reduction of 0.08 units FMD ($P = 0.004$). A similar association was demonstrated by multivariable regression modeling. When adjusted for age at visit, disease duration, SLEDAI score, t-PA/PAI-1 ratio, family history of cardiovascular disease, and body mass index, each increase in 1 ng/mL of PAI-1 was associated with a reduction of 0.07 units FMD ($P = 0.039$). PAI-1 was the only variable in the model that was significantly associated with FMD, and there was no evidence for interaction between variables.

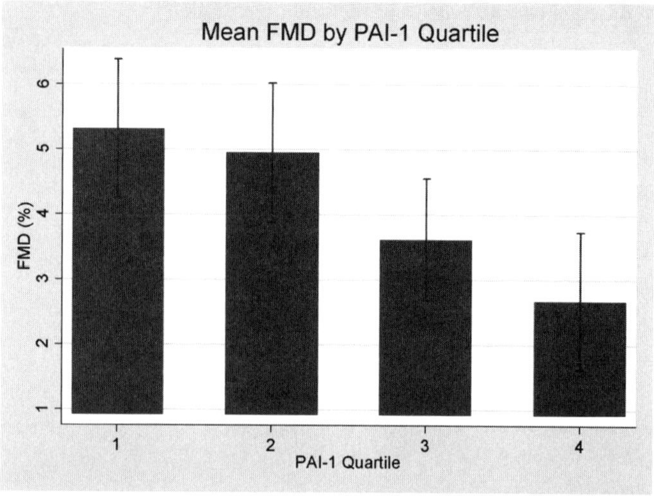

FIGURE 1. Increases in PAI-1 levels are associated with decreased flow-mediated dilatation. Bars represent mean FMD ± SEM, according to quartile of PAI-1 ($P_{trend} = 0.044$).

DISCUSSION

In this ongoing study, we found an inverse relationship between circulating PAI-1 levels and endothelial function, as measured by flow-mediated dilatation, in women under 55 years old with SLE. This relationship persisted after controlling for several potential confounders, including age, BMI, and lupus disease activity.

Relatively small reductions in brachial FMD, similar to those which we reported between the lowest and highest PAI-1 quartiles in this study, have been shown to be independently associated with worse cardiovascular prognosis.[21] Although formal cutoffs have not been established for normal versus abnormal FMD, and calibrations in various laboratories can be different, our research group considers less than 4% to represent impaired endothelial function. A full 47% of the SLE population in this study had an FMD value of less than 4%, indicating that a substantial proportion of these patients exhibit some degree of endothelial dysfunction. Within this group of patients exhibiting low FMD, further cardiovascular risk profiling may help identify pathogenic mechanisms and potential strategies to forestall development of clinically significant vascular damage.

A link between PAI-1 and endothelial dysfunction is biologically plausible. PAI-1 appears to play a crucial role in fibrin homeostasis, with diminished plasmin generation being the primary downstream mediator of PAI-1's effect.[22] PAI-1 has been hypothesized to play an important role in regulating thrombin activity in the blood vessel wall, an environment in which thrombin may stimulate VSMC proliferation.[23–26] Furthermore, PAI-1 could potentially promote interactions between vascular cells and the extracellular matrix.[22] In addition, it has been proposed that upregulation of PAI-1 expression after arterial injury favors atherosclerosis development.[22] Conversely, in mice that completely lack PAI-1, the lysis of arterial thrombi is accelerated and thrombus formation after arterial injury is delayed.[24,27,28]

A cause-and-effect relationship has not been established between vascular PAI-1 expression and the size and extent of atherosclerotic lesions. Elevated plasma PAI-1 levels are associated with complications of atherosclerosis. By affecting VSMC migration, PAI-1 could modulate the composition of plaques and their susceptibility to acute complications. Therefore, it is probable that PAI-1 promotes atherogenesis and/or its complications in humans, although there are insufficient data at this time to make definitive conclusions.[22]

PAI-1 and its regulation may have particular relevance in lupus. The PAI-1 4G/4G genotype has been proposed to influence the development of lupus nephritis. The 4G/5G polymorphism of the PAI-1 gene was reported to be associated with the activity but not the chronicity of lupus nephritis. The presence of the 4G4G genotype did not increase the risk of developing SLE or lupus nephritis, but predicted the development of higher nephritis activity and more extensive necrotizing lesions.[29] Further, the presence of the 4G allele of the 4G/5G polymorphism of the PAI-1 gene has been proposed as an additional risk factor for the development of arterial thrombosis in antiphospholipid antibody syndrome.[29,30] In addition, osteonecrosis in SLE has been reported to be significantly associated with elevated levels of PAI-1 activity and with elevated PAI-1/t-PA ratio.[31]

Glomerular PAI-1/t-PA balance is involved in extracellular matrix turnover, as well as fibrin deposition in glomeruli. PAI-1 mRNA levels are significantly increased in MRL/*lpr* and NZB/NZW animals compared with controls. PAI-1 mRNA or protein is not found in normal mouse or human kidney, but is strongly upregulated in MRL/*lpr* mouse kidneys, as well as many other experimental and human renal diseases. This and other studies have suggested that changes in the expression of these genes may promote the formation of microthrombi and thus contribute to the progression of lupus nephritis. Increased TGF-1 expression has been reported in murine and human lupus nephritis and this molecule stimulates PAI-1 synthesis. PAI-1 has been implicated in extracellular matrix accumulation in kidney by its effects to inhibit matrix degradation.[32–39]

The association between PAI-1 and depressed FMD that we have found in this study further implies a role for PAI-1 in endothelial function among lupus patients. Coupled with previous findings from our group demonstrating an association between apoptotic endothelial cells and both endothelial dysfunction and plasma tissue factor, multiple candidate risk factors for cardiovascular disease in SLE are emerging.[40] Whether abnormalities or interactions of these biomarkers are unique to SLE, and the degree to which they contribute to vascular injury and CVD risk, remain to be elucidated. It will be important within a larger series of lupus patients and controls to analyze all of these factors in concert, in order to more fully characterize the role of these markers and potential interactive effects.

The current study has several limitations. First, due to the cross-sectional design, we were not able to assess the temporality of the association between PAI-1 and FMD. Further, while the utility of FMD has been shown in other populations, we will need long-term follow-up to determine the predictive value of FMD in these lupus patients in terms of future cardiovascular events. It will also be informative to study the association of fibrinolysis and endothelial function in non-lupus controls. Due to the relatively small size of the population in this study, we were limited in terms of statistical power to perform more detailed subset analyses at this time.

We performed all study measurements during the morning hours to account for circadian variation in PAI-1 levels; plasma concentrations have been observed to be lower during the day versus night.[41] However, despite the fact that we performed vascular measurements in a controlled environment to the extent possible, for logistical reasons we were unable to time study assessments according to the menstrual cycle. This would have been preferable, as variation of PAI-1 and t-PA has been reported within the menstrual cycle, with higher values outside of days 2–7 of the menstrual cycle.[42]

Features underlying lupus pathology are hypothesized to play a key role in vascular injury. We have identified PAI-1 as a potential marker of increased risk, and future investigations should be performed to discern whether PAI-1 is directly involved in the etiology of CVD in lupus. We are continuing study enrollment, which will enable further subset analyses, and the characterization of additional biomarkers in a larger population. This may provide further elucidation of mechanisms of endothelial injury in systemic lupus, which would aid in the development of targeted interventions.

ACKNOWLEDGMENTS

This work was funded by the Arthritis Foundation, Lupus Research Institute, Herbert and Carol Amster Lupus Fund, Klein Lupus Research Fund, and the University of Michigan General Clinical Research Center (GCRC) (Grant M01-RR00042)

REFERENCES

1. WEISS, S. 1939. Diseases of the heart and the aorta which are not well recognized. Med. Clin. North Am. **5:** 1323–1344.
2. UROWITZ, M.B. & D.D. GLADMAN. 1980. Late mortality in SLE: "the price we pay for control." J. Rheumatol. **7:** 412–416.
3. MANZI, S., F. SELZER, K. SUTTON-TYRRELL, *et al.* 1999. Prevalence and risk factors of carotid plaque in women with systemic lupus erythematosus. Arthritis Rheum. **42:** 51–60.
4. FAY, W.P., D.T. EITZMAN, A.D. SHAPIRO, *et al.* 1994. Platelets inhibit fibrinolysis in vitro by both plasminogen activator inhibitor-1-dependent and -independent mechanisms. Blood **83:** 351–356.
5. LYON, C.J. & W.A. HSUEH. 2003. Effect of plasminogen activator inhibitor-1 in diabetes mellitus and cardiovascular disease. Am. J. Med. (Suppl.) **115**: 62S–68S.
6. THOGERSEN, A.M., J.H. JANSSON, K. BOMAN, *et al.* 1998. High plasminogen activator inhibitor and tissue plasminogen activator levels in plasma precede a first acute myocardial infarction in both men and women: evidence for the fibrinolytic system as an independent primary risk factor. Circulation **98:** 2241–2247.
7. GONG, R., Z. LIU, Z. CHEN, *et al.* 2002. [Genetic variations in plasminogen activator inhibitor-1 gene and beta fibrinogen gene associated with glomerular microthrombosis in lupus nephritis and the gene dosage effect]. Zhonghua Yi Xue Yi Chuan Xue Za Zhi **19:** 1–5.
8. BICK, R.L. 2000. Recurrent miscarriage syndrome due to blood coagulation protein/platelet defects: prevalence, treatment and outcome results. DRW Metroplex Recurrent Miscarriage Syndrome Cooperative Group. Clin. Appl. Thromb. Hemost. **6:** 115–125.

9. BATES, R.L., S.J. PAYNE, S.L. DRURY, *et al.* 2003. The prevalence and clinical significance of autoantibodies to plasminogen activator inhibitor 1 in systemic lupus erythematosus. Lupus **12:** 617–622.
10. SALAZAR-PARAMO, M., I. GARCIA DE LA TORRE, M.J. FRITZLER, *et al.* 1996. Antibodies to fibrin-bound tissue-type plasminogen activator in systemic lupus erythematosus are associated with Raynaud's phenomenon and thrombosis. Lupus **5:** 275–278.
11. RUIZ-ARGUELLES, A., E. ANGLES-CANO, B. PEREZ-ROMANO, *et al.* 1995. Serum antibodies to distinct epitopes of the tissue-type plasminogen activator (t-PA) in patients with systemic lupus erythematosus. Am. J. Hematol. **49:** 109–114.
12. TAN, E.M., A.S. COHEN, J.F. FRIES, *et al.* 1982. The 1982 revised criteria for the classification of systemic lupus erythematosus. Arthritis Rheum. **25:** 1271–1277.
13. HOCHBERG, M.C. 1997. Updating the American College of Rheumatology revised criteria for the classification of systemic lupus erythematosus. Arthritis Rheum. **40:** 1725.
14. SMEETH, L., S.L. THOMAS, A.J. HALL, *et al.* 2004. Risk of myocardial infarction and stroke after acute infection or vaccination. N. Engl. J. Med. **351:** 2611–2618.
15. BOMBARDIER, C., D.D. GLADMAN, M.B. UROWITZ, *et al.* 1992. Derivation of the SLEDAI. A disease activity index for lupus patients. The Committee on Prognosis Studies in SLE. Arthritis Rheum. **35**: 630–640.
16. GLADMAN, D., E. GINZLER, C. GOLDSMITH, *et al.* 1996. The development and initial validation of the Systemic Lupus International Collaborating Clinics/American College of Rheumatology damage index for systemic lupus erythematosus. Arthritis Rheum. **39:** 363–369.
17. EXPERT PANEL ON THE IDENTIFICATION, EVALUATION, AND TREATMENT OF OVERWEIGHT IN ADULTS. 1998. Clinical guidelines on the identification, evaluation, and treatment of overweight and obesity in adults: executive summary. Am. J. Clin. Nutr. **68:** 899–917.
18. RAJAGOPALAN, S., R. BROOK, R.H. MEHTA, *et al.* 2002. Effect of losartan in aging-related endothelial impairment. Am. J. Cardiol. **89:** 562–566.
19. BROOK, R.D., J.R. BROOK, B. URCH, *et al.* 2002. Inhalation of fine particulate air pollution and ozone causes acute arterial vasoconstriction in healthy adults. Circulation **105:** 1534–1536.
20. MYERS, G.L., G.R. COOPER, C.L. WINN, *et al.* 1989. The Centers for Disease Control-National Heart, Lung and Blood Institute Lipid Standardization Program: an approach to accurate and precise lipid measurements. Clin. Lab. Med. **9:** 105–135.
21. LERMAN, A. & A.M. ZEIHER. 2005. Endothelial function: cardiac events. Circulation **111:** 363–368.
22. FAY, W.P. 2004. Plasminogen activator inhibitor 1, fibrin, and the vascular response to injury. Trends Cardiovasc. Med. **14:** 196–202.
23. PENG, L., N. BHATIA, A.C. PARKER, *et al.* 2002. Endogenous vitronectin and plasminogen activator inhibitor-1 promote neointima formation in murine carotid arteries. Arterioscler. Thromb. Vasc. Biol. **22:** 934–939.
24. FARREHI, P.M., C.K. OZAKI, P. CARMELIET, *et al.* 1998. Regulation of arterial thrombolysis by plasminogen activator inhibitor-1 in mice. Circulation **97:** 1002–1008.
25. FAY, W.P., J.G. MURPHY W.G. OWEN. 1996. High concentrations of active plasminogen activator inhibitor-1 in porcine coronary artery thrombi. Arterioscler. Thromb. Vasc. Biol. **16:** 1277–1284.
26. ZHU, Y., P.M. FARREHI & W.P. FAY. 2001. Plasminogen activator inhibitor type 1 enhances neointima formation after oxidative vascular injury in atherosclerosis-prone mice. Circulation **103:** 3105–10.
27. ZHU, Y., P. CARMELIET & W.P. FAY. 1999. Plasminogen activator inhibitor-1 is a major determinant of arterial thrombolysis resistance. Circulation **99:** 3050–3055.
28. FAY, W.P., A.C. PARKER, L.R. CONDREY, *et al.* 1997. Human plasminogen activator inhibitor-1 (PAI-1) deficiency: characterization of a large kindred with a null mutation in the PAI-1 gene. Blood **90:** 204–208.
29. WANG, A.Y., P. POON, F.M. LAI, *et al.* 2001. Plasminogen activator inhibitor-1 gene polymorphism 4G/4G genotype and lupus nephritis in Chinese patients. Kidney Int. **59:** 1520–1528.

30. TASSIES, D., G. ESPINOSA, F.J. MUNOZ-RODRIGUEZ, *et al.* 2000. The 4G/5G polymorphism of the type 1 plasminogen activator inhibitor gene and thrombosis in patients with antiphospholipid syndrome. Arthritis Rheum. **43:** 2349–2358.
31. SHEIKH, J.S., G.S. RETZINGER & E.V. HESS. 1998. Association of osteonecrosis in systemic lupus erythematosus with abnormalities of fibrinolysis. Lupus **7:** 42–8.
32. BAO, L., J. ZHOU, V.M. HOLERS, *et al.* 2003. Excessive matrix accumulation in the kidneys of MRL/lpr lupus mice is dependent on complement activation. J. Am. Soc. Nephrol. **14:** 2516–2525.
33. HAMANO, K., M. IWANO, Y. AKAI, *et al.* 2002. Expression of glomerular plasminogen activator inhibitor type 1 in glomerulonephritis. Am. J. Kidney Dis. **39:** 695–705.
34. YAMAMOTO, T., N.A. NOBLE, A.H. COHEN, *et al.* 1996. Expression of transforming growth factor-beta isoforms in human glomerular diseases. Kidney Int. **49:** 461–469.
35. YAMAMOTO, K. & D.J. LOSKUTOFF. 1997. The kidneys of mice with autoimmune disease acquire a hypofibrinolytic/procoagulant state that correlates with the development of glomerulonephritis and tissue microthrombosis. Am. J. Pathol. **151:** 725–734.
36. YAMAMOTO, K. & D.J. LOSKUTOFF. 2000. Expression of transforming growth factor-beta and tumor necrosis factor-alpha in the plasma and tissues of mice with lupus nephritis. Lab. Invest. **80:** 1561–1570.
37. KEETON, M., C. AHN, Y. EGUCHI, *et al.* 1995. Expression of type 1plasminogen activator inhibitor in renal tissue in murine lupus nephritis. Kidney Int. **47:** 148-157.
38. TROYER, D.A., B. CHANDRASEKAR, T. THINNES, *et al.* 1995. Effects of energy intake on type 1 plasminogen activator inhibitor levels in glomeruli of lupus-prone B/W mice. Am. J. Pathol. **146:** 111–120.
39. MOLL, S., P.A. MENOUD, T. FULPIUS, *et al.* 1995. Induction of plasminogen activator inhibitor type 1 in murine lupus-like glomerulonephritis. Kidney Int. **48:** 1459–1468.
40. RAJAGOPALAN, S., E.C. SOMERS, R.D. BROOK, *et al.* 2004. Endothelial cell apoptosis in systemic lupus erythematosus: a common pathway for abnormal vascular function and thrombosis propensity. Blood **103:** 3677–3683.
41. ANGLETON, P., W.L. CHANDLER & G. SCHMER. 1989. Diurnal variation of tissue-type plasminogen activator and its rapid inhibitor (PAI-1). Circulation **79:** 101–106.
42. SOWERS, M., C. DERBY, M.L. JANNAUSCH, *et al.* 2003. Insulin resistance, hemostatic factors, and hormone interactions in pre- and perimenopausal women: SWAN. J. Clin. Endocrinol. Metab. **88:** 4904–4910.

Early Atherosclerosis in Rheumatoid Arthritis

Effects of Smoking on Thickness of the Carotid Artery Intima Media

ROBERTO GERLI,[a,e] YANIV SHERER,[b,e] GAETANO VAUDO,[c] GIUSEPPE SCHILLACI,[c] BORIS GILBURD,[b] ANDREA GIORDANO,[a] ELENA BARTOLONI BOCCI,[a] ROSITA ALLEGRUCCI,[a] SIMONA MARCHESI,[c] ELMO MANNARINO,[c] AND YEHUDA SHOENFELD[b,d]

[a]*Section of Internal Medicine and Oncological Sciences, Center for the Study of Rheumatic Diseases, University of Perugia, Perugia, Italy*

[b]*Department of Medicine "B" and Center of Autoimmune Diseases, Sheba Medical Center, Tel-Hashomer, and Sackler Faculty of Medicine, Tel Aviv University, Tel Aviv, Israel*

[c]*Section of Internal Medicine, Angiology and Atherosclerosis Diseases, Department of Clinical & Experimental Medicine, University of Perugia, Perugia, Italy*

ABSTRACT: This study was designed to compare intima media thickness (IMT) of the carotid arteries among rheumatoid arthritis (RA) patients and controls and to determine whether disease-associated characteristics, smoking, and other classic risk factors for atherosclerosis are associated with IMT values. IMT was measured in the carotid arteries of 101 RA patients and 75 control subjects. The IMT was evaluated in the common carotid (CC), carotid bifurcation (BI), and internal carotid (IC). Eight IMT values were calculated including four mean and four maximal values of CC, BI, IC, and carotid artery (C). The following data were obtained for every patient: age, sex, body mass index (BMI), presence of erosions, extra-articular manifestations, rheumatoid factor, medications, hypertension, hypercholesterolemia, diabetes mellitus, smoking status, daily number of cigarettes, number of smoking years, family history of cardiovascular diseases (CVD), and erythrocyte sedimentation rate (ESR) levels. RA patients had significantly higher mean-BI IMT than controls (1.02 mm vs. 0.89 mm; *P* < 0.01), higher incidence of increased mean-BI IMT and max-BI IMT, but lower incidence of increased max-IC IMT than controls. Factors significantly associated with IMT in the controls were age, BMI, and hypertension, whereas factors significantly associated with IMT in RA patients were age and smoking status. Mean carotid IMT was associated with all characteristics related to smoking in RA patients. Current smokers had higher mean carotid IMT and internal carotid artery IMT than former smokers. RA is associated with higher carotid artery bifurcation IMT. The profile of factors

Address for correspondence: Y. Shoenfeld, M.D., Department of Medicine "B," Sheba Medical Center, Tel Hashomer 52621, Israel. Voice: 972-3-530-2652; fax: 972-3-535-2855. shoenfel@post.tau.ac.il

[d]Incumbent of the Laura Schwartz Kipp Chair for Research of Autoimmune Diseases, Tel Aviv University, Tel Aviv, Israel.

[e]Both authors contributed equally to this work.

**Ann. N.Y. Acad. Sci. 1051: 281–290 (2005). © 2005 New York Academy of Sciences.
doi: 10.1196/annals.1361.069**

associated with IMT values is different between RA patients and controls. Smoking is an important factor augmenting early atherosclerosis in RA patients.

KEYWORDS: **rheumatoid arthritis; carotid artery; intima media thickness (IMT); smoking**

INTRODUCTION

Rheumatoid arthritis (RA) is an inflammatory and immune-mediated disease that is associated with excess cardiac mortality linked to premature atherosclerosis.[1–3] There is an increased body of evidence connecting the immune system, including infectious, inflammatory, and autoimmune factors, to atherosclerosis.[4] However, classic risk factors for cardiovascular diseases (CVD) might also have a role in promoting atherosclerosis and its consequences in RA patients. Ultrasound scans can detect intima-media thickness (IMT) of the carotid arteries and hence detect increased IMT and atherosclerotic plaques as early signs of carotid artery disease. Enhanced atherosclerosis as expressed by increased IMT in RA patients versus controls has been reported in several studies.[5–10] Several factors, such as dyslipidemia, inflammatory markers of RA, and disease activity, have been found in association with the thickness of the intima-media in RA patients. In this study, an investigation was carried out to search for differences in IMT of various parts of the carotid artery (common carotid, carotid bifurcation, internal carotid) between RA patients and controls. In addition, because smoking is an important risk factor for the incidence and severity of extra-articular RA,[11,12] and also for atherosclerosis and cardiovascular diseases, we aimed to determine whether smoking and other classic risk factors could augment atherosclerosis in RA patients.

METHODS

Patients

One hundred and one patients from the rheumatology outpatient clinic of the University of Perugia who fulfilled the American College of Rheumatology classification criteria for RA[13] were included in the study. All patients had a functional capacity at the I-III stages of the Steinbrocker disability index. Seventy-five age- and sex-matched subjects, seen at the same outpatient clinic and suffering from degenerative joint disease (localized at the knee, hand, and/or spine) or other non-inflammatory rheumatic disorders (non-articular and psychogenic musculoskeletal syndromes), acted as controls. Ischemic heart disease, heart failure, cerebrovascular disease, and peripheral artery disease represented exclusion criteria for both patients and controls. Clinical data and risk factors for cardiovascular diseases are presented in TABLE 1. TABLE 2 details the various medications taken by RA patients and other features of their disease including extra-articular manifestation, presence of rheumatoid factor, and bony erosions. Written informed consent was obtained from every subject included in the study.

TABLE 1. Clinical characteristics and risk factors for cardiovascular disease of 101 patients with rheumatoid arthritis and 75 control subjects

Data	Patients with RA	Control Subjects
Age (years)	63 ± 11	61 ± 14
Men	27 (27)	22 (29)
Body mass index (kg/m^2)	26 ± 4.8*	24 ± 4.9*
Hypertension	37 (37)**	17 (23)**
Hypercholesterolemia	13 (12.9)	6 (8)
Diabetes mellitus	7 (6.9)**	0 (0) **
Smoking status	33 (32.7)*	9 (7.3)*
Family history of CVD	8 (7.9)	10 (13.3)
ESR (mm/h)	27 ± 18*	14 ± 5.8*

NOTES: Data are presented as mean ± SD or as number and percentage at parentheses.

Hypertension was defined as systolic blood pressure ≥140 mm Hg, or diastolic BP ≥90 mm Hg, or antihypertensive drug treatment. Hypercholesterolemia was diagnosed if there was a serum of low-density lipoprotein concentration ≥160 mg/dL or hypolipidemic drug treatment. Diabetes mellitus was diagnosed if fasting glucose was ≥7.00 mmol/L (126 mg/dL) or there was a clinical diagnosis of diabetes with dietary, oral, or insulin treatment.

*$P < 0.01$.

**$P < 0.05$.

TABLE 2. Manifestations of disease, treatment, and clinical variables in 101 patients with rheumatoid arthritis

Manifestations of RA and Drug Therapy	Number of Patients (% or mean ± SD)
Disease duration (years)	11 ± 9
Rheumatoid factor +	56 (55)
Bony erosions	46 (45.5)
Extra-articular manifestations	3 (3)
Methotrexate	55 (54)
NSAIDs	50 (49.5)
Prednisone	46 (45.5)
Hydroxychloroquine	27 (26.7)
Cyclosporin A	10 (9.9)
Salazopirine	9 (8.9)
Leflunomide	7 (6.9)
Anti-TNFα	3 (3)
Azathioprine	3 (3)

Carotid Intima Media Thickness (IMT) Measurement

Carotid artery IMT was evaluated by a commercially available ultrasound device (HDI 3500, Advanced Technology Laboratories, USA) equipped with a linear multifrequency 5–12-MHz transducer.[14] Subjects were examined in the supine position, and all measurements were obtained at end-diastole by electrocardiographic triggering. The ultrasound images were stored on S-VHS videotape and analyzed using an image processing workstation (Kontron KS-200, Munich, Germany). On a longitudinal two-dimensional ultrasound image of the carotid artery, the near and far arterial walls are displayed as two bright white lines separated by a hypoechogenic space. The distance between the leading edge of the first bright line on the far wall (lumen–intima interface) and the leading edge of the second bright line (media–adventitia interface) indicated the IMT of the far wall. For the near wall, IMT was calculated as the distance between the trailing edge of the first bright line and the trailing edge of the second bright line. Distances were read by two observers who were unaware of patients' clinical data. The mean and maximal values of the following arterial segments were examined in each patient: the common carotid artery immediately caudal to the bulb (CC-mean, CC-max), carotid bifurcation (BI-mean, BI-max), and the proximal segment of the internal carotid artery (IC-mean, IC-max). The mean values were defined as the average of 12 IMT readings from three sampling points per segment on both the right and left sides of the far and near walls. The maximal value was the highest IMT reading from each site (CC, BI, and IC). In addition, mean carotid IMT (C-mean) and maximal carotid IMT (C-max) were calculated as the mean value of the three sites' mean and maximal values, respectively. Thickened intima-media was defined as IMT > 0.9 mm, and the presence of atherosclerotic plaque was defined as IMT >1.3 mm. The intra-observer coefficient of variation was 3.9%, while inter-observer values were 5.6%.

Statistical Analysis

Continuous variables were presented as mean ± standard deviation. Comparison between groups was carried out using *t*-tests and ANOVA tests. Comparison between groups of non-continuous variables was done using Chi-square tests. Pearson correlations were done between continuous variables. Significant differences were considered at $P < 0.05$ for two-tailed tests.

RESULTS

IMT in RA Patients versus Control Subjects

In a comparison of eight measurements of carotid IMT (CC-mean, BI-mean, IC-mean, C-mean, CC-max, BI-max, IC-max, C-max) there were no significant differences in the distribution of the 101 RA patients and 76 control subjects around most normal IMT, increased IMT, and atherosclerotic plaque levels. In addition, no significant differences were found in most average values between RA patients and controls, except for the average level of BI-mean IMT, which was significantly greater in RA patients (TABLE 3). Control patients included 44 (58.7%) with normal

TABLE 3. IMT values (mm; mean ± SD) in the carotid arteries in patients with rheumatoid arthritis and control subjects

IMT	RA Patients (N = 101)	Control Subjects (N = 75)
Common carotid–mean	0.85 ± 0.22	0.85 ± 0.26
Common carotid–maximal	0.93 ± 0.60	0.95 ± 0.26
Carotid bifurcation–mean	1.02 ± 0.24*	0.89 ± 0.26*
Carotid bifurcation–maximal	1.03 ± 0.23	0.99 ± 0.27
Internal carotid–mean	0.77 ± 0.20	0.82 ± 0.26
Internal carotid–maximal	0.81 ± 0.48	0.92 ± 0.26
Carotid artery–mean [a]	0.88 ± 0.18	0.86 ± 0.25
Carotid artery–maximal [b]	0.92 ± 0.31	0.95 ± 0.25

*P < 0.01.
[a]The values of carotid artery–mean are the average of CC-mean, BI-mean, and IC-mean.
[b]The values of carotid artery–maximal are the average of CC-max, BI-max, and IC-max.

BI-mean IMT, 28 (37.3%) with increased BI-mean IMT, and 3 (4.0%) with atherosclerotic plaque. The figures in RA patients were 34 (33.7%), 59 (58.4%), and 8 (7.9%), respectively (P < 0.01). Hence, most RA patients (62.3%) had increased BI-mean IMT, as compared with only 41.3% of control subjects.

Similar results were found regarding the maximal value of IMT at the bifurcation. Whereas 54.7% of control patients had normal BI-max IMT, only 31.7% of RA patients did not have thickened BI-max IMT or atherosclerotic plaque (P < 0.01). These figures were opposite to those found in the internal carotid maximal IMT measurements (IC-max), though not IC-mean. Among control subjects, 62.7% had normal IC-max IMT, in contrast to 83.2% among RA patients (P < 0.01). The former were also four times more likely to have atherosclerotic plaque according to IC-max IMT measurements when compared with RA patients (12% versus 3%).

Factors Associated with IMT among RA Patients and Controls

The associations between IMT values and the risk factors for cardiovascular diseases and other characteristics in TABLE 1 were studied in RA patients, controls, and the combined population of 176 subjects. In the entire population and control subjects, age was found in association with all eight IMT measurements. In RA patients, age was associated with six different IMT measurements, including all four mean IMT values. Whereas body mass index (BMI) was strongly associated with IMT values in the controls (it was associated with all eight IMT measurements), BMI was associated only with IC-max in RA patients (P = 0.03), and hence only with three IMT measurements in the entire population, not including C-mean IMT. With respect to IMT differences between males and females, even though a trend towards higher IMT values in males compared with females was noted in all comparisons, none reached a statistical significance in controls. In the entire population, only IC-max IMT levels were higher in males (P = 0.04), but among RA patients, males had higher IC-mean IMT, IC-max IMT, and C-mean IMT (C-mean IMT was 0.95 mm for males and 0.86 mm for females; $P = 0.02$).

Erythrocyte sedimentation rate (ESR) was not associated with IMT in RA patients or in the whole population. In the control subjects, an association was found only with IC-mean IMT ($P = 0.03$). No association between the presence of hypercholesterolemia and IMT could be demonstrated in any group, as was the case regarding diabetes and family history of CVD (except for increased IC-max IMT values in RA patients with family history of CVD). The various factors associated with RA, including disease duration, extra-articular manifestations, presence of rheumatoid factor, bony erosions, and the various medications taken by patients, were not associated with IMT.

Hypertension and Increased IMT in Normal Subjects

Hypertension was strongly associated with increased carotid IMT in the control subjects; indeed, the patients with hypertension had increased IMT values for all eight measurements. Similarly, seven of the eight IMT measurements (CC-max was the exception) were also increased in the whole population of 176 subjects. However, the contribution of hypertension to increased IMT in the whole population was mainly caused by the control subjects. Among hypertensive RA patients, only BI-mean IMT and BI-max IMT values were increased, while no significant differences were found in the other six IMT measurements (FIGURE 1).

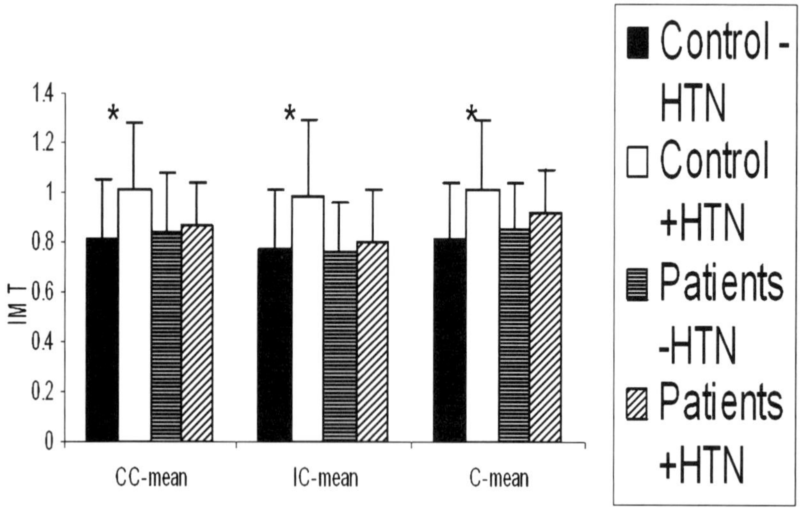

FIGURE 1. Comparison of mean values of IMT in the common carotid (CC), internal carotid (IC), and the carotid artery (C) between subjects with and without hypertension. Higher IMT among hypertensive patients was found only in controls ($P < 0.05$).

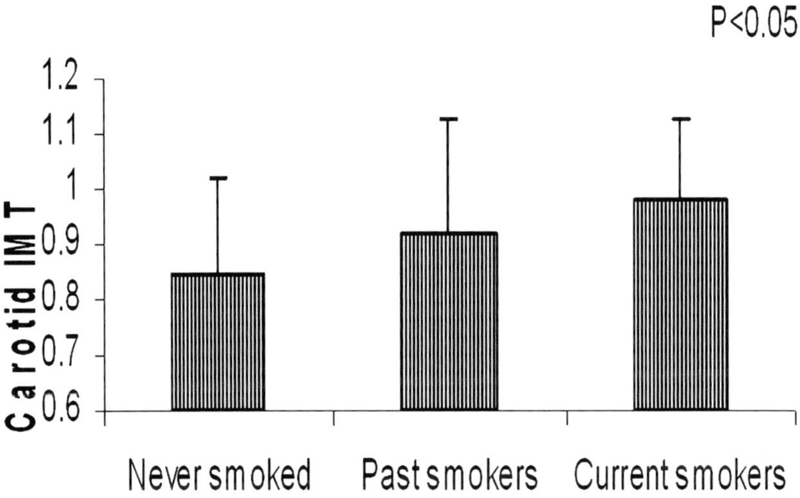

FIGURE 2. Mean value and standard deviation of carotid IMT in RA patients according to smoking status. Current smokers have higher IMT levels than former smokers. Former smokers have higher levels than those who never smoked.

Smoking and Increased IMT in RA Patients

Smoking was associated with increases in some IMT measurements in the whole population. Positive smoking status was associated with increases in three IMT measurements: number of smoking years was associated with increases in five measurements; number of daily cigarettes was associated with increases in three measurements; and "cigarette years" (the product of number of smoking years and number of daily cigarettes) were also associated with increases in three measurements. However, the association of smoking with carotid artery IMT was confined only to RA patients. None of the above variables related to smoking was found in association with any of the eight IMT measurements among controls. Among RA patients, smoking status, number of smoking years, number of daily cigarettes and "cigarette years" were all associated with increased C-mean IMT ($P < 0.05$ in all cases). In these patients, smoking was associated with increases in three IMT measurements, smoking years was associated with increases in five measurements, and "cigarette years" was associated with increases in four measurements. Moreover, in a comparison among RA patients of C-mean IMT levels between the 12 current smokers and the 21 former smokers, the current smokers had higher IMT levels than the former smokers, and both had higher IMT levels than non-smokers (FIGURE 2). Similar significant differences were also noted regarding IC-mean IMT.

DISCUSSION

IMT measured in the carotid arteries of both RA patients and normal subjects in this study was highest in the carotid bifurcation, lower in the common carotid artery, and lowest in the internal carotid artery. Differences between groups were found in the carotid bifurcation IMT measurements, where RA patients had higher mean levels, as well as a higher prevalence of increased IMT and atherosclerotic plaque. It is possible that enhanced atherosclerosis in RA is expressed only in the bifurcation, since both groups have the highest IMT values in that portion of the carotid artery. Age was strongly associated with IMT values both in patients and controls, whereas BMI was associated with IMT mainly among control subjects. This latter finding could be due to the significantly higher BMI of RA patients compared with controls. No positive correlation was found between IMT levels and the various medications consumed by patients, or other factors related to RA.

Among cardiovascular risk factors, hypertension was associated with higher IMT levels for all eight values measured in the controls. The contributing effect of hypertension to enhanced IMT has been described in several studies. Compared with normotensive subjects, the odds ratio of hypertensive patients developing carotid atherosclerosis has been reported to be 5.0 (range 3.0–8.4).[15] Among 1,781 asymptomatic subjects, age, systolic blood pressure, and fasting blood sugar levels were independent risk factors for thickened intima media and carotid atherosclerosis.[16] Chironi *et al.* also report that IMT was increased in hypertensive compared with normotensive subjects.[17] Hypertension had a smaller effect in RA patients, as it was associated only with higher IMT in the bifurcation area, possibly because of the high turbulence occurring in this region. According to the literature, IMT values among RA patients are associated with lipid levels, disease activity, disease duration, and inflammatory markers such as ESR and C-reactive protein (CRP).[6–8,10]

In the present cohort of 101 RA patients, smokers had higher mean carotid IMT than non-smokers. The effects of smoking are even more evident when it is noted that current smokers had higher mean carotid IMT levels than former smokers. Smoking has also been reported in several studies as a risk factor for carotid atherosclerosis and thickened intima-media.[18–20] Such an association was not found among controls, possibly because of the lower prevalence of smokers among them. This finding may also reflect a stronger contribution of smoking to early atherosclerosis in RA than outside the RA setting. Smoking is associated with increased susceptibility to some autoimmune diseases.[21] Accordingly, smoking was found by several studies as a risk factor for RA development and RA severity; occasionally, the duration and intensity of smoking were also associated with RA.[11,22–24] Smoking was also an independent risk factor for extra-articular RA.[12] As accelerated atherosclerosis has also been suggested as an extra-articular manifestation of RA,[3] we believe that smoking promotes this extra-articular feature of RA, namely early atherosclerotic changes of the carotid arteries. The lack of association between ESR and IMT in our study contradicts a previous work,[10] but in that work smokers were excluded. Thus it is possible that initial changes in IMT are reflected by inflammation manifested as ESR and CRP values, whereas smoking exerts greater damage to arterial walls that masks inflammation in RA patients.

In conclusion, RA patients have higher IMT of the carotid artery bifurcation than controls. The profile of risk factors associated with IMT values is different between RA patients and controls. Smoking appears to be an important factor augmenting IMT in RA patients, and therefore smoking should be regarded as a risk factor for RA but also as an important contributing factor to enhanced atherosclerosis and its associated morbidity and mortality, especially in RA.

REFERENCES

1. SOLOMON, D.H., E.W. KARLSON, E.B. RIMM, *et al.* 2003. Cardiovascular morbidity and mortality in women diagnosed with rheumatoid arthritis. Circulation **107:** 1303–1307.
2. WOLFE, F., B. FREUNDLICH & W.L. STRAUS. 2003. Increase in cardiovascular and cerebrovascular disease prevalence in rheumatoid arthritis. J. Rheumatol. **30:** 36–40.
3. VAN DOORNUM, S., G. MCCOLL & I.P. WICKS. 2002. Accelerated atherosclerosis: an extraarticular feature of rheumatoid arthritis? Arthritis Rheum. **46:** 862–873.
4. SHOENFELD, Y., Y. SHERER & D. HARATS. 2001. Atherosclerosis as an infectious, inflammatory and autoimmune disease. Trends Immunol. **22:** 293–295.
5. RODRIGUEZ, G, A. SULLI, M. CUTOLO, *et al.* 2002. Carotid atherosclerosis in patients with rheumatoid arthritis: a preliminary case-control study. Ann. N.Y. Acad. Sci. **966:** 478–482.
6. JONSSON, S.W., C. BACKMAN, O. JOHNSON, *et al.* 2001. Increased prevalence of atherosclerosis in patients with medium term rheumatoid arthritis. J. Rheumatol. **28:** 2597–2602.
7. KUMEDA, Y., M. INABA, H. GOTO, *et al.* 2002. Increased thickness of the arterial intima-media detected by ultrasonography in patients with rheumatoid arthritis. Arthritis Rheum. **46:** 1489–1497.
8. PARK, Y.B., C.W. AHN, H.K. CHOI, *et al.* 2002. Atherosclerosis in rheumatoid arthritis: morphologic evidence obtained by carotid ultrasound. Arthritis Rheum. **46:** 1714–1719.
9. ALKAABI, J.K., M. HO, R. LEVISON, *et al.* 2003. Rheumatoid arthritis and macrovascular disease. Rheumatology **42:** 292–297.
10. DEL RINCON, I., K. WILLIAMS, M.P. STERN, *et al.* 2003. Association between carotid atherosclerosis and markers of inflammation in rheumatoid arthritis patients and healthy subjects. Arthritis Rheum. **48:** 1833–1840.
11. ALBANO, S.A., E. SANTANA-SAHAGUN & M.H. WEISMAN. 2001. Cigarette smoking and rheumatoid arthritis. Semin. Arthritis Rheum. **31:** 146–159.
12. TURESSON, C., W.M. O'FALLON, C.S. CROWSON, *et al.* 2003. Extra-articular disease manifestations in rheumatoid arthritis: incidence trends and risk factors over 46 years. Ann. Rheum. Dis. **62:** 722–727.
13. AMETT, F.C., S.M. EDWORTHY, D.A. BLOCH, *et al.* 1988. The American Rheumatism Association 1987 revised criteria for the classification of rheumatoid arthritis. Arthritis Rheum. **31:** 315–324.
14. VAUDO, G., G. SCHILLACI, F. EVANGELISTA, *et al.* 2000. Arterial wall thickening at different sites and its association with left ventricular hypertrophy in newly diagnosed essential hypertension. Am. J. Hypertens. **13:** 324–331.
15. SU, T.C., J.S. JENG, K.L. CHIEN, *et al.* 2001. Hypertension status is the major determinant of carotid atherosclerosis: a community-based study in Taiwan. Stroke **32:** 2265–2271.
16. SUN, Y., C.H. LIN, C.J. LU, *et al.* 2002. Carotid atherosclerosis, intima media thickness and risk factors—an analysis of 1781 asymptomatic subjects in Taiwan. Atherosclerosis **164:** 89–94.
17. CHIRONI, G., J. GARIEPY, N. DENARIE, *et al.* 2003. Influence of hypertension on early carotid artery remodeling. Arterioscler. Thromb. Vasc. Biol. **23:** 1460–1464.
18. CSANYI, A., A. EGERVARI & Z. NAGY. 2001. Influence of hypertension and smoking as the single vascular risk factors on the intima-media thickness. Eur. J. Epidemiol. **17:** 855–861.
19. WEBER, F. 2002. Risk factors for subclinical carotid atherosclerosis in healthy men. Neurology **59:** 524–528.
20. KNOFLACH, M., S. KIECHL, M. KIND, *et al.* 2003. Cardiovascular risk factors and atherosclerosis in young males: ARMY study (Atherosclerosis Risk-Factors in Male Youngsters). Circulation **108:** 1064–1069.
21. GEORGE, J., Y. LEVY & Y. SHOENFELD. 1997. Smoking and immunity: an additional player in the mosaic of autoimmunity. Scand. J. Immunol. **45:** 1–6.
22. CRISWELL, L.A., L.A. MERLINO, J.R. CERHAN, *et al.* 2002. Cigarette smoking and the risk of rheumatoid arthritis among postmenopausal women: results from the Iowa Women's Health Study. Am. J. Med. **112:** 465–471.

23. MATTEY, D.L., D. HUTCHINSON, P.T. DAWES, *et al.* 2002. Smoking and disease severity in rheumatoid arthritis: association with polymorphism at the glutathione S-transferase M1 locus. Arthritis Rheum. **46:** 640–646.
24. STOLT, P., C. BENGTSSON, B. NORDMARK, *et al.* 2003. Quantification of the influence of cigarette smoking on rheumatoid arthritis: results from a population based case-control study, using incident cases. Ann. Rheum. Dis. **62:** 835–841.

Investigation of Arthritic Joint Destruction by a Novel Fibroblast-Based Model

U. SACK,[a] B. SEHM,[a] F. KAHLENBERG,[a] A. MURR,[a] J. LEHMANN,[b] A. TANNAPFEL,[c] K. UBERLA,[d] A. MOESSNER,[e] A. DIETRICH,[f] F. EMMRICH,[a] F. LANGE,[a] A. JUNGEL,[a] J-M. BRAUN,[a] AND U. ANDEREGG[g]

[a]*Medical Faculty, Institute of Clinical Immunology and Transfusion Medicine, University of Leipzig, Leipzig, Germany*

[b]*Labor Diagnostik GmbH Leipzig, Research and Development, Leipzig, Germany*

[c]*Institute of Pathology, University of Leipzig, Leipzig, Germany*

[d]*Medical Faculty, Department of Molecular and Medical Virology, University of Bochum, 44801 Bochum, Germany*

Departments of [e]*Ophthalmology,* [f]*Surgery, and the* [g]*Clinic of Dermatology, University of Leipzig, Leipzig, Germany*

ABSTRACT: The key pathologic mechanism in rheumatoid arthritis (RA) is the destruction of cartilage by fibroblasts. In a severe combined immunodeficient (SCID) mouse model, this process can be modulated by gene transfer using invasive LS48 fibroblasts. This study aims to investigate the effect of interleukins (IL) -11 and -12 on cartilage destruction when transferred into LS48, and of IL-15 when transfected into non-invasive 3T3 cells; to compare three transduction systems (a lentiviral vector system, a retroviral vector system, and a particle-mediated gene transfer); and to establish an *in vitro* cartilage destruction system based on LS48 cells. Transduced fibroblasts were injected into SCID mice knee joints, and disease progression assessed microscopically. Distinctive morphologic pattern revealed invasion of fibroblasts into the articular cartilage by transfected, as well as non-transfected, LS48 cells. IL-12 and IL-15 did not alter swelling or cartilage destruction. Animals treated with IL-11–transfected cells showed reduced cartilage damage but no changes in swelling. Efficacy of gene transfer to establish transfected fibroblasts was shown to be >85% for lentiviral transfer, compared to <10% for retroviral transfer and gene gun. Furthermore, cells were co-incubated with porcine cartilage. Transduction of IL-11 led to a reduction of apoptosis in chondrocytes. These findings suggest that cartilage destruction by invasive fibroblasts can be modulated by gene transfer. Lentiviral vector systems offer the most effective approach for gene transduction. *In vitro* fibroblast/cartilage co-cultures present a convenient system for the assessment of novel therapeutic strategies toward reduction of articular destruction.

KEYWORDS: arthritis; fibroblasts; gene therapy; joint destruction; animal model

Address for correspondence: Ulrich Sack, Institute of Clinical Immunology and Transfusion Medicine, University of Leipzig, Johannisallee 30, 04103 Leipzig, Germany. Voice: +49-341-97-25-500; fax: +49-341-97-25-828.
ulrich.sack@medizin.uni-leipzig.de

**Ann. N.Y. Acad. Sci. 1051: 291–298 (2005). © 2005 New York Academy of Sciences.
doi: 10.1196/annals.1361.070**

INTRODUCTION

In rheumatoid arthritis (RA), joint structures are destroyed primarily by invading inflammatory fibroblasts;[1] the process can be investigated in severe combined immunodeficient (SCID) mice using the novel invasive fibroblast line LS48.[2] Synovial membrane fibroblasts have been shown to be morphologically altered[3] and strongly activated[4] in human rheumatoid synovitis and in SCID mice transfer models of RA. By injecting RA fibroblasts into SCID mice, an incremental progredient destructive arthritis can be induced within 12 to 20 weeks.[5,6] To overcome two major disadvantages of this model—limited availability and delayed course—we have isolated the destructive murine fibroblast line LS48, which resembles the morphologic, ultrastructural, immunologic, and functional parameters of RA synovial fibroblasts, including inducible nitric oxide synthase (iNOS) activity and synthesis of IL-6.[2] Injection of 5×10^5 LS48 cells, but not of 3T3 fibroblasts, into the knee joint of SCID mice initiated cartilage destruction within 10 days. Morphologic studies revealed direct infiltration of LS48 cells into the cartilage.[2] Novel anti-destructive therapies for the treatment of RA should target these cells.[1] Here we describe the effect of interleukins (IL) -11 and -12 transferred into LS48 on cartilage destruction in mice and of IL-15 on non-invasive 3T3 cells. Because IL-15 has been shown to amplify cartilage destruction,[7] this cytokine was transfected into non-invasive 3T3 cells. To find an efficient method for gene transduction, we compared a lentiviral vector with a retroviral vector system and particle-mediated gene transfer. In addition, we investigated how to move this model from mice to an *in vitro* model.

MATERIAL AND METHODS

mIL-11

Whole RNA was purified from 3×10^6 mouse fibroblasts (NIH 3T3),[8] stimulated by TNF-α and IL-1α,[9] and transcribed into cDNA.[10] From this cDNA, the message coding for murine IL-11 (Met_1-Leu_{209}) was amplified using the following primers: IL-11fwd - 5′ GGT ACC ATG AAC TGT GTT TGT CGC CTG G 3′ and IL-11rev - 5′ GCG GCC GCT CAC AGT CGA GTC TTT AAC AAC AGC 3′. Restriction site sequences for *Kpn* I and *Not* I were added to the forward and reverse primers respectively. The cDNA was amplified using Taq-polymerase (Applied Biosystems, Mannheim, Germany) and the PCR product was cloned into a pCRII TOPO vector (Invitrogen, Carlsbad, CA). The specific sequence was cut off from insert-bearing plasmids with *Kpn* I and *Not* I and inserted subsequently into the expression vectors pTracerSV40, pSecTag2-B (Invitrogen, Karlsruhe, Germany) and VGΔBH.[11] The vector pTracerSV40 allows the visualization of transfected cells by co-expression of GFP, whereas the use of the vector pSecTag2-B ensures that the secretion of the protein is driven by an Ig κ-chain leader sequence. The cloned sequence and its correct in-frame position were verified by DNA sequencing (ABI Prism 377, Perkin Elmer, Mannheim, Germany).

mIL-12

pBluscript SK vectors containing the cDNA for mIL-12p40 or mIL-12p35 were obtained from the American Type Culture Collection (ATCC). The pRSC expression plasmid, a plasmid with two multiple cloning sites, was generously provided by E. Hersh (Arizona Cancer Center, University of Arizona, Tucson, AZ). The mIL-12p40 gene was cloned into the first multiple cloning site driven by a RSV promoter; mIL-12p35 was cloned into the second multiple cloning site driven by a CMV promoter.[12] The correct cloning was confirmed by DNA-sequencing (ABI Prism 377, Perkin Elmer).

mIL-15

The IL-15 cDNA originated from a plasmid (pRCCMV; a gift of Raffaela Meazza, Italy). The cDNA was cut off from the plasmid and re-ligated into VGΔBH vector.[11] The cloned sequence and its correct in-frame position were verified by DNA sequencing (ABI Prism 377, Perkin Elmer).

Lentiviral Gene Transfer

To produce the lentiviral vector, 1.5×10^6 293T cells were transfected by calcium phosphate co-precipitation with 5 μg of vesicular stomatitis virus glycoprotein G (VSV-G)-encoding pHIT-G plasmid, SIV gag-pol expression plasmid Sgp-2 and accessory genes, and VGΔBH[11] bearing IL-11 or IL-15 cDNA. Vector supernatants were harvested after 48 hours and filtrated through a 0.45 μm filter (Sartorius, Goettingen, Germany). A volume of 0.2 mL was used to infect 5×10^5 3T3 (IL-15) or LS48 (IL-11) cells.

Retroviral Gene Transfer

Plasmids pTracerSV40-mIL-11 and pSecTag2-B-mIL-11 containing the cDNA of mIL-11 were purified from transformed *E. coli* cultures (Quantum PrepTM, Bio-Rad, Munich, Germany). Twenty micrograms of the purified plasmid were transfected into LS48 (5×10^6 cells) through an optimized electroporation procedure (low voltage 340 V, capacity 1050 μF, shunt maximum) using an EasyjecT PLUS 450 V (Equibio, Belgium).

Particle-Mediated Gene Transfer

Plasmid DNA was precipitated onto 0.6-μm gold particles for *in vitro* gene transfer. DNA and gold were mixed to a gold–DNA loading rate of 0.5 mg gold and 1.5 μg plasmid DNA per shot. DNA–gold particles were coated onto the inner surface of a Tefzel tube (Bio-Rad, Munich, Germany). The tube was cut into 70 0.5-inch segments, which were used as bullets for the helium-driven Helios Gene Gun (Bio-Rad, Munich, Germany).[13] Cells were transfected with an expression plasmid containing the cDNA for mIL-12 or GFP. 5×10^6 LS48 cells in 20 μL culture medium were stretched out in a 15-mm circle in a six-well plate and shot with a 200 psi helium pulse. After 2 mL medium was added, the cells were collected, and either injected into SCID mice or cultured for 14 further days under standard conditions.

Control of Transfection Effects

To analyze transduction *efficacy*, 10^5 cells were analyzed for GFP fluorescence with a FACS Calibur flow cytometer (lentiviral transduced IL-11; BD Live Sciences, San Jose, CA) or grown on chamber slides for fluorescence microscopy (GFP fluorescence of IL-12– and IL-15–transduced cells). *Proliferation and viability* were compared to non-transfected cells by MTT assay[14] after 1 week. Supernatants of transfected cells were collected repeatedly until day 7 for ELISA (IL-12 and IL-15; R&D, Minneapolis, MN) or Western blot (IL-11). Experiments were performed in triplicate.

Cell Culture

Non-invasive 3T3 fibroblasts[8] (ATCC, CCL-92, Rockville, MD) and destructive LS48 cells[2] were cultured and used for *in vivo* and *in vitro* models. Cells were cultured with 1×10^5 cells/mL in a cell culture medium containing DMEM and RPMI 1640 (1:2), 10% FCS, 25 mM HEPES, penicillin (100 U/mL), and streptomycin (100 μg/mL) (all Gibco, Eggenstein, Germany); hereafter called culture medium. Cells were cultured using 75 cm^2 culture flasks (Greiner, Solingen, Germany). At confluency, the cells were trypsinized with trypsin-EDTA (0.25% trypsin/0.2% EDTA; Gibco), released by a cell scraper, washed, and 1:2-diluted.[2]

SCID Mice

Female CB-17/lcrCrl-scid mice (8–10 weeks of age; Charles River Wiga, Sulzfeld, Germany) were acclimatized for at least 1 week prior to any experimental manipulation (license of the local authority TVV 23/02) and kept in laminar-flow filter cabinets in the local animal care facility with free access to water and food under germ-free and stable conditions (27°C, 80% air humidity). To exclude SCID mice with incomplete expression of the immune deficiency ("leakyness"), murine immunoglobulin levels were examined by ELISA.[15] Mice with immunoglobulin levels > 10 μg/mL were considered leaky and were not included in our experiments.

Arthritis Induction

Mice were narcotized by an intraperitoneal application of a combination of metomidate (6 mg/100 g BW) and fentanyl (0.006 mg/100 g BW). Under sterile conditions, the left knee was shaved. 5×10^5 cells suspended in 20 μL PBS were instilled into the left knee joints through the patellar tendon. Swelling of both knee joints of each animal was monitored daily by measuring the diameter with a caliper. The mice were killed 10 days after injection, when cartilage destruction could be found and the mice would not suffer any disabilities or pain.[2]

In Vitro *Model*

Sterile porcine cartilage explants were fitted inside culture inserts (Nunc, Roskilde, Denmark) and co-cultured with 10^5 overlaid LS48 cells in 24-well microculture plates (Greiner) for 14 days in 500 μL culture medium. Final examination for cartilage infiltration and destruction by injected cells was performed histologically.

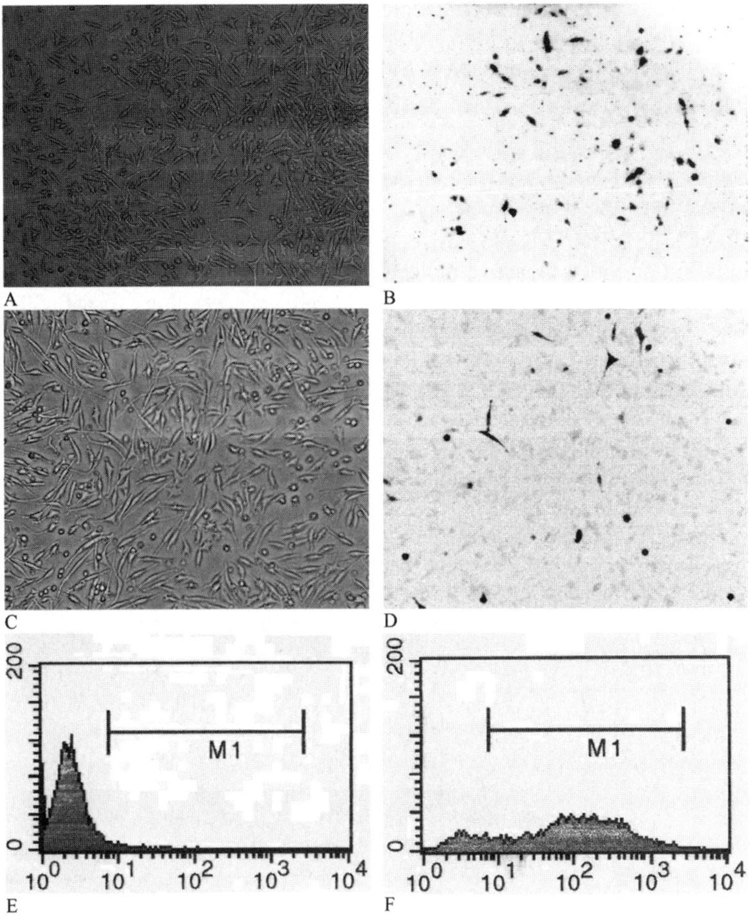

FIGURE 1. Transduction efficacy by using different vectors and infection protocols. After electroporation of pSecTag2-B, IL-11 was expressed by less than 5% of LS48 cells. (**A**) Phase-contrast; (**B**) GFP fluorescence, ×40. Particle-mediated transfer of the IL-12 expression plasmid induced less than 10% of LS48 cells to synthesize the protein. (**C**) Phase-contrast; (**D**) GFP fluorescence, ×40. In contrast, the lentiviral vector was able to infect more than 85% of 3T3 cells as shown by flow cytometry. (**E**) Negative control; (**F**) GFP.

Histology

To prepare serial paraffin sections, the isolated knee joints or cartilage explants were fixed in 4% paraformaldehyde for two days and transferred into a graded series of aqueous ethanol (70%, 80%, 96%, 100%). Dehydrated samples were placed successively in methylbenzoate (for 10 h), xylene (3 h), and liquid paraffin (20 h) prior to embedding into paraffin blocks. The extent of joint destruction was assessed histologically evaluating safranin O/fast green-stained paraffin sections (5–7 μm). All reagents were obtained from Merck (Darmstadt, Germany). Apoptosis in chondrocytes was detected by the Intergen in Situ Apoptosis Detection Kit (Chemicon, Temecula, CA).

RESULTS

All cytokine mRNAs could be isolated and cloned into eukaryotic expression plasmids and provided bioactive molecules when transfected into LS48 cells. Because pTracerSV40 inhibited proliferation of LS48 cells, we chose pSecTag2. None of the vectors used in the following experiments had any significant effects on vitality or proliferation of LS48 or 3T3 cells.

Transduction efficacy was highly variable because different vectors and transfer protocols were used. After electroporation of pSecTag2-B, IL-11 was expressed by less than 5% of LS48 cells (FIGS. 1A and B). Particle-mediated transfer of the IL-12 expression plasmid induced less than 10% of LS48 cells to synthesize the protein (FIGS. 1C and D). In contrast, the lentiviral vector was able to infect more than 85% of LS48 cells (IL-11) and 3T3 cells (IL-15; FIGS. 1E and F).

After injecting cells transduced by gene gun or lentiviral vector into SCID mouse knee joints, no reduction of LS48-induced and no increase of 3T3-induced knee joint swelling could be observed. In contrast, histologic examination revealed a slightly

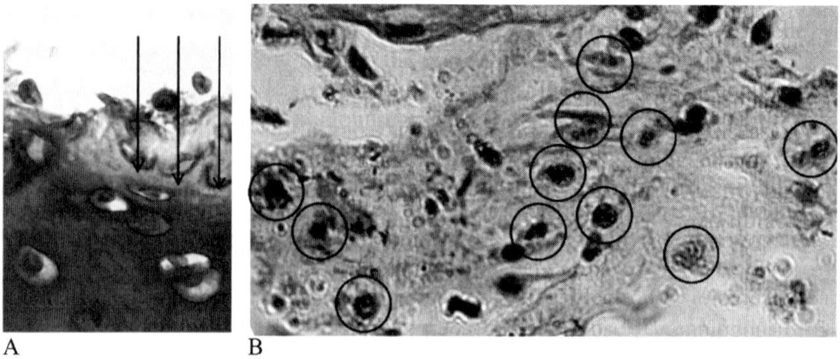

FIGURE 2. (**A**) Invasion of LS48 cells into the cartilage in an *in vitro* model. (**B**) IL-11 reduces cartilage damage by inhibiting apoptosis of chondrocytes (indicated by *circles*).

reduced degree of destruction of cartilage by IL-11-producing LS48 cells in comparison to non-transduced cells. Furthermore, when LS48 cells were injected into SCID mice, no adverse effects such as tumor induction or any other indicators of disease except for the LS48-induced cartilage destruction could be observed.

Generation of the *in vitro* model was successful. LS48 cells invaded the cartilage as shown in FIGURE 2A. Further examination revealed that IL-11 reduced cartilage damage by reducing the frequency of apoptotic chondrocytes (FIG. 2B).

DISCUSSION

Transduction of cytokine genes into destructive fibroblasts in an animal model of RA provides an excellent model for better understanding their role in cartilage destruction. Therefore a SCID mouse model was used to investigate the influence of IL-11, -12, and -15 when transferred into LS48 fibroblasts.

Previous data indicated that IL-11 plays an anti-inflammatory role in bone metabolism, inflammation, and acute-phase response in RA.[9,16] This could be confirmed in part through observation of reduced apoptosis in chondrocytes and lack of inflammation in the LS48-based SCID mouse model.

In contrast, IL-12, as a proinflammatory cytokine, failed to modulate the process in our experiments. Because its major biological activity is directed towards T and NK cells, and the differentiation of $CD4^+$ and $CD8^+$ type-1 cells, this lack of effect could be caused by the absence of target cells in immunodeficient SCID mice.[17]

IL-15 is another pro-inflammatory cytokine similar to IL-12 and with predominant activity on T- and NK cells.[7] This cytokine could play a role in activation of autoreactive T cells in RA and is thereby a candidate for novel agents. The finding that transfection of this cytokine into non-invasive 3T3 cells does not alter their activity in our model supports the relevance of immunoregulatory processes in RA.

Expression of transfected genes in target cells depends on efficient vector systems. The highest transduction efficacy was obtained by infecting cells with a self-inactivating (SIV)-based lentiviral vector.[11] In this limited study, potential side effects of lentiviral gene transfer were not observed. Expression vectors with retroviral promoter sequences that were introduced into cell lines by electroporation, such as pTracerSV40 and pSecTag2-B, did not provide significantly improved results. A gene gun that uses a shock wave to accelerate DNA-coated gold particles into target cells is cell surface receptor-independent and can deliver genes in a wide spectrum of mammalian cell types. Transgene expression and effective secretion of the proteins using this method has been well demonstrated.[13] In RA treatment, gene gun transfection may be helpful for therapy in small joints.

Induction of cartilage destruction by intra-articular application of LS48 cells into SCID mice[2] or *in vitro* represents a rapid and highly reproducible model for investigation of cartilage destruction as one important focus of RA therapy. This model provides excellent tools to investigate novel therapeutic strategies.

We conclude that the LS48 model can be used to investigate the influence of bioactive compounds on fibroblast-mediated joint destruction in RA. Highest efficacy was reached when using a lentiviral vector system. The activity of IL-11 in this model seems to be caused by a reduced sensitivity of chondrocytes to apoptotic stimuli.

ACKNOWLEDGMENTS

This work was supported by grants from the German Research Foundation (DFG; Sa 606/2), the Ernst-von-Weber-Stiftung, and the Interdisziplinäres Zentrum für Klinische Forschung Leipzig (IZKF) of the Medical Faculty, University of Leipzig, Germany (Project Z10).

REFERENCES

1. PAP, T., U. MULLER-LADNER, R.E GAY & S. GAY. 2000. Role of synovial fibroblasts in the pathogenesis of rheumatoid arthritis. Arthritis Res. **2:** 361–367.
2. SACK, U., A. HIRTH, B. FUNKE, *et al.* 2005. A novel model of fibroblast-mediated cartilage destruction. Scand. J. Immunol. **61:** 18–28.
3. FASSBENDER, H.G. 1983. The significance of inflammatory processes in osteoarthrosis. Z. Rheumatol. **42:** 145–152.
4. KINNE, R.W., E. PALOMBO-KINNE & F. EMMRICH. 1995. Activation of synovial fibroblasts in rheumatoid arthritis. Ann. Rheum. Dis. **54:** 501–504.
5. LEHMANN, J., A. JUNGEL, I. LEHMANN, *et al.* 2000. Grafting of fibroblasts isolated from the synovial membrane of rheumatoid arthritis (RA) patients induces chronic arthritis in SCID mice-A novel model for studying the arthritogenic role of RA fibroblasts in vivo. J. Autoimmun. **15:** 301–313.
6. GEILER, T., J. KRIEGSMANN, G.M. KEYSZER, *et al.* 1994. A new model for rheumatoid arthritis generated by engraftment of rheumatoid synovial tissue and normal human cartilage into SCID mice. Arthritis Rheum. **37:** 1664–1671.
7. MCINNES, I.B., J. AL-MUGHALES, M. FIELD, *et al.* 1996. The role of interleukin-15 in T-cell migration and activation in rheumatoid arthritis. Nat. Med. **2:** 175–182.
8. TODARO, G.J. & H. GREEN. 1963. Quantitative studies of the growth of mouse embryo cells in culture and their development into established lines. J. Cell. Biol. **17:** 299–313.
9. OKAMOTO, H., M. YAMAMURA, Y. MORITA, *et al.* 1997. The synovial expression and serum levels of interleukin-6, interleukin-11, leukemia inhibitory factor, and oncostatin M in rheumatoid arthritis. Arthritis Rheum. **40:** 1096–1105.
10. CHOMCZYNSKI, P. & N. SACCHI. Single-step method of RNA isolation by acid guanidinium thiocyanate-phenol-chloroform extraction. Anal. Biochem. **162:** 156–159.
11. SCHNELL, T., P. FOLEY, M. WIRTH, *et al.* 2000. Development of a self-inactivating, minimal lentivirus vector based on simian immunodeficiency virus. Hum. Gene Ther. **11:** 439–447.
12. DIETRICH, A., K. KRAUS, U. BRINCKMANN, *et al.* 2002. Complex cancer gene therapy in mice melanoma. Langenbecks Arch. Surg. **387:** 177–182.
13. CHENG, L., P.R. ZIEGELHOFFER & N.S. YANG. 1993. In vivo promoter activity and transgene expression in mammalian somatic tissues evaluated by using particle bombardment. Proc. Natl. Acad. Sci. USA **90:** 4455–4459.
14. WICHMANN, G., O. HERBARTH & I. LEHMANN. 2002. The mycotoxins citrinin, gliotoxin, and patulin affect interferon-gamma rather than interleukin-4 production in human blood cells. Environ. Toxicol. **17:** 211–218.
15. KUHN, H., J. ERMANN & U. SACK. 1997. Modulation of hu/mu severe combined immunodeficient (SCID) mouse arthritis by local application of human recombinant IL-1beta, IL- 2 and IL-6. Clin. Exp. Immunol. **107:** 96–102.
16. TRONTZAS, P., E.F. KAMPER, A. POTAMIANOU, *et al.* 1998. Comparative study of serum and synovial fluid interleukin-11 levels in patients with various arthritides. Clin. Biochem. **31:** 673–679.
17. LEHMANN, J. & G. ALBER. 1998. Murine leishmaniosis: a paradigm for the importance of T helper 1 and T helper 2 cells. Rev. Sci. Tech. **17:** 176–187.

Prevalence of Antiphospholipid and Antioxidized Low-Density Lipoprotein Antibodies in Rheumatoid Arthritis

YANIV SHERER,[a,e] ROBERTO GERLI,[b,e] GAETANO VAUDO,[c] GIUSEPPE SCHILLACI,[c] BORIS GILBURD,[a] ANDREA GIORDANO,[b] ELENA BARTOLONI BOCCI,[b] ROSITA ALLEGRUCCI,[b] SIMONA MARCHESI,[c] ELMO MANNARINO,[c] AND YEHUDA SHOENFELD[a,d]

[a]*Department of Medicine "B" and Center of Autoimmune Diseases, Sheba Medical Center, Tel Hashomer, and Sackler Faculty of Medicine, Tel Aviv University, Israel*

[b]*Section of Internal Medicine and Oncological Sciences, Center for the Study of Rheumatic Diseases, University of Perugia, Perugia, Italy*

[c]*Section of Internal Medicine, Angiology and Atherosclerosis Diseases, Department of Clinical & Experimental Medicine, University of Perugia, Perugia, Italy*

ABSTRACT: Antiphospholipid antibodies characterize the antiphospholipid syndrome (APS), but they can also be found in various autoimmune, infectious, and malignant conditions. This study's objectives were to detect the prevalence of antiphospholipid and antioxidized low-density lipoprotein (anti-oxLDL) antibodies among patients with rheumatoid arthritis (RA) who did not have clinical manifestations of APS. Using a standard enzyme-linked immunosorbent assay (ELISA), we evaluated the levels of immunoglobulin G (IgG) and IgM anticardiolipin, IgG, and IgM anti–beta-2-glycoprotein-I (anti-β_2GPI), and anti-oxLDL autoantibodies in 82 patients with RA. The cutoff levels for detecting these autoantibodies were 15 IgG phospholipid units (GPL), 15 IgM phospholipid units (MPL), and 25 ELISA units (EU)/mL, respectively. Elevated levels of IgG anticardiolipin antibodies were detected in 17 of 82 (21%) RA patients, including 10 with low levels of IgG anticardiolipin and 7 with medium to high levels of anticardiolipin autoantibodies. IgM anticardiolipin was found in only 1 (1%) patient, and both IgG and IgM anti-β_2GPI were found in 3 (4%) patients with RA. Elevated levels of anti-oxLDL antibodies were found in 8 (10%) patients, 4 of whom also had elevated levels of IgG anticardiolipin. We conclude that IgG anticardiolipin autoantibodies can be found in about one-fifth of RA patients who do not have clinical manifestations of APS. Whether the presence of anticardiolipin signifies increased risk for thrombosis and atherosclerosis in these patients should be studied further.

KEYWORDS: rheumatoid arthritis; antiphospholipid antibody; anticardiolipin

Address for correspondence: Y. Shoenfeld, M.D., Department of Medicine "B," Sheba Medical Center, Tel Hashomer 52621, Israel. Voice: 972-3-5302652; fax: 972-3-5352855.
shoenfel@post.tau.ac.il

[d]Incumbent of the Laura Schwartz Kipp Chair for Research of Autoimmune Diseases, Tel Aviv University, Tel Aviv, Israel.

[e]Both authors contributed equally to this work.

**Ann. N.Y. Acad. Sci. 1051: 299–303 (2005). © 2005 New York Academy of Sciences.
doi: 10.1196/annals.1361.071**

thrombosis; atherosclerosis; antiphospholipid syndrome; anti–beta-2 glycoprotein I

INTRODUCTION

The antiphospholipid syndrome (APS) is characterized by the presence of direct-binding antiphospholipid antibodies (aPLs), which target phospholipid molecules mainly via beta-2-glycoprotein-I (β_2GPI). APS can also be characterized by the presence of lupus anticoagulant, which is associated with recurrent fetal loss, thrombo-embolic phenomena, thrombocytopenia, neurological, heart, skin, and other organ disorders.[1–3] The antiphospholipid syndrome can be either primary or secondary to various conditions including autoimmune diseases. The disease most frequently associated with APS is systemic lupus erythematosus (SLE); nonetheless, other-autoimmune diseases, including rheumatoid arthritis (RA), reportedly have been associated with secondary APS.[4]

Antiphospholipid antibodies have been detected in many patients who do not fulfill the criteria for APS; hence, the aim of this study was to detect the prevalence of aPLs among patients with RA who did not have clinical manifestations of APS, as well as the prevalence of antioxidized low-density lipoprotein (anti-oxLDL) antibodies.

METHODS

Patients

Eighty-two patients who fulfilled the American College of Rheumatology classification criteria for RA[5] and who were without overt cardiovascular disease were included in the study. Written informed consent was obtained from every subject who participated in the study.

Antiphospholipid Antibody Measurement

The following autoantibodies were measured using an enzyme immunoassay (values in parentheses stand for cutoff levels): anticardiolipin (IgG <15 IgG phospholipid units [GPL]; IgM <15 IgM phospholipid units [MPL]) and anti-β_2GPI (<15 enzyme immunoassay [EIA] units for IgG and IgM isotypes). To do so, plastic microwell plate wells were coated with purified cardiolipin/β_2GPI and then stabilized. Upon incubation, serum samples from RA patients containing cardiolipin/β_2GPI isotype antibodies were bound with their respective autoantigens. Unbound protein was removed by washing and adding to the wells isotype-specific, enzyme-labeled anti-human alkaline phosphatase-labeled conjugate for cardiolipin, or anti-human horseradish peroxidase–labeled conjugate for β_2GPI. After incubation, the unbound conjugate was removed by washing. An alkaline phosphatase (for cardiolipin) or a peroxidase substrate (for β_2GPI) was then added, which undergoes a color change in the presence of the conjugated enzyme. The presence or absence of an autoantibody was determined by comparing sample optical density (OD) with that of a 6-point calibration curve.

Native and copper oxLDL was prepared as previously described.[6] The 96-well ELISA plates (Nunc, Copenhagen, Denmark) were coated with either oxLDL, native LDL (at a concentration of 10 mg/mL in phosphate buffered saline [PBS]), or PBS and incubated overnight at 4°C. After washing four times with PBS containing 0.05% Tween and 0.001% aprotinin (Sigma-Aldrich, St. Louis, MO), the plates were blocked with 2% bovine serum albumin (BSA) for 2 h at room temperature. Serum fractions were diluted to 1:50 in PBS containing 0.05% Tween and 0.2% BSA. After additional overnight incubation, the sera were washed, and alkaline phosphatase-conjugated mouse antihuman IgG (Jackson ImmunoResearch Laboratories Inc., West Grove, PA) was added, diluted 1:10,000 in PBS containing 0.05% Tween and 0.2% BSA, and incubated for 1 h at room temperature.

After extensive washing, 1 mg/mL *p*-nitro-phenyl-phosphate in 50 mmol/L carbonate buffer, containing 1 mmol/L $MgCl_2$ (pH 9.8), was added as a substrate. The reaction was stopped after 30 minutes by adding 1 mol/L of NaOH. The color was read at a 405 nm wavelength, and results were expressed as OD and converted to ELISA units per milliliter (EU/mL). The levels of anti-oxLDL antibodies were calculated by subtracting the value obtained by binding to native LDL from the value obtained by binding to oxLDL. Cutoff levels were greater than 35 EU/mL.

RESULTS

Elevated levels of IgG anticardiolipin antibodies were detected in 17 of 82 (21%) RA patients. These 17 patients included 10 with low levels of IgG anticardiolipin and 7 with medium to high levels of anticardiolipin autoantibodies (40–98 GPL). IgM anticardiolipin was found in only 1 (1%) patient, who was also positive for the IgM anti-β_2GPI antibody. Both IgG and IgM anti-β_2GPI were found in 3 (4%) patients with RA. Elevated levels of anti-oxLDL antibodies were found in 8 (10%) patients, 4 of whom also displayed elevated levels of IgG anticardiolipin. Positive correlations were found between levels of the different autoantibodies: 0.27 between IgG anti-β_2GPI and IgG anticardiolipin; 0.28 between IgM anti-β_2GPI and IgM anticardiolipin; and 0.19 between IgG anticardiolipin and anti-oxLDL antibodies.

DISCUSSION

The presence of aPLs in arthritis patients has been reported in a few studies. Merkel and colleagues[7] measured IgG, IgM, and IgA isotypes of anticardiolipin antibodies in 70 RA patients and found a 15.7% positivity rate for these antibodies in their cohort. Among their patients (which included patients with various autoimmune diseases), IgG or IgM anticardiolipin positivity was significantly associated with hemolytic anemia and a positive serologic test for syphilis, but negatively associated with Raynaud's phenomenon.[7] However, anticardiolipin positivity was not associated with other clinical manifestations of APS.

Several years later, Seriolo and colleagues[8] evaluated the presence of anticardiolipin and lupus anticoagulant in 168 female patients with RA, 30 of whom were found to be aPL positive. The authors described the possible contribution of high levels of homocysteine to the risk of thrombosis, because aPL-positive RA patients who had thrombosis had significantly higher homocysteine levels than did aPL-positive RA patients without thrombosis.[8] In another report, aPLs were induced in RA patients following tumor necrosis factor–blocker therapy in 21% of patients.[9] Of note is that among ankylosing spondylitis patients, a 27% induction rate for aPLs was observed.[9]

Other studies have described the presence of aPLs among patients with juvenile rheumatoid arthritis (JRA). Whereas Gedalia and colleagues[10] found anticardiolipin antibodies in only 2 of 28 JRA patients (the 2 positive patients exhibited no manifestation of APS), significantly higher rates have been reported in two other studies.[11,12] In the latter studies, serum anticardiolipin levels were detected in 28 of 86 JRA patients, none of whom exhibited the classical clinical manifestations of APS,[11] and in 28.6–46.4% of 28 juvenile idiopathic arthritis (JIA) patients during follow-up.[12] This second study also failed to find an association between either aPL presence and disease activity or APS manifestations. Anti-β_2GPI antibodies were also not found in higher frequency in the patient group compared with a healthy control group.[12] The presence of anti-oxLDL antibodies has been documented in 17% of JRA patients in whom a good correlation was found between anti-oxLDL and aPL levels.[13]

CONCLUSIONS

Our results emphasize that patients with RA have a relatively high prevalence of IgG anticardiolipin antibodies. Because these patients lack the clinical manifestations of APS, they cannot be regarded as having secondary APS. However, these patients may be at increased risk for thrombosis and other features of APS in the future. Alternatively, the high prevalence of observed anticardiolipin combined with the low prevalence of anti-β_2GPI antibodies supports the association of RA with infections (as found in many autoimmune diseases). These infections favor the production of anticardiolipin antibodies that are not β_2GPI dependent. aPLs are also considered proatherogenic and have been associated with enhanced atherosclerosis.[14] Moreover, because RA is also associated with excess cardiovascular mortality,[15] the presence of aPLs and anti-oxLDL antibodies possibly signifies a heightened risk of advanced atherosclerosis and its complications in RA. This assumption warrants further study.

REFERENCES

1. HARRIS, E.N., A.E. GAHARAVI, M.L. BOEY, *et al.* 1983. Anticardiolipin antibodies: detection by radioimmunoassay and association with thrombosis in systemic lupus erythematosus. Lancet **2:** 1211–1214.
2. HUGHES, G.R., N.N. HARRIS & A.E. GHARAVI. 1986. The anticardiolipin syndrome. J. Rheumatol. **13:** 486–489.
3. ASHERSON, R.A., R. CERVERA, J.C. PIETTE & Y. SHOENFELD. 2002. Milestones in the antiphospholipid syndrome. *In* The Antiphospholipid Syndrome II: Autoimmune Thrombosis. R.A. Asherson, R. Cervera, J.C. Piette & Y. Shoenfeld, Eds. Elsevier Science. Amsterdam.
4. SHERER, Y. & Y. SHOENFELD. 1999. The antiphospholipid (Hughes') syndrome: an entity to be expanded. Am. J. Reprod. Immunol. **41:** 113–116.

5. Arnett, F.C., S.M. Edworthy, D.A. Bloch, *et al.* 1988. The American Rheumatism Association 1987 revised criteria for the classification of rheumatoid arthritis. Arthritis Rheum. **31:** 315–324.
6. George, J., M. Blank, M. Hojnik, *et al.* 1997. Oxidized low-density lipoprotein (Ox-LDL) but not LDL aggravates the manifestations of experimental antiphospholipid syndrome (APS). Clin. Exp. Immunol. **108:** 227–233.
7. Merkel, P.A., Y. Chang, S.S. Pierangeli, *et al.* 1996. The prevalence and clinical associations of anticardiolipin antibodies in a large inception cohort of patients with connective tissue diseases. Am. J. Med. **101:** 576–583.
8. Seriolo, B., D. Fasciolo, A. Sulli & M. Cutolo. 2001. Homocysteine and antiphospholipid antibodies in rheumatoid arthritis patients: relationships with thrombotic events. Clin. Exp. Rheumatol. **19:** 561–564.
9. Ferraro-Peyret, C., F. Coury, J.G. Tebib, *et al.* 2004. Infliximab therapy in rheumatoid arthritis and ankylosing spondylitis–induced specific antinuclear and antiphospholipid autoantibodies without autoimmune clinical manifestations: a two-year prospective study. Arthritis. Res. Ther. **6:** R535–R543.
10. Gedalia, A., J.F. Molina, C.O. Garcia, *et al.* 1998. Anticardiolipin antibodies in childhood rheumatic disorders. Lupus **7:** 551–553.
11. Serra, C.R., S.H. Rodrigues, N.P. Silva, *et al.* 1999. Clinical significance of anticardiolipin antibodies in juvenile idiopathic arthritis. Clin. Exp. Rheumatol. **17:** 375–380.
12. Avcin, T., A. Ambrozic, B. Bozic, *et al.* 2002. Estimation of anticardiolipin antibodies, anti-beta2 glycoprotein I antibodies and lupus anticoagulant in a prospective longitudinal study of children with juvenile idiopathic arthritis. Clin. Exp. Rheumatol. **20:** 101–108.
13. Savolainen, A., R. von Essen, J. Leikola, *et al.* 1995. Antibodies against oxidised low-density lipoprotein in juvenile chronic arthritis. Scand. J. Rheumatol. **24:** 209–211.
14. Sherer, Y. & Y. Shoenfeld. 2001. Antiphospholipid syndrome, antiphospholipid antibodies, and atherosclerosis. Curr. Atheroscler. Rep. **3:** 328–333.
15. Solomon, D.H., E.W. Karlson, E.B. Rimm, *et al.* 2003. Cardiovascular morbidity and mortality in women diagnosed with rheumatoid arthritis. Circulation **107:** 1303–1307.

Mono-organic versus Multi-organic Involvement in Primary Antiphospholipid Syndrome

GABRIELA MEDINA,[a] OLGA VERA-LASTRA,[b,e] ULISES ANGELES,[c] AND LUIS J. JARA[d,e]

[a]Hospital General de Zona 76, [b]Internal Medicine Department, [c]Epidemiology Department, and [d]Rheumatology Department and Research Division, Hospital de Especialidades Centro Médico La Raza, Antonio Fraga Mouret, IMSS, Mexico City, Mexico

[e]Universidad Nacional Autónoma de México, Mexico City, Mexico

ABSTRACT: The prevalence of mono-organic and multi-organic involvement during long-term follow-up in patients with primary antiphospholipid syndrome (pAPS) was investigated. We studied 60 pAPS patients followed up at least 5 years. Patients with associated systemic lupus erythematosus were excluded. All patients received oral anticoagulant therapy. A diagnosis of mono-organic involvement was considered when one organ was affected exclusively, and multi-organic involvement was considered when two or more organs became affected during follow-up. Average age at diagnosis was 32.9 ± 12.4 years, 40 subjects were female and 20 male, and mean disease evolution totaled 11.5 ± 4.5 years. The mean number of clinical events was 3.75 ± 1.87. Among patients, immunoglobulin G anticardiolipin (IgM aCL) titers totaled 50 ± 40.3 IgG phospholipid units, and IgM aCL titers totaled 47.3 ± 35.4 IgM phospholipid units. The most frequent clinical manifestations at study onset were deep venous thrombosis, stroke, pulmonary thromboembolism, fetal loss, and pre-eclampsia. At the beginning of follow-up, 46 patients had mono-organic involvement and 14 had multi-organic involvement ($P = 0.0001$). In contrast, at the end of the study, only 8 patients still had mono-organic involvement, leading to deep venous thrombosis ($n = 3$), stroke ($n = 3$), and retinal thrombosis ($n = 2$) ($P = 0.0001$). Kaplan-Meier analysis showed that the probability of remaining with mono-organic involvement decreased throughout the cumulative years, especially during the first 3. The hazard risk ratio for developing multi-organic involvement was 1.47 patients per year. In conclusion, PAPS is a chronic disorder with unpredictable clinical course and multi-organic involvement, especially during the first years. The conversion to multi-organic involvement supports the concept that pAPS is a systemic autoimmune disease.

KEYWORDS: primary antiphospholipid syndrome; mono-organic involvement; multi-organic involvement; deep venous thrombosis

Address for correspondence: Luis J. Jara, M.D., Research Division, Hospital de Especialidades Centro Médico La Raza, Seris y Zaachila S/N Col. La Raza, México, CP. 02990. Voice/fax: +5255-56059968.

luis_jara_quezada@hotmail.com

Ann. N.Y. Acad. Sci. 1051: 304–312 (2005). © 2005 New York Academy of Sciences. doi: 10.1196/annals.1361.072

INTRODUCTION

In 1983, Hughes and colleagues[1] described a clinical syndrome characterized by venous and arterial thrombosis, recurrent pregnancy loss, neurologic disease, and the presence of antiphospholipid antibodies (aPLs). Primary antiphospholipid syndrome (pAPS) is defined by recurrent arterial or venous thrombosis, thrombocytopenia, and/or pregnancy morbidity in the presence of aPLs, without evidence of another definable condition.[2] This syndrome has become one of the commonest in the world; for example, 20–30% of all deep-vein thromboses (DVTs) are the result of the antiphospholipid syndrome (APS). From a triad of manifestations, it has also become one of the most systemic diseases reported in the literature so far, encompassing almost every organ and tissue in the body. Recently, Shoenfeld[3] proposed that the name APS be changed to the *systemic antiphospholipid syndrome,* because 17 organs and systems are involved in APS.

Although the etiology of this syndrome is unknown, several hypotheses have been proposed to explain the mechanism by which aPLs promote thrombosis. The first theory implicates the interaction of endothelial cells, aPLs, and anti–β_2-glycoprotein I, leading to subsequent activation of endothelial cells and induction of non-inflammatory thrombosis.[4] A second theory focuses on complement activation. Recent publications have shown that in mice, complement activation (particularly of C3, C5, and its cleavage product, C5a) and neutrophils are required for aPL-mediated thrombosis and pregnancy loss.[5]

In humans, hypocomplementemia was found in patients with pAPS and was associated with some APS features such as livedo reticularis, thrombocytopenia, and aPLs.[6] Many infections may be accompanied by aPL elevations, and in some these elevations may be related to clinical manifestations of APS.[7] Molecular mimicry mechanisms linking the pathogenic agent with phospholipids and β_2-glycoprotein I may be involved in the generation of pathogenic aPL.[8] In addition, these antibodies have other actions, such as antihormonal and anticytokine effects, expression of intracellular adhesion molecules, and induction of apoptosis.[3,9] This evidence suggests that pAPS may have an unpredictable clinical course with multi-organic involvement resulting from diverse pathogenic mechanisms.

Different clinical studies of pAPS have analyzed its pathogenesis, clinical course after the first thrombotic event, factors influencing recurrent thrombosis, long-term treatment, and functional outcome.[10–13] Nevertheless, information on the progression from mono-organic to multi-organic involvement is limited. Therefore, the aim of this study was to analyze the clinical characteristics of PAPS patients and to follow up their evolution from mono-organic to multi-organic involvement over the long term.

PATIENTS AND METHODS

This retrospective cohort study included 60 PAPS patients from a single referral center, the Hospital de Especialidades Centro Médico La Raza, part of the Mexican Social Security Institute (IMSS). The study used the following inclusion criteria: patients with PAPS were selected according to the Sapporo criteria,[14] having had at

TABLE 1. Characteristics of PAPS patients

Characteristic	
Male/female ratio	20/40
Mean age at diagnosis (y)	32.9 ± 12.4
Mean duration of disease evolution (y)	11.5 ± 4.5
Mean number of clinical events	3.75 ± 1.87 (1–8)
aCL IgG titer	50 ± 40.3 GPL U
aCL IgM titer	47.3 ± 35.4 MPL U
LA	28%

ABBREVIATIONS: aCL, anti-cardiolipin; Ig, immunoglobulin; LA, lupus anticoagulant; GPL= IgG phospholipid unit; MPL = IgM phospholipid unit; PAPS = primary antiphospholipid syndrome.

TABLE 2. Mono-organic involvement in PAPS at onset

Manifestation	Number of patients (n = 60) (%)
Deep venous thrombosis	14 (23)
Stroke	12 (20)
Pulmonary thromboembolism	11 (18)
Fetal loss, pre-eclampsia	8 (13)
Mesenteric thrombosis	1 (1.7)
Deep venous thrombosis	14 (23)
Total	46 (76.7)

least 5 years of previous follow-up; all patients were receiving oral anticoagulants. Patients with APS associated with systemic lupus erythematosus (SLE) were excluded.

Of the 60 PAPS patients studied, 20 were male and 40 were female; their mean disease evolution was 11.5 ± 4.5 years. Their clinical characteristics are summarized in TABLE 1. Initial manifestations are shown in TABLE 2. Almost one-fourth of the patients presented with DVT. The mean follow-up duration was 11.5 ± 4.5 years.

The diagnosis of DVT was based on clinical grounds and confirmed by Doppler ultrasonographic scans or venography. Pulmonary embolism was diagnosed by ventilation-perfusion lung scanning or pulmonary angiography. Cerebrovascular ischemic episodes were diagnosed by assessing the clinical picture and by computed tomographic (CT) scanning or magnetic resonance imaging (MRI). Angina or myocardial infarction were diagnosed according to clinical presentation, electrocardiographic changes, and elevated levels of cardiac enzymes in the blood. Endocardial valve disease was diagnosed using echocardiography. Thromboses at other sites were diagnosed by angiographic studies. A diagnosis of thrombocytopenia was considered when the platelet count was less than 150×10^9 on a minimum of two occasions: mild if the platelet count was $100–150 \times 10^9$/L, moderate if $50–100 \times 10^9$ L, or severe if less than 50×10^9/L.

Anticardiolipin antibodies (aCLs) were measured using a standardized enzyme-linked immunosorbent assay (ELISA) and were found in all patients on at least two occasions. We defined mono-organic involvement as only one organ being affected for at least 6 months, and multi-organic involvement as two or more organs being affected. Both conditions were analyzed at study onset and during follow-up.

Statistical Analysis

Descriptive statistics, chi-square testing, and life-table analysis using the product-limit (Kaplan-Meier) method were used to estimate the probability of the subject continuing with mono-organic involvement. Cox-proportional hazard models were employed to examine the association between disease evolution and multi-organic involvement. Statistical analysis was performed using the statistical package SPSS version 10.0 for Windows.

RESULTS

Mono-organic versus Multi-organic Involvement

At study onset, the majority of patients (46, or 76.7%) had mono-organic involvement, and only 14 patients (23.3%) had multi-organic involvement ($P = 0.0001$). In contrast, at the end of follow-up, the majority of patients (52, or 86.7%) had developed multi-organic involvement. Regarding the number of affected organs, 46 patients (76.7%) had 2 or 3 affected organs, and 6 patients (10.0%) had 4 or 5 affected organs. After follow-up, only 8 patients (13.3%) still had mono-organic involvement. These patients had DVT ($n = 3$), stroke ($n = 3$), and retinal thrombosis ($n = 2$) ($P = 0.0001$).

Clinical Course

After the first event, we found that 34 patients (56.7%) had disease recurrence (e.g., obstetric complications or thrombocytopenia) in different arterial, venous, or other anatomic territories. Only 26 patients (43.3 %) had recurrence in the same territory. Among the 60 patients, the subsequent clinical manifestations that evolved from mono-organic to multi-organic involvement during the disease's course are shown in TABLE 3. The time until conversion from mono-organic to multi-organic involvement ranged from 6 to 36 months.

Multi-organic Conversion Calculation

According to the Kaplan-Meier analysis, the actuarial probability of remaining with mono-organic involvement decreased throughout the cumulative years, especially during the first 3 (FIG. 1). At the beginning of the study, the probability calculation of conversion to multi-organic involvement was present in 19 of 60 patients (31.7%), and 68% of patients continued with mono-organic involvement. The probability of continuing with mono-organic involvement decreased over the next years. At the end of follow-up, the estimated percentage of subjects maintaining mono-

TABLE 3. Subsequent clinical manifestations evolving into multi-organic involvement in PAPS

Manifestation	Number of patients (%)
Deep venous thrombosis	15 (25)
Thrombocytopenia	10 (17)
Pulmonary thromboembolism	8 (13)
Renal involvement	3 (5)
Stroke	3 (5)
Fetal loss	2 (3)
Pre-eclampsia	2 (3)

TABLE 4. Kaplan-Meier analysis of patients maintaining mono-organic involvement in PAPS

Follow-up time (years)	Number of patients	Patients with probability of multi-organic conversion	Continued mono-organic involvement	95% CI
0	60	19	0.68	0.54–0.78
1	41	7	0.56	0.43–0.68
3	28	6	0.36	0.24–0.48
6	17	1	0.26	0.16–0.38
9	13	1	0.20	0.11–0.30
13	7	4	0.05	0.01–0.12
16	2	1	0.01	0.001–0.07

Note: At the beginning, the probability calculation of multi-organic conversion was present in 19 patients. At the end of follow-up (>5 years), only 1% of patients remained with mono-organic involvement.

organic involvement was only 1% (TABLE 4). Using the Cox regression test, we found that 1.47 PAPS patients are at risk of evolving to multi-organic disease per year (95%; CI = 0.63–2.31).

DISCUSSION

This study was the first to analyze the evolution from mono-organic to multi-organic involvement during a long-term follow-up of PAPS patients. Our findings show that initially, the majority of patients have mono-organic involvement, but at the end of five or more years of follow-up, the majority have evolved to multi-organic involvement. As to the number of affected organs, at baseline, more than 75% had a mono-organic involvement, and 23.3% had multi-organic involvement. However, after follow-up, only 8 patients (13.3%) remain with mono-organic involvement.

Among our PAPS patients, the major initial disease manifestations were DVT, stroke, pulmonary thromboembolism, and maternal and fetal complications. This

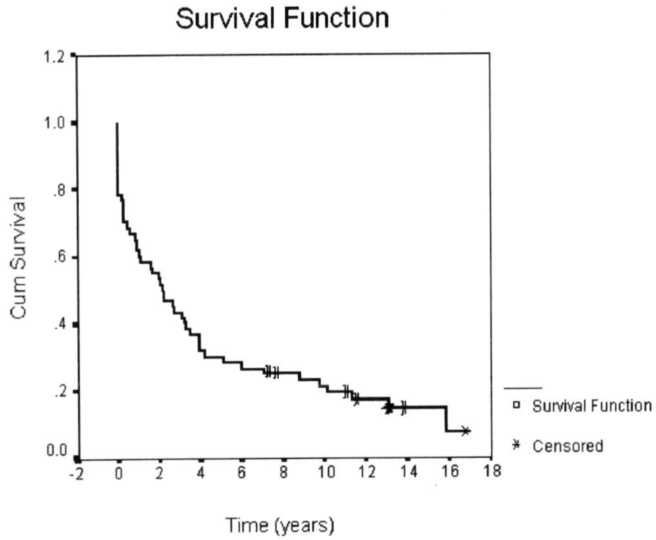

FIGURE 1. Actuarial probability of remaining with mono-organic involvement. This probability decreased throughout cumulative years.

initial clinical picture does not differ from those of other reported series.[15–17] During follow-up, these clinical manifestations, in addition to thrombocytopenia and renal dysfunction, subsequently evolved into multi-organic involvement.

The evolution from mono-organic to multi-organic involvement may give rise to a wide variety of presentations in PAPS. Initial reports have described the classic manifestations of PAPS: arterial and venous thrombosis, thrombocytopenia, fetal loss, leg ulcers, and livedo reticularis.[18,19] Both studies had similar follow-up duration (mean = 5 years) without evidence of SLE, and the authors described a variety of other manifestations: Budd-Chiari syndrome, multi-infarct dementia, multiple visceral arterial occlusions, renal infarction, transverse myelitis, perforation nasal septum, placental infarction, migraine, and others. These early reports suggested the systemic nature of PAPS and associated the disease with a single autoantibody. Nowadays, the expanding spectrum of clinical events in PAPS seems to associate the syndrome with multiple autoantibodies.[20,21]

Long-term follow-up studies showed that recurrent arterial or venous thrombotic events in different organs are common and that the time interval between them also varies considerably, from months to years.[17] However, research into PAPS has not systematically analyzed the mean time between mono-organic manifestations and subsequent manifestation in other organs (multi-organic conversion) as well as the risk of PAPS evolving from mono-organic into multi-organic disease. Our study demonstrated that the probability of converting to systemic disease is high—above all, during the first 3 years of follow-up. In fact, we found that 1.47 PAPS patients are likely to see their condition evolve into multi-organic disease each year.

Because PAPS was first described only 15 years ago, few reports have been published on the natural history of these patients. In relation to aPLs' natural history, Finazzi and colleagues discovered that high titers of aPL are independent predictors of subsequent vascular complications, adverse pregnancy outcomes, or hematologic neoplastic disease.[22] In relation to disease recurrence, Rosove and colleagues[10] described the clinical course after the first thrombotic event. In this study, the site of the first event (arterial or venous) tended to predict the site of subsequent events. Unlike the Rosove study finding, we observed that the site of the first event (arterial, venous, thrombocytopenic, or obstetric complications) did not predict the site of subsequent events. In fact, following the first event, 43.3% of our PAPS patients experienced recurrence in the same territory (arterial or venous), but more than half (56.7%) experienced recurrence in a different territory (arterial, venous, or other).

After 10 years of follow-up in a retrospective study, Shah and colleagues[15] reported a high chance of recurrence of new vascular events recurring in 52 patients (10 with PAPS), despite antithrombotic treatment. They observed no differences between PAPS and secondary APS with respect to chance of recurrence. However, the authors did not analyze changes of organ involvement during follow-up. In our study, independent of vascular pattern, the majority of patients evolved to multi-organic involvement. This result suggests that different factors are responsible for the conversion from mono-organic to multi-organic involvement than for vascular targeting.

The interaction among aPLs, anti-β2 glycoprotein-I, and endothelium may induce endothelial activation with associated vasculopathy.[23,24] *In vitro* and *in vivo* experimental models have demonstrated the induction of a pro-inflammatory or -coagulant phenotype.[25,26] Other mechanisms, including a wide variety of infections, have been associated with thrombotic events in patients with APS. Also possibly contributing to the systemic manifestations observed in our PAPS patients[21] were accelerated atherosclerosis[27,28] as well as new autoantibodies directed to laminin-I, thromboplastin, mitochondrial antibodies of the M5 type, corpus luteum, prolactin, poly (ADP-ribose), thyroglobulin, and others (which were also found in SLE and APS patients).

All these factors may play a role in the multiple clinical manifestations of PAPS, especially during the first years of disease evolution. This pattern has been described in other autoimmune diseases, such as SLE and rheumatoid arthritis. In SLE, the disease's heterogeneity pertains to the type of clinical manifestations at onset and to the time it takes for these manifestations to evolve, thus making the diagnosis of lupus possible.[29] In rheumatoid arthritis, a similar situation occurs: persistent arthritis and radiologic damage are often observed early in the course of disease, but joint erosion may take years to appear after symptom onset.[30]

The limitations of our study include its retrospective design, the relatively small number of patients, and bias towards the selection of certain patients.

CONCLUSIONS

This study suggests that PAPS is a chronic disorder with variable onset, course, and outcome. The conversion to multi-organic involvement supports the concept that PAPS is a systemic autoimmune disease that results from diverse pathogenic mechanisms.

REFERENCES

1. HUGHES, G.R.V. 1983. Thrombosis, abortion, cerebral disease, and the lupus anticoagulant. Br. Med. J. (Clin. Res. Ed.) **287:** 1088–1089.
2. MACKWORTH-YOUNG, C.G., J. DAVID, S. LOIZOU, *et al.* 1987. Primary antiphospholipid syndrome: features in patients with anticardiolipin antibodies and no other disorder. Br. J. Rheumatol. **26:** 94.
3. SHOENFELD, Y. 2003. Systemic antiphospholipid syndrome. Lupus **12:** 497–498.
4. LEVINE, J.S., D.W. BRANCH & J. RAUCH. 2002. The antiphospholipid syndrome. N. Engl. J. Med. **346:** 752–763.
5. GIRARDI, G., J. BERMAN, P. REDECHA, *et al.* 2003. Complement C5a receptors and neutrophils mediate fetal injury in the antiphospholipid syndrome. J. Clin. Invest. **112:** 1644–1654.
6. RAMOS-CASALS, M., M.T. CAMPOAMOR, A. CHAMORRO, *et al.* 2004. Hypocomplementemia in systemic lupus erythematosus and primary antiphospholipid syndrome: prevalence and clinical significance in 667 patients. Lupus **13:** 777–783.
7. CERVERA, R., R.A. ASHERSON, M.L. ACEVEDO, *et al.* 2004. Antiphospholipid syndrome associated with infections: clinical and microbiological characteristics of 100 patients. Ann. Rheum. Dis. **63:** 1312–1317.
8. GHARAVI, E.E., H. CHAIMOVICH, E. CUCURULL, *et al.* 1999. Induction of antiphospholipid antibodies by immunization with synthetic viral and bacterial peptides. Lupus **8:** 449–455.
9. HARRIS, E.N. & M. KHAMASHTA. 2004. Anticardiolipin test and the antiphospholipid (Hughes) syndrome: 20 years and counting! J. Rheumatol. **31:** 2099–2101.
10. ROSOVE, M.H. & P.M. BREWER. 1992. Antiphospholipid thrombosis: clinical course after the first thrombotic event in 70 patients. Ann. Intern. Med. **117:** 303–308.
11. KNRIC-BARRIE, S., C.R. O'CONNOR, S.W. LOONEY, *et al.* 1997. A retrospective review of 61 patients with antiphospholipid syndrome. Analysis of factors influencing recurrent thrombosis. Arch. Intern. Med. **157:** 2101–2108.
12. MUÑOZ-RODRÍGUEZ, F.J., J. FONT, R. CERVERA, *et al.* 1999. Clinical study and follow-up of 100 patients with the antiphospholipid syndrome. Semin. Arthritis Rheum. **29:** 182–190.
13. ERKAN, D., Y. YAZICI, R. SOBEL & M.D. LOCKSHIN. 2000. Primary antiphospholipid syndrome: functional outcome after 10 years. J. Rheumatol. **27:** 2817–2821.
14. WILSON, W.A., A.E. GHARAVI, T. KOIKE, *et al.* 1999. International consensus statement on preliminary classification criteria for definite antiphospholipid syndrome: report of an international workshop. Arthritis Rheum. **42:** 1309–1311.
15. SHAH, N.M., M.A. KHAMASHTA, T. ATSUMI & G.R. HUGHES. 1998. Outcome of patients with anticardiolipin antibodies: a 10 year follow-up of 52 patients. Lupus **7:** 3–6.
16. KHAMASHTA, M.A., M.J. CUADRADO, F. MUJIC, *et al.* 1995. The management of thrombosis in the antiphospholipid-antibody syndrome. N. Engl. J. Med. **332:** 993–997.
17. CERVERA, R., J.C. PIETTE, J. FONT, *et al.* 2002. Antiphospholipid syndrome: clinical and immunologic manifestations and patterns of disease expression in a cohort of 1,000 patients. Arthritis Rheum. **46:** 1019–1027.
18. ASHERSON, R.A., M.A. KHAMASHTA, J. ORDI-ROS, *et al.* 1989. The "primary" antiphospholipid syndrome: major clinical and serological features. Medicine (Balt.) **68:** 366–374.
19. ALARCON-SEGOVIA, D. & J. SANCHEZ-GUERRERO. 1989. Primary antiphospholipid syndrome. J. Rheumatol. **16:** 482–488.
20. ASHERSON, R.A. & R. CERVERA. 2003. Unusual manifestations of the antiphospholipid syndrome. Clin. Rev. Allergy Immunol. **25:** 61–78.
21. SHOENFELD, Y. & M. BLANK. 2004. Autoantibodies associated with reproductive failure. Lupus **13:** 643–648.
22. FINAZZI, G., V. BRANCACCIO, M. MOIA, *et al.* 1996. Natural history and risk factors for thrombosis in 360 patients with antiphospholipid antibodies: a four-year prospective study from the Italian Registry. Am. J. Med. **100:** 530–536.
23. GEORGE, J., M. BLANK, Y. LEVY, *et al.* 1998. Differential effects of anti-β2-glycoprotein I antibodies on endothelial cells and on the manifestations of experimental antiphospholipid syndrome. Circulation **97:** 900–906.

24. ALARCÓN-SEGOVIA, D., M.H. CARDIEL & E. REYES. 1989. Antiphospholipid arterial vasculopathy. J. Rheumatol. **16:** 762–767.
25. SALMON, J.E. & G. GIRARDI. 2004. The role of complement in the antiphospholipid syndrome. Curr. Dir. Autoimmun. **7:** 133–148.
26. BERMAN, J., G. GIRARDI & J.E. SALMON. 2005. TNF-alpha is a critical effector and a target for therapy in antiphospholipid antibody-induced pregnancy loss. J. Immunol. **174:** 485–490.
27. MEDINA, G., D. CASAOS, L.J. JARA, *et al.* 2003. Increased carotid artery intima-media thickness may be associated with stroke in primary antiphospholipid syndrome. Ann. Rheum. Dis. **62:** 607–610.
28. JARA, L.J., G. MEDINA, O. VERA-LASTRA & Y. SHOENFELD. 2003. Atherosclerosis and antiphospholipid syndrome. Clin. Rev. Allergy Immunol. **25:** 79–88.
29. ALARCON, G.S., G. MCGWIN, JR., J.M. ROSEMAN, *et al.* 2004. Systemic lupus erythematosus in three ethnic groups. XIX. Natural history of the accrual of the American College of Rheumatology criteria prior to the occurrence of criteria diagnosis. Arthritis Rheum. **51:** 609–615.
30. OLLIER, W.E., B. HARRISON, D. SYMMONS. 2001. What is the natural history of rheumatoid arthritis? Best Pract. Res. Clin. Rheumatol. **15:** 27–48.

OxLDL/β2GPI Complexes and Autoantibodies in Patients with Systemic Lupus Erythematosus, Systemic Sclerosis, and Antiphospholipid Syndrome

Pathogenic Implications for Vascular Involvement

LUIS R. LOPEZ,[a] DANIEL F. SIMPSON,[a] BETH L. HURLEY,[a] AND EIJI MATSUURA[b]

[a]*Corgenix Inc., Westminster, Colorado 80234, USA*

[b]*Okayama University Graduate School of Medicine and Dentistry, Okayama 700-8558, Japan*

ABSTRACT: **Oxidized low-density lipoprotein (oxLDL) interacts with β2GPI, forming oxLDL/β2GPI complexes. Autoimmune vascular inflammation (and oxidative stress) may promote the formation of these complexes. The coexistence of oxLDL/β2GPI complexes with autoantibodies to these complexes suggests an active pro-atherogenic role in vascular thrombosis and atherosclerosis. Immunoglobulin G (IgG) anti-oxLDL/β2GPI antibodies have been regarded as pro-atherogenic, whereas IgM antibodies are thought to be anti-atherogenic. For this study, oxLDL/β2GPI complexes, IgG, and IgM anti-oxLDL/β2GPI antibodies were measured using enzyme-linked immunosorbent assay (ELISA). Measurements were taken in two patient groups: (1) those with systemic lupus erythematosus (SLE), systemic sclerosis (SSc), and rheumatoid arthritis (RA); and (2) those with primary and secondary antiphospholipid syndrome (APS). For oxLDL/β2GPI complexes, SLE and SSc patients had the highest mean optical densities (ODs) (*P* <.001), followed by RA (*P* = .139) and healthy controls. IgG anti-oxLDL/β2GPI antibody distribution followed the same pattern observed with oxLDL/β2GPI complexes, SLE and SSc (*P* <.001), RA (*P* = .08), and controls. IgM antibodies showed a reverse pattern, with the highest mean OD in RA (*P* <.001), followed by SSc (*P* = .007) and SLE (*P* = 143). Both IgG and IgM anti-oxLDL/β2GPI antibodies were significantly higher in secondary APS patients compared with SLE controls without APS. In addition, the highest mean OD and prevalence of IgG anti-oxLDL/β2GPI antibodies were observed in APS patients with a history of arterial thrombosis. These results may reflect the widespread vascular involvement seen in SLE and SSc, in contrast to the relatively low vascular involvement in RA. In SLE and SSc, high serum levels and prevalence of circulating oxLDL/β2GPI complexes and IgG anti-oxLDL/β2GPI antibodies indicate significant vascular oxidative stress as well as a possible pathogenic role in autoimmune-mediated atherosclerosis.**

Address for correspondence: Luis R. Lopez, M.D., Corgenix Inc., 12061 Tejon Street, Westminster, Colorado 80234. Voice: 303-457-4345; fax: 303-457-4519.
llopez@corgenix.com

**Ann. N.Y. Acad. Sci. 1051: 313–322 (2005). © 2005 New York Academy of Sciences.
doi: 10.1196/annals.1361.073**

KEYWORDS: autoimmunity; antiphospholipid syndrome; atherosclerosis; oxidized low-density lipoprotein; β2-glycoprotein I; systemic lupus erythematosus; systemic sclerosis; rheumatoid arthritis

INTRODUCTION

The accelerated (or premature) occurrence of atherosclerosis in patients with systemic lupus erythematosus (SLE) is associated with significant cardiovascular morbidity and mortality.[1] Because atherosclerosis in SLE could not be fully explained by traditional risk factors for cardiovascular disease or by therapeutic intervention, the participation of disease-specific factors such as autoantibodies has been proposed.[2,3] The presence of oxidized low-density lipoprotein (oxLDL) and beta-2 glycoprotein-I (β2GPI), along with immunoreactive cells in human atherosclerotic plaques,[4] has suggested that autoimmune mechanisms play a direct role in the development of foam cells and atherosclerotic lesions.

Lipid peroxidation (oxidative stress) modifies LDL into oxidized forms. This process is thought to play a central role in the initiation and progression of atherosclerosis.[5] OxLDL triggers the production of pro-inflammatory and chemotactic factors, favoring the accumulation of immunoreactive cells (macrophages and lymphocytes) in the arterial wall.[6] Autoimmune vascular inflammation may alter antioxidant regulatory mechanisms, thereby contributing to oxidative stress and oxLDL formation.

OxLDL binds β2GPI via LDL-derived ligands (oxLig-1) to form stable (or nondissociable) and possibly pathogenic oxLDL/β2GPI complexes *in vitro*.[7,8] These complexes have been detected in patients with systemic autoimmune diseases that have vascular complications (i.e., SLE and antiphospholipid syndrome [APS]) and have been implicated as atherogenic autoantigens.[9] Immunoglobulin G (IgG) antibodies to oxLDL/β2GPI complexes have also been demonstrated in SLE patients with secondary APS and have shown a strong association with arterial thrombosis.[10,11] We now report on the presence of oxLDL/β2GPI complexes and IgG and IgM antibodies to these complexes in patients with systemic sclerosis (SSc; also known as scleroderma), another systemic autoimmune disease characterized by generalized vascular complications.

MATERIAL AND METHODS

Subjects

Serum samples were obtained from two patient populations. One consisted of 224 consecutive patients: 86 with SLE, 59 with SSc, and 79 with rheumatoid arthritis (RA). Serum from 100 healthy blood donors served as controls. A second patient population included in the study consisted of 74 selected SLE patients, 29 with a history of APS and 45 without one. These patients were used to study the relation between oxLDL/β2GPI antibodies and APS.

An additional 93 selected APS patients were used to study the relation between oxLDL/β2GPI antibodies and clinical manifestations of APS. Twenty of these patients had primary APS and 73 had secondary APS. Forty-two had a history of an arterial thrombotic event, 37 of venous thrombosis, and 14 of pregnancy morbidity. A diagnosis of APS was established according to the Sapporo criteria.[12]

ELISA for oxLDL/β2GPI Complexes

Murine IgG monoclonal antibodies against human β2GPI (WB-CAL-1) were coated onto Nunc MaxiSorp 96-MicroWell Plates (Nunc, Denmark). WB-CAL-1 monoclonal antibodies used in this assay bind only oxLDL/β2GPI complexes, but not free β2GPI.[7] Diluted serum samples in diluent containing 10 mM $MgCl_2$ were added to the coated microwells and incubated for 1 hour at room temperature. $MgCl_2$ dissociates intermediate or electrostatically bound oxLDL/β2GPI complexes, enabling the specific detection of nondissociable or stable covalently bound complexes, if the latter are present in serum samples.

Horseradish peroxidase (HRP)–conjugated anti-human Apo B100 murine monoclonal antibody (2E10) was added to the microwells and incubated for an additional hour. Color was developed with tetramethylbenzydine (TMB)/H_2O_2, and the reaction was stopped with 0.36N sulfuric acid. Optical density (OD) was read at a wavelength of 450 nm (650-nm reference). The reactivity of the assay was assessed with a curve built with oxLDL/β2GPI complex solution. The complexes were prepared in advance by incubating equal amounts of Cu^{2+}-oxLDL and purified human β2GPI. A normal cutoff value for the assay was established by testing serum samples from healthy blood donors (mean + 3 standard deviations).

ELISA for IgG and IgM Anti-oxLDL/β2GPI Antibodies

OxLDL/β2GPI complexes, prepared by incubating equal amounts of Cu^{2+}-oxLDL and purified human β2GPI, were coated onto Immunlon 1B 96-microwell plates (Dynex Technologies Inc., Chantilly, Virginia). These oxLDL/β2GPI complexes served as antigenic substrates to capture patients' antibodies. Diluted serum samples were added to the microwells and incubated for 1 hour at room temperature. HRP-conjugated anti-human IgG (or IgM) antibody was added to the microwells and incubated for 1 hour. Color was developed with TMB/H_2O_2 and the reaction was stopped with 0.36N sulfuric acid. OD was read at a wavelength of 450 nm (650 nm reference). The reactivity of the assay was evaluated with a curve built with serial dilutions of selected positive sera for IgG or IgM anti-oxLDL/β2GPI antibodies. A normal cutoff value for the assay was established by testing serum samples from healthy blood donors (mean + 3 standard deviations).

RESULTS

OxLDL/β2GPI Complexes in Consecutive Autoimmune Disease Patients

The mean ODs for SLE (0.851 ± 0.914) and SSc (0.504 ± 0.386) patients were significantly higher than the mean OD for healthy controls (0.061 ± 0.018; $P < .001$). The mean OD for RA patients (0.058 ± 0.023) was not statistically different from that of healthy controls ($P = .139$) (FIG. 1). Seventy-two percent of SLE and 95% of SSc patients reacted above the cutoff limit of the oxLDL/β2GPI complex assay (OD = 0.115). In contrast, only 1% of RA patients had positive levels of oxLDL/

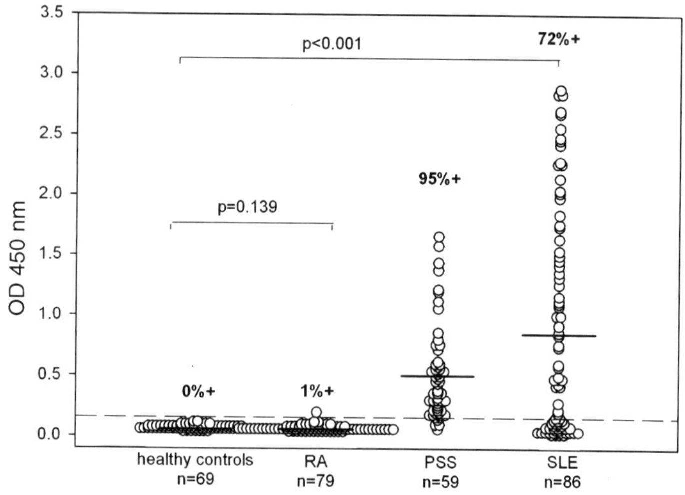

FIGURE 1. Serum levels of oxLDL/β2GPI complexes measured by ELISA in consecutive autoimmune disease patients (SLE, SSc, and RA) and healthy controls. The *horizontal broken line* represents the cutoff OD value of the assay (mean + 3 SD of 100 healthy controls). *Solid lines* represent the mean OD of each group. *P* value (Mann-Whitney rank test) of <.05 was deemed significant.

β2GPI complexes. Because serum levels of oxLDL/β2GPI complexes do not correlate with the presence or absence of APS or with any clinical manifestation of APS, this association was not evaluated further.[10,11]

IgG and IgM Anti-oxLDL/β2GPI Antibodies in Consecutive Autoimmune Patients

For IgG anti-oxLDL/β2GPI antibodies, SLE patients had the highest mean OD (0.235 ± 0.226), followed by RA patients (0.185 ± 0.210), SSc patients (0.177 ± 0.061), and healthy controls (0.135 ± 0.034) (FIG. 2). Both SLE and SSc patients' mean ODs were significantly higher than those of controls ($P < .001$). Thirty percent of SLE patients, 20% of SSc patients, 18% of RA patients, and 1% of the controls reacted above the cutoff level of the assay (OD = 0.241).

For IgM anti-oxLDL/β2GPI antibodies, the distribution pattern was altered. RA patients had the highest mean OD (0.516 ± 0.399), followed by SSc patients (0.279 ± 0.255), SLE patients (0.240 ± 0.224), and healthy controls (0.178 ± 0.129). The mean IgM antibody levels for RA patients (P <.001) and SSc patients ($P = .007$) were significantly different from those of healthy controls, whereas the mean IgM for SLE was not ($P = .143$).

The possibility that the assay was detecting IgM rheumatoid factor (RF) in patients with RA was investigated. An IgM RF reference preparation (Centers for Disease Control, Atlanta, Georgia) did not react (OD <0.197) when tested on the assay at 200, 100, and 50 U/mL dilutions, and IgM anti-oxLDL/β2GPI antibody levels did not correlate with the RF titers ($r = .046$) in this group of RA patients.

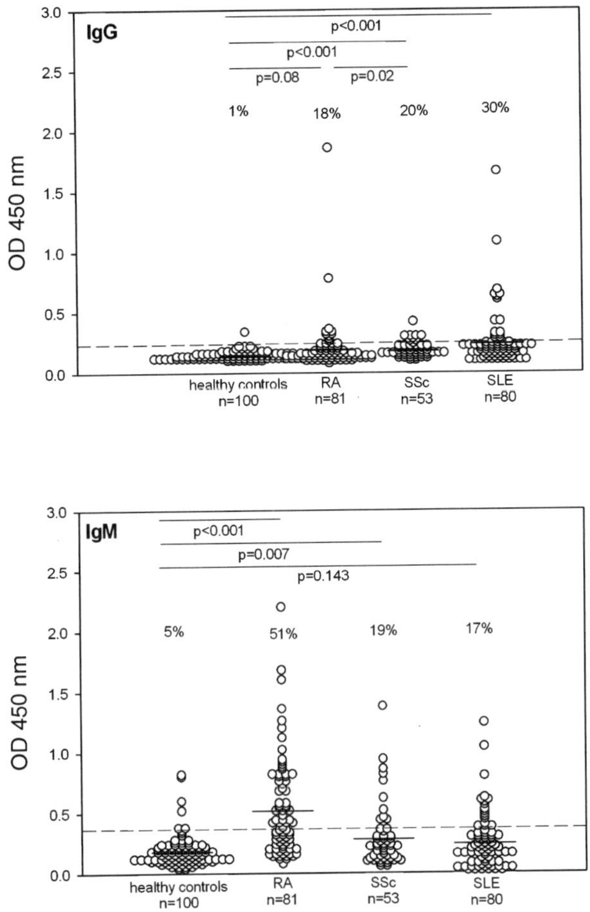

FIGURE 2. Serum levels of IgG and IgM anti-oxLDL/β2GPI antibodies measured by ELISA in consecutive autoimmune disease patients (SLE, SSc, and RA) and healthy controls. The *horizontal broken line* represents the cutoff OD value of the assay (mean + 3 SD of 100 healthy controls). *Solid lines* represent the mean OD of each group. *P* value (Mann-Whitney rank test) of <.05 was deemed significant.

IgG and IgM Anti-oxLDL/β2GPI Antibodies in APS Patients

For IgG anti-oxLDL/β2GPI antibodies, the mean OD for SLE patients with APS (0.521 ± 0.568) was significantly higher than that of SLE patients without APS (0.251 ± 0.069; *P* <.001) (FIG. 3). Seventy-five percent of SLE patients with APS had positive antibody levels compared with 37% of SLE patients without APS. The clinical performance of IgG anti-oxLDL/β2GPI antibodies was compared with IgG anticardiolipin (aCL) antibodies to predict APS in these SLE patients (2 × 2 contingency table analysis). IgG anti-oxLDL/β2GPI antibodies were found to be 45% sensitive and 93.7% specific for APS, with a predictive value of 90% (P <.001). IgG aCL antibodies were 62.5% sensitive and 80% specific, with a predictive value of 71.4% (P <.001).

For IgM anti-oxLDL/β2GPI antibodies, a similar distribution pattern to that of IgG antibodies was observed. The mean OD among SLE patients with APS (0.684 ± 0.709) was significantly higher than that of SLE patients without APS (0.265 ± 0.150; P = .007) (FIG. 3). Forty-one percent of SLE patients with APS had positive antibody levels compared with 20% of SLE patients without APS. The predictive value of IgM anti-oxLDL/β2GPI antibodies for APS was only 75%.

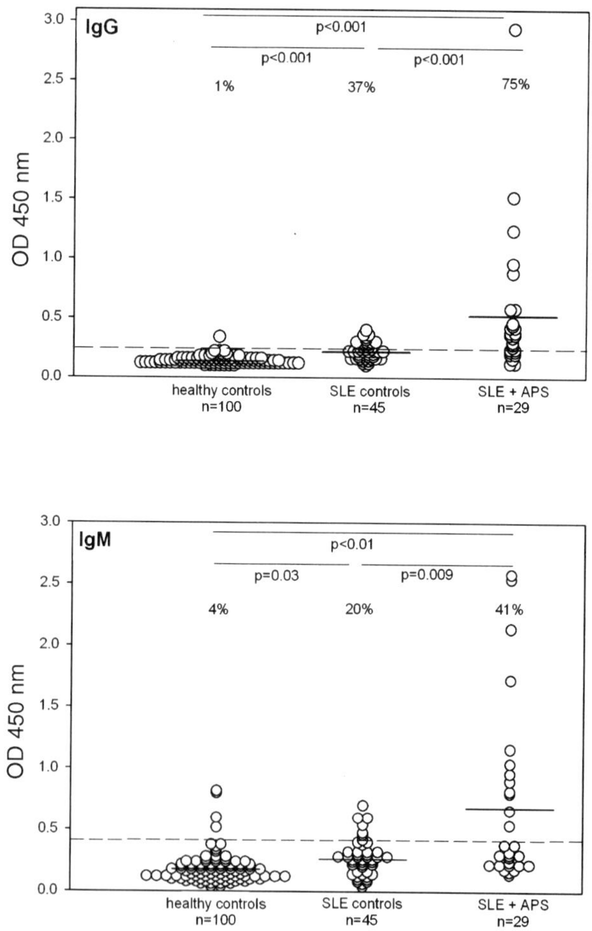

FIGURE 3. Serum levels of IgG and IgM anti-oxLDL/β2GPI antibodies measured by ELISA in patients with SLE and APS compared with SLE patients without a history of APS and healthy controls. The *horizontal broken line* represents the cutoff OD value of the assay (mean + 3 SD of 100 healthy controls). *Solid lines* represent the mean OD of each group. P value (Mann-Whitney Rank test) of <.05 was deemed significant.

A population of 93 selected APS patients was classified into subgroups according to clinical history of venous thrombosis, arterial thrombosis, and pregnancy morbidity. For IgG anti-oxLDL/β2GPI antibodies, the mean OD among APS patients with a history of arterial thrombosis was 0.802 ± 1.084, with 38% reacting above the cutoff limit. For APS patients with a history of venous thrombosis, OD was 0.544 ± 0.932, with 19% reacting above the cutoff. For APS patients with a history of pregnancy morbidity, OD was 0.137 ± 0.092, with none reacting above the cutoff (FIG. 4). The difference between the subgroups with arterial and venous thrombosis did not reach statistical significance (P = .262).

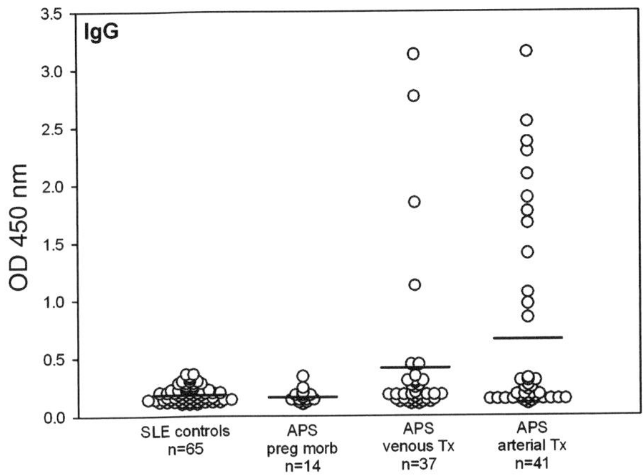

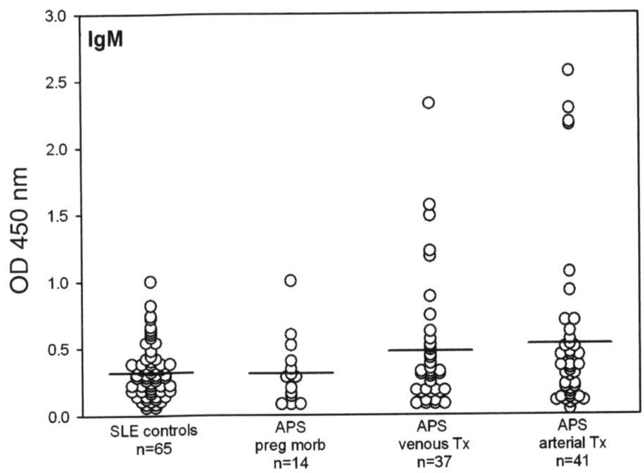

FIGURE 4. Serum levels of IgG and IgM anti-oxLDL/β2GPI antibodies, measured by ELISA in APS patients classified according to history of arterial, venous thrombosis, or pregnancy morbidity. SLE patients without a history of APS served as controls. *Solid horizontal lines* represent the mean OD of each group. P value (Mann-Whitney Rank test) of <.05 was deemed significant.

The clinical performance of IgG anti-oxLDL/β2GPI antibodies to predict thrombosis (arterial and venous, arterial only, or venous only) in these APS patients was studied (2×2 contingency table analysis). The predictive value of IgG anti-oxLDL/β2GPI antibodies for total (arterial and venous) thrombosis was 92% ($P = .018$), for arterial thrombosis 89% ($P = .004$), and for venous thrombosis 77% ($P = .168$).

For IgM anti-oxLDL/β2GPI antibodies, the mean OD for APS patients with a history of arterial thrombosis was 0.523 ± 0.633, with 39% reacting above the cutoff. For APS patients with a history of venous thrombosis, OD was 0.489 ± 0.501, with 38% reacting above the cutoff, and for patients with a history of pregnancy morbidity, OD was 0.310 ± 0.256, with 28% reacting above the cutoff (FIG. 4). No statistical differences were found when the subgroups were compared.

DISCUSSION

These results demonstrate significantly higher serum levels of oxLDL/β2GPI complexes in a population of consecutive patients with SLE and SSc compared with RA patients and healthy controls. We have previously shown that high serum levels of oxLDL/β2GPI complexes are frequent in SLE patients with vascular complications and proposed that these complexes play a pathogenic role in autoimmune-mediated thrombosis and atherosclerosis.[8,9] This is the first report describing oxLDL/β2GPI complexes in patients with SSc. Unlike RA, both SLE and SSc are characterized by generalized vascular complications.

Increased lipid peroxidation (oxidative stress), assessed by urinary isoprostane-$F_{2\alpha}$ production and decreased antioxidant activity of the enzyme paraoxonase (PON), has been reported in patients with SLE and APS.[13–15] Augmented susceptibility to Cu^{2+} LDL oxidation and increased isoprostane-$F_{2\alpha}$ production in SSc patients has also been reported.[16,17] Furthermore, *in vivo* markers of oxidation, measured in various systemic autoimmune diseases, have shown that SLE patients have the highest degree of oxidation, followed by SSc patients, RA patients, and healthy controls.[18] However, in the present study, the degree of oxidation in RA patients was similar to that found in healthy controls. If serum levels of oxLDL/β2GPI complexes are an indication of oxidative stress, our results correspond to the degree of autoimmune *in vivo* oxidation.[18] Widespread, chronic autoimmune vascular inflammation, together with decreased PON activity, may contribute to oxidative stress, LDL modification (oxLDL), and oxLDL/β2GPI complex formation. However, the exact mechanism(s) for vascular inflammation that triggers oxidative stress in patients with SSc remains to be identified.

OxLDL/β2GPI complexes may indeed function as atherogenic antigens.[8,9] In SLE and SSc patients, IgG anti-oxLDL/β2GPI antibodies were significantly higher than those in RA patients and healthy controls. These antibodies were also significantly higher among SLE patients with secondary APS, showing a predictive value for APS of 90%, whereas IgG aCL antibodies had a predictive value of only 71.4%. APS patients with arterial and venous thrombosis also had higher IgG antibody levels than did either patients with a history of pregnancy morbidity or SLE controls without APS. The predictive value of IgG anti-oxLDL/β2GPI antibodies for arterial thrombosis was 89%, better than the 77% value for venous thrombosis.

The distribution of IgM anti-oxLDL/β2GPI antibodies was different (opposite) from that of IgG antibodies, with higher levels in RA patients and lower levels in SLE patients. In patients with RA, the nature of the antigen that induces IgM antibody production in the absence of oxLDL/β2GPI complexes is puzzling. One possible explanation for this phenomenon is that IgM antibodies cross-react with oxLDL/β2GPI complexes. Another possibility is that natural antibodies (IgM isotype) may be anti-atherogenic,[19] so their absence (or decreased levels) may indirectly facilitate the development of atherosclerosis. Consistent with these findings, a negative association between IgM anti-oxLDL antibodies and atherosclerosis has been reported in healthy individuals.[20] Although some APS patients had both IgG and IgM antibodies, it is likely that the pro-atherogenic IgG overcomes IgM's protective effect.

Atherosclerotic plaque formation in autoimmune diseases requires the uptake by macrophages of immune complexes (e.g., oxLDL/β2GPI/IgG). In this study, the *in vitro* macrophage uptake of oxLDL/β2GPI complexes increased in the presence of anti-β2GPI antibodies, implying the participation of Fcγ receptors.[21] We also used enzyme-linked immunosorbent assay (ELISA) to test for IgG- and IgM-containing oxLDL/β2GPI immune complexes and found similar results to those of IgG and IgM anti-oxLDL/β2GPI antibodies.

It is possible that other autoantibodies further enhance platelet and endothelial activation. These antibodies would be produced by unidentified antigenic complexes created during chronic oxidative stress. Along with them, a range of metabolic and inflammatory abnormalities would result in severe autoimmune-mediated atherothrombotic disease.

Our results suggest that oxLDL/β2GPI complexes, and autoantibodies to these complexes, not only play a pathogenic role, but also may be used as serologic markers to assess a patient's risk for vascular complications. In addition, these results provide a rationale for developing vascular disease prevention programs and/or more targeted therapeutic interventions.

COMPETING INTEREST: Luis R. Lopez is CEO of Corgenix, Inc., a manufacturer of ELISA test kits.

REFERENCES

1. WARD, M.M. 1999. Premature morbidity from cardiovascular and cerebrovascular diseases in women with systemic lupus erythematosus. Arthritis Rheum. **42:** 338–346.
2. ESDAILE, J.M., M. ABRAHAMOWICZ, T. GRODZICKY, *et al.* 2001. Traditional Framingham risk factors fail to fully account for accelerated atherosclerosis in systemic lupus erythematosus. Arthritis Rheum. **44:** 2331–2337.
3. ROMAN, M.J., B.A. SHANKER, A. DAVIS, *et al.* 2003. Prevalence and correlates of accelerated atherosclerosis in systemic lupus erythematosus. N. Engl. J. Med. **349:** 2399–2406.
4. GEORGE, J., D. HARATS, B. GILBURD, *et al.* 1999. Immunolocalization of β2-glycoprotein I (apolipoprotein H) to human atherosclerotic plaques: potential implications for lesion progression. Circulation **99:** 2227–2230.
5. STEINBERG, D. 1997. Low density lipoprotein oxidation and its pathobiological significance. J. Biol. Chem. **272:** 20963–20966.
6. STEINBERG, D. 2002. Atherogenesis in perspective: hypercholesterolemia and inflammation as partners in crime. Nat. Med. **8:** 1211–1217.
7. KOBAYASHI, K., M. KISHI, T. ATSUMI, *et al.* 2003. Circulating oxidized LDL forms complexes with β2-glycoprotein I: implication as an atherogenic autoantigen. J. Lipid Res. **44:** 716–726.

8. MATSUURA, E., K. KOBAYASHI, T. KOIKE, *et al.* 2003. Atherogenic autoantigen: oxidized LDL complexes with β2-glycoprotein I. Immunobiol. **207:** 17–22.
9. MATSUURA, E. & L.R. LOPEZ. 2004. Are oxidized LDL/β2-glycoprotein I complexes pathogenic antigens in autoimmune-mediated atherosclerosis? Clin. Dev. Immunol. **11:** 103–111.
10. LOPEZ, D., I. GARCIA-VALLADARES, C.A. PALAFOX-SANCHEZ, *et al.* 2004. Oxidized low-density lipoprotein/β2-glycoprotein I complexes and autoantibodies to oxLig-1/β2-glycoprotein I in patients with systemic lupus erythematosus and antiphospholipid syndrome. Am. J. Clin. Pathol. **121:** 426–436.
11. LOPEZ, D., K. KOBAYASHI, J.T. MERRILL, *et al.* 2003. IgG autoantibodies against β2-glycoprotein I complexed with a lipid ligand derived from oxidized low-density lipoprotein are associated with arterial thrombosis in antiphospholipid syndrome. Clin. Dev. Immunol. **10:** 203–211.
12. WILSON, W.A., A.E. GHARAVI, T. KOIKE, *et al.* 1999. International consensus statement on preliminary classification criteria for definite antiphospholipid syndrome: report of an international workshop. Arthritis Rheum. **42:** 1309–1311.
13. AMES, P.R.J., J. ALVES, I. MURAT, *et al.* 1999. Oxidative stress in systemic lupus erythematosus and allied conditions with vascular involvement. Rheumatology (Oxf.) **38:** 529–534.
14. DELGADO ALVES, J., P.R.J. AMES, S. DONOHUE, *et al.* 2002. Antibodies to high-density lipoprotein and β2-glycoprotein I are inversely correlated with paraoxonase activity in systemic lupus erythematosus and primary antiphospholipid syndrome. Arthritis Rheum. **46:** 2686–2694.
15. FROSTEGARD, J., E. SVENUNGSSON, R. WU, *et al.* 2005. Lipid peroxidation is enhanced in patients with systemic lupus erythematosus and is associated with arterial and renal disease manifestations. Arthritis Rheum. **52:** 192–200.
16. BRUCKDORFER, K.R., J.B. HILLARY, T. BUNCE, *et al.* 1995. Increased susceptibility to oxidation of low-density lipoproteins isolated from patients with systemic sclerosis. Arthritis Rheum. **38:** 1060–1067.
17. STEIN, C.M., S.B. TANNER, J.A. AWAD, *et al.* 1996. Evidence of free radical–mediated injury (isoprostane overproduction) in scleroderma. Arthritis Rheum. **39:** 1146–1150.
18. BASU, S., M. WHITEMAN, D.L. MATTEY & B. HALLIWELL. 2001. Raised levels of F2-isoprostanes and prostaglandin $F2_{\alpha}$ in different rheumatic diseases. Ann. Rheum. Dis. **60:** 627–631.
19. BINDER, C.J., M.K. CHANG, P.X. SHAW, *et al.* 2002. Innate and acquired immunity in atherogenesis. Nat. Med. **8:** 1218–1226.
20. HULTHE, J., O. WIKLUND, E. HURT-CAMEJO & G. BONDJERS. 2001. Antibodies to oxidized LDL in relation to carotid atherosclerosis, cell adhesion molecules, and phospholipase A(2). Arterioscler. Thromb. Vasc. Biol. **21:** 269–274.
21. LIU, Q., K. KOBAYASHI, J. FURUKAWA, *et al.* 2002. ω-carboxyl variants of 7-ketocholesteryl esters are ligands for β2-glycoprotein I and mediate antibody-dependent uptake of oxidized LDL by macrophages. J. Lipid Res. **43:** 1486–1495.

Anti-HSP60 Immunity Is Already Associated with Atherosclerosis Early in Life

M. KNOFLACH,[a,b] D. BERNHARD,[a] AND G. WICK[a]

[a]*Division of Experimental Pathophysiology and Immunology, Biocenter, Innsbruck Medical University, Innsbruck, Austria*

[b]*University Hospital for Neurology, 6020 Innsbruck, Austria*

ABSTRACT: In this review, we first briefly introduce the reader to our autoimmune hypothesis for the development of atherosclerosis based on experimental and clinical data. This hypothesis postulates that humoral and cellular immunity against heat-shock protein 60 (HSP60), a phylogenetically highly conserved stress protein, is the mechanism that initiates atherogenesis. We then turn to our investigations of arterial specimens from children and young adults. These clearly show that mononuclear cell infiltrations of the intimal layer already occur before the emergence of clear-cut atherosclerotic lesions, a phenomenon we have termed *vascular-associated lymphoid tissue* (VALT). In early lesions analyzed within the framework of the Pathological Determinants of Atherosclerosis in Youth (PDAY) study, T lymphocytes proved to be a major cellular constituent. In the Bruneck Study, a large, prospective atherosclerosis-prevention study in adults aged 40 years and older, we found a highly significant correlation between serum anti-HSP60 antibody titers and the occurrence and extent of sonographically demonstrable atherosclerotic lesions. However, no such correlation emerged with respect to HSP60-reactive T cells in the peripheral blood. In contrast, the similar Atherosclerosis Risk-Factors in Male Youngsters (ARMY) study, performed on 17- to 18-year-old volunteers, showed a highly statistically significant correlation between arterial intima-media thickening and HSP60 reactivity among peripheral T cells and (less pronounced) anti-HSP60 antibodies, even at this young age. We take this as indirect evidence that both T cell and B cell immunity against HSP60 plays a major role in the earliest stages of the disease. Because VALT can already be observed in healthy children and young adults, we hypothesize that T cells initiate the disease and that humoral antibodies play a facilitating, accelerating role. Finally, we provide initial evidence that smoking, as the most important risk factor for atherogenesis, also exerts its disease-inducing and disease-promoting effects by inducing HSP60 expression by vascular endothelial cells.

KEYWORDS: atherogenesis; early atherosclerosis; autoimmunity; cardiovascular disease; infection; heat-shock protein 60; T cells; smoking; aging

Address for correspondence: Georg Wick, M.D., Professor and Director, Division of Experimental Pathophysiology and Immunology, Biocenter, Innsbruck Medical University, Fritz-Pregl-Strasse 3/IV, 6020 Innsbruck, Austria. Voice: +43-512-507-3100; fax: +43-512-507-2867.
georg.wick@uibk.ac.at

**Ann. N.Y. Acad. Sci. 1051: 323–331 (2005). © 2005 New York Academy of Sciences.
doi: 10.1196/annals.1361.074**

BACKGROUND

Cardiovascular diseases (CVDs) are the leading cause of death in the industrialized world. Although in clinical practice young victims of CVD seem few compared with the vast number of elderly who experience myocardial infarction or stroke, CVDs are already the leading cause of death in young adults aged 21–30 in these societies.[1] The large-scale postmortem and histopathologic Pathological Determinants of Atherosclerosis in Youth (PDAY) study and *in vivo* studies demonstrate that classic cardiovascular risk factors such as smoking, hypertension, or dyslipidemia are already important in this age group.[2–4]

A hypothesis that was initially formulated more than a century ago can now be considered firmly established: inflammation, in general, and the immune system, in particular, do play an important role in atherogenesis. Virchow, a 19th century German pathologist, described atherosclerosis as an inflammatory disorder based on the presence of mononuclear cells in atherosclerotic lesions.[5] In the early 20th century, Osler reintroduced this idea to the scientific community,[6] and more recently, Fabricant and colleagues provided the first experimental evidence that viral infections promote atherogenesis.[7] In the last 20 years, numerous publications have established inflammatory markers and chronic infections as risk factors for atherosclerosis.[8–11] However, most of these studies have concentrated on late stages and clinical end points of atherosclerosis, such as death from cardiovascular disorders. Comparatively little is known about the role of inflammation and the immune system in early atherogenesis. Therefore, this latter issue is the main focus of our work in this area.

PATHOPHYSIOLOGY OF ATHEROSCLEROSIS

Vascular-Associated Lymphoid Tissue

Infiltration of a healthy arterial intima (the innermost layer of the vessel wall) with mononuclear cells can be demonstrated in healthy juvenile vessels. This process takes place predominantly at arterial branching points and other vascular sites exposed to excessive mechanical (turbulent) stress. In a surprising observation made exclusively on immunohistologic grounds, our group recently characterized a network of dendritic cells in the arterial intima interlaced with lymphocytes (mostly activated T cells), macrophages, and mast cells. Analogous to what is termed mucosa-associated lymphoid tissue (MALT) of the gut, we called this accumulation of mononuclear cells in the arterial intima the *vascular-associated lymphoid tissue* (VALT).[12] When looking at the early lesions found in the PDAY study specimens (taken from 15- to 30-year-olds), mononuclear cell infiltrates were demonstrated in every single vessel segment. Here, too, activated T cells were the predominant cell type.[13] So far, the specificity of these T cells is not yet known. However, an oligoclonal origin of these cells has been demonstrated in early murine lesions[14] but not in late developing human lesions.[15]

Heat-Shock Proteins

Heat-shock proteins (HSPs) are stress proteins that are either constitutively expressed or induced in response to various environmental stress factors, such as heat (hence the name), mechanical stress, oxidants, and various cytokines.[16] Apart from their physiologic functions in the cell cycle, protein folding and intracellular transport, they act as chaperones under stressful conditions, protecting other proteins from denaturation.[17] HSPs are classified according to their molecular weight in subgroups: from less than 10 kD to 90–100 kD.

In rabbit experiments, HSP60 was first identified as the culprit autoantigen for the initiation of atherosclerosis.[18] Upon depletion of HSP60 immunized rabbits from mononuclear cells in the peripheral blood, this effect could be prevented.[19] Later, similar results were obtained in low-density lipoprotein (LDL)–receptor-deficient mice.[20] In this experimental setting, inducing tolerance by oral or nasal administration of recombinant HSP60 reduced lesion size.[21,22]

In the mouse model, immunity against HSPs is carried by B cells and T cells. Researchers have observed that the transfer of immunoglobulin G (IgG) or lymph-node cells (predominantly T cells) or splenocytes (predominantly B cells) from immunized mice to non-immunized littermates all enhanced atherosclerotic lesion formation.[23]

In vitro studies (mostly on human endothelial cells and macrophages) have shown that endogenous human HSP60 is produced upon stress (heat, cytokine, or oxidant), transported from the mitochondria into the cytosol, and expressed on the cell surface.[24–26]

AUTOIMMUNE HYPOTHESIS OF ATHEROSCLEROSIS

Based on the evidence reviewed above, we formulated our Autoimmune Hypothesis of Atherosclerosis,[27–29] as summarized in FIGURE 1.

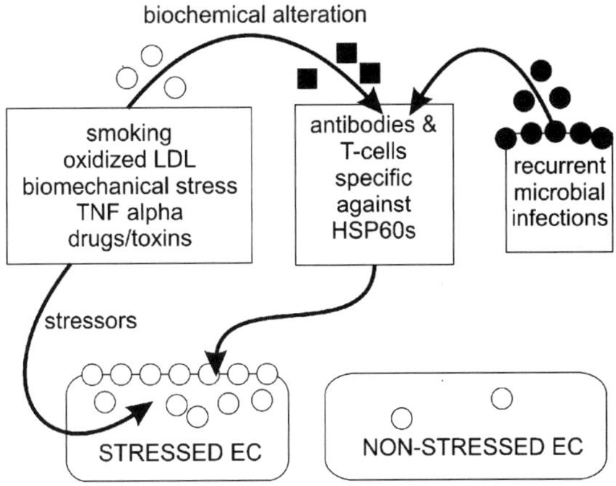

FIGURE 1. Antibodies and T cells that formed against microbial heat-shock protein 60 (HSP60, *filled circles*) owing to recurrent infections can cross-react with human HSP60 (*open circles*) expressed on stressed, but not on unstressed, endothelial cells (ECs). Stressors include biomechanical stress (e.g., hypertension and turbulent stress at vessel branching points), cytokines (such as tumor necrosis factor [TNF]–alpha) or even oxidized low-density lipoprotein (oxLDL). Some of these factors can chemically alter human HSP60 to become immunogenic (*filled squares*) and induce a bona fide autoimmune reaction.

Recurrent microbial infections activate the immune system, involving numerous specific antibodies and T cells against various antigens, among which HSP60 is also found. Because HSPs are highly conserved during evolution (bacterial and human HSP60 share more than 55% of their overall amino acid sequence[16]), this process leads to a cross-reaction between microbial and human HSP60s. Also, chemically altered autologous HSP60 leads to the formation of bona fide autoreactive antibodies and T cells.

As long as human endothelial cells are not stressed, they do not express a significant amount of HSP60 on their surface. However, *in vitro* experiments and histologic staining of human arterial walls have shown that different forms of stress (e.g., heat, tumor necrosis factor [TNF], turbulent biomechanical stress at arterial branching points, oxidized LDL) can lead to the presence of HSP60 on the cell surface.[24,30] In turn, the presence of HSP60 leads to an autoimmune reaction against the innermost vessel wall and to local inflammation of the artery. Adhesion molecules are simultaneously expressed, and mononuclear cells infiltrate the wall, predisposing it to more severe lesions, provided that the aforementioned classic risk factors continue to be present.

Evidence from the Bruneck Study

Although our main interest is in early atherosclerosis, we took the opportunity to participate in the prospective, population-based Bruneck Study for the prevention of carotid atherosclerosis.[31,32] In 1990, this study enrolled 1,000 men and women aged 40 and older and conducted follow-up examinations every 5 years. As just described, we had postulated a humoral and cellular cross-reaction of the immune system between human and bacterial HSP60. At baseline, the antibody titers against microbial HSP60 (in this study, mycobacterial HSP65) were higher in subjects with prevalent atherosclerotic plaques.[33] Five-year follow-up revealed not only that anti-HSP60 antibody titers remained constant over time, but also that they correlated with mortality due to cardiovascular diseases.[34] In the meantime, these results have been reproduced by numerous other groups (summarized in Wick *et al.*[29]).

Furthermore, the amount of soluble HSP60 (sHSP60) in the study population correlated with both prevalence and progression of atherosclerotic plaques.[35]

During the 2000 follow-up of the Bruneck Study participants, we selected a subsample of 50 males with sonographically demonstrable atherosclerosis and 50 without (at that time point, 50 years and older), isolated their blood lymphocytes, and challenged these cells *in vitro* with different kinds of microbial and human HSP60. As expected, a high correlation was seen between the proliferation of different HSP60s, yet no difference in the median stimulation index was seen between men with and those without atherosclerosis (data submitted for publication). However, because all of these subjects had late developing atherosclerotic lesions and we expected the immune reaction against HSPs to be important in early atherogenesis, the next logical step was to look at early atherosclerotic changes in young adults. In this context, our experience in the PDAY Study[13] and the discovery of VALT[12,36] were of great help.

Evidence from the ARMY Study

The Atherosclerosis Risk-Factors in Male Youngsters (ARMY) study[4] included 141 healthy 17- or 18-year-old male volunteers and applied a protocol established in the Bruneck Study.[31,32] Early atherosclerosis was evaluated by measuring the intima-media thickness (IMT), a good surrogate parameter for atherosclerotic load,[37] at eight sites in the peripheral vascular system. Within this young population, both the humoral and the cellular immune reactions against HSP60 emerged as significant predictors of early atherosclerotic wall thickening.[4] These results were independent of other classic cardiovascular risk factors (TABLE 1). Even in this young population, a high T-cell reaction against human HSP60 equaled the impact of smoking more than 20 cigarettes per day (FIG. 2).

TABLE 1. Stepwise logistic regression analysis of high intima-media thickness on potential cardiovascular risk factors

Variable	OR (95% CI)	*P* value
T cell reactivity against hHSP60	2.18 (1.32–3.60)	<0.01
Pulmonary function (MEF50)	0.52 (0.33–0.82)	<0.01
Smoking	3.58 (1.34–9.54)	<0.05
HDL cholesterol	0.56 (0.36–0.89)	<0.05
Antimicrobial HSP60 antibodies	1.52 (1.00–2.31)	<0.05
Alcohol consumption	0.51 (0.30–0.87)	<0.05
Diastolic blood pressure	1.61 (1.03–2.52)	<0.05

ABBREVIATIONS: HDL, high-density lipoprotein; hHSP60, human heat-shock protein 60; MEF50, maximum expiratory flow at 50% of vital capacity; OR, odds ratio; CI, confidence interval.

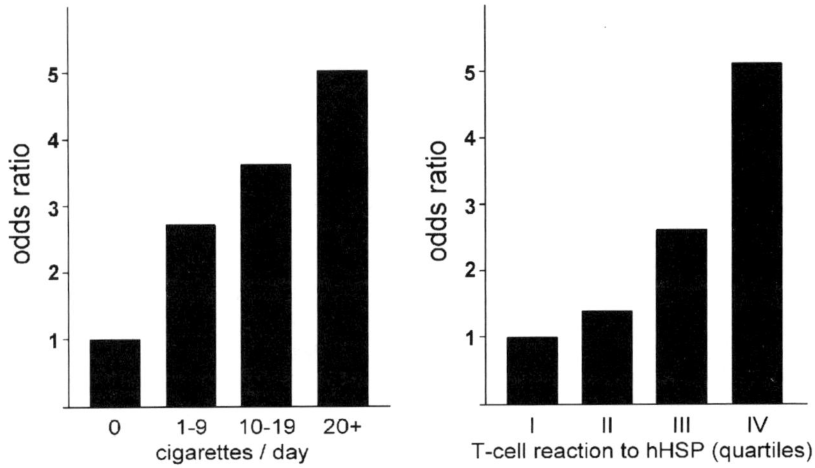

FIGURE 2. Dose-dependent rise in the risk for early atherosclerotic wall changes in clinically healthy 17- to 18-year-old males (results from the ARMY Study[4]). $P < 0.01$ for linear trend.

CONCLUSIONS

Humoral Immunity against HSP60 Is an Important Factor in Atherosclerosis

In summary, humoral immunity against HSP60 seems to be an important factor in early *and* late developing atherosclerosis, whereas cellular immune reaction seems to influence only early atherosclerotic changes in the young. As described, mononuclear cells are present in atherosclerotic lesions[12,13] and initially seem to be of oligoclonal origin.[14] Drawing an analogy with rabbit experiments, where reactivity against HSP was higher in T cells isolated from atherosclerotic lesions than in those from the peripheral blood,[38] we hypothesize that in early atherosclerosis, HSP60-specific T cells circulate in the peripheral blood and then accumulate in the atherosclerotic lesions, the site of maximal HSP60 expression. This sequence of events also holds true for other autoimmune disorders.[39]

In concluding thus, we do not deny the importance of classic cardiovascular risk factors that are the target of primary and secondary CVD prevention strategies. However, we have demonstrated *in vitro* (and partly *in vivo*) that multiple risk factors can act as primary stressors on the vessel wall and induce HSP60 expression; these risk factors include mechanical stress,[40] endotoxin/lipopolysaccarides (LPS),[41] cytokines such as TNF-α,[30] oxidized LDL,[30] and drugs such as cyclosporin A.[42]

Smoking Is Proatherogenic and Helps Release HSP60

Although smoking is among the most important risk factors for CVD, the pathophysiologic processes through which it causes atherosclerosis are not yet understood. However, it has been demonstrated in great detail on an epidemiologic and clinical basis that smoking is linked to atherogenesis. We were recently able to reveal some reasons for the proatherogenic activity of smoking by focusing on the effects of the hydrophilic cigarette-smoke fraction on vascular endothelial cells.[43–45] The hydrophilic fraction was analyzed because it had been shown to cause atherosclerosis in animal models.[46] In fact, the hydrophilic compounds of cigarette smoke exert dramatic effects on vascular endothelial cells. Vascular endothelial cells exposed to cigarette smoke extract (CSE) contract, resulting in increased permeability of the vessel endothelium, which is thought to be an important step in atherogenesis. In addition, CSE induces a necrotic and, hence, pro-inflammatory type of death among vascular endothelial cells that involves the release of HSP60 and other cytosolic constituents into the environment.

We also observed a release of P-selectin, interleukin (IL)-6, and IL-8[45] from endothelial cells, which reflects the interference of smoking with platelet aggregation, inflammatory signaling, and leukocyte chemotaxis. Our studies also provided evidence for a potential link between immunity to HSP60 and smoking. Upon exposing vascular endothelial cells to CSE, HSP60 translocates from the mitochondria into the cytosol. Surprisingly, HSP60 was released after treating endothelial cells not only with high CSE concentrations, but also with low, noncytotoxic CSE concentrations (Bernhard *et al.*, unpublished observations).

So far, the mechanisms involved in these processes have not been defined. However, the data agree well with the *in vivo* observation that the serum level of sHSP60 is associated with more rapid progression of atherosclerosis.[35] Finally, we could also show in further studies that CSE causes a modification of proteins, which might lead to the generation of biochemically altered and possibly autoantigenic HSP60.[45]

ACKNOWLEDGMENTS

The work summarized in this paper has been supported by the Austrian Science Fund (project no. 14741 to G.W.), a grant from the Austrian Ministry of Defense (to G.W.), and the Jubiläumsfonds of the Austrian National Bank (project no. 10869 to D.B.).

REFERENCES

1. BURKE, A.P., A. FARB, R. VIRMANI, *et al.* 1991. Sports-related and non-sports-related sudden cardiac death in young adults. Am. Heart J. **121**(2 Pt 1)**:** 568–575.
2. WISSLER, R.W. & J.P. STRONG. 1998. Risk factors and progression of atherosclerosis in youth. PDAY Research Group. Pathological Determinants of Atherosclerosis in Youth. Am. J. Pathol. **153:** 1023–1033.
3. BERENSON, G.S., S.R. SRINIVASAN, W. BAO, *et al.* 1998. Association between multiple cardiovascular risk factors and atherosclerosis in children and young adults. The Bogalusa Heart Study. N. Engl. J. Med. **338:** 1650–1656.
4. KNOFLACH, M., S. KIECHL, M. KIND, *et al.* 2003. Cardiovascular risk factors and atherosclerosis in young males: ARMY study (Atherosclerosis Risk-Factors in Male Youngsters). Circulation **108:** 1064–1069.
5. VIRCHOW, R. 1858. Die Cellularpathologie in ihrer Begründung auf Physiologische und Pathologische Gewebelehre. Zwanzig Vorlesungen. Berlin.
6. OSLER, W. 1908. Diseases of the arteries. *In* Modern Medicine. Its Theory and Practice in Original Contributions by Americans and Foreign Authors. Vol. 4. W. Osler & T. MacCrae, Eds. Lea & Febiger. Philadelphia.
7. FABRICANT, C.G., J. FABRICANT, M.M. LITRENTA & C.R. MINICK. 1978. Virus-induced atherosclerosis. J. Exp. Med. **148:** 335–340.
8. ROSS, R. 1999. Atherosclerosis—an inflammatory disease. N. Engl. J. Med. **340:** 115–126.
9. HANSSON, G.K. 2001. Immune mechanisms in atherosclerosis. Arterioscler. Thromb. Vasc. Biol. **21:** 1876–1890.
10. LIBBY, P. 2002. Inflammation in atherosclerosis. Nature **420:** 868–874.
11. KIECHL, S., G. EGGER, M. MAYR, *et al.* 2001. Chronic infections and the risk of carotid atherosclerosis: prospective results from a large population study. Circulation **103:** 1064–1070.
12. MILLONIG, G., C. SCHWENTNER, P. MUELLER, *et al.* 2001. The vascular-associated lymphoid tissue: a new site of local immunity. Curr. Opin. Lipidol. **12:** 547–553.
13. MILLONIG, G., G.T. MALCOM & G. WICK. 2002. Early inflammatory-immunological lesions in juvenile atherosclerosis from the Pathobiological Determinants of Atherosclerosis in Youth (PDAY)-study. Atherosclerosis **160:** 441–448.
14. PAULSSON, G., X. ZHOU, E. TORNQUIST & G.K. HANSSON. 2000. Oligoclonal T cell expansions in atherosclerotic lesions of apolipoprotein E-deficient mice. Arterioscler. Thromb. Vasc. Biol. **20:** 10–17.
15. STEMME, S., L. RYMO & G.K. HANSSON. 1991. Polyclonal origin of T lymphocytes in human atherosclerotic plaques. Lab. Invest. **65:** 654–660.
16. YOUNG, D.B. 1992. Heat-shock proteins: immunity and autoimmunity. Curr. Opin. Immunol. **4:** 396–400.
17. BENJAMIN, I.J. & D.R. MCMILLAN. 1998. Stress (heat shock) proteins: molecular chaperones in cardiovascular biology and disease. Circ. Res. **83:** 117–132.
18. XU, Q., H. DIETRICH, H.J. STEINER, *et al.* 1992. Induction of arteriosclerosis in normocholesterolemic rabbits by immunization with heat shock protein 65. Arterioscler. Thromb. **12:** 789–799.

19. METZLER, B., M. MAYR, H. DIETRICH, *et al.* 1999. Inhibition of arteriosclerosis by T-cell depletion in normocholesterolemic rabbits immunized with heat shock protein 65. Arterioscler. Thromb. Vasc. Biol. **19:** 1905–1911.
20. AFEK, A., J. GEORGE, B. GILBURD, *et al.* 2000. Immunization of low-density lipoprotein receptor deficient (LDL-RD) mice with heat shock protein 65 (HSP-65) promotes early atherosclerosis. J. Autoimmun. **14:** 115–121.
21. HARATS, D., N. YACOV, B. GILBURD, *et al.* 2002. Oral tolerance with heat shock protein 65 attenuates *Mycobacterium tuberculosis*–induced and high-fat-diet-driven atherosclerotic lesions. J. Am. Coll. Cardiol. **40:** 1333–1338.
22. MARON, R., G. SUKHOVA, A.M. FARIA, *et al.* 2002. Mucosal administration of heat shock protein-65 decreases atherosclerosis and inflammation in aortic arch of low-density lipoprotein receptor-deficient mice. Circulation **106:** 1708–1715.
23. GEORGE, J., A. AFEK, B. GILBURD, *et al.* 2001. Cellular and humoral immune responses to heat shock protein 65 are both involved in promoting fatty-streak formation in LDL-receptor deficient mice. J. Am. Coll. Cardiol. **38:** 900–905.
24. SCHETT, G., Q. XU, A. AMBERGER, *et al.* 1995. Autoantibodies against heat shock protein 60 mediate endothelial cytotoxicity. J. Clin. Invest. **96:** 2569–2577.
25. SOLTYS, B.J. & R.S. GUPTA. 1997. Cell surface localization of the 60 kDa heat shock chaperonin protein (hsp60) in mammalian cells. Cell Biol. Int. **21:** 315–320.
26. MAYR, M., B. METZLER, S. KIECHL, *et al.* 1999. Endothelial cytotoxicity mediated by serum antibodies to heat shock proteins of *Escherichia coli* and *Chlamydia pneumoniae*: immune reactions to heat shock proteins as a possible link between infection and atherosclerosis. Circulation **99:** 1560–1566.
27. WICK, G., R. KLEINDIENST, H. DIETRICH, *et al.* 1992. Is atherosclerosis an autoimmune disease? Trends Food Sci. Technol. **3:** 114–119.
28. WICK, G., H. PERSCHINKA & G. MILLONIG. 2001. Atherosclerosis as an autoimmune disease: an update. Trends Immunol. **22:** 665–669.
29. WICK, G., M. KNOFLACH & Q. XU. 2004. Autoimmune and inflammatory mechanisms in atherosclerosis. Annu. Rev. Immunol. **22:** 362–403.
30. AMBERGER, A., C. MACZEK, G. JURGENS, *et al.* 1997. Co-expression of ICAM-1, VCAM-1, ELAM-1 and Hsp60 in human arterial and venous endothelial cells in response to cytokines and oxidized low-density lipoproteins. Cell Stress & Chaperones **2:** 94–103.
31. KIECHL, S. & J. WILLEIT. 1999. The natural course of atherosclerosis. Part I: incidence and progression. Arterioscler. Thromb. Vasc. Biol. **19:** 1484–1490.
32. KIECHL, S. & J. WILLEIT. 1999. The natural course of atherosclerosis. Part II: vascular remodeling. Bruneck Study Group. Arterioscler. Thromb. Vasc. Biol. **19:** 1491–1498.
33. XU, Q., J. WILLEIT, M. MAROSI, *et al.* 1993. Association of serum antibodies to heat-shock protein 65 with carotid atherosclerosis. Lancet **341:** 255–259.
34. XU, Q., S. KIECHL, M. MAYR, *et al.* 1999. Association of serum antibodies to heat-shock protein 65 with carotid atherosclerosis: clinical significance determined in a follow-up study. Circulation **100:** 1169–1174.
35. XU, Q., G. SCHETT, H. PERSCHINKA, *et al.* 2000. Serum soluble heat shock protein 60 is elevated in subjects with atherosclerosis in a general population. Circulation **102:** 14–20.
36. MILLONIG, G., H. NIEDEREGGER, W. RABL, *et al.* 2001. Network of vascular-associated dendritic cells in intima of healthy young individuals. Arterioscler. Thromb. Vasc. Biol. **21:** 503–508.
37. PIGNOLI, P., E. TREMOLI, A. POLI, *et al.* 1986. Intimal plus medial thickness of the arterial wall: a direct measurement with ultrasound imaging. Circulation **74:** 1399–1406.
38. XU, Q., R. KLEINDIENST, W. WAITZ, *et al.* 1993. Increased expression of heat shock protein 65 coincides with a population of infiltrating T lymphocytes in atherosclerotic lesions of rabbits specifically responding to heat shock protein 65. J. Clin. Invest. **91:** 2693–2702.
39. KROEMER, G., N. NEU, T. KUEHR, *et al.* 1989. Immunogenetic analysis of spontaneous autoimmune thyroiditis of obese strain chickens. Clin. Immunol. Immunopathol. **52:** 202–213.

40. HOCHLEITNER, B.W., E.O. HOCHLEITNER, P. OBRIST, *et al.* 2000. Fluid shear stress induces heat shock protein 60 expression in endothelial cells in vitro and in vivo. Arterioscler. Thromb. Vasc. Biol. **20:** 617–623.
41. SEITZ, C.S., R. KLEINDIENST, Q. XU & G. WICK. 1996. Coexpression of heat-shock protein 60 and intercellular-adhesion molecule-1 is related to increased adhesion of monocytes and T cells to aortic endothelium of rats in response to endotoxin. Lab. Invest. **74:** 241–252.
42. AMBERGER, A., M. HALA, M. SAURWEIN-TEISSL, *et al.* 1999. Suppressive effects of anti-inflammatory agents on human endothelial cell activation and induction of heat shock proteins. Mol. Med. **5:** 117–128.
43. BERNHARD, D., G. PFISTER, C.W. HUCK, *et al.* 2003. Disruption of vascular endothelial homeostasis by tobacco smoke: impact on atherosclerosis. FASEB J. **17:** 2302–2304.
44. BERNHARD, D., C.W. HUCK, T. JAKSCHITZ, *et al.* 2004. Development and evaluation of an in vitro model for the analysis of cigarette smoke effects on cultured cells and tissues. J. Pharmacol. Toxicol. Methods **50:** 45–51.
45. BERNHARD, D., A. CSORDAS, B. HENDERSON, *et al.* 2005. Cigarette smoke metal catalyzed protein oxidation leads to vascular endothelial cell contraction by depolymerization of microtubules. FASEB J. In press.
46. PENN, A., K. KELLER, C. SNYDER, *et al.* 1996. The tar fraction of cigarette smoke does not promote arteriosclerotic plaque development. Environ. Health Perspect. **104:** 1108–1113.

Determinants of Vessel Targeting in Vasculitis

GARY S. HOFFMAN

Department of Rheumatic and Immunologic Diseases and Center for Vasculitis Care and Research, Cleveland Clinic Foundation A50, Cleveland, Ohio 44195, USA

ABSTRACT: Studies of autoimmune diseases have not yet elucidated why certain organs or vessels become the objects of injury while others are spared. This paper explores the hypothesis that important differences exist in regions of the aorta; these regional variations determine vulnerability to such diseases as atherosclerosis, aortitis, giant-cell arteritis, and Takayasu's disease. The reader is invited to reassess two issues: (1) whether the aorta is indeed a single homogeneous structure; and (2) whether the initial stage of aortitis (and indeed other diseases considered "autoimmune") may primarily be the result of acquired alterations of substrate that influence unique immune profiles, but that by themselves may not be pathogenic. Disease susceptibility and patterns are influenced by many factors that are either inborn or acquired. Examples include genetic background, gender, ethnicity, aging, prior and concomitant illnesses, habits, diet, and exposure to toxins and other environmental hazards. Studies of vascular diseases must assess how such variables affect regional anatomic differences in endothelial cells, subendothelial matrix, and vascular smooth muscle, as well as the response of each to a variety of stimuli.

KEYWORDS: aging; vasculitis; idiopathic aortitis; giant-cell arteritis; Takayasu's disease; atherosclerosis; aortitis

GIANT-CELL ARTERITIS, TAKAYASU'S DISEASE, AND IDIOPATHIC AORTITIS

Giant-cell arteritis (GCA) and Takayasu's arteritis (TA, also known as Takayasu's disease) are granulomatous inflammatory diseases of the large arteries that share similar and, some would argue, identical profiles of vessel targets with regard to size and distribution. Both may be complicated by inflammatory aneurysms that are predominantly thoracic.[1] However, in GCA, the mean age at presentation is greater than 70 years, whereas in TA, it is about 25 years.[2] In patients with idiopathic aortitis (IA), which may or may not have granulomatous histopathology, age at onset is less polarized, and often systemic illness is absent.[3] Such a diagnosis may come to the attention of physicians only because of the hemodynamic effects of aortic regurgitation and root dilatation. Aortitis may be recognized only after specimens are reviewed from aortic aneurysm surgeries (FIG. 1).

Address for correspondence: Gary S. Hoffman M.D., Harold C. Schott Chair of Rheumatic and Immunologic Diseases, Center for Vasculitis Care and Research, Cleveland Clinic Foundation A50, Cleveland, OH 44195. Voice: 216-445-6996; fax: 216-445-7569.
hoffmag@ccf.org

**Ann. N.Y. Acad. Sci. 1051: 332–339 (2005). © 2005 New York Academy of Sciences.
doi: 10.1196/annals.1361.075**

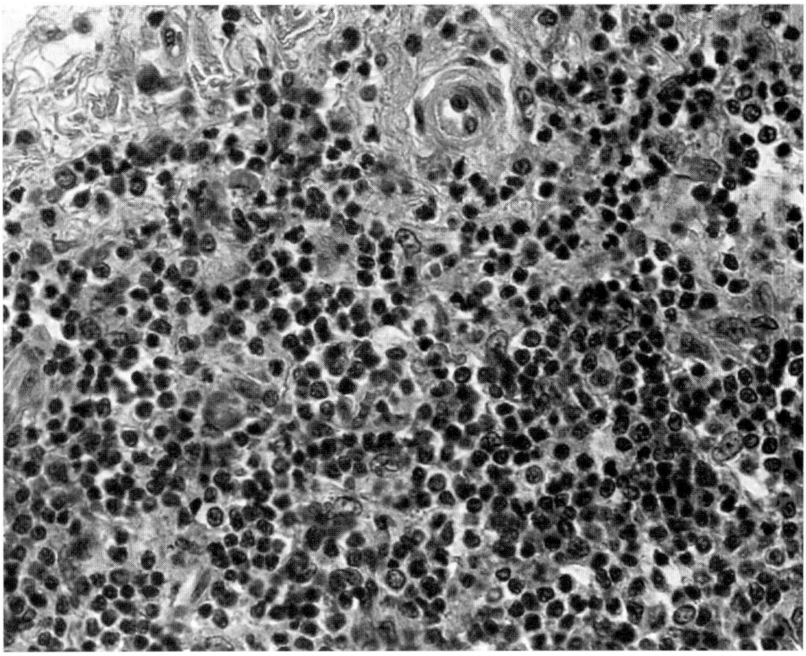

FIGURE 1. Aortitis was discovered after surgery in a 67-year-old man who did not have symptoms of a systemic inflammatory illness. Surgical intervention was required for aortic root dilatation and consequent severe aortic regurgitation (300× magnification).

Herein we report on the characteristics of patients with IA and compare them to those of patients with atherosclerosis, cystic medial necrosis, GCA, and TA. Of 48 inflammatory aneurysms in our IA cohort, 96% were thoracic. In contrast, among 798 non-inflammatory aortic aneurysms, 69% were in the abdominal region and were caused principally by atherosclerosis (i.e., inflammation around only atheromatous plaques, not diffuse). This striking trend for inflammatory aneurysms to be located in the thoracic region has been confirmed in surveys of large-vessel pathology from postmortem examinations. Aortitis of uncertain etiology has been recognized in up to 8% of all postmortem examinations. However, when authors have restricted their analyses to aortitis with aneurysms, inflammatory aneurysms were almost always noted in the thoracic region.[4–6]

The most common cause of thoracic aortic aneurysms is not aortitis; rather, it is cystic medionecrosis.[7] In the absence of atherosclerosis, cystic medionecrosis is far more common in the thoracic than in the abdominal aorta, where it generally coexists with and may, in part, result from atherosclerotic injury. Patchy atherosclerosis may be common in postmortem thoracic aorta specimens in the elderly, but atherosclerosis alone is an uncommon cause of thoracic aneurysm formation.

These observations emphasize variations in vulnerability to different diseases within the same vessel, which is not homogeneous throughout its course.

TABLE 1. Relative differences between the thoracic and abdominal aorta

Feature	Thoracic region	Abdominal region
Wall thickness	Greater	
Wall diameter	30–40% greater	
Elastic fiber	Greater concentration (decreases distal to root)	
Derivation SMCs	Neural crest ectoderm	Mesoderm
Smooth muscle cells—media^{inner}	Greater concentration	
Vasa vasorum (media)	Numerous	Few to absent
Disease predilections	Inflammatory	Diffuse atherosclerosis
	Cystic medial necrosis	

VARIABILITY OF THE AORTA THROUGHOUT ITS REGIONS

The foregoing discussion implies that the aorta, this single tubular structure, must have inherent variations in its content and/or responsiveness to injury to account for regional differences in disease patterns. In addition, apart from Takayasu's arteritis, inflammatory aortic aneurysms are found mainly in older adults. Does advanced age instigate changes within regions of the aorta that make it more vulnerable to inflammatory injury? Are elements of immunologic senescence present that may respond to altered substrate to produce aortitis? What are the implications for younger patients with aortitis? Although answers to these questions are not readily available, regional differences within the aorta are well known and therefore will be considered (TABLE 1).

Anatomic Differences

The thoracic aorta is wider and has a thicker wall diameter than that of more distal regions. In humans, the aortic arch wall is about 1.5 mm thick, whereas the abdominal aortic wall is 1 mm thick or less.[8]

Vessel-Wall Perfusion and the Vasa Vasorum

The concentration of aortic vasa vasorum is about 9.4 vessels/mm^2 in the thick-walled thoracic region but only 1.9 vessels/mm^2 in the abdominal region (FIG. 2). As wall thickness increases owing to disease, especially atherosclerosis, a concordant penetration of the vasa vasorum takes place that extends into the vascular media and even into the intima.[8,9]

Aorta Collagen and Elastin

The synthesis of collagen and elastin[10] as well as the thickness of elastic membranes and the number of elastic laminae[11] diminishes with increased distance from the aortic root. Elastin, the main extracellular matrix component in arteries, is synthesized by vascular smooth muscle cells (SMCs) and plays both a structural and a

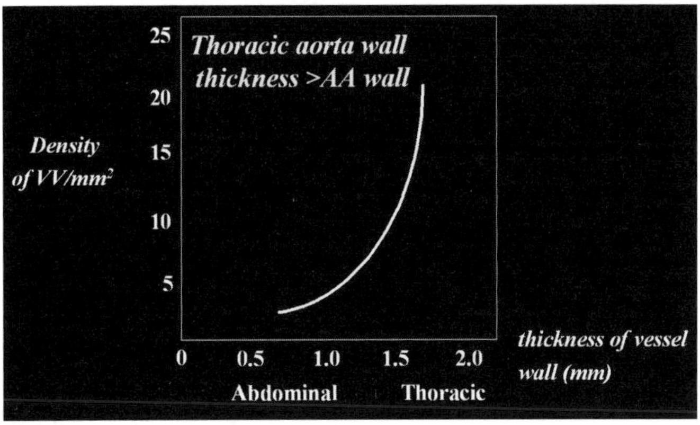

FIGURE 2. In concert with decreased thickness of the aortic wall, the vasa vasorum (vv) becomes less dense from proximal to distal aorta. *Source*: Okuyama *et al.*[8]

developmental role in arterial morphogenesis. Animals that lack the gene for elastin have abnormal vascular SMC proliferation and neointimal thickening. Elastin is therefore considered a regulatory protein, influencing the proliferation and migration of its cell of origin, the SMC.[12] During the aging process, the aorta develops increasing degrees of elastin fragmentation and degeneration, concurrent with increased collagen content. The functional consequences are well understood: loss of elasticity and stiffening.[13] However, whether changes in elastin influence immunogenicity is less certain.

AN ANIMAL MODEL OF ATHEROSCLEROSIS

In a study reported in 1966, Haimovici and Maier[14] addressed the issue of aortic heterogeneity. They studied dogs given a diet intended to induce atherosclerosis, a process that is most obvious in the abdominal aorta. Prior to giving them the atherogenic diet, the authors switched segments of thoracic and abdominal aorta between these inbred dogs. Although the abdominally located thoracic aorta did not develop atherosclerosis, the thoracically located abdominal aorta still did. Thus, inherent differences in aortic wall anatomy and physiology determined disease vulnerability, apart from location and properties of flow.

Embryologic Differences

Studies of aortic embryogenesis in animals have revealed that neural crest cells contribute to the formation of SMCs in the aortic trunk, proximal arch, and pulmonary artery trunk, but not in the more distal parts of the aorta. In contrast, abdominal aortic SMCs derive primarily from mesoderm. These basic differences imply that unique genetic programs may be responsible for the variable responses of SMCs in the thoracic and abdominal aorta to a variety of stimuli.[15]

Understanding Differences at the Genetic Level

Absi and colleagues[16] recently utilized gene expression techniques to more fully explore the issue of regional variation. They asked why aortic aneurysms in the thoracic region are usually the result of cystic medial necrosis, whereas abdominal aortic aneurysms are caused primarily by atherosclerosis. The authors identified striking differences in gene expression patterns between areas of unaffected thoracic and abdominal aorta as well as between segments of aneurysms from both regions.[16]

Role of Exogenous Pathogens

The possible role that undiscovered infection plays in GCA, TA, and IA is an area of great controversy. Nonetheless, in other settings, infection is a known cause of aortitis and demonstrates site selectivity. Aortitis may result from *Staphylococcus aureus,* Salmonella, fungi, tuberculosis, or other organisms.[17] Furthermore, the patterns of idiopathic aortitis and infectious aortitis are often similar. For example, syphilitic aortitis involves the thoracic aorta in approximately 75% of cases (ascending 46%, transverse arch 25%) but affects the aorta distal to the renal arteries only infrequently.[18]

Pathogens possess adhesion molecules and may produce unique by-products that display selective tissue affinities. This selective adhesion may account for differences in targeting end-organs.[19] Because products of pathogens may act at sites remote from their origin, injury can occur in the absence of the pathogen itself. Alternatively, pathogens may be effectively cleared from the body but have already induced a response to self-Ag (molecular mimicry) or caused alterations in self-Ag that lead it to be perceived as foreign (i.e., a neoantigen). It is also possible that if an infectious agent triggers autoimmunity, the critical factor leading to illness may not be the body's ability to clear the agent but its inability to downregulate the immune response.

Variations in immune response are likely to explain the broad range of outcomes observed following a variety infections. For example, hepatitis viruses, parvovirus B19, and Epstein-Barr virus (EBV) are well known for causing a diversity of illness phenotypes. Also, in children, parvovirus B19 may cause erythema infectiosum, but in other individuals it produces red-cell aplasia, aplastic anemia, a Still's disease-like illness, a rheumatoid arthritis-like illness, or hydrops fetalis during pregnancy. The virus appears to be the same, but the results are extraordinarily different.

AGE-RELATED IMMUNE SYSTEM DECLINE

Although acquired changes in the vessel wall likely play a role in determining patterns in vasculitis, acquired changes in immune function are probably required for disease expression. In addition, certain vasculitides are clearly influenced by age and gender, and related factors including changes in hormone production and function. For instance, 80% of patients with Kawasaki disease are less than 5 years old, and boys are affected 1.5 times as often as girls. Takayasu's arteritis affects mostly women of reproductive age, and GCA is seen in individuals whose mean age is 74 years, women being affected about twice or three times as often as men. Immune senescence may be especially relevant in the etiology of GCA. Increasing age is associated with a decline in thymic function, impairment of T-cell activation, defective generation of T-cell memory, a decline in specific antibody responses, and defects in apoptosis and antigen presentation and processing.[20]

CONCLUSIONS

Certain basic pathogenic components of "vasculitis" require greater study. There is a need to acquire more complete knowledge of the sites that are the object of injury before injury actually occurs. Although studying the cells and their products within the affected sites is important, this approach alone is unlikely to reveal the etiology of these disorders. Studies of the "target" might include distinguishing molecular and genetic differences between controls and patients with regard to elements of tissue structure, antigens, and response to injury.

If the initial events in the pathogenesis of certain vasculitides are related to changes in the vessel wall, and not primarily the result of aberrations in immune function, then microarray and proteomics techniques may provide unique insights into susceptibility factors imparted by age, ethnicity, and gender. For example, GCA is frequent among people whose origins are Northern European or Icelandic but is

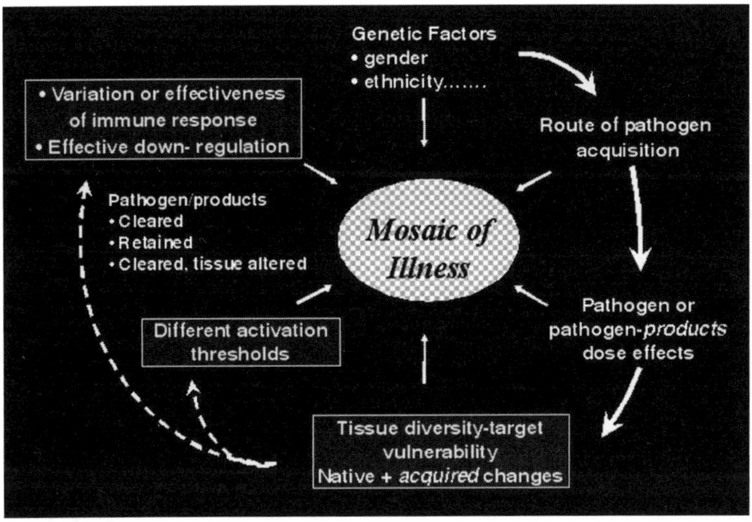

FIGURE 3. Conceptual mosaic for organ targeting. Pathogenic factors in immune-mediated diseases may be endogenous and/or exogenous. Whether disease results may be related, in part, to general or tissue-specific host susceptibility factors. Determinants of organ targeting may reside within the target itself and include unique native or acquired characteristics (e.g., ligands for pathogens, age-related changes, postinfectious changes). These characteristics influence a pathogen's (organism's or molecule's) adhesion, retention, and penetration. In health, pathogenic factors would be cleared from the body, the immune response would be appropriately downregulated, and normal structure and function would be restored. *Source*: Reprinted from Hoffman[1] with permission of John Wiley & Sons.

relatively uncommon in African Americans and Asians. Important differences in the "targeted" vessels in these populations may enhance or even determine disease susceptibility. The big picture that emerges in considering all factors that influence the expression of large vessel vasculitis is a mosaic of an illness. As with many diseases, the mosaic comprises factors that are genetic, environmental, and acquired (FIG. 3). Microarray and proteomics techniques are now being applied to study pattern variations within temporal arteries in GCA and normal controls. These tools are providing the opportunity to better understand the role of targeted tissue in the mosaic of large vessel vasculitis.

ACKNOWLEDGMENT

This work was supported in part by the Harold C. Schott Foundation.

REFERENCES

1. HOFFMAN, G.S. 2003. Large-vessel vasculitis: unresolved issues. Arthritis Rheum. **48:** 2406–2414.
2. KERR, G.S., C.W. HALLAHAN, J. GIORDANO, *et al.* 1994. Takayasu arteritis. Ann. Intern. Med. **120:** 919–929.
3. ROJO-LEYVA, F., N.B. RATLIFF, D.M. COSGROVE, III & G.S. HOFFMAN. 2000. Study of 52 patients with idiopathic aortitis from a cohort of 1,204 surgical cases. Arthritis Rheum. **43:** 901–907.
4. SVENSJO, S., H. BENGTSSON & D. BERGQVIST. 1996. Thoracic and thoracoabdominal aortic aneurysm and dissection: an investigation based on autopsy. Br. J. Surg. **83:** 68–71.
5. OSTBERG, G. 1973. An arteritis with special reference to polymyalgia rheumatica. Acta Pathol. Microbiol. Scand. **237** (Suppl. 237): 1–59.
6. BICKERSTAFF, L.K., P.C. PAIROLERO, L.H. HOLLIER, *et al.* 1982. Thoracic aortic aneurysms: a population-based study. Surgery **92:** 1103–1108.
7. POMERANCE, A., M.H. YACOUB & G. GULA. 1977. The surgical pathology of thoracic aortic aneurysms. Histopathology **1:** 257–276.
8. OKUYAMA, K., G. YAGINUMA, T. TAKAHASHI, *et al.* 1988. The development of vasa vasorum of the human aorta in various conditions. A morphometric study. Arch. Pathol. Lab. Med. **112:** 721–725.
9. SCHUTTE, H.E. 1968. Changes in the vasa vasorum of the atherosclerotic aortic wall. Angiologica **5:** 210–222.
10. FISCHER, G.M., M.L. SWAIN & K. CHERIAN. 1980. Increased vascular collagen and elastin synthesis in experimental atherosclerosis in the rabbit. Variation in synthesis among major vessels. Atherosclerosis **35:** 11–20.
11. SOKOLIS, D.P., H. BOUDOULAS, N.G. KAVANTZAS, *et al.* 2002. A morphometric study of the structural characteristics of the aorta in pigs using an image analysis method. Anat. Histol. Embryol. (Vet. Med. Series C) **31:** 21–30.
12. KARNIK, S.K., B.S. BROOKE, A. BAYES-GENES, *et al.* 2003. A critical role for elastin signaling in vascular morphogenesis and disease. Development **130:** 411–423.
13. SCHLATMANN, T.J. & A.E. BECKER. 1977. Pathogenesis of dissecting aneurysm of the aorta. Comparative histopathologic study of significance of medial changes. Am. J. Cardiol. **39:** 21–26.
14. HAIMOVICI, H. & N. MAIER. 1966. Role of arterial tissue susceptibility in experimental canine atherosclerosis. J. Atherosclerosis Res. **6:** 62–74.
15. GADSON, P.F., JR., M.L. DALTON, E. PATTERSON, *et al.* 1997. Differential response of mesoderm- and neural crest–derived smooth muscle to TGF-beta1: regulation of c-myb and alpha1 (I) procollagen genes. Exp. Cell Res. **230:** 169–180.

16. Absi, T.S., T.M. Sundt, III, W.S. Tung, *et al.* 2003. Altered patterns of gene expression distinguishing ascending aortic aneurysms from abdominal aortic aneurysms: complementary DNA expression profiling in the molecular characterization of aortic disease. J. Thor. Cardiovasc. Surg. **126:** 344–357.
17. Oz, M.C., B.J. Brener, J.A. Buda, *et al.* 1989. A ten year experience with bacterial aortitis. J. Vasc. Surg. **10:** 439–449.
18. Heggtveit, H.A. 1964. Syphilitic aortitis. A clinicopathologic autopsy study of 100 cases, 1950–1960. Circulation **29:** 346–355.
19. Patti, J.M., B.L. Allen, M.J. McGavin & M. Hook. 1994. MSCRAMM-mediated adherence of microorganisms to host tissues. Annu. Rev. Microbiol. **48:** 585–617.
20. Weyand, C.M. & J.J. Goronzy. 1997. Multisystem interactions in the pathogenesis of vasculitis. Curr. Opin. Rheumatol. **9:** 3–11.

Lymphocyte Activation as a Possible Measure of Atherosclerotic Risk in Patients with Sleep Apnea

LARISSA DYUGOVSKAYA, PERETZ LAVIE, AND LENA LAVIE

The Lloyd Rigler Sleep Apnea Research Laboratory, Unit of Anatomy and Cell Biology, The Bruce Rappaport Faculty of Medicine, Technion-Israel Institute of Technology, Haifa, Israel

ABSTRACT: Obstructive sleep apnea (OSA), a breathing disorder in sleep characterized by intermittent hypoxia and sleep fragmentation, constitutes an independent risk factor for cardiovascular morbidity. Investigating how this breathing disorder modulates immune responses may facilitate understanding one of the risk factors for atherosclerosis. T cells play a significant role in atherogenesis and plaque development via cytokine production and by directly contributing to vascular injury. Using flow cytometry and chromium release assays, we found that CD4 and CD8 T cells of OSA patients undergo phenotypic and functional changes and acquire cytotoxic capabilities. Thus, a shift in CD4 and CD8 T cells toward type 2 cytokine dominance with increased IL-4 expression was noted. IL-10 expression in T cells was negatively correlated with the severity of OSA, as determined by the apnea–hypopnea index (AHI), whereas TNF-α was positively correlated. CD8 T cells of OSA patients expressed a fourfold increase in TNF-α and CD40 ligand (CD40L), and exhibited an increased OSA severity–dependent cytotoxicity against endothelial cells. The percentage of $CD4^{+}CD28^{null}$ and cytotoxicity of CD4 T lymphocytes were also significantly higher in OSA patients than in controls. Nasal continuous positive airway pressure (nCPAP) treatment, which ameliorated the severity of OSA, significantly lowered TNF-α and CD40L expression, and decreased cytotoxicity in CD8 T cells. In conclusion, increased cytotoxicity and cytokine imbalance in CD4 and CD8 T cells may be involved in atherogenesis in OSA. Nasal CPAP treatment ameliorates some lymphocyte dysfunctions and thus may moderate some atherogenic pathways.

KEYWORDS: T lymphocytes; sleep apnea; nCPAP; cytokines; atherosclerosis

INTRODUCTION

Obstructive sleep apnea syndrome (OSA), which is characterized by intermittent and recurrent pauses in respiration during sleep, leading to a decrease in oxygen saturation and sleep fragmentation, constitutes an independent risk factor for car-

Address for correspondence: Dr. Lena Lavie, Unit of Anatomy and Cell Biology, The Ruth and Bruce Rappaport Faculty of Medicine, Technion, POB 9649, 31096 Haifa, Israel. Voice: +972-4-8295234; fax: +972-4-8295403 or +972-4-8343934.
lenal@techunix.technion.ac.il

**Ann. N.Y. Acad. Sci. 1051: 340–350 (2005). © 2005 New York Academy of Sciences.
doi: 10.1196/annals.1361.076**

diovascular morbidity.[1–4] As yet, the underlying mechanisms are poorly understood. Atherogenesis is determined by multiple factors, of which innate and acquired immunity and inflammatory pathways are critical.[5–8] Moreover, modification of immune responses could prevent or alleviate atherosclerosis.[9,10] We have recently shown increased oxidative stress[11–14] and immune cell activation in OSA patients, as attested by increased free-radical production in monocytes and overexpression of adhesion molecules, followed by increased adhesion and cytotoxicity of monocytes and γδ T lymphocytes against endothelial cells.[12,15] These may exacerbate atherogenesis in OSA patients, as T cell immunity plays a significant role in plaque formation and in the development of acute coronary syndrome.[7,16–18] Upon activation, T cells differentiate into effector cells with tissue-damaging potential, or secrete cytokines that may affect such atherogenic pathways as macrophage activation, oxygen free radical production, adhesion molecule expression, smooth muscle proliferation, and vascular contractility.[17,19] T cells exist in functionally polarized populations, depending on the cytokines they produce—those secreting type 1 cytokines (IL-2 and IFN-γ), and those secreting type 2 cytokines (IL-4, IL-5, IL-6, and IL-10). Type 1/type 2 imbalance has adverse effects on health and disease. Type 1, for example, has been implicated in cardiovascular disease.[20] Besides the definition of type 1 and type 2, the cytokines are also classified by their proinflammatory and anti-inflammatory activity.[21] Among the proinflammatory cytokines, TNF-α has a powerful effect on the initiation and progression of cardiovascular pathology.[19,22–24] IL-10, on the other hand, is a potent inhibitor of proinflammatory cytokines in T cells,[25] and interaction between IL-10 and TNF-α production may influence the outcome of several cardiovascular disorders.[19,26–30]

The cytokines are known to be regulated by altered oxygen tension and high oxygen–free radical production,[31] which are prominent features of OSA pathology.[11] Accordingly, plasma levels of IL-6 and TNF-α were found to be elevated in OSA patients.[32] Moreover, a significant increase in plasma TNF-α was measured immediately after the first obstructive apnea causing a SaO2 desaturation <85%.[33] Hence, treatment with nasal continuous positive air pressure (nCPAP) that normalizes breathing in sleep of OSA patients decreased IL-6 production by OSA monocytes.[34] Unlike most clinical investigations in OSA, in which circulating cytokine levels were determined, we focused on the inflammatory cells producing these cytokines.

The purpose of this study was to evaluate the balance between TNF-α/IL-10 and IL-2/IL-4 cytokine expression, as well as to characterize the presence of activating markers such as CD40 ligand (CD40L) and CD28 in CD4 and CD8 T cells of patients with OSA. CD4 and CD8 T cell cytotoxicity against endothelial cells was investigated as well. In order to ensure that the observed changes are due to sleep apnea and not to other concurrent factors, we also investigated the expression of these markers after a single night of treatment with nCPAP.

METHODS

Patients and Controls

Both patients and controls were recruited from the patient population of the Technion Sleep Medicine Center, Haifa. The protocol was approved by the local Human

Rights Committee, and all participants signed an informed consent form. A diagnosis of OSA was based on in-laboratory polysomnographic recording. The apnea–hypopnea index (AHI) was calculated as the total number of apneas plus hypopneas divided by hours of sleep; percent sleep time spent with oxygen saturation below 90% was also determined. Inclusion criteria for the patient group ($n = 23$) were absence of comorbidities such as hypertension, ischemic heart disease, and diabetes; a sleep laboratory finding of AHI > 15; and absence of acute illness during the week before the study. The control group ($n = 15$) was recruited from subjects who were referred for polysomnographic monitoring because of suspected sleep apnea, but were found to have AHI < 10, provided that most of the disordered breathing events were hypopneas not associated with arterial oxygen desaturation. Earlier, we found that there was no difference in inflammatory and cellular markers between participants with an AHI between 5 and 15.[35] A separate group of 16 moderate-to-severe OSA patients treated for one night with nCPAP was also studied simultaneously with the untreated patients and the controls. This group, which was similar to the untreated patients with respect to pretreatment severity of OSA, differed from patients after the single-night treatment only with respect to AHI. TABLE 1 provides clinical and demographic data.

Flow Cytometry

Blood samples were drawn at 6:00 to 6:30 AM just after awakening. The cell-surface phenotype was determined in whole blood using mouse IgG monoclonal antibody (mAb) reacting with the following human markers: CD8-FITC (clone LT8), CD4-FITC (clone RPA-T4), CD28-RPE (clone YTH 913.12), and CD40L-RPE (CD154, clone TRAP1) (Dako A/S, Glostrup Denmark). Intracellular cytokines were detected in freshly isolated nonstimulated FITC-labeled CD4/CD8 T cells in Ficoll-separated peripheral blood mononuclear cells by using Cytofix/Cytoperm Kit (PharMingen, San Diego, CA) according to the manufacturer's instructions. RPE-conjugated rat anti–human IL-2, IL-4, IL-10, and TNF-α (Serotec, Ltd., Kidlington, UK) mAbs were used. The results are expressed as the percentage of $CD4^+$ and $CD8^+$ T cells that contain each of the cytokines investigated, identified according to isotypic control background staining. Lymphoid cells were gated by forward and side light scatter using a minimum of 30,000 cells for each analysis. Cell samples were analyzed by FACS Calibur (Becton Dickinson, Lincoln Park, NJ) by employing a dual-staining protocol.

Isolation of T Cells and Cytotoxicity Assay

Enriched $CD4^+$ T cells were prepared by RosetteSep Ab cocktail (StemCell Technologies, Inc., Vancouver, Canada). Importantly, $CD4^+$ monocytes were not copurified. Enriched fractions of $CD8^+$ and $\gamma\delta$ T cells were prepared using magnetic microbeads conjugated with anti-FITC, and a magnetic field system (Miltenyi Biotec GmbH, Bergisch Gladbach, Germany). All procedures were performed according to the manufacturer's instructions.

Cytotoxicity against human umbilical vein endothelial cells (HUVECs) was measured by ^{51}Cr-release assay.[15] HUVECs were kindly provided by Dr. N. Lanir (Rambam Medical Center, Haifa, Israel) and were treated as previously described.[12,15]

HUVECs were loaded overnight with ^{51}Cr (1 μCi/mL). Following washing, purified T cells were added to the ^{51}Cr-labeled HUVECs at effector/target (E/T) ratios of 5:1, 10:1, and 20:1. After 16 h of coculture, radioactivity (cpm) was determined and calculated.[15]

TABLE 1. Demographic, sleep, and flow cytometry data of patients with OSA and control subjects participating in different experiments

	Control	OSA	OSA nCPAP	Control vs. OSA	Control vs. nCPAP	OSA vs. nCPAP
Age (yr)	42.1 ± 9.5	46.4 ± 10.3	51.9 ± 11.5	0.2	0.02	0.14
Males (%)	79	82	88	NS	NS	NS
BMI (kg/m^2)	27.4 ± 6.5	28.1 ± 4.9	29.0 ± 5.6	NS	NS	NS
AHI	7.4 ± 3.6	30.5 ± 14.2	11.1 ± 4.5[a]	0.000001	0.02	0.000001
O_2 Sat.	0.9 ± 2.0	6.9 ± 13.2	0.3 ± 1.2[a]	0.0001	0.003	0.0001
Smokers (%)	25	27.8	20	NS	NS	NS
CD8 TNF-α (%)[b]	1.3 ± 1.4	5.2 ± 6.2	2.3 ± 1.4	0.008	0.07	0.04
CD8 IL-10 (%)[b]	8.5 ± 9.7	11.2 ± 9.6	9.7 ± 6.5	NS	NS	NS
CD4 TNF-α (%)[b]	2.3 ± 3.2	3.4 ± 5.9	4.1 ± 5.6	NS	NS	NS
CD4 IL-10 (%)[b]	2.4 ± 1.3	11.8 ± 10.7	12.0 ± 6.1	0.001	0.001	NS
CD4 IL-4 (%)[b]	3.5 ± 3.4	15.1 ± 12.9	24.4 ± 24.0	0.004	0.03	NS
CD4 IL-2 (%)[b]	2.8 ± 3.2	4.5 ± 6.1	9.5 ± 11.2	NS	0.09	NS
CD8 IL-4 (%)[b]	2.0 ± 1.5	12.5 ± 9.4	11.2 ± 10.2	0.0001	0.008	NS
CD8 IL-2 (%)[b]	2.2 ± 2.7	5.6 ± 6.4	5.1 ± 3.5	0.07	0.05	NS
$CD8^+CD40L^+$ (%)[b]	3.4 ± 2.5	14.4 ± 10.5	4.0 ± 2.8	0.006	NS	0.02
$CD4^+CD28^{null}$ (%)[b]	6.8 ± 1.3	19.9 ± 5.0	ND	0.0006	ND	ND

ABBREVIATIONS: AHI, apnea/hypopnea index; BMI, body mass index; ND, not determined; NS, nonsignificant; O_2 Sat., percent time with <90% arterial O_2 saturation.

[a]Before nCPAP: AHI = 29.9 ± 11.3; O_2 Sat. = 7.0 ± 6.3.

[b]Percentage of double-stained cells among $CD8^+$ or $CD4^+$ T lymphocytes.

Statistical Analysis

Data are expressed as mean ± SD. Differences between the OSA, control, and nCPAP-treated groups were evaluated by analysis of the covariance using age, gender, and body mass index (BMI) as covariates, followed by planned post hoc comparisons. The relationship between OSA severity, as determined by AHI, and cytokine expression was analyzed by Spearman correlations.

RESULTS

TNF-α and IL-10 Expression in CD8 and CD4 Lymphocytes of OSA Patients

A fourfold increase in the percentage of CD8 T cells expressing intracellular TNF-α was observed in OSA patients as compared with controls (TABLE 1). The percentage of IL-10–expressing CD8 cells varied greatly in controls and did not differ between groups. Within the sleep apnea group AHI was negatively correlated with percentage of $CD8^+$/IL-10^+ T lymphocytes and was positively correlated with percentage of $CD8^+$/TNF-α^+ T cells (FIGS. 1A and 1B). In addition, increased TNF-α expression was positively correlated with BMI ($r = 0.49$, $P = .018$). The individual analysis of CD8 T cells revealed that, depending on the ratio of cells expressing TNF-α/IL-10, OSA patients could be divided into two subgroups (FIG. 2). The major subgroup had a TNF-α IL-10 ratio <1, which was characterized by high IL-10 and low TNF-α expression. The smaller subgroup (17.4%; FIG. 2, solid line rectangle) was characterized by a decrease in the percentage of IL-10–expressing and increase in the percentage of TNF-α–expressing CD8 cells. This resulted in a TNF-α IL-10 ratio ranging from 1.2 to 11.5. All patients in this subgroup had an AHI > 25, and three-quarters of the patients were obese.

In contrast to the $CD8^+$ T cells, the percentage of $CD4^+$ cells expressing IL-10 was 4.9-fold higher in OSA patients as compared with controls (TABLE 1), whereas

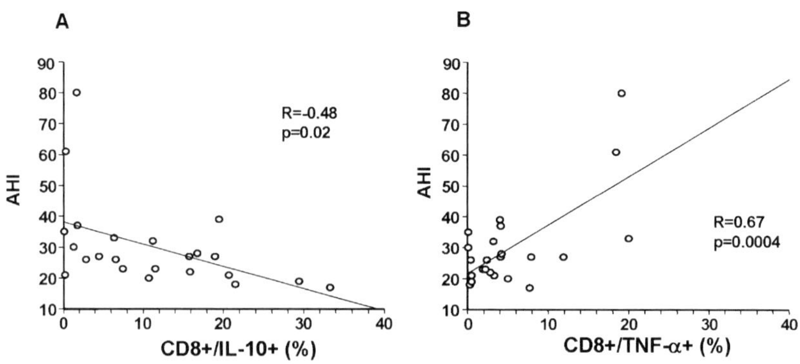

FIGURE 1. Correlation between AHI and percentage of $CD8^+$ T cells from OSA patients expressing cytokines. (**A**) $CD8^+$/IL-10^+; (**B**) $CD8^+$/TNF-α^+. Intracellular cytokines were detected in $CD8^+$ T cells from OSA patients using the Cytofix/Cytoperm Kit. The results are expressed as the percentage of $CD8^+$ T cells that contain each of the cytokines investigated.

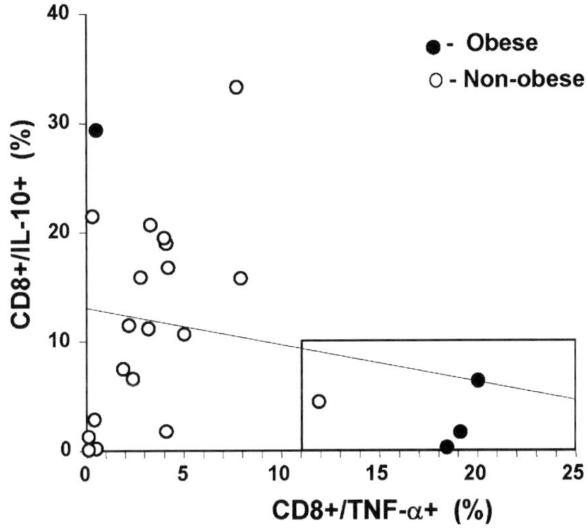

FIGURE 2. Correlation between the percentages of CD8 T cells expressing IL-10 versus TNF-α in OSA patients. The *solid line rectangle* represents a subgroup of OSA patients (17.4%) with TNF-α/IL-10 ratio > 1.

the expression of TNF-α in $CD4^+$ T cells was not significantly different than in controls.

Similar to the CD8 subset, within the OSA group AHI was negatively correlated with the percentage of $CD4^+$/IL-10^+ T lymphocytes ($r = -0.48$, $P = .046$) and was positively correlated with percentage of $CD4^+$/TNF-α^+ T cells ($r = 0.83$, $P = .00001$).

Type 2 Dominance in CD4 and CD8 Lymphocytes in OSA Patients

Type 2 and Type 1 cytokine expression were analyzed depending on IL-4 and IL-2 cytokine expression, respectively. The percentage of IL-4–positive T cells was significantly higher in OSA patients as compared with controls (4.3-fold higher for $CD4^+$ and 6.3-fold higher for $CD8^+$ subsets; TABLE 1). The results were less clear for IL-2; only some of the OSA patients demonstrated increased expression of IL-2 in both CD4 and CD8 T cells, but because of large variability the differences were only of borderline significance. Notably, the increase in the percentage of IL-4–expressing T cells was more pronounced than in the T cells expressing IL-2, suggesting a type 2–dominant cytokine expression. Type 1 dominance was found in only 2 out of 23 OSA patients (8.7%).

Cytotoxicity against HUVECs

Because killing of endothelial cells is of great relevance to atherosclerosis, HUVECs were utilized as target cells. The cytotoxicity of OSA CD8 T cells against HUVECs at an E/T ratio of 10:1 was found to be significantly higher in moderate-to-severe OSA patients with AHI > 25 (71.1 ± 7.0%) as compared with controls

(41.1 ± 6.4%; $P = .0002$) or to patients with mild OSA with AHI < 25 (37.6 ± 6.4%; $P = .0001$).

Lysis of HUVECs by OSA CD4$^+$ T cells was also significantly higher than in controls, but only at an E/T ratio of 20:1 and with a large variability between subjects (range 6.4% to 48.3%, mean 31.96 ± 16.8% vs. range 7.5% to 22.7%, mean 13.5 ± 0.8%, respectively, $P = .03$). For comparison, at the same experimental conditions in the same patients (n = 4), significant cytotoxicity of γδ T lymphocytes against HUVECs was noted at an E/T ratio of 5:1.[15]

CD4$^+$CD28^{null} T Cells in OSA Patients and Controls

Because CD4$^+$CD28^{null} T cells induce killing of endothelial cells,[36–38] we investigated whether this subset is involved in CD4-mediated cytotoxicity in OSA patients. We found that the frequencies of CD4$^+$CD28^{null} T cells were low in controls (TABLE 1), as previously demonstrated for normal individuals.[38] In OSA patients, however, this subset was found to be increased by 2.9-fold (TABLE 1). In addition, by depleting CD4$^+$CD28^{null} T cells from the CD4$^+$ population, the lysis of HUVECs was significantly decreased (data not shown).

CD40L Expression on Circulating CD8 T Lymphocytes

CD40L is an important T cell activation marker, and CD40-CD40L interactions are involved in inflammatory cell activation in atherogenesis.[39] Furthermore, cytotoxic T cell responses are mediated by CD40 signaling.[40,41] Therefore, we investigated whether CD40L is upregulated in T cells of OSA patients. Indeed, despite the large variability in patient data, the percentage of CD8$^+$ T cells expressing CD40L was significantly higher in OSA patients as compared with controls (TABLE 1). In CD4$^+$ T cells, however, CD40L expression varied greatly (range 2% to 34.4% in patients with OSA) and was not significantly different from controls.

Effects of Single-Night nCPAP Treatment on Cytokine Expression and Phenotype in CD8 and CD4 Lymphocytes

To demonstrate further that sleep apnea and not any other associated variables affected lymphocyte function we compared OSA patients and controls simultaneously with a group of OSA patients after their first night of treatment with nCPAP, which normalized their breathing in sleep as evidenced by decreased AHI and percent time below 90% arterial O_2 saturation (TABLE 1).

Treatment with a single night of nCPAP did not affect the percentage of CD8 T cells expressing IL-2, IL-4, or IL-10 , but the percentage of TNF-α–expressing CD8 T cells was decreased by 2.3-fold (TABLE 1). In addition, in nCPAP-treated patients, CD40L expression was dramatically decreased (3.6-fold), and cytotoxicity of CD8$^+$ T lymphocytes against HUVECs was only 30% to 40% that of untreated OSA patients and was comparable to that of controls (24.8 ± 9.7%). These data are consistent with a previous study demonstrating decreased cytotoxicity against K562 target cells of CD8 T cells from nCPAP-treated OSA patients compared with control values.[42]

DISCUSSION

In the current communication, $CD4^+$ and $CD8^+$ T cells of patients with OSA were shown to be activated phenotypically and functionally. Moreover, this is consistent with our previous studies demonstrating increased activation in patients with OSA of monocytes and γδ T cells,[12,15,42] both implicated in atherosclerotic and cardiovascular consequences. Specifically, we found a shift in type 1/type 2 cytokine expression towards type 2 dominance in patients with OSA. A similar balance in favor of type 2 dominance has been associated with insomnia,[43] demonstrating a possible relationship between sleep disturbances and immune disorders. Furthermore, catecholamines, which have been shown to be increased in OSA patients, [44] have also been shown to inhibit the production of type 1 cytokines by T cells and to stimulate the production of type 2 cytokines such as IL-4 and IL-10, possibly through stimulation of the β_2-adrenoreceptor–cAMP–protein kinase A pathway.[45] The shift towards type 2 dominance may represent a protective mechanism in OSA to attenuate or moderate hypoxia-induced atherogenesis by increasing IL-4 production, as IL-4 has also been shown to possess antiatherogenic properties [46,47] via suppression of proinflammatory cytokine production. It should be noted, however, that IL-4 has also been reported to possess proatherogenic properties, particularly in the early stages of the disease.[19] Thus, IL-4 may participate in the progression of early 'inflammatory' atherosclerotic lesions[48] by upregulating P-selectin[49] and VCAM-1[50] in human endothelial cells. In such an event, it could aggravate proatherogenic pathways in OSA.

Interestingly, the IL-10/TNF-α distribution among the different lymphocyte subsets varied considerably in patients with OSA. In γδ T lymphocytes we observed an increase in the content of TNF-α and a decrease in IL-10,[15] indicating that γδ T lymphocytes of patients with OSA were activated. In CD4 T cells, on the other hand, a higher percentage IL-10–expressing cells was detected. This may represent a compensatory mechanism to downregulate TNF-α overexpression and to balance proinflammatory versus anti-inflammatory cytokine release. In contrast to CD4 cells, the percentage of IL-10–expressing CD8 T cells in OSA was similar to controls, and the altered IL-10/TNF-α balance was apparent by the increase in the percentage of TNF-α–expressing CD8 T cells. All in all, IL-10 expression in the various T cell subsets was negatively correlated with the severity of OSA, whereas TNF-α expression was positively correlated.

Based on the TNF-α/IL-10 ratio in CD8 T cells, OSA patients could be subdivided into two groups: the major group, with a TNF-α/IL-10 ratio < 1, and a smaller group of moderate-to-severe OSA patients ($AHI > 25$) that, similar to OSA γδ T lymphocytes, exhibited decreased levels of IL-10 contrasted with high expression of TNF-α. IL-10 has been reported to inhibit proinflammatory signal-induced NF-κB activation in peripheral T lymphocytes and to prevent the release of oxygen free radicals by monocytes and macrophages. This suggests that it may serve as a protective mechanism to prevent or moderate the progression of atherosclerosis.[51,52] In addition, we found increased cytotoxicity of OSA CD8 T cells against endothelial cells. The presence of such highly cytotoxic lymphocytes with increased TNF-α expression and low IL-10 levels may have significant implications to cardiovascular pathology. These data suggest that OSA patients with low IL-10 and high TNF-α could be at a higher risk for cardiovascular morbidity. Thus, such an analysis at the cellular level may help to identify patients at cardiovascular risk. Additionally, the expression of CD40L was also expanded in OSA CD8 T cells. Because CD40-CD40L interactions can influence T cell–mediated MHC-unrestricted cytotoxicity[53] and participate in organ-specific autoimmune disease and atherosclerosis,[39–41] our results suggest that the $CD40L^+CD8^+$ T cells may enhance inflammatory and autoimmune processes in OSA patients. The impact of nCPAP treatment is clearly evident, as it was followed by a drastic decrease in the percentage of CD40L–expressing cells among the $CD8^+$ T subset.

A significant elevation of cytotoxicity was also noted in OSA CD4 T cells, possibly owing to the increase in the $CD4^+CD28^{null}$ subset, which could be involved directly in plaque rupture,[36,38] and which is distinct from the classical $CD4^+CD28^+$ T cells that can induce cytolysis of endothelial cells.[36–38]

On the basis of our data, it is reasonable to assume that not all lymphocyte subpopulations of OSA patients are affected in a similar manner by the intermittent hypoxia and/or sleep fragmentation that results in catecholamine release. For example, increased cytotoxicity of CD8 T cells in OSA directly depends on the presence of perforin and CD56CD16 NK receptors,[42] whereas in $\gamma\delta$ T cells, CD16CD56 has only a minor effect on HUVEC killing, and their cytotoxicity is mainly attributed to increased TNF-α.[15] Moreover, it appears that $\gamma\delta$ T cells are more highly affected than CD8 T lymphocytes,[15,42] whereas CD4 T lymphocytes are less affected. This possibility is strongly supported by data showing differential effects of exposure to hypoxia *in vitro* on the functions of $\gamma\delta$ versus $\alpha\beta$ T cells and CD8 versus CD4 T lymphocytes.[54]

In conclusion, despite differences in various T cell mechanisms of cytotoxicity, all T cell populations in OSA patients could contribute to endothelial activation and damage through their uniquely enhanced cytotoxic abilities and through cytokine imbalance. Nasal CPAP treatment could moderate some lymphocyte dysfunctions and thus could attenuate some atherogenic pathways.[55]

REFERENCES

1. LAVIE, P., P. HERER & V. HOFFSTEIN. 2000. Obstructive sleep apnoea syndrome as a risk factor for hypertension: population study. Br. Med. J. **320:** 479–482.
2. ROUX, F., C. D'AMBROSIO & V. MOHSENIN. 2000. Sleep-related breathing disorders and cardiovascular disease. Am. J. Med. **108:** 396–402.
3. SHAHAR, E. *et al.* 2001. Sleep-disordered breathing and cardiovascular disease cross-sectional results of the Sleep Heart Health Study. Am. J. Respir. Crit. Care Med. **163:** 19–25.
4. PARISH, J.M. & V.K. SOMERS. 2004. Obstructive sleep apnea and cardiovascular disease. Mayo. Clin. Proc. **79:** 1036–1046.
5. WICK, G., M. KNOFLACH & Q. XU. Autoimmune and inflammatory mechanisms in atherosclerosis. 2004. Annu. Rev. Immunol. **22:** 361–403.
6. HANSSON, G.K. 2001. Immune mechanisms in atherosclerosis. Arterioscler. Thromb. Vasc. Biol. **21:** 1876–1890.
7. LIBBY, P. 2002. Inflammation in atherosclerosis. Nature **420:** 868–874.
8. FAN, J. & T. WATANABE. 2003. Inflammatory reactions in the pathogenesis of atherosclerosis. J. Atheroscler. Thromb. **10:** 63–71.
9. SHERER, Y. & Y. SHOENFELD. 2002. Immunomodulation for treatment and prevention of atherosclerosis. Autoimmun. Rev. **2:** 21–27.
10. ZHOU, X. & G.K. HANSSON. 2004. Immunomodulation and vaccination for atherosclerosis. Expert Opin. Biol. Ther. **4:** 599–612.

11. LAVIE, L. 2003. Obstructive sleep apnoea syndrome—an oxidative stress disorder. Sleep Med. Rev. **7:** 35–51.
12. DYUGOVSKAYA, L., P. LAVIE & L. LAVIE. 2002. Increased adhesion molecules expression and production of reactive oxygen species in leukocytes of sleep apnea patients. Am. J. Respir. Crit. Care Med. **165:** 934–939.
13. LAVIE, L. *et al.* 2003. Plasma level of nitric oxide and L-arginine in sleep apnea patients. J. Mol. Neurosci. **21:** 57–62.
14. LAVIE, L., A. VISHNEVSKY & P. LAVIE. 2004. Evidence for lipid peroxidation in obstructive sleep apnea. Sleep **27:** 123–128.
15. DYUGOVSKAYA, L., P. LAVIE & L. LAVIE. 2003. Phenotypic and functional characterization of blood γδ T cells in sleep apnea. Am. J. Respir. Crit. Care Med. **168:** 242–249.
16. SONG, L., C. LEUNG & C. SCHINDLER. 2001. Lymphocytes are important in early atherosclerosis. J. Clin. Invest. **108:** 251–259.
17. WEYAND, C.M. *et al.* 2001. T-cell immunity in acute coronary syndromes. Mayo. Clin. Proc. **76:** 1011–1020.
18. NAKAJIMA, T. *et al.* 2002. T-cell-mediated lysis of endothelial cells in acute coronary syndromes. Circulation **105:** 570–575.
19. VON DER THUSEN, J.H. *et al.* 2003. Interleukins in atherosclerosis: molecular pathways and therapeutic potential. Pharmacol. Rev. **55:** 133–166.
20. SOEJIMA, H. *et al.* 2003. Preference toward a T-helper type 1 response in patients with coronary spastic angina. Circulation **107:** 2196–2200.
21. MANTOVANI, A. *et al.* 1998. Regulation of endothelial cell function by pro- and anti-inflammatory cytokines. Transplant Proc. **30:** 4239–4243.
22. FERRARI, R. 1999. The role of TNF in cardiovascular disease. Pharmacol. Rev. **40:** 97–105.
23. RIDKER, P.M. *et al.* 2000. Elevation of tumor necrosis factor-alpha and increased risk of recurrent coronary events after myocardial infarction. Circulation **101:** 2149–2153.
24. SACK, M. 2002. Tumor necrosis factor-alpha in cardiovascular biology and the potential role for anti-tumor necrosis factor-alpha therapy in heart disease. Pharmacol. Ther. **94:** 123–135.
25. MOORE, K.W. *et al.* 2003. Interleukin-10 and the interleukin-10 receptor. Annu. Rev. Immunol. **19:** 683–765.
26. STUMPF, C. *et al.* 2003. Decrease of serum levels of the anti-inflammatory cytokine interleukin-10 in patients with advanced chronic heart failure. Clin. Sci (Lond.) **105:** 45–50.
27. MALLAT, Z. *et al.* 1999. Protective role of interleukin-10 in atherosclerosis. Circ. Res. **85:** 17–24.
28. TENGUI, A. & Z. MALLAT. 2001. Interleukin-10: an anti-atherogenic cytokine? Eur. J. Clin. Invest. **31:** 1–2.
29. PINDERSKI, L.J. *et al.* 2002. Overexpression of interleukin-10 by activated T lymphocytes inhibits atherosclerosis in LDL receptor-deficient mice by altering lymphocyte and macrophage phenotypes. Circ. Res. **90:** 1064–1071.
30. PEREZ FERNANDEZ, R. & J.C. KASKI. 2002. Interleukin-10 and coronary disease. Rev. Esp. Cardiol. **55:** 738–750.
31. HADDAD, J. & C. FAHLMAN. 2002. Redox- and oxidant-mediated regulation of interleukin-10: an inflammatory, antioxidant cytokine? Biochem. Biophys. Res. Commun. **297:** 163–176.
32. TERAMOTO, S., H. YAMAMOTO & O. YASUYOSHI. 2003. Increased C-reactive protein and increased plasma interleukin-6 may synergistically affect the progression of coronary atherosclerosis in obstructive sleep apnea syndrome. Circulation **107:** 1129–1134.
33. ALBERTI, A. *et al.* 2003. Plasma cytokine levels in patients with obstructive sleep apnea syndrome: a preliminary study. J. Sleep Res. **12:** 305–311.
34. YOKOE, T. *et al.* 2003. Elevated levels of C-reactive protein and interleukin-6 in patients with obstructive sleep apnea syndrome are decreased by nasal continuous positive airway pressure. Circulation **107:** 1129–1134.
35. LAVIE, L. 2004. Sleep apnea syndrome, endothelial dysfunction, and cardiovascular morbidity. Sleep **27:** 1053–1055.

36. NAKAJIMA, T. *et al.* 2003. De novo expression of killer immunoglobulin-like receptors and signaling proteins regulates the cytotoxic function of CD4 T cells in acute coronary syndromes. Circ. Res. **93:** 106–113.
37. LIUZZO, G. *et al.* 2000. Monoclonal T-cell proliferation and plaque instability in acute coronary syndromes. Circulation **101:** 2883–2888.
38. SCHMIDT, D., J.J. GORONZY & C.M. WEYAND. 1996. CD4+ CD7– CD28– T cells are expanded in rheumatoid arthritis and are characterized by autoreactivity. J. Clin. Invest. **97:** 2027–2037.
39. MARX, N. *et al.* 2000. Effect of rosiglitazone treatment on soluble CD40L in patients with type 2 diabetes and coronary artery disease. Circulation **107:** 1954–1957.
40. BENNETT, S.R. *et al.* 1998. Help for cytotoxic-T-cell responses is mediated by CD40 signalling. Nature **393:** 478–480.
41. SCHOENBERGER, S.P. *et al.* 1998. T-cell help for cytotoxic T lymphocytes is mediated by CD40–CD40L interactions. Nature **393:** 480–483.
42. DYUGOVSKAYA, L., P. LAVIE & L. LAVIE. 2004. Elevated cytotoxicity and cytokine imbalance as markers of pro-atherogenic activation of lymphocytes in sleep apnea patients. Effects of nCPAP treatment [abstract]. Sleep **27:** A203–204.
43. SAKAMI, S. *et al.* 2002. Coemergence of insomnia and a shift in the Th1/Th2 balance toward Th2 dominance. Neuroimmunomodulation **10:** 337–343.
44. PELED, N. *et al.* 1998. Contributions of hypoxia and respiratory disturbance index to sympathetic activation and blood pressure in obstructive sleep apnea syndrome. Am. J. Hypertens. **11:** 1284–1289.
45. ELENKOV, I.J. & G.P. CHROUSOS. 1999. Stress, cytokine patterns and susceptibility to disease. Bailliere's Best Pract. Res. Clin. Endocrinol. Metab. **13:** 583-595.
46. SASAGURI, T. *et al.* 1998. A role for interleukin 4 in production of matrix metalloproteinase 1 by human aortic smooth muscle cells. Atherosclerosis **138:** 247–253.
47. ELLIOTT, M.J. *et al.* 1991. Inhibition of human monocyte adhesion by interleukin-4. Blood **77:** 2739–2745.
48. GEORGE, J. *et al.* 2000. Requisite role for interleukin-4 in the acceleration of fatty streaks induced by heat shock protein 65 or Mycobacterium tuberculosis. Circ. Res. **86:** 1203–1210.
49. KHEW-GOODALL, Y. *et al.* 1999. Stat6 activation is essential for interleukin-4 induction of P-selectin transcription in human umbilical vein endothelial cells. Arterioscler. Thromb. Vasc. Biol. **19:** 1421–1429.
50. LEE, Y.W. *et al.* 2001. IL-4-induced oxidative stress upregulates VCAM-1 gene expression in human endothelial cells. J. Mol. Cell. Cardiol. **33:** 83–94.
51. TERKELTAUB, R.A. 1999. IL-10: An "immunologic scalpel" for atherosclerosis? Arterioscler. Thromb. Vasc. Biol. **19:** 2823–2825.
52. PARK, S.H. *et al.* 2003. Regulatory effect of SOCS on NF-kappaB activity in murine monocytes/macrophages. DNA Cell Biol. **22:** 131–139.
53. SARTORIUS, R. *et al.* 2003. Induction of human NK cell-mediated cytotoxicity by CD40 triggering on antigen presenting cells. Cell. Immunol. **221:** 81–88.
54. CALDWELL, C.C. *et al.* 2001. Differential effects of physiologically relevant hypoxic conditions on T lymphocyte development and effector functions. J. Immunol. **167:** 6140–6149.
55. MILLERON, O. *et al.* 2004. Benefits if obstructive sleep apnoea treatment in coronary artery disease: a long-term follow-up study. Eur. Heart. J. **25:** 728–734.

Systemic Lupus Erythematosus, Atherosclerosis, and Autoantibodies

SANDRA ZAMPIERI,[a] LUCA IACCARINO,[a] ANNA GHIRARDELLO,[a] ELENA TARRICONE,[a] SILVIA ARIENTI,[a] PIERCARLO SARZI-PUTTINI,[b] PIERFRANCA GAMBARI,[a] AND ANDREA DORIA[a]

[a]*Division of Rheumatology, Department of Medical and Surgical Science, University of Padova, Padova, Italy*

[b]*Hospital L. Sacco, University of Milano, Milano, Italy*

ABSTRACT: Over the past number of years numerous data have been published regarding increased atherosclerosis in patients with systemic lupus erythematosus (SLE), and it has been shown that premature or accelerated atherosclerosis is an important cause of morbidity and mortality in these patients. Besides the traditional risk factors for cardiovascular disease, the association between SLE and atherosclerosis can be attributed to additional risk factors closely related to inflammation and autoimmunity. In particular, several autoantibodies and their respective autoantigens have been identified as possible factors in the development and progression of the atherosclerotic process in SLE. The understanding of SLE-related risk factors for enhanced atherosclerosis could shed more light on disease mechanisms, leading to new therapeutic strategies for the treatment of cardiovascular diseases in SLE patients. In the present paper, the biological characteristics and possible pathogenetic role of the oxidized low-density lipoprotein (oxLDL) and anti-oxLDL, β_2-glycoprotein I (β_2GPI) and anti-β_2GPI, and heat-shock protein 60/65 (HSP60/65) and anti-HSP60/65 autoantibody systems are summarized.

KEYWORDS: systemic lupus erythematosus; atherosclerosis; cardiovascular disease; autoantibodies; oxidized low-density lipoprotein; heat-shock proteins; phospholipid proteins; β_2-glycoprotein I; risk factors

INTRODUCTION

Systemic lupus erythematosus (SLE) is a chronic inflammatory disease characterized by a perturbed immune response against self with the consequent production of autoantibodies. Some of these autoantibodies form immune complexes that are responsible for tissue inflammation directly contributing to the development of different clinical manifestations of the disease.

It has been suggested that the local inflammatory and autoimmune processes can promote atherosclerosis in SLE patients.[1] In fact, an increased prevalence of cardio-

Address for correspondence: Andrea Doria, M.D., Division of Rheumatology, University of Padova, Via Giustiniani, 2, I-35128 Padova, Italy. Voice: +39-049-8212202; fax: +39-049-8212191.

adoria@unipd.it

**Ann. N.Y. Acad. Sci. 1051: 351–361 (2005). © 2005 New York Academy of Sciences.
doi: 10.1196/annals.1361.077**

vascular disease related to premature or accelerated atherosclerosis, which has been indicated as an important cause of morbidity and mortality in SLE,[2,3] has been reported in these patients.

Premature atherosclerosis in association with SLE was first described in 1975 by Bulkley *et al.*[4] in necroscopy cases and was later confirmed by Urowitz *et al.*[5] in a survival study. Several subsequent studies reported that SLE is strongly associated with coronary artery diseases and with atherosclerosis.[6–8] This association is only partially linked to the traditional risk factors for cardiovascular disease such as hyperlipidemia, hypertension, diabetes mellitus, smoking, and genetic background, which seem to be similar to those observed in the general population.

Systemic inflammation and autoantibodies, circulating immune complexes and complement products, dyslipidemia, and nephritis can be considered SLE-related risk factors, in addition to standard risk factors, that may explain the enhanced atherogenesis in these patients.[9] Moreover, steroid therapy at certain dosages can impair the lipid profile, with a possible influence on cardiovascular events.[10]

ATHEROSCLEROSIS, INFLAMMATION, AND IMMUNE RESPONSE

Although it was initially considered a bland lipid storage disease, atherosclerosis is now considered to be a process closely related to inflammation.[11] Advances in basic and experimental science have actually underlined the pivotal role of inflammatory mechanisms in the induction, progression, and rupture of the atherosclerotic plaque.

Besides the importance of the inflammatory process, recent studies have demonstrated that the immune system plays a key role in the pathogenesis of atherosclerosis by involving effectors of both cellular and humoral immunity. Studies on transgenic mice have shown that $CD4^+$ and $CD8^+$ T cells are important in the development and progression of atherosclerosis.[12,13] In particular, atherosclerosis seems to be a Th1-mediated disease, as Th1 response induces plaque formation.[14,15]

Moreover, several data have been published regarding the association between autoantibodies and atherosclerosis. The possible mechanisms by which these autoantibodies participate in the development and progression of atherosclerosis have largely been investigated,[9,12,16,17] and have also been studied in animals, providing broad evidence of autoantibody-mediated atherosclerosis.[18–20]

The present paper is focused on the characteristics of the most investigated autoantibodies, and their respective autoantigens, involved in the atherosclerotic process. In particular, the role of such autoantibodies in the development and progression of atherosclerosis in SLE patients is summarized.

AUTOANTIGENS AND AUTOANTIBODIES

Numerous autoantigens and their respective autoantibodies are involved in the pathogenesis of atherosclerosis,[21] but for some a dual function has been hypothesized, because a protective role against atherosclerosis has also been described.[22]

The three major autoantigen-autoantibody systems involved in the atherosclerotic process are oxidized low-density lipoprotein (oxLDL) and anti-oxLDL, β_2-glycoprotein I (β_2GPI) and anti-β_2GPI, and heat-shock protein 60/65 (HSP60/65) and anti-HSP60/65.

Anti-oxLDL Antibodies

Modified forms of low-density lipoprotein (LDL) are among the targeted autoantigens in atherosclerosis. LDL is constituted by molecules of phospholipids, triglycerides, and cholesterol, and accumulates in macrophages. During early atherogenesis, LDL become trapped in the subendothelial space and is subsequently oxidized.[17] This oxLDL is thought to be responsible for triggering inflammatory responses in macrophages and vascular wall cells. It increases the adhesive properties of endothelial cells[23] and induces the activation of monocytes and T cells.[24,25] oxLDL can be actively taken up by scavenger receptor-mediated endocytosis, transforming macrophages into so-called foam cells.[26]

Epitopes generated by LDL oxidation have been implicated as targets for autoantibodies. Some anti-oxLDL antibodies can enhance oxidized-LDL uptake by macrophages through the involvement of the Fc receptors rather than via the usually employed scavenger receptor, favoring foam cell formation and macrophage activation.[27]

Consistent with this finding, several groups have found an association between increased anti-oxLDL antibodies and some conditions linked to coronary artery diseases in humans.[28–32] However, recent studies showed that immunization with oxLDL resulted in induction of anti-oxLDL antibodies, but suppression rather than aggravation of early atherogenesis.[33,34] In addition, in animal models the infusion of anti-oxLDL monoclonal antibody inhibits the uptake of oxLDL by macrophages.[35]

Therefore, the repertoire of anti-oxLDL in humans may include both "protective" and "pathogenic" autoantibodies. Under normal circumstances, anti-oxLDL may help to clear high levels of oxLDL. However, upon enhanced oxidation of LDL (e.g., because of smoking, or lack of anti-oxidants), anti-oxLDL with higher affinity or different target epitopes is generated and may aid the uptake of oxLDL by macrophages, turning them into foam cells within atherosclerotic plaques. The protective antibodies most likely belong to the IgM class, whereas the pathogenetic autoantibodies are most likely IgG.

Increased levels of anti-oxLDL have been found in SLE patients[9,10,36,37] (TABLE 1). However, in SLE, the association between anti-oxLDL and cardiovascular disease (CVD) is still being debated.[36,37] OxLDL could be considered a common pathogenetic factor in SLE and atherosclerosis,[38] but additional prospective studies are needed to clearly identify anti-oxLDL autoantibodies as a nontraditional risk factor for atherosclerosis in SLE.

Antiphospholipid Antibodies

Antiphospholipid antibodies are a heterogeneous group of autoantibodies, including, anticardiolipin antibody (aCL) and lupus anticoagulant (LA), generally directed to phospholipid binding proteins; in this regard, β_2GPI represents the major antigenic target.

Human β_2GPI is a 50 kDa plasma glycoprotein that binds to negatively charged components.[39] Anti-β_2GPI antibodies may react directly with their antigens, expressed on endothelial cell membranes, inducing a proinflammatory and a procoagulant endothelial phenotype that is also proatherogenic.[16]

Moreover, it has been shown that IgG anti–high-density lipoprotein (HDL) and IgG anti-β_2GPI are associated with reduced paraoxonase (PON) activity in SLE and primary antiphospholipid syndrome (APS).[40] PON is an enzyme with antioxidant activity that circulates in plasma attached to HDL. Its physiological role is to prevent oxidation of LDL. Therefore, anti-HDL and anti-β_2GPI may be responsible for LDL oxidation via an inhibitory effect on PON activity.[40]

Beta$_2$GPI has been found to bind oxLDL, and this complex inhibits the uptake of oxLDL by macrophages through scavenger receptors, therefore providing a sort of protection against atherosclerosis.[27] However, the binding of anti-β_2GPI antibodies to oxLDL/β_2GPI complexes makes the uptake of oxLDL by macrophages even more efficient through Fc receptors, leading to an increase of foam cell formation.[41] Stable oxLDL/β_2GPI complexes have been detected in the sera of SLE and APS patients. Both the presence of these complexes and IgG antibodies directed against them have been found to be strongly associated with arterial thrombosis.[16]

Recently, it has been shown that high-sensitivity C-reactive protein (hsCRP), a useful marker for detecting subclinical atherosclerosis, forms circulating immune complexes with oxLDL and β_2GPI.[16] Of note, only CRP from SLE, APS, and diabetes mellitus (DM) patients interacts with oxLDL/β_2GPI, whereas CRP from rheumatoid arthritis (RA) patients does not have this property.[16] CRP of SLE, APS and DM patients is synthesized by activated macrophages in arterial intima, allowing the direct formation of CRP/oxLDL/β_2GPI immune complexes in the intima of atherogenic arteries.[16]

It is noteworthy that β_2GPI can also be found in human atherosclerotic lesions obtained from carotid endoarterectomies. It is expressed abundantly within the subendothelial regions and the intimal-medial border of human atherosclerotic plaques, and it localizes with CD4$^+$ lymphocytes.[42]

The proatherosclerotic effect of anti-β_2GPI is also supported by studies on animals.[19,43,44] In LDL receptor–deficient mice or in apo E knockout mice, immunization with β_2GPI enhances atherosclerotic lesions, which contain abundant CD4$^+$ cells.[19] The transfer of lymphocytes from mice immunized with β_2GPI to mice of similar genetic background increases atherosclerotic lesions compared with those occurring in animals transferred with lymphocytes from control mice.[44] Finally, T cell depletion impairs reproduction of the experimental model. Therefore, T cells specific to β_2GPI are capable of increasing atherosclerosis, suggesting that β_2GPI is a target autoantigen in atherosclerosis.

The presence of antiphospholipid antibodies has been found to be a risk factor for various manifestations of coronary artery disease, such as angina, myocardial infarction, or cardiac death, as well as being associated with subclinical atherosclerosis.[17,45–47] It has also been shown that patients with APS have a high prevalence of increased carotid intima-media thickness or plaque.[48–50] As seen with anti-oxLDL antibodies, some antiphospholipid antibodies may play a protective role in atherogenesis. In fact, it has been shown that these antibodies, which cross-react with native and oxLDL, significantly reduced plaque formation in atherosclerosis-prone LDL receptor–deficient rabbits.[18]

In SLE patients both antiphospholipid antibodies as well as APS are frequently observed.[51] However, despite all these observations, most studies on subclinical ath-

TABLE 1. Cross-sectional studies on the relationship between autoantibodies and atherosclerosis (ATS) in SLE patients

Antibody	SLE vs. Controls	Association with ATS	Reference
Anti-oxLDL	Increased	ND	9
Anti-oxLDL	Increased	No	36
Anti-oxLDL	Increased	Yes	37
aCL	Increased	No	8
LA	Increased	No	8
aCL	Increased	No (protective)	54
LA	Increased	No	54
aCL	Increased	No	52
LA	Increased	No	52
Anti-HSP60/65	Increased	ND	9
Anti-HSP60/65	Marginally increased	ND	62
Anti-HSP60/65	Not increased	ND	63

ABBREVIATIONS: ND, not determined; aCL, anticardiolipin; LA, lupus anticoagulant; HSP60/65, heat-shock protein 60/65; oxLDL, oxidized low-density lipoprotein.

erosclerosis in SLE have failed to find an association with antiphospholipid antibodies[8,52–54] (TABLE 1). A protective role of these antibodies was found in only one recent study.[54] In this case-control study, anticardiolipin antibodies were found to be present less frequently in SLE patients with carotid plaque than in those without plaque, confirming the lack of association between anticardiolipin antibody and carotid plaque or cardiovascular disease as reported by other authors.[8,37]

Anti–Heat-Shock Protein Antibodies

The human HSPs are a group of proteins that are involved in maintaining the folding of several cell components. They are expressed at high levels on endothelial cells in response to stressors such as hypertension, smoking, lipoproteins, and oxidants.[55] They are classified on the basis of their molecular weight. The 60-kDa family has been identified as a candidate autoantigen in early atherosclerosis. HSP60 in mammals and in *chlamydiae*, and the mycobacterial homologue mHSP65 are members of this family.[56]

The members of 60-kDa family are evolutionarily highly conserved proteins, thus facilitating cross-reactivity between human and bacterial species.[56] As mentioned above, they are overexpressed in response to stressors in order to maintain the viability of targeted cells. Under such circumstances, HSPs offer a target for autoimmunity. Due to high sequence homology, antibodies directed against human HSP60 as well as bacterial HSP65 can be found easily in patient sera mediating a proatherogenic effect.

There are clinical, subclinical, and experimental data that anti-HSP60/65 has a proatherogenic role. Patients with high levels of anti-HSP65 were found to be at increased risk of subsequent cardiovascular events and cardiovascular mortality.[57,58]

TABLE 2. Prospective study on the relationship between autoantibodies and atherosclerosis in SLE patients at baseline and after five-year follow-up

Antibody	Association with ATS
Anti-oxPAPC	
Baseline	No
5-year follow-up	Yes
aCL	
Baseline	No
5-year follow-up	No
LA	
Baseline	No
5-year follow-up	No
Anti-b2GPI	
Baseline	No
5-year follow-up	No
Anti-HSP60/65	
Baseline	No
5-year follow-up	No

ABBREVIATIONS: aCL, anticardiolipin; β_2GPI, β_2-glycoprotein 1; HSP60/65, heat-shock protein 60/65; LA, lupus anticoagulant; oxPAPC, oxidized palmitoyl arachidonoyl phosphocholine.

Subjects with sonographic evidence of carotid atherosclerotic lesions had significantly elevated levels of anti-HSP65 compared with controls.[59]

It has been shown that immunization of normocholesterolemic rabbits with HSP65 induces atherosclerosis.[60] Moreover, immunization with mycobacterial or recombinant HSP65 also induces early atherosclerosis in LDL receptor–deficient mice,[20] and enhances fatty-streak formation in C57BL/6J mice fed a high cholesterol diet.[61]

In SLE patients, data on the serum concentration of anti-HSP65 antibodies are heterogeneous. In three different studies, serum levels of these autoantibodies were found to be increased, only marginally increased, or not increased compared with normal subjects[9,62,63] (TABLE 1). Moreover, to date, no data on the relationship between anti-HSP60/65 and atherosclerosis in SLE patients have been available.

RISK FACTORS FOR ATHEROSCLEROSIS IN A COHORT OF SLE PATIENTS FOLLOWED PROSPECTIVELY

Recently, we investigated traditional and nontraditional risk factors for atherosclerosis in a cohort of SLE patients followed prospectively over five years.[10] These patients had no evidence of overt atherosclerotic disease at baseline evaluation. All prominent clinical and laboratory features were recorded at baseline and after five-year follow-up, including SLE disease activity as measured by the European Consensus Lupus Activity Measurement (ECLAM) score, and cumulative damage using

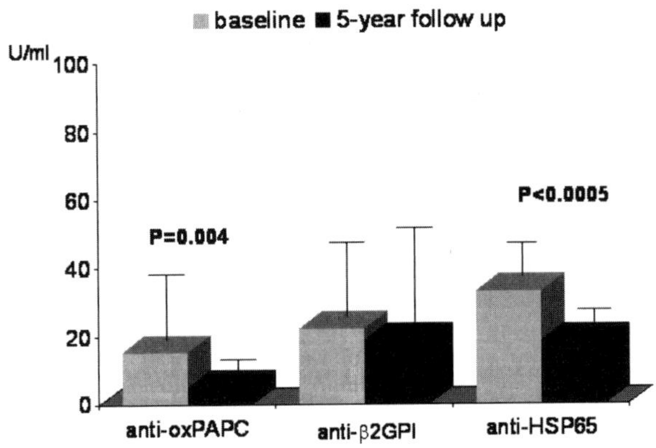

FIGURE 1. Serum levels of anti-oxPAPC, anti-HPS65, and anti-β_2GPI antibodies in 78 SLE patients. Autoantibodies directed against oxPAPC, HPS65, and β_2GPI were detected in patient sera by ELISA at baseline and after five-year follow-up. Values are reported as mean ± SD.

the Systemic Lupus International Collaborating Clinics (SLICC) damage index. At baseline and after five-year follow up, we also tested for several autoantibodies, including anti–oxidized palmitoyl arachidonoyl phosphocholine (oxPAPC), anti-β_2GPI, and anti-HSP65 (TABLE 2). (OxPAPC is an important antigenic epitope of oxLDL. They have similar bioactivities, but oxPAPC as an antigen is more stable than oxLDL during preparation and storage.[64]) Moreover, traditional risk factors for atherosclerosis and treatment taken during the study period were monitored regularly and recorded at each clinical evaluation. Finally, at the end of follow-up, carotid ultrasound examination was performed.

The mean serum levels of anti-oxPAPC, anti-HPS65, and anti-β_2GP1 antibodies were lower in the second sample in comparison with the first (FIG. 1). However, differences were significant only for anti-HSP65 and anti-oxPAPC antibody levels (FIG. 1). It is possible that in SLE patients, disease treatment, especially immunosuppressants, reduces the serum levels of such antibodies.

With univariate analysis, we did not observe any significant relationship between these autoantibodies and carotid parameters, apart from the correlation between anti-oxLDL levels at the time of ultrasound examination and maximum intima-media thickness (IMT; FIG. 2). Moreover, with multivariate analysis, anti-oxPAPC levels at the time of ultrasound examination were associated with increased maximum (M) and mean (m) IMT.

Therefore, our data show that anti-oxPAPC may play a role in the accelerated atherosclerotic process observed in SLE patients, whereas the role of anti-β_2GPI and anti-HSP65 seems to be masked by some disease-related features, particularly cumulative prednisone dosage and renal involvement.

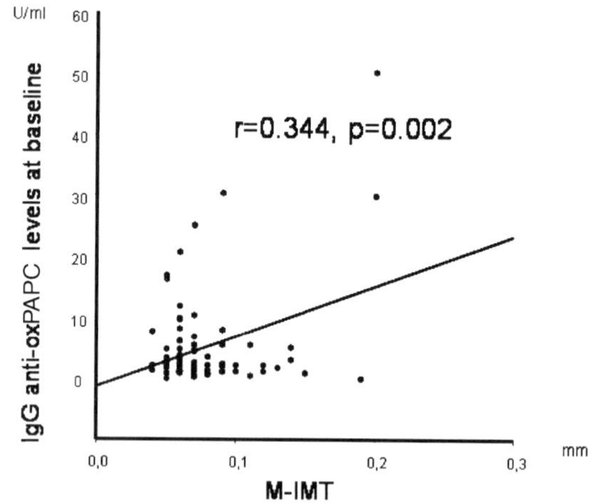

FIGURE 2. Correlation between maximum intima-media thickness (M-IMT) and IgG anti-oxPAPC levels at baseline.

CONCLUSIONS

SLE patients are at high risk of cardiovascular disease, and premature or accelerated atherosclerosis has been demonstrated in these patients. Several studies have identified traditional and nontraditional risk factors for atherosclerosis in these patients, and among them enhanced titers of autoantibodies against antigens involved in the atherosclerotic process provide evidence of the association between SLE and atherosclerosis.

However, studies on clinical features or markers as predictors for atherosclerosis in SLE are heterogeneous, and apparently conflicting results have been reported. A major part of this inconsistency probably is due to the cross-sectional design of these studies. Differences in laboratory parameters and techniques used to measure immune and inflammatory biomarkers must be considered as well.

Therefore, further prospective studies are needed to understand in depth the mechanisms involved in the development and progression of atherosclerosis in SLE patients so as to identify predictive markers and to develop therapeutic options to treat these patients.

REFERENCES

1. Wick, G., G. Schett, A. Amberger, *et al.* 1995. Is atherosclerosis an immunological mediated disease? Immunol. Today **16:** 27–33.
2. Ward, M.M. 1999. Premature morbidity from cardiovascular and cerebrovascular diseases in women with systemic lupus erythematosus. Arthritis Rheum. **42:** 338–346.
3. Gladman, D.D. & M.B. Urowitz. 1987. Morbidity in systemic lupus erythematosus. J. Rheumatol. **14:** 223–226.

4. BULKLEY, B.H. & W.C. ROBERTS. 1975. The heart in systemic lupus erythematosus and the changes induced in it by corticosteroid therapy: a study of 36 necroscopy cases. Am. J. Med. **53:** 243–264.
5. UROWITZ, M.B., A.A. BOOKMAN, B.E. KOEHLER, *et al.* 1976. The bimodal mortality pattern of SLE. Am. J. Med. **60:** 221–225.
6. PETRI, M., S. PEREZ-GUTTHANN, D. SPENCE, *et al.* 1992. Risk factors for coronary artery disease in patients with systemic lupus erythematosus. Am. J. Med. **93:** 513–519.
7. ESDAILE, J.M., M. ABRAHAMOWICZ, T. GRODZICKY, *et al.* 2001. Traditional Framingham risk factors fail to fully account for accelerated atherosclerosis in systemic lupus erythematosus. Arthritis Rheum. **44:** 2231–2237.
8. MANZI, S., F. SELZER, K. SUTTON-TYRRELl, *et al.* 1999. Prevalence and risk factors of carotid plaque in women with systemic lupus erythematosus. Arthritis Rheum. **42:** 51–60.
9. GEORGE, J., D. HARATS, B. GILBURD, *et al.* 1999. Atherosclerosis-related markers in systemic lupus erythematosus patients: the role of humoral immunity in enhanced atherogenesis. Lupus **8:** 220–226.
10. DORIA, A., Y. SHOENFELD, R. WU, *et al.* 2003. Risk factors for subclinical atherosclerosis in a prospective cohort of patients with systemic lupus erythematosus. Ann. Rheum. Dis. **62:** 1071–1077.
11. ROSS, R. 1999. Atherosclerosis—an inflammatory disease. N. Engl. J. Med. **340:** 115–126.
12. SHERER, Y. & Y. SHOENFELD. 2002. Is atherosclerosis a cellular or humoral mediated autoimmune disease? Ann. Rheum. Dis. **61:** 97–99.
13. MACH, F., U. SCHONBECK, G.K. SUKHOVA, *et al.* 1998. Reduction of atherosclerosis in mice by inhibition of CD40 signalling. Nature **394:** 200–203.
14. EMESON, E.E., M.L. SHEN, C.G. BELL, *et al.* 1996. Inhibition of atherosclerosis in CD4 T-cell-depleted and nude (nu/nu) C57BL/6 hyperlipidemic mice. Am. J. Pathol. **149:** 675–685.
15. HANSSON, G.K., P. LIBBY, U. SCHONBECK & Z.Q. YAN. 2002. Innate and adaptive immunity in the pathogenesis of atherosclerosis. Circ. Res. **91:** 281–291.
16. KOBAYASHI, K., M. KISHI, T. ATSUMI, *et al.* 2003. Circulating oxidized LDL forms immune complexes with beta2-glycoprotein I: implication as an atherogenic autoantigen. J. Lipid Res. **44:** 716–726.
17. SHOENFELD, Y., Y. SHERER, J. GEORGE & D. HARATS. 2000. Autoantibodies associated with atherosclerosis. Ann. Med. **32:** 37–40.
18. PALINSKI, W., E. MILLER & J.L. WITZTUM. 1995. Immunization of low density lipoprotein (LDL) receptor-deficient rabbits with homologous malondialdehyde-modified LDL reduces atherogenesis. Proc. Natl. Acad. Sci. USA **92:** 821–825.
19. GEORGE, J., A. AFEK, B. GILBURD, *et al.* 1998. Induction of early atherosclerosis in LDL-receptor-deficient mice immunized with beta2-glycoprotein I. Circulation **98:** 1108–1115.
20. AFEK, A., J. GEORGE, B. GILBURD, *et al.* 2000. Immunization of low-density lipoprotein receptor deficient (LDL-RD) mice with heat shock protein 65 (HSP-65) promotes early atherosclerosis. J. Autoimmun. **14:** 115–121.
21. NICOLO, D. & M. MONESTIER. 2004. Antiphospholipid antibodies and atherosclerosis. Clin. Immunol. **112:** 183–189.
22. SHOENFELD, Y., R. WU, D.L. DEARING & E. MATSUURA. 2004. Are anti-oxidized low-density lipoprotein antibodies pathogenic or protective? Circulation **110:** 2552–2558.
23. FROSTEGARD, J., A. HAEGERSTRAND, M. GIDLUND & J. NILSSON. 1991. Biologically modified LDL increases the adhesive properties of endothelial cells. Atherosclerosis **90:** 119–126.
24. STEMME, S., B. FABER, J. HOLM, *et al.* 1995. T lymphocytes from human atherosclerotic plaques recognize oxidized low density lipoprotein. Proc. Natl. Acad. Sci. USA **92:** 3893–3897.
25. FROSTEGARD, J., Y.H. HUANG, J. RONNELID & L. ELINDER-SCHAFER. 1997. Platelet-activating factor and oxidized LDL induce immune activation by a common mechanism. Arterioscler. Thromb. Vasc. Biol. **17:** 963–968.

26. BROWN, M.S. & J.L. GOLDSTEIN. 1986. A receptor-mediated pathway for cholesterol homeostasis. Science **232:** 34–47.
27. LOPES-VIRELLA, M.F., N. BINZAFAR, S. RACKLEY, *et al.* 1997. The uptake of LDL-IC by human macrophages: predominant involvement of the FcgRI receptor. Atherosclerosis **135:** 161–170.
28. LEHTIMAKI, T., S. LEHTINEN, T. SOLAKIVI, *et al.* 1999. Autoantibodies against oxidized low density lipoprotein in patients with angiographically verified coronary artery disease. Arterioscler. Thromb. Vasc. Biol. **19:** 23–27.
29. MAGGI, E., R. CHIESA, G. MELISSANO, *et al.* 1994. LDL oxidation in patients with severe carotid atherosclerosis. A study of in vitro and in vivo oxidation markers. Arterioscler. Thromb. **14:** 1892–1899.
30. SALONEN, J.T., S. YLA-HERTTUALA, R. YAMAMOTO, *et al.* 1992. Autoantibodies against oxidised LDL and progression of carotid atherosclerosis. Lancet **339**: 883–887.
31. MERAVIGLIA, M.V., E. MAGGI, G. BELLOMO, *et al.* 2002. Autoantibodies against oxidatively modified lipoproteins and progression of carotid restenosis after carotid endarterectomy. Stroke **33:** 1139–1141.
32. GEORGE, J., D. HARATS, E. BAKSHI, *et al.* 1999. Anti-oxidized low density lipoprotein antibody determination as a predictor of restenosis following percutaneous transluminal coronary angioplasty. Immunol. Lett. **68:** 263–266.
33. GEORGE, J., A. AFEK, B. GILBURD, *et al.* 1998. Hyperimmunization of apo-E mice with homologous malondialdehyde low-density lipoprotein suppresses early atherogenesis. Atherosclerosis **138:** 147–152.
34. AMELI, S., A. HULTGARDH-NILSSON, J. REGNSTROM, *et al.* 1996. Effect of immunization with homologous LDL and oxidized LDL on early atherosclerosis in hypercholesterolemic rabbits. Atheroscler. Thromb. Vasc. Biol. **16:** 1074–1079.
35. SHAW, P.X., S. HORKKO, S. TSIMIKAS, *et al.* 2001. Human-derived anti-oxidized LDL autoantibody blocks uptake of oxidized LDL by macrophages and localizes to atherosclerotic lesions in vivo. Atheroscler. Thromb. Vasc. Biol. **21:** 333–339.
36. HAYEM, G., P. NICAISE-ROLAND, E. PALAZZO, *et al.* 2001. Anti-oxidized low-density-lipoprotein (OxLDL) antibodies in systemic lupus erythematosus with and without antiphospholipid syndrome. Lupus **10:** 346–351.
37. SVENUNGSSON, E., K. JENSEN-URSTAD, M. HEIMBÜRGER, *et al.* 2001. Risk factors for cardiovascular disease in systemic lupus erythematosus. Circulation **104:** 1887–1893.
38. FROSTEGARD, J. 2002. Autoimmunity, oxidized LDL and cardiovascular disease. Autoimmun. Rev. **1:** 233–237.
39. SCHWARZENBACHER, R., K. ZETH, K. DIEDERICHS, *et al.* 1999. Crystal structure of human beta 2-glycoprotein I: implications for phospholipid binding and the antiphospholipid syndrome. EMBO J. **18:** 6228–6239.
40. DELGADO ALVES, A.J., P.R. AMES, S. DONOHUE, *et al.* 2002. Antibodies to high-density lipoprotein and β_2-glycoprotein I are inversely correlated with paraoxonase activity in systemic lupus erythematosus and primary antiphospholipid syndrome. Arthritis Rheum. **46:** 2686–2694.
41. HASUNUMA, Y., E. MATSUURA, Z. MAKITA, *et al.* 1997. Involvement of beta 2-glycoprotein I and anticardiolipin antibodies in oxidatively modified low-density lipoprotein uptake by macrophages. Clin. Exp. Immunol. **107:** 569–573.
42. GEORGE, J., D. HARATS, B. GILBURD, *et al.* 1999. Immunolocalization of b2-glycoprotein I (apolipoprotein H) to human atherosclerotic plaques: potential implications for lesion progression. Circulation **99:** 2227–2230.
43. AFEK, A., J. GEORGE, Y. SHOENFELD, *et al.* 1999. Enhancement of atherosclerosis in beta-2-glycoprotein I-immunized apolipoprotein E-deficient mice. Pathobiology **67:** 19–25.
44. GEORGE, J., D. HARATS, B. GILBURD, *et al.* 2000. Adoptive transfer of beta-2-glycoprotein-I-reactive lymphocytes enhances early atherosclerosis in LDL receptor-deficient mice. Circulation **102:** 1822–1827.
45. VAARALA, O., M. MANTTARI, V. MANNINEN, *et al.* 1995. Anti-cardiolipin antibodies and risk of myocardial infarction in a prospective cohort of middle-aged men. Circulation **91:** 23–27.

46. SHERER, Y., J. SHEMESH, A. TENENBAUM, *et al.* 2000. Coronary calcium and anti-cardiolipin antibody are elevated in patients with typical chest pain. Am. J. Cardiol. **86:** 1306–1311.
47. SHERER, Y., A. TENENBAUM, M. BLANK, *et al.* 2001. Coronary artery disease but not coronary calcification is associated with elevated levels of cardiolipin, β–2-glycoprotein-I, and oxidized-LDL antibodies. Cardiology **95:** 20–24.
48. AMES, P.R., A. MARGARITA, J. DELGADO ALVES, *et al.* 2002. Anticardiolipin antibody titre and plasma homocysteine level independently predict intima media thickness of carotid arteries in subjects with idiopathic antiphospholipid antibodies. Lupus **11:** 208–214.
49. MEDINA, G., D. CASAOS, L.J. JARA, *et al.* 2003. Increased carotid artery intima-media thickness may be associated with stroke in primary antiphospholipid syndrome. Ann. Rheum. Dis. 42: 607–610.
50. VLACHOYIANNOPOULOS, P.G., P.G. KANELLOPOULOS, J.P. IOANNIDIS, *et al.* 2003. Atherosclerosis in premenopausal women with antiphospholipid syndrome and systemic lupus erythematosus: a controlled study. Rheumatology **42:** 645–651.
51. GHIRARDELLO A., A. DORIA, A. RUFFATTI, *et al.* 1994. Antiphospholipid antibodies (aPL) in systemic lupus erythematosus: are they specific tools for the diagnosis of aPL syndrome? Ann. Rheum. Dis. **54:** 140–142.
52. SELZER, F., K. SUTTON-TYRRELL & S.G. FITZGERALD, *et al.* 2004. Comparison of risk factors for vascular disease in the carotid artery and aorta in women with systemic lupus erythematosus. Arthritis Rheum. **50:** 151–159.
53. PHADKE, K.V., R.A. PHILLIPS, D.T. CLARKE, *et al.* 1993. Anticardiolipin antibodies in ischemic heart disease: marker or myth? Br. Heart J. **69:** 391–394.
54. ROMAN, M.J., B.A. SHAKER, A. DAVIS, *et al.* 2003. Prevalence and correlates of accelerated atherosclerosis in systemic lupus erythematosus. N. Engl. J. Med. **349:** 2399–2406.
55. XU, Q. & G. WICK. 1996. The role of heat shock proteins in protection and pathophysiology of the arterial wall. Mol. Med. Today **2:** 372–379.
56. YOUNG, R.A. & T.J. ELLIOTT. 1989 Stress proteins, infection and immune surveillance. Cell **59:** 5–8.
57. SORELLE R. 2002. Blood containing high levels of antibodies to heat shock protein 65 (hsp65) were found to be at increased risk of subsequent cardiovascular events. Circulation **106:** 9052–9058.
58. XU, Q., S. KIECHL, M. MAYR, *et al.* 1999. Association of serum antibodies to heat-shock protein 65 with carotid atherosclerosis: clinical significance determined in a follow-up study. Circulation **100:** 1169–1174.
59. XU, Q., J. WILLEIT, M. MAROSI, *et al.* 1993. Association of serum antibodies to heat-shock protein 65 with carotid atherosclerosis. Lancet **341:** 255–259.
60. XU, Q., H. DIETRICH, H.J. STEINER, *et al.* 1992. Induction of arteriosclerosis in normocholesterolemic rabbits by immunization with heat shock protein 65. Arterioscler. Thromb. **12:** 789–799.
61. GEORGE, J., Y. SHOENFELD, A. AFEK, *et al.* 1999. Enhanced fatty streak formation in C57BL/6J mice by immunization with heat shock protein-65. Arterioscler. Thromb. Vasc. Biol. **19:** 505–510.
62. GRUBER, R., S. LEDERER, U. BECHTEL, *et al.* 1996. Increased antibody titers against mycobacterial heat-shock protein 65 in patients with vasculitis and arteriosclerosis. Int. Arch. Allergy Immunol. **110:** 95–98.
63. HORVATH, L., L. CZIRJAK, B. FEKETE, *et al.* 2001. Levels of antibodies against C1q and 60 kDa family of heat shock proteins in the sera of patients with various autoimmune diseases. Immunol. Lett. **75:** 103–109.
64. WU, R. 2001. Autoantibodies against oxidized palmitoyl arachidonoyl phosphocholine in atherosclerosis. *In* Atherosclerosis and autoimmunity. Y. Shoenfeld, D. Harats & G. Wick, Eds.: 151–159. Elsevier. Amsterdam.

Accelerated Atherosclerosis in Patients with Systemic Autoimmune Diseases

KARINA DE LEEUW, CEES KALLENBERG, AND MARC BIJL

Department of Internal Medicine, Division of Clinical Immunology, University Hospital, Groningen, the Netherlands

ABSTRACT: Systemic autoimmune diseases such as systemic lupus erythematosus and Wegener's granulomatosis are associated with a significantly increased prevalence of cardiovascular disease (CVD) compared with age- and sex-matched controls. Many risk factors are involved in the pathogenesis of atherosclerosis, the major underlying cause of CVD. In patients with systemic autoimmune diseases, it has been shown that traditional risk factors for CVD cannot completely explain the prevalence of atherosclerosis. Therefore, in addition to these traditional factors, nontraditional risk factors are suggested to contribute to atherogenesis. All risk factors, traditional and nontraditional, contribute to endothelial activation that, followed by endothelial dysfunction, is seen as one of the first steps in this process. This review updates information on the factors that contribute to accelerated atherosclerosis in patients with systemic autoimmune diseases, such as disease-related factors, inflammatory mediators, and advanced glycation end products.

KEYWORDS: atherosclerosis; systemic autoimmune diseases; endothelial activation; endothelial dysfunction

INTRODUCTION

Atherosclerosis can be considered a progressive process that starts as early as in adolescence, becoming manifest clinically at a much later age. Accumulating evidence suggests that inflammation plays a fundamental role in each stage of atherogenesis, from the initial phases, starting with endothelial cell (EC) activation, to eventual rupture of the vulnerable atherosclerotic plaque. EC activation results in upregulation of adhesion molecules such as P-selectin, E-selectin, intercellular adhesion molecule-1 (ICAM-1), and vascular cell adhesion molecule-1 (VCAM-1) on the EC surface, leading to attachment and, finally, migration of circulating leukocytes. Differentiation of migrated monocytes into macrophages, and the subsequent uptake of lipids by these cells, results in foam cell generation and fatty streak formation. Further recruitment of inflammatory cells and proliferation of smooth muscle cells lead to the development of an atherosclerotic plaque.[1,2]

Address for correspondence: Karina de Leeuw, Department of Internal Medicine, Division of Clinical Immunology, University Hospital, P.O. Box 30.001, 9700 RB Groningen, the Netherlands. Voice: +31-50-3613851; fax: +31-50-3619069.
k.de.leeuw@int.umcg.nl

Ann. N.Y. Acad. Sci. 1051: 362–371 (2005). © 2005 New York Academy of Sciences.
doi: 10.1196/annals.1361.078

TABLE 1. Traditional and nontraditional risk factors in atherosclerosis in patients with systemic autoimmune diseases

Traditional risk factors	Nontraditional risk factors in systemic autoimmune diseases
Age	Autoantibodies against phospholipids, endothelial cells, dsDNA or ANCA
Gender	Systemic inflammation
Dyslipidemia	Enhanced lipid oxidation
Smoking	Altered vascular remodeling?
Hypertension	Levels of HSPs and antibodies against HSPs?
Diabetes	Renal impairment?
Obesity	Elevated levels of homocysteine?
Positive family history for CVD	Medication, especially steroids?
	Exhaustion of endothelial progenitor cells?
	Advanced glycation end products?

ABBREVIATIONS: ANCA, anti-neutrophil cytoplasmic antibody; CVD, cardiovascular disease; dsDNA, double-stranded DNA; HSP, heat shock protein.

Despite growing knowledge of the pathogenesis of atherosclerosis, the exact cause is not known yet. Many traditional risk factors, such as hypercholesterolemia, hypertension, and smoking, can injure and activate the endothelium. Infectious agents, such as bacteria and viruses have also been indicated as potential triggering pathogens that start the cascade resulting in plaque formation.[3]

In some situations the development of atherosclerosis is accelerated, for example in systemic autoimmune diseases. Increased prevalence of cardiovascular morbidity and mortality due to atherosclerosis, which cannot fully be explained by traditional risk factors, has been observed in patients with systemic autoimmune disease, indicating that additional "nontraditional" factors also are involved.[4–11] A simplified overview of factors contributing to atherosclerosis in systemic autoimmune diseases is presented in TABLE 1. In this review atherosclerosis in systemic autoimmune diseases is discussed. In addition, a selection of more or less established nontraditional risk factors and, last, the role of other hypothetical contributing factors in the pathogenesis of atherosclerosis will be discussed.

SYSTEMIC AUTOIMMUNE DISEASES

Systemic autoimmune diseases such as systemic lupus erythematosus (SLE) and Wegener's granulomatosis (WG) are characterized by inflammation of many organ systems. The course of these diseases is very variable among patients. The disease can be quiescent for years after an inflammatory period, but also can have a relapsing/remitting course. The long-term outcome of these diseases is receiving increasing focus now that the ability to control recurrences has improved remarkably. In 1976 Urowitz *et al.* reported that mortality in SLE follows a bimodal pattern.[12] Due to the better treatment modalities now available, more patients die late instead of early in the course of their disease. Early death is associated with active disease, large doses of steroids, and a marked incidence of infection, whereas in the late stage death is associated with inactive lupus, long duration of steroid therapy, and a striking incidence of myocardial infarction due to atherosclerotic heart disease.

In SLE as well as in WG this increased prevalence of cardiovascular disease (CVD) cannot be explained by the presence of traditional risk factors such as hypertension, hyperlipidemia, diabetes mellitus, and smoking.[4–11] To determine other factors that participate in the development of atherosclerosis, the initial steps of the process should be investigated. EC activation and EC dysfunction precede atherosclerosis. Whereas in systemic autoimmune diseases vessels are often involved in the inflammatory process, increased EC activation may be expected. Indeed, EC activation has been demonstrated indirectly by the elevation of circulating soluble adhesion molecules and thrombomodulin.[13,14] Also, in skin biopsy specimens of SLE patients, endothelial expression of E-selectin, VCAM-1 and ICAM-1 is increased, most markedly in active disease.[15] The next step in the process is EC dysfunction, which is considered crucial in the early stages of atherogenesis. Indeed, EC dysfunction is described in CVD,[16] as well as in systemic autoimmune diseases.[17–22] EC dysfunction can be measured by different methods. The most commonly used is flow-mediated dilation, but increasingly, laser Doppler fluxmetry in combination with iontophoresis is used.[23,24] To determine endothelial function, both methods compare the ability for endothelium-dependent vasodilatation with the ability for endothelium-independent vasodilatation. Thus, considering the presence of diffuse EC dysfunction in autoimmune diseases, it can be assumed that these patients have a higher risk of developing CVD. This hypothesis is supported by several studies that demonstrated increased prevalence of clinical and subclinical atherosclerosis in patients with SLE and WG.[4–11]

The contribution in this process of nontraditional risk factors is discussed in the remainder of this review.

AUTOANTIBODIES

A hallmark of systemic autoimmune diseases is the presence of autoantibodies. In SLE, many autoantibodies can be found, such as autoantibodies directed to phospholipids, endothelial cells, or double-stranded DNA. Anti-neutrophil cytoplasmic antibodies (ANCAs), particularly those directed to proteinase 3 (PR3-ANCA), are characteristic autoantibodies for WG. Binding to and subsequent activation of ECs by these antibodies has been shown in several studies,[25–27] giving a direct explanation for the presence of accelerated atherosclerosis.[13,25,28]

Furthermore, systemic low-grade inflammation, which is reflected by increased levels of high-sensitivity C-reactive protein (hsCRP), even when disease activity is low, is present in systemic autoimmune diseases. CRP has been found to be an independent prognostic marker for CVD.[29] Several studies have suggested that CRP may contribute directly to development of atherosclerosis, as it induces expression of adhesion molecules on the endothelial surface and promotes the adherence of leukocytes.[30,31] Note that EC dysfunction in systemic vasculitis is related to inflammation, as reflected by CRP levels and the Birmingham Vasculitis Activity Score.[18,19,32]

Furthermore, heat shock proteins (HSPs) have been suggested to contribute to the cascade that leads to atherosclerosis. It has been demonstrated that classic atherosclerosis risk factors, such as high blood pressure, smoking, diabetes, and chemically altered lipoproteins, act as stress factors for ECs, which express HSPs upon activation.[33,34] Owing to activation, ECs may die, resulting in release of HSPs, then called soluble HSPs (sHSPs), into intercellular spaces. These sHSPs seem to be directly proatherogenic, as they stimulate macrophages to produce proinflammatory cytokines and ECs to express adhesion molecules.[35] Simultaneously, macrophages present antigens to B cells, which may induce the production of autoantibodies against HSPs, which, in turn, can react with HSPs expressed on activated ECs. Increases in both HSPs and autoantibodies against HSPs have been associated with atherosclerosis.[33,36,37] Also, in systemic autoimmune diseases a defective HSP response could accelerate the development of atherosclerosis. However, data on this latter effect are controversial, for example, Cederholm *et al.* could not find any differences in levels of HSP60, HSP70, or antibodies against HSP60, HSP65, and HSP70 between controls and SLE patients with or without a history of CVD.[38]

Another disease-related factor, especially in SLE, is suggested to be the enhanced oxidation of lipids.[39,40] Oxidized LDL (oxLDL) plays an important role in atherogenesis and may contribute to the immune activation and inflammation present in atherosclerotic lesions, because it is chemotactic, activates T cells, and is taken up by macrophages in the atherosclerotic plaque.[41] OxLDL could, therefore, be a common pathogenic factor in SLE and atherosclerosis. Furthermore, autoantibodies to oxLDL have been found to be related to atherosclerosis.[42–45] Elevated antibodies against oxLDL are found in atherosclerotic lesions[46] and in the plasma of patients with atherosclerosis.[46,47] Also, SLE patients have elevated anti-oxLDL antibodies.[40,48,49] However, several studies have suggested that antibodies against oxLDL prevent plaque formation. The precise mechanisms remain unclear. Some authors have suggested that autoantibodies to oxLDL may act as scavengers and clear oxLDL from the circulation.[50] So far, it has not been well established whether the immune response to oxLDL is predominantly proatherogenic or antiatherogenic.[44,45]

MATRIX METALLOPROTEINASES

Vascular remodeling, in which matrix metalloproteinases (MMPs) play a major role, is important in atherosclerosis.[51] Excessive tissue remodeling and increased MMP activity have been demonstrated during atherosclerotic lesion progression, including plaque disruption. Increased MMP-1, MMP-3, MMP-9, and one of their inhibitors, TIMP-1, were found in human atherosclerotic plaques.[52] Also, in acute coronary syndromes, increased serum MMPs have been detected.[53–55] Various cells present in plaques produce MMPs, including smooth muscle cells and basophils, but the major source is the activated macrophage. Production is stimulated by cytokines, such as inflammatory mediators. Therefore, some studies suggest that MMPs can also be used as markers for disease activity, for example, in Takayasu arteritis[56] and giant cell arteritis.[57] Also, in WG and SLE patients, increases in MMPs and their inhibitors are found.[8,58,59] Whether this is a reflection of atherosclerotic changes of the vessel wall or of smoldering disease activity in these patients, which results in endothelial activation and, eventually, in atherosclerosis, is unknown at present.

MEDICATION

Treatment, especially the use of steroids, also influences the process of atherosclerosis. Steroid treatment is often believed to be atherogenic, because of effects on plasma lipoproteins. Because inflammation is implicated in atherosclerosis, steroid treatment could actually prevent atherosclerosis as well. Indeed, there are conflicting studies. Several studies did not find an association between long-term treatment with glucocorticoids and atherosclerosis.[60,61] Wei *et al.* demonstrated in a large group of patients that those who received high-dose glucocorticoids, defined as more than 7.5 mg daily for 1 year or more, were more than twice as likely to have had a cardiovascular event than patients who used no glucocorticoids.[62] In contrast, Roman *et al.* found a negative association between carotid plaque and a high mean daily dose of prednisolone in SLE patients.[10] Clearly, the role of prednisolone treatment in development of CVD in SLE deserves further study.

OTHERS

Last, two factors that may play a role in induction of EC activation and dysfunction in systemic autoimmune diseases are discussed briefly, namely, renal impairment and homocysteine. It has been demonstrated that EC dysfunction is related to renal impairment.[63] However, this is debatable, as in SLE no relationship could be found between renal function and presence of plaque, and in WG patients no relationship could be detected between renal function and EC dysfunction.[10,18] Also, elevated levels of homocysteine have been associated with CVD in the general population,[64,65] as well as in SLE patients, who have even higher levels of homocysteine compared with controls.[40,60,66,67]

HYPOTHETICAL NONTRADITIONAL RISK FACTORS: ADVANCED GLYCATION END PRODUCTS

Recently, the accumulation of advanced glycation end products (AGEs) has been recognized as a contributing factor in the progression of atherosclerosis.[68] AGEs are a class of compounds resulting from glycation and oxidation of proteins, lipids, or nucleic acids. Glycation is the nonenzymatic addition or insertion of saccharide derivatives to these molecules. This leads to the formation of intermediary Schiff bases and Amadori products, and, finally, to irreversible AGEs. The formation of AGEs occurs ubiquitously and irreversibly in patients with diabetes mellitus, and the presence of these compounds contribute to the pathogenesis of accelerated atherosclerosis found in diabetes.[69–71] Apart from AGE formation in the extracellular matrix, resulting in decreased elasticity and increased thickness and rigidity of the vascular wall, the interaction of AGEs with their receptors (RAGEs) has been implicated in endothelial dysfunction.[72] The interaction between AGEs and RAGEs on macrophages induces oxidative stress and activation of intracellular signaling, causing secretion of cytokines and mediators of inflammation, vasoconstriction because of reduced production of nitric oxide, and coagulation.[73] Furthermore, in a model of accelerated and advanced atherosclerosis in diabetic mice, treatment with soluble RAGE completely suppressed diabetic atherosclerosis.[74]

Although the primary causal factor leading to the formation of AGEs and their pathophysiologic effects in diabetes is chronic exposure to high blood levels of glucose, in recent years it has been suggested that AGEs can be formed in multiple milieus, such as in inflammation and renal failure.[75,76] In systemic autoimmune diseases, such as SLE and WG, where inflammation of vessels is common, increased AGE formation at these sites can be expected, which could contribute to accelerated atherogenesis. Currently, this hypothesis is under investigation in our laboratory.

ENDOTHELIAL PROGENITOR CELLS

A healthy endothelium is important to prevent atherogenesis. Therefore, disturbances in the equilibrium between vascular injury and vascular repair will be followed by atherosclerosis.

Recent insights suggest that injured endothelium can be regenerated by circulating bone marrow–derived endothelial progenitor cells (EPCs). Exhaustion of these cells in number, function, or both, due to chronic exposure to cardiovascular risk factors, can result in atherosclerosis.[77,78] In apolipoprotein $E^{-/-}$ mice after transplantation with wild-type bone marrow from younger animals, reduction in atherosclerotic lesions was found, because of regeneration by the transferred cells.[79] Furthermore, possible anti-inflammatory effects of these cells have been suggested. After transfer, interleukin-6 (IL-6) levels were decreased. Considering that atherosclerosis is an inflammatory disease, these anti-inflammatory effects of EPCs, next to vascular repair, could prevent development or progression of atherosclerosis.

In animal studies, as in humans, it has been demonstrated that the number of EPCs correlates negatively with established risk factors for atherosclerosis and endothelial function.[77,78] However, not only number, but also functionality is important. It has been shown that in diabetes, which is characterized by accelerated atherosclerosis, the capacity of EPCs to adhere is compromised.[80]

How might EPCs be a link between accelerated atherosclerosis and systemic autoimmune disease? It is possible that in SLE and WG, both characterized by chronic vascular and systemic inflammation that cause continuous vascular injury, the pool of EPCs is exhausted. Furthermore, because of this continuous demand on EPCs, quality and functionality of these cells could be compromised, resulting in decreased capacity to repair vascular damage, thereby disturbing the equilibrium between vascular injury and repair.

CONCLUSION

In summary, in systemic autoimmune diseases, which are associated with increased EC activation, EC dysfunction, and accelerated development of atherosclerosis, not only traditional risk factors, but also nontraditional factors play an important role in atherogenesis. Clearly, at present, questions remain as to whether all nontraditional risk factors have already been elucidated and which factors play the most important role in the accelerated development of atherosclerosis in these patients. Further insights into the pathophysiological role of these factors may result in new strategies for interference in these pathological processes.

REFERENCES

1. LIBBY, P., P.M. RIDKER & A. MASERI. 2002. Inflammation and atherosclerosis. Circulation **105:** 1135–1143.
2. ROSS, R. 1999. Atherosclerosis–an inflammatory disease. N. Engl. J. Med. **340:** 115–126.
3. SHOENFELD, Y., D. HARATS & J. GEORGE. 2000. Heat shock protein 60/65, beta 2-glycoprotein I and oxidized LDL as players in murine atherosclerosis. J. Autoimmun. **15:** 199–202.
4. AHMAD, Y. & I.N. BRUCE. 2004. Subclinical atherosclerosis in systemic lupus erythematosus. J. Rheumatol. **31:** 841–843.
5. MANZI, S., F. SELZER, K. SUTTON-TYRRELL, *et al.* 1999. Prevalence and risk factors of carotid plaque in women with systemic lupus erythematosus. Arthritis Rheum. **42:** 51–60.
6. SELZER, F., K. SUTTON-TYRRELL, S.G. FITZGERALD, *et al.* 2004. Comparison of risk factors for vascular disease in the carotid artery and aorta in women with systemic lupus erythematosus. Arthritis Rheum. **50:** 151–159.
7. DORIA, A., Y. SHOENFELD, R. WU, *et al.* 2003. Risk factors for subclinical atherosclerosis in a prospective cohort of patients with systemic lupus erythematosus Ann. Rheum. Dis. **62:** 1071-1077.
8. DE LEEUW, K., J.S. SANDERS, C.A. STEGEMAN, *et al.* 2005. Accelerated atherosclerosis in patients with Wegener's granulomatosis. Ann. Rheum. Dis. **64:** 753–759.
9. ESDAILE, J.M., M. ABRAHAMOWICZ, T. GRODZICKY, *et al.* 2001. Traditional Framingham risk factors fail to fully account for accelerated atherosclerosis in systemic lupus erythematosus. Arthritis Rheum. **44:** 2331–2337.
10. ROMAN, M.J., B.A. SHANKER, A. DAVIS, *et al.* 2003. Prevalence and correlates of accelerated atherosclerosis in systemic lupus erythematosus. N. Engl. J. Med. **349:** 2399–2406.
11. VLACHOYIANNOPOULOS, P.G., P.G. KANELLOPOULOS, J.P. IOANNIDIS, *et al.* 2003. Atherosclerosis in premenopausal women with antiphospholipid syndrome and systemic lupus erythematosus: a controlled study. Rheumatology (Oxford) **42:** 645–651.
12. UROWITZ, M.B., A.A. BOOKMAN, B.E. KOEHLER, *et al.* 1976. The bimodal mortality pattern of systemic lupus erythematosus. Am. J. Med. **60:** 221–225.
13. SPRONK, P.E., H. BOOTSMA, M.G. HUITEMA, *et al.* 1994. Levels of soluble VCAM-1, soluble ICAM-1, and soluble E-selectin during disease exacerbations in patients with systemic lupus erythematosus (SLE); a long term prospective study. Clin. Exp. Immunol. **97:** 439–444.
14. STEGEMAN, C.A., J.W. TERVAERT, M.G. HUITEMA, *et al.* 1994. Serum levels of soluble adhesion molecules intercellular adhesion molecule 1, vascular cell adhesion molecule 1, and E-selectin in patients with Wegener's granulomatosis. Relationship to disease activity and relevance during followup. Arthritis Rheum. **37:** 1228–1235.
15. BELMONT, H.M., J. BUYON, R. GIORNO & S. ABRAMSON. 1994. Up-regulation of endothelial cell adhesion molecules characterizes disease activity in systemic lupus erythematosus. The Shwartzman phenomenon revisited. Arthritis Rheum. **37:** 376–383.
16. HEITZER, T., T. SCHLINZIG, K. KROHN, *et al.* 2001. Endothelial dysfunction, oxidative stress, and risk of cardiovascular events in patients with coronary artery disease. Circulation **104:** 2673–2678.
17. BIJL, M. 2003. Endothelial activation, endothelial dysfunction and premature atherosclerosis in systemic autoimmune diseases. Neth. J. Med. **61:** 273–277.
18. FILER, A.D., J.M. GARDNER-MEDWIN, J. THAMBYRAJAH, *et al.* 2003. Diffuse endothelial dysfunction is common to ANCA associated systemic vasculitis and polyarteritis nodosa. Ann. Rheum. Dis. **62:** 162–167.

19. BOOTH, A.D., D.R. JAYNE, R.K. KHARBANDA, *et al.* 2004. Infliximab improves endothelial dysfunction in systemic vasculitis: a model of vascular inflammation. Circulation **109:** 1718–1723.
20. EL-MAGADMI, M., H. BODILL, Y. AHMAD, *et al.* 2004. Systemic lupus erythematosus: an independent risk factor for endothelial dysfunction in women. Circulation **110:** 399–404.
21. LIMA, D.S., E.I. SATO, V.C. LIMA, *et al.* 2002. Brachial endothelial function is impaired in patients with systemic lupus erythematosus. J. Rheumatol. **29:** 292–297.
22. RAZA, K., J. THAMBYRAJAH, J.N. TOWNEND, *et al.* 2000. Suppression of inflammation in primary systemic vasculitis restores vascular endothelial function: lessons for atherosclerotic disease? Circulation **102:** 1470–1472.
23. SERNE, E.H., C.D. STEHOUWER, J.C. TER MAATEN, *et al.* 1999. Microvascular function relates to insulin sensitivity and blood pressure in normal subjects. Circulation **99:** 896–902.
24. FARKAS, K., E. KOLOSSVARY, Z. JARAI, *et al.* 2004. Non-invasive assessment of microvascular endothelial function by laser Doppler flowmetry in patients with essential hypertension. Atherosclerosis **173:** 97–102.
25. MULLER KOBOLD, A.C., R.T. VAN WIJK, C.F. FRANSSEN, *et al.* 1999. In vitro up-regulation of E-selectin and induction of interleukin-6 in endothelial cells by autoantibodies in Wegener's granulomatosis and microscopic polyangiitis. Clin. Exp. Rheumatol. **17:** 433–440.
26. MERONI, P.L., E. RASCHI, C. TESTONI & M.O. BORGHI. 2004. Endothelial cell activation by antiphospholipid antibodies. Clin. Immunol. **112:** 169–174.
27. SIMANTOV, R., S.K. LO, A. GHARAVI, *et al.* 1996. Antiphospholipid antibodies activate vascular endothelial cells. Lupus **5:** 440–441.
28. PERRY, G.J., T. ELSTON, N.A. KHOURI, *et al.* 1993. Antiendothelial cell antibodies in lupus: correlations with renal injury and circulating markers of endothelial damage. Q. J. Med. **86:** 727–734.
29. RIDKER, P.M., N. RIFAI, L. ROSE, *et al.* 2002. Comparison of C-reactive protein and low-density lipoprotein cholesterol levels in the prediction of first cardiovascular events. N. Engl. J. Med. **347:** 1557–1565.
30. KHREISS, T., L. JOZSEF, L.A. POTEMPA & J.G. FILEP. 2004. Conformational rearrangement in C-reactive protein is required for proinflammatory actions on human endothelial cells. Circulation **109:** 2016–2022.
31. PASCERI, V., J.T. WILLERSON & E.T. YEH. 2000. Direct proinflammatory effect of C-reactive protein on human endothelial cells. Circulation **102:** 2165–2168.
32. BOOTH, A.D., S. WALLACE, C.M. MCENIERY, *et al.* 2004. Inflammation and arterial stiffness in systemic vasculitis: a model of vascular inflammation. Arthritis Rheum. **50:** 581–588.
33. WICK, G., M. KNOFLACH, M. KIND, *et al.* 2004. Heat shock proteins and stress in atherosclerosis. Autoimmun. Rev. **3** (Suppl. 1): S30–S31.
34. AMBERGER, A., C. MACZEK, G. JURGENS, *et al.* 1997. Co-expression of ICAM-1, VCAM-1, ELAM-1 and Hsp60 in human arterial and venous endothelial cells in response to cytokines and oxidized low-density lipoproteins. Cell Stress Chaperones **2:** 94–103.
35. KOL, A., T. BOURCIER, A.H. LICHTMAN & P. LIBBY. 1999. Chlamydial and human heat shock protein 60s activate human vascular endothelium, smooth muscle cells, and macrophages. J. Clin. Invest. **103:** 571–577.
36. SCHETT, G., Q. XU, A. AMBERGER, *et al.* 1995. Autoantibodies against heat shock protein 60 mediate endothelial cytotoxicity. J. Clin. Invest. **96:** 2569–2577.
37. XU, Q., G. SCHETT, H. PERSCHINKA, *et al.* 2000. Serum soluble heat shock protein 60 is elevated in subjects with atherosclerosis in a general population. Circulation **102:** 14–20.
38. CEDERHOLM, A., E. SVENUNGSSON, D. STENGEL, *et al.* 2004. Platelet-activating factor-acetylhydrolase and other novel risk and protective factors for cardiovascular disease in systemic lupus erythematosus. Arthritis Rheum. **50:** 2869–2876.
39. FROSTEGARD, J., E. SVENUNGSSON, R. WU, *et al.* 2005. Lipid peroxidation is enhanced in patients with systemic lupus erythematosus and is associated with arterial and renal disease manifestations. Arthritis Rheum. **52:** 192–200.

40. SVENUNGSSON, E., K. JENSEN-URSTAD, M. HEIMBURGER, *et al.* 2001. Risk factors for cardiovascular disease in systemic lupus erythematosus. Circulation **104:** 1887–1893.
41. BINDER, C.J., M.K. CHANG, P.X. SHAW, *et al.* 2002. Innate and acquired immunity in atherogenesis. Nat. Med. **8:** 1218–1226.
42. HULTHE, J. 2004. Antibodies to oxidized LDL in atherosclerosis development–clinical and animal studies. Clin. Chim. Acta **348:** 1–8.
43. NICOLO, D. & M. MONESTIER. 2004. Antiphospholipid antibodies and atherosclerosis. Clin. Immunol. **112:** 183–189.
44. HORKKO, S., C.J. BINDER, P.X. SHAW, *et al.* 2000. Immunological responses to oxidized LDL. Free Radic. Biol. Med. **28:** 1771–1779.
45. ROSE, N. & M. AFANASYEVA. 2003. Autoimmunity: busting the atherosclerotic plaque. Nat. Med. **9:** 641–642.
46. YLA-HERTTUALA, S., W. PALINSKI, S.W. BUTLER, *et al.* 1994. Rabbit and human atherosclerotic lesions contain IgG that recognizes epitopes of oxidized LDL. Arterioscler. Thromb. **14:** 32–40.
47. SALONEN, J.T., S. YLA-HERTTUALA, R. YAMAMOTO, *et al.* 1992. Autoantibody against oxidised LDL and progression of carotid atherosclerosis. Lancet **339:** 883–887.
48. VAARALA, O., G. ALFTHAN, M. JAUHIAINEN, *et al.* 1993. Crossreaction between antibodies to oxidised low-density lipoprotein and to cardiolipin in systemic lupus erythematosus. Lancet **341:** 923–925.
49. GEORGE, J., D. HARATS, B. GILBURD, *et al.* 1999. Atherosclerosis-related markers in systemic lupus erythematosus patients: the role of humoral immunity in enhanced atherogenesis. Lupus **8:** 220–226.
50. HORKKO, S., D.A. BIRD, E. MILLER, *et al.* 1999. Monoclonal autoantibodies specific for oxidized phospholipids or oxidized phospholipid-protein adducts inhibit macrophage uptake of oxidized low-density lipoproteins. J. Clin. Invest. **103:** 117–128.
51. NEWBY, A.C. 2005. Dual role of matrix metalloproteinases (matrixins) in intimal thickening and atherosclerotic plaque rupture. Physiol Rev. **85:** 1–31.
52. ORBE, J., L. FERNANDEZ, J.A. RODRIGUEZ, *et al.* 2003. Different expression of MMPs/TIMP-1 in human atherosclerotic lesions. Relation to plaque features and vascular bed. Atherosclerosis **170:** 269–276.
53. KAI, H., H. IKEDA, H. YASUKAWA, *et al.* 1998. Peripheral blood levels of matrix metalloproteases-2 and -9 are elevated in patients with acute coronary syndromes. J. Am. Coll. Cardiol. **32:** 368–372.
54. NOMOTO, K., S. OGUCHI, I. WATANABE, *et al.* 2003. Involvement of inflammation in acute coronary syndromes assessed by levels of high-sensitivity C-reactive protein, matrix metalloproteinase-9 and soluble vascular-cell adhesion molecule-1. J. Cardiol. **42:** 201–206.
55. TZIAKAS, D.N., G.K. CHALIKIAS, J.T. PARISSIS, *et al.* 2004. Serum profiles of matrix metalloproteinases and their tissue inhibitor in patients with acute coronary syndromes. The effects of short-term atorvastatin administration. Int. J. Cardiol. **94:** 269–277.
56. MATSUYAMA, A., N. SAKAI, M. ISHIGAMI, *et al.* 2003. Matrix metalloproteinases as novel disease markers in Takayasu arteritis. Circulation **108:** 1469–1473.
57. SORBI, D., D.L. FRENCH, G.J. NUOVO, *et al.* 1996. Elevated levels of 92-kd type IV collagenase (matrix metalloproteinase 9) in giant cell arteritis. Arthritis Rheum. **39:** 1747–1753.
58. RIBBENS, C., M. PORRAS, N. Franchimont, *et al.* 2002. Increased matrix metalloproteinase-3 serum levels in rheumatic diseases: relationship with synovitis and steroid treatment. Ann. Rheum. Dis. **61:** 161–166.
59. KEYSZER, G., I. LAMBIRI, R. NAGEL, *et al.* 1999. Circulating levels of matrix metalloproteinases MMP-3 and MMP-1, tissue inhibitor of metalloproteinases 1 (TIMP-1), and MMP-1/TIMP-1 complex in rheumatic disease. Correlation with clinical activity of rheumatoid arthritis versus other surrogate markers. J. Rheumatol. **26:** 251–258.
60. ASANUMA, Y., A. OESER, A.K. SHINTANI, *et al.* 2003. Premature coronary-artery atherosclerosis in systemic lupus erythematosus. N. Engl. J. Med. **349:** 2407–2415.

61. TOLOZA, S.M., A.G. URIBE, G. MCGWIN, JR., *et al.* 2004. Systemic lupus erythematosus in a multiethnic US cohort (LUMINA). XXIII. Baseline predictors of vascular events. Arthritis Rheum. **50:** 3947–3957.
62. WEI, L., T.M. MACDONALD & B.R. WALKER. 2004. Taking glucocorticoids by prescription is associated with subsequent cardiovascular disease. Ann. Intern. Med. **141:** 764–770.
63. VAN GULDENER, C., M.J. JANSSEN, J. LAMBERT, *et al.* 1998. Endothelium-dependent vasodilatation is impaired in peritoneal dialysis patients. Nephrol. Dial. Transplant. **13:** 1782–1786.
64. RIDKER, P.M., J.E. MANSON, J.E. BURING, *et al.* 1999. Homocysteine and risk of cardiovascular disease among postmenopausal women. JAMA **281:** 1817–1821.
65. CLARKE, R., L. DALY, K. ROBINSON, *et al.* 1991. Hyperhomocysteinemia: an independent risk factor for vascular disease. N. Engl. J. Med. **324:** 1149–1155.
66. PETRI, M., R. ROUBENOFF, G.E. DALLAL, *et al.* 1996. Plasma homocysteine as a risk factor for atherothrombotic events in systemic lupus erythematosus. Lancet **348:** 1120–1124.
67. REFAI, T.M., I.H. AL-SALEM, D. NKANSA-DWAMENA & M.H. AL-SALEM. 2002. Hyperhomocysteinaemia and risk of thrombosis in systemic lupus erythematosus patients. Clin. Rheumatol. **21:** 457–461.
68. STITT, A.W., C. HE, S. FRIEDMAN, *et al.* 1997. Elevated AGE-modified ApoB in sera of euglycemic, normolipidemic patients with atherosclerosis: relationship to tissue AGEs. Mol. Med. **3:** 617–627.
69. BASTA, G., A.M. SCHMIDT & R. DE CATERINA. 2004. Advanced glycation end products and vascular inflammation: implications for accelerated atherosclerosis in diabetes. Cardiovasc. Res. **63:** 582–592.
70. SCHMIDT, A.M., S.D. YAN, J.L. WAUTIER & D. STERN. 1999. Activation of receptor for advanced glycation end products: a mechanism for chronic vascular dysfunction in diabetic vasculopathy and atherosclerosis. Circ. Res. **84:** 489–497.
71. SIMS, T.J., L.M. RASMUSSEN, H. OXLUND & A.J. BAILEY. 1996. The role of glycation cross-links in diabetic vascular stiffening. Diabetologia **39:** 946–951.
72. SMIT, A.J. & H.L. LUTGERS. 2004. The clinical relevance of advanced glycation endproducts (AGE) and recent developments in pharmaceutics to reduce AGE accumulation. Curr. Med. Chem. **11:** 2767–2784.
73. WAUTIER, J.L. & A.M. SCHMIDT. 2004. Protein glycation: a firm link to endothelial cell dysfunction. Circ. Res. **95:** 233–238.
74. PARK, L., K.G. RAMAN, K.J. LEE, *et al.* 1998. Suppression of accelerated diabetic atherosclerosis by the soluble receptor for advanced glycation endproducts. Nat. Med. **4:** 1025–1031.
75. WEISS, M.F., P. ERHARD, F.A. KADER-ATTIA, *et al.* 2000. Mechanisms for the formation of glycoxidation products in end-stage renal disease. Kidney Int. **57:** 2571–2585.
76. ANDERSON, M.M., J.R. REQUENA, J.R. CROWLEY, *et al.* 1999. The myeloperoxidase system of human phagocytes generates Nepsilon-(carboxymethyl)lysine on proteins: a mechanism for producing advanced glycation end products at sites of inflammation. J. Clin. Invest. **104:** 103–113.
77. HILL, J.M., G. ZALOS, J.P. HALCOX, *et al.* 2003. Circulating endothelial progenitor cells, vascular function, and cardiovascular risk. N. Engl. J. Med. **348:** 593–600.
78. VASA, M., S. FICHTLSCHERER, A. AICHER, *et al.* 2001. Number and migratory activity of circulating endothelial progenitor cells inversely correlate with risk factors for coronary artery disease. Circ. Res. **89:** E1–E7.
79. RAUSCHER, F.M., P.J. GOLDSCHMIDT-CLERMONT, B.H. DAVIS, *et al.* 2003. Aging, progenitor cell exhaustion, and atherosclerosis. Circulation **108:** 457–463.
80. TEPPER, O.M., R.D. GALIANO, J.M. CAPLA, *et al.* 2002. Human endothelial progenitor cells from type II diabetics exhibit impaired proliferation, adhesion, and incorporation into vascular structures. Circulation **106:** 2781–2786.

Nocturnal Hormones and Clinical Rhythms in Rheumatoid Arthritis

MAURIZIO CUTOLO,[a] KATI OTSA,[b] OIVI AAKRE,[b] AND ALBERTO SULLI[a]

[a]*Research Laboratory and Division of Rheumatology, Department of Immunology and Endocrinology, University of Genova, Genova, Italy*

[b]*Department of Rheumatology, Central Hospital, Tallinn, Estonia*

ABSTRACT: It is well known that some clinical signs and symptoms of rheumatoid arthritis (RA) vary within a day and between days; the morning stiffness that is observed in patients who have RA has become one of the diagnostic criteria of the disease. The circadian changes in the metabolism or nocturnal secretion of endogenous corticosteroids is certainly responsible, in part, for the time-dependent changes that are observed in the inflammatory response and related clinical symptoms. More recently, melatonin (mLT), another circadian nocturnal hormone that is the secretory product of the pineal gland, has been implicated in time-dependent inflammatory reactions, with effects that are opposite of those of corticosteroids. Therefore, altered functioning of the hypothalamic-pituitary-adrenocortical axis (reduced corticosteroid production) and of the pineal gland (increased mLT production) found in RA patients seem to be important factors in the perpetuation and clinical circadian symptoms of the disease. Consistently, human proinflammatory Th1-type cytokine production (related to mLT stimulation) exhibits a diurnal rhythmicity, with peak levels during the night and early morning, at a time when plasma cortisol (inducing Th2-type cytokine production) is lowest and mLT is highest. Reduced daily light exposure as observed in northern Europe (Estonia), at least during the winter, might explain the higher and more prolonged mLT concentrations as well as some epidemiological features that are observed in northern European patients with RA versus southern European patients.

KEYWORDS: rheumatoid arthritis; circadian rhythms; cytokines; melatonin; cortisol; Europe

INTRODUCTION: THE BIOLOGIC RHYTHMS

It is well known that some clinical signs and symptoms of rheumatoid arthritis (RA) vary within a day and between days; the morning stiffness that is observed in patients with RA has become one of the diagnostic criteria of the disease.[1] These circadian rhythms are driven by biologic clocks and are endogenous in origin, which suggests that clinical signs and symptoms in RA follow a biologic clock (biologic rhythms).

Address for correspondence: Maurizio Cutolo, Research Laboratory and Division of Rheumatology, Department of Immunology and Endocrinology, University of Genova, Viale Benedetto XV, 16132 Genova-I, Italy.
mcutolo@unige.it

Ann. N.Y. Acad. Sci. 1051: 372–381 (2005). © 2005 New York Academy of Sciences.
doi: 10.1196/annals.1361.079

Interestingly, the intensity of pain varies as a function of the hour of the day; pain is greater after awakening in the morning than in the afternoon or evening.[2] Circadian changes also are observed in joint swelling and finger circumference. The circadian pattern of joint stiffness of a patient with RA is in phase with the circadian rhythm of pain. In addition, these biologic rhythms differ inversely by approximately 12 h from the circadian changes in left- and right-hand grip strength. Greater grip strength is demonstrated when joint circumferences and the subjective ratings of stiffness and pain are least, and vice versa.[3]

BIOLOGIC RHYTHMS AND INFLAMMATION

The presence of biologic rhythms has been detected with different animal models of inflammation.

For example, one study showed that maximal inflammation occurred during the activity period of the animals (i.e., between midnight and 8 AM).[4] In contrast, in humans, maximal inflammatory reactivity was present before awakening. Biologic rhythms with a periodicity longer than 24 h also have been detected in a rodent model. In addition, a circaseptan rhythm (~7 days) of paw edema was observed over a period of 30 days, with peak inflammation every 6 to 7 days.[5]

Circannual variations have been identified in different models of inflammation, and showed that maximal articular edema was significantly greater in spring and was lowest in winter.[6] A time-dependent change of blood flow to an inflammatory site also could explain circadian variations in experimental edema, and data in rats showed that the blood flow was greater in the night and less in the morning.[2]

The mechanisms of the time-dependent variations of the inflammatory reaction are complex, and include several systems of mediators, for example, histamine, bradykinin, prostaglandins, and, mainly, proinflammatory and anti-inflammatory cytokines.

Circadian changes in the metabolism or secretion of endogenous corticosteroids are certainly responsible, in part, for the time-dependent changes that are observed in the inflammatory response. This assumption is supported by the finding that adrenalectomy abolishes the circadian variation in the rate of formation of experimental edema, and that this pattern is restored by hydrocortisone administration.[7] Further studies have shown that the inflammatory response produced by different agents is in phase opposition with the nocturnal corticosterone rhythm, with less edema observed when plasma corticosterone levels are higher, and vice versa.[4,6]

More recently, melatonin (mLT), another circadian nocturnal hormone and the secretory product of the pineal gland, has been implicated in time-dependent inflammatory reactions, with effects that are opposite of those of cortisol.[8] In several species, pinealectomy—or any other experimental procedure that inhibits mLT synthesis and secretion—induces a state of immunodepression that is counteracted by mLT replacement.[9–11]

In general, mLT displays an immunoenhancing effect.[12] Melatonin is able to activate T lymphocytes, monocytes, natural killer cells, neutrophils, and antibody-dependent cellular cytotoxicity and enhances antibody responses *in vivo*.[10] In animal models, humans, and *in vitro* experiments, mLT enhances inflammatory cytokine and nitric oxide (NO) production.[13,14] Recently, a high mLT dose (30 μg/mL) that resulted in a 50- to 60-fold increase in plasma mLT was shown to augment the inflammatory and immune response in Freund's adjuvant arthritis in rats.[15] These results should be considered in light of recent reports that RA patients have increased nocturnal plasma levels of mLT, and that their synovial macrophages respond to mLT with increased cytokine production.[16,17]

NOCTURNAL HORMONES (CORTISOL AND mLT) REGULATE CIRCADIAN CYTOKINE PRODUCTION

In adult primates, only visible light (400–700 nm) is perceived by the retina. This photic energy is transduced and delivered to the visual cortex and, by an alternative pathway, to the suprachiasmatic nucleus, and then to the hypothalamic region that directs circadian rhythms. Visible light exposure also modulates the pituitary and pineal glands and leads to neuroendocrine changes. Melatonin, norepinephrine, and acetylcholine decrease with light activation, whereas cortisol, serotonin, γ-aminobutyric acid, and dopamine increase.

Ocular light exposure appears to be the predominant time cue and major determinant of circadian rhythm for many neuroendocrine hormones. Cortisol and mLT show an opposite response to light. The increasing light conditions in the early morning have a strong impact on the morning cortisol peak, whereas mLT is synthesized in a strictly nocturnal pattern. Direct inhibitory effects of light on pineal activity may contribute to phasing of the onset and termination of mLT production.[9,18]

Recently, in healthy humans, a diurnal rhythmicity was found between cellular (Th1 type) and humoral (Th2 type) immune responses and was found to be related to immune modulatory actions of cortisol and mLT (FIG. 1).[19] Specifically, lipopolysaccharide (LPS)– or tetanus-stimulated human whole-blood interferon (IFN)–γ (type 1) and interleukin (IL)–10 (type 2) production, and the IFN-γ to IL-10 ratio, exhibited significant diurnal rhythmicity. The IFN-γ/IL-10 ratio peaked during the early morning and correlated positively with plasma mLT but correlated negatively with plasma cortisol. IFN-γ production and, to a lesser extent, IL-10 production were sensitive to inhibition by exogenous cortisone. The IFN-γ/IL-10 ratio decreased by more than 70% after the administration of oral cortisone acetate (25 mg). These findings support the concept that plasma cortisol, and possibly mLT, regulate diurnal variation in the IFN-γ/IL-10 ratio. IFN-γ and IL-10 have opposing effects on cellular (type 1) immunity; changes in their balance would be anticipated to impose diurnal rhythmicity on cellular immunity.

In normal subjects, mLT peaks at approximately 3 AM, whereas cortisol peaks at approximately 9 AM[20] IL-1, IL-6, and soluble IL-2 receptors peak between 1 AM and 4 AM, and decrease throughout the day.[19] Melatonin stimulates IL-1 and IFN-γ production by human monocytes, and serum IL-2 increases during the night, concomitant with the mLT increase. Also, mLT seems to enhance IL-2 immunomodulating effects.[21–24] Melatonin increases the production of IL-12 and NO by human synovial macrophages, enhances IL-2, IL-6, and IFN-γ production by human circulating $CD4^+$ lymphocytes, and upregulates the level of gene expression of tumor necrosis factor (TNF)–α and macrophage–colony-stimulating factor.[14,25,26]

In contrast, cortisol correlates negatively with the IFN-γ/IL-10 ratio, and cortisone administration markedly reduces the ratio with a clear causal relationship.[19]

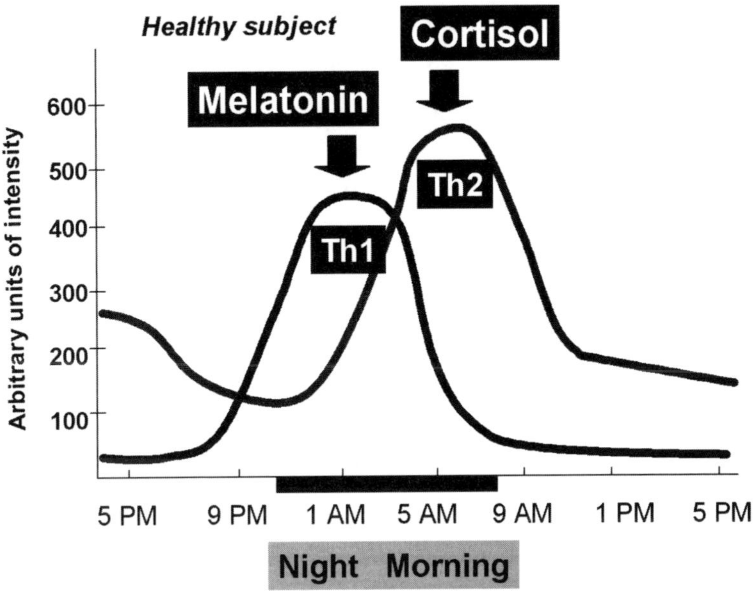

FIGURE 1. Th1 and Th2 cytokine peaks are driven by the nocturnal hormones melatonin and cortisol, respectively.

Besides IFN-γ and IL-1, TNF-α and IL-12 also exhibit distinct diurnal rhythms that peak in the early morning and are related inversely to the plasma cortisol rhythm.[27] Because IFN-γ and IL-10 might be considered to be markers of cellular (type 1) and humoral (type2) immunity, respectively, these studies suggest a bias toward increased cellular immunity during the night and the early morning (peak of mLT), when the IFN-γ/IL-10 ratio is high (FIG. 1). Conversely, a relative bias toward increased humoral (type 2) immunity during the day is suggested.[28]

CIRCADIAN RHYTHMS AND CORTISOL IN RHEUMATOID ARTHRITIS

The activation of the immune system induces inflammatory cytokines (e.g., IL-6, IL-1, TNF-α) as soluble products that stimulate the production of corticotropin-releasing hormone (CRH) in the hypothalamus. CRH release leads to pituitary production of corticotropin, followed by glucocorticoid secretion by the adrenal cortex.[29,30] These components constitute the hypothalamic-pituitary-adrenocortical (HPA) axis. Impaired cortisol response to ACTH in patients with active RA has been described, supporting the concept of a coexisting relative adrenal glucocorticoid insufficiency, already suggested 40 years ago.[31,32]

Increased HPA axis function is a normal response to the stress of inflammation and may be mediated by central and peripheral actions of circulating cytokines. IL-6 seems to be a major cytokine that mediates interactions between the activated immune system and the anterior pituitary cells and adrenal steroidogenesis.

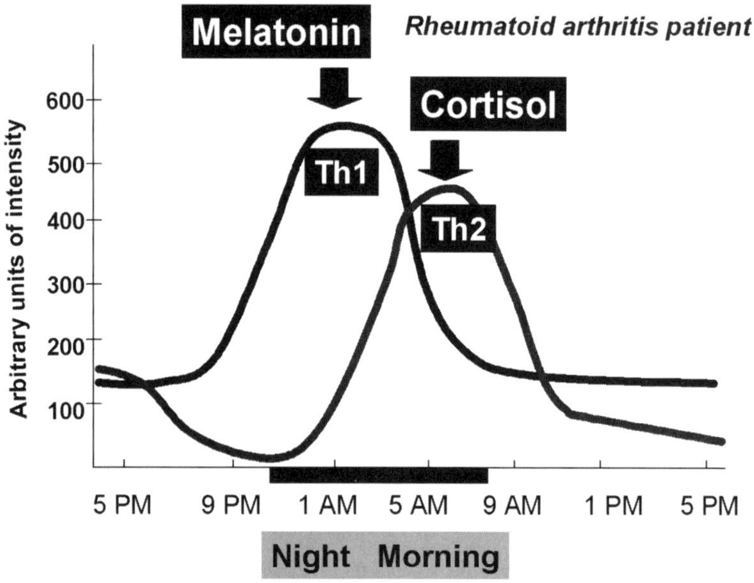

FIGURE 2. Altered Th1 and Th2 cytokine peaks follow altered nocturnal production of melatonin and cortisol in rheumatoid arthritis patients.

Recent studies in patients with RA, however, show that overall activity of the HPA axis remains inappropriately normal (or relatively low) and apparently is insufficient to inhibit ongoing inflammation, at least in patients with early, untreated arthritis (FIG. 2).[33,34] In particular, in the early morning hours, an earlier surge of plasma corticotropin and cortisol was observed in patients with RA; significantly increased IL-6 levels and a pronounced circadian variation of plasma levels were detected when compared with healthy subjects.[35] In addition, a positive temporal correlation was found between plasma IL-6 levels and the corticotropin/cortisol ratio; elevation of IL-6 occurring 1 and 2 h before elevations of corticotropin and cortisol, respectively, was found in patients with RA.[35]

In the same patients, a negative correlation between cortisol and IL-6 was found, with a delay of 5 h, indicating that HPA function in RA apparently is insufficient to inhibit ongoing inflammation. Decreased plasma levels of the adrenal androgen (AA) dehydroepiandrosterone (DHEA) and its sulfate metabolite were found in another study.[36] Also, these levels correlated significantly with decreased early morning cortisol concentrations and increased basal levels of IL-6 in patients with RA.[36] Early morning IL-6 peak values were greater in patients with RA than in controls, and correlated significantly with morning C-reactive protein (CRP) levels and the Ritchie's index.[36,37]

Another observation, of reduced DHEA production combined with normal cortisol production during ovine corticotropin-releasing hormone (oCRH) and corticotropin testing, further supports the concept of adrenal–androgen hypofunction in patients with active RA.[38] IL-6 has a strong central effect on steroid production and may be one of the factors that control the long-term adrenal response to stress. This cytokine also is able to act synergistically with corticotropin on adrenal cells to stimulate the release of corticosterone.[39,40] Accordingly, the reduced secretion of cortisol and AA that are observed during testing in patients with RA and are not treated with glucocorticoids may be regarded as evidence of "relative adrenal insufficiency" in the setting of a sustained inflammatory process, as shown by increased IL-6 levels.[36]

In a recent investigation on salivary cortisol levels in patients with early RA, afternoon concentrations in patients with high disease activity did not decrease, as did the cortisol levels in healthy controls or patients with RA and low disease activity.[41] These findings and others further indicate that activation of the HPA axis occurs in RA, but is insufficient.[42] The observed less-than-adequate production of cortisol supports the use of low-dose corticosteroid "replacement therapy" in patients with RA.[43]

CIRCADIAN RHYTHMS OF MELATONIN IN RHEUMATOID ARTHRITIS

Recent studies have evaluated mLT levels in patients with RA, with a focus on analyses of circadian variations.[44] Melatonin serum levels at 8 PM and 8 AM were significantly greater in patients with RA than in controls ($P < 0.05$; FIGS. 1 and 2). The differences were more evident in patients who were older than 60 years.

In patients with RA and in healthy subjects, mLT levels increased progressively from 8 PM to the early morning hours. However, they reached peak levels at midnight in patients with RA, that is, at least 2 h earlier than in controls. Subsequently, mLT concentrations in patients with RA reached a plateau that lasted for 2 to 3 h; this was not observed in controls. After 2 AM, mLT levels decreased similarly in patients with RA and in healthy subjects. The study confirmed that nocturnal rhythm of mLT occurs also in patients with RA, but with an earlier peak level and a longer duration in the early morning.[44] IFN-γ, IL-1, IL-2, IL-6, IL-12, and TNF-α production (Th1 cytokines) reach their peak during the night and early morning, at the same time that serum mLT is highest and plasma cortisol is lowest.

Accordingly, among the symptoms of joint inflammation in patients with RA, the intensity of pain varies as a function of the hour of the day; pain is greater after awakening in the morning than in the afternoon or evening.[2,3] Circadian changes also are observed in joint swelling and finger size in the early morning in patients with RA.[1] Therefore, mLT could be involved in activating the inflammatory response during the night, at least in RA, which is considered to be a Th1-cytokine–driven immune disease.[45] In addition, mLT was found in high concentration in synovial fluids from patients with RA, and binding sites for mLT have been detected in synovial macrophages.[46,47]

Recent studies and reviews have examined epidemiologic evidence that suggests that ultraviolet radiation may play a protective role in RA. A gradient of increasing incidence of RA with latitude and seasonal variation also has been reported.[48–50] Therefore, we evaluated serum mLT, cortisol, TNF-α, and IL-6 circadian rhythm in patients with RA from a northern European country (Estonia). In particular, we compared the mLT and cortisol levels in this group with patients from a southern

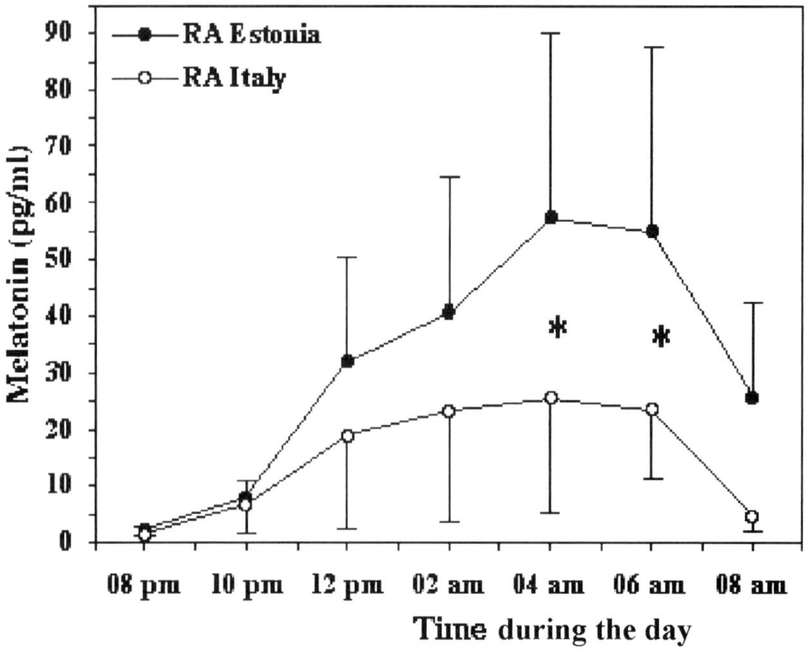

FIGURE 3. Circadian production of melatonin in Estonian rheumatoid arthritis patients as compared with age- and sex-matched Italian rheumatoid arthritis patients.

European country (Italy), to detect a possible influence of different daily winter photoperiods.[51]

Patients with RA from Estonia and Italy were characterized by similar RA disease severity and duration, and both groups were compared with age- and sex-matched healthy controls. Blood samples were obtained at 8 PM, 10 PM, 12 AM, 2 AM, 4 AM, 8 AM, and 3 PM during the months of January and February. Starting with the 10 PM mLT measurement, a significantly ($P < 0.01$) greater mLT concentration and earlier peaking in mLT were observed in Estonian patients with RA compared with age- and sex-matched controls. At the midnight measurement, serum mLT was significantly higher in Estonian patients than in Italian patients, and the difference was even greater over the study duration (FIG. 3). No significant difference in serum cortisol was observed between Estonian patients with RA and controls.[16,51] TNF-α serum levels were significantly higher in Estonian patients with RA than in controls. Significantly higher serum IL-6 and TNF-α were observed at 10 PM and midnight in Estonian patients with RA than in Italian patients with RA.[49,50]

This important study shows, for the first time, that in a northern European country (Estonia), the circadian serum concentrations of mLT and TNF-α are significantly higher than in matched patients with RA from a southern European country (Italy). In addition, mLT and TNF-α were increased in patients with RA.

Reduced daily light exposure as observed in northern Europe, at least during the winter, might explain the higher and more prolonged mLT concentrations that were observed in northern patients with RA. The increased prevalence of autoimmune diseases such as RA that is observed in northern Europe also may be related to increased immunostimulatory effects that are exerted during the night by mLT, and to reduced neuroendocrine stimulation during the light phase of the photoperiod.

CONCLUSIONS

The clinical symptoms of RA show a circadian variation; joint stiffness and pain are more prominent in the early morning. Altered functioning of the HPA axis and of the pineal gland seem to be important factors in the perpetuation and clinical circadian symptoms of RA.[16]

Human proinflammatory Th1-type cytokine production consistently exhibits diurnal rhythmicity, with peak levels during the night and early morning at a time when plasma cortisol is lowest and mLT is highest.

Inappropriately decreased secretion of cortisol is a typical feature of the inflammatory disease in patients with RA. Conversely, the nocturnal rhythm of mLT in patients with RA shows an earlier peak level and a longer duration in the early morning compared with the pattern of serum mLT normal subjects. Therefore, an imbalance between the anti-inflammatory effects of cortisol and the proinflammatory effects of mLT during the night seems evident in patients with RA. This imbalance may play an important pathogenetic role in RA and may also drive the circadian rhythm of the clinical symptoms (i.e., morning stiffness and pain).

ACKNOWLEDGMENTS

This research was supported in part by the first executive program of the cultural, educational, scientific, and technological cooperation between Italy and Estonia, and by the Ministries for Foreign Affairs of Italy and for Culture, Education, and Research of Estonia.

REFERENCES

1. Cutolo, M. & A.T. Masi. 2005. Circadian rhythms and arthritis. Rheum. Dis. Clin. North. Am. **31:** 115–129.
2. Labrecque, G., J.P. Bureau & A.E. Reinberg. 1995. Biological rhythms in the inflammatory response and in the effects of non-steroidal anti-inflammatory drugs. Pharmac. Ther. **66:** 285–300.
3. Harkness, J.A., M.B. Richter, G.S. Panayi, *et al.* 1982. Circadian variation in disease activity in rheumatoid arthritis. Br. Med. J. **284:** 551–554.
4. Latman, N.S. 1983. Relation of menstrual cycle phase to symptoms of rheumatoid arthritis. Am. J. Med. **74:** 957–960.
5. Muir, V.Y. & R. Pownall. 1983. Identification of a seven day biological cycle in the rat. J. Pharm. Pharmac. **35:** 186–188.
6. Loubaris, N., G. Cros, J.J. Serrano & M. Boucard. 1983. Circadian and circannual variation of the carrageenan inflammatory effect in the rat. Life Sci. **32:** 1349–1354.
7. Labreque, G., F. Dore & P.M. Berlanger. 1981. Circadian variation of carrageenan-paw edema in the rat. Life Sci. **28:** 1337–1343.
8. Maestroni, G.J., A. Conti & W. Pierpaoli. 1986. Role of the pineal gland in immunity: circadian synthesis and release of melatonin modulates the antibody response

and antagonizes the immunosuppressive effect of corticosterone. J. Neuroimmunol. **13:** 19–30.
9. REITER, R.J. 1991. Pineal melatonin: cell biology of its synthesis and of its physiological interactions. Endocr. Rev. **12:** 151–180.
10. MAESTRONI, G.J. 1993. The immunoneuroendocrine role of melatonin. J. Pineal Res. **14:** 1–10.
11. MAESTRONI, G.J. 1995. T-helper-2 lymphocytes as a peripheral target of melatonin. J. Pineal Res. **18:** 84–89.
12. BARRIGA, C., M.I. MARTIN, E. ORTEGA & A.B. RODRIGUEZ. 2002. Physiological concentrations of melatonin and corticosterone in stress and their relationship with phagocytic activity. J. Neuroendocrinol. **14:** 691–695.
13. ESQUIFINO, A.I. & D.P. CARDINALI. 1999. Effects of melatonin on 24-h rhythms of neuroendocrine and immune changes in Freund's adjuvant-induced arthritis. Neuro. Endocrinol. Lett. **20:** 163–166.
14. GARCIA-MAURINO, S., M.G. GONZALEZ-HABA, J.R. CALVO, *et al.* 1997. Melatonin enhances IL-2, IL-6 and IFN-gamma production by human circulating CD4+ cells: a possible nuclear receptor-mediated mechanism involving T helper type 1 lymphocytes and monocytes. J. Immunol. **159:** 574–581.
15. CARDINALI, D.P., A.P. GARCIA, P. CANO & A.I. ESQUIFINO. 2004. Melatonin role in experimental arthritis. Curr. Drug Targets Immune Endocr. Metabol. Disord. **4:** 1–10.
16. CUTOLO, M., G.J. MAESTRONI, K. OTSA, *et al.* 2005. Circadian melatonin and cortisol levels in rheumatoid arthritis patients in winter time: a north and south Europe comparison. Ann. Rheum. Dis. **64:** 212–216.
17. CUTOLO, M., B. VILLAGGIO, F. CANDIDO, *et al.* 1999. Melatonin influences interleukin-12 and nitric oxide production by primary cultures of rheumatoid synovial macrophages and THP-1 cells. Ann. N.Y. Acad. Sci. **876:** 246–254.
18. SCHEER, F.A. & R.M. BUIJS. 1999. Light affects morning salivary cortisol in humans. J. Clin. Endocrinol. **84:** 3395–3398.
19. PETROVSKY, N., P. MCNAIR & L. HARRISON. 1998. Diurnal rhythms of pro-inflammatory cytokines: regulation by plasma cortisol and therapeutic implications. Cytokine **10:** 307–312.
20. MIYATAKE, A., Y. MORIMOTO, T. OISHI, *et al.* 1980. Circadian rhythm of serum testosterone and its relation to sleep: comparison with the variation in serum luteinizing hormone, prolactin, and cortisol in normal men. J. Clin. Endocrinol. Metab. **51:** 1365–1371.
21. GUDEWILL, S., I. POLLMACHER, H. VEDDER, *et al.* 1992. Nocturnal plasma levels of cytokines in healthy men. Eur. Arch. Psychiatry Clin. Neurosci. **242:** 53–56.
22. MORREY, K.M., J.A MCLACHLAN, C.D. SERKIN & O. BAKOUCHE. 1994. Activation of human monocytes by the pineal hormone melatonin. J. Immunol. **153:** 2671–2680.
23. LISSONI, P., F. ROVELLI, F. BRIVIO, *et al.* 1998. Circadian secretions of IL-2, IL-12, IL-6 and IL-10 in relation to light/dark rhythm of the pineal hormone melatonin in healthy humans. Nat. Immun. **16:** 1–5.
24. LISSONI, P. 2000. Modulation of anticancer cytokines IL-2 and IL-12 by melatonin and the other pineal indoles 5-methoxytryptamine and 5-methoxytrypholol in the treatment of human neoplasms. Ann. N.Y. Acad. Sci. **917:** 560–567.
25. MAESTRONI, G.J., D.P. CARDINALI, A.I. ESQUIFINO, *et al.* 2005. Does melatonin play a disease-promoting role in rheumatoid arthritis? J. Neuroimmunol. **158:** 106–111.
26. LIU, F., T.B. NG & M.C. FUNG. 2001. Pineal indoles stimulate the gene expression of immunomodulating cytokines. J. Neural Transm. **108:** 397–405.
27. PETROVSKY, N. & L.C. HARRISON. 1998. The chronobiology of human cytokine production. Int. Rev. Immunol. **16:** 635–649.
28. PETROVSKY, N. 2001. Towards a unified model of neuroendocrine-immune interaction. Immunol. Cell Biol. **79:** 350–357.
29. MASI, A.T., S.L. FEIGENBAUM, R.T. CHATTERTON & M. CUTOLO. 1995. Integrated hormonal-immunological-vascular (H-I-V triad) systems interactions in the rheumatic diseases. Clin. Exp. Rheumatol. **13:** 203–216.
30. CHROUSOS, G.P. 1995. The hypothalamic-pituitary-adrenal axis and immune-mediated inflammation. N. Engl. J. Med. **332:** 1351–1362.

31. Gudbjornsson, B., B. Skogseid, B. Oberg, *et al.* 1996. Intact adrenocorticotropic hormone secretion but impaired cortisol response in patients with active rheumatoid arthritis. Effect of glucocorticoids. J. Rheumatol. **23:** 596–602.
32. West, H.F. 1996. Corticosteroid metabolism and rheumatoid arthritis. Ann. Rheum. Dis. **16:** 173–181.
33. Masi, A.T. & G.P. Chrousos. 1996. Hypothalamic-pituitary-adrenal-glucocorticoid axis function in rheumatoid arthritis. J. Rheumatol. **23:** 577–581.
34. Straub, R.H. & M. Cutolo. 2001. Involvement of the hypothalamic–pituitary–adrenal/gonadal axis and the peripheral nervous system in rheumatoid arthritis: viewpoint based on a systemic pathogenetic role. Arthritis Rheum. **44:** 493–507.
35. Crofford, L.J., K.T. Kalogeras, G. Mastorakos, *et al.* 1997. Circadian relationships between interleukin IL-6 and hypothalamic-pituitary-adrenal axis hormones: failure of IL-6 to cause sustained hypercortisolism in patients with early untreated rheumatoid arthritis. J. Clin. Endocrinol. Metab. **82:** 1279–1283.
36. Cutolo, M., L. Foppiani, C. Prete, *et al.* 1999. Hypothalamic-pituitary-adrenocortical axis function in premenopausal women with rheumatoid arthritis not treated with glucocorticoids. J. Rheumatol. **26:** 282–288.
37. Arvidson, N.G., G. Gudbjornsson, L. Elfman, *et al.* 1994. Circadian rhythm of serum interleukin-6 in rheumatoid arthritis. Ann. Rheum. Dis. **53:** 521–524.
38. Templ, E., M. Koeller, M. Riedl, *et al.* 1996. Anterior pituitary function in patients with newly diagnosed rheumatoid arthritis. Br. J. Rheumatol. **35:** 350–356.
39. Mastorakos, G., G.P. Chrousos & J.S. Weber. 1993. Recombinant interleukin-6 activates the hypothalamic pituitary-adrenal axis in human. J. Clin. Endocrinol. Metab. **77:** 1690–1694.
40. Ehrhart-Bornstein, M., J.P. Hinson, S.R. Bornstein, *et al.* 1998. Intraadrenal interactions in the regulation of adrenocortical steroidogenesis. Endocr. Rev. **19:** 101–104.
41. Dekkers, J.C., R. Geenen, G.L. Godaert, *et al.* 2000. Diurnal rhythm of salivary cortisol levels in patients with recent onset rheumatoid arthritis. Arthritis Rheum. **43:** 465–467.
42. Straub, R.H., L. Paimela, R. Peltomaa, *et al.* 2002. Inadequately low serum levels of steroid hormones in relation to IL-6 and TNF in untreated patients with early rheumatoid arthritis and reactive arthritis. Arthritis Rheum. **46:** 654–662.
43. van Everdingen, A.A., J.W. Jacobs, D.R. Siewertsz van Reesema & J.W. Bijlsma. 2002. Low-dose prednisone therapy for patients with early active rheumatoid arthritis: clinical efficacy, disease-modifying properties, and side effects: a randomized, double-blind, placebo-controlled clinical trial. Ann. Intern. Med. **136:** 1–12.
44. Sulli, A., G.J. Maestroni, B. Villaggio, *et al.* 2002. Melatonin serum levels in rheumatoid arthritis. Ann. N.Y. Acad. Sci. **966:** 276–283.
45. Schulze-Koops, H., P.E. Lipsky, A.F. Kavanaugh & L.S. Davis. 1995. Elevated Th1 or Th2-like cytokine mRNA in peripheral circulation of patients with rheumatoid arthritis. J. Immunol. **155:** 5029–5037.
46. Maestroni, G.J., A. Sulli, C. Pizzorni, *et al.* 2002. Melatonin in rheumatoid arthritis: synovial macrophages show melatonin receptors. Ann. N.Y. Acad. Sci. **966:** 271–275.
47. Maestroni, G.J., A. Sulli, C. Pizzorni, *et al.* 2002. Melatonin in rheumatoid arthritis: a disease promoting and modulating hormone? Clin. Exp. Rheumatol. **20:** 872–873.
48. Cantorna, M.T. 2000. Vitamin D and autoimmunity: is vitamin D status an environmental factor affecting autoimmune disease prevalence? Proc. Soc. Exp. Biol. Med. **223:** 230–233.
49. Rozin, A., A. Balbir-Gurman & D. Shapira. 2003. Seasonal distribution of relapse onset in rheumatoid arthritis and spondyloarthropathy: the possible effect of solar factor. Clin. Exp. Rheumatol. **21:** 161–169.
50. Cutolo, M. 2003. Solar light effects on onset/releases and circannual/circadian symptomatology in rheumatoid arthritis. Clin. Exp. Rheum. **21:** 148–150.
51. Otsa, K., T. Peets, G. Maestroni, *et al.* 2004. Circadian rhythms of melatonin in Estonian rheumatoid arthritis patients. Ann. Rheum. Dis. **63:** S139.

Xenobiotic-Induced Recruitment of Autoantigens to Nuclear Proteasomes Suggests a Role for Altered Antigen Processing in Scleroderma

MIN CHEN AND ANNA VON MIKECZ

Institut für umweltmedizinische Forschung at Heinrich-Heine-University Duesseldorf, Duesseldorf, Germany

ABSTRACT: **The cell nucleus is a prominent target of autoantibodies in systemic autoimmune disorders. Approximately 2% of the population in Europe and North America suffers from systemic rheumatic diseases, such as rheumatoid arthritis, systemic lupus erythematosus (SLE), and scleroderma. The molecular mechanisms of systemic autoimmunity are largely unknown despite its high prevalence. Contributing factors that have been considered include (1) genetic predisposition, (2) influence of hormones, and (3) environmental factors. The latter are mainly correlated with the generation of scleroderma, as xenobiotic-induced subsets of this disease have been observed in individuals exposed to silica (SiO_2) dusts, organic solvents, heavy metals, and certain drugs. In addition to the epidemiological relevance, animal models of xenobiotic-induced autoimmunity serve as elegant tools for controlled induction of antigen-driven autoimmune responses. Because antigen processing and presentation constitute the basis for every antigen-driven autoimmune response, effects of xenobiotics on degradation of nuclear autoantigens have been characterized to elucidate molecular mechanisms of autoimmunity that target the cell nucleus. By means of a cell-based disease model, it has been shown that xenobiotics such as mercuric chloride, platinum salts, and silica (nano)particles specifically alter structure, function, and proteolysis in the cell nucleus. Signature proteins of the cell nucleus redistribute to aberrant, nucleoplasmic clusters, where they colocalize with proteasomes and are subjected to proteasomal proteolysis. Recruitment of nuclear autoantigens to proteasomal degradation is correlated with autoimmune responses that specifically target these antigens in both animal models of xenobiotic-induced autoimmunity and patients with idiopathic scleroderma.**

KEYWORDS: **antigen processing; proteasomes; nuclear autoantigens; scleroderma**

Address for correspondence: Min Chen, M.D., Institut für umweltmedizinische Forschung at Heinrich-Heine-University Duesseldorf, Auf'm Hennekamp 50, D-40225 Duesseldorf, Germany. Voice: +49-211-3389245; fax: +49-211-3190910.
chenmin@uni-duesseldorf.de

Ann. N.Y. Acad. Sci. 1051: 382–389 (2005). © **2005 New York Academy of Sciences.**
doi: 10.1196/annals.1361.080

INTRODUCTION

Systemic rheumatic diseases such as systemic lupus erythematosus (SLE) and scleroderma (systemic sclerosis, SSc) are chronic, life-threatening multiorgan disorders that affect approximately 2% of the population in Europe and North America.[1] A hallmark of these disorders is the production of autoantibodies against "self" proteins that localize to the cell nucleus. Despite the high prevalence of these disorders, the molecular mechanisms underlying systemic autoimmune responses largely remain unclear.

Autoantibodies against nucleolus-associated proteins such as DNA topoisomerase I (topo I, Scl-70), centromeres (CENP-A, CENP-B, CENP-C), RNA polymerase I, and fibrillarin have been identified as disease-specific autoantibodies and diagnostic markers in scleroderma, whereas nucleoplasmic proteins, for example, histones, and spliceosomal components such as U1-70k and SmB/B′, are marker proteins for SLE.[2,3] Patients with scleroderma produce a monospecific autoimmune response that is directed against a limited number of nuclear proteins, which are unified by their enrichment within the cell nucleus under unique physiological conditions.[3–5] Thus, the idea was put forward that alteration of the molecular context of nuclear proteins by environmental factors might lead to aberrant processing and presentation of previously cryptic proteins. It has been shown that exposure to a variety of different environmental substances may lead to the development of disease that mimics clinical and histopathological features of idiopathic scleroderma.[6] Chronic administration of mercuric chloride, for example, induces scleroderma-like autoimmunity in susceptible mouse strains. The main target of mercury-induced antinuclear autoantibodies (ANAs) is the nucleolar protein fibrillarin, which also represents an autoantigen in a subset of patients with scleroderma.[7–11] A striking occupational clustering of scleroderma was observed in miners and workers exposed to silica dust. In the case of silica-induced scleroderma, topoisomerase I is the main target.[12,13] Together, these observations provide a framework within which to investigate the potential role of the environment in the pathogenesis of autoimmunity in scleroderma. Administration of xenobiotics to cell culture and to susceptible animals can be considered valuable tools for studying the influence of the environment on the initiation of autoimmunity, and for studying the molecular mechanisms for the initial steps, such as antigen processing, in xenobiotic-induced autoimmunity and scleroderma, as well.

ANTIGEN PROCESSING AND PRESENTATION PATHWAYS OVERLAP

Antigen processing and presentation is the prerequisite for generation of antigen-driven immune responses. The immune system utilizes generalized catabolic processes and transport mechanisms within the cell to perform the very basic functions of proteolysis and transport of antigenic peptides. The conventional binary notion of antigen processing and presentation holds that endogenous antigens are processed by proteasomes via a nonlysosomal pathway and presented to $CD8^+$ T cells in the context of cell surface MHC class I molecules, whereas exogenous antigens typically are processed by the lysosomal pathway and presented to $CD4^+$ T cells in the context of cell surface MHC class II molecules.[14,15]

However, an increasing number of studies have provided solid evidence that these two classic major antigen-processing and presentation pathways are less restrictive than originally recognized. In fact, endogenous antigens are presented in the context of MHC class II molecules to activate CD4$^+$ T cells, and exogenous antigens that are phagocytosed by antigen-presenting cells do gain access to the MHC class I pathway.[16–21] Although the cellular mechanisms allowing such crisscross pathways are not clear, chaperones such as heat shock proteins might mediate both cross-presentation pathways for exogenous antigens on MHC class I molecules, and for endogenous antigens on MHC class II molecules.[22,23]

Consistent with this new concept of crisscross pathways, antigenic peptides generated intracellularly by proteasomal processing from endogenous antigens such as nucleoplasmic proteins and nucleolar proteins may normally be presented on MHC class I molecules for continual surveillance by CD8$^+$ T cells. However, under certain circumstances, they may also be presented on MHC class II molecules to activate CD4$^+$ T cells and induce the process of autoantigen-specific antibody production.

XENOBIOTIC-INDUCED RECRUITMENT OF SCLERODERMA NUCLEAR AUTOANTIGENS TO NUCLEAR PROTEASOMAL PROCESSING IN CELL CULTURE

It is well known that the cell nucleus is a prominent target in systemic autoimmune diseases such as scleroderma. However, to date it has not been clear where and how proteolysis of nuclear autoantigens takes place within the cell. A prerequisite for protein interaction in a cell is localization in the same intracellular regions. Now that proteasomes are known to be involved in antigen processing of endogenous antigens, and their location has been identified not only in the cytosol but also in the nucleoplasm of normal eukaryotic cells, it is of importance to determine the subcellular localization of proteasomes in relation to nuclear autoantigens. Dual-labeling studies by indirect immunofluorescence and confocal microscopy revealed that nucleoplasmic autoantigens such as histone protein H2A, splicing factor SC35, and spliceosomal components U1-70k and SmB/B′ colocalize with proteasomes in distinct nuclear proteasomal processing centers (NPPCs), where these SLE-specific autoantigens are degraded by proteasomes.[24] However, nucleolus-associated marker proteins for scleroderma such as DNA topoisomerase I, fibrillarin, and centromeres do not colocalize with proteasomes under normal conditions. Because degradation of nuclear proteins via the proteasomal pathway is correlated with their subnuclear colocalization with proteasomes, the question occured whether scleroderma autoantigens change their subcellular distribution and overlap with proteasomes under unique conditions?

Because environmental substances such as chemicals are associated with scleroderma, effects of xenobiotics on intracellular localization and degradation of scleroderma nuclear autoantigens have been analyzed in cell culture. Xenobiotics such as mercuric chloride and the anticancer drugs camptothecin and topotecan specifically alter structure, function, and proteolysis within the cell nucleus. Mercuric chloride induces redistribution of the scleroderma autoantigen fibrillarin from the nucleolus to nucleoplasmic clusters, owing to specific inhibition of RNA polymerase I–dependent transcription of ribosomal RNAs (rRNAs) in the nucleolus.[25] Specific colocal-

TABLE 1. Recruitment of nuclear autoantigens to nuclear proteasomal processing centers by xenobiotics in cell culture and *in vivo*

Xenobiotic	Autoantigen	In cell culture in NPPC localization/ degradation	*In vivo* correlation with antibody specificity
$HgCl_2$	Fibrillarin (SSc Ag)	+/+	+
Camptothecin	Topo I (SSc Ag)	+/+	ND
Topotecan	Topo I (SSc Ag)	+/+	+
Silica nanoparticles	Topo I (SSc Ag)	+/ND	+
Platinum salts	Undefined nucleo- plasmic antigen	+/ND	+

ABBREVIATIONS: NPPC, nuclear proteasomal processing center; SSc Ag, scleroderma-specific autoantigen; topo I, topoisomerase I; ND, not determined.

ization of fibrillarin with proteasomes in mercury-induced aberrant nucleoplasmic clusters correlates with degradation of fibrillarin by the ubiquitin-proteasome system.[26] Similarly, camptothecin and topotecan specifically induce the formation of aberrant nuclear proteasomal processing centers consisting of topoisomerase I and proteasomes.[27,28] Redistribution of topoisomerase I to aberrant nucleoplasmic clusters has also been observed upon treatment with silica nanoparticles (FIG. 1F). Thus, formation of nucleoplasmic clusters of scleroderma nuclear autoantigens represents an indication of xenobiotic-induced alteration of the subnuclear structure of the cells, which leads to formation of subnuclear domains dedicated to aberrant proteasomal antigen processing (TABLE 1). In other words, scleroderma nuclear autoantigens require xenobiotic induction to be processed by the ubiquitin-proteasome system.

RECRUITMENT OF SCLERODERMA AUTOANTIGENS TO NUCLEAR PROTEASOMAL PROCESSING *IN VIVO*

To determine whether recruitment of scleroderma autoantigens to proteasomal degradation is correlated with autoimmune responses against the specific autoantigens, we extended investigations to animal models and to patients. Chronic administration of subtoxic doses of mercuric chloride to susceptible H-2^S mice showed that fibrillarin redistributes from the nucleolus to nucleoplasmic clusters (FIG. 1C) and colocalizes with proteasomes in distinct nucleoplasmic domains in splenic cells. This recruitment of fibrillarin to subnuclear domains of proteasomal antigen processing *in vivo* in mercury-treated mice correlates with the generation of autoantibodies against fibrillarin (TABLE 1).[26] Similarly, redistribution of the scleroderma autoantigen topoisomerase I to nucleoplasmic clusters has been observed in dendritic cells isolated from scleroderma patients with anti–topoisomerase I antibodies (FIG. 1G). Consistent with the results from animal models, topoisomerase I colocalizes with proteasomes within nucleoplasmic clusters of dendritic cells from scleroderma patients, and such colocalization correlates with a specific autoimmune response against topoisomerase I.[28] In contrast, scleroderma-specific autoantigens,

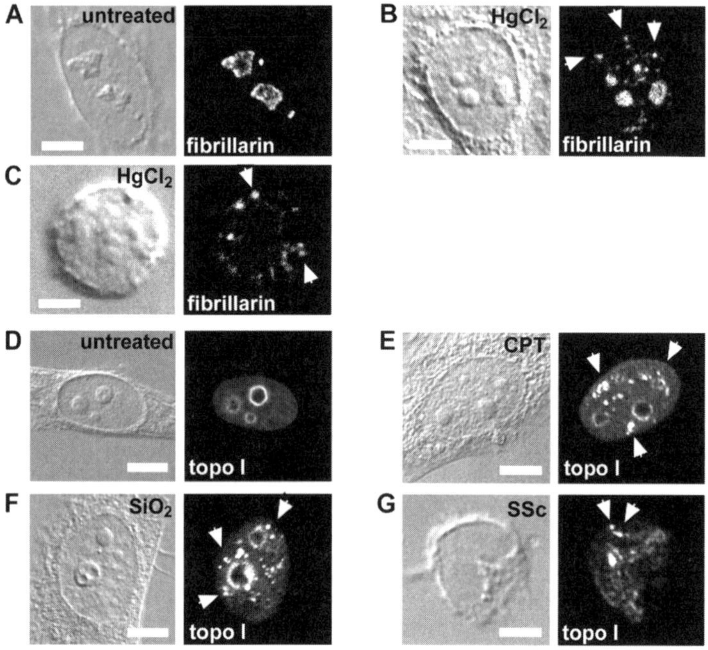

FIGURE 1. Redistribution of scleroderma autoantigens to aberrant nucleoplasmic clusters. (**A**) Confocal immunofluorescence of the nucleolar autoantigen fibrillarin in untreated HEp-2 cells shows exclusive staining of nucleoli and coiled bodies. (**B**) Confocal immunofluorescence of the nucleolar autoantigen fibrillarin in mercury-treated HEp-2 cells shows redistribution of fibrillarin from the nucleolus to aberrant nucleoplasmic clusters. (**C**) Confocal immunofluorescence of the nucleolar autoantigen fibrillarin in a representative dendritic cell from a mercury-treated, anti-fibrillarin–positive mouse shows redistribution of fibrillarin from the nucleolus to aberrant nucleoplasmic clusters. (**D**) Confocal immunofluorescence of the nucleolus-associated autoantigen topoisomerase I in untreated HEp-2 cells shows nucleolar staining and homogenous staining in the nucleoplasm. Confocal immunofluorescence shows redistribution of topoisomerase I to aberrant nucleoplasmic clusters in camptothecin-treated HEp-2 cells (**E**), in silica-treated HEp-2 cells (**F**), and in a representative dendritic cell from an anti–topoisomerase I–positive scleroderma patient (**G**). CPT, camptothecin; SSc, scleroderma; topo I, topoisomerase I. *Arrows* indicate aberrant nuclear clusters. Bars = 5 μm.

including topoisomerase I and centromeres, did not colocalize with proteasomes in dendritic cells from scleroderma patients who were negative for ANAs or positive for other autoantibody specificities. Correlation between colocalization of nuclear autoantigens with proteasomes and autoimmune responses against the respective autoantigens was confirmed by the observation that platinum salts induce production of autoantibodies against as-yet-undefined nucleoplasmic autoantigens and recruitment of these autoantigens to proteasomes in dendritic cells from platinum-treated mice.[29] Taken together, these data confirm that recruitment of scleroderma autoantigens to proteasomal degradation correlates with specific autoimmune responses against the respective autoantigens.

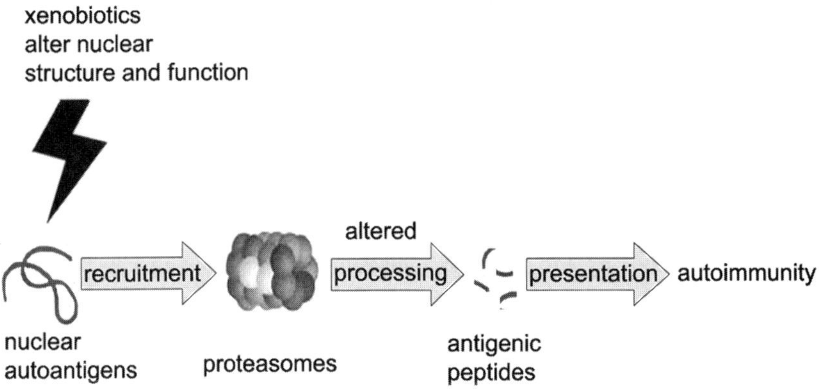

FIGURE 2. Molecular mechanisms of xenobiotic-induced autoimmunity (hypothesis).

CONCLUSION

Antigenic proteins need to be processed proteolytically to generate ligands for MHC-molecule binding. Aberrant proteasomal antigen processing of scleroderma autoantigens can be induced by xenobiotics such as heavy metals, drugs, and viruses.[26,30] According to a new concept of antigen-processing and presentation pathways,[31] the resulting peptides are subsequently loaded on MHC class I and/or class II molecules and presented on the cell surface to activate specific autoimmune responses. As aberrant antigen processing of scleroderma autoantigens by proteasomes also contributes to the production of anti–topoisomerase I antibodies in scleroderma, we conclude that scleroderma autoantigens are recruited to proteasomes for altered antigen processing to initiate the process of autoimmune reactions in xenobiotic-induced autoimmunity and scleroderma (FIG. 2, TABLE 1). However, different mechanisms may be involved in generating autoantibodies against other scleroderma autoantigens such as centromeres, and against SLE-specific autoantigens. The specificity of alteration of nuclear structure, function and proteolysis may induce particular autoimmune responses, for example, various autoantibody specificities.

The cell's nucleus represents a key player in eukaryotic lives, because it harbors the genetic information and the first steps in gene expression, namely, replication, transcription, and mRNA processing. Its importance for the development of multicellular organisms was already appreciated in the nineteenth century by Robert Brown and other cell biologists. Consistent with this idea, it seems obvious that disturbances of nuclear structure and function cause developmental defects and/or disease.[32,33] This review describes a subnuclear pathology that may contribute to systemic autoimmunity against the cell nucleus. Nucleoplasmatic protein aggregates/clusters are formed in response to xenobiotics such as mercuric chloride ($HgCl_2$) and silica (SiO_2), which are well-known inducers of systemic autoimmune responses against distinct nuclear proteins/autoantigens. The nucleus represents a dynamic, self-organizing structure consisting of substructures (domains, compartments) that form in response to the requirements of gene expression. A paradigm for the formation of nuclear substructures is the nucleolus, which is assembled when transcription of genes encoding ribosomal RNA (rRNA) resumes after cell division, and is disassembled when transcription ceases during prophase. Similar function-dependent clusters of nuclear proteins have been observed during transcription of mRNA in the nucleoplasm, DNA replication/recombination/repair, and processing of mRNA. Because clusters of nuclear proteins are also found in pathological conditions, a major challenge of future research on nuclear structure and function and on subnuclear pathology will be to distinguish functional protein clusters from such pathological clusters.

Recently, SiO_2-nanoparticles (nano-SiO_2) have been identified as novel xenobiotics that specifically alter nuclear structure and function.[34] Nano-SiO_2 induce aberrant nucleoplasmic clusters that contain signature proteins of subnuclear domains, the ubiquitin-proteasome pathway, and protein aggregation, such as cellular poly(Q) proteins and huntingtin. Because these clusters are composed of prominent nuclear autoantigens and resemble nucleoplasmic aggresomes, it has been proposed that xenobiotics induce a subnuclear pathology that might play a role in generation of both xenobiotic-induced autoimmune responses and protein aggregation diseases such as Huntington chorea.[33]

ACKNOWLEDGMENTS

This work was supported by grants from the German Scleroderma Foundation, the German Research Council through SFB 503, and the Federal Ministry of Eduction and Research through “MedNet Rheuma” awarded to A. von Mikecz.

REFERENCES

1. Jacobson, D.L., S.J. Gange, N.R. Rose & N.M. Graham. 1997. Epidemiology and estimated population burden of selected autoimmune diseases in the United States. Clin. Immunol. Immunopathol. **84:** 223–243.
2. Tamby, M.C., Y. Chanseaud, L. Guillevin & L. Mouthon. 2003. New insights into the pathogenesis of systemic sclerosis. Autoimmun. Rev. **2:** 152–157.
3. Tan, E.M. 1989. Antinuclear antibodies: diagnostic markers for autoimmune diseases and probes for cell biology. Adv. Immunol. **44:** 93–151.
4. Rothfield, N.F. 1992. Autoantibodies in scleroderma. Rheum. Dis. Clin. North Am. **18:** 483–498.
5. Tan, E.M. 1991. Autoantibodies in pathology and cell biology. Cell **67:** 841–842.
6. Silman, A.J. & M.C. Hochberg. 1996. Occupational and environmental influences on scleroderma. Rheum. Dis. Clin. North Am. **22:** 737–749.
7. Hultman, P., S. Enestrom, K.M. Pollard & EM. Tan. 1989. Anti-fibrillarin antibodies in mercury-treated mice. Clin. Exp. Immunol. **78:** 470–477.
8. Reuter, R. *et al.* 1989. Mercuric chloride induces autoantibodies against U3 small nuclear ribonucleoprotein in susceptible mice. Proc. Natl. Acad. Sci. USA **86:** 237–241.
9. Pollard, K.M. *et al.* 1997. The autoimmunity-inducing xenobiotic mercury interacts with the autoantigen fibrillarin and modifies its molecular and antigenic properties. J. Immunol. **158:** 3521–3528.
10. Lee, B. & J.E. Craft. 1995. Molecular structure and function of autoantigens in systemic sclerosis. Int. Rev. Immunol. **12:** 129–144.

11. ARNETT, F.C. *et al.* 1996. Autoantibodies to fibrillarin in systemic sclerosis (scleroderma). An immunogenetic, serologic, and clinical analysis. Arthritis Rheum. **39:** 1151–1160.
12. HAUSTEIN, U.F. & V. ZIEGLER. 1985. Environmentally induced systemic sclerosis-like disorders. Int. J. Dermatol. **24:** 147–151.
13. FOX, R.I. & H.I. KANG. 1992. Genetic and environmental factors in systemic sclerosis. Curr. Opin. Rheumatol. **4:** 857–861.
14. YEWDELL, J.W. & J.R. BENNINK. 1990. The binary logic of antigen processing and presentation to T cells. Cell **62:** 203–206.
15. GERMAIN, R.N. & D.H. MARGULIES. 1993. The biochemistry and cell biology of antigen processing and presentation. Annu. Rev. Immunol. **11:** 403–450.
16. ALBERT, M.L. *et al.* 1998. Immature dendritic cells phagocytose apoptotic cells via alphavbeta5 and CD36, and cross-present antigens to cytotoxic T lymphocytes. J. Exp. Med. **188:** 1359–1368.
17. GUERMONPREZ, P. *et al.* 2003. ER-phagosome fusion defines an MHC class I cross-presentation compartment in dendritic cells. Nature **425:** 397–402.
18. HOUDE, M. *et al.* 2003. Phagosomes are competent organelles for antigen cross presentation. Nature **425:** 402–406.
19. LEHNER, P.J. & P. CRESSWELL. 2004. Recent developments in MHC-class-I-mediated antigen presentation. Curr. Opin. Immunol. **16:** 82–89.
20. MALNATI, M.S. *et al.* 1992. Processing pathways for presentation of cytosolic antigen to MHC class II-restricted T cells. Nature **357:** 702–704.
21. MUNZ, C. *et al.* 2000. Human CD4(+) T lymphocytes consistently respond to the latent Epstein-Barr virus nuclear antigen EBNA1. J. Exp. Med. **191:** 1649–1460.
22. REED, R.C. & C.V. NICCHITTA. 2000. Chaperone-mediated cross-priming: a hitchhiker's guide to vesicle transport. Int. J. Mol. Med. **6:** 259–264.
23. HEATH, W.R. & F.R. CARBONE. 2001. Cross-presentation in viral immunity and self-tolerance. Nature Rev. Immunol. **1:** 126–134.
24. ROCKEL, T. & A. VON MIKECZ. 2002. Proteasome-dependent processing of nuclear proteins is correlated with their subnuclear localization. J. Struct. Biol. **140:** 189–199.
25. CHEN, M. & A. VON MIKECZ. 2000. Specific inhibition of rRNA transcription and dynamic re-location of fibrillarin induced by mercury. Exp. Cell Res. **259:** 225–238.
26. CHEN, M. *et al.* 2002. Subcellular recruitment of fibrillarin to nucleoplasmic proteasomes: implications for processing of a nucleolar autoantigen. Mol. Biol. Cell **13:** 3576–3587.
27. DESAI, S.D., L.F. LIU, D. VAZQUEZ-ABAD & P. D'ARPA. 1997. Ubiquitin-dependent destruction of topoisomerase I is stimulated by the antitumor drug camptothecin. J. Biol. Chem. **272:** 24159–24164.
28. CHEN, M. *et al.* 2005. Recruitment of topoisomerase I (Scl-70) to nucleoplasmic proteasomes in response to xenobiotics suggests a role for altered antigen processing in scleroderma. Arthritis Rheum. **52:** 877–884.
29. CHEN, M., P. HEMMERICH & A. VON MIKECZ. 2002. Platinum-induced autoantibodies target nucleoplasmic antigens related to active transcription. Immunobiology **206:** 474–483.
30. LOMONTE, P., K.F. SULLIVAN & R.D. EVERETT. 2001. Degradation of nucleosome-associated centromeric histone H3-like protein CENP-A induced by herpes simplex virus type 1 protein ICP0. J. Biol. Chem. **276:** 5829–5835.
31. CHEN, M. & A. VON MIKECZ. 2005. Proteasomal processing of nuclear autoantigens in systemic autoimmunity. Autoimmun. Rev. **4:** 117–122.
32. VON MIKECZ, A. & P. HEMMERICH. 2004. Subnuclear pathology. *In* Visions of the Cell Nucleus. P. Hemmerich & S. Diekmann, Eds.: 184–203. American Scientific Publishers. Stevenson Ranch, CA.
33. VON MIKECZ, A. 2005. Xenobiotic-induced autoimmunity and protein aggregation diseases share a common subnuclear pathology. Autoimmun. Rev. **4:** 214–218.
34. CHEN, M. & A. VON MIKECZ. 2005. Formation of nucleoplasmic protein aggregates impairs nuclear function in response to SiO_2 nanoparticles. Exp. Cell Res. **305:** 51–62.

Humoral Antigenic Targets of the Ribosomal P0 Lupus Autoantigen Are Not Limited to the Carboxyl Region

BENJAMIN F. BRUNER,[a,b] DONNY M. WYNN,[a,b] MORRIS REICHLIN,[a] JOHN B. HARLEY,[a,b] AND JUDITH A. JAMES[a,b]

[a]*Arthritis and Immunology Program, Oklahoma Medical Research Foundation, Oklahoma City, Oklahoma 73104, USA*

[b]*Departments of Medicine and Pathology, University of Oklahoma Health Sciences Center, Oklahoma City, Oklahoma, USA*

ABSTRACT: Autoantibodies binding the ribosomal P phosphoproteins are highly specific for systemic lupus erythematosus (SLE) and can be found in precipitating levels in approximately 15% of these patients. Anti–ribosomal P antibodies are directed against three proteins, and the primary autoimmune target of this response has been described as a common 22–amino acid sequence. Sera from 31 anti–ribosomal P immunodiffusion–positive SLE patients were tested for C-terminal P-peptide reactivity by ELISA. Sera from three patients (9.7%) were negative for the peptide ELISA, despite having anti–ribosomal P by immunodiffusion and Western blot. In addition, inhibition experiments showed that the common P-peptide response accounts for a variable amount of anti–ribosomal P0 reactivity (52–89% of the response dependent upon the patient serum). Based upon these findings, fine-specificity sequential humoral epitope mapping of ribosomal P0 was performed. Several common sequential antigenic targets were defined dispersed throughout the molecule. The most commonly targeted epitopes included RDMLLANKVPAAARA (amino acids 99–113, 11 of 12 patients reactive) and QALGITTKISRGT (amino acids 139–151, 9 of 12 patients reactive). This study confirms that the P22 ribosomal peptide is commonly targeted in SLE and accounts for a variable percentage of the anti–ribosomal P response. Additional anti–ribosomal P humoral epitopes are described.

KEYWORDS: autoantibodies; lupus; anti–ribosomal P; ribosomal P0; epitope

INTRODUCTION

The autoimmune response observed in systemic lupus erythematosus (SLE) is characterized by the production of antibodies to self-proteins. Alongside this induction of autoantibodies, distinct clinical manifestations, such as inflammatory rashes

Address for correspondence: Judith A. James, M.D., Ph.D., Oklahoma Medical Research Foundation, 825 NE 13th Street, Oklahoma City, OK 73104. Voice: 405-271-4987; fax: 405-271-7063.
jamesj@omrf.ouhsc.edu

**Ann. N.Y. Acad. Sci. 1051: 390–403 (2005). © 2005 New York Academy of Sciences.
doi: 10.1196/annals.1361.081**

and arthritis, can be seen. The resulting autoimmunity can cause systemic organ damage with fatal consequences if untreated.

Autoantibodies are a nearly universal hallmark of SLE, with sera from more than 95% of untreated SLE patients having antinuclear antibodies (ANAs).[1] One interesting subset of SLE patients forms autoantibodies to the ribosomal P phosphoproteins. Approximately 15% of SLE patients have precipitating levels of anti–ribosomal P antibodies, although recent work shows that up to 30% of patients may have antibodies by ELISA and Western blot combined.[2] Prevalence rates have been reported to be much higher in pediatric lupus patients than in adult-onset SLE patients, with 42% of pediatric SLE patients having anti–ribosomal P antibodies by Western blot.[3] The specificities of these autoantibodies seem to be confined to three proteins of the 60S subunit of the ribosomal complex. Ribosomal P0, P1, and P2 (38 kDa, 19 kDa, 17 kDa, respectively) are associated together in a pentameric complex (one P0 bound to two P1s and two P2s). These three proteins share the same 22–amino acid carboxyl-terminal sequence. The elucidation of this region as the main antigenic target in anti–ribosomal P–positive patients has resulted in the clinically adapted diagnostic testing of ELISAs against the 22–amino acid C-terminal peptide for ribosomal P autoantibody detection.[4]

The presence of anti–ribosomal P–specific antibodies may predispose SLE patients toward specific clinical manifestations. Koscec *et al.* have studied the role of anti–ribosomal P in hepatitis and have observed an antigen-mediated internalization of anti–ribosomal P antibodies inside hepatocytes that suggests a possible role of the autoantibodies in the disruption of normal cellular function, which could lead to hepatitis.[5] Anti–ribosomal P antibodies have also been associated with lupus nephritis; anti–ribosomal P antibodies in this subset of patients are highly correlated with double-stranded (ds) DNA and increased disease activity.[2,6] Anti–ribosomal P antibodies have also been variably implicated in central nervous system involvement in a certain subset of SLE patients, although debate remains.[7–9] Anti–ribosomal P0 antibodies have also been shown to cross-react with other antigens on the surface of lymphocytes, possibly inducing SLE lymphopenia.[10] Interestingly, potential cross-reactivity of anti–ribosomal P autoantibodies with various common lupus autoantigens, such as SmD1, SmB′, and dsDNA, has also been shown.[6,11–13]

Primary work on the targets of anti-ribosomal antibodies was performed by Elkon *et al.* with the characterization of antibody specificity to three ribosomal proteins, P0, P1, and P2, from the more than 80 possible ribosomal proteins.[4] Proteolytic digestion epitope mapping narrowed the antibody reactivity to the carboxyl-terminal 22 amino acids, which are homologous in all three ribosomal proteins.[4] After an antigenic determinant was found on the ribosomal P proteins, it was verified in a cohort of 102 SLE patients that the 22–amino acid C-terminal peptide, constructed on a four-branch polylysine (multiple antigenic peptide (MAP)) backbone, could be used to detect anti–ribosomal P antibodies accurately (sensitivity 0.80, specificity 0.97).[14]

Present clinical testing relies on the assumption that all anti–ribosomal P–positive SLE patient sera bind the C22 peptide. However, evolving evidence suggests that the humoral immune response is more diverse than originally suspected.[15–17] Based upon the variable clinical associations of anti–ribosomal P autoantibodies within SLE, this study seeks specifically to map the sequential targets of anti–ribosomal P autoantibodies and to identify previously undescribed regions of antigenicity to provide new insight into the role of these antibodies in SLE. To achieve these goals, this study compares clinical testing methods for anti–ribosomal P reactivity, assesses the percentage of the anti–ribosomal P response against C22, and defines additional anti–ribosomal P–specific sequential epitopes.

MATERIALS AND METHODS

Selection of Patient Sera

Deidentified serum samples containing anti–ribosomal P precipitins were obtained from the Clinical Immunology Serum Repository at the Oklahoma Medical Research Foundation. Fourteen patients had two samples, one from the earliest date and one from the latest date showing ribosomal P antibodies (on average spanning 3.04 ± 3.41 years). Twenty frequency-matched controls (selected on the basis of age, ethnicity, and sex) were assayed in parallel. Sera were kept at –20°C for storage until testing.

Autoantibody Screening

Human sera were tested for ANAs against Hep-2 cells by a standard immunofluorescence test (INOVA, San Diego, CA, USA), and for antibodies to native dsDNA by an immunofluroescent *Crithidia lucillae* assay (Helix Diagnostics, West Sacramento, CA, USA) using the methods previously published.[18,19] Samples were also tested for precipitating levels of autoantibodies against such autoantigens as Ro, La, Sm, nRNP, and ribosomal P by immunodiffusion, as previously described.[3]

Western Blot Assay and Inhibition

Each serum sample was verified to contain anti–ribosomal P antibodies by Western blot analysis.[20] In brief, rabbit ribosomal extract was electrophoresed through a 12.5% polyacrylamide gel, transferred to nitrocellulose and probed for anti–ribosomal P antibodies at a dilution of 1:100, and then incubated with secondary anti–human IgG conjugated to alkaline phosphatase (Jackson Immunoresearch Laboratories, West Grove, PA). Finally, the nitrocellulose strips were exposed to an NBT/BCIP substrate to detect anti–ribosomal P antibodies. Sera from 6 of the 31 patients were selected for linear carboxyl-peptide inhibition to determine the percentage of the ribosomal P response directed against this common antigenic peptide. The samples were preincubated with 10 μg/mL of the peptide for 2 h at room temperature and then tested as previously described.[20] The Western blots were then analyzed using UVP Labworks version 4.0 to measure the intensities of the bands and to calculate inhibition levels.

Ribosomal P0 Carboxyl Peptide ELISA

The 22–amino acid carboxyl terminus of ribosomal P0 (R5HUP0) was constructed on a 4-mer branching polylysine backbone (MAP) and used as the coating antigen on a 96-well polystyrene ELISA plate with 1 μg of antigen per well. Assays were performed as previously described.[14,21] In brief, the polystyrene plates were first coated with the ribosomal P0 carboxyl-peptide–MAP antigen for 3 h, washed, and then blocked with 0.1% BSA solution for 1 h. Next, sera diluted 1:100 and 1:1000 in 0.1% bovine serum albumin–Tween solution were added to the wells and incubated for 3 h. Plates were washed and incubated with anti–human IgG whole-molecule secondary antibody conjugated to alkaline phosphatase (Jackson Immunoresearch Laboratories) for 3 h. P-nitrophenyl phosphate disodium solution was used as substrate, and the plates were read at 410 nm on a microELISA plate reader. All assays were standardized to a common positive standard.

Solid-Phase Peptide Synthesis and ELISA Assay

The 310 possible overlapping octapeptides of ribosomal P0 were constructed on solid-phase supports to be used for sequential epitope mapping.[22] The peptides were synthesized using Fmoc amino acid chemistry on the ends of radiation-derivatized polyethylene supports (Mimotopes Pty. Ltd., San Diego, CA) arranged in the format of 96-well microtiter plates.[20,23] Positive control peptides were synthesized on each plate using an octapeptide sequence with reactivity to a known positive control sample.

Humoral epitope mapping of 12 of the 31 anti–ribosomal P–positive SLE patients, based on serum availability, was conducted using the solid-phase peptide ELISA previously described in detail.[20,23] After blocking serum dilution of 1:100 was tested and detected by a 1:10,000 dilution of anti–human IgG conjugated to alkaline phosphatase (Jackson ImmunoResearch Laboratories). Results were normalized with the positive control having an OD of 1.0. Common epitopes were defined by mean patient binding >2 SD above the normal mean and with reactivity by more than one patient.

RESULTS

Demographics of the Anti–Ribosomal P–Positive SLE Patients

Serum samples from 31 SLE patients[24] were selected based upon precipitating levels of anti–ribosomal P autoantibodies. These patients varied in age, race, sex, and clinical manifestations. Interestingly, 29% of the patients were male, and the mean age at the time of the specimen was 39.8 ± 15.9 years (range 13–68). Patients were of a wide variety of ethnic origins, including African American (35%), European American (26%), American Indian (13%), Hispanic (10%), and Asian (6%). Two patients came from ethnically mixed origins, and the race of one patient was unknown.

Concomitant Autoantibody Specificities in Anti–Ribosomal P–Positive Patients

Other common lupus autoantibodies were also tested in these sera. To decrease the possibility of cross-reactivity from other specificities, patients with anti–ribosomal P but no other precipitating levels of common RNA-protein autoantibodies were selected for fine-specificity humoral epitope mapping. Surprisingly, serum from only one of these 12 patients had low-positive anti-dsDNA reactivity. Normal control sera tested showed no evidence of autoantibodies by these methods. Eleven of the 12 patients had positive ANAs with similar binding patterns.

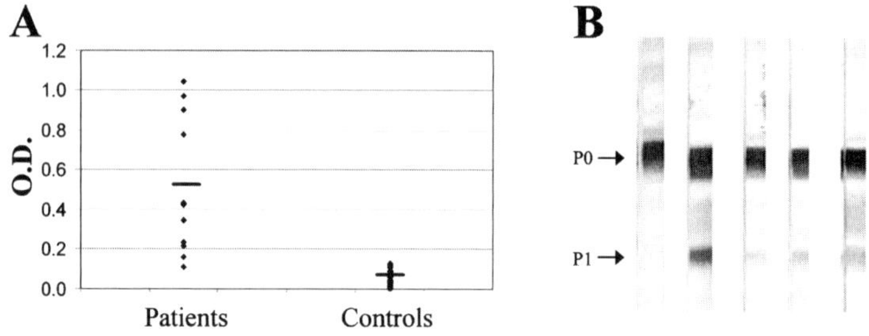

C

C-22 ELISA	anti-P ppt +	anti-P ppt -
+	29	0
-	2	20

p<0.0001

D

Western Blot	anti-P ppt +	anti-P ppt -
+	28	0
-	3	20

p<0.0001

FIGURE 1. Comparison of anti–ribosomal P reactivity by various assays. (**A**) C22 ELISA binding of patients (average 0.504 ± 0.331) and controls (average 0.053 ± 0.038) (Student's *t*-test, $P < 0.0001$). (**B**) Reactivity of five positive anti–ribosomal P patients detected by Western blot; *arrow* marks the band that represents the P0 protein. When C22 ELISA (**C**) and Western blot (**D**) results are compared with the immunodiffusion results to determine the reliability of each particular assay, both the Western blot (sensitivity 0.90, specificity 1.00) and the C22 ELISA (sensitivity 0.93, specificity 1.00) showed a small variation versus immunodiffusion.

Ribosomal P Carboxyl Terminus Peptide Reactivity

The 22–amino acid C-terminal peptide (4-mer MAP ELISA) reactivity (C22) was tested in the sera from the 31 identified patients. Sera from 29 of the 31 patients (93.5%) were positive (at least three standard deviations above the normal mean) for antibodies to the C22 MAP peptide as compared with the mean reactivity of sera from 20 normals tested with the same peptide ELISA. Comparison of patient serum responses to the C22 MAP peptide ELISA with control responses is shown in FIGURE 1A. The mean OD of patient samples was 0.504 (±0.331), whereas for controls the average OD was 0.053 (±0.038). Sera from the 31 patients were also tested for reactivity to two variants of this polypeptide. Sera from 25 of the 31 patients (80.6%) had reactivity to a linear 22-mer carboxyl-terminal peptide at least three standard deviations above the normal mean (sensitivity 0.806, specificity 1.00). In addition, the patient sera were tested for antibody binding to a core 11–amino acid sequence (SDEDMGFGLFD) constructed on a 4-mer MAP branching polylysine backbone. Sera from 29 of the 31 patients (93.5%) were positive for P antibodies with the assay using this 11–amino acid carboxyl-terminal sequence (sensitivity 0.935, specificity 1.00).

Sera from 11 scleroderma and 11 rheumatoid arthritis patients were tested as controls using the C11 MAP and the C22 MAP ELISAs to determine the ability of these assays to distinguish between patients with and without anti–ribosomal P antibodies. Sera from 2 of 11 scleroderma patients (18.2%) and 1 of 11 rheumatoid arthritis (RA) patients (9.1%) were positive when tested on the 22–amino acid carboxyl-terminal sequence. However, sera from 7 of the 11 scleroderma (63.6%) and 5 of the 11 RA patients (45.5%) had reactivity to the 11–amino acid carboxyl-terminal sequence peptide ELISA, decreasing the usefulness of this truncated peptide.

Prevalence of Anti–Ribosomal P Reactivity by Western Blot Analysis

Sera from the 31 immunodiffusion anti–ribosomal P–positive patients were confirmed for anti–ribosomal P specificity by Western blot analysis using rabbit ribosomal extract. Twenty-eight of the 31 patients (90%) were positive for any anti–ribosomal P antibodies as shown by serum binding to the 38, 19, and/or 17 kDa bands (ribosomal P0, P1, P2, respectively). The serum reactivity of five of these patients to the 38 kDa ribosomal P0 band is shown in FIGURE 1B. All 20 normal controls tested negative for anti–ribosomal P antibodies by Western blot.

C-Terminal Peptide Inhibition of Anti–Ribosomal P Antibodies

Based upon reactivity by Western blot and peptide ELISA, sera from six patients were selected for carboxyl–terminal peptide inhibition with the carboxyl 22–amino

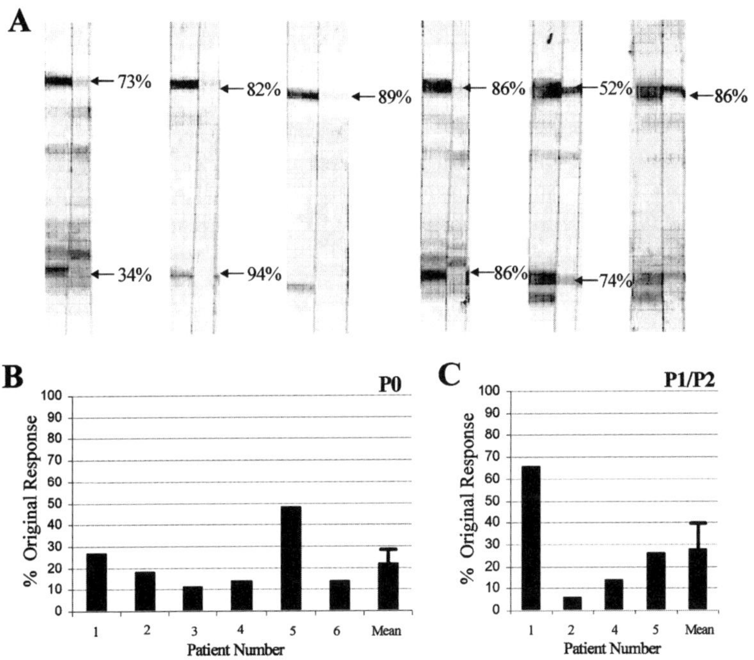

FIGURE 2. Percentage of anti–ribosomal P reactivity directed against the C-terminal common antigenic peptide. (**A**) Serum inhibition Western blot results for six patients with their paired native sera and peptide-inhibited responses to the ribosomal P proteins. (**B**) Inhibition of the anti–ribosomal P0 response. (**C**) Inhibition of the anti–ribosomal P1/P2 responses.

TABLE 1. Autoantibody information for the 12 anti–ribosomal P–positive patients used for humoral epitope mapping

Patients	Ribo P Ppt	Ribo P WB	Ribo P0 C-22 Pep	Ribo P0 Octapeptide ELISA	dsDNA	ANA
1	+	+	–	+	–	1080
2	+	+	+	+	–	3240
3	+	+	+	+	–	–
4	+	+	–	+	30	1080
5	+	+	–	+	–	80
6	+	+	+	+	–	1080
7	+	+	–	+	–	360
8	+	+	+	+	–	360
9	+	+	–	+	–	1080
10	+	+	+	+	–	80
11	+	+	–	–	–	1080
12	+	+	+	+	–	80

NOTE: The first four experimental columns show presence of anti–ribosomal P0 antibody as determined by four different assays (Ppt = immunodiffusion, WB = Western blot against rabbit ribosomal P extract, C22 Pep = carboxyl 22–amino acid peptide on 4-mer MAP backbone). The last two columns show other SLE-specific antibody data tested by immunofluorescence. Other precipitins tested include Ro, La, Sm, nRNP, Jo-1, and PM-Scl. Patients without other precipitins were selected for this study.

acid linear peptide (FIG. 2A). Inhibition of the anti–ribosomal P0 response ranged from 52% to 89%, with mean inhibition of 77 ± 13.4% (FIG. 2B). Inhibition of the anti–ribosomal P1/P2 response was measurable in only four of the patient sera tested. Inhibition of the P1/P2 response ranged from 34% to 94%, with mean inhibition of 72 ± 26.6% (FIG. 2C). Interestingly, within the same patient sample, inhibition of the P0, P1, and P2 responses did not occur in parallel, as might have been expected.

Sequential Ribosomal P0 Epitope Mapping

Of the 31 SLE patients found to be positive for anti–ribosomal P antibodies by immunodiffusion, 12 patients were selected for epitope mapping based on anti–ribosomal P titer, absence of other autoantibodies, and serum availability. Each of the 12 patients selected had similar autoantibody profiles (TABLE 1). Overlapping octapeptides spanning the ribosomal P0 protein were tested with samples from the 12 patients, as well as with control samples. The octapeptide binding of the anti–ribosomal P patient sample with the lowest level of anti–ribosomal P reactivity by peptide ELISA (FIG. 3B) showed a diversified response exclusive of the C terminus. On the other hand, FIGURE 3A shows the octapeptide data of the patient sample that had the highest reactivity against the C-terminal peptide by ELISA (five standard deviations above the mean). Representative normal overlapping octapeptide control binding is also shown (FIG. 3C).

Average antibody reactivity for samples from all 12 patients demonstrated common antibody binding to seven separate regions throughout the protein, not solely

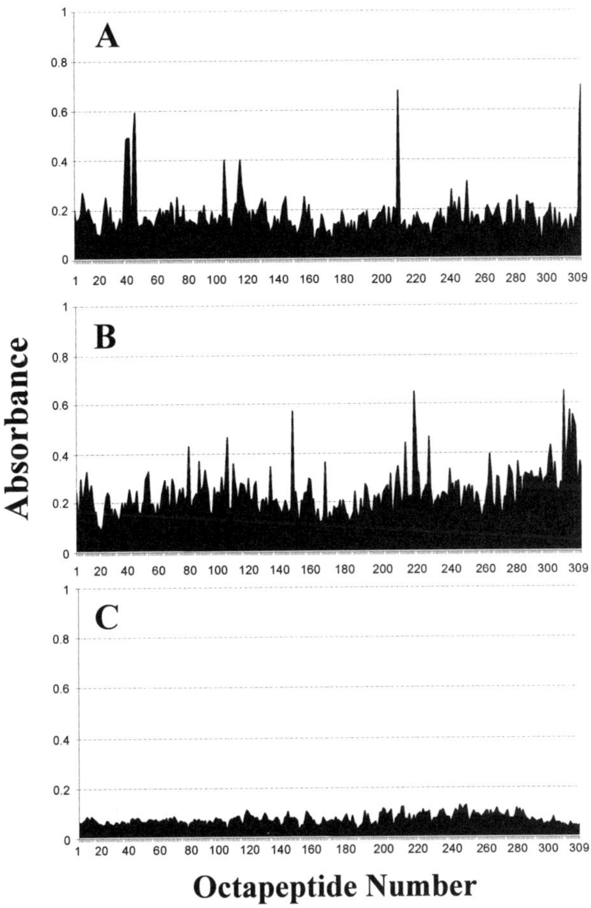

FIGURE 3. Ribosomal P0 octapeptide binding by anti–ribosomal P–positive SLE patient sera and by control sera. Patient responses that exhibit a reactivity (**A**) including and (**B**) excluding the C-terminal peptide. (**C**) Normal human negative control binding.

localized to the C terminus (FIG. 4). Most notably, these data showed an average binding to the C terminus only two standard deviations above the normal mean, whereas binding to the epitope at amino acids 99–113 was four standard deviations above the normal mean. In fact, more patient samples were determined to have statistically relevant binding to sequences found in the beginning and middle portions of the protein than to the C-terminal region. For example, samples from 11 of the 12 patients had statistically relevant antibody binding to the span of amino acids from 99 to 113, yet only 5 of the 12 patient samples had autoantibody binding two standard deviations above the mean to the C terminus of the protein. Note that all five patient samples with binding to the C terminus also bound the internal epitope at amino acids 99–113. Two other sequences (amino acids 6–13 and 139–151) were

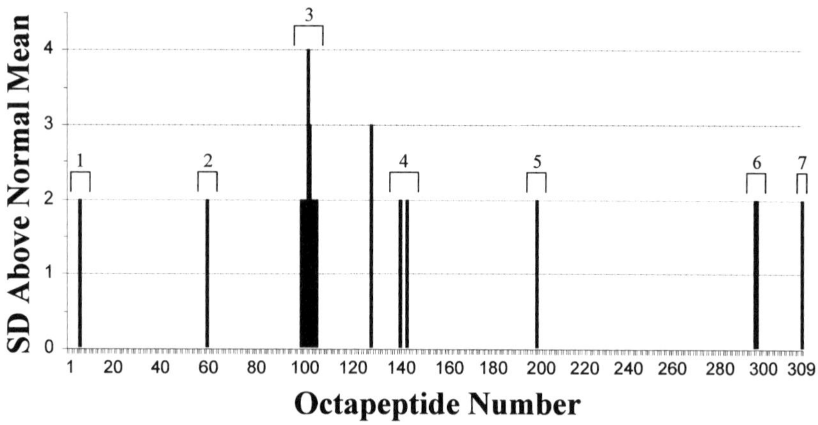

FIGURE 4. Average patient binding in standard deviations (SDs) above the normal average for each individual octapeptide of the ribosomal P0 protein. The seven major antigenic regions are bracketed.

also bound by a greater number of patient samples than was the C-terminal portion of the peptide. Only one patient sample was negative on the C-terminal peptide ELISA but had binding at the C terminus via the solid-phase peptide assay two standard deviations above the mean. Serum from one patient was noted to have binding to ribosomal P0 by Western blot but had no antibodies specific to the 99–113 epitope or to the C-terminal epitope by peptide ELISA, suggesting that binding two other sequential epitopes was sufficient to provide a positive response by Western blot.

The variable reactivity identified when comparing results from the solid-phase peptide ELISA and the C-terminal MAP ELISA is likely the product of distinct differences in peptide presentation and experimental preparation. The length and presentation of peptides by the MAP backbone seems to promote the higher sensitivity seen within the C-terminal ELISA. Other factors include differences in experimental procedures and reagents used during the solid-phase peptide assay when compared with the standard peptide ELISA.

Characteristics of the Epitopes

The characteristics of the individual epitopes revealed in this study are summarized in TABLE 2. One noticeable trend is that the average isoelectric point (pI) of 8.25 for dominant epitopes is substantially higher than the average pI of 6.39 of nonantigenic regions ($t = -3.09$, $P = 0.001$). Subsequent analysis of the Parker antigenicity index also showed nonsignificant minimal increase in antigenicity of dominant epitopes versus that of the remaining protein, 1.405 and 1.151, respectively ($t = -1.0549$, $P = 0.146$). Therefore, this antigenicity index is not as strong a determinant for the identification of these particular epitopes as is the isoelectric point alone.[25] An amino acid analysis comparing amino acid usage differences between epitopes and the remaining sequence showed little change except for a 10.3% increase in the occurrence of alanine residues ($P = 0.002$) within antigenic sequences.

TABLE 2. Sequences of the seven common antigenic regions of ribosomal P0.

Epitope	a.a Sequence	a.a #	pI
1	RATWKSNY	6–13	10.0
2	MMRKAIRG	60–67	12.0
3	RDMLLANKVPAAARA	99–113	10.8
4	QALGITTKISRGT	139–151	11.0
5	GSIYNPEVILD	196–205	4.0
6	AAAAAPAK	290–297	8.8
7	DMGFGLFD	310–317	3.9

DISCUSSION

Based upon the specificity of anti–ribosomal P0 antibodies for SLE and their association with specific subpopulations (pediatric) and disease manifestations such as hepatic and renal involvement, significant work has been devoted to understanding the role of this autoantibody in disease pathogenesis. Previous work to establish the specificity of anti-ribosomal antibodies narrowed the reactivity to the homologous 22–amino acid C-terminal of the three ribosomal P proteins, P0, P1, and P2.[4,14] Our tasks in this study were to determine the percentage of the anti–ribosomal P response directed against the common carboxyl epitope and to accurately identify additional common antigenic targets of these proteins.

Currently, most researchers agree that antibody binding occurs most frequently at the C terminus. Therefore, the 22–amino acid peptide–MAP ELISA protocol is the most common clinical technique used to identify anti–ribosomal P autoantibodies in SLE patients. Although the sensitivity of this technique has proved to be quite good, some discrepancies have arisen, suggesting that the C-terminal sequence may not be the only epitope targeted by anti–ribosomal P sera. One study showed that not all anti–ribosomal P patient sera bound all three P proteins, suggesting that anti–ribosomal P autoantibodies do not necessarily bind the common C-terminal sequence.[15] This same study also observed that binding by monoclonal antibodies isolated from mice immunized with the P1 ribosomal protein is not limited to the C terminus of the three ribosomal P proteins.[15] Other experiments have shown that sera from P peptide–immunized rabbits, as well as human anti–ribosomal P–positive SLE sera, were not completely inhibited by binding against whole ribosomes after incubation with the C-terminal peptide.[16] In addition, Mahler *et al.*, using peptide array, reported ribosomal P epitopes other than the C terminus that bound ribosomal P autoantibodies.[17] All of these observations suggest that ribosomal P antibody specificity may extend beyond the C terminus.

Our data have confirmed that other humoral epitopes exist within the ribosomal P0 protein. In fact, seven epitopes on ribosomal P0 are targeted by anti–ribosomal P antibodies in SLE sera, one of which is the C terminus of the protein at amino acids 310–317 (epitope 7: DMGFGLFD). Eleven of the 12 patient sera tested for sequential peptide binding had antibodies that strongly bound the ribosomal P0 protein at amino acids 99–113 (epitope 3: RDMLLANKVPAAARA). Other significant common epitopes were defined at various locations throughout the protein (TABLE 2). In

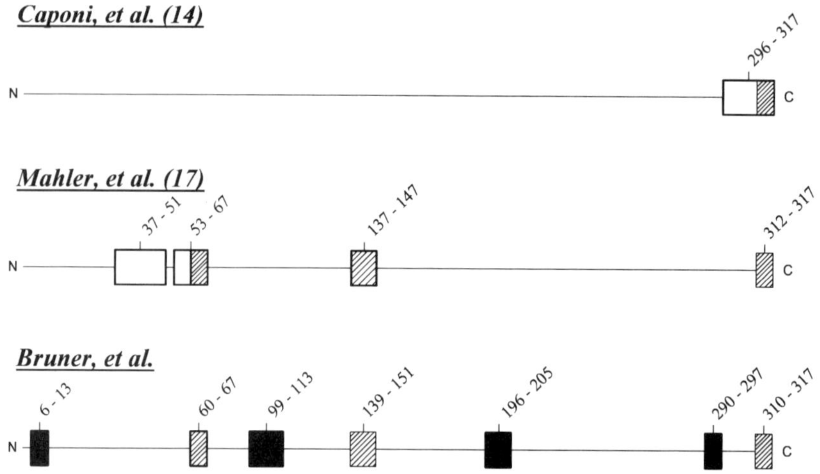

FIGURE 5. Correlation of epitopes between this and previous studies, showing a variety of responses toward the ribosomal P0 protein. *Solid boxes* represent newly described epitopes, *clear boxes* represent previously described epitopes that are not common within subsequent studies, and *hatched boxes* represent epitopes common to two or more studies.[14,17]

the solid-phase epitope mapping, only 5 of the 12 patients had antibodies reactive to the octapeptides representing the carboxyl terminus, whereas on the peptide ELISA with the full 22–amino acid peptide, 11 patients were positive.

Using the SPOT method of epitope mapping, Mahler *et al.* showed that anti–ribosomal P antibodies in SLE patients can bind other epitopes beyond the C terminus.[17] This group showed that sera from 20 patients also bound epitopes on the ribosomal P0 protein other than the 22–amino acid carboxyl terminus, including the regions 37–51, 53–67, and 137–147 (FIG. 5). Despite the additional binding to other epitopes, this group maintains that most anti–ribosomal P binding, as shown by the SPOT method, is to the C terminus.

When comparing our study and the work of Mahler *et al.*[17] and Caponi *et al.*,[14] all three studies distinguish the significance of the reactivity in the C-terminal sequence of the P0 protein. In our study, as well as in the work of Mahler *et al.*,[17] two additional antigenic regions were found in the beginning (amino acids 53–67) and middle (amino acids 137–147) portions of the P0 protein that display high reactivity to anti–ribosomal P antibodies. A comparison of the ribosomal P0 epitopes identified in our study and the epitopes that previously have been described is shown in FIGURE 5.

With sera from 93.5% of patients testing positive on the 22-mer and 11-mer MAP ELISA, the ELISA appears to be a screening method essentially comparable to, but technically easier than, the Western blot, which resulted in a 90% positivity rate ($n = 31$; FIG. 1C, D). Although these results might suggest that either the 22-mer or 11-mer MAP ELISA method could be an equally effective screening method, the binding of these sequences by sera from scleroderma and rheumatoid arthritis patients presents issues of patient specificity. The number of positive other-disease patients increased to 46% in scleroderma and 36% in RA patients with the 11-mer MAP ELISA when compared with the 22-mer MAP ELISA. This shows a possible correlation between the specificity of patient binding and the length of the tested peptide.

The diversity of response shown within the 12 patients analyzed by the solid-phase peptide assay lends strong support to the idea that antibody response to the ribosomal P0 protein is much more diverse than simple binding to the C terminus. Unlike previous work, our study includes patient sera that did not bind to the C-terminal sequence but showed significant binding elsewhere on the protein. One potential problem caused by this lack of binding to the C-terminal sequence is the strong possibility that these patients could be missed on screening with a C22 or C11 MAP ELISA. The difference in diversity between our patients and previous studies is likely in part the result of different patient screening and selection processes, as well as different experimental approaches.

Although the exact role that ribosomal P0 plays in the onset and progression of SLE is yet undetermined, the common specific occurrence of anti–ribosomal P antibodies in SLE warrants further investigation. These experiments have identified seven major antigenic targets of the ribosomal P0 protein that have high affinity to anti–ribosomal P antibodies, as well as increased surface probability and pI, which are indicative of epitopes in other common lupus autoantigens. The C-terminal epitope is currently the only one of these epitopes that is being used as a clinical indicator for patients with anti–ribosomal P antibodies. If screening methods that currently fail to allow for the diversity of response toward the ribosomal P proteins were to be modified to account for such diversity, more sensitive assays could be introduced to ensure antibody detection. These results extend our current knowledge of the specificity with which ribosomal P0 contributes to SLE and will advance future research to determine the pathogenic mechanisms in this disease.

ACKNOWLEDGMENTS

We thank Haraldine Stafford, Ph.D., M.D., Kenneth Kaufman, Ph.D., and Micah McClain, M.D., Ph.D., for scientific assistance; and Camille Andersen, Bryan Young, Derek Handke, and Amie Spears for technical assistance. We also thank the Clinical Immunology Serum Repository at the Oklahoma Medical Research Foundation and the Oklahoma Molecular Biology Core Facility for providing essential resources necessary for the completion of this work. This work was supported in part by the following grants: AR45451, AR45231, AR47575, AR48940, RR15577, and AR48045.

REFERENCES

1. KLIPPEL, J.H. 1997. Primer on the rheumatic diseases. Arthritis Foundation. Atlanta, GA.
2. CHINDALORE, V., B. NEAS & M. REICHLIN. 1998. The association between anti-ribosomal P antibodies and active nephritis in systemic lupus erythematosus. Clin. Immunol. Immunopathol. **87:** 292–296.

3. REICHLIN, M., T.F. BROYLES, O. HUBSCHER, *et al.* 1999. Prevalence of autoantibodies to ribosomal P proteins in juvenile-onset systemic lupus erythematosus compared with the adult disease. Arthritis Rheum. **42:** 69–75.
4. ELKON, K., S. SKELLY, A. PARNASSA, *et al.* 1986. Identification and chemical synthesis of a ribosomal protein antigenic determinant in systemic lupus erythematosus. Proc. Natl. Acad. Sci. USA **83:** 7419–7423.
5. KOSCEC, M., E. KOREN, M. WOLFSON-REICHLIN, *et al.* 1997. Autoantibodies to ribosomal P proteins penetrate into live hepatocytes and cause cellular dysfunction in culture. J. Immunol. **159:** 2033–2041.
6. TAKEDA, I., K. RAYNO, M. WOLFSON-REICHLIN & M. REICHLIN. 1999. Heterogeneity of anti-dsDNA antibodies in their cross-reaction with ribosomal P protein. J. Autoimmun. **13:** 423–428.
7. TZIOUFAS, A.G., N.G. TZORTZAKIS, E. PANOU-POMONIS, *et al.* 2000. The clinical relevance of antibodies to ribosomal-P common epitope in two targeted systemic lupus erythematosus populations: a large cohort of consecutive patients and patients with active central nervous system disease. Ann. Rheum. Dis. **59:** 99–104.
8. ISSHI, K. & S. HIROHATA. 1996. Association of anti-ribosomal P protein antibodies with neuropsychiatric systemic lupus erythematosus. Arthritis Rheum. **39:** 1483–1490.
9. BONFA, E., S.J. GOLOMBEK, L.D. KAUFMAN, *et al.* 1987. Association between lupus psychosis and anti-ribosomal P protein antibodies. N. Engl. J. Med. **317:** 265–271.
10. STAFFORD, H.A., A.E. CHEN, C.J. ANDERSON, *et al.* 1997. Anti-ribosomal and "P-peptide"-specific autoantibodies bind to T lymphocytes. Clin. Exp. Immunol. **109:** 12–19.
11. ELKON, K.B., E. BONFA, R. LLOVET & R.A. EISENBERG. 1989. Association between anti-Sm and anti-ribosomal P protein autoantibodies in human systemic lupus erythematosus and MRL/lpr mice. J. Immunol. **143:** 1549–1554.
12. CAPONI, L., S. BOMBARDIERI & P. MIGLIORINI. 1998. Anti-ribosomal antibodies bind the Sm proteins D and B/B′. Clin. Exp. Immunol. **112:** 139–143.
13. SUN, K.H., W.T. LIU, C.Y. TSAI, *et al.* 1995. Anti-dsDNA antibodies cross-react with ribosomal P proteins expressed on the surface of glomerular mesangial cells to exert a cytostatic effect. Immunology **85:** 262–269.
14. CAPONI, L., S. PEGORARO, V. DI BARTOLO, *et al.* 1995. Autoantibodies directed against ribosomal P proteins: use of a multiple antigen peptide as the coating agent in ELISA. J. Immunol. Methods **179:** 193–202.
15. FABIEN, N., A. MOREIRA, J.P. LAVERGNE, *et al.* 1999. Autoantibodies directed against the ribosomal P proteins are not only directed against a common epitope of the P0, P1 and P2 proteins. J. Autoimmun. **13:** 103–110.
16. GORDON, T.P., M. WOLFSON-REICHLIN, D. BLALOCK, *et al.* 1996. Humoral response in spontaneous and experimental autoimmunity to the ribosomal P proteins. Lupus **5:** 340–341.
17. MAHLER, M., K. KESSENBROCK, J. RAATS, *et al.* 2003. Characterization of the human autoimmune response to the major C-terminal epitope of the ribosomal P proteins. J. Mol. Med. **81:** 194–204.
18. GONZALEZ, E.N. & N.F. ROTHFIELD. 1966. Immunoglobulin class and pattern of nuclear fluorescence in systemic lupus erythematosus. N. Engl. J. Med. **274:** 1333–1338.
19. AARDEN, A., E.R. DE GROOT & T.E. FELTKAMP. 1975. Immunology of DNA. III. *Crithidia lucilia*, a simple substrate for the determination of anti-dsDNA with the immunofluorescence technique. Ann. N.Y. Acad. Sci. **254:** 505–515.
20. MCCLAIN, M.T., P.A. RAMSLAND, K.M. KAUFMAN & J.A. JAMES. 2002. Anti-Sm autoantibodies in systemic lupus target highly basic surface structures of complexed spliceosomal autoantigens. J. Immunol. **168:** 2054–2062.
21. JAMES, J.A., T. GROSS, R.H. SCOFIELD & J.B. HARLEY. 1995. Immunoglobulin epitope spreading and autoimmune disease after peptide immunization: Sm B/B′-derived PPPGMRPP and PPPGIRGP induce spliceosomal autoimmunity. J. Exp. Med. **181:** 453–461.
22. RICH, B.E. & J.A. STEITZ. 1987. Human acidic ribosomal phosphoproteins P0, P1, and P2: analysis of cDNA clones, in vitro synthesis, and assembly. Mol. Cell. Biol. **7:** 4065–4074.

23. James, J.A. & J.B. Harley. 1996. Human lupus anti-spliceosome A protein autoantibodies bind contiguous surface structures and segregate into two sequential epitope binding patterns. J. Immunol. **156:** 4018–4026.
24. Hochberg, M.C. 1997. Updating the American College of Rheumatology revised criteria for the classification of systemic lupus erythematosus. Arthritis Rheum. **40:** 1725.
25. Parker, J.M., D. Guo & R.S. Hodges. 1986. New hydrophilicity scale derived from high-performance liquid chromatography peptide retention data: correlation of predicted surface residues with antigenicity and X-ray-derived accessible sites. Biochemistry **25:** 5425–5432.

Clinical Correlations of Potential Activity Markers in Systemic Sclerosis

R. BEČVÁŘ,[a] J. ŠTORK,[b] V. PEŠÁKOVÁ,[a] A. STÁŇOVÁ,[a] H. HULEJOVÁ,[a] L. RYSOVÁ,[a] A. ZATLOUKALOVÁ,[c] P. ZATLOUKAL,[d] M. JÁCHYMOVÁ,[e] AND L. POUROVÁ[e]

[a]*Institute of Rheumatology, Prague, Czech Republic*

[b]*Clinic of Dermatovenerology,* [e]*Clinic of Medicine 2, General Teaching Hospital, Prague, Czech Republic*

[c]*Private Pneumological Practice, Prague, Czech Republic*

[d]*Clinic of Pneumology and Thoracic Surgery, Teaching Hospital Bulovka, Prague Czech Republic*

ABSTRACT: The objectives of the project were the following: (1) to establish a group of patients with a confirmed diagnosis of systemic sclerosis (Ssc), (2) to perform a detailed entrance examination of each patient, (3) to determine concentrations of potential activity markers, and (4) to make a comprehensive examination of each patient 1 year after inclusion into the study. A total of 49 patients were examined, 36 with a limited form of SSc, 9 with diffuse SSc, and 4 with other forms of SSc. We determined plasma or serum levels of the N-terminal propeptide of procollagen type III (NPIIIP), interleukin-6 (IL-6), soluble receptor for interleukin-2 (sIL-2r), soluble intercellular adhesion molecule-1 (sICAM-1), soluble vascular adhesion molecule–1 (sVCAM-1), von Willebrand factor antigen (vWFAg), and big endothelin-1 (BET-1) using commercial kits, and urinary excretion of pyridinoline (PYR) and deoxypyridinoline (D-PYR) using high-performance liquid chromatography. Correlations of these markers with selected clinical data were calculated. The mean levels of all potential activity markers were increased compared with normal values, but differences were not significant. The levels of NPIIIP, D-PYR, and IL-6 were normal. The measured values after 1 year did not differ from the entry values. At entry, NPIIIP concentrations correlated with the finger-to-palm distance, and D-PYR corresponded with findings on a simplified health assessment questionnaire (FQ). IL-6 levels correlated with the leukocyte count, sIL-2r with the FQ, and ET-1 with the diffuse lung capacity for carbon monoxide. In general, we found only a few clinical correlates of potential activity markers. Our data confirmed the correlations of collagen metabolism markers with skin involvement and FQ, as was reported previously. Larger studies in this field are needed.

KEYWORDS: systemic sclerosis; activity; collagen metabolism; adhesion molecules; interleukins

Address for correspondence: Radim Bečvář, M.D., Na slupi 4, 128 50 Praha 2, Czech Republic. Voice: +420-234-075-101.
becv@revma.cz

Ann. N.Y. Acad. Sci. 1051: 404–412 (2005). © 2005 New York Academy of Sciences.
doi: 10.1196/annals.1361.082

INTRODUCTION

Systemic sclerosis (SSc) is a generalized connective tissue disease that presents as thickening and fibrosis of the skin with typical involvement of internal organs, gastrointestinal (GI) tract, lungs, heart, and kidneys. The etiology and pathogenesis of SSc are so far unknown. The causes of variability in the extent and progression of the disease, the rapid accumulation of extracellular matrix components in different organs, the irregular alternation of acute and chronic inflammatory stages, and the characteristic changes in the vessel wall and function remain unexplained.[1]

Among the cytokines, fibronectin[2] plays an important role in pathogenesis of SSc. Fibronectin is produced by fibroblasts, endothelial cells, and other cells, and binds to extracellular matrix components. In SSc, fibroblasts synthesize more fibronectin when stimulated by transforming growth factor–beta (TGF-β),[3] and similar activity is observed in lung macrophages. Interleukin-1 (IL-1), which is produced by macrophages, also stimulates proliferation of fibroblasts and, thus, synthesis of collagen types I and III. Another proinflammatory cytokine, IL-2, is produced by T lymphocytes and acts simultaneously as their growth factor. Increased serum IL-2 and soluble IL-2 receptors have been found in patients with SSc, and they correlate with disease progression.[4]

In general, the N-terminal propeptide of procollagen type III (NPIIIP)[5] is considered to be a useful marker of collagen synthesis, and pyridinoline (PYR) and deoxypyridinoline (D-PYR)[6] are markers of collagen degradation. PYR and D-PYR are cross-links that are excreted by the kidneys into urine in the form of cyclic compounds with typical fluorescence.

The aims of this study were to establish a group of patients with a definite diagnosis of SSc; to perform a detailed entrance examination on each patient; to determine concentrations of selected potential activity markers (TABLE 1), soluble intercellular adhesion molecule–1 (sICAM-1), soluble vascular adhesion molecule-1 (sVCAM-1), von Willebrand factor antigen (vWFAg), interleukin-6 (IL-6), soluble receptor for interleukin-2 (sIL-2r), precursor of endothelin-1 (big endothelin-1, BET-1), NPIIIP, PYR, and D-PYR; and to perform a comprehensive examination of each patient 1 year after inclusion into the study. Further, we correlated the obtained data with the results of routine clinical tests and examinations.

TABLE 1. Potential activity markers examined

Immunological markers	Endothelial activation markers	Collagen metabolism markers
IL-6	sICAM-1	NPIIIP
sIL2r	SVCAM-1	PYR
	BET-1	D-PYR
	VWFAg	

ABBREVIATIONS: BET-1, big endothelin-1; D-PYR, deoxypyridinoline; IL-6, interleukin-6; NPIIIP, N-terminal propeptide of procollagen type III; PYR, pyridinoline; sICAM-1, soluble intercellular adhesion molecule–1; sIL-2r, soluble interleukin-2 receptor; sVCAM-1, soluble vascular adhesion molecule–1; vWFAg; von Willebrand factor antigen.

TABLE 2. Basic demographic characteristics of systemic scleroderma patients in the study

Total	49
M/F	3/46
Age, years (SD)	51.61 (12.86)
Height, cm (SD)	165.82 (5.39)
Weight, kg (SD)	67.18 (11.87)

ABBREVIATIONS: BET-1, big endothelin-1; D-PYR, deoxypyridinoline; IL-6, interleukin-6; NPIIIP, N-terminal propeptide of procollagen type III; PYR, pyridinoline; sICAM-1, soluble intercellular adhesion molecule–1; sIL-2r, soluble interleukin-2 receptor; sVCAM-1, soluble vascular adhesion molecule–1; vWFAg, von Willebrand factor antigen.

PATIENTS AND METHODS

Patients

A total of 49 patients with SSc within different subsets of the disease were enrolled in this study, 36 with limited disease, 9 with diffuse disease, 3 with scleroderma *sine* scleroderma, 1 with overlap syndrome, and 1 with undifferentiated connective tissue disease. The diagnosis of scleroderma was made according to skin changes and, in the unclear cases, based on histological findings from skin biopsy. The patients were further characterized according to accepted classification criteria.[7] The basic demographic characteristics of our cohort are given in TABLE 2. Individuals with systemic or pulmonary hypertension or with overt signs of atherosclerosis were excluded.

In all patients, Raynaud's phenomenon was the starting symptom. According to the protocol used, selected symptoms and signs important in the diagnosis of SSc were followed, and differences 1 year after study entry were recorded. On average, dyspnea on exertion and synovitis worsened, whereas other symptoms and signs remained unchanged (lung rales) and even improved.

METHODS

Routine hematological and biochemical tests were performed. Complete blood counts were obtained on an automatic analyzer, erythrocyte sedimentation rate (ESR) was measured according Fahraeus and Westergren, and C-reactive protein (CRP) concentration was assessed using turbidimetry. Clinical chemistry was measured on an automatic analyzer.

Among immunological tests, antinuclear antibodies (ANAs) were detected using indirect immunofluorescence on HEP2 cells. Further, the antibodies of the ENA complex (anti-U1RNP, anti-NRNP, anti-Ro, anti-La, anti–topoisomerase I, anti–Jo-1, anti–P protein, anti-Sm, ACA) were assayed by immunoblot. IgG and IgM anticardiolipin antibodies were measured using ELISA.

Assays for Potential Activity Markers

Plasma IL-6 and IL-2r were estimated by ELISA using commercial kits (Novitec, Austria). Assay sensitivities were 1.4 pg/mL for IL-6 and 36 pg/mL for IL-2r. Quantitative measurements of adhesion molecules plasma levels were performed by "sandwich" enzyme-immunosorbent analysis using commercial kits (Bender MedSystems, Austria).

For sICAM-1, the cutoff value was 3.3 ng/mL and the interassay coefficient was 7.7%; for sVCAM-1 these values were 0.9 ng/mL and 5.2%, respectively. BET-1 concentrations were measured using a commercial competitive ELISA kit (Big Endothelin-1 kit; Peninsula Laboratories, Inc., San Carlos, CA, USA); the assay cutoff value was 0.06 ng/mL and interassay coefficient 14%. Plasma VWFAg was measured using an ELISA commercial kit (Immundiagnostika, Berlin, Germany).

Serum NPIIIP was measured by radioimmunoassay using a commercial procollagen III kit (Orion Diagnostica, Espoo, Finland). PYR and D-PYR were estimated using high-performance liquid chromatography (HPLC) as described previously.[8]

Examination of Individual Organ Systems

Severity of skin involvement was assessed by a modified skin-scoring method according to Rodnan,[9] finger-to-palm distance in full flexion and extension (FTP), and measurement of mouth aperture. Furthermore, ulcerations on fingertips were recorded.

The cardiovascular evaluation included nail fold capillaroscopy of the second to the fifth finger on the nondominant hand, performed according to Maricq *et al.*[10] using a stereomicroscope (Leitz, Austria). The findings were evaluated as follows: normal, slight abnormalities, nonspecific pathological changes, and pathological changes specific for SSc. In all patients, standard ECG and echocardiography were performed; in those with a high frequency of extrasystoles, Holter monitoring was performed.

For respiratory system evaluation, all patients underwent physical examination, lung function tests, and diffuse lung capacity for carbon monoxide (DLCO). Later, chest x-ray and high-resolution chest tomography (HRCT) were performed. The degree of alveolitis and interstitial fibrosis were scored as follows: 0, no changes; 1, mild changes; 2, moderate changes; and 3, severe changes.

For the examination of esophagus, scintigraphy with technetium radionuclide was performed. The observed changes were scored as follows: 0, normal finding; 1, slightly slowed peristalsis; 2, moderately slowed peristalsis; 3, severely slowed peristalsis.

To measure overall quality of life and functional abilities, we used a special questionnaire (FQ), a simplified health assessment questionnaire[11] of 11 questions.

For statistical evaluation, Student's t-test and Pearson's correlation coefficient were applied.

RESULTS

Routine Laboratory Tests

All patients had normal complete blood counts, as well as ESR, at entry and after 1 year. Similarly, the values of selected biochemical tests were within the normal range, and any differences were insignificant.

TABLE 3. Concentrations of potential activity markers

Marker	Normal values	At study entry		At 1 year		Difference
		Mean	SD	Mean	SD	
sIL-2r (ng/mL)	1–4.2	5.39	2.26	5.40	3.03	0
IL-6 (pg/mL)	1.4–14.1	8.25	8.45	10.03	11.75	1.78
sICAM-1 (ng/mL)	675	953.71	381.84	920.93	293.55	–32.79
sVCAM-1 (ng/mL)	1602	1999.27	648.83	2203.98	874.89	204.71
BET-1 (pg/mL)	12.76	114.66	154.68	93.28	102.69	–21.38
vWFAg (U/mL)	0.7–1.5	10.11	8.52	13.84	9.68	3.73
NPIIIP (μg/L)	1.5–4.0	2.69	1.18	2.87	1.27	0.18
PYR (nmol/mmol)	50	63.18	43.92	39.97	20.97	–23.21
D-PYR (nmol/mmol)	13	12.06	10.36	5.98	2.82	–6.08

ANAs were detected in 93.78% patients, mostly with a speckled immunofluorescence pattern (46.94%). ACAs were found in 6 individuals (12.24%), and anti-Scl70 was positive in 21 (42.86%). In 11 patients (22.45%), antibodies to ENA were found, and in 8 (16.33%) immunoblotting showed an unknown antibody.

Clinical Examinations

The mean skin scores were relatively low (6.69) and did not change substantially after one year. FTP in both hands increased insignificantly (difference +1.23) after 1 year.

The finger ulceration ratio showed a certain tendency to decrease; on the other hand, the capillaroscopic findings worsened after one year.

The mean lung function parameters were normal at entry and did not change after one year. HRCT was normal in half of the patients, but the frequency of individual findings at control revealed substantial worsening both of alveolitis (difference +2) and especially fibrosis (difference +7) at 1 year.

Both the initial and one-year scintigraphic examinations of the esophagus showed a slight impairment of motility in the majority of our patients.

The mean FQ values were 5.41 at entry and 5.20 after one year. The difference was not significant.

Potential Activity Markers

The mean plasma IL-2r was increased at entry and at one year, but the differences were statistically insignificant, whereas the mean plasma IL-6 was within the normal range in both evaluations (TABLE 3).

TABLE 4. Correlation of immunological markers and of endothelial activation markers with routine laboratory tests, DLCO, capillaroscopy, and functional questionnaire at study entry

Marker	sIL-2r	BET-1	IL-6
Capillaroscopy	n.s.	n.s.	0.05
DLCO	n.s.	0.005	n.s.
ESR	n.s.	n.s.	n.s.
Erythrocytes	0.05	n.s.	0.01
Leukocytes	0.1	n.s.	0.001
Thrombocytes	n.s.	n.s.	n.s.
Albumin	n.s.	n.s.	n.s.
FQ	0.001	n.s.	0.01

ABBREVIATIONS: BET-1, big endothelin-1; DLCO, diffuse lung capacity for carbon monoxide; ESR, erythrocyte sedimentation rate; FQ, functional questionnaire; IL-6, interleukin-6; n.s., not significant; sIL-2r, soluble interleukin-2 receptor.

TABLE 5. Correlation of immunological markers and of endothelial activation markers with routine laboratory tests, DLCO, capillaroscopy, and functional questionnaire at 1 year after study entry

Marker	sIL-2r	BET-1	IL-6
Capillaroscopy	0.1	n.s.	0.05
DLCO	n.s.	0.001	n.s.
ESR	n.s.	n.s.	0.1
Erythrocytes	0.005	n.s.	0.05
Leukocytes	0.1	n.s.	0.001
Thrombocytes	n.s.	n.s.	n.s.
Albumin	n.s.	n.s.	n.s.
FQ	0.001	n.s.	0.005

ABBREVIATIONS: BET-1, big endothelin-1; DLCO, diffuse lung capacity for carbon monoxide; FQ, functional questionnaire; IL-6, interleukin-6; n.s., not significant; sIL-2r, soluble interleukin-2 receptor.

Serum ICAM-1 was increased compared with reference values at entry and after one year, but without statistical significance. Similarly, serum VCAM-1 in both measurements exceeded normal range. At one year, a certain increase compared with entry was observed. The mean BET-1 concentrations were increased compared with the normal range, but the difference was not statistically significant. After one year the measured values even decreased. Plasma vWFAg concentrations exceeded the reference values in both measurements, but without statistical significance.

Mean serum NPIIIP was within the normal range given with the assay kit, and after one year the mean value did not change. PYR urinary excretion was only slightly enhanced, whereas D-PYR levels were within the normal range at any time. At one year, levels of both cross-link elements decreased insignificantly compared with entry data.

TABLE 6. Correlation of collagen metabolism markers with skin involvement and functional questionnaire at study entry

Marker	FTP: flexion Right	FTP: flexion Left	Skin score	FQ
NPIIIP	0.01	0.005	0.05	0.01
PYR	n.s.	n.s.	n.s.	n.s.
D-PYR	0.001	0.001	0.001	0.001

ABBREVIATIONS: D-PYR, deoxypyridinoline; FTP, finger-to-palm distance; FQ, functional questionnaire; NPIIIP, N-terminal propeptide of procollagen type III; PYR, pyridinoline.

TABLE 7. Correlation of collagen metabolism markers with skin involvement and functional questionnaire at 1 year after study entry

Marker	FTP: flexion Right	FTP: flexion Left	Skin score	FQ
NPIIIP	0.01	0.005	n.s.	0.01
PYR	n.s.	n.s.	n.s.	n.s.
D-PYR	0.001	0.001	0.001	0.001

ABBREVIATIONS: D-PYR, deoxypyridinoline; FTP, finger-to-palm distance; FQ, functional questionnaire; NPIIIP, N-terminal propeptide of procollagen type III; n.s., not significant; PYR; pyridinoline.

Correlation of Potential Activity Markers with Selected Clinical Findings

Among the immunological markers evaluated, we found significant correlations at entry of only sIL-2r with FQ ($P = 0.001$) and IL-6 with leukocyte count ($P = 0.001$) (TABLE 4). After one year, sIL-2r correlated with erythrocyte count and FQ, whereas IL-6 levels correlated with leukocyte count and FQ (TABLE 5).

In the set of endothelial activation markers, only BET-1 correlated with DLCO at entry ($P = 0.005$) and after one year ($P = 0.001$) (TABLE 4 and TABLE 5). Serum vWFAg and plasma concentrations of adhesion molecules did not correlate with any clinical test or sign at either time point.

In the group of collagen metabolism markers, at entry NPIIIP concentrations correlated with the FTP ($P = 0.005$), whereas D-PYR correlated with skin score and the FQ ($P = 0.001$) (TABLE 6). The one-year measurements showed the same correlations for NPIIIP and D-PYR (TABLE 7). PYR excretion did not correlate with any clinical test or sign at either time point.

DISCUSSION AND CONCLUSIONS

In our study, all immunological markers assessed except IL-6 were increased insignificantly at entry; similar data were obtained after 1 year. Endothelial activation markers were increased compared with the normal range, and after 1 year only an insignificant increase in vWFAg and decrease in BET-1 were found as compared with entry values.

For the calculation of possible clinical correlations, we used the SSc activity criteria proposed by Valentini *et al.*:[12] skin score, scleredema, ulcerations and necrosis of fingertips, arthritis, proximal muscle weakness, DLCO, echocardiography findings, and ESR. To these variables, we added several clinical signs, organ-specific findings, results of selected routine laboratory tests, and FQ results.

In several studies[13] looking for new laboratory markers of activity for SSc various correlations with clinical signs, routine activity markers (acute phase reactants), and markers of disease severity (degree of organ damage) were calculated, and we used a similar approach. In these studies, disease activity usually has not been distinguished from disease severity, perhaps because of the lack of standardized clinical markers of activity for SSc.

Our data are consistent with the results of Zachariae *et al.*,[14] who found a significant correlation between ET-1 concentration and DLCO decrease. Stuart *et al.*[15] measured serum IL-6 levels in patients with limited and diffuse SSc and correlated their findings with disease activity, as defined by arthritis, proximal muscle weakness, and subfebrilia. They found a correlation in the subgroup with active disease. The significant correlations of collagen metabolism markers with skin changes obtained are consistent with the findings of other authors.[16] Clements[17] tried to identify several relevant candidate activity markers much resembling our set, but the clinical correlations differ from our results and associations.

The endothelial activation markers examined correlated with neither the clinical signs and findings nor the results of routine tests. The importance of these and other markers should be verified by new studies on larger cohorts of patients using multinational databases.

ACKNOWLEDGMENTS

This study was supported by the research grant of Czech Ministry of Health #000 000 23728.

REFERENCES

1. Medsger, T.A. 1985. Comment on scleroderma criteria cooperative study. *In* Systemic sclerosis (Scleroderma). C.M. Black & A.R. Myers, Eds.: 235–249. Gower Med. New York.
2. Xu, W., E.C. LeRoy & E.A. Smith. 1991. Fibronectin release by systemic sclerosis and normal dermal fibroblasts in response to TGF beta. J. Rheumatol. **18:** 241–246.
3. Roberts, A.B., M.B. Sporn, R.K. Assoian, *et al.* 1986. Transforming growth factor type beta: rapid induction of fibrosis and angiogenesis *in vivo* and stimulation of collagen formation *in vitro.* Proc. Natl. Acad. Sci. USA **83:** 4167–4171.
4. Kahaleh, M.B. & E.C. LeRoy. 1989. Interleukin-2 in scleroderma: correlation of serum levels with extent of skin involvement and disease duration. Ann. Intern. Med. **110:** 446–450.
5. Black, C.M., A. McWhirter, N.K. Harrison, *et al.* Serum type III procollagen peptide concentrations in systemic sclerosis and Raynaud's phenomenon: relationship to disease duration. Br. J. Rheumatol. **28:** 98–103.

6. IŠTOK, R., L. CZIRJÁK, J. LUKÁČ, *et al.* 2001. Increased urinary pyridinoline cross-link compound of collagen in patients with systemic sclerosis and Raynaud's phenomenon. Rheumatology **40:** 140–146.
7. LEROY, E.C., C.M. BLACK, R. FLEISCHMAJER, *et al.* 1988. Scleroderma (systemic sclerosis): classification, subsets and pathogenesis. J. Rheumatol. **15:** 202–205.
8. TANIMOTO, K., S. OHNO, M. IMADA, *et al.* 2004. Utility of urinary pyridinoline and deoxypyridinoline ratio for diagnosis of osteoarthritis at temporomandibular joint. J. Oral. Pathol. Med. **33:** 218–223.
9. RODNAN, G.P., E. LIPINSKI & J. LUKSICK. 1979. Skin thickness and collagen content in progressive systemic sclerosis and localized scleroderma. Arthritis Rheum. **22:** 130–140.
10. MARICQ, H.R. 1984. Nailfold capillaroscopy and biopsy in scleroderma and related disorders. Dermatologica **168:** 73–77.
11. SILMAN, A.J., A. AKESSON, J. NEWMAN, *et al.* 1998. Assessment of functional ability in patients with scleroderma: a proposed new disability assessment instrument. J. Rheumatol. **25:** 79–83.
12. VALENTINI, G., A. DELLA ROSSA, S. BOMBARDIERI, *et al.* 2001. European multicentre study to define disease activity criteria for systemic sclerosis. II. Identification of disease activity variables and development of preliminary activity indexes. Ann. Rheum. Dis. **60:** 592–598.
13. DEGIANNIS, D., J.R. SEIBOLD & M. CZARNECKI. 1990. Soluble and cellular markers of immune activation in patients with systemic sclerosis. Clin. Immunol. Immunopathol. **56:** 259–266.
14. ZACHARIAE, H., P. BJERRING, L. HALKIER-SØRENSEN, *et al.* 1994. Skin scoring in systemic sclerosis: a modification—relations to subtypes and aminoterminal propeptide of type III procollagen (PIIINP). Acta Derm. Venereol. **74:** 444–446.
15. STUART, R.A., A.J. LITTLEWOOD, P.J. MADDISON & N.D. HALL. 1995. Elevated serum interleukin-6 levels associated with active disease in systemic connective tissue disorders. Clin. Exp. Rheumatol. **13:** 17–22.
16. HEICKENDORFF, L., H. ZACHARIAE, P. BJERRING, *et al.* 1995. The use of serologic markers for collagen synthesis and degradation in systemic sclerosis. J. Am. Acad. Dermatol. **32:** 584–588.
17. CLEMENTS, P.J. 1995. Measuring disease activity and severity in scleroderma. Curr. Opin. Rheumatol. **7:** 517–521.

Complement Activation

A Novel Pathogenic Mechanism in the Antiphospholipid Syndrome

SILVIA S. PIERANGELI,[a] MARIANO VEGA-OSTERTAG,[a] XIAOWEI LIU,[a] AND GUILLERMINA GIRARDI[b]

[a]*Department of Microbiology, Biochemistry and Immunology, Morehouse School of Medicine, Atlanta, Georgia 30310, USA*

[b]*Hospital for Special Surgery, New York, New York, USA*

ABSTRACT: Antiphospholipid antibodies (aPLs) have been shown to induce thrombosis, activate endothelial cells, and induce fetal loss. The pathogenesis of aPL-induced thrombosis is incompletely understood, but it is thought to involve platelet and endothelial cell activation as well as pro-coagulant effects of aPL antibody directly on clotting pathway components. Recent studies have shown that uncontrolled complement activation leads to fetal death in aPL-antibody treated mice. We hypothesized that aPL antibodies activate complement, generating split products that induce thrombosis. To test this hypothesis, we used an *in vivo* model of thrombosis in which aPL antibodies induce a significant increase in thrombus size and a mouse model of endothelial cell activation in which aPLs induce significant adhesion of leukocytes (WBCs) to endothelial cells. We found that mice deficient in complement components C3 and C5 were resistant to enhanced thrombosis and endothelial cell activation induced by aPL antibodies. Furthermore, inhibition of C5 activation using anti-C5 mAb prevented thrombophilia induced by aPL antibodies. Our data show that complement activation mediates two important effectors of aPL antibodies: induction of thrombosis and endothelial activation.

KEYWORDS: antiphospholipid antibodies; thrombosis; endothelial cells; and complement activation

INTRODUCTION

Antiphospholipid syndrome (APS) is a disorder of recurrent thrombosis, pregnancy loss, and thrombocytopenia associated with persistently positive anticardiolipin (aCL) and/or lupus anticoagulant (LA) tests.[1,2] APS is a multisystem disorder that may or may not be associated with systemic lupus erythematosus (SLE).

Studies have shown that antiphospholipid (aPL) antibodies cause pregnancy loss, thrombosis, and endothelial cell activation *in vivo* in mice.[3–5] However, the mecha-

Address for correspondence, Silvia S. Pierangeli, Ph.D., Gloster Building Room 332, Department of Microbiology, Biochemistry and Immunology, Morehouse School of Medicine, 720 Westview Dr., S.W. Atlanta, GA 30310-1495. Voice: 404-752-1882; fax: 404-752-1644. spierangeli@msm.edu

Ann. N.Y. Acad. Sci. 1051: 413–420 (2005). © 2005 New York Academy of Sciences. doi: 10.1196/annals.1361.083

nisms by which these antibodies mediate disease are only partially understood, and our understanding is limited by the apparent polyspecificity of the antibodies, the multiple potential end-organ targets, and the variability of clinical context that disease may present.

APL antibodies are heterogenous and it is likely than more than one mechanism may be involved in causing thrombosis.[6,7] In fact, *in vitro* studies have reported that aPL may cause thrombosis by interfering with activation of protein C (or inactivation of factor V by activated protein C), inhibit endothelial prostacyclin production, impair fibrinolysis, and exert stimulatory effect on platelet function.[6–19]

Recently convincing evidence has shown that activation of complement mediates thrombogenic effects of aPL and fetal loss in APS.[20–24] This paper discusses specifically those new and exciting findings with respect to the involvement of the complement cascade in pathogenic effects of aPL antibodies. Understanding molecular mechanisms by which these antibodies cause thrombosis and pregnancy loss is important and may help in devising new targeted modalities for the treatment of patients with APS.

ACTIVATION OF THE COMPLEMENT CASCADE AND ANTIPHOSPHOLIPID ANTIBODIES

As indicated, passive transfer of IgG from antiphospholipid antibody-positive sera (IgG-APS) has been found to induce fetal loss and thrombosis in mice, suggesting a direct pathogenic role for of aPL antibodies.[3–5] Recent studies have suggested that activation of the complement cascade is necessary for aPL-mediated thrombophilia and fetal loss.[20–24] First, in a study by our group, we found that inhibition of the complement cascade *in vivo*, using the C3 convertase inhibitor complement receptor 1-related gene protein y (Crry)-Ig, blocks aPL-induced fetal loss and growth retardation and inhibits aPL-mediated thrombosis.[20] Furthermore, mice deficient in complement C3 and C5 were resistant to fetal injury induced by aPL antibodies.[21] It was also shown that the interaction of complement component 5a (C5a) with its receptor (C5aR) is necessary for thrombosis of placental vasculature.[22] Moreover, Girardi and coworkers proposed that heparin, the current standard treatment in patients with APS, seems to prevent obstetric complications by blocking activation of complement and not by preventing placental thrombosis.[23]

Recently, Berman *et al.* showed that TNF-α is a critical effector and a target for therapy in antiphospholipid antibody-induced pregnancy loss.[24] The authors showed that aPL Abs are specifically targeted to decidual tissue and cause a rapid increase in decidual and systemic TNF-α levels. They also identified the release of TNF-α as a critical intermediate that acts downstream of C5 activation, based on the fetal protective effects of TNF-α deficiency and TNF blockade and on the absence of increased TNF-α levels in C5-deficient mice treated with aPL. The study concluded that TNF-α links pathogenic aPL to fetal damage and identifies TNF blockade as a potential therapy for the pregnancy complications of APS.[24] It is then concluded that in this murine model, complement activation is a necessary intermediary event in the pathogenesis of fetal loss associated with aPL antibodies.

It is well established that activated complement fragments themselves have the capacity to bind and activate inflammatory and endothelial cells as well as to induce a prothrombotic phenotype, either directly through C5b-9 (membrane attack complex (MAC) or through C5a receptor-mediated effects.[25,26] Endothelial cells can release tissue factor in response to C5a activation.[27] Inflammatory cells, when triggered by complement proteolytic products C5a and C3a, respond with the production of selected procoagulant activities, thereby initiating the coagulation pathways. MAC has also been associated with thrombosis. Studies performed in rats showed that CD59, an inhibitor of C5b-9 assembly and insertion, serves a protective role in a rat model of thrombotic microangiopathy, demonstrating that C5b-9 plays a critical pathogenic role in thrombosis.[28]

Hence, we tested the hypothesis that C3 and C5 activation mediates endothelial cell activation and thrombogenic effects of IgG-APS; we used C3- and C5-deficient mice ($C3^{-/-}$ and $C5^{-/-}$, respectively) and a specific anti-C5 monoclonal antibody (C5MoAb).

C3- AND C5-DEFICIENT MICE ARE PROTECTED FROM APL-INDUCED THROMBOPHILIA AND ENDOTHELIAL CELL ACTIVATION *IN VIVO*

We tested the hypothesis whether $C3^{-/-}$ and $C5^{-/-}$ mice are protected from aPL-induced thrombophilia and endothelial cell activation *in vivo*. C3-deficient mice were obtained from Dr. V.M. Holers' laboratory (University of Colorado Health Sciences, Denver, CO).[29] They were generated by intercrossing $C3^{+/-}$ mice at F1 during a backcross to C57BL/6 and then propagating $C3^{-/-}$ progeny. $C5^{-/-}$ (B10.D2-$H2^dH2$-$T18^c$ Hc^o/o2Sn) and the $C5^{+/+}$ background-strain mice (B10.D2-$H2^dH2$-$T18^c$ Hc^o/oSnJ) were obtained from the Jackson Laboratories (Bar Harbor, Maine, USA). CD1 male mice (weighing approximately 30 g) were obtained from Charles River Laboratories (Wilmington, DE). All animals were housed in the Animal Care (American Association of Laboratory Animal Care-Approved) facilities of the Morehouse School of Medicine. Animals were handled by trained personnel according to Institutional Animal Care and Use Committee guidelines.

To investigate the role of C3 and C5 in thrombophilia induced by aPL antibodies, $C3^{+/+}$ and $C3^{-/-}$ mice (7–10 animals) and $C5^{+/+}$ and $C5^{-/-}$ mice ($n = 7$–10) were injected intraperitoneally with 500 μg of IgG from a patient with APS (IgG-APS) IgG-APS or with 500 μg of control IgG (IgG-NHS) twice (at time 0 and 48 hours later). Surgical procedures to study thrombus dynamics and adhesion of leukocytes to the endothelium of postcapillary venules (number of adhering WBCs) in the exposed cremaster muscle were performed 72 hours after the first IgG-APS or IgG-NHS injection as described.[4,5] The mouse model of thrombosis formation employed in this study has been described in detail.[4,5] In brief: mice were anesthetized, and the right femoral vein was exposed, resulting in a 0.5-cm segment of vein free for manipulation and observation. The vein was pinched with a pressure of 1500 g/mm^2 to introduce a standardized injury that induced a clot. Clot formation and dissolution in the transilluminated vein were visualized with a microscope equipped with a closed-circuit video system (including a color monitor and a recorder). Thrombus size (in square micrometers) was measured 1 min after the pinch injury by freezing the digitized image and tracing the outer margin of the thrombus. Three to five thrombi were successfully induced in each animal, and mean values were computed. The number of leukocytes (WBCs) adhering (sticking) within five different venules in the cremaster muscle was determined and adhesion was defined as WBCs remained stationary for at least 30 seconds.[5]

As previously reported, IgG-APS significantly enhanced thrombus size in $C3^{+/+}$ mice compared to thrombus size in $C3^{+/+}$ mice treated with IgG-NHS (3.3-fold increase). $C3^{-/-}$ mice treated with IgG-APS showed a significant reduction in thrombi size as compared to $C3^{+/+}$ mice (67%, $P = 0.0002$). Thrombus size in $C3^{-/-}$ mice treated with IgG-APS was not different from that of $C3^{-/-}$ mice treated with IgG-NHS or that of $C3^{+/+}$ mice treated with IgG-NHS.

Similarly, IgG-APS induced a significant 2.3-fold increase in thrombus size in $C5^{+/+}$ mice when compared to $C5^{+/+}$ mice treated with IgG-NHS ($P = 0.003$). This increase in thrombus size was reduced by 63% in $C5^{-/-}$ mice treated with IgG-APS. Thrombus size in $C5^{-/-}$ mice injected with IgG-APS was not different from thrombi induced in $C5^{-/-}$ treated with IgG-NHS or $C5^{+/+}$ mice treated with IgG-NHS.

We then examined WBC adhesion to endothelium of cremaster muscle. IgG-APS induced an increase in WBC adhesion in both $C3^{+/+}$ and $C5^{+/+}$ mice (2.5- and 4.6-fold, respectively ($P = 0.01$ and 0.0025) when compared to treatment with IgG-NHS. This increase in IgG-APS–induced WBC adhesion was not observed in $C3^{-/-}$ and $C5^{-/-}$ mice treated with IgG-APS.

The titer of aCL antibodies in $C3^{+/+}$ mice injected with IgG-APS was not different from titers in $C3^{-/-}$ mice (78 ± 8.6 GPL units vs. 86.3 ± 10.4 GPL units). Similarly, the levels of aCL antibodies in $C5^{+/+}$ mice treated with IgG-APS were not different from $C5^{-/-}$ mice (115.7 ± 74.2 GPL vs. 102.3 ± 12.2 GPL). This excludes the possibility that the protection observed against thrombogenic effects of IgG-APS observed in $C3^{-/-}$ and in $C5^{-/-}$ mice was related to lower aCL titers in the serum of the mice.

ANTI-C5 MONOCLONAL ANTIBODY PREVENTS IgG-APS–INDUCED THROMBOSIS

It has been described that anti-C5 mAb prevents C5 activation and protects from aPL-antibody–induced pregnancy loss in mice.[22] To further investigate the role of C5 in thrombophilia induced by aPL antibodies, male CD1 mice (25–30 g) (Charles River Breeding Laboratories, Wilmington, MA) were injected intraperitoneally with 500 μg of IgG-APS or IgG-NHS (10–15 mice) at time 0 and 48 hours. Half of the mice in each group received 1 mg anti-C5 mAb (30) or 1 mg of murine IgG control, 30 minutes before each injection with IgG-APS or IgG-NHS. Surgical procedures to study thrombus dynamics were performed 72 hours after the first IgG-APS (or IgG-NHS) injection as previously described.[4]

A significant increase in thrombus size was observed in mice treated with IgG-APS compared to mice treated with IgG-NHS (3577 ± 1129 μm^2 vs. 712.0 ± 272 μm^2; $P = 0.0001$) (FIG. 1). In contrast, when IgG-APS-treated mice were treated with anti C5 mAb, thrombus size was significantly smaller (838 ± 222 μm^2 ($P = 0.00005$) compared to mice treated with IgG-APS and mouse IgG (FIG. 1). Mouse IgG treatment did not affect thrombus size in animals treated with IgG-APS or IgG-NHS. The aCL titer in IgG-APS–treated mice was 152.2 ± 14.8 GPL units and was not different from the aCL titer of mice treated with IgG-APS and anti-C5 mAb (135.3 ± 20.3 GPL units), excluding the possibility that the protective

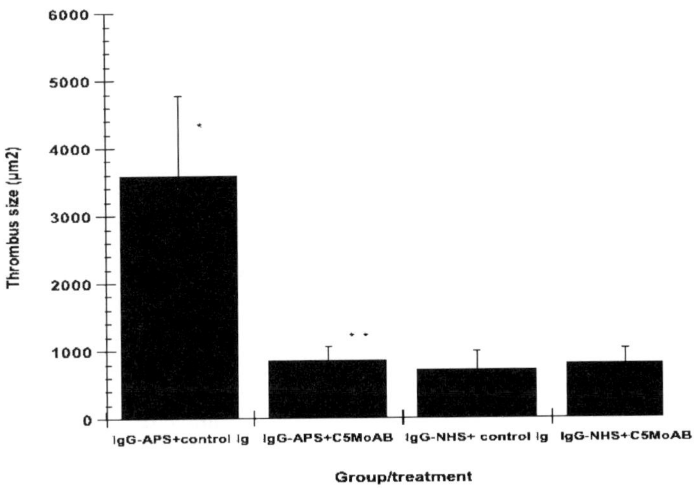

FIGURE 1. Effects of anti-C5 mAb on IgG-APS–induced thrombosis. CD1 mice in groups of 5 were injected with IgG-APS or with IgG-NHS 30 minutes after the injection of 1 mg of C5MoAb or 1 mg of murine IgG (control) at time 0 and 48 hours later, and the size of induced thrombus was measured. Results are expressed in μm^2 as mean ± SD. *Statistically significantly different from IgG-NHS + control Ig-treated mice; **statistically significantly different from IgG-APS + control Ig-treated mice.

effects of anti-C5 mAb can be due to a diminution in aCL titers because of interferences between IgG-APS and anti-C5 mAb.

DISCUSSION

The data clearly indicate that aPL proinflammatory and thrombogenic effects are abrogated in C3- and in C5-deficient mice. Furthermore, a monoclonal antibody anti-C5 reversed thrombogenic properties of aPL *in vivo*, confirming that complement activation is involved in aPL-induced thrombosis. We concluded that in mice complement activation not only is a necessary intermediate in the pathogenesis of fetal loss,[20–24] but also is involved in endothelial cell activation and thrombosis mediated by aPL. We postulate that activated complement fragments themselves have the capacity to bind and activate inflammatory and endothelial cells as well as induce a prothrombotic phenotype, either directly through the membrane attack complex (MAC) or through C5a receptor (CD88)–mediated effects.[21] We then propose the following mechanism for the pathogenic effects of aPL antibodies on thrombosis. First aPL antibodies bind to endothelial cells and induce their activation and a procoagulant state, as demonstrated *in vivo* and *in vitro* studies.[5,16–19,30] These include upregulation of adhesion molecules and tissue factor expression. APL antibodies also induce platelet activation and interact with elements of the coagulation cascade.[8,9,10–15] This activity, however, does not seem to be sufficient to cause thrombosis. Activation of the complement cascade by aPL may amplify these effects by stimulation of the generation of potent mediators of platelet and endothelial cell activation, including C3a and C5a and the C5b-MAC.[22,25,26,31,32] The addition of these complement activation products has been shown to cause thrombosis, tissue hypoxia, and inflammation.[27,33,34] Furthermore, C5a is a potent soluble inflammatory anaphylotoxic and chemotactic molecule that promotes recruitment and activation of neutrophils (PMN) and monocytes and mediates endothelial cell activation through its receptor (C5R, CD88).[22,25,27,31] Binding of C5b to the target initiates the non-enzymatic assembly of the C5b-9MAC. Insertion of important effects of C5b-9MAC in disease is on nucleated cells, where it activates proinflammatory signaling pathways through the interaction of membrane-associated MAC proteins with heterotrimeric G proteins.[22,25,31]

In summary, pathogenic aPL antibodies bind to target cells and then bind complement. The complement system in turn damages the endothelial cells, leading to a procoagulant state and undesirable thrombosis. We hypothesize that in APS patients, owing to aPL deposition targeted to the endothelium, complement activation may be increased locally and may overwhelm normally adequate inhibitory mechanisms. Hence activation of complement may be a critical proximal effector mechanism in aPL-associated thrombosis.

The treatment of the APS can be directed towards preventing thromboembolic events by using antithrombotic medications or towards modulating the immune response with immunotherapy. In the case of thrombotic manifestations, both approaches have been used. In both cases, the treatments have considerable side effects.[35–37] On the one hand, current treatment recommendations are clear. In patients with a history of thrombosis, there is a high risk of recurrence, and oral anticoagulation at a relative high INR is frequently used for a long period of time. In patients with aPL antibodies without a previous thrombotic event, most clinicians would recommend prophylaxis with low-dose aspirin.[35–37] On the other hand the risk of bleeding with oral anticoagulation is high. Furthermore, there is a need for frequent monitoring and patient compliance with diet and lifestyle to minimize risk of recurrence of thrombosis. Hence, there is need for new, more efficient and less harmful modalities of treatment for APS.

It is possible to speculate that inhibition of complement activation should ameliorate vascular thrombosis in individuals with APS. Therefore, complement may be an important new target for therapy in patients with thrombotic and vascular complications in APS. Complement inhibitors are now being tested in patients with inflammatory, ischemic, and autoimmune diseases.[38,39] Complement activation can be an important target that will allow us to create interventions that prevent, arrest, or modify the thrombogenic effects of aPL antibodies. For this reason, therapeutic strategies that include C5a and its receptor are considered an especially promising approach to complement inhibition.[38,39]

ACKNOWLEDGMENTS

This study was partially funded by a Research Center in Minority Institution Grant (NIH Grant No. G12-RR03034) and a Minority Biomedical Research Support Grant No. S02GMM08248 from the NIH.

REFERENCES

1. HARRIS, E.N. 1987. Syndrome of the black swan. Br. J. Rheumatol. **26:** 324–326.
2. WILSON, W.A., A.E. GHARAVI, T. KOIKE, *et al.* 1999. International consensus statement on preliminary classification criteria for definite antiphospholipid syndrome: report of an international workshop. Arthritis Rheum. **42:** 1309–1311.
3. BRANCH, D.W., D.J. DUDLEY, M.D. MITCHELL, *et al.* 1990. Immunoglobulin G fractions from patients with antiphospholipid antibodies cause fetal death in BALB/c mice: a model for autoimmune fetal loss. Am. J. Obstet. Gynecol. **163:** 210–216.
4. PIERANGELI, S.S., X. LIU, G.H. ANDERSON, *et al.* 1995. Induction of thrombosis in a mouse model by IgG, IgM and IgA immunoglobulins from patients with the antiphospholipid syndrome. Thromb. Haemost. **74:** 1361–1367.
5. PIERANGELI, S.S., M. COLDEN-STANFIELD, X. LIU, *et al.* 1999. Antiphospholipid antibodies from antiphospholipid syndrome patients activate endothelial cells *in vitro* and in *vivo*. Circulation **99:** 1997–2000.
6. ROUBEY, R.A.S. 1998. Mechanisms of autoantibody-mediated thrombosis. Lupus **7:** S114–119.
7. MERONI, P.L. & P. RIBOLDI. 2001. Pathogenic mechanisms mediating antiphospholipid syndrome. Curr. Opin. Rheumatol. **13:** 377–382.
8. ESMON, N.L., O. SAFA, M. SMIRNOV & C.T. ESMON. 2000. Antiphospholipid antibodies and the protein C pathway. J. Autoimmun. **15:** 221–225.
9. CAMPBELL, A.L., S.S. PIERANGELI, S. WELLHAUSEN & E.N. HARRIS. 1995. Comparison of the effect of anticardiolipin antibodies from patients with the antiphospholipid syndrome and with syphilis on platelet activation and aggregation. Thromb. Haemost. **73:** 529–534.
10. HARRIS, E.N., R.A. ASHERSON, A.E. GHARAVI, *et al.* 1985. Thrombocytopenia in SLE and related autoimmune disorders: association with anti-cardiolipin antibody. Br. J. Haematol. **59:** 227–230.
11. KHAMASHTA, M.A., E.N. HARRIS, A.E. GHARAVI, *et al.* 1988. Immune mediated mechanism for thrombosis: antiphospholipid antibody binding to platelet membranes. Ann. Rheum. Dis. **47:** 849–854.
12. OUT, H.J., P. DEGROOT, M. VAN VLIET, *et al.* 1991. Antibodies to platelets in patients with antiphospholipids antibodies. Blood **77:** 2655–2659.
13. ARVIEUX, J., B. ROUSELL, P. POUZOL & M.G. COLOMB. 1993. Platelet activating properties of murine monoclonal antibodies to $\beta_2$glycoprotein I. Thromb. Haemost. **70:** 336–341.
14. ESPINOLA, R.G., S.S. PIERANGELI, A.E. GHARAVI & E.N. HARRIS. 2002. Hydroxychloroquine reverses platelet activation induced by human IgG antiphospholipid antibodies. Thromb. Haemost. **87:** 518–522.
15. LIN, Y.L. & C.T. WANG, 1992. Activation of human platelets by the rabbit anticardiolipin antibodies. Blood **80:** 3135–3143.
16. MERONI, P.L., E. RASCHI, M. CAMERA, *et al.* 2000. Endothelial activation by aPL: a potential pathogenetic mechanism for the clinical manifestations of the syndrome. J. Autoimmun. **15:** 237–240.
17. SIMANTOV, R., S.K. LO, A. GHARAVI, *et al.* 1996. Antiphospholipid antibodies activate vascular endothelial cells. Lupus **5:** 440-441.
18. AMENGUAL, O., T. ATSUMI, M.A. KHAMASHTA & G.R.V. HUGHES. 1998. The role of the tissue factor pathway in the hypercoagulable state in patients with the antiphospholipid syndrome. Thromb. Haemost. **79:** 276–281.
19. FERRARA, D.E., R. SWERLICK, K. CASPER, *et al.* 2004. Fluvastatin inhibits upregulation of tissue factor expression by antiphospholipid antibodies on endothelial cells. J. Thomb. Haemost. **2:** 1558–1563.
20. HOLERS, V.M., G. GIRARDI, L. MO, *et al.* 2002. C3 Activation is required for anti-phospholipid antibody-induced fetal loss. J. Exp. Med. **195:** 211–220.
21. SALMON, J.E., G. GIRARDI & V.M. HOLERS. 2002. Complement activation as a mediator of antiphospholipid antibody induced pregnancy loss and thrombosis. Ann. Rheum. Dis. **61:** 46–50.

22. GIRARDI, G., J. BERMAN, P. REDECHA, *et al.* 2003. Complement C5a receptors and neutrophils mediate fetal injury in the antiphophospholipid syndrome. J. Clin. Invest. **112:** 1644–1654.
23. GIRARDI, G., P. REDECHA & J. SALMON. 2004. Heparin prevents antiphospholipid antibody-induced fetal loss by inhibiting complement activation. Nature Med. **10:** 1222–1226.
24. BERMAN, J., G. GIRARDI & J.E. SALMON. 2005. TNF-α is a critical effector and a target for therapy in antiphospholipid antibody-induced pregnancy loss. J. Immunol. **174:** 485–490.
25. WETSEL, R.A. 1995. Structure, function and cellular expression of complement anaphylotoxin receptors. Curr. Opin. Immunol. **7:** 48–53.
26. SHIN, M.L., H.G. RUS & F.I. NICOLESCU. 1996. Membrane attack by complement: assembly and biology of terminal complement complexes. Biomembranes **4:** 123–114
27. HATTORI, E., K.K. HAMILTON, R.P. MCEVER & P.J. SIMS. 1989. Complement proteins C5b-9 induce secretion of high molecular weight multimers of endothelial von Willebrand factor and translocation of granule membrane protein GMP-140 to the cell surface. J. Biol. Chem. **264:** 9053–9060.
28. NANGAKU, M., C.E. ALPERS, J. PIPPIN, *et al.* 1998. CD59 protects glomerular endothelial cells from immune-mediated thrombotic microangiopathy in rats. J. Am. Soc. Nephrol. **9:** 590–597.
29. CIRCOLO, A., G. GARNIER, W. FUKUDA, *et al.* 1999. Genetic disruption of the murine complement C3 promoter region generates deficient mice with extrahepatic expression of C3 mRNA. Immunopharmacology **42:** 135–149.
30. FREI, Y., J.D. LAMBRIS & B. STOCKINGER. 1987. Generation of a monoclonal antibody to mouse C5 application in an ELISA assay for detection of anti-C5 antibodies. Mol. Cell Probes. **1:** 141–149.
31. WOJTA, J., C. KAUN, G. ZORN, *et al.* 2002. C5a stimulates production of plasminogen activator inhibitor-1 in human mast cells and basophils. Blood **100:** 517–523.
32. KONDO, C., M. MIZUNO, K. NISHIKAWA, *et al.* 2001. The role of C5a in the development of thrombotic glomerulonephritis in rats. Clin. Exp. Immunol. **124:** 323–329.
33. DAVIS, W.D. & R.L. BREY. 1992. Antiphospholipid antibodies and complement activation in patients with cerebral ischemia. Clin. Exp. Immunol. **10:** 455–460.
34. MUNAKATA, Y., T. SAITO, K. MATUSA, *et al.* 2000. Detection of complement-fixing antiphospholipid antibodies in association with thrombosis. Thromb. Haemost. **83:** 728–731.
35. KHAMASHTA, M.A., M.J. CUADRADO, T. MUJIC, *et al.* 1995. The management of thrombosis in the antiphospholipid antibody syndrome. N. Engl. J. Med. **332:** 993–997.
36. KRNIC-BARRIE, S., C.R. O'CONNOR, S.W. LOONEY, *et al.* 1997. A retrospective review of 61 patients with antiphospholipid syndrome. Arch. Intern. Med. **157:** 2101–2108.
37. CROWTHER, M.A., J.S. GINSBERG, J. JULIAN, *et al.* 2003. A comparison of two intensities of warfarin for the prevention of recurrent thrombosis in patients with the antiphospholipid antibody syndrome. N. Engl. J. Med. **349:** 1133–1138.
38. QUIGG, R.J. 2002. Use of complement inhibitors in tissue injury. Trends Mol. Med. **8:** 430–436.
39. TESSER, J. *et al.* 2001. Safety and efficacy of the humanized anti-C5a antibody h5G1.1 in patients with rheumatoid arthritis [abstract]. Arthritis Rheum. **44:** s274.

The Interplay of Chemokines and Dendritic Cells in the Pathogenesis of Lupus Nephritis

MARCO TUCCI,[a] NICOLA CALVANI,[a] HANNO B. RICHARDS,[b]
COSIMA QUATRARO,[a] AND FRANCO SILVESTRIS[a]

[a]*DIMO, Department of Internal Medicine and Clinical Oncology, University of Bari, Bari, Italy*

[b]*Department of Medicine, Division of Rheumatology and Clinical Immunology, University of Florida, Gainesville, Florida 32610, USA*

ABSTRACT: Lupus nephritis (LN) occurs in more that one-third of patients with systemic lupus erythematosus. Production of nephritogenic autoantibodies, glomerular immune complex deposition, and cytokine overproduction have been postulated to contribute to the pathogenesis of LN. However, overexpression of chemokines and imbalance of dendritic cell (DC) homeostasis may contribute to the development of nephritis in SLE. We present evidence that monocyte chemoattractant protein (MCP)-1 promotes renal disease in experimental glomerulonephritis, while its increased urinary levels reflect the severity of the disease in humans. Although macrophages are the prevalent infiltrating population within the kidney, it has been recently proposed that several chemokines and related receptors expressed by DCs may divide this cell population into myeloid (mDC) and plasmacytoid (pDC) subsets. However, the chemokine receptors expressed by pDCs are not functional, and other molecules are involved in the chemoattraction of these cells. We found increased expression of interleukin (IL)-18 in glomeruli of patients with active LN along with glomerular infiltration by pDCS. Since pDCs bear IL-18 receptor (IL-18R), it is conceivable that circulating pDCs may migrate toward glomeruli by IL-18/IL-18R interactions. Therefore, the relative depletion of circulating pDCs reflects the severity of inflammatory disease in LN.

KEYWORDS: lupus nephritis; interleukin-18; dendritic cells; SLE

INTRODUCTION

Lupus nephritis (LN) contributes substantially to morbidity and mortality in patients with systemic lupus erythematosus (SLE). LN is generally considered to be caused by the glomerular deposition of immune complexes (ICs) that induce a cascade of inflammatory events ultimately leading to severe tissue damage. It is popular opinon that ICs trigger the production of key mediators of inflammation, including

Address for correspondence: Franco Silvestris, M.D., DIMO, University of Bari, Section of Internal Medicine and Oncology, P.za Giulio Cesare, 11, 70124 Bari, Italy. Voice: +39-080-5478-771; fax: +39-080-5478-820
f.silvestris@dimo.uniba.it

Ann. N.Y. Acad. Sci. 1051: 421–432 (2005). © 2005 New York Academy of Sciences.
doi: 10.1196/annals.1361.084

cytokines, chemokines, and adhesion molecules, resulting in glomerular infiltration by mononuclear cells, tissue damage, and renal failure in murine models of LN.[1,2]

Chemokines secreted by cells within inflammatory sites enable chemotaxis of other inflammatory cells which are attracted and migrate by a concentration gradient of the particular chemokine toward the site of its production. Several chemokines have been implicated in renal inflammatory diseases,[3] such as both MCP-1 and macrophage inflammatory protein (MIP)-1α,[4,5] which play a key role in the pathogenesis of either human or experimental LN. Increased urinary levels of these chemokines have been found in active nephritis.[6]

Macrophages are the prevalent cellular population that infiltrates the glomeruli and promotes renal injury after their activation by both MCP-1 and MIP-1α molecules.[7] However, other cells, such as dendritic cells (DCs) and autoreactive T cells have also been suspected to promote renal disease in SLE.[8] DCs are almost unique in their capability to initiate either primary or secondary immune response upon innate stimulation or activation, resulting in cell maturation and alteration of their chemokine and cytokine profile, respectively. DCs are responsive to a wide range of inflammatory molecules since they express a number of receptors for cytokines and chemokines and are able to migrate toward peripheral sites where chemoattractants are being produced. On the basis of cell surface molecule expression, two distinct subsets—plasmacytoid (p) and myeloid (m) DCs—have been described.[9] Both subsets show different functions and migrate toward both lymphoid and non-lymphoid sites. Current evidence suggests that pDCs express specific receptors promoting their migratory properties, which include selectins, CXCR4, CCR7 and α_4-integrins.[10] The mechanisms by which pDCs are trafficked toward inflamed peripheral tissues are not well defined, although unlike mDCs, they are refractory to inflammatory chemokines such as CCR5 and CXCR3.[11] Therefore, additional factors must be involved in their recruitment and recent studies have suggested that IL-18 may be instrumental in attracting pDCs to the site of inflammation.[12]

Here, we report recent data on the role of MCP-1, as a key molecule in the pathogenesis of LN. Furthermore, we describe the potential pathogenic properties of both mDCs and pDCs with respect to glomerular infiltration in the context of local chemokine overproduction and upregulation of IL-18 expression in diffuse proliferative glomerulonephritis.

MCP-1 AND LUPUS NEPHRITIS

LN is an immune-mediated inflammatory disease triggered by IC deposition promoting both glomerular and tubular infiltration by activated macrophages, autoreactive T-cells, and DCs. The study of experimental models of LN, such as MRL/lpr and NZB/WF$_1$, showed that in response to glomerular IC deposition, inflammatory chemokine and cytokine production promotes the development of nephritis in SLE and occurs prior to cellular infiltration, proteinuria, and kidney damage.[13]

MCP-1 is a member of the CC chemokine group with a size of about 11 kDa. The MCP-1 gene is located on the long arm of chromosome 17 adjacent to CCL1, CCL7, CCL8, and CCL13. Since the first cloning of the gene for MCP-1,[14] several studies elucidated the role of this chemokine. MCP-1 secretion was formerly demonstrated to be induced by ICs[15] since urinary levels of MCP-1 are remarkably elevated in patients with LN.[16] However, MCP-1 production by human proximal tubular epithelial cells is stimulated by interleukin (IL)-1 and tumor necrosis factor (TNF)-α whereas peripheral blood mononuclear cells produce MCP-1 in response to IL-6 stimulation.[17] Although MCP-1–deficient mice show normal number of circulating leukocytes and resident macrophages, they are unable to recruit monocytes after intraperitoneal thioglycollate administration.[18] Accumulation of monocytes in delayed-type hypersensitivity lesions is impaired and the development of secondary pulmonary granulomas in response to *Schistosoma mansoni* is blunted in MCP-1 knockout mice along with a relative defect in IL-4, IL-5, and interferon (IFN)-γ production.[18] In addition, MCP-1–deficient mice show a defect in both macrophage and T cell recruitment within the kidney, despite high levels of circulating ICs and glomerular deposition of complement fractions, thus suggesting that the latter are unable to promote leukocyte recruitment and drive the renal pathology without MCP-1.[3] Furthermore, administration of anti-MCP-1 antibodies to MRL/lpr mice decreases the extent of both proteinuria and glomerulosclerosis and ameliorates the extent of the renal disease,[19] whereas the neutralizing MCP-1 in a gene therapy approach also reduces nephritis in MRL/lpr mice.[20] However, conflicting data exist with regard to the tubular, glomerular (or both) localization of MCP-1 within the nephritic lupus kidney. Previous studies identified the location of MCP-1 secretion in patients with LN as primarily tubular and suggested that many cytokines may stimulate MCP-1 production. Moreover, urinary levels correlated with its tubular content and number of interstitial infiltrating macrophages ($CD68^+$) in biopsies from patients with active LN.[3] By contrast, other investigators demonstrated a predominant concentration of MCP-1 in glomeruli in experimental models of nephritis.[5] MCP-1 is essential for monocyte recruitment in several inflammatory models *in vivo* and influences the expression of cytokines related to T helper response,[18] and in experimental models of LN[20] the chemokine is apparently involved in developing the tubular rather than the glomerular damage.[21] Increased expression of MCP-1 on peripheral blood monocytes is associated with the presence of LN in patients with SLE and is related to a promoter polymorphism that confers increased susceptibility to LN.[22]

The main receptor for MCP-1 is CCR2, a 374 amino acid protein with its genetic locus on the short arm of chromosome 3 in close proximity to the CCR3 and CCR5 genes.[23] The gene encodes two functional isoforms of CCR2 formed by alternative splicing.[24] The A isoform binds predominantly MCP-,1 whereas the B isoform can bind both MCP-1 and MCP-3 (CCL7). Mice lacking CCR2 show a relative defect in interferon (IFN)-γ production in response to antigen-specific stimulation in parallel with a relative impairment in the recruitment of antigen-presenting cells (APCs) to draining lymph nodes.[25] This suggests that CCR2 is required for trafficking of APCs to sites of interaction with T cells such as germinal centers, and specifically in eliciting T helper (Th)1 responses. Moreover CCR2-deficient mice are unable to clear infection with *Mycobacterium tuberculosis* owing to lack of macrophage and DC recruitment in the initial stages of infection.[26] CCR2 also appears essential for monocyte recruitment, an early process in atherogenesis in apolipoprotein E–deficient mice that spontaneously develop accelerated atherosclerosis.[27] Several chemokine receptors act as co-receptors to CD4 for HIV infection and certain CCR2 polymorphisms confer a relative protective effect to viral infection.[28] Taken together, MCP-1 and CCR2 are critical for the recruitment of both monocytes and DCs in a wide array of inflammatory and infectious diseases and appear particularly important for the development of Th1-mediated responses. There is good evidence that interaction of MCP-1 in the kidney with CCR2 on circulating monocytes is involved in the pathogenesis of lupus nephritis.

We investigated the role of MCP-1 in SLE with a particular focus on LN[22] and found that urinary MCP-1 levels were significantly higher in SLE patients (968 ± 388.2) when compared to controls (46.8 ± 3.5 units, $P < 0.0001$) (FIG. 1, panel A). SLE patients with LN had higher MCP-1 (1732 + 388.8 units) than those without LN (161.3 + 35.4 units, $P < 0.0001$), indicating that the difference in urinary MCP-1

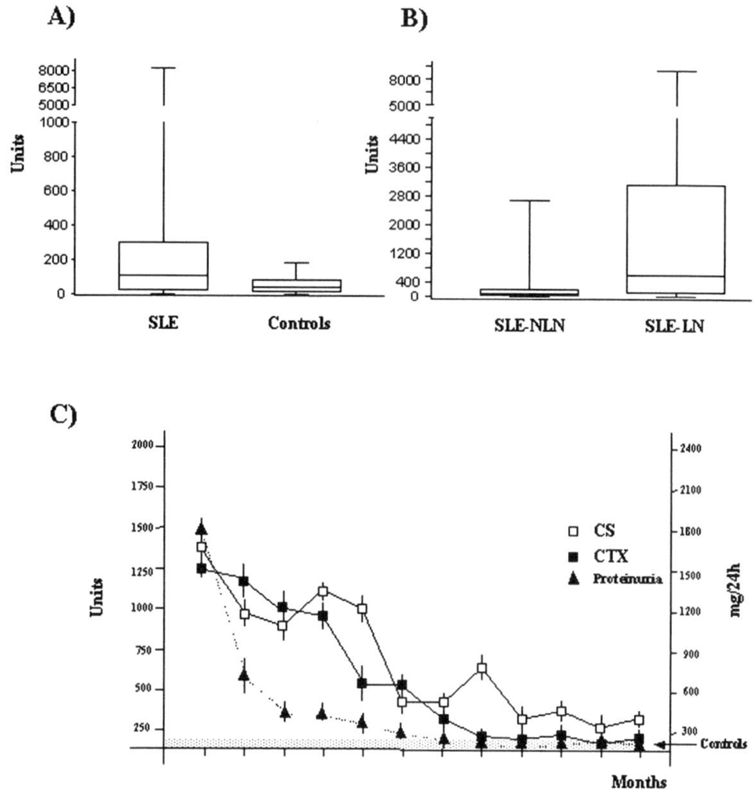

FIGURE 1. Correlation of urinary MCP-1 with occurrence of nephritis in SLE. Urinary levels of MCP-1 were measured by ELISA and corrected for urine volume by measuring urinary creatinine. Values are expressed as units indicating the MCP-1/creatinine ratio. SLE patients produced more urinary MCP-1 compared to normal controls (mean ± SD: 968.8 ± 388.2 units versus 46.8 ± 3.5 units, $P < 0.0001$; panel **A**), and this elevation was associated with LN when patients were stratified for the presence or absence of nephritis (1.732 ± 388.8 versus 161.3 ± 35.4 units, $P < 0.0001$; panel **B**). In panel **C**, the longitudinal measurement of urinary MCP-1 after either steroids alone or intravenous cyclophosphamide associated with oral prednisolone is shown. Steroids (*open squares*) reduced urinary MCP-1 levels, but the association with cyclophosphamide (*solid squares*) induced a stable decrease of the chemokine higher than steroids alone. MCP-1 decrement paralleled with the progressive amelioration of renal function measured as total urinary proteins (*solid triangles*).

detected between the entire SLE cohort and controls was primarily due to those with LN (FIG.1, panel B). Also, further analysis provided evidence that MCP-1 was inversely correlated with urinary creatinine ($P < 0.0001$) and serum albumin ($P = 0.0007$), while showing a positive correlation with serum creatinine ($P < 0.0001$), urinary microalbumin ($P < 0.05$), and proteinuria ($P < 0.0001$). Furthermore, serum MCP-1 levels were significantly higher in many patients with SLE (626 ± 147.5 pg/mL, mean ± SD) when compared to controls (100.7 ± 8.8 pg/mL, mean ± SD, $P < 0.05$), but there was no association between serum MCP-1 levels and the presence of LN. Similarly, there was no correlation between urinary and serum MCP-1 titers, indicating that urinary MCP-1 levels reflect predominantly the local production of this chemokine rather than simply filtration of MCP-1. It is also noteworthy that there was no correlation between serum MCP-1 and any other laboratory parameters such as serum creatinine, serum albumin, urinary creatinine, and urinary microalbumin.

Steroids are known to suppress MCP-1 and the reduction of urinary levels of MCP-1 after steroid therapy has been described.[16] To further study the role of immunosuppressive therapy on urinary MCP-1 excretion in patients with LN we completed several longitudinal studies. We found that urinary MCP-1 levels in selected patients treated with monthly intravenous cyclofosfamide plus oral prednisolone showed a peculiar and progressive decrement of MCP-1 concentrations as compared to patients receiving steroids alone. In addition, the urinary MCP-1 reduction paralleled the improvement of renal function (FIG. 1, panel C). Overall patients with complete remission after immune suppression showed MCP-1 levels comparable to normal controls, whereas those who relapsed during the treatment produced an increment of the urinary chemokine, which correlated with both proteinuria and other parameters of renal function. These data strongly support the use of MCP-1 as potential biomarker for both diagnosis and follow-up of patients with LN.

Chemokines other than MCP-1 are also involved in the recruitment of mononuclear cells to the kidney in inflamed sites. Data from human renal biopsies have demonstrated a high number of CCR5-positive infiltrating mononuclear cells whereas CCR2, CCR1, and CXCR3 receptors were found upregulated in nephritic mice.[29] CCR5 is the natural ligand of both MIP-1α and MIP-1β and the presence of large amounts of CCR5-positive cells within glomeruli confirms the role of MIP-1α in LN.[30] In addition, similarly to MCP-1, high urinary levels of MIP-1α have been reported to correlate with the severity of the disease. Therefore, urinary measurement of MIP-1α has been proposed as a tool for the management of nephritis in SLE.

LN is an intriguing disease and chemokine/chemokine receptor interactions are integral to its pathogenesis. In this context, our data provide evidence that chemokines produced by resident renal cells in response to ICs deposition may initially recruit mononuclear cells that undergo definite activation by local inflammatory cytokines. Thus, the invading cells release large amounts of additional molecules to recruit other mononuclear cells, leading to amplification of the initial response. Subsequent events may include downregulatory mechanisms mediated through phagocytosis of apoptotic cells as well as the defective release of anti-inflammatory cytokines such as IL-10 and TGF-β driving the ultimately extensive tissue damage. In particular, MCP-1 appears to extensively contribute to the initiating events in the pathogenesis of LN, and novel therapeutic strategies devoted to its suppression are at present in progress.

DENDRITIC CELL SUBSETS DIFFERENTLY MIGRATE TOWARD THE KIDNEY

A number of studies in human and murine SLE suggest that humoral autoimmunity exists in conjunction with abnormal T cell function, thus reflecting either an intrinsic defect or a consequence of an underlying default of APCs. DCs are the most powerful APC in exposing various antigens to T cells during the induction of an immune response. DCs circulate at low number in peripheral blood and although their functions in autoimmune diseases are not completely understood, different hypotheses have been postulated. For instance, immature progenitors might be inhibited or their differentiation into DCs might be altered, despite the fact that hematopoietic $CD34^+$ cells are not decreased in autoimmune disorders. Also, an accelerated turnover due to increased apoptosis has been described and, lastly, activated DCs might be recruited by abnormal peripheral stimuli to inflammatory tissues while their final maturation is in progress.

DCs are differentiated in relation to their antigen expression as well as the migratory behavior in response to chemotactic stimuli.[31] Both myeloid and plasmacytoid subsets show a similar pattern of chemokine receptors, but a different response to chemokine stimuli.[10] *In vitro* experiments have demonstrated an increased migration of mDCs after stimulation with MCP-1, RANTES, SDF-1, and CXCL12, whereas pDCs are only responsive to CXCL12 mediated by its cognate ligand CXCR4, despite the considerable expression of other receptors such as CCR5, CCR7, and CXCR3 that do not appear functional.[32] However, pDCs are currently found in lymphoid tissues in differential sites of inflammation and lymphocytic infiltrates, such as the inflamed nasal mucosa as well as other skin lesions correlated with SLE[33] or in inflammatory infiltrates in muscles during dermatomyositis.[34] Since circulating pDCs do not respond to the majority of inflammatory chemokines, it is conceivable that additional chemoattractants might be involved in their trafficking from peripheral blood to extra-lymphoid tissues.

IL-18, a cytokine that promotes Th1 polarization, synergizes with IL-12 in inducing IFN-γ production in T lymphocytes. It is produced by both DCs and activated macrophages. mDCs are the major producer of IL-18 though they are defective of the relative receptor (IL-18R), which, on the contrary, is largely expressed by pDCs.[12] Interestingly, IL-18 is a strong chemoattractant for pDCs in a dose-dependent manner that exceeds that induced by CXCL12 stimulation. Blocking of IL-18 by anti-IL-18 monoclonal antibody abrogates migration of pDCs, thus suggesting the specific role of IL-18–induced chemotaxis as an alternative mechanism to chemokine attraction.[12] Mature DCs produce several cytokines and promote a Th1 or Th2 immune predominance as a function of their myeloid versus plasmacytoid differentiation, respectively. Excess of IL-18 increases the allostimulatory capacity of pDCs by inducing the production of IFN-γ by stimulated T cells and by a putative switch of their differentiation pathway toward the Th1 phenotype through the modulation of pDC functions. With respect to LN, the overexpression of IL-12, IFN-γ, and IL-18 in the context of lesser production of Th2 cytokines strongly aggravates the renal disease.[35–37]

These findings led us to investigate IL-18 levels in patients with SLE with a particular focus on LN. We have recently demonstrated that serum concentration of IL-18 is significantly increased in SLE patients compared to normal controls and that

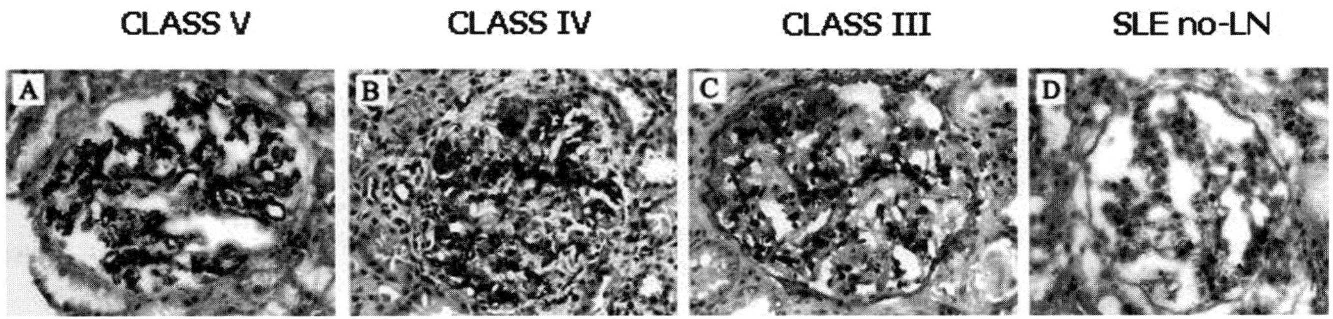

FIGURE 2. Representative pattern of glomerular expression of IL-18 in LN. A prominent expression of IL-18 (dark gray) occurred in patients with class V (**A**) and IV (**B**) of LN, whereas a mild expression in those with class III (**C**) was documented. Glomerular sections from SLE patients without LN were IL-18 negative (**D**). The mononuclear infiltrating cells represented the prevalent IL-18–positive population (**A, B,** and **C**). Original magnification ×40.

this elevation was associated with LN.[38] Analysis of peripheral Th1/Th2 cellular balance confirmed the predominance of a Th1 immune response detected as percent of IFN-γ/IL-4–positive cells in patients with LN with respect to those without nephritis. Since data from SLE patients from our study support a role for IL-18 in LN, we examined its local expression in glomeruli from patients with different histologic classes of LN.[38] We found a high prevalence of IL-18–positive cells within glomeruli from patients with active class IV and V when compared to those with class III or minor glomerular lesions. In contrast, IL-18 was absent in patients with SLE that underwent biopsy for a mild-to-moderate proteinuria without histologic evidence of glomerular damage (FIG. 2). The excess of IL-18 within nephritic glomeruli supports its pathogenic role in LN. These observations suggest that the locally produced IL-18 may promote glomerular damage and may raise the peripheral levels of IL-18 in patients with ongoing LN.

Since IL-18 may apparently drive the Th1 polarization of the immune system and influences the migration of pDCs, we reasoned that it may uniquely contribute to the propagation of inflammation in LN. Therefore, pDCs are putatively recruited at high rates from peripheral blood and migrate to sites of renal inflammation.

To examine this hypothesis in our patients with SLE, we analyzed the phenotypic characteristics of peripheral circulating DCs. mDCs were defined as $CD11c^+/CD4^+/Lin^-$ ($CD3^+/CD19^+/CD14^+$), whereas the $CD123^+/BDCA2^+/Lin^-$ cells were defined as plasmacytoid. Flow-cytometry analysis showed a decrease of both myeloid (1.91 ± 0.38%) and plasmacytoid (0.79 ± 0.19%) cells in SLE patients compared to controls (2.31 ± 0.2% versus 1.98 ± 0.3). However, as shown in FIGURE 3 (panels A and B), when SLE patients were stratified by either presence or absence of LN, we observed a remarkable reduction of circulating pDCs in those with active nephritis as compared to patients without LN or to those with inactive disease (pDCs: 0.29 ± 0.07% *versus* 1.57 ± 0.4%). The number of mDCs in LN (FIG. 3, panel D; 1.61 ± 0.11%) was slightly lower as compared to patients without LN (panel C; 2.2 ± 0.3%). Both subsets appeared highly activated with respect to intensity of staining for HLA-DR, but differed in IL-18 and IL-18R expression. In concordance with previous reports,[39] mDCs were $IL\text{-}18^+/IL\text{-}18R^-$, whereas pDCs expressed IL-18R at high levels, further supporting their potential response to IL-18. Patients with LN showed predominance of a Th1 immune response since they produced higher levels of serum IL-12, IFN-γ, and IL-18 when compared to patients without renal disease, whereas IL-4 and IL-6 levels were similar in both groups. The number of circulating pDCs was characteristically decreased in patients with active LN, thus suggesting that these cells migrate to inflammatory sites. To further examine this issue, we investigated the presence of both myeloid and plasmacytoid DCs in glomerular sections from eighteen patients with different classes of nephritis by immunohistochemistry. Two markers have been described to distinguish plasmacytoid DCs, known as BDCA2 and BDCA4 antigens. The BDCA2 molecule is identified as a type-II lectin that may be involved in ligand internalization, processing, and presentation.[40] Since pDCs are the major producer of IFN-α in peripheral blood of patients with SLE, it has been shown that, by using antibodies directed against the BDCA2 molecule, the production of IFN-α can be dramatically inhibited. Thus, BDCA2 may be used as specific marker of pDCs. We detected a preponderance of $BDCA2^+$ cells in glomeruli from SLE patients with either class IV or V of glomerulonephritis. Interestingly, renal sections from patients with class III showed fewer $BDCA2^+$ cells, whereas

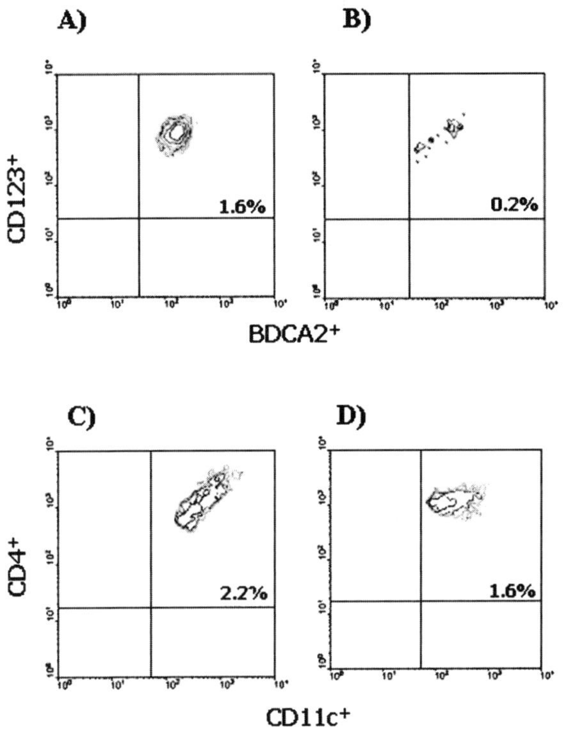

FIGURE 3. Flow cytometry analysis of circulating DCs in representative SLE patients. DC subsets were differentiated with regard to antigen specificity by flow cytometry. Both subsets were Lin$^-$ (CD3$^+$, CD14$^+$, CD19$^+$), and myeloid cells were characterized for both CD11c and CD4 expression, whereas CD123$^+$/BDCA2$^+$ cells identified the plasmacytoid subset. Circulating DCs were decreased in peripheral blood of patients with SLE compared to normal controls. pDCs were markedly reduced in patients with LN (0.29 ± 0.07%, panel **B**) when compared to those without nephritis (1.57 ± 0.4%, panel **A**), whereas the number of mDCs was slightly higher in patients with LN compared to those without renal disease (panels **D** and **C**).

almost no evidence of these cells was found in both class I and II of LN as well as in SLE with normal renal histology. In contrast, mDCs expression measured as number of CD11c-positive cells, was substantially low or absent in all class of nephritis with some positive cells observed in glomeruli from patients with class V of LN. TABLE 1 shows the comparative analysis between both BDCA2$^+$ and CD11c$^+$ as well as IL-18$^+$ cells in patients with different classes of nephritis expressed as mean number of mononuclear cells/gcs.

The presence of pDCs within nephritic glomeruli supports their pathogenic role in LN. It is conceivable that during the initiation phases of an immune response, resident activated macrophages might recruit pDCs and alter their properties in relation to the high concentrations of IL-18. Our observations support the importance of the cytokine microenvironment and its influence on DCs with subsequent induction of Th1 cytokines.

TABLE 1. Correlative analysis between IL-18–positive cells and different subsets of DCs in glomerular sections in lupus nephritis

	Class of Lupus Nephritis				
	I	II	III	IV	V
IL-18$^+$ (cells/gcs)	1.2 ± 0.2	2.7 ± 0.5	7.8 ± 1	21.5 ± 8*	14.3 ± 2*
BDCA-2$^+$ (cells/gcs)	0.8 ± 0.2	1.4 ± 0.2	5.2 ± 2**	15.1 ± 6**	11.1 ± 4**
CD11c (cells/gcs)	0	0	0	1.4 ± 0.5	2.1 ± 0.7

NOTE: LN, lupus nephritis; class of LN was based on biopsy according to WHO classification for LN. Number of glomerular infiltrating mononuclear cells (IL-18$^+$), plasmacytoid DCs (BDCA2$^+$), and myeloid DCs (CD11$^+$) are expressed as mean value/glomerular section (gcs) and indicated as mean ± SD.

*$P < 0.05$ among class of LN.

**$P < 0.05$ between BDCA2$^+$ and CD11c$^+$ cells in each class of LN.

CONCLUSIONS

Data from experimental and human SLE have provided more insight into the role of chemokines in the pathogenesis of LN. Time-course analysis of MCP-1 and MIP-1α production suggests that they are early mediators for the recruitment of activated macrophages into the kidney. Our results provide evidence that urinary elevation of MCP-1 is associated with LN and might be used for evaluating patients undergoing treatment for LN. Furthermore, LN appears to be a Th1 immune-mediated disorder characterized by high levels of circulating IL-12 and IL-18, and in our work the glomerular cells from patients with active nephritis have been proved to produce large amounts of IL-18 acting as a potent chemoattractant for IL-18R–positive cells. In the context of decreased circulating pDCs in patients with active LN and their accumulation in glomeruli, we postulate that IL-18 contributes substantially to the propagation of renal disease in SLE through its interaction with IL-18R expressed by pDCs.

REFERENCES

1. KELLEY, V.R. & R.P. WUTHRICH. 1999. Cytokines in the pathogenesis of systemic lupus erythematosus. Semin. Nephrol. **19:** 57–66.
2. HANDWERGER, B.S., V. RUS, L. DA SILVA & C.S. VIA. 1994. The role of cytokines in the immunopathogenesis of lupus. Springer Semin. Immunopathol. **16:** 153–180.
3. PEREZ DE LEMA, G., H. MAIER, E. NIETO, *et al.* 2001. Chemokine expression precedes inflammatory cell infiltration and chemokine receptor and cytokine expression during the initiation of murine lupus nephritis. J. Am. Soc. Nephrol. **12:** 1369–1382.
4. WADA, T., K. FURUICHI, C. SEGAWA-TAKAEDA, *et al.* 1999. MIP-1alpha and MCP-1 contribute to crescents and interstitial lesions in human crescentic glomerulonephritis. Kidney Int. **56:** 995–1003.
5. TESCH, G.H., S. MAIFERT, A. SCHWARTING, *et al.* 1999. Monocyte chemoattractant protein 1-dependent leukocytic infiltrates are responsible for autoimmune disease in MRL-Fas(lpr) mice. J. Exp. Med. **190:** 1813–1824.
6. WADA, T., H. YOKOYAMA, S.B. SU, *et al.* 1996. Monitoring urinary levels of monocyte chemotactic and activating factor reflects disease activity of lupus nephritis. Kidney Int. **49:** 761–767.

7. KLUTH, D.C., L.P. ERWIG & A.J. REES. 2004. Multiple facets of macrophages in renal injury. Kidney Int. **66:** 542–557.
8. BALABANIAN, K., J. COUDERC, L. BOUCHET-DELBOS, *et al.* 2003. Role of the chemokine stromal cell-derived factor 1 in autoantibody production and nephritis in murine lupus. J. Immunol. **170:** 3392–3400.
9. SCHEINECKER, C., B. ZWOLFER, M. KOLLER, *et al.* 2001. Alterations of dendritic cells in systemic lupus erythematosus: phenotypic and functional deficiencies. Arthritis Rheum. **44:** 856–865.
10. PENNA, G., M. VULCANO, S. SOZZANI & L. ADORINI. 2002. Differential migration behavior and chemokine production by myeloid and plasmacytoid dendritic cells. Hum. Immunol. **63:** 1164–1171.
11. PENNA, G., S. SOZZANI & L. ADORINI. 2001. Cutting edge: selective usage of chemokine receptors by plasmacytoid dendritic cells. J. Immunol. **167:** 1862–1866.
12. KASER, A., S. KASER, N.C. KANEIDER, *et al.* 2004. Interleukin-18 attracts plasmacytoid dendritic cells (DC2s) and promotes Th1 induction by DC2s through IL-18 receptor expression. Blood **103:** 648–655.
13. LLOYD, C.M., A.W. MINTO, M.E. DORF, *et al.* 1997. RANTES and monocyte chemoattractant protein-1 (MCP-1) play an important role in the inflammatory phase of crescentic nephritis, but only MCP-1 is involved in crescent formation and interstitial fibrosis. J. Exp. Med. **185:** 1371–1380.
14. YOSHIMURA, T., E.A. ROBINSON, S. TANAKA, *et al.* 1989. Purification and amino acid analysis of two human monocyte chemoattractants produced by phytohemagglutinin-stimulated human blood mononuclear leukocytes. J. Immunol. **142:** 1956–1962.
15. HORA, K., J.A. SATRIANO, A. SANTIAGO, *et al.* 1992. Receptors for IgG complexes activate synthesis of monocyte chemoattractant peptide 1 and colony-stimulating factor 1. Proc. Natl. Acad. Sci. USA **89:** 1745–1749.
16. NORIS, M., S. BERNASCONI, F. CASIRAGHI, *et al.* 1995. Monocyte chemoattractant protein-1 is excreted in excessive amounts in the urine of patients with lupus nephritis. Lab. Invest. **73:** 804–809.
17. BISWAS, P., F. DELFANTI, S. BERNASCONI, *et al.* 1998. Interleukin-6 induces monocyte chemotactic protein-1 in peripheral blood mononuclear cells and in the U937 cell line. Blood **91:** 258–265.
18. LU, B., B.J. RUTLEDGE & L. GU, *et al.* 1998. Abnormalities in monocyte recruitment and cytokine expression in monocyte chemoattractant protein 1-deficient mice. J. Exp. Med. **187:** 601–608.
19. TANG, W.W., M. QI & J.S. WARREN. 1996. Monocyte chemoattractant protein 1 mediates glomerular macrophage infiltration in anti-GBM Ab GN. Kidney Int. **50:** 665–671.
20. HASEGAWA, H., M. KOHNO, M. SASAKI, *et al.* 2003. Antagonist of monocyte chemoattractant protein 1 ameliorates the initiation and progression of lupus nephritis and renal vasculitis in MRL/lpr mice. Arthritis Rheum. **48:** 2555–2566.
21. TESCH, G.H., A. SCHWARTING, K. KINOSHITA, *et al.* 1999. Monocyte chemoattractant protein-1 promotes macrophage-mediated tubular injury, but not glomerular injury, in nephrotoxic serum nephritis. J. Clin. Invest. **103:** 73–80.
22. TUCCI, M., E.V. BARNES, E.S. SOBEL, *et al.* 2004. Strong association of a functional polymorphism in the monocyte chemoattractant protein 1 promoter gene with lupus nephritis. Arthritis Rheum **50:** 1842–1849.
23. DAUGHERTY, B.L. & M.S. SPRINGER. 1997. The beta-chemokine receptor genes CCR1 (CMKBR1), CCR2 (CMKBR2), and CCR3 (CMKBR3) cluster within 285 kb on human chromosome 3p21. Genomics **41:** 294–295.
24. WONG, L.M., S.J. MYERS, C.L. TSOU, *et al.* 1997. Organization and differential expression of the human monocyte chemoattractant protein 1 receptor gene: evidence for the role of the carboxyl-terminal tail in receptor trafficking. J. Biol. Chem. **272:** 1038–1045.
25. PETERS, W., M. DUPUIS & I.F. CHARO. 2000. A mechanism for the impaired IFN-gamma production in C-C chemokine receptor 2 (CCR2) knockout mice: role of CCR2 in linking the innate and adaptive immune responses. J. Immunol. **165:** 7072–7077.

26. PETERS, W., H.M. SCOTT, H.F. CHAMBERS, *et al.* 2001. Chemokine receptor 2 serves an early and essential role in resistance to Mycobacterium tuberculosis. Proc. Natl. Acad. Sci. USA **98:** 7958–7963.
27. BORING, L., J. GOSLING, M. CLEARY & I.F. CHARO. 1998. Decreased lesion formation in CCR2-/- mice reveals a role for chemokines in the initiation of atherosclerosis. Nature **394:** 894–897.
28. SMITH, M.W., M. DEAN, M. CARRINGTON, *et al.* 1997. Contrasting genetic influence of CCR2 and CCR5 variants on HIV-1 infection and disease progression. Hemophilia Growth and Development Study (HGDS), Multicenter AIDS Cohort Study (MACS), Multicenter Hemophilia Cohort Study (MHCS), San Francisco City Cohort (SFCC), ALIVE Study. Science **277:** 959–965.
29. SEGERER S., K.M. MAC, H. REGELE H., *et al.* 1999. Expression of the C-C chemokine receptor 5 in human kidney diseases. Kidney Int. **56:** 52–64.
30. NATORI, Y., M. SEKIGUCHI & Z. OU. 1997. Gene expression of CC chemokines in experimental crescentic glomerulonephritis (CGN). Clin. Exp. Immunol. **109:** 143–148.
31. BLOMBERG, S., M.L. ELORANTA, M. MAGNUSSON, *et al.* 2003. Expression of the markers BDCA-2 and BDCA-4 and production of interferon-alpha by plasmacytoid dendritic cells in systemic lupus erythematosus. Arthritis Rheum. **48:** 2524–2532.
32. PENNA, G., M. VULCANO, A. RONCARI, *et al.* 2002. Cutting edge: differential chemokine production by myeloid and plasmacytoid dendritic cells. J. Immunol. **169:** 6673-6676.
33. FARKAS, L., K. BEISKE, F. LUND-JOHANSEN, *et al.* 2001. Plasmacytoid dendritic cells (natural interferon- alpha/beta-producing cells) accumulate in cutaneous lupus erythematosus lesions. Am. J. Pathol. **159:** 237–243.
34. PAGE, G., G. CHEVREL & P. MIOSSEC. 2004. Anatomic localization of immature and mature dendritic cell subsets in dermatomyositis and polymyositis: interaction with chemokines and Th1 cytokine-producing cells. Arthritis Rheum. **50:** 199–208.
35. CALVANI N., SATOH M., CROKER B. P., *et al.* 2003. Nephritogenic autoantibodies but absence of nephritis in Il-12p35-deficient mice with pristane-induced lupus. Kidney Int. **64:** 897–905.
36. RICHARDS, H.B., M. SATOH, J.C. JENNETTE, *et al.* 2001. Interferon-gamma is required for lupus nephritis in mice treated with the hydrocarbon oil pristane. Kidney Int. **60:** 2173–2180.
37. AKAHOSHI, M., H. NAKASHIMA, Y. TANAKA Y., *et al.* 1999. Thl/Th2 balance of peripheral T helper cells in systemic lupus erythematosus. Arthritis Rheum. **42:** 1644–1648.
38. CALVANI, N., H.B. RICHARDS, M. TUCCI, *et al.* 2004. Up-regulation of IL-18 and predominance of a Th1 immune response is a hallmark of lupus nephritis. Clin. Exp. Immunol. **138:** 1711–1718.
39. DE JONG, E.C., P.L. VIEIRA, P. KALINSKI, *et al.* 2002. Microbial compounds selectively induce Th1 cell-promoting or Th2 cell-promoting dendritic cells in vitro with diverse th cell-polarizing signals. J. Immunol. **168:** 1704–1709.
40. DZIONEK, A., Y. SOHMA, J. NAGAFUNE, *et al.* 2001. BDCA-2, a novel plasmacytoid dendritic cell-specific type II C-type lectin, mediates antigen capture and is a potent inhibitor of interferon alpha/beta induction. J. Exp. Med. **194:** 1823–1834.

Cellular and Molecular Mechanisms of Regulation of Autoantibody Production in Lupus

BEVRA H. HAHN,[a] FANNY EBLING,[a] RAM R. SINGH,[a,b] RAM P. SINGH,[a] GEORGE KARPOUZAS,[a,c] AND ANTONIO LA CAVA[a]

[a]*Division of Rheumatology, David Geffen School of Medicine at the University of California Los Angeles, Los Angeles, California 91436, USA*

[b]*Department of Internal Medicine, University of Cincinnati, Cincinnati, Ohio, USA*

[c]*Harbor UCLA Medical Center, Torrance, California, USA*

ABSTRACT: The hyperactive interaction between helper T cells and autoimmune B cells in individuals predisposed to systemic lupus erythematosus (SLE) can be interrupted by induction of regulatory and suppressor T cells. Using two strategies—high dose tolerance to an immunoglobulin-derived peptide, and minigene vaccination with DNA encoding T cell epitopes presented by MHC class I molecules—our group has induced at least three types of regulatory/suppressive T cells. They include CD8$^+$ T cells that suppress helper T cells by cytokine secretion, CD8$^+$ T suppressors that kill B cells making anti-DNA antibodies, and peptide-binding CD4$^+$CD25$^+$ regulatory T cells that suppress B cells by direct cell contact. Each of these lymphocyte subsets suppresses anti-DNA antibody production and delays the onset of nephritis in BWF1 lupus-prone mice. Patients with SLE have amino acid sequences similar to those from murine anti-DNA antibodies used in these studies, and at similar locations in the VH regions of anti-DNA immunoglobulins. Therefore, strategies described here might ultimately be useful in therapy of the human disease.

KEYWORDS: systemic lupus erythematosus; CD8$^+$ T cells; regulatory T cells; suppressor T cells

INTRODUCTION

Because systemic lupus erythematosus (SLE) depends on the production of autoantibodies by B cells driven by helper T cells—a process that occurs in a milieu of permissive cytokines, chemokines, and sex hormones influencing interactions between cell surface receptors and their ligands—interruptions of any of these circuits are likely to alter disease. Our laboratory has focused on interrupting helper T cell–B cell interactions in the (NZB/NZW)F1 (BWF1) murine lupus model via induction

Address for correspondence: Bevra H. Hahn, M.D., Professor of Medicine, UCLA Division of Rheumatology, 1000 Veteran Ave., Los Angeles, CA 90095. Voice: 310-825-7992; fax: 310-206-9707.
bhahn@mednet.ucla.edu

**Ann. N.Y. Acad. Sci. 1051: 433–441 (2005). © 2005 New York Academy of Sciences.
doi: 10.1196/annals.1361.085**

of immune tolerance to immunoglobulin-based peptides, which calls up regulatory and suppressive T cells.

CONTROL MECHANISMS THAT PREVENT AUTOREACTIVITY IN HEALTHY INDIVIDUALS

In recent years there has been great interest in the role of regulatory/suppressive T cells in preventing and controlling autoimmunity.[1] There are several natural mechanisms for controlling autoreactivity. Many T cells with high avidity for self-antigens are deleted in the thymus (negative selection). T cells with relatively low avidity for self are likely to enter the peripheral immune system (positive selection), where they are closely regulated by peripheral tolerance mechanisms in healthy individuals. Although such cells have the potential upon contact with self or cross-reactive antigens to expand, activate, and cause autoreactivity ultimately leading to autoimmune disease, several inactivating mechanisms exist to prevent this. The mechanisms of peripheral tolerance include (a) activation-induced death, which occurs in T and B lymphocytes that receive very strong activating signals, capable of activating Fas/FasL interactions or tumor necrosis factor receptor (TNFR)-family death receptors; (b) anergy—a state in which T and B cells cannot secrete cytokines or immunoglobulins after activation, particularly if they receive signals only through their T cell receptor (TCR) or B cell receptor (BCR) without second signals through CD40/CD40 ligand (CD40L) pathways or CD28/CD80:CD86; (c) cytokine production that suppresses autoimmunity, including IL-4, IL-10, and transforming growth factor (TGF); and (d) active suppression by antigen-specific T cells.[1,2] Our work has focused on this last mechanism, the induction of T cells that actively suppress autoimmunity.

T CELLS INVOLVED IN SUPPRESSION

T cells that can suppress T and/or B cells include NK T cells, $CD4^+CD25^+$ regulatory T cells, and $CD8^+$ suppressors (TABLE 1). Many $CD8^+$ T cells suppress responses in a largely antigen-nonspecific manner, but recent data have suggested that some subsets can operate via mechanisms that involve antigen recognition.[1,3] The induction of $CD8^+$ suppressor/effectors from precursor cells requires interaction with certain $CD4^+$ T cell subsets, which in certain cases can be activated T cells expressing Qa-1 (an MHC class Ib molecule that can present autologous or exogenous peptides to $CD8^+$ T cells).[1,4,5] In turn, the target cells downregulated by $CD8^+$ suppressors probably include $CD4^+Qa\text{-}1^+$ antigen-specific CD4 recognized by the TCR of the $CD8^+$ suppressors.[6] There are several different types and/or mechanisms of action of $CD8^+$ T cell suppressor/effectors (Ts). These include cytotoxic T cells that require cell–cell contact, cells that secrete cytokines (TGF-β, interferon [INF]-γ) that induce apoptosis or death in their targets, and Ts cells that interact with antigen-presenting cells (APCs) to render them "tolerogenic," that is, capable of producing anergy in $CD4^+$ helper T cells and of inducing $CD4^+CD25^-$ T regulatory cells.[3,6–8] There are examples of two types of $CD8^+$ Ts cells protecting against SLE-like disease in NZB/NZW F1 (BWF1) lupus-prone mice, as discussed below. Further-

TABLE 1. Characteristics of T cells that control autoimmunity

Cell Types	Characteristics	Pathways of Effector Functions
NK T Cells	Coexpress NK markers and TCR. Scant in blood, abundant in certain tissues such as liver. Recognize CD1-restricted glycolipid antigens. Usually $CD4^+$ and $CD4^-CD8^-$. Centain subsets are regulatory, including those with surface Vα24-Jα18 TCR in humans. Participate in tumor rejection, early response to infections and downregulation of autoimmunity.[29–31]	1. Secretion of IFN-γ, Il-4, TGF-β, IL-10. 2. May be cytotoxic for immature immune cells. 3. May regulate autoimmunity by supporting immune deviation in $CD4^+$ T cells from Th1 to Th2.
$CD4^+CD25^+$ T cells	Suppress self-reactive T or B cells. Educated in the thymus. Prevent "natural" autoimmunity (organ-specific and systemic) induced by other $CD4^+$ T cells. Other surface molecules include CD45RBlow, CTLA4 and GITR, all of which are induced by activation but may be present constitutively on some Tr cells. Some Tr cells express membrane-bound TGF-β. Some express Toll-like receptors that allow antigen non-specific activation in innate immunity. Tr cells proliferate poorly. When activated they express high levels of the transcription factor Foxp3, which represses transcription factors that regulate T cell activation.	1. Secretion of TGF-β, IL-10, IL-4, IFN-γ. 2. Suppression of $CD4^+CD25^-$ proliferation and of B cells may be contact dependent and may be mediated by lap-TGF-β, GITR, and/or CTLA4. 3. Suppressive effects may depend on Foxp3.
$CD8^+$ cytotoxic/ inhibitory T (Ti) cells	Antigen-specific $CD8^+$ T cells can kill target immune cells. Naive cytotoxic $CD8^+$ cells are not effectors; they express CD45RA. Memory $CD8^+$ T cells are effectors and express CD45RO. When antigen-primed, $CD8^+$ Ti cells regulate $CD4^+$ T cells activated by the same antigen, this may depend on CD8 TCR recognition of antigen presented by Qa-1 molecules expressed on activated $CD4^+$ T cells. Superantigen also induces suppressor $CD8^+$ cells through the Qa-1 restriction MHC element presented by $CD4^+$ T cells.	1. Direct cytotoxicity toward T and B cells and APCs. This may be mediated by release of Ca^{2+}, perforin, and granzyme polarized toward the target after $CD8^+$TCR recognize antigen, or by activation of apoptosis in the target via Fas/FasL receptors. 2. Cytokine secretion: TGF-β, IL-10, IFN-γ, TNF-α.

more, recent experiments in our laboratory have shown that as BWF1 mice age, their peripheral $CD8^+$ T cells become increasingly defective.[9] $CD8^+$ T cell populations in these mice do not expand as dramatically as do $CD4^+$ cells, and only small proportions of $CD8^+$ T cells express activation and memory surface markers. In contrast, such markers are found on the majority of BWF1 $CD4^+$ T cells. When activated, significantly higher proportions of BWF1 CD8$^+$ T cells from older mice undergo apoptosis compared with CD8$^+$ T cells from young, healthy BWF1 mice or other nonlupus murine strains. Therefore, abnormal elimination of activated CD8$^+$ suppressor cells probably contributes to the failure of BWF1 mice to regulate autoantibody production and to their predisposition to SLE.

Murine CD4$^+$ T cells contain not only helper cells and suppressor-inducers, but also direct suppressors.[1,10–14] These cells, now termed "regulatory T cells" (Tr cells) were first discovered by Sakaguchi *et al.* in thymectomized mice that developed organ-specific autoimmunity.[10] Tr cells are CD4$^+$CD25$^+$CTLA4$^+$ and depend on the DNA-binding Foxp3 gene to exert suppressive activity.[13,14] They are educated in the thymus and then migrate to the periphery. The target of these Tr cells in some experimental systems is other CD4$^+$ T cells (CD4$^+$CD25$^-$), which cannot proliferate in the presence of Tr; data from our laboratory (discussed below) suggests that some Tr cells also directly suppress B cells. Their mechanism of action is complex and differs in different systems. In some experimental systems (particularly colitis and diabetes) suppression depends at least in part on the CTLA4 surface molecule;[14–16] the "suppressive" cytokines IL-10 and TGF-β may also be involved.[16] In other systems, including the BWF1 mouse, interactions between the target cells and membrane-bound TGF-β or glucocorticoid-induced TNFR-related gene (GITR) on Tr cells have been implicated.[17,18]

POTENTIAL IMPORTANCE OF REGULATORY/SUPPRESSIVE T CELLS IN HUMAN SLE

Although Tr and CD8$^+$ Ts cells were originally defined in mice, and much of the information discussed above was derived from studies in mice, similar cells exist in the peripheral lymphoid compartments and circulation of healthy humans, as well as in abnormal human tissues (inflamed synovium, tumor masses, virally infected tissues).[19–22] In patients with SLE, one study reported that the numbers of circulating CD4$^+$CD25$^+$ T cells during periods of disease activity are significantly lower than in normal individuals.[21] Another group of investigators has shown that during periods of disease activity, CD8$^+$ T cells in the circulation of SLE patients have impaired ability to suppress autologous CD4$^+$ T cell proliferation; this proliferation returns toward normal when disease is controlled.[22,23] Impairing the function of IFN-γ and IL-6 impairs the suppressive effects of SLE CD8$^+$ Ts cells, and IL-10 is required to generate Ts cells from CD8$^+$CD28$^-$ precursors. Because Tr and Ts cells can control autoimmunity, we performed several interventions in lupus-prone mice to establish the *in vivo* utility of this approach to treatment.

INDUCTION OF REGULATORY/SUPPRESSIVE T CELLS TO CONTROL LUPUS-LIKE DISEASE

Regulatory/suppressor CD4$^+$ and CD8$^+$ T cells become defective in unmanipulated BWF1 mice as they age, probably permitting sustained helper T/B interactions that drive disease.[9] We developed strategies to induce Tr and Ts cells. To induce both, we administered intravenously high doses of a tolerogenic peptide, pCON-

SENSUS (pCONS), to young, healthy BWF1 females. Spleen cells were harvested one week later; different populations were studied for their ability to influence autoantibody production and clinical lupus-like nephritis. The pCONS peptide is an artificial 15-mer peptide based on amino acid sequences in the first hypervariable/second constant region of the V_H region of a BWF1 monoclonal IgG antibody to DNA. Similar sequences are found in the same regions of human anti-DNA monoclonal antibodies (mAbs) from SLE patients.[24] We have previously shown that monthly administration of pCONS, either to young mice or mice with established nephritis, prolongs survival by significantly delaying or suppressing autoantibodies and nephritis.[25]

CD4$^+$ Tr cells are induced by this tolerance regimen. As shown in FIGURE 1, these Tr cells suppress anti-DNA antibody production.[17] In these experiments,

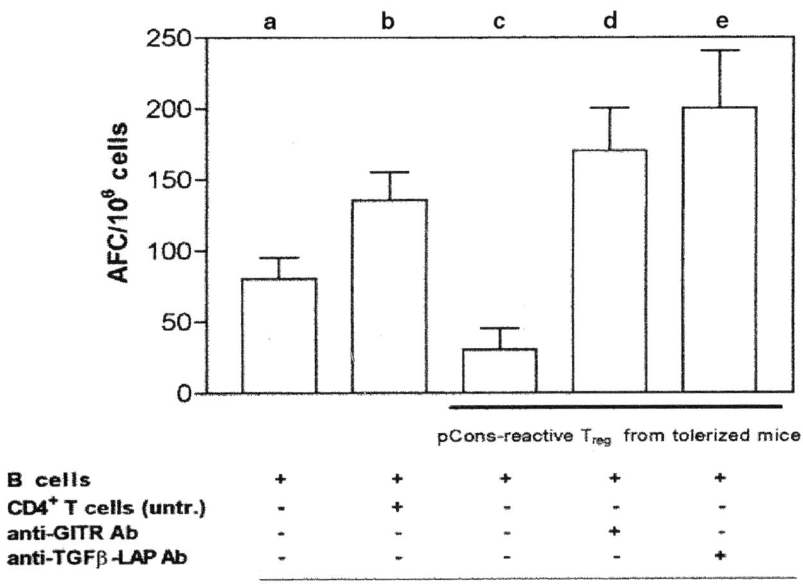

FIGURE 1. CD4$^+$CD25$^+$ regulatory T cells from tolerized NZB/NZW F1 mice suppress the ability of syngeneic B cells to synthesize IgG anti-DNA antibody *in vitro*, and that suppression depends upon membrane-associated TGF and/or GITR. 1×10^5 B cells from spleens of unmanipulated old BWF1 females were cocultured with 1×10^6 CD4$^+$ splenic helper T cells from naive young mice and 1×10^6 pCONS-binding CD4$^+$CD25$^+$ spleen cells from young BWF1 mice tolerized with 1 mg pCONS i.v. one week prior to harvest. Various cell combinations are shown on the *x*-axis, as well as inhibition with anti-GITR or anti-TGF-β-LAP antibody. Antibody-forming cells (AFC) per 10^6 B cells are shown on the *y*-axis. Information below the graphic indicates the contents of cultures labeled **a, b, c, d, e.** CD4$^+$CD25$^+$ T cells were selected by binding with a soluble dimer of I-Ed and pCONS. Note that in **c**, AFC formation is suppressed compared with **b** ($P < 0.0004$), and the suppression is abolished by inhibiting either GITR (**d**) or TGF-lap (**e**). Addition of CTLA4-Ig to the culture to inhibit surface CTLA4 on Tr cells did not inhibit suppression (data not shown). Statistical analysis by ANOVA showed that the following comparisons were significantly different at $P < 0.0004$: **a** vs. **b**, **a** vs. **c**, **b** vs. **c**, **c** vs. **d**, **c** vs. **e**.

$CD4^+CD25^+$ T cells isolated from spleens of BWF1 mice one week following injection of pCONS were divided into peptide-binding and nonbinding populations (using labeled soluble dimers of I-Ed containing pCONS to identify binders). The suppression was confined to the peptide-binding $CD4^+CD25^+$ cells, and they required cell-cell contact to function. Their targets were B cells. Tr cells obtained *ex vivo* from tolerized mice prevented B cells from unmanipulated BWF1 mice from secreting immunoglobulin (including anti-DNA antibodies) *in vitro*. This regulation was interrupted by adding to B + Tr cell culture antibodies to membrane-bound TGF-β (LAP-TGF-β) or antibodies to GITR. In contrast, CTLA4 immunoglobulin did not impair the regulation. As expected, the pCONS-binding Tr cells expressed Foxp3.

We have also characterized the $CD8^+$ Ts cells found in spleen cells one week after a single injection of 1 mg of pCONS (Ref. 26 and manuscript in preparation). These cells suppress anti-DNA antibody production and nephritis *in vivo*, and anti-DNA antibody production *in vitro* (FIG. 2). They do not depend on cell-cell contact, but suppress primarily by production of TGF-β. Preliminary work suggests that the suppressive capacity of these $CD8^+$ Ts cells also involves expression of Foxp3. These Ts cells are similar to those induced by repeatedly immunizing normal, non–lupus-prone mice with heavy chains or V_H peptides from BWF1 anti-DNA autoantibodies.[27] In immunized normal mice, anti-DNA antibodies can be induced by such immunizations, and proteinuria occurs. However, the autoimmune state is short-lived, and disappears in conjunction with the appearance of both Tr and Ts cells. Similar to the experiments in pCONS-induced tolerance the $CD8^+$ Ts cells in those experiments suppressed anti-DNA antibody production and nephritis via secretion of TGF-β.

In a second method of inducing $CD8^+$ Ts cells in BWF1 mice,[7] mice were inoculated with DNA encoding each of three MHC class I–binding peptides found in a

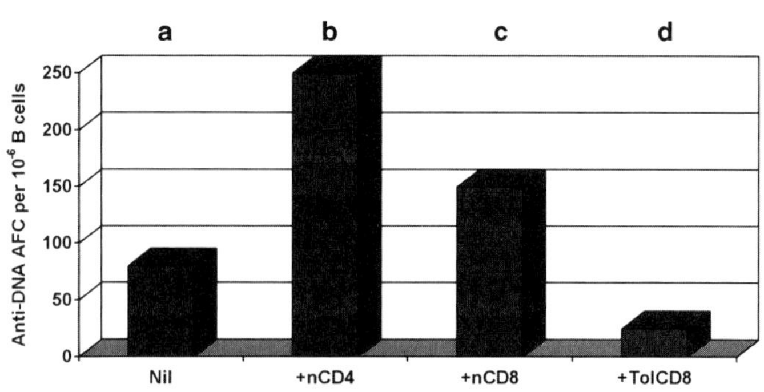

FIGURE 2. $CD8^+$ T cells from BWF1 mice tolerized with 1 mg pCONS suppress anti-DNA antibody production by syngeneic B cells. Data shown are representative of four experiments. Cultures contain 1×10^5 B cells from spleens of unmanipulated old BWF1 females, and pCONS. $CD4^+$ T cells are from unmanipulated young BWF1 mice and give help for the B cell production of anti-DNA antibody (**b**). To $CD4^+$ B are added $CD8^+$ cells from unmanipulated young syngeneic mice (**c**), or $CD8^+$ cells harvested from spleens one week after administration of pCONS (**d**). CD8 to CD4 ratios are 1:1. Note that the tolerized $CD8^+$ T cells suppress anti-DNA antibody production 10-fold (compare **d** vs. **b**).

wild murine antibody to DNA (A6.1 from a nephritic BWF1 mouse). The treatment induced CD8$^+$ Ts cells that were cytotoxic for anti-DNA antibody–producing B cells with surface immunoglobulin (sIg) containing the epitopes against which the CD8$^+$ Ts were targeted. This strategy was effective in delaying the appearance of anti-DNA antibodies and nephritis, and in prolonging survival.

DISCUSSION

In recent years, the importance of regulatory CD4$^+$ Tr cells and suppressive CD8$^+$ Ts cells in preventing autoimmunity in normal individuals has been recognized. In our hands, two methods have been effective in inducing Tr and Ts cells that can suppress anti-DNA antibodies and nephritis in BWF1 mice. The methods include a peptide-based tolerizing regimen and DNA vaccination. Both methods use the principle that autoantibodies to DNA, the hallmark of SLE, contain amino acid sequences that are T cell epitopes. We and others have identified several regions in the V_H region of both murine and human autoantibodies to DNA that induce T cells to proliferate or secrete cytokines.[24,25,28] These sequences are similar in location and in amino acid content in different anti-DNA antibodies from patients of different ethnic backgrounds and from mice of different strains. Individuals predisposed to SLE may have biased selection of B cells bearing surface immunoglobulin containing these amino acid sequences.

To induce effector Ts cells, we induced immune tolerance in young BWF1 mice by intravenous administration of high doses of an artificial peptide, pCONS, that contains amino acid sequences that bind the MHC class II molecule I-Ed and induce proliferation in BWF1 T cells;[25,28] pCONS contains at least one epitope that binds the MHC class I molecule Kd.[7] Thus, administration of pCONS as tolerogen can induce both CD4$^+$ Tr and CD8$^+$ Ts cells. One of these sets, the CD8$^+$ effectors that help suppress antibody production, becomes defective spontaneously in BWF1 mice near the time of disease onset.[9] However, when treated with our regimens, the animals are perfectly capable of raising both Tr and at least two types of CD8$^+$ Ts cells that downregulate autoantibody production and delay the onset of nephritis. Similar strategies might be used to develop therapeutic interventions in patients with SLE or other autoantibody-mediated diseases.

ACKNOWLEDGMENTS

This work was supported by The National Institutes of Health (AI/AR 46776 to B.H.H., AR47322 and DK69282 to R.R.S.), the Arthritis Foundation (Southern California Chapter), the Lupus Foundation of America, the Arthritis National Research Foundation, the Dorough Foundation, the Paxson Family, the California Community Foundation, The Bertram Maltz Laboratory, and Jeanne Rappaport.

REFERENCES

1. JIANG, H. & L. CHESS. 2004. An integrated model of immunoregulation mediated by regulatory T cell subsets. Adv. Immunol. **83:** 253–288.

2. KUCHROO, V.K., A.C. ANDERSON, H. WALDNER, *et al.* 2002. T cell response in experimental autoimmune encephalomyelitis (EAE): role of self and cross-reactive antigens in shaping, tuning and regulating the autopathogenic T cell repertoire. Annu. Rev. Immunol. **20:** 101–123.
3. SCOTTO, L., A.J. NAIYER, S. GALLUZZO, *et al.* 2004. Overlap between molecular markers expressed by naturally occurring CD4+CD25+ regulatory T cells and antigen specific CD4+CD25+ and CD8+CD28– suppressor cells. Hum. Immunol. **65:** 1297–1306.
4. CONNOLLY, D.J., L.A. COTTERILL, R.A. HEDERER, *et al.* 1993. A cDNA clone encoding the mouse Qa-1a histocompatibility antigen and proposed structure of the putative peptide binding site. J. Immunol. **151:** 6089–6098.
5. JIANG, H. & L. CHESS. 2000. The specific regulation of immune responses by CD8+ T cells restricted by the MHC class Ib molecule QA-1. Annu. Rev. Immunol. **18:** 185–216.
6. JIANG, H., S. CURRAN, E. RUIZ-VAZQUEZ, *et al.* 2003. Regulatory CD8+ T cells finetune the myelin basic protein-reactive T cell receptor V beta repertoire during experimental autoimmune encephalomyelitis. Proc. Natl. Acad. Sci. USA **100:** 8378–8383.
7. FAN, G.C. & R.R. SINGH. 2002. Vaccination with minigenes encoding V(H)-derived major histocompatibility complex class I-binding epitopes activates cytotoxic T cells that ablate autoantibody-producing B cells and inhibit lupus. J. Exp. Med. **196:** 731–741.
8. SUCIU-FOCA, N., J.S. MANAVALAN, L. SCOTTO, *et al.* 2005. Molecular characterization of allospecific T suppressor and tolerogenic dendritic cells: review. Int. Immunopharmacol. **5:** 7–11.
9. KARPOUZAS, G.A., R.R. SINGH, F.M. EBLING, *et al.* 2004. Defects in CD8+ cell inhibitory function characterize lupus-prone but not non-autoimmune mice. Eur. J. Immunol. **34:** 2489–2499.
10. SAKAGUCHI, S., K. FUKUMA, K. KURIBAYASHI & T. MASUDA. 1985. Organ-specific autoimmune diseases induced in mice by elimination of T cell subset. I. Evidence for the active participation of T cells in natural self-tolerance; deficit of a T cell subset as a possible cause of autoimmune diseases. J. Exp. Med. **161:** 72–87.
11. SAKAGUCHI, S. 2000. Regulatory T cells: key controller of immunologic self-tolerance. Cell **101:** 455–458.
12. SHEVACH, E.M. 2000. Regulatory cells in autoimmunity. Annu. Rev. Immunol. **18:** 423–449.
13. HORI, S., T. NOMURA & S. SAKAGUCHI. 2003. Control of regulatory T cell development by the transcription factor Foxp3. Science **299:** 1057–1061.
14. SHEVACH, E.M. 2002. CD4+CD25+ suppressor T cells: more questions than answers. Nat. Rev. Immunol. **2:** 389–400.
15. BODEN, E., Q. TANG, H. BOUR-JORDAN, *et al.* 2003. The role of CD28 and CTLA4 in the function and homeostasis of CD4+CD25+ regulatory T cells. Novartis Found. Symp. **252:** 55–63.
16. LIU, H., B. HU, D. XU & F.Y. LIEW, *et al.* 2003. CD4+CD25+ regulatory T cells cure murine colitis: the role of IL-10, TGF-beta and CTLA4. J. Immunol. **171:** 5012–5017.
17. LA CAVA, A., F.M. EBLING & B.H. HAHN. 2004. Ig-reactive CD4+CD25+ T cells from tolerized (New Zealand Black × New Zealand White)F1 mice suppress in vitro production of antibodies to DNA. J. Immunol. **173:** 3542–3548.
18. STEPHENS, G.L., R.S. MCHUGH, M.J. WHITTERS, *et al.* 2004. Engagement of glucocorticoid-induced TNFR family-related receptor on effector T cells by its ligand mediates resistance to suppression by CD4+CD25+ T cells. J. Immunol. **173:** 5008–5020.
19. VAN AMELSFORT, J.M., K.M. JACOBS, J.W. BIJLSMA, *et al.* 2004. CD4(+)CD25(+) regulatory T cells in rheumatoid arthritis: differences in the presence, phenotype, and function between peripheral blood and synovial fluid. Arthritis Rheum. **50:** 2775–2785.
20. MOTTONEN, M, J. HEIKKINEN, L. MUSTONEN, *et al.* 2005. $CD4^+CD25^+$ T cells with the phenotypic and functional characteristics of regulatory T cells are enriched in the synovial fluid of patients with rheumatoid arthritis. Clin. Exp. Immunol. **140:** 360–367.
21. CRISPIN, J.C., A. MARTINEZ, & J. ALCOCER-VARELA. 2003. Quantification of regulatory T cells in patients with systemic lupus erythematosus. J. Autoimmunity **21:** 273–276.

22. Filaci, G., S. Bacilieri, M. Fravega, *et al.* 2001. Impairment of CD8+ T suppressor cell function in patients with active systemic lupus erythematosus. J. Immunol. **166:** 6452–6457.
23. Filaci, G., M. Fravega, S. Negrini, *et al.* 2004. Nonantigen specific CD8+ T suppressor lymphocytes originate from CD8+CD28– T cells and inhibit both T-cell proliferation and CTL function. Hum. Immunol. **65:** 142–156.
24. Kalsi, J.K., J. Grossman, J. Kim, *et al.* 2004. Peptides from antibodies to DNA elicit cytokine release from peripheral blood mononuclear cells from patients with systemic lupus erythematosus: relation of cytokine pattern to disease duration. Lupus **13:** 490–500.
25. Hahn, B.H., R.R. Singh, W.K. Wong, *et al.* 2001. Treatment with a consensus peptide based on amino acid sequences in autoantibodies prevents T cell activation by autoantigens and delays disease onset in murine lupus. Arthritis Rheum. **44:** 432–441.
26. Singh, R.R., F.M. Ebling, D.A. Albuquerque, *et al.* 2002. Induction of autoantibody production is limited in nonautoimmune mice. J. Immunol. **169:** 587–594.
27. Hahn, B.H., R.R. Singh, B.P. Tsao & F.M. Ebling. 1997. Peptides from Vh regions of antibodies to DNA activate T cell help to upregulate autoantibody synthesis. Lupus **6:** 330–332.
28. Singh, R.P., F. Ebling, D. Elashoff, *et al.* 2004. Genome analysis in whole blood cells, CD4 and CD8 cell subsets in tolerized with a peptide (pCONS) vs non-tolerized animals in experimental mouse model (BWF1) of SLE [abstract]. Arthritis Rheum. **50:** S418.
29. Yang, J.Q., A.K. Singh, M.T. Wilson, *et al.* 2003. Immunoregulatory role of CD1d in the hydrocarbon oil-induced model of lupus nephritis. J. Immunol. **171:** 2142–2153.
30. Yang, J.Q., V. Saxena, H. Xu, *et al.* 2003. Repeated alpha-galactosylceramide administration results in expansion of NK T cells and alleviates inflammatory dermatitis in MRL-lpr/lpr mice. J. Immunol. **171:** 4439–4446.
31. Yang, J.Q., T. Chun, H. Liu, *et al.* 2004. CD1d deficiency exacerbates inflammatory dermatitis in MRL-lpr/lpr mice. Eur. J. Immunol. **34:** 1723–1732.

The Role of Innate and Adaptive Immunity to Oxidized Low-Density Lipoprotein in the Development of Atherosclerosis

KAZUKO KOBAYASHI,[a] LUIS R. LOPEZ,[b] YEHUDA SHOENFELD,[c] AND EIJI MATSUURA[a]

[a]*Department of Cell Chemistry, Okayama University Graduate School of Medicine and Dentistry, Okayama, Japan*

[b]*Corgenix, Inc., Westminster, Colorado, USA*

[c]*Department of Medicine B, Sheba Medical Center, Tel-Hashomer, Israel*

ABSTRACT: Atherosclerosis is a chronic inflammatory process of the arterial wall associated with systemic and local immune responses to various antigens, oxidized low-density lipoprotein (oxLDL) being the most significant. Both IgM and IgG antibodies to oxLDL are produced during atherosclerosis. Some studies have shown that elevated levels of antibody to oxLDL correlate with the degree of atherosclerosis. Other studies reported that immunization of experimental animals with oxLDL induces high levels of antibodies to oxLDL, with decreased atherosclerosis, suggesting that the immune response to oxLDL may be antiatherogenic. The accelerated development of atherosclerosis has been observed in patients with systemic autoimmune diseases. In patients with antiphospholipid syndrome (APS), β2-glycoprotein I (β2GPI) is a major antigenic target for anticardiolipin antibodies (aCLs). We recently reported that oxLDL interacts with β2GPI via oxLDL-derived specific ligands, such as 7-ketocholesteryl-9-caboxynonanoate (oxLig-1) to form complexes. *In vitro*, anti-β2GPI autoantibodies bind to oxLDL/β2GPI complexes that are actively taken up by macrophages via Fcγ receptors. Circulating oxLDL/β2GPI complexes were detected in patients with systemic lupus erythematosus (SLE) and APS, at higher levels than in healthy individuals. Autoantibodies against these complexes were also present; however, IgG anti-oxLig-1/β2GPI antibody levels in SLE patients with APS were significantly higher than those in SLE patients without APS and those in healthy individuals.

KEYWORDS: oxidized low-density lipoprotein; antiphospholipid syndrome; β2-glycoprotein I

INTRODUCTION

Atherosclerosis is a major health concern of worldwide importance. Traditional risk factors for atherosclerosis include hypercholesterolemia, hypertension, diabetes,

Address for correspondence: Eiji Matsuura, Ph.D., Associate Professor, Department of Cell Chemistry, Okayama University Graduate School of Medicine and Dentistry, 2-5-1 Shikata-cho, Okayama 700-8558, Japan. Voice: +81-86-235-7402; fax: +81-86-235-7404.
eijimatu@md.okayama-u.ac.jp

Ann. N.Y. Acad. Sci. 1051: 442–454 (2005). © 2005 New York Academy of Sciences.
doi: 10.1196/annals.1361.086

and smoking, but newer inflammatory and immunologic mechanisms are emerging as relevant factors not only for the initiation but for the progression of atherosclerotic lesions. In the last few years, much experimental evidence has been accumulated indicating that oxidation of low-density lipoproteins (LDL) plays a central role in early proatherogenic events that promote the formation of macrophage-derived foam cells.[1–3]

Oxidized LDL (oxLDL) is highly immunogenic. Oxidation of LDL generates a variety of oxidatively modified lipids and proteins that may activate the immune system. Autoantibodies to specific epitopes of oxLDL occur in plasma and may contribute to atherogenesis in humans and animals.[4,5] The potential role of these antibodies in the atherogenic process is complex and remains unresolved. A positive correlation between titers of anti-oxLDL antibodies and the extent of atherosclerosis was found in some studies,[6] whereas other studies showed that immunization of animals with oxLDL induced high levels of antibodies to oxLDL with decreased atherosclerosis.[7]

Accelerated atherosclerosis has been detected in patients with prototypic systemic autoimmune disease such as systemic lupus erythematosus (SLE). Some patients with antiphospholipid syndrome (APS) also develop premature atherosclerosis in the absence of other risk factors. A contributing role of autoimmunity in the development of atherosclerosis has been suggested. APS is characterized by the presence of a group of heterogenous antiphospholipid antibodies, such as anticardiolipin antibodies (aCL) and lupus anticoagulants (LA), and by the occurrence of thromboembolic complications in the arterial and/or venous vasculatures. The exact mechanism(s) by which aCL, LA, and/or other antiphospholipid antibodies promote thrombosis is not completely understood. However, it is now widely agreed that β2-glycoprotein I (β2GPI) plays a central role in APS, and, more important, represents a major antigenic target for antiphospholipid antibodies.[8–12]

In this paper, we review the possible role of autoantibodies (anti-oxLDL and other autoantibodies, i.e., anti-β2GPI) in the atherogenic process of autoimmune diseases.

ANTIPHOSPHOLIPID SYNDROME AND OXIDIZED LDL

Large amounts of oxLDL accumulate in atherosclerotic lesions that colocalize with β2GPI and immunoreactive lymphocytes.[13] It has also been reported that aCL antibodies from patients with SLE cross-react with malondialdehyde (MDA)-modified LDL,[14] and that anti-β2GPI antibodies are associated with arterial thrombosis.[15,16] These findings further indicate the participation of antiphospholipid antibodies in atherogenesis. More recently, we have demonstrated that oxLDL binds to β2GPI, and that these complexes (oxLDL/β2GPI) can be found in the blood stream of patients with various autoimmune and chronic inflammatory diseases, such as SLE, APS, chronic renal disease, and diabetes mellitus, as well as in some patients with acute myocardial infarction.[17]

IgG antibodies to oxLDL/β2GPI were detected only in SLE and APS patients and were strongly associated with arterial thrombosis. Further, immune complexes containing oxLDL, β2GPI, and IgG anti-β2GPI antibodies have also been detected in SLE and APS patients.[17] Our recent *in vitro* experiments showed that oxLDL/β2GPI complexes are internalized by macrophages via an anti-β2GPI antibody–mediated phagocytosis.[17–20] Thus, circulating IgG immune complexes containing oxLDL and β2GPI may be atherogenic.

OXIDATION OF LDL AND ATHEROGENESIS

The causal relationship between atherosclerosis and blood cholesterol has been established. The cholesterol that accumulates in macrophage-derived foam cells is derived from circulating lipoproteins, mainly from the proatherogenic oxLDL.[2–3] Native (unmodified) LDL and, perhaps, minimally modified LDL are removed from circulation by LDL receptors located on endothelial and monocyte-macrophage cells. These LDL receptors are downregulated to prevent excessive intracellular lipid accumulation. By contrast, oxLDL is removed at a higher rate by macrophage scavenger receptors. Scavenger receptors are not downregulated, making possible an excessive intracellular accumulation of oxLDL that leads to foam cell formation.

Several studies have demonstrated an inflammatory component in atherosclerosis that involves the dysregulation of cholesterol homeostasis by aberrant interactions between lipid-modulating elements and mediators of inflammation.[21] More recently, the active participation of antibodies in atherogenesis has been proposed.[22]

OxLDL plays an important pathogenic role in early events leading to atherosclerosis,[3,23] acting as a proinflammatory chemotactic agent for macrophages and T lymphocytes,[24] being cytotoxic for endothelial cells, and stimulating the release of soluble inflammatory molecules. In addition, oxLDL has been found in both human and rabbit atherosclerotic lesions.[25] Oxidation of LDL may generate immunogenic epitopes capable of producing autoantibodies. These autoantibodies have been demonstrated in patients with autoimmune disorders, such as SLE and APS.[6,14,26] Further, β2GPI has been localized with oxLDL in human atherosclerotic lesions by immunohistochemical staining,[13] a finding that suggests a role of β2GPI (and antiphospholipid antibodies, i.e., anti-β2GPI antibodies) in atherosclerosis.

ANTI-oxLDL ANTIBODIES IN EXPERIMENTAL MODELS

Oxidation of LDL generates a variety of oxidatively modified lipids and proteins that present highly immunogenic neoepitopes. In atherosclerosis-prone apoE-deficient (apoE$^{-/-}$) mice, the autoimmune response to epitopes of oxLDL is vigorous. Palinski and colleagues isolated a panel of B cell hybridomas with specificity for oxLDL neoepitopes from the spleens of diseased apoE$^{-/-}$ mice that had not received experimental immunization or *in vitro* stimulation.[27] These produced IgM autoantibodies, termed "EO" antibodies, that bound strongly to MDA-LDL and Cu^{2+}-oxLDL. These antibodies specifically bound to the phosphorylcholine (PC) moiety of oxidized PC-containing phospholipids, such as 1-palmitoyl-2-(5-oxovaleroly)-*sn*-glycerol-3-phosphorylcholine (POVPC), an oxidation product derived from 1-palmitoyl-2-arachidonyl-*sn*-glycero-3-phosphorylcholine (PAPC). However, EO antibodies did not bind to the PC moiety of nonoxidized phospholipids, as found in native LDL, even though they contain the same PC moiety. The genes encoding the antigen-binding site of EO6 antibody were found to be genetically and structurally identical to those of T15 antibodies.[28] T15 is a classic antiphospholylcholine B cell clone, and protects against common infectious pathogens, including pneumococci. The EO antibodies blocked the binding and degradation of oxLDL by macrophages *in vitro*.[29]

Because antibodies may protect against or neutralize pathogens and immunogens,[30,31] humoral immunity to oxLDL can reduce the incidence of atherosclerosis. The protective role of T cell–dependent antibody has been demonstrated in rabbits and mice immunized with oxLDL. The reduced atherosclerosis correlated with the levels of immunoglobulin G (IgG) anti-oxLDL antibodies.[30–33] Transfer of B cells from atherosclerotic apoE$^{-/-}$ mice to young, disease-prone apoE$^{-/-}$ mice appeared to protect the latter from developing advanced disease. Protection to a lesser extent was observed when B cells from young apoE$^{-/-}$ mice were transferred, implying a role for development of adaptive immunity as a protective response. Interleukin-10 (IL-10) may also play a crucial role in anti-oxLDL pathogenicity because IL-10–deficient mice had significantly more advanced disease.[34] The above-mentioned experiments demonstrate that anti-oxLDL antibodies potentially bear an immunoprotective function against the development of atherosclerosis.

PROTECTIVE ROLE OF ANTI-oxLDL ANTIBODIES

Human anti-oxLDL antibodies play an important role in the regulation of oxLDL levels. These antibodies have been found in children,[35] healthy adults, and patients with coronary heart disease.[36] Circulating antibodies recognizing oxLDL are present in cardiovascular risk–free children. Antibody levels in children are significantly higher than in adults,[35] suggesting that these antibodies may not necessarily be related to atherosclerosis and cardiovascular diseases (CVD). It is probable that high levels of antibodies in children modulate the antigen and thus protect against the development of atherosclerosis and CVD. A study investigating anti-oxLDL antibodies in patients with early CVD found that anti-oxLDL antibodies were decreased in patients with borderline hypertension.[37] Results of a survey on complications of diabetic coronary artery disease (CAD) support this finding.[38]

In another study that explored the relationship between oxLDL and its antibody, the plasma oxLDL concentration in 130 healthy subjects was inversely correlated with the level of anti-oxLDL antibodies.[39] Yet another study in a healthy population with no clinical signs of atherosclerosis showed that anti-oxLDL antibody levels were inversely related to the intima-media thickness of carotid arteries.[40] As mentioned previously, the binding activity of IgG anti-oxLDL is significantly higher in children than in adults.[35] These studies seem to support the idea that anti-oxLDL antibodies have a protective function against the development of atherosclerosis and CVD in healthy individuals.

The role of anti-oxLDL antibodies in hypertension has also been analyzed. The levels of anti-oxLDL antibodies were significantly lower in borderline stages, whereas the concentrations of oxLDL were not. The concentration of oxLDL was higher in subjects with hypertension than in those who were normotensive. There was no difference between the levels of anti-oxLDL antibodies in hypertensive subjects and controls.[38,41]

PATHOGENIC ROLE OF ANTI-oxLDL ANTIBODIES IN HUMANS

Atherosclerotic lesions contain immunoglobulins that specifically recognize oxLDL.[42] Elevated anti-oxLDL antibody concentrations may be a predictor for the development of atherosclerosis and CVD.[6,43,44] These antibodies are the most effective parameters for predicting the extent of coronary atherosclerosis.[45] Their presence is also associated with a higher risk for coronary restenosis after percutaneous transluminal coronary angioplasty.[46] Higher levels of the antibodies in patients with peripheral occlusive arterial disease portend more extensive atherosclerotic lesions.[47] Elevated levels of anti-oxLDL antibody are related to hypertension, systemic vasculitis, peripheral arterial disease, endothelial dysfunction, atherosclerosis, and CVD.[6,43,44,47]

Conversely, antibodies can induce other immune effects, such as immune opsonin-associated antigen binding to phagocytes, complement activation, and presentation of antigens to T lymphocytes, to trigger an adaptive immune response. Anti-oxLDL antibodies involved in these immune functions can induce immunological injury.[42,48–50]

Human anti-oxLDL antibodies[49,51] may belong to different classes and subclasses, including IgA, IgG1, IgG2, IgG3, and IgM, as well as having specific idiotypes.[52] Multiple classes and subclasses of anti-oxLDL antibodies may result in heterogeneous responses: IgG2 is the dominant subclass to respond to oxLDL epitopes containing phospholipids; and the IgG3 subclass fixes complement better and binds Fc receptors more avidly and thus has more pathogenic properties than the IgG2 subclass.[53,54] However, these differences in anti-oxLDL antibody characteristics and their correlation with clinical manifestations have not yet been fully analyzed.

Anti-oxLDL antibodies are extensively prevalent in diseases except CVD. Elevated levels of anti-oxLDL antibodies have been found in patients with autoimmune diseases, including rheumatoid arthritis, SLE, and APS,[56–61] as well as in other conditions such as diabetes mellitus.

oxLDL/β2GPI COMPLEXES AND THEIR UPTAKE BY MACROPHAGES

β2GPI is a 50 kDa single-chain polypeptide composed of 326 amino acid residues, arranged in five homologous repeats known as complement control protein domains. β2GPI's fifth domain contains a patch of positively charged amino acids that likely represents the binding region for phospholipids.[62,63] β2GPI binds strongly to negatively charged molecules, such as phospholipids, heparin, and certain lipoproteins, as well as to activated platelets and apoptotic cell membranes. This binding may aid the clearance of apototic cells from circulation.[64] Further, β2GPI may have anticoagulant properties, as it has been shown to inhibit the intrinsic coagulation pathway, prothrombinase activity, and ADP-dependent platelet aggregation.[65] It has also been reported to interact with several components of the protein C/protein S anticoagulant system.[66]

We recently demonstrated[17–20] the specific interaction between Cu^{2+}-oxLDL and β2GPI by ELISA, optical biosensor, and ligand blot analysis on a silica gel plate for thin-layer chromatography (TLC). Thus, oxLDL, but not native LDL, binds β2GPI and anti-β2GPI autoantibodies. Two chloroform-extractable lipids (oxLig-1 and

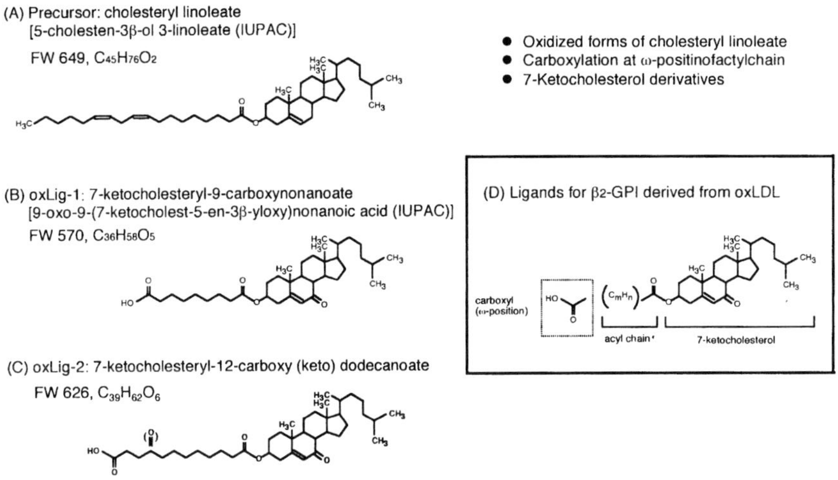

FIGURE 1. Structures of oxLDL-derived ligands specific for β2GPI. (**A**) Cholesteryl linoleate (as a precursor). Major ligands for β2GPI: (**B**) oxLig-1 and (**C**) oxLig-2. (**D**) A common structure for the β2GPI ligands (e.g., oxLig-1).

oxLig-2) were identified as the ligands for the specific interaction between oxLDL and β2GPI. These oxLDL-derived β2GPI specific ligands were purified further by reverse-phase high-performance liquid chromatography (HPLC) and their structures were identified as 7-ketocholesteryl-9-carboxynonanoate [9-oxo-9-(7-ketocholest-5-en-3β-yloxy) nonanoic acid (IUPAC)] and 7-ketocholesteryl-12-carboxy (keto) dodecanoate, respectively (FIG. 1). Cholesteryl linoleate present in LDL is a major core lipid and represents the most probable candidate for a precursor of these ligands.

The initial *in vitro* interaction of Cu^{2+}-oxLDL with β2GPI is due to electrostatic interactions between ω-carboxyl functions and lysine residues of β2GPI, and is reversible by Mg^{2+} treatment. This interaction later progresses to a much more stable bond such as Schiff base formation with an ω-aldehyde. Interestingly, the negative charges generated by Cu^{2+}-oxLDL were neutralized by the interaction with β2GPI. These complexes are occasionally present in APS and SLE patients as IgG immune complexes with anti-β2GPI antibodies.[17] The strength of the bond formed and the neutralization of the charges by the complexes may contribute to their stability in the blood stream.

We first demonstrated in 1997 that the *in vitro* macrophage uptake of ^{125}I-Cu^{2+}-oxLDL was significantly enhanced in the presence of β2GPI and IgG anti-β2GPI autoantibodies.[18] Further, the macrophage uptake of liposomes containing β2GPI ligands (oxLig-1 and oxLig-2) was also enhanced, confirming the previous results.[17,19,20] These findings indicate that IgG anti-β2GPI autoantibodies may be proatherogenic. The *in vivo* oxLDL uptake is likely mediated by Fcγ receptors, rather than by scavenger receptors. By contrast, Fcμ receptors have poor phagocytic properties, possibly making the IgM class of autoantibodies and/or natural antibodies antiatherogenic (or protective).

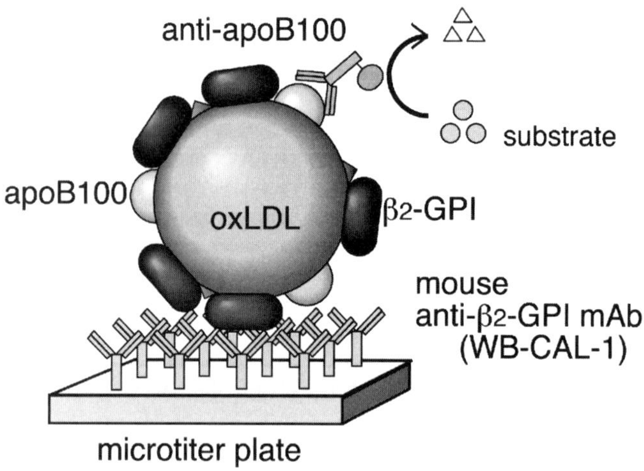

FIGURE 2. Detection system (ELISA) for oxLDL/β2GPI complexes. OxLDL/β2GPI complexes in serum samples are detected in a sandwich ELISA using WB-CAL-1 (anti-β2GPI monoclonal antibody) coated plate and labeled anti-apoB100 as probe antibody.

Both a ketone function at the 7 position (not at the 22 position) on the sterol backbone and the ω-carboxyl function on the acyl chain of the ligands are responsible either for the interaction between oxLDL and β2GPI or the β2GPI/anti-β2GPI–mediated uptake of oxLDL by macrophages.[20]

oxLDL/β2GPI AND ANTI-oxLDL/β2GPI COMPLEX ELISA

We have established a novel ELISA system for oxLDL/β2GPI complexes using an anti-β2GPI monoclonal antibody, WB-CAL-1, derived from an NZW × BXSB F1 mouse[67] (FIG. 2). Microwells were coated with WB-CAL-1, diluted serum samples applied, and bound oxLDL/β2GPI complexes determined with an enzyme-labeled anti-apoB antibody. WB-CAL-1 antibody only captured β2GPI when it was complexed with oxLDL, and did not react with free β2GPI in solution. ELISA for anti-oxLDL/β2GPI antibodies used oxLDL/β2GPI complexes as the antigenic substrate. oxLDL/β2GPI–coated microwells were reacted with diluted samples, and bound antibodies were determined with an enzyme-labeled anti-human antibody.[17,19,20]

oxLDL/β2GPI COMPLEXES IN AUTOIMMUNE DISEASES

Lipid peroxidation resulting in oxLDL is a common occurrence in patients with some systemic autoimmune diseases.[68] OxLDL, but not native LDL, binds β2GPI *in vitro*, initially forming dissociable electrostatic complexes followed by more stable complexes bound by covalent interactions. Circulating oxLDL/β2GPI complexes have been detected in patients with autoimmune diseases.[17] High serum levels of stable oxLDL/β2GPI complexes were detected by ELISA in 75% to 80% of patients with SLE and systemic sclerosis (SSc). OxLDL/β2GPI complex levels of patients with rheumatoid arthritis (RA) were slightly elevated compared with healthy controls, but this difference did not reach statistical significance. Unlike RA, both SLE and SSc are characterized by widespread vascular abnormalities. Serum levels of oxLDL/β2GPI complexes were also significantly elevated in patients with secondary APS and in SLE patients without APS, compared with healthy controls. However, these complexes were not associated with SLE disease activity or any major clinical manifestation of APS.[69] Although it can be hypothesized that this interaction might be related to chronic inflammation of the vasculature that occurs in autoimmune patients, the exact mechanism(s) for the increased oxidation of LDL and formation of oxLDL/β2GPI complexes are not fully understood. It is possible that the interaction between oxLDL and β2GPI may promote the clearance of oxLDL from the circulation to prevent thrombus formation. Serum levels of oxLDL/β2GPI complexes fluctuated widely when measured in samples obtained at different time intervals over a 12-month follow-up from six SLE patients. This suggests that LDL oxidation and the formation of complexes are very active processes under the control of unknown regulatory mechanism(s). Stable oxLDL/β2GPI complexes may be clinically relevant, as they have been implicated as atherogenic autoantigens, and their presence may represent a risk factor or an indirect but significant contributor for thrombosis and atherosclerosis in patients with an autoimmune background.[17]

ANTI-oxLDL/β2GPI ANTIBODIES IN AUTOIMMUNE DISEASES

Serum levels of IgG anti-oxLDL/β2GPI antibodies were measured in the same group of SLE, SSc, and RA patients. SLE and SSc patients had significantly higher levels of anti-oxLDL/β2GPI antibodies compared with controls (FIG. 3A). RA patients showed higher antibody levels than controls, but this difference was not statistically significant. When IgG anti-oxLDL/β2GPI antibodies were evaluated for their association with the major clinical manifestations of APS,[17,69] a stronger correlation with arterial thrombosis was observed, compared with the correlation with venous thrombosis and pregnancy morbidity (FIG. 3B). Further, the positive predictive value of IgG anti-oxLDL/β2GPI antibodies for total thrombosis (arterial and venous) in patients with secondary APS was 92% and for arterial thrombosis was 88.9%. In contrast, the positive predictive value for venous thrombosis was not statistically significant at 77.7%. In addition, anti-oxLDL/β2GPI antibodies were present in three of four SLE patients with active disease followed over a 12-month period, whereas two patients with inactive disease and oxLDL/β2GPI complexes did not have these antibodies.[68]

The coexistence of oxLDL /β2GPI autoantibodies with oxLDL/β2GPI complexes suggests that these two elements interact, perhaps forming circulating immune complexes (oxLDL/β2GPI/antibody). Such immune complexes have recently been detected in patients with SLE and/or APS.[17] These observations, along with the increased *in vitro* uptake of oxLDL/β2GPI complexes by macrophages in the presence of anti-oxLDL/β2GPI antibodies,[15,18–20] provide an explanation for the accelerated (premature) development of atherosclerosis in autoimmune patients. Although evidence is preliminary, IgG anti-oxLDL/β2GPI antibodies represent a

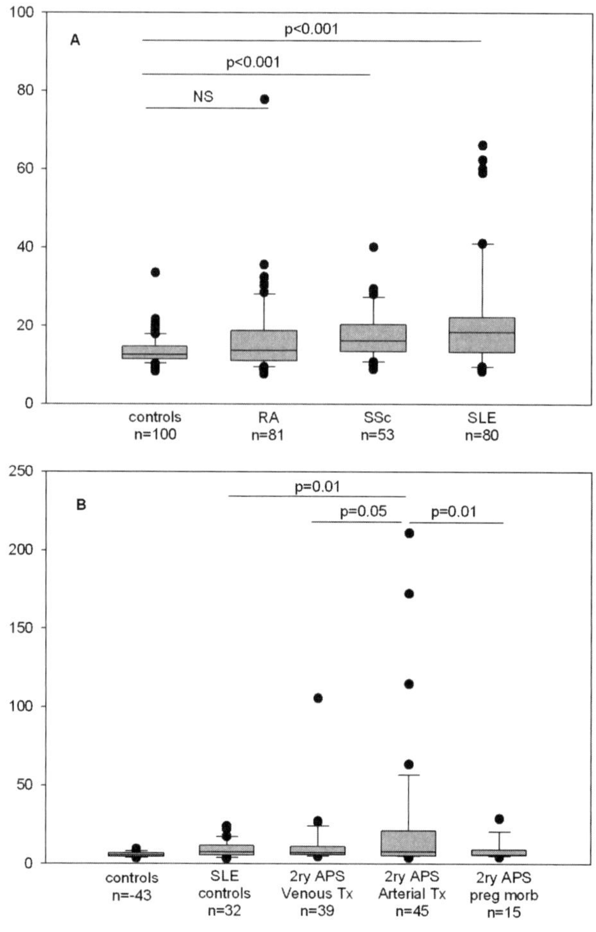

FIGURE 3. Box plot for serum levels of IgG anti-oxLDL/β2GPI antibodies measured by ELISA (**A, top**) in patients with systemic autoimmune diseases and in healthy controls, and (**B, bottom**) in secondary antiphospholipid syndrome (APS) patients classified into venous thrombosis (venous Tx), arterial thrombosis (arterial Tx), or pregnancy morbidity (preg morb) subgroups. In **B**, patients with SLE without APS and healthy individuals served as controls. IgG anti-oxLDL/β2GPI antibody levels (y-axis) are expressed in arbitrary units (U/mL). *Boxes* represent 75th and 25th percentiles and horizontal line the median for the group. *Dots* are samples reacting outside the 90th and 10th percentile bars. P values of 0.05 or less were considered significant (Mann-Whitney Rank Sum test). APS, antiphospholipid syndrome; RA, rheumatoid arthritis; SLE, systemic lupus erythematosus; SSc, systemic sclerosis.

distinct subset of antiphospholipid antibodies (i.e., anti-β2GPI) that coexist with other antiphospholipid antibodies. Thus, IgG anti-oxLDL/β2GPI antibodies appear to be useful serologic markers for atherosclerotic risk in autoimmune patients with high specificity for antiphospholipid syndrome.

REFERENCES

1. STEINBRECHER, U.P., S. PARTHASARATHY, D.S. LEAKE, *et al.* 1984. Modification of low density lipoprotein by endothelial cells involves lipid peroxidation and degradation of low density lipoprotein phospholipids. Proc. Natl. Acad. Sci. USA **81:** 3883–3887.
2. STEINBERG, D., S. PARTHASARATHY, T.E. CAREW, *et al.* 1989. Beyond cholesterol. Modifications of low-density lipoprotein that increase its atherogenicity. N. Engl. J. Med. **320:** 915–924.
3. STEINBERG, D. 1997. Low density lipoprotein oxidation and its pathobiological significance. J. Biol. Chem. **272:** 20963–20966.
4. HAMMER, A., G. KAGER, G. DOHR, *et al.* 1995. Generation, characterization, and histochemical application of monoclonal antibodies selectively recognizing oxidatively modified apoB-containing serum lipoproteins. Arterioscler. Thromb. Vasc. Biol. **15:** 704–713.
5. PALINSKI, W., V.A. ORD, A.S. PLUMP, *et al.* 1994. ApoE-deficient mice are a model of lipoprotein oxidation in atherogenesis. Demonstration of oxidation-specific epitopes in lesions and high titers of autoantibodies to malondialdehyde-lysine in serum. Arterioscler. Thromb. **14:** 605–616.
6. SALONEN, J.T., S. YLA-HERTTUALA, R. YAMAMOTO, *et al.* 1992. Autoantibody against oxidis ed LDL and progression of carotid atherosclerosis. Lancet **339:** 883–887.
7. PALINSKI, W., E. MILLER & J.L. WITZTUM. 1995. Immunization of low density lipoprotein (LDL) receptor-deficient rabbits with homologous malondialdehyde-modified LDL reduces atherogenesis. Proc. Natl. Acad. Sci. USA **92:** 821–825.
8. MCNEIL, H.P., R.J. SIMPSON, C.N. CHESTERMAN & S.A. KRILIS. 1990. Anti-phospholipid antibodies are directed against a complex antigen that includes a lipid-binding inhibitor of coagulation: β2-glycoprotein I (apolipoprotein H). Proc. Natl. Acad. Sci. USA **87:** 4120–4124.
9. GALLI, M., P. COMFURIUS, C. MAASSEN, *et al.* 1990. Anticardiolipin antibodies (ACA) directed not to cardiolipin but to a plasma protein cofactor. Lancet **335:** 1544–1547.
10. MATSUURA, E., Y. IGARASHI, M. FUJIMOTO, *et al.* 1990. Anticardiolipin cofactor(s) and differential diagnosis of autoimmune disease. Lancet **336:** 177–178.
11. MATSUURA, E., Y. IGARASHI , M. FUJIMOTO, *et al.* 1992. Heterogeneity of anticardiolipin antibodies defined by the anticardiolipin cofactor. J. Immunol. **148:** 3885–3891.
12. MATSUURA, E., Y. IGARASHI, T. YASUDA, *et al.* 1994. Anticardiolipin antibodies recognize β2-glycoprotein I structure altered by interacting with an oxygen modified solid phase surface. J. Exp. Med. **179:** 457–462.
13. GEORGE, J., D. HARATS, B. GILBURD, *et al.* 1999. Immunolocalization of β2-glycoprotein I (apolipoprotein H) to human atherosclerotic plaques: potential implications for lesion progression. Circulation **99:** 2227–2230.
14. VAARALA, O., G. ALFTHAN, M. JAUHIAINEN, *et al.* 1993. Crossreaction between antibodies to oxidised low-density lipoprotein and to cardiolipin in systemic lupus erythematosus. Lancet **341:** 923–925.
15. TINAHONES, F.J., M.J. CUADRADO, M.A. KHAMASHTA, *et al.* 1998. Lack of cross-reaction between antibodies to β2-glycoprotein-I and oxidized low-density lipoprotein in patients with antiphospholipid syndrome. Br. J. Rheumatol. **37:** 746–749.
16. ROMERO, F.I., O. AMENGUAL, T. ATSUMI, *et al.* 1998. Arterial disease in lupus and secondary antiphospholipid syndrome: a ssociation with anti-β2-glycoprotein I antibodies but not with antibodies against oxidized low-density lipoprotein. Br. J. Rheumatol. **37:** 883–888.

17. KOBAYASHI, K., M. KISHI, T. ATSUMI, *et al.* 2003. Circulating oxidized LDL forms complexes with β2-glycoprotein I: implication as an atherogenic autoantigen. J. Lipid Res. **44:** 716–726.
18. HASUNUMA, Y., E. MATSUURA, Z. MAKITA, *et al.* 1997. Involvement of β2-glycoprotein I and anticardiolipin antibodies in oxidatively modified low-density lipoprotein uptake by macrophages. Clin. Exp. Immunol. **107:** 569–573.
19. KOBAYASHI, K., E. MATSUURA, Q. LIU. *et al.* 2001. A specific ligand for β2-glycoprotein I mediates autoantibody-dependent uptake of oxidized low density lipoprotein by macrophages. J. Lipid Res. **42:** 697–709.
20. LIU, Q., K. KOBAYASHI, J. INAGAKI, *et al.* 2002. ω-carboxyl variants of 7-ketocholesteryl esters are ligands for β2-glycoprotein I and mediate antibody-dependent uptake of oxidized LDL by macrophages. J. Lipid Res. **43:** 1486–1495.
21. STEINBERG, D. 2002. Atherogenesis in perspective: hypercholesterolemia and inflammation as partners in crime. Nat. Med. **8:** 1211–1217.
22. VIRELLA, G., D.H. ATCHLEY, S. KOSKINEN, *et al.* 2002. Pro-atherogenic and pro-inflammatory properties of immune complexes prepared with purified human oxLDL antibodies and human oxLDL. Clin. Immunol. **105:** 81–92.
23. BERLINER, J.A. & J.W. HEINECKE. 1996. The role of oxidized lipoproteins in atherogenesis. Free Radical Biol. & Med. **20:** 707–727.
24. MCMURRAY, H.F., S. PARTHASARATHY & D. STEINBERG. 1993. Oxidatively modified low density lipoprotein is a chemoattractant for human T lymphocytes. J. Clin. Invest. **92:** 1004–1008.
25. YLA-HERTTUALA, S., W. PALINSKI, M.E. ROSENFELD, *et al.* 1989. Evidence for presence of oxidatively modified low density lipoprotein in atherosclerotic lesions of rabbit and man. J. Clin. Invest. **85:** 1086–1095.
26. VAARALA, O. 1996. Antiphospholipid antibodies and atherosclerosis. Lupus **5:** 442–447.
27. PALINSKI, W., S. HORKKO, E. MILLER, *et al.* 1996. Cloning of monoclonal autoantibodies to epitopes of oxidized lipoproteins from apolipoprotein E-deficient mice. Demonstration of epitopes of oxidized low density lipoprotein in human plasma. J. Clin. Invest. **98:** 800– 814.
28. SHAW P.X., S. HORKKO, M.K. CHANG, *et al.* 2000. Natural antibodies with the T15 idiotype may act in atherosclerosis, apoptotic clearance, and protective immunity. J. Clin. Invest. **105:** 1731–1740.
29. HORKKO, S., N.A. BIRD, E. MILLER, *et al.* 1999. Monoclonal autoantibodies specific for oxidized phospholipids or oxidized phospholipid-protein adducts inhibit macrophage uptake of oxidized low-density lipoproteins. J. Clin. Invest. **103:** 117–128.
30. ZHOU, X., G. CALIGIURI, A. HAMSTEN, *et al.* 2001. LDL immunization induces T-cell-dependent antibody formation and protection against atherosclerosis. Arterioscler. Thromb. Vasc. Biol. **21:** 108–114.
31. CALIGIURI, G., A. NICOLETTI, B. POIRIER & G.K. HANSSON. 2002. Protective immunity against atherosclerosis carried by B cells of hypercholesterolemic mice. J. Clin. Invest. **109:** 745–753.
32. GEORGE, J., A. AFEK, B. GILBURD, *et al.* 1998. Hyperimmunization of apo-E deficient mice with homologous malondialdehyde low-density lipoprotein suppresses early atherogenesis. Atherosclerosis **138:** 147–152.
33. SHOENFELD, Y., D. HARATS & J. GEORGE. 2000. Heat shock protein 60/50, beta 2-glycoprotein I and oxidized LDL as players in murine atherosclerosis. J. Autoimmun. **15:** 199–202.
34. CALIGIURI, G., M. RUDLING, V. OLLIVIER, *et al.* 2003. Interleukin-10 deficiency increases atherosclerosis, thrombosis, and low-density lipoproteins in apolipoprotein E knockout mice. Mol. Med. **9:** 10–17.
35. IUGHETTI, L., C. VOLTA, E. MAGGI, *et al.* 1999. Circulating antibodies recognizing oxidatively modified low-density lipoprotein in children. Pediatr. Res. **45:** 94–99.
36. VIRELLA, G., I. VIRELLA, R.B. LEMAN, *et al.* 1993. Anti-oxidized low-density lipoprotein antibodies in patients with coronary heart disease and normal healthy volunteers. Int. J. Clin. Lab. Res. **23:** 95–101.
37. WU, R., U. DE FAIRE, C. LEMNE, *et al.* 1999. Autoantibodies to oxLDL are decreased in individuals with borderline hypertension. Hypertension **33:** 53–59.

38. Lopes-Virella, M.F., G. Virella, T.J. Orchard, *et al.* 1999. Antibodies to oxidized LDL and LDL-containing immune complexes as risk factors for coronary artery disease in diabetes mellitus. Clin. Immunol. **90:** 165–172.
39. Shoji, T., Y. Nishizawa, M. Fukumoto, *et al.* 2000. Inverse relationship between circulating oxidized low density lipoprotein (oxLDL) and anti-oxLDL antibody levels in healthy subjects. Atherosclerosis **148:** 171–177.
40. Fukumoto, M., T. Shoji, M. Emoto, *et al.* 2000. Antibodies against oxidized LDL and carotid artery intima-media thickness in a healthy population. Arterioscler. Thromb. Vasc. Biol. **20:** 703–707.
41. Frostegard, J., R. Wu, C. Lemne, *et al.* 2003. Circulating oxidized low-density lipoprotein is increased in hypertension. Clin. Sci. **105:** 615–620.
42. Yla-Herttuala, S., W. Palinski, S.W. Butler, *et al.* 1994. Rabbit and human atherosclerotic lesions contain IgG that recognizes epitopes of oxidized LDL. Arterioscler. Thromb. **14:** 32–40.
43. Wu, R., S. Nityanand, L. Berglund, *et al.* 1997. Antibodies against cardiolipin and oxidatively modified LDL in 50-year-old men predict myocardial infarction. Arterioscler. Thromb. Vasc. Biol. **17:** 3159–3163.
44. Puurunen, M., M. Manttari, V. Manninen, *et al.* 1994. Antibody against oxidized low-density lipoprotein predicting myocardial infarction. Arch. Intern. Med. **154:** 2605–2609.
45. George, J., A. Ahmed, M. Patnaik, *et al.* 2000. The prediction of coronary atherosclerosis employing artificial neural networks. Clin. Cardiol. **23:** 453–456.
46. George, J., D. Harats, E. Bakshi, *et al.* 1999. Anti-oxidized low density lipoprotein antibody determination as a predictor of restenosis following percutaneous transluminal coronary angioplasty. Immunol. Lett. **68:** 263–266.
47. Bergmark, C., R. Wu, U. de Faire, *et al.* 1995. Patients with early-onset peripheral vascular disease have increased levels of autoantibodies against oxidized LDL. Arterioscler. Thromb. Vasc. Biol. **15:** 441–445.
48. Libby, P. 2002. Inflammation in atherosclerosis. Nature **420:** 868–874.
49. Wu, R. & A.K. Lefvert. 1995. Autoantibodies against oxidized low density lipoproteins (oxLDL): characterization of antibody isotope, subclass, affinity and effect on the macrophage uptake of oxLDL. Clin. Exp. Immunol. **102:** 174–180.
50. Virella, G., D. Atchley, S. Koskinen, *et al.* 2002. Proatherogenic and proinflammatory properties of immune complexes prepared with purified human oxLDL antibodies and human oxLDL. Clin. Immunol. **105:** 81–92.
51. Mironova, M., G. Virella & M.F. Lopes-Virella. 1996. Isolation and characterization of human antioxidized LDL autoantibodies. Arterioscler. Thromb. Vasc. Biol. **16:** 222–229.
52. Wu, R., Y. Shoenfeld, Y. Sherer, *et al.* 2003. Anti-idiotypes to oxidized LDL antibodies in intravenous immunoglobulin preparations—possible immunomodulation of atherosclerosis. Autoimmunity **36:** 91–97.
53. Devey, M.E. & D. Voak. 1974. A critical study of the IgG subclasses of Rh anti-D antibodies formed in pregnancy and in immunized volunteers. Immunology **27:** 1073–1079.
54. Henriksen, T., E.M. Mahoney & D. Steinberg. 1981. Enhanced macrophage degradation of low density lipoprotein previously incubated with cultured endothelial cells: recognition by receptors for acetylated low density lipoproteins. Proc. Natl. Acad. Sci. USA **78:** 6499–6503.
55. Wu, R., E. Svenungsson, I. Gunnarsson, *et al.* 1999. Antibodies to adult human endothelial cells cross-react with oxidized low-density lipoprotein and beta 2-glycoprotein I (beta 2-GPI) in systemic lupus erythematosus. Clin. Exp. Immunol. **115:** 561–566.
56. Zhao, D., H. Ogawa, X. Wang, *et al.* 2001. Oxidized low-density lipoprotein and autoimmune antibodies in patients with antiphospholipid syndrome with a history of thrombosis. Am. J. Clin. Pathol. **116:** 760–767.
57. Cvetkovic, J.T., S. Wallberg-Jonsson, E. Ahmed, *et al.* 2002. Increased levels of autoantibodies against copper-oxidized low density lipoprotein, malondialdehyde-modified low density lipoprotein and cardiolipin in patients with rheumatoid arthritis. Rheumatology (Oxford) **41:** 988–995.

58. Wu, R., E. Svenungsson, I. Gunnarsson, *et al.* 1999. Antibodies against lysophosphatidylcholine and oxidized LDL in patients with SLE. Lupus **8:** 142–150.
59. Wu, R., E. Svenungsson, I. Gunnarsson, *et al.* 1999. Antibodies to adult human endothelial cells cross-react with oxidized low-density lipoprotein and beta 2-glycoprotein I (beta 2-GPI) in systemic lupus erythematosus. Clin. Exp. Immunol. **115:** 561–566.
60. Hayem, G., P. Nicaise-Roland, E. Palazzo, *et al.* 2001. Anti-oxidized low-density-lipoprotein (OxLDL) antibodies in systemic lupus erythematosus with and without antiphospholipid syndrome. Lupus **10:** 346–351.
61. Orchard, T.J., G. Virella, K.Y. Forrest, *et al.* 1999. Antibodies to oxidized LDL predict coronary artery disease in type 1 diabetes: a nested case-control study from the Pittsburgh Epidemiology of Diabetes. Diabetes **48:** 1454–1458.
62. Bouma, B., P.G. de Groot, J.M van den Elsen, *et al.* 1999. Adhesion mechanism of human β2-glycoprotein I to phospholipids based on its crystal structure. EMBO J. **18:** 5166–5174.
63. Hoshino, M., Y. Hagihara, I. Nishii, *et al.* 2000. Identification of the phospholipid-binding site of human β2-glycoprotein I domain V by heteronuclear magnetic resonance. J. Mol. Biol. **304:** 927–939.
64. Inanc, M., E.L. Radway-Bright & D.A. Isenberg. 1997. β2-glycoprotein I and anti-β2-glycoprotein I antibodies: where are we now? Br. J. Rheumatol. **36:** 1247–1257.
65. Sheng, Y., D.A. Kandiah & S.A. Krilis. 1998. β2-glycoprotein I: target antigen for 'antiphospholipid' antibodies. Immunological and molecular aspects. Lupus **7:** S5–9.
66. Merrill, J.T., H.W. Zhang, C. Shen, *et al.* 1999. Enhancement of protein S anticoagulant function by β2-glycoprotein I, a major target antigen of antiphospholipid antibodies: β2-glycoprotein I interferes with binding of protein S to its plasma inhibitor, C4β-binding protein. Thromb. Haemost. **81:** 748–757.
67. Hashimoto, Y., M. Kawamura, K. Ichikawa, *et al.* 1992. Anticardiolipin antibodies in NZW x BXSB F1 mice. A model of antiphospholipid syndrome. J. Immunol. **149:** 1063–1068.
68. Lopez, D., I. Garcia-Valladares, C. Palafox-Sanchez, *et al.* 2004. Oxidized low-density lipoprotein/β2-glycoprotein I complexes and autoantibodies to oxLig-1/β2-glycoprotein I in patients with systemic lupus erythematosus and antiphospholipid syndrome. Am. J. Clin. Pathol. **121:** 426–436.
69. Lopez, D., K. Kobayashi, J.T. Merrill, *et al.* 2003. IgG Autoantibodies against b2-glycoprotein I complexed with a lipid ligand derived from oxidized low-density lipoprotein are associated with arterial thrombosis in antiphospholipid syndrome. Clin. Dev. Immunol. **10:** 203–211.

Predictive Markers for Development of Severe Organ Involvement in Patients with Systemic Sclerosis

LAURE YSEBRANT DE LENDONCK,[a] ANNICK OCMANT,[b] FLORENCE ROUFOSSE,[a] AND ELIE COGAN[a]

[a]*Department of Internal Medicine, Hôpital Erasme, Université Libre de Bruxelles, Brussels, Belgium*

[b]*Department of Immunology-Hematology-Transfusion, Hôpital Erasme, Université Libre de Bruxelles, Brussels, Belgium*

ABSTRACT: Prognosis of systemic sclerosis (SSc) is associated with the extent of skin involvement and the presence of lung, heart, kidney, and/or digestive tract damage. Most patients do not require disease-modifying therapy. However, to avoid irreversible tissue injury, early detection of visceral involvement is crucial for prompt initiation of therapy. The aim of this study is to identify, among initial investigations performed at time of diagnosis, predictive markers for the development of severe organ involvement (SOI). We retrospectively reviewed the medical records of 41 patients with SSc who were followed for 5 years after diagnosis, including those who died because of SSc within this 5-year period. We considered 68 clinical, biological, and technical parameters obtained at time of diagnosis and studied their association with development of SOI during this 5-year period, using a multivariate logistic regression. Eighteen patients (44%) developed SOI, with a median delay of 1.5 years following diagnosis. Three independent markers were identified: reduced vital capacity, fulfilment of American College of Rheumatology criteria at diagnosis, and presence of rheumatoid factor. To identify patients at risk for developing severe disease, given the short delay between diagnosis of SSc and development of SOI, we recommend monitoring these markers at diagnosis.

KEYWORDS: systemic sclerosis; scleroderma

INTRODUCTION

Systemic sclerosis (SSc) is a complex, life-threatening connective tissue disease that targets the skin, lungs, heart, gastrointestinal tract, peripheral circulation, and musculoskeletal system. It is characterized by tissue fibrosis and small-vessel vasculopathy due to an autoimmune response associated with very specific autoantibodies.[1]

Address for correspondence: Prof. Elie Cogan, Department of Internal Medicine, Hôpital Erasme, 808, route de Lennik, 1070 Brussels, Belgium. Voice: +32-2-555-3806; fax: +32-2-555-3211.

ecogan@ulb.ac.be

Ann. N.Y. Acad. Sci. 1051: 455–464 (2005). © 2005 New York Academy of Sciences.
doi: 10.1196/annals.1361.087

The digestive tract, lungs, kidneys, and heart are involved in 90%, 70%, 50%, and 10%, respectively, of affected subjects.[2] The heterogeneity of the disease requires the development of a classification system that, ideally, takes into account the potential complications, prognoses, and management of the patients.

The first classification system was developed in 1980 by a subcommittee of the American Rheumatism Association;[3] these are now known as the American College of Rheumatology (ACR) criteria. The purpose of this classification was not to aid in diagnosis, but rather to establish a standard to differentiate patients affected by systemic sclerosis from those affected by other connective tissue diseases, such as systemic lupus erythematosus, polymyositis/dermatomyositis, or simple Raynaud's phenomenon.

Currently, the most widely used classification is the two-subset model proposed by Leroy *et al.* in 1988, which is based on the extent of skin involvement: the localized and diffuse systemic sclerosis. The aim of this classification was to identify two subgroups of patient with different characteristics (clinical and serological patterns) and different clinical outcome.[1] Unfortunately, the classification fails to identify patients with favorable or bad prognosis.

Although there is no cure for scleroderma, therapeutic advances have produced benefits for several organ-specific manifestations, for example, scleroderma renal crisis (angiotensin-converting enzyme inhibitors), gastrointestinal reflux disease (proton pump inhibitors), Raynaud's phenomenon (vasodilator therapy, calcium channel blockers), active alveolitis (cyclophosphamide), and pulmonary hypertension (vasodilator therapy with epoprostenol or bosentan).[4]

To modify the natural history of SSc and to improve survival, therapy must be initiated as soon as possible. Therefore, it is critical to identify predictive markers for the development of severe organ involvement (SOI) among initial investigations performed at time of diagnosis.

PATIENTS AND METHODS

Study Design

We retrospectively studied the medical files of 86 patients with systemic sclerosis followed in our institution (an 858-bed academic hospital) during the last 10 years. The patients were identified using different data sources: (1) outpatient clinic listings ($n = 56$); (2) immunology laboratory database ($n = 42$) ; (3) nailfold capillaroscopy records ($n = 19$) ; (4) records from the Department of Pathology ($n = 6$).

Patients

After rechecking the data in each case, the diagnosis of SSc was confirmed in 77 patients. Nine patients were excluded: four patients had mixed connective tissue disease, and five patients had a localized form of scleroderma. Among these 77 patients, we included only those patients followed for 5 years since diagnosis or who died because of systemic sclerosis before the five-year period had elapsed. Patients with cardiac, pulmonary, digestive, or renal abnormalities not related to systemic sclerosis were also excluded. After the above exclusions, we finally studied medical files of 41 patients.

Data Collection

A standardized procedure was used to collect 324 data in each case, including the extent of skin involvement (limited or diffuse), some clinical characteristics, the fulfilment of ACR criteria, the pattern of auto-antibodies, and the results of other investigations performed at diagnosis and during the yearly follow-up.

End Point

The occurrence of SOI was determined 5 years after diagnosis by reviewing clinical records, using the definition proposed by Steen and Medsger:[5]

(1) Kidneys: malignant arterial hypertension and/or rapidly progressive renal failure and/or microangiopathic hemolytic anemia.

(2) Heart: cardiomyopathy with decrease in left ventricular ejection fraction and symptoms of congestive heart failure, symptomatic pericarditis, or an arrhythmia attributable to scleroderma heart disease requiring treatment.

(3) Lungs: pulmonary fibrosis on chest radiograph, with a forced vital capacity <55% of predicted.

(4) Gastrointestinal tract: malabsorption syndrome, intestinal pseudo-obstruction.

Statistical Analysis

Univariate analysis of the relationship between the risk factors considered and the subsequent development of SOI was undertaken using a univariate logistic regression. All the variables associated with the development of SOI with a $P < 0.1$ were processed with a multivariable logistic regression. After that we proceeded by retrograde elimination to identify independent variables associated with the development of SOI (statistical significance assessed for $P < 0.05$).

RESULTS

Baseline Characteristics

The female-to-male ratio was 35 to 6. At diagnosis, the median age was 52 years and the median disease duration at study entry was 18 months. Baseline characteristics of the subjects are shown in TABLE 1. Twenty-three patients had SSc with limited cutaneous involvement (lcSSc), nine patients had diffuse cutaneous involvement (dcSSc), four had systemic sclerosis sine scleroderma (ssSSc) and five were considered to have prescleroderma. Twenty-two patients satisfied ACR criteria for SSc at diagnosis: 9 patients with dc SSc (100%), and 12 patients with lc SSc (56%). None of the patients with ssSSc or prescleroderma satisfied ACR criteria. The frequency distributions of the other clinical and laboratory variables are shown in TABLE 1.

Follow-up

Five years after diagnosis, 18 patients had developed at least one SOI: 6 (68%) with dc-SSc, 10 (43%) with lcSSc, 2 (50%) with ss SSc, and none with prescleroderma. Eight patients had developed severe lung involvement, five had developed severe digestive tract involvement, four severe heart involvement, and three severe kidney

TABLE 1A. Baseline disease characteristics (n = 41)

Variables	Event	Percentage	M
General			
dcSSc	9/41	22%	0
lcSSc	23/41	56.1%	0
ssSSc	4/41	9.76%	0
preSSc	5/41	12.2%	0
ACR criteria	22/41	53.66%	0
Sex (female)	35/41	85%	0
Presentation			
First symptom = Raynaud	25/41	60.98%	0
First symptom = other one	16/41	39.2%	0
Symptom			
Telangiectasia	19/41	46.34%	0
Calcinosis	10/41	24.39%	0
Raynaud	38/41	92.68%	0
Digital tip pitting scars	12/41	29.27%	0
Dyspnea	10/41	24.39%	0
Orthopnea	0/41	0%	0
Dyspnea on exertion	23/41	56.1%	0
Chest pain	5/41	12.2%	0
Palpitations	3/41	7.32%	0
Lightheadedness	1/41	2.44%	0
Pedal edema	0/41	0%	0
Neck vein dilatation	0/41	0%	0
Pyrosis	12/41	29.27%	0
Dysphagia	12/41	29.27%	0
Diarrhea	3/41	7.32%	0
Constipation	0/41	0%	0
Joint pain	24/41	58.54%	0
Stiffness	10/41	24.39%	0
Biological parameters			
Antinuclear antibodies	37/41	90.24%	0
Anticentromere antibodies	18/41	43.9%	0
Antinuclear antibodies unidentified	9/41	21.95%	0
Anti-Scl70 antibodies	5/41	12.2%	0
Anti-DNAds antibodies	3/41	7.32%	0
Anti-SSA antibodies	5/41	12.2%	0
Anti-SSB antibodies	2/41	4.88%	0
Anti-PmScl antibodies	2/41	4.88%	0
Rheumatoid factor	10/41	24.39%	0
Antimitochondrial antibodies	7/41	17.07%	21
Antiphospholipid antibodies	5/41	12.2%	0
Lupus anticoagulant	4/41	9.76%	0

TABLE 1A. Baseline disease characteristics (n = 41)

Variables	Event	Percentage	M
Circulating immune complexes	6/41	14.64%	8
Cryoglobulins	4/41	9.76%	4
Decreased complement	4/41	9.76%	9
Gammaglobulins >1.2 g/dL	8/41	19.51%	1
Abnormal capillaroscopy	33/41	80.4%	0
Abnormal ECG	11/41	26.82%	7
Abnormal chest radiograph	10/41	24.39%	3
Fibrosis on chest CT scanner	5/41	12.2%	17
Alveolitis on chest CT scanner	8/41	19.51%	17
Abnormal hand radiograph	16/41	39.02%	8
Skin biopsy	4/41	9.76%	—
Kidney biopsy	1/41	2.44%	—

ABBREVIATIONS: M, missing values; %, percentages are based on total number of subjects; dcSSc, diffuse cutaneous systemic sclerosis; lcSSc, limited cutaneous systemic sclerosis; ssSSc,, sine scleroderma systemic sclerosis; preSsc, prescleroderma; ACR criteria, criteria proposed by the American College of Rheumatology 1980; ECG, electrocardiogram.

TABLE 1B. Baseline disease characteristics (n = 41)

Variables	Median	Percentile 25–75	M
Age at entry (years)	52.00	39.5–60.5	0
Disease duration at entry (years)	1.50	0.5–8.0	5
Vital capacity (% predicted)	93.00	74.5–102.0	9
Low carbon monoxide diffusing capacity (% predicted)	53.50	45.0–67.5	11
Erythrocyte sedimentation rate (mm/h)	15.00	10.0–24.0	2
C-reactive protein (mg/dL)	0.80	0.0–1.67	11
Serum creatinin (mg/dL)	0.90	0.8–1.0	0
Serum urea (mg/dL)	28.00	24.2–37.75	1
Proteinemia (g/L)	7.25	6.7–7.5	5
Proteinuria (g/24 h)	0.10	0.0–0.2	16
Hemoglobinemia (g/dL)	13.00	11.80–13.75	0

ABBREVIATIONS: M, missing values; %, percentages are based on total number of subjects; dcSSc, diffuse cutaneous systemic sclerosis; lcSSc, limited cutaneous systemic sclerosis; ssSSc, sine scleroderma systemic sclerosis; preSsc, prescleroderma; ACR criteria, criteria proposed by the American College of Rheumatology 1980; ECG, electrocardiogram.

involvement. Two patients had developed more than one SOI. Five years after the diagnosis of SSc, three patients had died due to SSc.

Findings of Univariate Analysis

Univariate analysis was performed for all variables (TABLE 2). Nine variables were associated with the development of SOI ($P < 0.05$): dyspnea, dyspnea on exertion, rheumatoid factor, ECG abnormalities, chest radiograph abnormalities, hand

TABLE 2. Assessing the relationship between severe organ involvement and 68 variables collected at time of diagnosis by univariate analysis

Variable	n^a	Coefficient[b]	SE	P
Sex (female)	41	−9.2163	17.9477	0.6076
Age	41	−0.0105	0.02346	0.8176
Classification				
dcSSc	41	1.2040	0.7955	0.1302
lcSSc	41	−0.0392	0.6340	0.9507
ssSSc	41	0.2719	1.0536	0.7963
preSSc	41	−7.5652	11.9293	0.5260
ACR criteria	41	1.3973	1.5145	0.0391
Presentation				
First symptom = Raynaud	41	−0.4055	0.6455	0.5301
First symptom = others	41	0.4055	0.6455	0.5301
Symptom				
Telangiectasia	41	−0.5390	0.6387	0.3987
Calcinosis	41	1.4451	0.7851	0.0657
Raynaud	41	−1.0116	1.2675	0.4248
Digital tip pitting scars	41	0.3483	0.6895	0.6135
Dyspnea	41	2.1282	0.8785	0.0154
Orthopnea	41	Dropped		
Dyspnea on exertion	41	2.2380	0.7691	0.0036
Chest pain	41	0.7419	0.9734	0.446
Palpitation	41	Dropped		
Lightheadedness	41	6.8661	16.1841	0.6714
Pedal edema	41	Dropped		
Neck vein distention	41	Dropped		
Pyrosis	41	0.8289	0.6995	0.2360
Dysphagia	41	0.8289	0.6995	0.2360
Diarrhea	41	−0.4818	1.2669	0.7037
Constipation	41	Dropped		
Joint pain	41	0.1869	0.6408	0.7673
Stiffness	41	0.3254	0.7297	0.6556
Biology				
Erythrocyte sedimentation rate	39	0.0563	0.0303	0.0630
C-reactive protein	30	0.1472	0.1619	0.3632
Proteinemia	36	−0.5678	0.5176	0.2726
BUN	40	0.0326	0.0395	0.2689
Creatininemia	41	1.0103	1.3382	0.4502
Eosinophils	40	−1.0943	1.6133	0.4976
Lymphocytes	41	−0.1070	0.4665	0.8186
Hemoglobin	41	−0.2460	0.2615	0.3468
Proteinuria	25	Dropped		
Antinuclear antibodies	41	−0.2719	1.5036	0.7963

TABLE 2. (*continued*) Assessing the relationship between severe organ involvement and 68 variables collected at time of diagnosis by univariate analysis

Variable	n^a	Coefficient[b]	SE	P
Anticentromere antibodies	41	–2.9060	0.8730	0.0009
Antinuclear antibodies unidentified	41	1.2040	0.7955	0.1302
Anti-Scl70 antibodies	41	0.7419	0.9734	0.4459
Anti-DNAds antibodies	41	–0.4818	1.2669	0.7037
Anti-SSA antibodies	41	1.8383	1.1686	0.1157
Anti-SSB antibodies	41	6.9267	11.446	0.5451
Anti-PmScl antibodies	41	6.9267	11.446	0.5451
Rheumatoid factor	41	1.8994	0.8833	0.0315
Antimitochondrial antibodies	20	–0.4418	0.9449	0.6401
Antiphospholipid antibodies	41	–1.2751	1.1663	0.2743
Lupus anticoagulant	41	–0.9361	1.1999	0.4353
Complement reduced	32	0.2877	1.0704	0.7881
Cryoglobulinemia	37	8.0125	13.3371	0.5424
Circulating immune complexes	33	–1.3863	1.1619	0.2328
Gammaglobulinemia	40	–0.9734	0.88934	0.2737
Technical examinations				
Abnormal capillaroscopy	41	0.0102	0.64521	0.9874
Electrocardiogram	34	2.1326	0.8958	0.0173
Vital capacity	32	–0.0741	0.0287	0.0097
Low carbon monoxide diffusing capacity	30	–0.0441	0.0250	0.0778
Abnormal hand radiograph	33	1.9671	0.7854	0.0123
Abnormal chest radiograph	38	1.9741	0.8831	0.0254
Fibrosis on chest CT scanner	24	1.0678	1.2107	0.3780
Alveolitis on chest CT scanner	24	Dropped		

[a]n = Number of observation for each variable.
[b]Logistic regression coefficient.
ABBREVIATIONS: SE, standard deviation; dcSSc, diffuse cutaneous systemic sclerosis; lcSSc, limited cutaneous systemic sclerosis; ssSSc, sine scleroderma systemic sclerosis; preSsc, prescleroderma; ACR criteria, criteria proposed by the American College of Rheumatology 1980.

X-ray abnormalities, and fulfilment of ACR criteria at diagnosis. Vital capacity (VC) and the presence of anti-centromere antibodies at diagnosis were inversely correlated with the development of SOI 5 years later ($P < 0.05$).

Three variables were associated with development of SOI with a $P < 0.1$: elevated erythrocyte sedimentation rate (ESR) >25 mm/first hour, calcinosis, and low carbon monoxide diffusing capacity.

Findings of Multivariate Analysis

Using multivariable logistic regression and retrograde elimination, three independent predictive markers of SOI were identified (TABLE 3): (1) vital capacity (OR: 0.9); (2) fulfilment of ACR criteria (OR: 21); and (3) rheumatoid factor (OR: 40). An odds ratio lower than that for VC implies that patients with lower VC have more SOI.

TABLE 3. Multivariate analysis of 68 variables: identification of independent predictive markers for developement of severe organ involvement

Variables	Coefficient	SE	Coeff./SE	P	Odds ratio	CI at 95%
Vital capacity	–0.10630	0.04139	–2.57	0.0102	0.90	0.83–0.98
ACR criteria	3.04813	1.49887	2.03	0.0420	21.08	1.12–397.79
Rheumatoid factor	3.70580	1.64513	2.25	0.0243	40.68	1.62–1022.75

NOTE: SE, standard error; CI, confidence interval.

Timing of Development of SOI

The median time of development of SOI was 1.5 years (6 months to 3.2 years) following diagnosis and 3.5 years (1.5 years to 9 years) following the first symptom of disease.

DISCUSSION

Using medical files of 41 scleroderma patients who were newly diagnosed, we have identified three predictive markers for development of severe organ involvement among initial investigations performed at time of diagnosis: fulfilment of ACR criteria, reduced vital capacity, and rheumatoid factor positivity.

A finding at diagnosis of reduced vital capacity, a nonspecific marker of pulmonary involvement, has been demonstrated in previous studies to be a predictor of reduced survival,[6] and Bryan *et al.* showed that mortality can be predicted by elevated ESR, low carbon monoxide diffusing capacity, and proteinuria.[7]

The second predictive marker of SOI is the presence of rheumatoid factor (RF), with a strong predictive power (OR: 40). In a French study, RF was reported to be present in 20% of SSc patients.[8] RF was present at low titer in 21% of patients in the present study. We are not aware of previous data on RF as predictor of severity in SSc.

In other connective tissue diseases, RF is a predictor of severe disease: patients with rheumatoid arthritis and very increased RF present with severe erosions and more systemic involvement, and in Sjögren syndrome RF is an indicator of severe salivary gland damage.[9,10] In these diseases, RF could be considered as a marker of polyclonal activation of B lymphocytes resulting in a more important humoral immune stimulation.[9] It should be noted that in our patients the presence of RF was not correlated with the level of gammaglobulins. RF could also have a pathogenic role by formation of circulating immune complexes, complement activation, and liberation of chemokines attracting inflammatory cells in tissue.[9]

Unlike several previous studies, we chose to include patients for which a diagnosis of SSc was established, whatever the fulfilment of ACR criteria, given the lack of sensitivity of ACR criteria in identifying patients with lcSSc and ssSSc.[6,7] Actually, in one previous study by Medsger on 48 patients with ssSSc, only six satisfied ACR criteria.[11] Another study showed that some patients with lcSSc did not satisfy the ACR criteria for definite SSc.[12]

In our study, no patient with ssSSc and only 53% of patients with lcSSc satisfied ACR criteria at diagnosis. In addition, we show that satisfaction of ACR criteria at entry is associated with development SOI. We suggest that the use of ACR criteria for selecting patients in other studies may overestimate the prevalence of severe complications. It is important to emphasize that our study also differs from previous ones by the primary end point, which focuses on the development of SOI and not on survival.[6,7,13] We are not aware of other studies that have identified predictive markers of SOI in SSc.

In summary, among the medical files of 41 patients with SSc followed up for 5 years after diagnosis, we identified the presence of rheumatoid factor, a decreased vital capacity, and fulfilment of ACR criteria as associated with development of severe visceral damage. Given the short delay between diagnosis and development of SOI, early detection of organ involvement and specific therapeutic intervention is mandatory. In addition, we emphasize the limitations of both the ACR criteria and the Leroy classification for systemic sclerosis: the ACR criteria lack sensitivity for detecting lcSSc and ssSSc, and the two-subset classification of Leroy and Black is limited by the fact that clinical outcome within each major subset is so varied. Although the prevalence of SOI is higher for dcSSc, some patients with lcSSc develop SOI with a similarly poor prognosis. A new classification that takes into account clinical findings, serological markers (e.g., rheumatoid factor), and genetic markers is necessary to identify subsets of patients at increased risk for life-threatening complications.

REFERENCES

1. LeRoy, E.C. *et al.* 1988. Scleroderma (systemic sclerosis): classification, subsets and pathogenesis. J. Rheumatol. **15:** 202–205.
2. Ferri, C. *et al.* 2002. Systemic sclerosis: demographic, clinical, and serologic features and survival in 1,012 Italian patients. Medicine (Baltimore) **81:** 139–153.
3. Subcommittee for scleroderma criteria of the American Rheumatism Association Diagnostic and Therapeutic Criteria Committee. 1980. Preliminary criteria for the classification of systemic sclerosis (scleroderma). Arthritis Rheum. **23:** 581–590.
4. Denton, C.P. *et al.* 1996. Systemic sclerosis: current pathogenetic concepts and future prospects for targeted therapy. Lancet **347:** 1453–1458.
5. Steen, V.D. & T.A. Medsger, Jr. 2000. Severe organ involvement in systemic sclerosis with diffuse scleroderma. Arthritis Rheum. **43:** 2437–2444.
6. Altman, R.D., T.A. Medsger, Jr., D.A. Bloch & B.A. Michel. 1991. Predictors of survival in systemic sclerosis (scleroderma). Arthritis Rheum. **34:** 403–413.
7. Bryan, C., C. Knight, C.M. Black & A.J. Silman. 1999. Prediction of five-year survival following presentation with scleroderma: development of a simple model using three disease factors at first visit. Arthritis Rheum. **42:** 2660–2665.
8. Dourdan, P. *et al.* 1983. Antinuclear, anti-DNA and anti-lymphocyte antibodies in systemic scleroderma. 62 cases. Rev. Rhum. Mal. Osteoartic **50:** 521–524.
9. Dorner, T., K. Egerer, E. Feist & G.R. Burmester. 2004. Rheumatoid factor revisited. Curr. Opin. Rheumatol. **16:** 246–253.
10. Newkirk, M.M. 2002. Rheumatoid factors: host resistance or autoimmunity? Clin. Immunol. **104:** 1–13.
11. Poormoghim, H., M. Lucas, N. Fertig & T.A. Medsger, Jr. 2000. Systemic sclerosis sine scleroderma: demographic, clinical, and serologic features and survival in forty-eight patients. Arthritis Rheum. **43:** 444–451.

12. LONZETTI, L.S. *et al.* 2001. Updating the American College of Rheumatology preliminary classification criteria for systemic sclerosis: addition of severe nailfold capillaroscopy abnormalities markedly increases the sensitivity for limited scleroderma. Arthritis Rheum. **44:** 735–736.
13. SCUSSEL-LONZETTI, L. *et al.* 2002. Predicting mortality in systemic sclerosis: analysis of a cohort of 309 French Canadian patients with emphasis on features at diagnosis as predictive factors for survival. Medicine (Baltimore) **81:** 154–167.

Hughes Syndrome, the Antiphospholipid Syndrome

A New Chapter in Neurology

GIOVANNI SANNA,[a,b] MARIA LAURA BERTOLACCINI,[b]
AND GRAHAM R. V. HUGHES[b]

[a]*Department of Rheumatology, Homerton University Hospital, London, United Kingdom*

[b]*Lupus Research Unit, The Rayne Institute, St. Thomas' Hospital, London, United Kingdom*

ABSTRACT: **The importance of cerebral disease in patients with the antiphospholipid (Hughes) syndrome (APS) is now becoming more widely recognized. The range of neuropsychiatric manifestations of APS is comprehensive and includes focal symptoms attributable to lesions in a specific area of the brain as well as diffuse or global dysfunction. Patients with APS frequently present with strokes and transient ischemic attacks, but a wide spectrum of other neurologic features, also including nonthrombotic neurological syndromes, has been described in association with the presence of antiphospholipid antibodies. In this review, we attempt to highlight the large variety of the neurological features of APS.**

KEYWORDS: **central nervous system; cerebral ischemia; thrombosis; MRI; antiphospholipid antibodies; anticardiolipin antibodies; lupus anticoagulant**

INTRODUCTION

The antiphospholipid (Hughes) syndrome (APS) is a common autoimmune prothrombotic condition characterized by arterial and/or venous thrombosis and pregnancy morbidity associated with persistently positive anticardiolipin antibodies (aCLs) and/or lupus anticoagulant (LA).[1,2] APS can occur in association with other autoimmune disease (secondary APS), most frequently systemic lupus erythematosus (SLE), or as an isolated disorder (primary APS).[3] APS may affect any size of vessel and any organ of the body. A broad spectrum of clinical features that includes peripheral venous and arterial thrombosis, obstetric manifestations and pregnancy morbidity, skin disease, cardiac and pulmonary manifestations, renal involvement, hematologic manifestations, and neurological disorders can be seen in patients with APS.[4]

Address for correspondence: Graham R.V. Hughes, M.D., F.R.C.P., Lupus Research Unit, The Rayne Institute, St. Thomas' Hospital, London SE1 7EH, United Kingdom. Voice: +44-0-207-188-3570; fax: +44-0-207-620-2658.
graham.hughes@kcl.ac.uk

**Ann. N.Y. Acad. Sci. 1051: 465–486 (2005). © 2005 New York Academy of Sciences.
doi: 10.1196/annals.1361.088**

TABLE 1. Neuropsychiatric manifestations associated with the presence of antiphospholipid antibodies

Cerebrovascular disease
Transient ischemic attacks
Ischemic stroke
Sneddon's syndrome
Acute ischemic encephalopathy
Moyamoya disease
Cerebral venous thrombosis
Seizures
Headache
Chorea
Multiple sclerosis–like syndrome
Transverse myelitis
Idiopathic intracranial hypertension
Sensorineural hearing loss
Guillain-Barré syndrome
Transient global amnesia
Ocular syndromes
Dystonia-Parkinsonism
Cognitive dysfunction
Dementia
Depression
Psychosis

The full impact of APS on neurology was foreseen in the original description of the syndrome in 1983.[5–7] In the early 1980s, Hughes and his group reported the association of antiphospholipid antibodies (aPLs) with a large number of neuropsychiatric manifestations including cerebrovascular accidents, dementia, migraine, epilepsy, chorea, transverse myelitis, and Guillain-Barré syndrome.[6–9]

Today, more than 20 years later, APS is fully recognized as a major neurological disease.[10] Although cerebral ischemia is the most common manifestation, several other neuropsychiatric features, including chronic headache, dementia, cognitive dysfunction, psychosis, depression, transverse myelitis, multiple sclerosis–like disease, chorea, and seizures have been associated with aPL.[11–16] TABLE 1 summarizes the wide spectrum of central nervous system (CNS) manifestations associated with the presence of aPL.

Mechanisms of cerebral involvement in APS are not completely understood. Animal models are providing important insights in some of the underlying mechanisms for CNS dysfunction.[17–19] Interestingly, although the mechanism of neurological involvement in APS is considered to be primarily thrombotic, there is an increasing body of evidence that supports the hypothesis that aPLs may also have more direct pathogenetic effects.[20] It has been shown that aPLs bind neurons, glial cells, and myelin and disrupt their function.[21,22] aPLs may also interfere with endothelial cells and promote their procoagulant activity.[23–26]

CEREBROVASCULAR DISEASE

Strokes and transient ischemic attacks (TIAs) are considered the most common arterial thrombotic event in patients with APS.[4,13,27–29] Our own experience suggests a strong association between the presence of aPLs and cerebrovascular disease in a large series of patients with SLE.[30] Amaurosis fugax, transient paresthesia, ataxia, motor weakness, vertigo, and transient global ischemia can all be expressions of TIAs.[31] Khamashta *et al.*[32] showed that the prevalence of valvular abnormalities is higher in SLE patients with aPL than in those without. Left-sided valve lesion, in particular, can be a source for emboli and a possible cause of ischemic stroke in aPL patients.[33–35]

Many studies have found that aPLs are associated with an increased risk for cerebral ischemia in the general population,[36–47] although some have not.[48–52] Brey *et al.*[45] reported a prospective association between aCL and stroke over a 20-year period of follow-up in men enrolled in the Honolulu Heart program. They found that the presence of β2GPI-dependent aCL of the IgG class was significantly associated with both incident ischemic stroke and myocardial infarction. Janardhan *et al.*[47] recently published the results of a large prospective population-based cohort study with a 11-year period of follow-up in the context of the Framingham Heart Study. They showed that aCLs are an independent risk factor for ischemic stroke and TIA in women after multivariate adjustment for other cardiovascular risk factors, including age, systolic blood pressure, diabetes, cigarette smoking, and plasma C-reactive protein and cholesterol levels.

However, it is still controversial whether the presence of aPL at the time of initial stroke increases the risk of recurrence in an unselected population. In 1997, Levine *et al.*[53] showed that the risk for recurrent stroke was higher in patients with aPL after the first cerebral ischemic episode. These results were not confirmed in two studies by the Antiphospholipid Antibodies and Stroke Study (APASS) Group.[54,55] Levine and the APASS investigators[55] recently reported that the presence of either LA or aCL among patients with ischemic stroke did not predict an increased risk for further thrombo-occlusive events. The authors concluded that routine screening for aPL did not appear warranted in patients with ischemic stroke. Several important limitations of this study have raised serious concerns[56–58]: (1) the average age of patients (62.5 years) was significantly higher than that of those in previous studies of APS (34 years)[4]; (2) only a single measurement of aCL and LA was obtained; (3) a high proportion of patients was found positive for aPL (41%), but only 0.2% had high IgG levels and only 6.7% tested positive for both aCL and LA. Interestingly, the group of patients positive for both aCL and LA had a tendency to develop recurrent events. Although this recent study doubted whether the presence of aPL increases the risk factors for a recurrent stroke or other thromboembolic events, most data point to persistent medium/high-titer aCL and/or LA as a risk factor for recurrence. A recent systematic review of the literature showed LA to be a risk factor of thrombosis, independent of the site (venous or arterial) and the type of event (first or recurrence). aCLs were not such strong risk factors, unless the IgG isotype and medium and high titers were considered.[59]

Another recent study failed to find a higher incidence of recurrent cerebral ischemia in children positive for aPL.[60] This study included 185 children surviving first ischemic stroke or TIA who were tested for aCL and followed up for a median of 2.8 years. Although a higher rate of recurrent arterial ischemic stroke/TIA was observed (36%), no differences were found in rates of recurrent thromboembolism between aCL-positive and aCL-negative groups. The main limitation of this study is the fact that aCL-positive children were more likely to be treated with antithrombotic agents than those negative for aCL. Those receiving treatment had, in turn, a reduced risk of recurrent ischemic stroke or TIA.

Sneddon's Syndrome

Cerebrovascular disease in association with widespread livedo reticularis is also known as Sneddon's syndrome. The pathogenesis of Sneddon's syndrome has remained largely unclear since Sneddon's original description of four cases in 1965.[61] There has been an increasing number of reports of an association between Sneddon's syndrome and aPL, leading to the understanding that at least some cases diagnosed as Sneddon's syndrome can also be diagnosed as APS.[62,63]

Sneddon's syndrome is not a unique entity and aPL may play a pathogenic role in a subset of patients with this disorder. Some authors suggested including this condition among the neurologic manifestations of APS.[64,65] Frances and Piette[66] found a prevalence of aPL of approximately 41% in patients diagnosed with Sneddon's syndrome, and Kalashnikova *et al.*[67] reported a more severe progression of the neurologic disease in patients with Sneddon's syndrome and high levels of aCL. Recently, Gomez-Puerta *et al.*[16] confirmed these observations in their study on the clinical and radiological characteristics of dementia associated with APS. They found that 10 of 30 patients (33%) with APS and dementia also had Sneddon's syndrome.

Less Common Cerebral Thrombotic Disease

Acute ischemic encephalopathy is a rare manifestation recognized in only 1.1% of APS patients in the largest cohort described to date.[4] This condition has been reported in association with aPL since 1989.[68] These patients can present acutely ill, confused, disoriented, and obtunded. MRI often shows abnormalities and cerebral atrophy.

There are a few reports of an association of aPL with moyamoya disease.[69–74] This rare disorder of uncertain cause is characterized by progressive vascular stenosis and blockage involving the supraclinoid segment of the internal carotid arteries and the first part of the middle or anterior cerebral arteries and, to a lesser extent, the posterior cerebral arteries. The name moyamoya comes from the Japanese and it means "puff of smoke," which is the angiographic appearance of the extensive collateral circulation due to the extensive vascular blockage. Patients may present clinically with seizures, TIA, or stroke. This condition tends to affect children younger than 10 years of age but has also been described in adults (third to fourth decade). The association between APS and moyamoya disease has been reported only in children.[74] Booth *et al.*[71] have reported a 7-year-old child with ischemic stroke and persistently raised levels of aCL in the presence of moyamoya-like vascular changes. Treatment with warfarin and aspirin was followed by improvement in blood flow and reduction in the stenosis of the left internal carotid artery. Recently, Yamashita *et al.*[74] reported the case of a 12-year-old Japanese female who presented with choreic movements and thrombocytopenia. Tests for aCL and LA were persistently positive and angiogram showed typical moyamoya changes. The authors suggested considering the possibility of APS in children with moyamoya disease.

A less common form of cerebral thrombotic disease associated with aPL is sagittal venous sinus thrombosis.[13,75] This manifestation occurs at a younger age and with more extensive superficial and deep cerebral venous system involvement in patients with aPL than in those without.[76–81] Deschiens *et al.*[82] showed that aPLs often present in association with other concomitant risk factors for thrombophilia in patients with venous sinus thrombosis. The prevalence of cerebral venous thrombosis was 0.7% in the Euro-Phospholipid Project Group study.[4]

EPILEPSY

Seizures are one of the most prominent and common neurologic features of APS. All ages may be affected, and different forms of epilepsy are seen in association with aPL.[14] Generalized tonic-clonic seizures are the most common, but simple partial and complex seizures have also been described.[30,83,84] Several studies have confirmed the original observation of Mackworth-Young and Hughes in 1985[83] of the association between aPL and seizures.[3,30,84–91]

Most of the studies regarding epilepsy are related to SLE or to APS secondary to SLE, and limited data are available regarding epilepsy in primary APS. A recent article from the Euro-Phospholipid Project Group reported seizures in 7% of 1,000 patients with APS,[4] but this figure is probably an underestimate. Shoenfeld *et al.*[15] recently reported epilepsy in 8.6% of 538 patients with APS. Epilepsy was more prevalent among patients with APS secondary to systemic lupus erythematosus (SLE) (13.7%) when compared with those with primary APS (6%). They also found that patients with epilepsy had a higher prevalence of focal ischemic events, suggesting that in many cases seizures may be the expression of an underlying ischemic event occurring as a result of hypercoagulability.

The concomitance of cerebrovascular disease and positivity for aPL when analyzing risk factors for seizures may represent a confounding factor.[84] In fact, seizures are a well-known symptom of cerebral ischemia.[92] It is possible that aPLs cause ischemic events secondary to hypercoagulability and that these are, in turn, directly responsible for the occurrence of seizures in aPL-positive patients. However, this explains only part of the increased occurrence of epilepsy in APS, and a primary immunological basis for seizures in APS also has been postulated. Although the pathogenetic mechanisms underlying the association of seizures with aPL remain uncertain, there is increasing evidence supporting the hypothesis of a direct interaction of aPL with neuronal tissue as a possible alternative mechanism to hypercoagulability.[20,93,94] It has been demonstrated that aCLs obtained from patients with SLE who had seizures reduce a gamma-aminobutyric acid (GABA) receptor–mediated chloride current in snail neurons,[93] suggesting that aPL might lower the seizure threshold with a direct and reversible mechanism. Also, aPLs have been shown to bind directly to ependyma and myelin of fixed cat[95] and rat brain.[96] The finding that aPL depolarize brain nerve terminals[94] has provided further evidence that these antibodies may play a role in the pathogenesis of seizures in APS.

In a population-based cross-sectional study, Ranua *et al.*[97] found an association between the presence of aCL and long duration of partial epilepsy as well as an association between the presence of these antibodies and poor seizure control despite antiepileptic treatment, supporting the hypothesis that these antibodies may play a role at least in certain types of epilepsy. In a previous study from our group, seizures were found to be associated with moderate-to-high titers of aCL, supporting the possibility of a role for aPL in the etiopathogenesis of epilepsy in SLE.[87] In a 5-year-duration prospective study of 252 patients with SLE, Liou *et al.*[98] confirmed an association between epilepsy and high titers of aCL. The odds ratio of developing seizure was 3.7 for SLE patients who had a high baseline serum level of aCL when compared with those without a detectable level of these antibodies.

Our more recent experience confirmed a strong association between the presence of aPL and seizures in a large series of SLE patients.[30] We applied the new American College of Rheumatology (ACR) nomenclature for neuropsychiatric systemic lupus erythematosus [99] to determine the prevalence of the different neuropsychiatric syndromes in 323 patients with SLE and evaluated which of these manifestations correlated with the presence of aPL. In total, 185 patients (57.3%) with neuropsychiatric manifestations were identified. Prevalence of seizures was 8.3%. Both IgG and IgM aCL were more frequently found in patients with seizures than in those without. Interestingly, the association of seizures with aCL remained significant after excluding 47 patients with stroke and/or TIAs. Multivariate analysis confirmed that aCL were independently associated with cerebrovascular accidents and seizures.

Mikdashi and Handwerger[100] recently evaluated a cohort of 130 SLE patients to identify factors predictive of neuropsychiatric damage. Seizures, cerebrovascular accidents, and cognitive impairment were independently associated with the presence of IgG aCL and LA. This study further supports the importance of aPL as risk factor associated with significant neuropsychiatric damage, as has been shown by others.[30,101]

Appenzeller *et al.*[84] recently analyzed frequency and risk factors of epileptic seizures in a cohort of 519 SLE patients. Seizures were observed in 60 (11.6%) patients. Stroke and presence of moderate to high titers of IgG aCL were associated with epileptic seizures at disease onset. Patients with renal flares, presence of epileptic seizures at disease onset, and patients with positivity for aPL were at greater risk for seizures during follow-up. Recurrent unprovoked epileptic seizures were observed in 7 of 60 (11.7%) SLE patients, and, interestingly, all 7 patients had APS. This finding, which suggests that the risk of recurrent seizures is greater in SLE patients with APS than in those without, can have therapeutic consequences in the decision-making analysis regarding antiepileptic drug therapy.

Antiepileptic medications (e.g., phenytoin, carbamazepine, and valproate) have been reported to cause a drug-induced SLE and to trigger clinical exacerbation of SLE.[102] The increased prevalence of autoantibodies in patients with epilepsy has also been attributed to the use of antiepileptic drugs.[103] However, recent studies showed no associations between the presence of autoantibodies, including aPL, and antiepileptic medications in patients with epilepsy.[89,97,104,105]

HEADACHE

Chronic headache, including migraine, is common in patients with APS.[4,106] They may be migrainous and can last for days or weeks. The headaches are often intractable, unresponsive to narcotic analgesics, and can antedate the diagnosis by many years. Surprisingly, despite the overwhelmingly strong clinical association, the published data on the association of headache with aPL are still controversial,[107–109] and the exact prevalence of headache in patients with APS is unknown. Several problems contribute to these differences, especially the use of different classification for headache in the different studies. In our recent study in 323 SLE patients, we found that although the prevalence of headache was similar to that reported for the general population, aPL were more significantly prevalent in the group of patients with headache compared with those without. However, we failed to find an association between the presence of aPL and any particular type of headache, including migraine.[30]

CHOREA

Chorea is a rare manifestation, with an estimated prevalence of 1.3% in patients with APS.[4] Although rare, chorea has been strongly associated with the presence of aPL from the earliest descriptions of the syndrome.[5,7,110,111] The etiology of chorea is still unknown. A vascular pathogenesis is probable. In many patients with chorea, focal lesions on brain imaging have often been absent,[110,111] throwing doubt on a purely thrombotic cause. It has also been suggested that aPL can cause chorea by an antigen/antibody mechanism binding phospholipid in the basal ganglia.[112]

Cervera *et al.*[113] reviewed the clinical, radiological, and immunologic characteristics of 50 patients with chorea and the APS. Fifty-eight percent of patients had defined SLE, 12% "lupus-like" syndrome, 30% had PAPS. Twelve percent of patients developed chorea soon after they started taking estrogen-containing oral contraceptives, 6% developed chorea gravidarum, and 2% of patients developed chorea shortly after delivery. Most patients (66%) had only one episode of chorea. Chorea was bilateral in 55% of patients. Computed tomography and MRI scans reported cerebral infarcts in 35% of patients.

MULTIPLE SCLEROSIS–LIKE SYNDROME

Some patients with APS exhibit features often seen in multiple sclerosis (MS).[114,115] Ischemic changes in white matter may be difficult to differentiate from those of MS, making the differential diagnosis extremely difficult. Some APS patients can be misdiagnosed as having MS, making this a crucial point for the therapeutic approach.[14] Cuadrado *et al.*[11] in a study from our unit, analyzed 27 APS patients in whom an original diagnosis of MS was made, in an attempt to identify parameters that might differentiate the two entities. Neurologic symptoms and physical examination of the patients were not different from those common in MS patients.

A previous history of thrombosis or pregnancy morbidity in female patients may contribute to the differential diagnosis, favoring APS.[11,14] The abruptness of onset and resolution of symptoms, especially in regard to visual symptoms (i.e., amaurosis fugax), and atypical neurological features for MS, such as headache or epilepsy, strongly suggest APS rather than MS.[116] Moreover, in the majority of the patients ultimately correctly diagnosed with APS and appropriately anticoagulated, there were no further neurological events.[14] We think that, if not all, at least a subgroup of patients with "nonclassic" MS should be tested for aPL.

TRANSVERSE MYELITIS

This is a rare manifestation, with a recently estimated prevalence of less than 1% in patients with APS.[4,117] The first case of transverse myelitis associated with aPL was described in 1985 by our group[8] in a 45-year-old woman with a lupus-like illness and high-titer positivity for aCL of the IgM isotype. Later on, many other authors confirmed the association between aPL and transverse myelitis. The prevalence of aPL had been shown to be higher in SLE patients with transverse myelitis compared with SLE patients in general.[118] Lavalle *et al.*[119] reported 10 of 12 patients with transverse myelitis and SLE as having aCL, with the other 2 patients showing evidence of VDRL-positive and prolonged APTT. Both IgG and IgM isotype aCL were detected in 8 of 10 patients. The authors concluded that there is a strong association between transverse myelitis in SLE and the presence of aPL. Ruiz-Arguelles *et al.*[120] described a patient with refractory hiccup as the heralding symptom of transverse myelitis in association with aCL.

The pathophysiology of spinal cord damage in aPL-associated myelopathy is uncertain; however, both ischemia and antibody-mediated interaction have been postulated. Kovacs *et al.*[121] evaluated 14 patients with SLE and transverse myelitis and 91 additional cases published in the literature. Forty three percent of their patients and 64% of the patients reported in the literature were aPL-positive. More recently, D'Cruz *et al.*[122] described a series of 15 patients with transverse myelitis as the presenting manifestation of SLE or lupus-like disease. Interestingly, 73% of the patients were aPL-positive, supporting the view of a strong association of transverse myelitis with aPL.

IDIOPATHIC INTRACRANIAL HYPERTENSION

Idiopathic intracranial hypertension (IIH) can be the presenting symptom of APS, and the available evidence support the hypothesis that aPLs may play a role in the pathogenesis of this manifestation. However, the true incidence of IIH in APS patients is still unknown. After a few anecdotal reports on the presence of aPL in patients with IIH,[123,124] more recent studies confirmed that these antibodies are strongly associated with this neurologic complication. Sussman *et al.*[125] found that a substantial number of patients with intracranial hypertension were positive for aCL (11/38, 29%), but only four of them had aCL without evidence of underlying sinus thrombosis or any other associated prothrombotic risk factor. More interesting were the findings of Leker and Steiner,[75] who found persistently elevated titers of aCL in 6 of 14 patients (43%) with IIH. The association between aPL and IIH was more recently confirmed by Kesler *et al.*[126] in a retrospective study.

OTHER NEUROLOGICAL SYNDROMES

Sensorineural Hearing Loss

The association between sensorineural hearing loss and aPL, first anecdotally reported,[127–129] has been recently confirmed by several authors.[130–132] Toubi *et al.*[130]

found that 27% of 30 patients with sudden sensorineural hearing loss were positive for aCL compared with 0% of the control group, suggesting that aPLs may play a primary role in the pathogenesis of this condition. Naarendorp and Spiera[131] also described six patients with SLE or a lupus-like syndrome, who developed sudden sensorineural hearing loss and had elevated serum levels of aCL or positivity for LA. More recently, Green and Miller[132] described a case of sudden sensorineural hearing loss in association with aPL as a first manifestation of SLE and suggested anticoagulant treatment for these patients.

Guillain-Barré Syndrome

Guillain-Barré syndrome is a transient neurological disorder characterized by an inflammatory demyelination of peripheral nerves. Although the pathogenesis of this disorder has not been elucidated, there is increasing evidence pointing to an autoimmune etiology. This demyelinating neuropathy, also uncommon in SLE patients, was associated with aPL in the original descriptions of the Hughes syndrome.[6] Gilburd *et al.*[133] studied the reactivity of Guillain-Barré syndrome sera with various phospholipids which are known to be important constituents of myelin and serve as autoantigens in other autoimmune conditions, demonstrating that some Guillain-Barré syndrome patients produce autoantibodies to various phospholipid and nuclear antigens. However, these autoantibodies are probably produced as a result of the myelin damage rather than cause the demyelination.

Transient Global Amnesia

Transient global amnesia, a syndrome of sudden unexplained short-term memory loss in association with aPL was reported by Montalban *et al.*[134] Some regard this disturbance as migrainous in origin, but other mechanisms such as epileptic seizure have been advocated as involved in its pathogenesis.[135]

Ocular Syndromes

Ophthalmologic features are present in 15–88% of the patients with APS. An ophthalmic assessment should be part of the clinical evaluation of any patients with suspected or confirmed APS.[136] Amaurosis fugax suggests cerebral ischemia and is one of the most common ocular manifestations in APS. Other visual disturbances have been associated with the presence of aPL. Ischemic optic neuropathy is less frequently described in APS when compared with SLE patients.[137,138] Frohman *et al.*[139] recently reported the association between primary APS and autoimmune optic neuropathy in a 4-year-old child who presented four consecutive episodes of bilateral optic neuritis, one episode of unilateral optic neuritis, weakness, and ataxia in the presence of persistently raised aCL and abnormal skin biopsy showing microthrombosis. Papais-Alvarenga *et al.*[140] described clinical features and outcome of 24 Brazilian patients with optic neuromyelitis syndrome. Interestingly, three patients with recurrent optic neuropathy also had APS. Vaso-occlusive retinopathy has also been described in the presence of aPL.[141] This is a rare but severe form of retinopathy characterized by microthrombosis and often associated with other CNS manifestations.[142] Poor visual outcome with visual loss has been reported in 80% of cases, with neovascularization occurring in 40% of cases.[142] aPL have also been noted in a patient with acute multifocal posterior placoid pigment epitheliopathy, a disorder that has been associated with retinal vascular occlusive disease.[143]

Dystonia-Parkinsonism

There are a few anecdotal reports of Parkinsonism in association with APS.[144,145] Milanov et al.[145] recently reported the combination of dystonia with Parkinsonian-like symptoms as a presenting clinical manifestation of APS in a 60-year-old man who had ischemic lesions in the basal ganglia on MRI and positive aPL. Reiblat *et al.*[146] recently reported a 52-year-old man with Parkinson's disease who developed severe headache, progressive dementia, ataxia, downgaze palsy, and axial and limb rigidity. Treatment with levodopa was introduced without any improvement in his condition. Neurologic diagnosis was modified to supranuclear palsy. Subsequently, he developed livedo reticularis and thrombocytopenia and was found positive for aCL and LA. It has been suggested that anticoagulation should be considered in patients with aPL and dystonia-Parkinsonism to prevent further deterioration in case of lack of clinical improvement with levodopa, bromocriptine, and anticholinergics.[147]

COGNITIVE DYSFUNCTION

Cognitive deficits are an important feature of APS, but its epidemiology and pathogenesis are still unclear. They may vary from mild neurocognitive disorders to severe vascular dementia. Patients affected by mild cognitive dysfunction often complain of poor concentration or forgetfulness. Most published data are related to SLE patients, with limited data regarding cognitive dysfunction in APS patients. In the largest published series of APS to date, a prevalence of 2% was reported for multi-infarct dementia, but no data were provided on different types of cognitive dysfunction.[4] The recognition of subtle forms of cognitive dysfunction has been facilitated by the application of formal neuropsychological assessment mainly in patients with SLE.[30,148–152]

The relationship of cognitive dysfunction with aPL has been investigated in cross-sectional[153,154] and prospective/longitudinal studies.[155,156] Verbal and non-verbal memory, including working memory, verbal fluency, psychomotor speed, and cognitive flexibility, and decreased overall productivity have been correlated with aPL.[154–156] In the studies from Menon *et al.*[156] and Hanly *et al.*,[155] SLE patients persistently positive for aCL (medium to high titer) had significantly lower scores on a variety of neuropsychologic tests than SLE patients negative for aPL. There was no association between results of neuropsychologic tests and levels of anti-DNA or C3 fraction levels.

Denburg *et al.*[154] also found that LA-positive patients performed worse in measures of verbal memory, cognitive flexibility, and psychomotor speed. This pattern of deficits was compatible to a subcortical involvement, possibly on the basis of ongoing LA-related microthrombotic events or vasculopathy. Because many of these patients had no previous history of any neuropsychiatric involvement, the authors also suggested a direct relationship between the presence of aPL and cognitive impairment.

Whether these cognitive deficits are related to recurrent cerebral ischemia or whether there is any other underlying mechanism is not clear. Subtle cognitive dysfunction indicates a probable subclinical nervous system compromise, possibly on the basis of ongoing aPL-related microthrombotic events or vasculopathy. It is also possible that aPL may play a more direct pathogenetic role in causing cognitive dysfunction, as shown by recent experimental studies. It has been demonstrated that aPL may gain access to the CNS,[157] disrupt neuronal function,[94] and play a direct role in the pathogenesis of behavioral impairment in animal models of APS.[18–20,158]

Clinical implications of these findings are that, although the current evidence does not support the introduction of aggressive anticoagulation as a strategy to prevent subclinical cognitive impairment, there may be a role for more benign therapies such as low-dose aspirin or antimalarials. On the other hand, anecdotal reports of improvement of these symptoms after anticoagulation therapy commenced for other reasons in APS patients[159] may provide some support for the theory that arterial thrombosis and/or ischemia represent the primary cause of this type of central nervous system dysfunction, supporting the utility of further longitudinal case–control trials to answer the question of whether an anticoagulation treatment with low targeted international normalized ratio (INR) could be superior to aspirin in these patients.

DEMENTIA

A chronic multifocal disease, defined as a recurrent or progressive neurological deterioration attributable to cerebrovascular disease, can produce multi-infarct dementia. Dementia is an unusual manifestation of APS but has a high disability impact in a patient's daily life. In the largest published series of APS to date, a prevalence of 2% was reported for multi-infarct dementia.[4] Our group first described this manifestation in 1987.[9] We went on to describe in 1989[31] the clinical and serologic features of 35 patients with aPL and cerebrovascular disease. Strokes were often multiple and were followed by multi-infarct dementia in nine patients. This dementia, generally associated with a loss of cognitive functions and impairment of skills, concentration, memory dysfunction, language impairment, and judgmental defects, does not present with peculiar characteristics. It cannot be differentiated from other kinds of dementia such as in Alzheimer's disease, senile dementia, or metabolic/toxic conditions involving the brain. Many other authors have since reported this complication in patients with recurrent strokes.[160–162]

Mosek *et al.*[163] examined the relationship of aPL to dementia in the elderly in a case-controlled study. They found that 5 of the 87 demented patients (6%), but none of the 69 controls, had significantly elevated aCL IgG levels (>20 GPL). All the patients with high aCL IgG levels were diagnosed clinically as having dementia of the Alzheimer type, except for one who had mixed dementia, and none had features of an immune-mediated disease. This study showed that a small but significant number of patients with dementia having high levels of aPL. The role of the aPL in these patients, with apparently diffuse brain disease, is currently unknown. Chapman *et al.*[164] recently confirmed the association of APS with dementia in a hospital-based study. They found that 13 of 23 patients (56%) with primary APS were demented, with higher levels of aPL and significantly older when compared with the nondemented APS patients. The authors suggested that the length of exposure to aPL may play an important role, as well the presence of high levels of aPL, in determining the development of dementia. A recent article by Gomez-Puerta *et al.*[16] reviewed the clinical and radiologic characteristics of 30 patients with dementia associated with APS. Most of the cases (25 patients) were identified by a search of the literature; 5 were included from their own center. The mean age of patients was 49 ± 15 years. Forty-seven percent of patients had primary APS, 30% had SLE, and 23% had "lupus-like" syndrome. Thirty-seven percent of patients had cerebrovascular accidents, 33% had cerebrovascular disease in association with livedo reticularis (Sneddon's syndrome), and 27% had heart valve lesions. Computed tomography and MRI scans identified cortical infarcts in 63% of patients, subcortical infarcts in 30%, basal ganglia infarcts in 23%, and cerebral atrophy in 37%. Sixty-three percent of patients presented APS manifestations previously to the diagnosis of dementia, but only a minority of them (37%) was receiving anticoagulation. The mean time of evolution from the initial manifestation of APS to the diagnosis of dementia in these patients was 3.5 years. The authors recommended testing for aPL in young subjects with no explicable cause of dementia to rule out the possibility of APS. They also recommended considering MRI and echocardiographic evaluation in all patients with APS, and appropriate antithrombotic prophylaxis once the diagnosis of APS is made to prevent disease progression.

OTHER PSYCHIATRIC DISORDERS

Psychiatric problems such as mood alterations and psychosis may be present in patients with APS, although both the frequency and the pathophysiological relationship to APS remain controversial. It is also possible that these findings are complicated by the development in some cases of drug-induced aPL.[165] It is also difficult to establish whether or not the psychiatric symptoms are caused by a psychological reaction of suffering from a chronic disorder.[166]

SMALL HIGH-DENSITY LESIONS ON BRAIN MRI

Brain MRI in aPL patients with ischemic stroke typically shows cortical abnormalities consistent with large vessel occlusion. However, small high-density lesions on the brain MRI are frequently found in patients with aPL and, in our experience, also in SLE patients with or without overt neuropsychiatric manifestations[167] (FIG. 1). The significance of these lesions is not completely understood. They are often defined as consistent with the presence of small vessel disease by the neuroradiologists. It has been suggested that they may be caused by multiple small infarcts. There is also evidence that the presence of similar lesions is associated with a higher risk for stroke,[168] dementia, and cognitive decline in the elderly population.[169] The finding of white matter hyperintensities on the brain MRI may represent a diagnostic and therapeutic dilemma especially when recognized in young patients. In our experience, subclinical cognitive disorders, usually undetected in the absence of a formal neuropsychological assessment, are frequent in these patients. In a recent study, we also found that small high-density lesions on the brain MRI were associated with the

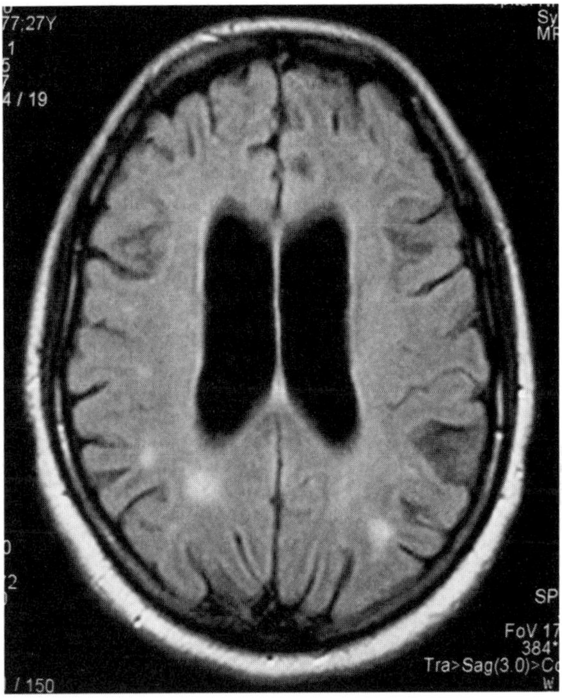

FIGURE 1. Brain MRI showing white matter hyperintensity lesions in a 27-year-old woman with systemic lupus erythematosus, severe cognitive dysfunction, and high-titer IgG anticardiolipin antibodies and positive lupus anticoagulant.

presence of LA,[30] supporting the hypothesis of an underlying ischemic/thrombotic mechanism for these lesions.

SPECT STUDIES

Abnormality in regional cerebral blood flow by SPECT study has been reported in APS patients.[170–174] Two recent studies[170,173] have reported brain SPECT abnormalities in patients with primary APS and mild diffuse neuropsychiatric manifestations (headache, memory loss, or other cognitive function deficits) in the presence of a normal brain MRI study. Focal and diffuse hypoperfusion brain lesions were found in 73–80% of the patients, mainly over the territory of the medial cerebral arteries. These studies demonstrated that brain SPECT is a sensitive diagnostic tool useful in identifying early neuropsychiatric involvement in patients with APS. Sun *et al.*[174] recently used brain SPECT to assess the effects of anticoagulant therapy on regional cerebral blood flow in 16 patients with primary APS and neuropsychiatric manifestations. All the patients presented with minor neuropsychiatric manifestations (headaches, cognitive dysfunction, depression) and had a normal brain MRI but abnormal findings on SPECT scan at the time of study entry. A follow-up SPECT study was repeated 1 month after anticoagulant therapy. All patients had a complete clinical recovery. Improvement in cerebral blood flow was demonstrated in all 16 patients, with a complete normalization of the hypoperfusion lesions in 70% of the cases. The authors suggested that brain SPECT is useful to assess the effects of anticoagulant therapy by determining changes on regional blood flow in APS patients with brain involvement.

CONCLUSION

The description of APS has had a profound impact on the understanding and management of the treatment of CNS manifestations associated with connective tissue diseases, in particular, SLE. Many patients with focal neurological manifestations and aPL, who a few years ago would have received a high dose of corticosteroids and/or immunosuppression, are now successfully treated with anticoagulation.[175] In our opinion, testing for aPL may have a major diagnostic and therapeutic impact not only in patients with autoimmune diseases and neuropsychiatric manifestations, but also in young individuals who develop cerebral ischemia, and in those with atypical multiple sclerosis, transverse myelitis, and atypical seizures. We would also recommend testing for aPL for young individuals found with multiple hyperintensity lesions on brain MRI in the absence of other possible causes, especially when younger than the age of 40. It is our practice to anticoagulate patients with aPL suffering from cerebral ischemia with a target INR of 3.0 to prevent recurrences. Low-dose aspirin alone (with occasional exceptions) does not seem helpful to prevent recurrent thrombosis in these patients. Our recommendation once the patient has had a proven thrombosis associated with aPL is long-term (possibly life-long) warfarin therapy.[13,176] Oral anticoagulation carries a risk of hemorrhage, but in our experience the risk of fatal bleeding in patients with APS and previous thrombosis treated with oral anticoagulation to a target INR of 3.5 was similar to that in groups of patients treated to lower target ratios.[177] In our experience, anticoagulation treatment has proved of benefit also in selected cases of patients with aPL and other neuropsychiatric manifestations, such as seizures and intractable headache unresponsive to conventional treatment.[159] However, a double-blind crossover trial comparing low-molecular weight heparin with placebo in patients with aPL and chronic incapacitating headache did not show any beneficial effect.[178]

REFERENCES

1. WILSON, W.A., A.E. GHARAVI, T. KOIKE, *et al.* 1999. International consensus statement on preliminary classification criteria for definite antiphospholipid syndrome: report of an international workshop. Arthritis Rheum. **42:** 1309–1311.
2. KHAMASHTA, M.A., M.L. BERTOLACCINI & G.R.V. HUGHES. 2004. Antiphospholipid (Hughes) syndrome. Autoimmunity **37:** 309–312.
3. MACKWORTH-YOUNG, C.G., S. LOIZOU & M.J. WALPORT. 1989. Primary antiphospholipid syndrome: features of patients with raised anticardiolipin antibodies and no other disorder. Ann. Rheum. Dis. **48:** 362–367.

4. CERVERA, R., J.C. PIETTE, J. FONT, *et al.* 2002. Antiphospholipid syndrome: clinical and immunologic manifestations and patterns of disease expression in a cohort of 1,000 patients. Arthritis Rheum. **46:** 1019–1027.
5. HUGHES, G.R.V. 1983. Thrombosis, abortion, cerebral disease and the lupus anticoagulant. Br. Med. J. **287:** 1088–1089.
6. HARRIS, E.N., H. ENGLERT, G. DERUE, *et al.* 1983. Antiphospholipid antibodies in acute Guillain-Barré syndrome. Lancet **ii:** 1361–1362.
7. HUGHES, G.R.V. 1984. The Prosser-White oration 1983. Connective tissue disease and the skin. Clin. Exp. Dermatol. **9:** 535–544.
8. HARRIS, E.N., A.E. GHARAVI, C.G. MACKWORTH-YOUNG, *et al.* 1985. Lupoid sclerosis: a possible pathogenetic role for antiphospholipid antibodies. Ann. Rheum. Dis. **44:** 281–283.
9. ASHERSON, R., D. MERCEY, G. PHILLIPS, *et al.* 1987. Recurrent stroke and multi-infarct dementia in systemic lupus erythematosus: association with antiphospholipid antibodies. Ann. Rheum. Dis. **46:** 605–611.
10. LAMPROPOULOS, C.E. & G.R.V. HUGHES. 2004. The antiphospholipid (Hughes') syndrome: changing the face of neurology. Eur. J. Intern. Med. **15:** 147–150.
11. CUADRADO, M.J., M.A. KHAMASHTA, A. BALLESTEROS, *et al.* 2000. Can neurologic manifestations of Hughes (antiphospholipid) syndrome be distinguished from multiple sclerosis? Analysis of 27 patients and review of the literature. Medicine (Baltimore) **79:** 57–68.
12. CUADRADO, M.J., M.A. KHAMASHTA, D. D'CRUZ, *et al.* 2001. Migraine in Hughes syndrome. Heparin as a therapeutic trial? Q. J. Med. **94:** 114–115.
13. SANNA, G., M.L. BERTOLACCINI, M.J. CUADRADO, *et al.* 2003. Central nervous system involvement in the antiphospholipid (Hughes) syndrome. Rheumatology (Oxford) **42:** 200–213.
14. HUGHES, G.R.V. 2003. Migraine, memory loss, and "multiple sclerosis." Neurological features of the antiphospholipid (Hughes') syndrome. Postgrad. Med. J. **79:** 81–83.
15. SHOENFELD, Y., S. LEV, I. BLATT, *et al.* 2004. Features associated with epilepsy in the antiphospholipid syndrome. J. Rheumatol. **31:** 1344–1348.
16. GOMEZ-PUERTA, J.A., R. CERVERA, L.M. CALVO, *et al.* 2005. Dementia associated with the antiphospholipid syndrome: clinical and radiological characteristics of 30 patients. Rheumatology (Oxford) **44:** 95–99.
17. BLANK, M., I. KRAUSE, M. FRIDKIN, *et al.* 2002. Bacterial induction of autoantibodies to beta2-glycoprotein-I accounts for the infectious etiology of antiphospholipid syndrome. J. Clin. Invest. **109:** 797–804.
18. SHROT, S., A. KATZAV, A.D. KORCZYN, *et al.* 2002. Behavioral and cognitive deficits occur only after prolonged exposure of mice to antiphospholipid antibodies. Lupus **11:** 736–743.
19. SHOENFELD, Y., A. NAHUM, A.D. KORCZYN, *et al.* 2003. Neuronal-binding antibodies from patients with antiphospholipid syndrome induce cognitive deficits following intrathecal passive transfer. Lupus **12:** 436–442.
20. KATZAV, A., J. CHAPMAN & Y. SHOENFELD. 2003. CNS dysfunction in the antiphospholipid syndrome. Lupus **12:** 903–907.
21. SUN, K.H., W.T. LIU, C.Y. TSAI, *et al.* 1992. Inhibition of astrocyte proliferation and binding to brain tissue of anticardiolipin antibodies purified from lupus serum. Ann. Rheum. Dis. **51:** 707–712.
22. KHALILI, A. & R.C. COOPER. 1991. A study of immune responses to myelin and cardiolipin in patients with systemic lupus erythematosus (SLE). Clin. Exp. Immunol. **85:** 365–372.
23. OOSTING, J.D., R.H. DERKSEN, L. BLOKZIJL, *et al.* 1992. Antiphospholipid antibody positive sera enhance endothelial cell procoagulant activity—studies in a thrombosis model. Thromb. Haemost. **68:** 278–284.
24. SIMANTOV, R., J.M. LASALA, S.K. LO, *et al.* 1995. Activation of cultured vascular endothelial cells by antiphospholipid antibodies. J. Clin. Invest. **96:** 2211–2219.
25. DEL PAPA, N., L. GUIDALI, A. SALA, *et al.* 1997. Endothelial cells as target for antiphospholipid antibodies. Human polyclonal and monoclonal anti-beta 2-glycoprotein I antibodies react in vitro with endothelial cells through adherent beta 2-glycoprotein I and induce endothelial activation. Arthritis Rheum. **40:** 551–561.

26. MERONI, P., A. TINCANI, N. SEPP, *et al.* 2003. Endothelium and the brain in CNS lupus. Lupus **12:** 919–928.
27. KRNIC-BARRIE, S., C.R. O CONNOR, S.W. LOONEY, *et al.* 1997. A retrospective review of 61 patients with antiphospholipid syndrome. Analysis of factors influencing recurrent thrombosis. Arch. Intern. Med. **157:** 2101–2108.
28. SHAH, N.M., M.A. KHAMASHTA, T. ATSUMI, *et al.* 1998. Outcome of patients with anticardiolipin antibodies: a 10 year follow-up of 52 patients. Lupus **7:** 3–6.
29. SASTRE-GARRIGA, J. & X. MONTALBAN. 2003. APS and the brain. Lupus **12:** 877–882.
30. SANNA, G., M.L. BERTOLACCINI, M.J. CUADRADO, *et al.* 2003. Neuropsychiatric manifestations in systemic lupus erythematosus: prevalence and association with antiphospholipid antibodies. J. Rheumatol. **30:** 985–992.
31. ASHERSON, R.A., M.A. KHAMASHTA, A. GIL, *et al.* 1989. Cerebrovascular disease and antiphospholipid antibodies in systemic lupus erythematosus, lupus-like disease, and the primary antiphospholipid syndrome. Am. J. Med. **86:** 391–399.
32. KHAMASHTA, M.A., R. CERVERA, R.A. ASHERSON, *et al.* 1990. Association of antibodies against phospholipids with heart valve disease in systemic lupus erythematosus. Lancet **335:** 1541–1544.
33. DEVINSKY, O., C.K. PETITO & D.R. ALONSO. 1988. Clinical and neuropathological findings in systemic lupus erythematosus: the role of vasculitis, heart emboli, and thrombotic thrombocytopenic purpura. Ann. Neurol. **23:** 380–384.
34. FORD, S.E., D. LILLICRAP, D. BRUNET, *et al.* 1989. Thrombotic endocarditis and lupus anticoagulant. A pathogenetic possibility for idiopathic "rheumatic type" valvular heart disease. Arch. Pathol. Lab. Med. **113:** 350–353.
35. NESHER, G., J. ILANY, D. ROSENMANN, *et al.* 1997. Valvular dysfunction in antiphospholipid syndrome: prevalence, clinical features, and treatment. Semin. Arthritis Rheum. **27:** 27–35.
36. BREY, R.L., R.G. HART, D.G. SHERMAN, *et al.* 1990. Antiphospholipid antibodies and cerebral ischemia in young people. Neurology **40:** 1190–1196.
37. LEVINE, S.R., M.J. DEEGAN, N. FUTRELL, *et al.* 1990. Cerebrovascular and neurologic disease associated with antiphospholipid antibodies: 48 cases. Neurology **40:** 1181–1189.
38. NENCINI, P., M.C. BARUFFI, R. ABBATE, *et al.* 1992. Lupus anticoagulant and anticardiolipin antibodies in young adults with cerebral ischemia. Stroke **23:** 189–193.
39. THE ANTIPHOSPHOLIPID ANTIBODIES IN STROKE STUDY (APASS) GROUP. 1993. Anticardiolipin antibodies are an independent risk factor for first ischemic stroke. Neurology **43:** 2069–2073.
40. CAMERLINGO, M., L. CASTO, B. CENSORI, *et al.* 1995. Anticardiolipin antibodies in acute non-hemorrhagic stroke seen within six hours after onset. Acta Neurol. Scand. **92:** 69–71.
41. LEVINE, S.R., R.L. BREY, K.L. SAWAYA, *et al.* 1995. Recurrent stroke and thrombo-occlusive events in the antiphospholipid syndrome. Ann. Neurol. **38:** 119–124.
42. TUHRIM, S., J.H. RAND, X.X. WU, *et al.* 1999. Elevated anticardiolipin antibody titer is a stroke risk factor in a multiethnic population independent of isotype or degree of positivity. Stroke **30:** 1561–1565.
43. ZIELINSKA, J., D. RYGLEWICZ, E. WIERZCHOWSKA, *et al.* 1999. Anticardiolipin antibodies are an independent risk factor for ischemic stroke. Neurol. Res. **21:** 653–657.
44. KENET, G., S. SADETZKI, H. MURAD, *et al.* 2000. Factor V Leiden and antiphospholipid antibodies are significant risk factors for ischemic stroke in children. Stroke **31:** 1283–1288.
45. BREY, R.L., R.D. ABBOTT, J.D. CURB, *et al.* 2001. beta(2)-Glycoprotein 1-dependent anticardiolipin antibodies and risk of ischemic stroke and myocardial infarction: the honolulu heart program. Stroke **32:** 1701–1706.
46. BREY, R.L., C.L. STALLWORTH, D.L. MCGLASSON, *et al.* 2002. Antiphospholipid antibodies and stroke in young women. Stroke **33:** 2396–2400.
47. JANARDHAN, V., P.A. WOLF, C.S. KASE, *et al.* 2004. Anticardiolipin antibodies and risk of ischemic stroke and transient ischemic attack: the Framingham cohort and offspring study. Stroke **35:** 736–741.
48. GINSBURG, K.S., M.H. LIANG, L. NEWCOMER, *et al.* 1992. Anticardiolipin antibodies and the risk for ischemic stroke and venous thrombosis. Ann. Intern. Med. **117:** 997–1002.

49. MUIR, K.W., I.B. SQUIRE, W. ALWAN, *et al.* 1994. Anticardiolipin antibodies in an unselected stroke population. Lancet **344:** 452–456.
50. MONTALBAN, J., J. RIO, M. KHAMASHTA, *et al.* 1994. Value of immunologic testing in stroke patients. A prospective multicenter study. Stroke **25:** 2412–2415.
51. METZ, L.M., S. EDWORTHY, R. MYDLARSKI, *et al.* 1998. The frequency of phospholipid antibodies in an unselected stroke population. Can. J. Neurol. Sci. **25:** 64–69.
52. AHMED, E., B. STEGMAYR, J. TRIFUNOVIC, *et al.* 2000. Anticardiolipin antibodies are not an independent risk factor for stroke: an incident case-referent study nested within the MONICA and Vasterbotten cohort project. Stroke **31:** 1289–1293.
53. LEVINE, S.R., L. SALOWICH-PALM, K.L. SAWAYA, *et al.* 1997. IgG anticardiolipin antibody titer > 40 GPL and the risk of subsequent thrombo-occlusive events and death. A prospective cohort study. Stroke **28:** 1660–1665.
54. THE ANTIPHOSPHOLIPID ANTIBODIES AND STROKE STUDY GROUP (APASS). 1997. Anticardiolipin antibodies and the risk of recurrent thrombo-occlusive events and death. Neurology **48:** 91–94.
55. LEVINE, S.R., R.L. BREY, B.C. TILLEY, *et al.* 2004. Antiphospholipid antibodies and subsequent thrombo-occlusive events in patients with ischemic stroke. JAMA **291:** 576–584.
56. RUIZ-IRASTORZA, G., M.A. KHAMASHTA & G.R.V. HUGHES. 2004. Antiphospholipid antibodies and risk for recurrent vascular events. JAMA **291:** 2701.
57. WAHL, D., V. REGNAULT, P. DE MOERLOOSE, *et al.* 2004. Antiphospholipid antibodies and risk for recurrent vascular events. JAMA **291:** 2701–2702.
58. CABRAL, A.R. 2004. Antiphospholipid antibodies and risk for recurrent vascular events. JAMA **291:** 2701.
59. GALLI, M., D. LUCIANI, G. BERTOLINI, *et al.* 2003. Lupus anticoagulants are stronger risk factors for thrombosis than anticardiolipin antibodies in the antiphospholipid syndrome: a systematic review of the literature. Blood **101:** 1827–1832.
60. LANTHIER, S., F.J. KIRKHAM, L.G. MITCHELL, *et al.* 2004. Increased anticardiolipin antibody IgG titers do not predict recurrent stroke or TIA in children. Neurology **62:** 194–200.
61. SNEDDON, I.B. 1965. Cerebro-vascular lesions and livedo reticularis. Br. J. Dermatol. **77:** 180–185.
62. LEVINE, S.R., S.L. LANGER, J.W. ALBERS, *et al.* 1988. Sneddon's syndrome: an antiphospholipid antibody syndrome? Neurology **38:** 798–800.
63. ALEGRE, V.A., R.K. WINKELMANN & D.A. GASTINEAU. 1990. Cutaneous thrombosis, cerebrovascular thrombosis, and lupus anticoagulant—the Sneddon syndrome. Report of 10 cases. Int. J. Dermatol. **29:** 45–49.
64. SINHARAY, R. 2003. Sneddon's syndrome: additional neurological feature in antiphospholipid (Hughes') syndrome. Postgrad. Med. J. **79:** 550.
65. ASHERSON, R.A. & R. CERVERA. 2003. Unusual manifestations of the antiphospholipid syndrome. Clin. Rev. Allergy Immunol. **25:** 61–78.
66. FRANCES, C. & J.C. PIETTE. 2000. The mystery of Sneddon syndrome: relationship with antiphospholipid syndrome and systemic lupus erythematosus. J. Autoimmun. **15:** 139–143.
67. KALASHNIKOVA, L.A., E.L. NASONOV, A.E. KUSHEKBAEVA, *et al.* 1990. Anticardiolipin antibodies in Sneddon's syndrome. Neurology **40:** 464–467.
68. BRILEY, D.P., B.M. COULL & S.H. GOODNIGHT, JR. 1989. Neurological disease associated with antiphospholipid antibodies. Ann. Neurol. **25:** 221–227.
69. SCHONING, M., R. KLEIN, I. KRAGELOH-MANN, *et al.* 1994. Antiphospholipid antibodies in cerebrovascular ischemia and stroke in childhood. Neuropediatrics **25:** 8–14.
70. TAKANASHI, J., K. SUGITA, S. MIYAZATO, *et al.* 1995. Antiphospholipid antibody syndrome in childhood strokes. Pediatr. Neurol. **13:** 323–326.
71. BOOTH, F., R. YANOFSKY, I.B. ROSS, *et al.* 1999. Primary antiphospholipid syndrome with moyamoya-like vascular changes. Pediatr. Neurosurg. **31:** 45–48.
72. BONDUEL, M., G. SCIUCCATI, M. HEPNER, *et al.* 1999. Prethrombotic disorders in children with arterial ischemic stroke and sinovenous thrombosis. Arch. Neurol. **56:** 967–971.
73. BAKDASH, T., A.R. COHEN, J.M. HEMPEL, *et al.* 2002. Moyamoya, dystonia during hyperventilation, and antiphospholipid antibodies. Pediatr. Neurol. **26:** 157–160.

74. YAMASHITA, Y., A. KUSAGA, Y. KOGA, *et al.* 2004. Noonan syndrome, moyamoya-like vascular changes, and antiphospholipid syndrome. Pediatr. Neurol. **31:** 364–366.
75. LEKER, R.R. & I. STEINER. 1998. Anticardiolipin antibodies are frequently present in patients with idiopathic intracranial hypertension. Arch. Neurol. **55:** 817–820.
76. CARHUAPOMA, J.R., P. MITSIAS & S.R. LEVINE. 1997. Cerebral venous thrombosis and anticardiolipin antibodies. Stroke **28:** 2363–2369.
77. LEVINE, S.R., S. KIERAN, K. PUZIO, *et al.* 1987. Cerebral venous thrombosis with lupus anticoagulants. Report of two cases. Stroke **18:** 801–804.
78. PROVENZALE, J.M. & H.A. LOGANBILL. 1994. Dural sinus thrombosis and venous infarction associated with antiphospholipid antibodies: MR findings. J. Comput. Assist. Tomogr. **18:** 719–723.
79. CAMAITI, A., A. DEL ROSSO, D. CHECCUCCI, *et al.* 1995. Venous dural sinus thrombosis in a middle-aged woman with anticardiolipin antibodies. Acta Neurol. Belg. **95:** 92–95.
80. DAIF, A., A. AWADA, S. AL-RAJEH, *et al.* 1995. Cerebral venous thrombosis in adults. A study of 40 cases from Saudi Arabia. Stroke **26:** 1193–1195.
81. BOGGILD, M.D., R.V. SEDHEV, D. FRASER, *et al.* 1995. Cerebral venous sinus thrombosis and antiphospholipid antibodies. Postgrad. Med. J. **71:** 487–489.
82. DESCHIENS, M.A., J. CONARD, M.H. HORELLOU, *et al.* 1996. Coagulation studies, factor V Leiden, and anticardiolipin antibodies in 40 cases of cerebral venous thrombosis. Stroke **27:** 1724–1730.
83. MACKWORTH-YOUNG, C.G. & G.R.V. HUGHES. 1985. Epilepsy: an early symptom of systemic lupus erythematosus. J. Neurol. Neurosurg. Psychiatry **48:** 185.
84. APPENZELLER, S., F. CENDES & L.T. COSTALLAT. 2004. Epileptic seizures in systemic lupus erythematosus. Neurology **63:** 1808–1812.
85. MACKWORTH-YOUNG, C.G., S. LOIZOU & M.J. WALPORT. 1989. Antiphospholipid antibodies and disease. Q. J. Med. **72:** 767–777.
86. INZELBERG, R. & A.D. KORCZYN. 1989. Lupus anticoagulant and the late onset seizures. Acta Neurol. Scand. **79:** 114–118.
87. HERRANZ, M.T., G. RIVIER, M.A. KHAMASHTA, *et al.* 1994. Association between antiphospholipid antibodies and epilepsy in patients with systemic lupus erythematosus. Arthritis Rheum. **37:** 568–571.
88. TOUBI, E., M.A. KHAMASHTA, A. PANARRA, *et al.* 1995. Association of antiphospholipid antibodies with central nervous system disease in systemic lupus erythematosus. Am. J. Med. **99:** 397–401.
89. VERROT, D., M. SAN-MARCO, C. DRAVET, *et al.* 1997. Prevalence and signification of antinuclear and anticardiolipin antibodies in patients with epilepsy. Am. J. Med. **103:** 33–37.
90. SHRIVASTAVA, A., S. DWIVEDI, A. AGGARWAL, *et al.* 2001. Anti-cardiolipin and anti-beta2 glycoprotein I antibodies in Indian patients with systemic lupus erythematosus: association with the presence of seizures. Lupus **10:** 45–50.
91. GIBBS, J.W. III & A.M. HUSAIN. 2002. Epilepsy associated with lupus anticoagulant. Seizure **11:** 207–209.
92. COCITO, L., E. FAVALE & L. RENI. 1982. Epileptic seizures in cerebral arterial occlusive disease. Stroke **13:** 189–195.
93. LIOU, H.H., C.R. WANG, H.C. CHOU, *et al.* 1994. Anticardiolipin antisera from lupus patients with seizures reduce a GABA receptor-mediated chloride current in snail neurons. Life Sci. **54:** 1119–1125.
94. CHAPMAN, J., M. COHEN-ARMON, Y. SHOENFELD, *et al.* 1999. Antiphospholipid antibodies permeabilize and depolarize brain synaptoneurosomes. Lupus **8:** 127–133.
95. KENT, M., F. ALVAREZ, E. VOGT, *et al.* 1997. Monoclonal antiphosphatidylserine antibodies react directly with feline and murine central nervous system. J. Rheumatol. **24:** 1725–1733.
96. KENT, M.N., F.J. ALVAREZ, A.K. NG, *et al.* 2000. Ultrastructural localization of monoclonal antiphospholipid antibody binding to rat brain. Exp. Neurol. **163:** 173–179.
97. RANUA, J., K. LUOMA, J. PELTOLA, *et al.* 2004. Anticardiolipin and antinuclear antibodies in epilepsy—a population-based cross-sectional study. Epilepsy Res. **58:** 13–18.
98. LIOU, H.H., C.R. WANG, C.J. CHEN, *et al.* 1996. Elevated levels of anticardiolipin antibodies and epilepsy in lupus patients. Lupus **5:** 307–312.

99. ACR Ad-Hoc Committee on Neuropsychiatric Lupus Nomenclature. 1999. The American College of Rheumatology nomenclature and case definitions for neuropsychiatric lupus syndromes. Arthritis Rheum. **42:** 599–608.
100. Mikdashi, J. & B. Handwerger. 2004. Predictors of neuropsychiatric damage in systemic lupus erythematosus: data from the Maryland lupus cohort. Rheumatology (Oxford) **43:** 1555–1560.
101. Karassa, F.B., J.P. Ioannidis, K.A. Boki, *et al.* 2000. Predictors of clinical outcome and radiologic progression in patients with neuropsychiatric manifestations of systemic lupus erythematosus. Am. J. Med. **109:** 628–634.
102. Jain, K.K. 1991. Systemic lupus erythematosus (SLE)-like syndromes associated with carbamazepine therapy. Drug Saf. **6:** 350–360.
103. Echaniz-Laguna, A., A. Thiriaux, I. Ruolt-Olivesi, *et al.* 1999. Lupus anticoagulant induced by the combination of valproate and lamotrigine. Epilepsia **40:** 1661–1663.
104. Peltola, J.T., A. Haapala, J.I. Isojarvi, *et al.* 2000. Antiphospholipid and antinuclear antibodies in patients with epilepsy or new-onset seizure disorders. Am. J. Med. **109:** 712–717.
105. Eriksson, K., J. Peltola, T. Keranen, *et al.* 2001. High prevalence of antiphospholipid antibodies in children with epilepsy: a controlled study of 50 cases. Epilepsy Res. **46:** 129–137.
106. Cuadrado, M.J., M.A. Khamashta & G.R. Hughes. 2001. Sticky blood and headache. Lupus **10:** 392–393.
107. Cuadrado, M.J. & G. Sanna. 2003. Headache and systemic lupus erythematosus. Lupus **12:** 943–946.
108. Montalban, J., R. Cervera, J. Font, *et al.* 1992. Lack of association between anticardiolipin antibodies and migraine in systemic lupus erythematosus. Neurology **42:** 681–682.
109. Tietjen, G.E., M. Day, L. Norris, *et al.* 1998. Role of anticardiolipin antibodies in young persons with migraine and transient focal neurologic events: a prospective study. Neurology **50:** 1433–1440.
110. Asherson, R.A., R.H. Derksen, E.N. Harris, *et al.* 1987. Chorea in systemic lupus erythematosus and “lupus-like” disease: association with antiphospholipid antibodies. Semin. Arthritis Rheum. **16:** 253–259.
111. Khamashta, M.A., A. Gil, B. Anciones, *et al.* 1988. Chorea in systemic lupus erythematosus: association with antiphospholipid antibodies. Ann. Rheum. Dis. **47:** 681–683.
112. Asherson, R.A. & G.R.V. Hughes. 1988. Antiphospholipid antibodies and chorea. J. Rheumatol. **15:** 377–379.
113. Cervera, R., R.A. Asherson, J. Font, *et al.* 1997. Chorea in the antiphospholipid syndrome. Clinical, radiologic, and immunologic characteristics of 50 patients from our clinics and the recent literature. Medicine (Baltimore) **76:** 203–212.
114. Scott, T.F., D. Hess & J. Brillman. 1994. Antiphospholipid antibody syndrome mimicking multiple sclerosis clinically and by magnetic resonance imaging. Arch. Intern. Med. **154:** 917–920.
115. Ijdo, J., A.M. Conti-Kelly, P. Greco, *et al.* 1999. Anti-phospholipid antibodies in patients with multiple sclerosis and MS-like illnesses: MS or APS? Lupus **8:** 109–115.
116. Ferreira, S., D.P. D’Cruz & G.R.V. Hughes. 2005. Multiple sclerosis, neuropsychiatric lupus and antiphospholipid syndrome: where do we stand? Rheumatology (Oxford) **44:** 434–442.
117. Kim, J.H., S.I. Lee, S.I. Park, *et al.* 2004. Recurrent transverse myelitis in primary antiphospholipid syndrome—case report and literature review. Rheumatol. Int. **24:** 244–246.
118. Alarcon-Segovia, D., M. Deleze, C.V. Oria, *et al.* 1989. Antiphospholipid antibodies and the antiphospholipid syndrome in systemic lupus erythematosus. A prospective analysis of 500 consecutive patients. Medicine (Baltimore) **68:** 353–365.
119. Lavalle, C., S. Pizarro, C. Drenkard, *et al.* 1990. Transverse myelitis: a manifestation of systemic lupus erythematosus strongly associated with antiphospholipid antibodies. J. Rheumatol. **17:** 34–37.

120. Ruiz-Arguelles, G.J., J. Guzman-Ramos, J. Flores-Flores, *et al.* 1998. Refractory hiccough heralding transverse myelitis in the primary antiphospholipid syndrome. Lupus **7:** 49–50.
121. Kovacs, B., T.L. Lafferty, L.H. Brent, *et al.* 2000. Transverse myelopathy in systemic lupus erythematosus: an analysis of 14 cases and review of the literature. Ann. Rheum. Dis. **59:** 120–124.
122. D'Cruz, D., S. Mellor-Pita, B. Joven, *et al.* 2004. Transverse myelitis as the first manifestation of systemic lupus erythematosus or lupus-like disease: good functional outcome and relevance of antiphospholipid antibodies. J. Rheumatol. **31:** 280–285.
123. Falcini, F., G. Taccetti, S. Trapani, *et al.* 1991. Primary antiphospholipid syndrome: a report of two pediatric cases. J. Rheumatol. **18:** 1085–1087.
124. Orefice, G., G. De Joanna, M. Coppola, *et al.* 1995. Benign intracranial hypertension: a non-thrombotic complication of the primary antiphospholipid syndrome? Lupus **4:** 324–326.
125. Sussman, J., M. Leach, M. Greaves, *et al.* 1997. Potentially prothrombotic abnormalities of coagulation in benign intracranial hypertension. J. Neurol. Neurosurg. Psychiatry **62:** 229–233.
126. Kesler, A., M.H. Ellis, T. Reshef, *et al.* 2000. Idiopathic intracranial hypertension and anticardiolipin antibodies. J. Neurol. Neurosurg. Psychiatry **68:** 379–380.
127. Hisashi, K., S. Komune, T. Taira, *et al.* 1993. Anticardiolipin antibody-induced sudden profound sensorineural hearing loss. Am. J. Otolaryngol. **14:** 275–277.
128. Casoli, P. & B. Tumiati. 1995. Cogan's syndrome: a new possible complication of antiphospholipid antibodies? Clin. Rheumatol. **14:** 197–198.
129. Tumiati, B. & P. Casoli. 1995. Sudden sensorineural hearing loss and anticardiolipin antibody. Am. J. Otolaryngol. **16:** 220.
130. Toubi, E., J. Ben-David, A. Kessel, *et al.* 1997. Autoimmune aberration in sudden sensorineural hearing loss: association with anti-cardiolipin antibodies. Lupus **6:** 540–542.
131. Naarendorp, M. & H. Spiera. 1998. Sudden sensorineural hearing loss in patients with systemic lupus erythematosus or lupus-like syndromes and antiphospholipid antibodies. J. Rheumatol. **25:** 589–592.
132. Green, L. & E.B. Miller. 2001. Sudden sensorineural hearing loss as a first manifestation of systemic lupus erythematosus: association with anticardiolipin antibodies. Clin. Rheumatol. **20:** 220–222.
133. Gilburd, B., M. Stein, Y. Tomer, *et al.* 1993. Autoantibodies to phospholipids and brain extract in patients with the Guillain-Barre syndrome: cross-reactive or pathogenic? Autoimmunity **16:** 23–27.
134. Montalban, J., A. Arboix, H. Staub, *et al.* 1989. Transient global amnesia and antiphospholipid syndrome. Clin. Exp. Rheumatol. **7:** 85–87.
135. Brey, R.L., A.E. Gharavi & M.D. Lockshin. 1993. Neurologic complications of antiphospholipid antibodies. Rheum. Dis. Clin. North Am. **19:** 833–850.
136. Durrani, O.M., C. Gordon & P.I. Murray. 2002. Primary anti-phospholipid antibody syndrome (APS): current concepts. Surv. Ophthalmol. **47:** 215–238.
137. Reino, S., F.J. Munoz-Rodriguez, R. Cervera, *et al.* 1997. Optic neuropathy in the "primary" antiphospholipid syndrome: report of a case and review of the literature. Clin. Rheumatol. **16:** 629–631.
138. Giorgi, D., C.B. Gabrieli & L. Bonomo. 1998. The clinical-ophtalmological spectrum of antiphospholipid syndrome. Ocular Immunol. Inflamm. **6:** 269–273.
139. Frohman, L., R. Turbin, L. Bielory, *et al.* 2003. Autoimmune optic neuropathy with anticardiolipin antibody mimicking multiple sclerosis in a child. Am. J. Ophthalmol. **136:** 358–360.
140. Papais-Alvarenga, R.M., C.M. Miranda-Santos, M. Puccioni-Sohler, *et al.* 2002. Optic neuromyelitis syndrome in Brazilian patients. J. Neurol. Neurosurg. Psychiatry **73:** 429–435.
141. Wiechens, B., J.O. Schroder, B. Potzsch, *et al.* 1997. Primary antiphospholipid antibody syndrome and retinal occlusive vasculopathy. Am. J. Ophthalmol. **123:** 848–850.

142. AU, A. & J. O'DAY. 2004. Review of severe vaso-occlusive retinopathy in systemic lupus erythematosus and the antiphospholipid syndrome: associations, visual outcomes, complications and treatment. Clin. Exp. Ophthalmol. **32:** 87–100.
143. UTHMAN, I., D.M. NAJJAR, S.S. KANJ, *et al.* 2003. Anticardiolipin antibodies in acute multifocal posterior placoid pigment epitheliopathy. Ann. Rheum. Dis. **62:** 687–688.
144. MILANOV, I.G., R. RASHKOV, M. BALEVA, *et al.* 1998. Antiphospholipid syndrome and parkinsonism. Clin. Exp. Rheumatol. **16:** 623–624.
145. MILANOV, I. & D. BOGDANOVA. 2001. Antiphospholipid syndrome and dystonia-parkinsonism. A case report. Parkinsonism Relat. Disord. **7:** 139–141.
146. REIBLAT, T., I. POLISHCHUK, E. DORODNIKOV, *et al.* 2003. Primary antiphospholipid antibody syndrome masquerading as progressive supranuclear palsy. Lupus **12:** 67–69.
147. ADHIYAMAN, V., R.J. MEARA & B.K. BHOWMICK. 2002. Antiphospholipid syndrome and dystonia-parkinsonism: need for anticoagulation. Parkinsonism Relat. Disord. **8:** 215; author reply 217.
148. AINIALA, H., J. LOUKKOLA, J. PELTOLA, *et al.* 2001. The prevalence of neuropsychiatric syndromes in systemic lupus erythematosus. Neurology **57:** 496–500.
149. BREY, R.L., S.L. HOLLIDAY, A.R. SAKLAD, *et al.* 2002. Neuropsychiatric syndromes in lupus: prevalence using standardized definitions. Neurology **58:** 1214–1220.
150. LOUKKOLA, J., M. LAINE, H. AINIALA, *et al.* 2003. Cognitive impairment in systemic lupus erythematosus and neuropsychiatric systemic lupus erythematosus: a population-based neuropsychological study. J. Clin. Exp. Neuropsychol. **25:** 145–151.
151. AFELTRA, A., P. GARZIA, A.P. MITTERHOFER, *et al.* 2003. Neuropsychiatric lupus syndromes: relationship with antiphospholipid antibodies. Neurology **61:** 108–110.
152. HANLY, J.G., G. MCCURDY, L. FOUGERE, *et al.* 2004. Neuropsychiatric events in systemic lupus erythematosus: attribution and clinical significance. J. Rheumatol. **31:** 2156–2162.
153. HANLY, J.G., N.M. WALSH, J.D. FISK, *et al.* 1993. Cognitive impairment and autoantibodies in systemic lupus erythematosus. Br. J. Rheumatol. **32:** 291–296.
154. DENBURG, S.D., R.M. CARBOTTE, J.S. GINSBERG, *et al.* 1997. The relationship of antiphospholipid antibodies to cognitive function in patients with systemic lupus erythematosus. J. Int. Neuropsychol. Soc. **3:** 377–386.
155. HANLY, J.G., C. HONG, S. SMITH, *et al.* 1999. A prospective analysis of cognitive function and anticardiolipin antibodies in systemic lupus erythematosus. Arthritis Rheum. **42:** 728–734.
156. MENON, S., E. JAMESON-SHORTALL, S.P. NEWMAN, *et al.* 1999. A longitudinal study of anticardiolipin antibody levels and cognitive functioning in systemic lupus erythematosus. Arthritis Rheum. **42:** 735–741.
157. CARONTI, B., C. CALDERARO, C. ALESSANDRI, *et al.* 1998. Serum anti-beta2-glycoprotein I antibodies from patients with antiphospholipid antibody syndrome bind central nervous system cells. J. Autoimmun. **11:** 425–429.
158. KATZAV, A., C.G. PICK, A.D. KORCZYN, *et al.* 2001. Hyperactivity in a mouse model of the antiphospholipid syndrome. Lupus **10:** 496–499.
159. HUGHES, G., M. CUADRADO, M. KHAMASHTA, *et al.* 2001. Headache and memory loss: rapid response to heparin in the antiphospholipid syndrome. Lupus **10:** 778.
160. KUSHNER, M. & N. SIMONIAN. 1989. Lupus anticoagulants, anticardiolipin antibodies, and cerebral ischemia. Stroke **20:** 225–229.
161. MONTALBAN, J., J. FERNANDEZ, A. ARDERIU, *et al.* 1989. Multi-infarct dementia associated with antiphospholipid antibodies. Presentation of 2 cases. Med. Clin. (Barc.) **93:** 424–426.
162. KURITA, A., T. HASUNUMA, S. MOCHIO, *et al.* 1994. A young case with multi-infarct dementia associated with lupus anticoagulant. Intern. Med. **33:** 373–375.
163. MOSEK, A., I. YUST, T.A. TREVES, *et al.* 2000. Dementia and antiphospholipid antibodies. Dement. Geriatr. Cogn. Disord. **11:** 36–38.
164. CHAPMAN, J., M. ABU-KATASH, R. INZELBERG, *et al.* 2002. Prevalence and clinical features of dementia associated with the antiphospholipid syndrome and circulating anticoagulants. J. Neurol. Sci. **203-204:** 81–84.
165. SCHWARTZ, M., M. ROCHAS, B. WELLER, *et al.* 1998. High association of anticardiolipin antibodies with psychosis. J. Clin. Psychiatry. **59:** 20–23.

166. BODANI, M. & M.D. KOPELMAN. 2003. A psychiatric perspective on the therapy of psychosis in systemic lupus erythematosus. Lupus **12:** 947–949.
167. SANNA, G., M. PIGA, J.W. TERRYBERRY, *et al.* 2000. Central nervous system involvement in systemic lupus erythematosus: cerebral imaging and serological profile in patients with and without overt neuropsychiatric manifestations. Lupus **9:** 573–583.
168. VERMEER, S.E., T. DEN HEIJER, P.J. KOUDSTAAL, *et al.* 2003. Incidence and risk factors of silent brain infarcts in the population-based Rotterdam Scan Study. Stroke **34:** 392–396.
169. VERMEER, S.E., N.D. PRINS, T. DEN HEIJER, *et al.* 2003. Silent brain infarcts and the risk of dementia and cognitive decline. N. Engl. J. Med. **348:** 1215–1222.
170. KAO, C.H., J.L. LAN, J.F. HSIEH, *et al.* 1999. Evaluation of regional cerebral blood flow with 99mTc-HMPAO in primary antiphospholipid antibody syndrome. J. Nucl. Med. **40:** 1446–1450.
171. ROMANOWICZ, G., P. LASS, M. KOSEDA-DRAGAN, *et al.* 2000. Technetium-99mTc-HMPAO brain SPECT in antiphospholipid syndrome—preliminary data. Nucl. Med. Rev. Cent. East. Eur. **3:** 17–20.
172. TOKUMARU, S., T. YOSHIKAI, A. UCHINO, *et al.* 2001. Technetium-99m-ECD SPECT in antiphospholipid antibody syndrome: a drastic improvement in brain perfusion by antiplatelet therapy. Eur. Radiol. **11:** 2611–2615.
173. CHEN, J.J., Y.C. SHIAU, J.J. WANG, *et al.* 2002. Abnormal regional cerebral blood flow in primary antiphospholipid antibody syndrome patients with normal magnetic resonance imaging findings. A preliminary report. Scand. J. Rheumatol. **31:** 89–93.
174. SUN, S.S., F.Y. LIU, J.J. TSAI, *et al.* 2003. Using 99mTc HMPAO brain SPECT to evaluate the effects of anticoagulant therapy on regional cerebral blood flow in primary antiphospholipid antibody syndrome patients with brain involvement—a preliminary report. Rheumatol. Int. **23:** 301–304.
175. SANNA, G., M.L. BERTOLACCINI & A. MATHIEU. 2003. Central nervous system lupus: a clinical approach to therapy. Lupus **12:** 935–942.
176. KHAMASHTA, M.A., M.J. CUADRADO, F. MUJIC, *et al.* 1995. The management of thrombosis in the antiphospholipid-antibody syndrome. N. Engl. J. Med. **332:** 993–997.
177. RUIZ-IRASTORZA, G., M.A. KHAMASHTA, B.J. HUNT, *et al.* 2002. Bleeding and recurrent thrombosis in definite antiphospholipid syndrome: analysis of a series of 66 patients treated with oral anticoagulation to a target international normalized ratio of 3.5. Arch. Intern. Med. **162:** 1164–1169.
178. CUADRADO, M.J., G. SANNA, M. SHARIEF, *et al.* 2003. Double blind, crossover, randomised trial comparing low molecular weight heparin versus placebo in the treatment of chronic headache in patients with antiphospholipid antibodies. Arthritis Rheum. **48:** S364 (abstract).

New Facet of Antiphospholipid Antibodies

GUIDO VALESINI AND CRISTIANO ALESSANDRI

Cattedra e Divisione di Reumatologia, Università La Sapienza, Rome, Italy

ABSTRACT: Since the aCL test was first described, several reports have described the heterogeneity of aPL, which binds to different anionic phospholipids, proteins, or to a phospholipid–protein complex. It has been recently reported that antiphospholipids (aPLs) from the sera of patients with the antiphospholipid syndrome (APS) are able to bind some newly identified antigens, the lyso(bis)phosphatidic acid (LBPA), lipid restricted to the late endosomes, and the sulfatides, acidic glycosphingolipids involved in the hemostatic process. Of interest, aLBPAs are present in the sera of a large number of patients with APS showing similar sensitivity and specificity compared to anti-β_2 glycoprotein I antibodies (aβ_2-GPIs) and close association with lupus anticoagulant. Moreover, β_2-GPI binds to sulfatides and the majority of the aPL reacting with cardiolipin–β_2-GPI complex also react with the sulfatide–β_2-GPI complex. Different mechanisms involved in the production of autoantibodies in autoimmune diseases have been proposed and, among them, apoptosis or programmed cell death seems to play a leading role. The relocation of CL and its metabolites during apoptosis may represent an *in vivo* trigger for the generation of aCL, and the higher reactivity of sera from APS patients to monolysocardiolipin, the immediate degradation product of mitochondrial CL validates this hypothesis. Finally, increasing evidence suggests that oxidative stress could be a pathogenic link between aPL and thrombosis, and antioxidant treatment may have some efficacy in preventing the clinical manifestations of this syndrome.

KEYWORDS: antiphospholipid antibodies; antiphospholipid syndrome; lyso(bis)phosphatidic acid; monolysocardiolipin; sulfatides; β_2-GPI; apoptosis

INTRODUCTION

Patients with antiphospholipid syndrome (APS) are prone to arterial and venous thrombosis, recurrent abortions, and/or fetal loss in association with high levels of antiphospholipid antibodies (aPLs); in the great majority of cases aPLs are detected using cardiolipin (CL) as solid-phase antigen.[1–3] Today, APS is assumed to be the most common cause of acquired systemic thrombotic disorders and the commonest treatable cause of recurrent pregnancy losses.[4] Several animal models suggest a pathogenic role of aPLs in APS, and aPLs are widely associated with the clinical spectrum of the syndrome *in vivo*. Moreover, recent findings suggest that the pres-

Address for correspondence: Prof. Guido Valesini, Dipartimento di Clinica e Terapia Medica Applicata, Cattedra di Reumatologia, Università "La Sapienza," V.le del Policlinico 155, 00161 Rome, Italy. Voice: +39-0649974631; fax +39-0649974642.
guido.valesini@uniroma1.it

Ann. N.Y. Acad. Sci. 1051: 487–497 (2005). © 2005 New York Academy of Sciences.
doi: 10.1196/annals.1361.089

ence of circulating anticardiolipin antibodies (aCLs) tend to precede clotting events by several years in patients with primary APS (PAPS) as well as in those with systemic lupus erythematosus (SLE).[5] Nevertheless, since the first description of the aCL test,[6] a huge number of reports have described the heterogeneity of aPL, which binds to different anionic phospholipids, proteins, or to a phospholipid–protein complex. Furthermore, it has been reported that aPLs also occur in infectious diseases and cancer even if, in these cases, the autoantibodies are present at low levels and are not usually associated with the clinical manifestations of APS. Therefore, it is commonly accepted that aPLs represent a heterogeneous group of autoantibodies and that their fine specificity remains a matter of debate. In this review, we analyze briefly what is known about the new target antigens of aPLs, focusing in particular on the role of apoptosis, oxidation, and infection for the generation of aPL.

NEW TARGET ANTIGENS IN APS

Although aPLs were initially thought to bind CL, in 1990 different reports described the requirement of β_2-glycoprotein I (β_2-GPI)—the phospholipid-binding protein—for the binding of aCLs in solid-phase immunoassays.[7–9] Since then, other phospholipid-binding proteins such as prothrombin, annexin V, proteins S and C, high- and low-molecular-weight kininogens, and factor XI have been described as phospholipid cofactors.[10] An accumulating body of evidence suggests β_2-GPI and prothrombin as the most relevant antigens in APS.[11,12] Nevertheless, it has also been recently reported that aPLs from APS sera are able to bind some newly identified antigens; Kobayashi and co-workers discovered autoantibodies specific for a phospholipid, the lyso(bis)phosphatidic acid (LBPA),[13] restricted to the late endosomes. Furthermore, these authors suggested a direct pathogenic role for anti-LBPA antibodies (aLBPA) because of their effects on altering endosomal sorting and vesicular trafficking. We observed that sera from patients with APS label late endosomes containing LBPA and induce a redistribution of intracellular β_2-GPI.[14] We have demonstrated that aLBPA are able to exert lupus anticoagulant activity *in vitro*, supporting the view that aLBPA may have a pathogenic role in APS. More recently, we have carried out another study showing a high prevalence of aLBPA in APS in striking correlation with positivity for lupus anticoagulant (LAC).[15] The results of all these studies clearly indicate that aLBPAs, as well as aβ_2-GPIs, have higher specificity but lower sensitivity for APS when compared to aCLs. The β_2-GPIs may mediate the binding of antibodies to LBPA, but it has been demonstrated in β_2-GPI-free experiments that a population of aCLs and aLBPAs also exist and are able to bind directly to lipids in the absence of β_2-GPIs.[15,16] On the basis of these findings it is possible to speculate that aPL reactivity in autoimmune diseases such as APS and SLE, is highly heterogeneous. Nonetheless, the finding of aLBPA in APS sera is intriguing because an accumulation of the LBPA precursors has been demonstrated in mouse mitochondrial membranes concomitantly with the rapid degradation of CL during apoptosis triggered by Fas stimulation.[17] Longitudinal studies are needed to clarify the putative clinical value of these antibodies in the diagnosis and management of patients with APS. Results from our previous study clearly demonstrated that aLBPAs are present in the sera of a large number of APS patients showing similar sensitivity and specificity as compared to aβ_2-GPI and close association with

LAC.[15] Our preliminary observation that aLBPA antibodies are detectable in β_2-GPI-free conditions (by immunostaining on thin-layer chromatography[18]) in two out of five sera from patients with clinical features of the syndrome, but without detectable titer of aCLs or aβ_2-GPIs (by standard tests), appears very promising (unpublished data).

Recently a new specificity has been identified in APS sera; autoantibodies that are able to bind to sulfatides, acidic glycosphingolipids involved in the hemostatic process, have been characterized.[19] Sulfatides are present in various tissues and cells (nervous tissue, kidney, testis, erythrocytes, platelets, and granulocytes), and they are one of the major lipids in serum. Several sulfatide-binding proteins are present in plasma, such as von Willebrand factor, thrombospondin, and P-selectin. β_2-GPI binds to surface-bound sulfatides, but not to other glycolipids, such as ceramide, cerebrosides, sphingomyelin, or ganglioside, and forms a complex (β_2-GPI/sulfatides), thereby becoming a target for antiphospholipid antibodies associated with thrombosis. The majority of the anti-phospholipid antibodies reacting with cardiolipin–β_2-GPI complex also react with the sulfatide–β_2-GPI complex. However, in at least some patients, there are separate antibodies specific to each of these complexes.[19] The reaction of these antibodies with sulfatide may contribute not only to the hemostatic abnormalities but also to other clinical features, such as neurologic symptoms and abortions, because sulfatides are present in nerve tissue and in the female genital tract.[19] This may represent another aspect of the nonvasculopathic mechanism of tissue damage induced by aPLs; we had previously demonstrated that astrocytes and neurons synthesize β_2-GPI, suggesting the direct antigenic function of this molecule within the central nervous system (CNS) and, consequently, the putative role of APS-associated autoantibodies in CNS damage.[20] Moreover, anti β_2-GPIs might contribute to CNS pathologies by interaction with brain cytotypes, as well as by interaction with cerebral vessel endothelium.[21,22]

Since the aCL test was first described in 1983,[6] great efforts were made to standardize the aPL routine screening tests.[23] Nevertheless, in some cases, when other known coagulopathies are excluded, the diagnosis of seronegative APS may be considered, even if the current classification criteria of APS[3] do not allow the diagnosis of classical APS in the absence of serologic markers (i.e., aPL ELISA and/or lupus anticoagulant positive tests). In a preliminary study, Hughes and co-workers have recently reported an increasing prevalence of pregnancy loss in 52 patients negative for aPLs who had livedo reticularis; the authors suggest the intriguing possibility of an undiscovered new autoantibody for seronegative APS.[24]

ROLE OF APOPTOSIS IN APS

Different mechanisms involved in the production of autoantibodies in autoimmune diseases have been proposed and, among them, apoptosis or programmed cell death seems to play a leading role. Since apoptosis was first described, increasing evidence has been provided about this implication in autoimmunity.[25] The particular defect of apoptosis may lead to the breaking of immunologic tolerance with survival of lymphocytes involved in autoimmune response. Moreover, during apoptosis there is an abnormal exposure of self-antigens in cytoplasmic surface blebs which may drive an autoimmune reaction, especially in the presence of an impaired clearance of apoptotic bodies. Furthermore, apoptosis may generate neoantigens by post-transcriptional modification such as phosphorylation/dephosphorylation, trans-glutamination, and deamination.[26]

Several analyses of apoptotic cells have shown a dramatic modification of the lipid bilayer on cellular membranes, such as the exposure of phosphatidylserine (PS) on the outer cytoplasmic membrane,[27] and the relocation of cardiolipin and its metabolites from mitochondria to another cellular membrane.[17] Cardiolipin is a unique anionic phospholipid predominantly associated with the inner mitochondrial membrane, where CL synthase is located. Once synthesized in mitochondria, CL is rapidly remodeled into its highly unsaturated species. This remodeling involves relocation of CL to the outer mitochondrial membrane, as well as to extra-mitochondrial compartments,[28,29] such as the endoplasmic reticulum (ER), for efficient re-acylation to mature forms of CL. This translocation onto the cell surface implies a leakage of CL (and/or of its metabolites) from the normal remodeling cycle,[30] probably as a consequence of an apoptosis-mediated increase in the traffic of endosomal and ER membranes. Interestingly, Degli Esposti and colleagues have recently demonstrated an early degradation of mitochondrial CL during Fas-induced apoptosis by means of mass spectroscopy analysis,[31] a finding we have now confirmed in human pro-monocytic U937 cells.[17] These findings prompt us to suggest that relocation of CL and its metabolites during apoptosis may represent an *in vivo* trigger for the generation of aCLs, as previously reported for other autoantigens.[26] Notably, Casciola and coworkers have shown aCL binding to surface blebs of apoptotic cells,[32] which would be consistent with the clustering of aCL immunostaining in focal surface regions, which we detected in apoptotic cells. To further evaluate our hypothesis, using ELISA, we tested the sera of patients with APS and SLE attending our department to detect autoantibodies toward CL and its derivatives (i.e., monolysocardiolipin (MCL), dilysocardiolipin and hydrocardiolipin). Interestingly, we observed a strong reactivity toward MCL, a key metabolite of CL (unpublished material). MCL is the immediate product of CL degradation, a process that has been shown to occur either in mitochondria (both membranes) as part of the remodeling cycle of the mature lipid or in lysosomes.[30,33] Significant concentration of MCL exist in healthy tissues and it increase after stimulation of physiological apoptotic pathways such as Fas/FasL, which are relevant to white blood cells and immunologic response.[17,31] In this context, our finding of autoantibodies that strongly react with MCL (in conjunction with CL) could provide a pathologically relevant link between the metabolic cell cycle, membrane traffic of CL, and apoptosis. Cardiolipin is known indeed to undergo degradation (including peroxidation) during many pathways of cell death.[33] Antibodies to lysophosphatidylethanolamine (LPE) and lysophosphatidylcholine (LPC) have been more recently identified in patients' sera, indicating that lysophospholipids may also contribute to the antigenicity of oxidized low-density lipoproteins (oxLDL).[34,35] Moreover, a strong correlation between antibodies directed to LPC and CL was found. It is noteworthy that LPC is a by-product of CL remodeling, PC being the predominant acyl donor for MCL during remodeling.[30] On the other hand, it has also been suggested that CL, after oxidation, could be hydrolyzed by serum phospholipase, thus creating molecular structures similar to either LPC or MCL.[35,36] Phospholipase A2 activity is enhanced in both autoimmune and inflammatory diseases,[37,38] as well as during apoptosis.[30] Consistent with our study, it is thus possible that CL hydrolysis of one fatty acid chain to yield MCL enhances CL antigenicity. In addition,

MCL has hybrid properties between a diacyl-lipid (bilayer-forming) and a lyso-lipid (micelle-forming), which may physically facilitate autoantibody reactivity.

In conclusion, we observe a higher reactivity of sera from APS and SLE patients to MCL, the immediate degradation product of mitochondrial CL. Indeed, it is possible that apoptosis or an inflammatory process enhances the hydrolysis (and membrane traffic) of CL into its metabolite MCL, which can then escape the mitochondrial cycle of lipid remodeling and become available to the cell surface, and consequently to the immune system. In this way, aPL binds to these lipids expressed on the cell surface directly or complexed with plasma proteins like β_2-GPIs that rapidly associate with anionic phospholipid on the membrane of apoptotic cells. It has also been suggested that some B cell receptor may recognize a protein–phospholipid complex on the apoptotic cell and secrete antibodies that opsonize apoptotic cells.[39] Further studies are under way to ascertain the etiologic and clinical relevance of aMCL in SLE and APS patients.

ROLE OF OXIDATION IN APS

Increasing evidence suggests that oxidative stress could be a pathogenic link between aPLs and thrombosis. Hydroperoxidation of CL has been shown to be essential for enhancing the binding of aPL autoantibodies to the lipids.[40,41] New findings suggest a role for oxidative damage in the development of aPLs in patients with alcoholic liver disease.[42] Hörkkö and colleagues clearly demonstrated that epitopes of aPLs might be adducts of oxLDL and β_2-GPI.[43] In particular, cardiolipin is an anionic phospholipid constituted by two phosphate groups and four fatty acid chains and represents the most unsaturated (i.e., susceptible of oxidation) lipid of the body.[29,30] In this context, we were unable to detect autoantibodies against a fully hydrogenated CL derivative (i.e., reduced CL; unpublished material) in sera of patients with APS or SLE. Enhancement of lipid peroxidation in aPL-positive SLE patients has been demonstrated by our previous studies showing increased urinary excretion of a marker of lipid peroxidation[44] in association with endothelial perturbation.[45] Oxidation of LDL also induces the expression of immunogenic neoepitopes with the production of autoantibodies able to bind the oxLDL and to enhance the uptake of oxLDL by macrophages.[35,46] Frostegård and colleagues demonstrated a higher level of oxidized phospholipids on LDL in SLE patients, mainly in those with arterial disease.[47] These authors have clearly shown that aCL recognizes oxidized CL and they have suggested a possible antioxidant therapy in these patients. Our group has previously demonstrated a significant reduction of thrombin generation with antioxidants *in vivo*.[48] Ferro and co-workers found a significant decrease of isoprostane and monocyte TF antigen in aPL-positive patients who received antioxidant supplementation.[49] In addition, it has been demonstrated *in vitro* that the increased production of superoxide anion and TF from monocytes stimulated with aβ_2-GPI, was inhibited by pretreatment with vitamin E. We also observed a reduction of aCL titer after antioxidant therapy in patients with APS and SLE.[50]

An elegant study has demonstrated that several aPLs appear and disappear in the blood of normal subjects after oxidation–reduction reactions.[51] McIntyre has come to the conclusion that the autoantibodies detected in autoimmune patients represent the same kind of autoantibodies detected in normal individuals after oxidation.

These findings suggest an important role of these autoantibodies in immunologic homeostatasis.[51]

In conclusion, enhanced lipid peroxidation seems to play an important role in the pathogenesis of APS, and antioxidant treatment may have some efficacy in preventing the clinical manifestations of this syndrome.

ROLE OF INFECTION IN APS

Understanding the relationship between autoimmune disease and infection has been a topic of interest for several decades. It is noteworthy that autoimmune diseases may be caused or triggered by infections. Accumulated evidence suggests that several mechanisms are involved in autoimmune reaction due to infectious disease. First, similarity between microbial and host antigens (molecular mimicry) may account for production of autoantibodies in APS, as recently reviewed by Blank and Shoenfeld.[52] Second, microbial infections may be related to the release of sequestered self-antigens or may stimulate the self-antigen-presenting cells by engaging Toll-like receptors (TLRs) on these cells.[53] Intriguingly, β_2-GPI shows a homology with the microbial agents that represent the natural ligands for TLR-4. Raschi and co-workers[54] showed that aβ_2-GPI antibodies activate endothelial cells in a way comparable to lipolysaccharide or IL-1, suggesting an interaction between autoantibodies and the β_2-GPI/TLR-4 complex.

Concerning a direct role of infections in inducing APS, catastrophic APS may be induced by an infection in about 30% of patients[55] and aPL has been found to be raised in several infectious diseases such as syphilis, HCV and HIV infections, mononucleosis, leprosy, and malaria.[56] On the contrary, in these cases aPLs are not usually associated with the clinical manifestation of APS and their prevalence may largely differ in relation to the infectious disease and the patient assortment, as well as the methods of detection. Taken together these findings suggest a different pattern of aPL specificity in autoimmune and infectious diseases. Using TLC immunostaining we have shown pure aCL (i.e., β_2-GPI independent antibodies) in infectious mononucleosis (IM) as well as anti-β_2-GPI in IM. In the last case their prevalence was significantly lower than in primary APS.[57] Thus, it is well recognized that β_2-GPI-dependence of aPL is the most relevant difference between autoimmune and infectious disease.[58–60]

In conclusion, although the role of infections, if any, in the pathogenesis of APS is yet to be well established, it is a reasonable hypothesis that APS, at least in some cases, may be induced by an autoimmune response triggered by an infectious disease in susceptible subjects with a particular genetic background. Nevertheless, given that aPL may be frequently associated with infectious disease without clinical relevance, a clear distinction should be made between autoimmunity and autoimmune disease such as APS.

CONCLUSIONS

Large bodies of evidence demonstrate that aPLs represents a heterogeneous group of autoantibodies with partially overlapping specificities and characteristics

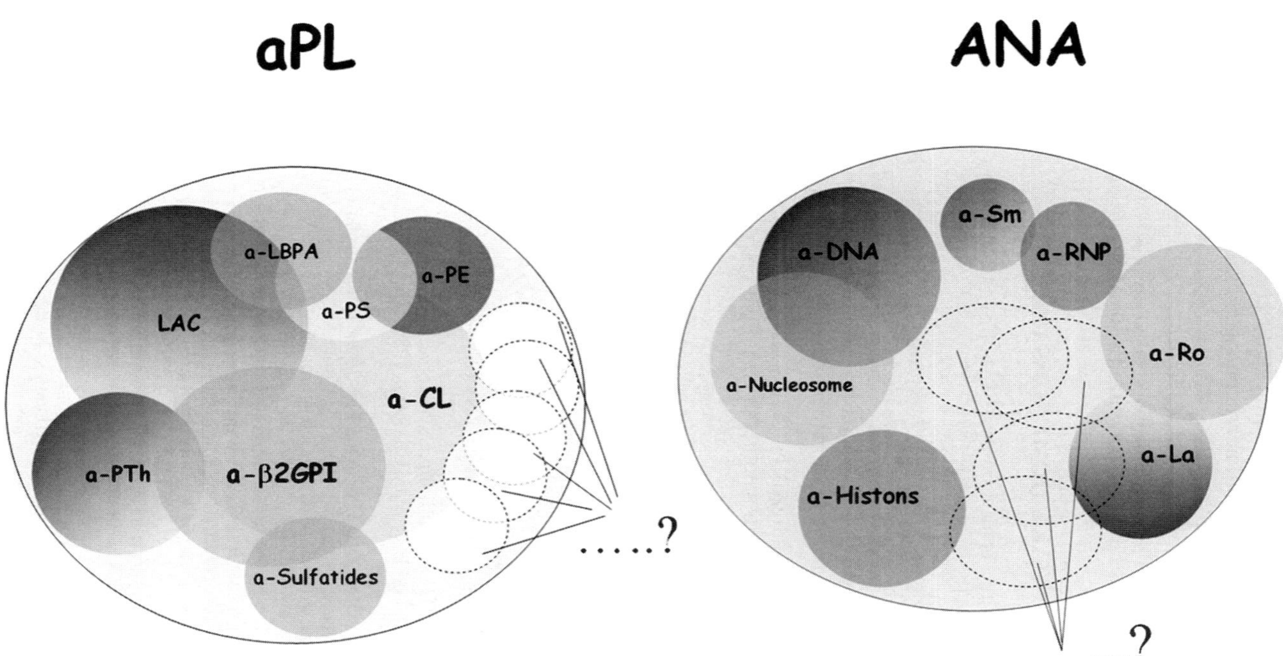

FIGURE 1. Antiphospholipid antibodies (aPLs) represent a heterogeneous family of autoantibodies directed to several antigens; they have partially overlapping specificities and characteristics similar to another well-recognized cluster of autoantibodies, such as antinuclear antibodies (ANAs). Several findings suggest β_2-glycoprotein I and prothrombin as the most relevant antigens in antiphosholipid antibody syndrome (APS). Nevertheless, new target antigens, such as lyso(bis)phosphatidic acid and sulfatides, have recently been described. New findings suggest the intriguing possibility of an undiscovered new autoantibody for seronegative APS. aLBPAs: anti–lyso(bis)phosphatidic acid antibodies; aPSs: anti-phosphatidylserine antibodies; aPEs: anti-phosphatidylethanolamine antibodies; aCLs: anti-cardiolipin antibodies; aPThs: anti-prothrombin antibodies; aβ_2 GPIs: anti-β_2 glycoprotein I antibodies; LAC: lupus anticoagulant.

similar to another well-recognized cluster of autoantigens, the target of antinuclear antibodies (ANA) (FIG. 1).

The aPLs as well as ANAs recognize intracellular complex antigens, and the target epitopes are usually not exposed, nonimmunogenic; they can become exposed and modified during apoptosis. The aPLs may be associated with various clinical manifestations and, as well as antinuclear antibodies (ANAs), are linked to very protean clinical signs. Further studies could identify some disease-restricted specificities in between the aPLs, as has been recognized in the ANA group.

TAKE-HOME MESSAGES

- Lyso(bis)phosphatidic acid, monolysocardiolin, and sulfatides represent new target antigens in APS.
- Diagnosis of seronegative APS may be considered when the other known congenital or acquired coagulopathies are excluded.
- During apoptosis cardiolipin and its immediate degradation product, monolysocardiolipin, move from mitochondria to other cellular membranes.
- aPLs can bind to their antigens on the surface of cells directly or by β_2-GPI that rapidly associates with anionic phospholipid on the membrane of apoptotic cells.
- Lipid peroxidation plays an important role in the pathogenesis of APS.
- Autoimmune response in APS may be triggered by an infection in susceptible subjects with an appropriate genetic background.
- aPLs detected during infectious disease are usually β_2-GPI independent and are not associated with the clinical manifestation of APS.

REFERENCES

1. HUGHES, G.R. 1985. The anticardiolipin syndrome. Clin. Exp. Rheumatol. **3:** 285–286.
2. HUGHES, G.R., E.N. HARRIS & A.E. GHARAVI. 1986. The anticardiolipin syndrome. J. Rheumatol. **13:** 486–489.
3. WILSON, W.A., A.E. GHARAVI, T. KOIKE, *et al.* 1999. International consensus statement on preliminary classification criteria for definite antiphospholipid syndrome: report of an international workshop. Arthritis Rheum. **42:** 1309–1311.
4. HARRIS, E.N. & M. KHAMASHTA. 2004. Anticardiolipin test and the antiphospholipid (Hughes) syndrome: 20 years and counting! J. Rheum. **31:** 2099–2101.
5. MCCLAIN, M.T., M. ARBUCKLE, L.D. HEINLEN, *et al.* 2004. The prevalence, onset, and clinical significance of antiphospholipid antibodies prior to diagnosis of systemic lupus erythematosus. Arthritis Rheum. **50:** 1226–1232.
6. HARRIS, E.N., A.E. GHARAVI, M.L. BOEY, *et al.* 1983. Anticardiolipin antibodies: detection by radioimmunoassay and association with thrombosis in systemic lupus erythematosus. Lancet **2:** 1211–1214.
7. GALLI, M., P. COMFURIUS, C. MAASSEN, *et al.* 1990. Anticardiolipin antibodies (ACA) directed not to cardiolipin but to a plasma protein cofactor. Lancet **355:** 1544–1547.
8. MCNEIL, H.P., R.J. SIMPSON, C.N. CHESTERMAN, *et al.* 1990. Anti-phospholipid antibodies are directed against a complex antigen that includes a lipid-binding inhibitor of coagulation: beta 2-glycoprotein I (apolipoprotein H). Proc. Natl. Acad. Sci. USA **87:** 4120–4124.

9. MATSUURA, E., Y. IGARASHI, M. FUJIMOTO, *et al.* 1990. Anticardiolipin cofactor(s) and differential diagnosis of autoimmune disease. Lancet **336:** 177–178.
10. MCINTYRE, J.A., D.R. WAGENKNECHT & T. SUGI. 1997. Phospholipid binding plasma proteins required for antiphospholipid antibody detection–an overview. Am. J. Reprod. Immunol. **37:** 101–110.
11. COCKERILL, K.A., M.D. LINNIK & G.M. IVERSON. 2004. Detection and characterization of B cell epitopes on beta2-glycoprotein I. Clin. Immunol. **112:** 129–135.
12. AMENGUAL, O., T. ATSUMI & T. KOIKE. 2004. Antiprothombin antibodies and the diagnosis of antiphospholipid syndrome. Clin. Immunol. **112:** 144–149.
13. KOBAYASHI, T., E. STANG, K.S. FANG, *et al.* 1998. A lipid associated with the antiphospholipid syndrome regulates endosome structure and function. Nature **392:** 193–197.
14. SORICE, M., D. FERRO, R. MISASI, *et al.* 2002. Evidence of anticoagulant activity and B2-GPI accumulation in late endosomes of endothelial cells induced by anti-LBPA antibodies. Thromb. Haemost. **87:** 735–741.
15. ALESSANDRI, C., M. BOMBARDIERI, L. DI PROSPERO, *et al.* 2005. Anti-LBPA in APS and SLE patients. Clin. Exp. Immunol. (online publication date 7 February 2005).
16. GALVE-DE ROCHEMONTEIX, B., T. KOBAYASHI, C. ROSNOBLET, *et al.* 2000. Interaction of anti-phospholipid antibodies with late endosomes of human endothelial cells. Arterioscler. Thromb. Vasc. Biol. **20:** 563–574.
17. SORICE, M., A. CIRCELLA, I. M. CRISTEA, *et al.* 2004. Cardiolipin and its metabolites move from mitochondria to other cellular membranes during death receptor-mediated apoptosis. Cell Death Differ. **xx:** 1–13.
18. SORICE, M., T. GRIGGI, A. CIRCELLA, *et al.* 1994. Detection of antiphospholipid antibodies by immunostaining on thin layer chromatography plates. J. Immunol. Methods **173:** 49–54.
19. MERTEN, M., S. MOTAMEDY, S. RAMAMURTHY, *et al.* 2003. Sulfatides targets for antiphospholipid antibodies. Circulation **108:** 2082–2087.
20. CARONTI, B., C. CALDERARO, C. ALESSANDRI, *et al.* 1999. Beta2-glycoprotein I (beta2-GPI) mRNA is expressed by several cell types involved in anti-phospholipid syndrome-related tissue damage. Clin. Exp. Immunol. **115:** 214–219.
21. DEL PAPA, N., L. GUIDALI, A. SALA, *et al.* 1997. Endothelial cells as target for antiphospholipid antibodies. Human polyclonal and monoclonal anti-beta 2-glycoprotein I antibodies react in vitro with endothelial cells through adherent beta 2-glycoprotein I and induce endothelial activation. Arthritis Rheum. **40:** 551–561.
22. CARONTI, B., V. PITTONI, G. PALLADINI, *et al.* 1998. Anti-b2-glycoprotein I antibodies bind to central nervous system. J. Neurol. Sci. **156:** 211–219.
23. TINCANI, A., F. ALLEGRI, G. BALESTRIERI, *et al.* 2004. Minimal requirements for antiphospholipid antibodies ELISAs proposed by the European forum on antiphospholipid antibodies. Thromb. Res. **114:** 553–558.
24. SANGLE, S., D.P. D'CRUZ & G.R. HUGHES. 2005. Livedo reticularis and pregnancy morbidity in patients negative for antiphospholipid antibodies. Ann. Rheum. Dis. **64:** 147–148.
25. PITTONI, V. & G. VALESINI. 2002. The clearance of apoptotic cells: implications for autoimmunity. Autoimmun. Rev. **1:** 154–161.
26. UTZ, P.J., T.J. GENSLER & P. ANDERSON. 2000. Death, autoantigen modifications, and tolerance. Arthritis Res. **2:** 101–114.
27. FADOK, V.A. & P.M. HENSON. 2003. Apoptosis: giving phosphatidylserine recognition an assist–with a twist. Curr. Biol. **13:** R655–R657.
28. HATCH, G.M. 1998. Cardiolipin: biosynthesis, remodeling and trafficking in the heart and mammalian cells. Int. J. Mol. Med. **1:** 33–41.
29. SCHLAME, M. & B. RUSTOW. 1990. Lysocardiolipin formation and reacylation in isolated rat liver mitochondria. Biochem. J. **272:** 589–595.
30. DEGLI ESPOSTI, M. 2002. Lipids, cardiolipin and apoptosis: a greasy licence to kill. Cell Death Differ. **9:** 234–236.
31. DEGLI ESPOSTI, M., I.M. CRISTEA S.J. GASKELL, *et al.* 2003. Proapoptotic Bid binds to monolysocardiolipin, a new molecular connection between mitochondrial membranes and cell death. Cell Death Differ. **10:** 1300–1309.

32. CASCIOLA-ROSEN, L.A., G. ANHALT & A. ROSEN. 1994. Autoantigens targeted in systemic lupus erythematosus are clustered in two populations of surface structures on apoptotic keratinocytes. J. Exp. Med. **179:** 1317–1330.
33. MCMILLIN, J.B. & W. DOWHAN. 2002. Cardiolipin and apoptosis. Biochim. Biophys. Acta **1585:** 97–107.
34. QAMAR, T., A.E. GHARAVI, R.A. LEVY, *et al.* 1990. Lysophosphatidylethanolamine is the antigen to which apparent antibody to phosphatidylethanolamine binds. J. Clin. Immunol. **10:** 200–203.
35. WU, R., Y.H. HUANG, L.S. ELINDER, *et al.* 1998. Lysophosphatidylcholine is involved in the antigenicity of oxidized LDL. Arterioscler. Thromb. Vasc. Biol. **18:** 626–630.
36. WU, R., E. SVENUNGSSON, I. GUNNARSSON, *et al.* 1999. Antibodies against lysophosphatidylcholine and oxidized LDL in patients with SLE. Lupus **8:** 142–150.
37. PRUZANSKI, W., E.C. KEYSTONE, B. STERNBY, *et al.* 1988. Serum phospholipase A2 correlates with disease activity in rheumatoid arthritis. J. Rheumatol. **15:** 1351–1355.
38. PRUZANSKI, W., N.J. GOULDING, R.J. FLOWER, *et al.* 1994. Circulating Group II phospholipase A2 activity and antilipocortin antibodies in systemic lupus erythematosus. Correlative study with disease activity. J. Rheumatol. **21:** 252–257.
39. COCCA, B.A., S.N. SEAL, P. D'AGNILLO, *et al.* 2001. Structural basis for autoantibody recognition of phosphatidylserine-beta 2 glycoprotein I and apoptotic cells. Proc. Natl. Acad. Sci. USA **98:** 13826–13831.
40. HORKKO, S., E. MILLER, E. DUDL, *et al.* 1996. Antiphospholipid antibodies are directed against epitopes of oxidized phospholipids. Recognition of cardiolipin by monoclonal antibodies to epitopes of oxidized low density lipoprotein. J. Clin. Invest. **98:** 815–825.
41. HORKKO, S., T. OLEE, L. MO, *et al.* 2001. Anticardiolipin antibodies from patients with the antiphospholipid antibody syndrome recognize epitopes in both beta(2)-glycoprotein 1 and oxidized low-density lipoprotein. Circulation **103:** 941–946.
42. ROLLA, R., D. VAY, E. MOTTARAN, *et al.* 2001. Antiphospholipid antibodies associated with alcoholic liver disease specifically recognise oxidised phospholipids. Gut **49:** 852–859.
43. HORKKO, S., E. MILLER, D.W. BRANCH, *et al.* 1997. The epitopes for some antiphospholipid antibodies are adducts of oxidized phospholipid and beta2 glycoprotein 1 (and other proteins). Proc. Natl. Acad. Sci. USA **94:** 10356–10361.
44. IULIANO, L., D. PRATICO, D. FERRO, *et al.* 1997. Enhanced lipid peroxidation in patients positive for antiphospholipid antibodies. Blood **90:** 3931–3935.
45. FERRO, D., V. PITTONI, C. QUINTARELLI, *et al.* 1997. Coexistence of anti-phospholipid antibodies and endothelial perturbation in systemic lupus erythematosus patients with ongoing prothrombotic state. Circulation **95:** 1425–1432.
46. HORKKO, S., D.A. BIRD, E. MILLER, *et al.* 1999. Monoclonal autoantibodies specific for oxidized phospholipids or oxidized phospholipid-protein adducts inhibit macrophage uptake of oxidized low-density lipoproteins. J. Clin. Invest. **103:** 117–128.
47. FROSTEGARD, J., E. SVENUNGSSON, R. WU, *et al.* 2005. Lipid peroxidation is enhanced in patients with systemic lupus erythematosus and is associated with arterial and renal disease manifestations. Arthritis Rheum. **52:** 192–200.
48. PRATICO, D., D. FERRO, L. IULIANO, *et al.* 1999. Ongoing prothrombotic state in patients with antiphospholipid antibodies: a role for increased lipid peroxidation. Blood **93:** 3401–3407.
49. FERRO, D., M. SALIOLA, P.L. MERONI, *et al.* 2003. Enhanced monocyte expression of tissue factor by oxidative stress in patients with antiphospholipid antibodies: effect of antioxidant treatment. J. Thromb. Haemost. **1:** 523–531.
50. FERRO, D., L. IULIANO, F. VIOLI, *et al.* 2002. Antioxidant treatment decreases the titer of circulating anticardiolipin antibodies: comment on the article by Sambo *et al.* Arthritis Rheum. **46:** 3110–3112.
51. MCINTYRE, J.A. 2004. The appearance and disappearance of antiphospholipid autoantibodies subsequent to oxidation-reduction reactions. Thromb. Res. **114:** 579–587.
52. BLANK, M. & Y. SHOENFELD. 2004. B2-glycoprotein I, infections, antiphospholipid syndrome and therapeutic considerations. Clin. Immunol. **112:** 190–199.

53. WRAITH, D. 2003. Vaccination and autoimmune disease: what is the evidence? Lancet **362:** 1659–1666.
54. RASCHI, E., C. TESTONI, D. BOSISIO, *et al.* 2003. Role of the MyD88 transduction signaling pathway in endothelial activation by antiphospholipid antibodies. Blood **101:** 3495–3500.
55. ASHERSON, R.A. & R. CERVERA. 2003. Antiphospholipid antibodies and infections. Ann. Rheum. Dis. **62:** 388–393.
56. LOIZOU, S., S. SINGH, E. WYPKEMA, *et al.* 2003. Anticardiolipin, anti-beta(2)-glycoprotein I and antiprothrombin antibodies in black South African patients with infectious disease. Ann. Rheum. Dis. **62:** 1106–1111.
57. SORICE, M., V. PITTONI, T. GRIGGI, *et al.* 2000. Specificity of anti-phospholipid antibodies in infectious mononucleosis: a role for anti-cofactor protein antibodies. Clin. Exp. Immunol. **120:** 301–306.
58. MATSUURA, E., Y. IGARASHI, M. FUJIMOTO, *et al.* 1992. Heterogeneity of anticardiolipin antibodies defined by the anticardiolipin cofactor. J. Immunol. **148:** 3885–3891.
59. CELLI, C.M., A.E. GHARAVI & H. CHAIMOVICH. 1999. Opposite beta2-glycoprotein I requirement for the binding of infectious and autoimmune antiphospholipid antibodies to cardiolipin liposomes is associated with antibody avidity. Biochim. Biophys. Acta **1416:** 225–238.
60. GHARAVI, A.E., W. WILSON & S. PIERANGELI. 2003. The molecular basis of antiphospholipid syndrome. Lupus **12:** 579–583.

Inhibitor Development in Patients with Hemophilia A after Continuous Infusion of FVIII Concentrates

CH. VON AUER,[a] J. OLDENBURG,[b] M. VON DEPKA,[c]
C. ESCURIOLA-ETTINGHAUSEN,[d] K. KURNIK,[e] H. LENK,[f]
AND I. SCHARRER[a]

[a]*Haemostaseology, Internal Medicine III,* [d]*Department of Paediatric Haematology and Oncology, Johann Wolfgang Goethe University Hospital, Frankfurt/Main, Germany*

[b]*Institute of Transfusion Medicine and Immune Haematology of the DRK Blood Donor Service Hessen, Frankfurt/Main, Germany*

[c]*Werlhof Institute for Haemostasis and Thrombosis, Hannover, Germany*

[e]*Dr. von Haunersches Kinderspital, Paediatric Hospital, Munich, Germany*

[f]*Haemophilia Center, Paediatric Hospital University of Leipzig, Germany*

ABSTRACT: Continuous infusion (CI) of coagulation factor concentrates has been used since the early 1990s. Recent reports of the occurrence of an inhibitor after CI have raised concerns about this method of treatment. We conducted a retrospective study to investigate the development of inhibitors after CI of Factor VIII concentrates in Germany. So far, 13 hemophilia centers have been contacted, and data have been collected by a questionnaire. Of the 13 centers, CI had never been performed in three, no inhibitors had been detected in five, and inhibitor development after CI was recorded in 10 patients in the remaining five centers. Of these 10 patients (ages 7 months to 57 years), five were suffering from severe, one from moderate, and four from mild hemophilia. Indications for treatment were major bleeds and surgical procedures. Plasma-derived (6 cases) and recombinant (4 cases) factor concentrates were given in various infusion sets. Data concerning amount infused (4300 to >100,000 IU), number of days of exposure to factor concentrates (1 to >100), and inhibitor characteristics (alloantibodies, 3 LR, 7 HR) were collected. Regarding hemophilia genotype, we found missense mutations in four patients, intron-22 inversions in two, and one small deletion in one; the genotype in three was unknown. In conclusion, only 3 out of 10 patients who developed an inhibitor after CI showed the typical risk profile for inhibitor formation, which is severe hemophilia A with a severe gene defect and less than 50 days of exposure to coagulation factor concentrates. Especially striking was the finding that 50% of the patients who developed inhibitors had mild to moderate hemophilia A. Our data point to the existence of a so-far unknown factor, related to CI, that might lead to inhibitor formation.

Address for correspondence: Charis von Auer, M.D., Haemostaseology, Department of Internal Medicine III, Johann Wolfgang Goethe University Hospital, Theodor-Stern-Kai 7, 60590 Frankfurt/Main, Germany. Voice: +49-69-6301-5051; fax: +49-69-6301-6738.
charis.auer@kgu.de

**Ann. N.Y. Acad. Sci. 1051: 498–505 (2005). © 2005 New York Academy of Sciences.
doi: 10.1196/annals.1361.094**

KEYWORDS: hemophilia A; inhibitor development; continuous infusion; missense mutation

INTRODUCTION

Bleeding in patients with hemophilia A is prevented or treated by factor replacement therapy with plasma-derived or recombinant factor VIII (FVIII) concentrates. Administration can be done either with intermittent intravenous bolus infusion (BI) or with continuous infusion (CI). Most hemophilia-treating centers traditionally use the well-established BI to replace the missing factor.

CI was first described by McMillan *et al.* in 1970[1] but did not receive much attention at that time. Since the early 1990s, CI has been used to a greater extent since basic questions about technical issues, stability of factor concentrates, and hygienic aspects have been resolved. Portable minipumps or common infusion sets are used for delivering the factor concentrate during prolonged periods, with exchange of infusion bags at daily intervals. The advantage of CI is seen in maintaining a steady factor level in the patient's circulation, thus avoiding critical low levels and unnecessary high peaks. Mathematically, it was shown that 30% of factor concentrate could be saved, pointing to an economic benefit of CI.[2] Indications for CI include the management of major bleeds and surgical procedures. Disadvantages of CI are the possible development of thrombophlebitis at the infusion site, assumed bacterial overgrowth inside the infusion bags, and lack of data and guidelines for CI. In addition, recent reports about inhibitors developing after CI of FVIII have raised concerns about this method of administration.

Today, the development of an inhibitor, a polyclonal IgG alloantibody directed against FVIII, represents the most serious complication of hemophilia therapy.[3] It poses a diagnostic and therapeutic challenge for the clinician, as patients may present with an uncontrolled bleeding episode involving, for example, intracerebral or gastrointestinal organs, soft tissue, or other organs. By neutralizing exogenous FVIII, the inhibitor leads to treatment failure and requires alternative treatment options that are likely to be more expensive and have a less predictable outcome.

The spontaneous occurrence of FVIII inhibitors in hemophiliacs is very rare, and almost always follows replacement therapy with exogenous FVIII.[4] The pathogenesis of inhibitor development is still not fully understood. There seems to be an interaction of several elements considered as risk factors. We know about patient-related factors (e.g., FVIII gene mutation, immunological response, concomitant immunological challenges, ethnicity, family history of inhibitor development) and therapy-related factors (e.g., FVIII product, number of exposures, pattern of exposures, change of product, and method of administration). Generally, it can be said that the risk for inhibitor development is highest in previously untreated patients (PUPs) with severe hemophilia having no endogenous FVIII.

In our comprehensive care center for hemophilia treatment we started to use CI during orthopedic surgery for patients with hemophilia A in the late 1990s. We conducted 14 CIs in 11 patients who had been treated with exogenous FVIII before (previously treated patients, PTPs). Two of them developed FVIII inhibitors during or shortly after CI. In comparison, we carried out 81 major orthopedic surgeries in the same time period with BI and no inhibitor development. Therefore, we stopped the

TABLE 1. Issues addressed in the questionnaire sent to hemophilia treatment centers

Age of patient	Infusion sets
Severity of hemophilia	Factor concentrate used for CI
Days of exposure throughout lifetime	Thrombophlebitis during CI
FVIII gene mutation	Inhibitor characteristic
Family history	ITT
Month and year of CI	ITT, duration
Indication for CI	ITT, success
Amount of FVIII infused	Prophylaxis/on-demand therapy

use of CI in our center. To find out about experiences at other centers we decided together with the Scientific Council of the German Hemophilia Society to conduct a retrospective study on the development of inhibitors after CI of FVIII in Germany.

METHODS

A questionnaire was developed and sent to 13 hemophilia centers that are members of the Scientific Council of the German Hemophilia Society and represent most of the largest hemophilia treatment centers in Germany. The questionnaire contained specific questions concerning patients who developed the inhibitor and about specific treatment modalities in each case (TABLE 1). All centers answered and reported their data to our center. Data were collected and documented, and open questions or ambiguous answers were checked by telephone calls.

RESULTS

In 10 of the 13 hemophilia centers CI regimens were used for the treatment of hemophilia A patients. Indications for FVIII replacement therapy were serious bleeding and surgical procedures. In total, approximately 250 CIs were conducted. Five of the 10 hemophilia centers recorded a total of 10 patients with inhibitor development after CI. These patients were between ages 7 months and 57 years (median 15 years) when CI was given. Five patients were suffering from severe hemophilia, one from moderate hemophilia, and four from mild hemophilia. Before inhibitor development the patients had lifetime exposures between one and >100 days (days on which at least one FVIII infusion was given), with a median of 22 days. Only two patients were PUPs who had never had FVIII replacement therapy before; the rest of the patients (8/10) were PTPs. A concomitant thrombophlebitis was found in two patients, and one patient had a positive family history of inhibitor development (in a cousin). The following FVIII gene mutations were reported for the 10 inhibitor patients: missense mutations (4), intron-22 inversions (2), a small deletion

TABLE 2. Patient data relevant for risk assessment of inhibitor formation

No.	Age	Hemophilia Severity	Former Treatment	Inhibitor Titer	Inhibitor Permanent/ Transient	Exposure Days	FVII Gene Mutation
1	7 months	severe	PUP	high	permanent	13	small deletion
2	3.5 years	severe	PTP	high	transient	1	intron-22 inversion
3	5.5 years	severe	PTP	low	transient	10	intron-22 inversion
4	8 years	mild	PTP	high	permanent	5	missense mutation
5	11 years	mild	PUP	low	permanent	28	missense mutation
6	19 years	mild	PTP	high	transient	16	missense mutation
7	35 years	mild	PTP	high	permanent	30	unknown
8	45 years	severe	PTP	high	permanent	>100	no intron-22 inversion
9	45 years	severe	PTP	low	permanent	>100	missense mutation
10	57 years	moderate	PTP	high	permanent	>100	unknown

(1), unknown (3). Infused amounts of FVIII concentrate before inhibitor development ranged between 4300 and >100,000 IU. The infusion sets varied from minipumps (2/10) to common infusion sets (7/10); one was unknown. The detected inhibitors were alloantibodies, three low-responding (3/10) and seven high-responding (7/10), three transient and seven permanent. Immune tolerance therapy (treatment with high FVIII concentrations) was done in seven patients for inhibitor suppression, with successful outcome in four patients. Several factor concentrates were used for CI before inhibitor development: six plasma-derived (6/10) and four recombinant (4/10) products. A summary of our results is shown in TABLE 2.

DISCUSSION

The appearance of inhibitors in 10 patients out of approximately 250 receiving CI is striking. Furthermore, the patient-related risk factors show an interesting, uncommon pattern in our 10 inhibitor patients. Consider, for example the FVIII gene mutations we found: the so-called null mutations (here intron-22 inversion and a small frame shift deletion), which cause severe hemophilia with no endogenous FVIII synthesis, were present in only three patients. Due to lack of endogenous FVIII, such patients have the highest risk for inhibitor development when first exposed to exogenous FVIII. They generally exhibit an inhibitor prevalence with a range of 21% to 88 percent.[5]

In our study, we found an unexpectedly high proportion of patients with missense mutations (4/10), mostly causing mild or moderate hemophilia. These patients have circulating endogenous FVIII, therefore the occurrence of inhibitors is not easily explained. In this patient group inhibitor development is thought to be uncommon, with a prevalence of <10%.[5] Looking at the distribution of FVIII gene mutations in a common inhibitor patient collective we find 4% of the patients with missense mutations (FIG. 1B, personal communication, J. Oldenburg). In our patient collective with inhibitor development after CI, patients with missense mutations amount to 40% (FIG. 1A), an unexpectedly high number.

Second, we found most of the patients to be PTPs, who are considered to be at low risk for inhibitor development. Having been exposed to exogenous FVIII before, without inhibitor development, these patients are thought to be tolerant to FVIII. Inhibitor detection in such a patient should raise concerns about therapy-related variables, such as product immunogenicity or method of administration.[6] This is especially the case for the four reported PTPs (4/8) with severe hemophilia A. The other four reported PTPs (4/8) had mild or moderate hemophilia with less severe bleeding. In these patients treatment episodes tend to occur later in life and less frequently than in those with severe hemophilia. Therefore, the first intense FVIII exposure, for example, for operative intervention, may take place at an older age and the patient still may have only a few exposure days. Thus, he still may be at a higher risk for inhibitor development, even at an older age.

Concerning further patient-related factors, we saw no correlation with a positive family history. Only one patient had inhibitor development in his family, underlining the low-risk profile for inhibitor development in that cohort. Other patient-related factors such as ethnicity, immunological challenges at time of CI, or immunological

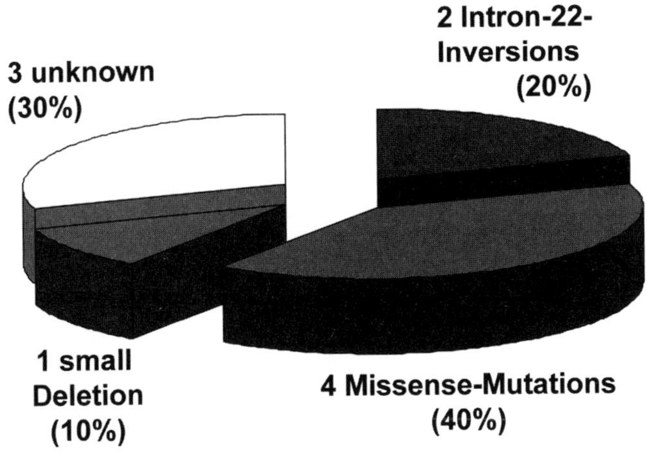

FIGURE 1A. Distribution of mutation types in 10 patients with inhibitor development during CI.

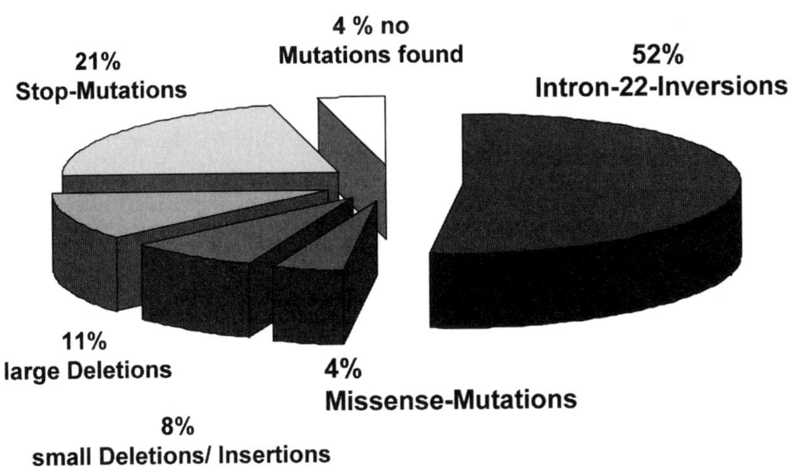

FIGURE 1B. Distribution of mutation types in a typical cohort of hemophilia A patients with inhibitor formation (personal communication with J. Oldenburg).

response characteristics were not questioned in our study, but should be considered in future studies.

In summary, we found inhibitor development after using CI for FVIII replacement therapy unexpectedly in many patients with missense mutations or mild to moderate hemophilia, and unexpectedly in many PTPs with severe hemophilia A. One could suggest that patients with mild hemophilia might exhibit a much higher prevalence of inhibitor development when treated with an intense FVIII treatment such as CI. These findings agree with published results on inhibitor detection in mild hemophilia, usually after a period of intense replacement treatment.[7–10]

On the other hand, our investigation suggests that there may be therapy-related risk factors for CI. This could be, for example, an uncommon inhibitor pathomechanism, resulting in a peculiar group of patients developing the inhibitor after CI. In general, the pathomechanisms leading to inhibitor development during or shortly after CI are still unknown. Possible explanations could be a modification of FVIII protein into a more antigenic form during storage *ex vivo* in infusion pumps, or by prolonged contact with plastic materials or inflamed veins. The latter could not be confirmed in our study, where only two patients had concomitant thrombophlebitis at the infusion site. Other explanations could be some subcutaneous leakage during infusion, or the context in which FVIII is given, such as significant bleeds or major surgery with probable tissue damage and associated inflammation. This could result in a more immunogenic type of FVIII exposure, or trigger an antibody response against exogenous FVIII. In one of our own patients we documented extravasation several times during CI; for the other patients this was not documented. In our study we cannot draw any conclusions concerning product immunogenicity. Patient numbers are still too small and both product types were used in almost equal numbers of patients, six plasma-derived versus four recombinant concentrates. To date, there is no definitive evidence in the literature to indicate a higher risk with recombinant or plasma-derived concentrates. Again, collection of further data on therapy-related risk factors should be considered in future studies: duration of acute replacement treatment until inhibitor development or time to inhibitor development postexposure, exact amount infused from beginning of current therapy episode until inhibitor development, and overall amount infused during patient lifetime.

In the literature, we found similar reports on inhibitor development after CI. So far, we have counted 34 reported cases. Most of these patients were PTPs and/or had mild hemophilia.[11–14]

In further investigations, it would be interesting to compare the inhibitor development after CIs with the inhibitor development after BIs carried out at the same center, in the same time frame, and for similar indications. Due to different documentation systems in the hemophilia centers, retrospective data collection appears to be difficult and time consuming. We also have to consider aggravated data collection in a retrospective study, or possible lack of documentation. Therefore, a prospective multicenter study to investigate inhibitor development after CI should be conducted.

ACKNOWLEDGMENTS

This work was presented in part at the 46th Annual Meeting of the American Society of Hematology, San Diego, 2004.

REFERENCES

1. McMillan, C.W., W.P. Webster, H.R. Roberts & W.B. Blythe. 1970. Continuous intravenous infusion of factor VIII in classic haemophilia. Br. J. Haematol. **18:** 659–667.
2. Hermens, W.T.H. 1975. Dose calculation of human factor VIII and factor IX concentrates for infusion therapy. *In* Handbook of Hemophilia. K.M. Brinkhouse & H.C. Hemker, Eds.: 569–589. American Elsevier Publishing. New York.
3. Scharrer, I., G.L. Bray & O. Neutzling. 1999. Incidence of inhibitors in haemophilia A patients—a review of recent studies of recombinant and plasma-derived factor VIII concentrates. Haemophilia **5:** 145–154.
4. Yee, T.T. & C.A. Lee. 2002. Incidence and prevalence of inhibitors and type of blood product in haemophilia A. *In* Inhibitors in Patients with Haemophilia. E.C. Rodriguez-Merchan & C.A. Lee, Eds.: 14–20. Blackwell Publishing. Oxford, UK.
5. Oldenburg, J. & E. Tuddenham. 2002. Genetic basis of inhibitor development in severe haemophilia A and B. *In* Inhibitors in Patients with Haemophilia. E.C. Rodriguez-Merchan & C.A. Lee, Eds.: 21–26. Blackwell Publishing. Oxford, UK.
6. White, G.C., D. DiMichele, K. Mertens, *et al.* 1999. Utilization of previously treated patients (PTPs), noninfected patients (NIPs), and previously untreated patients (PUPs) in the evaluation of new factor VIII and factor IX concentrates. Recommendation of the Scientific Subcommittee on Factor VIII and Factor IX of the Scientific and Standardization Committee of the International Society on Thrombosis and Haemostasis. Thromb. Haemost. **81:** 462.
7. Hay, C.R.M. & C.A. Lee. 2002. Inhibitors in mild and moderate haemophilia A. *In* Inhibitors in Patients with Haemophilia. E.C. Rodriguez-Merchan & C.A. Lee, Eds.: 92–97. Blackwell Publishing. Oxford, UK.
8. Carcao, M.D. 2004. More on: intensive factor VIII exposure and inhibitor development in mild hemophilia A. J. Thromb. Haemost. **2:** 677.
9. Koestenberger, M. 2004. More on: mild hemophilia A and inhibitor development. J. Thromb. Haemost. **2:** 676.
10. Sharathkumar, A., D. Lillicrap, V.S. Blanchette, *et al.* 2003. Intensive exposure to factor VIII is a risk factor for inhibitor development in mild hemophilia A. J. Thromb. Haemost. **1:** 1228–1236
11. Schulman, S. 2003. Continuous infusion. Haemophilia **9:** 368–375.
12. Suzuki, T., M. Arai, S. Miyasaka, *et al.* 1995. Factor VIII inhibitor developed in a 60-year-old patient with mild hemophilia A after surgery for colon cancer. Int. J. Hematol. **62:** 127–132.
13. Hermans, C. *et al.* 2002. Collected abstracts of the XXV International Congress of the World Federation of Hemophilia (Seville): no. 12PO35. Haemophilia **8:** 541.
14. Batorova, A. & U. Martinowitz. 2002. Continous infusion of coagulation factors. Haemophilia **8:** 170–77.

Increased Spontaneous Apoptosis of $CD4^+CD25^+$ T Cells in Patients with Active Rheumatoid Arthritis Is Reduced by Infliximab

E. TOUBI,[a] A. KESSEL,[a] Z. MAHMUDOV,[a] K. HALLAS,[a] M. ROZENBAUM,[b] AND I. ROSNER[b]

[a]*Division of Allergy and Clinical Immunology,* [b]*Rheumatology Unit, Bnai-Zion Medical Center, Technion, Rapaport Faculty of Medicine, Haifa, Israel*

ABSTRACT: Increased secretion of tumor necrosis factor-alpha (TNF-α), along with interleukin-1 (IL-1) and interleukin-6 (IL-6), is important in the pathogenesis of rheumatoid arthritis (RA). T regulatory $CD4^+CD25^+$ cells play a role in maintaining self-tolerance by downregulating Th1-induced proinflammation. This function has been found to be altered in active RA, whereas anti–TNF-α therapy has been found to improve the suppressive abilities of these cells. Our objectives were to investigate whether T regulatory cells in patients with active RA display a higher sensitivity to spontaneous apoptosis than in normals, and to look into the potential of infliximab (anti–TNF-α therapy) to reduce the sensitivity of these cells to spontaneous apoptosis. Seventeen patients suffering from active RA, having failed multiple disease-modifying antirheumatic drug (DMARD) therapies, were treated with infliximab. Spontaneous apoptosis (as detected by annexin V binding) was determined in all patients and compared with a group of normal individuals at baseline and after three months on infliximab treatment. Peripheral blood mononuclear cells were incubated in 24-well plates at 1×10^6 cells/mL for 48 hours. Annexin V binding on $CD4^+CD25^+$ was assessed using three-color assay by flow cytometry. Prior to infliximab initiation, spontaneous apoptosis of T regulatory cells from active RA patients was found to be increased in comparison with controls (26 ± 4.2% vs. 19.8 ± 4.8%, respectively; $P = 0.01$). Three months later (while still on infliximab) spontaneous apoptosis was comparable in the two groups (20.7 ± 5.2% vs. 20.9 ± 3.4%; $P = 0.8$). The absolute number of $CD4^+CD25^+$ cells/mL in the peripheral blood at baseline was reduced in 11 out of 17 active RA patients when compared with that of the control group (24 ± 7 vs. 32 ± 11, respectively; $P = 0.02$). Following anti–TNF-α therapy, $CD4^+CD25^+$ cell counts of patients were equivalent to those of normals. The alteration and reversal in both spontaneous apoptosis and cell count of T regulatory cells was found to correlate with RA disease activity. $CD4^+CD25^+$ T regulatory cells display increased proclivity to undergo spontaneous apoptosis in active RA. Alterations in $CD4^+CD25^+$ cell apoptosis and cell count were found to correlate with RA disease activity. Reversal of these deviations from normal was documented in association with the beneficial outcome of infliximab therapy.

Address for correspondence: Elias Toubi, M.D., Division of Allergy and Clinical Immunology, Bnai-Zion Medical Center, Golomb Str. 47, P. O. Box 4, Haifa, Israel.
elias.toubi@b-zion.org.il

**Ann. N.Y. Acad. Sci. 1051: 506–514 (2005). © 2005 New York Academy of Sciences.
doi: 10.1196/annals.1361.095**

KEYWORDS: **rheumatoid arthritis; apoptosis; anti-TNF; T regulatory cells**

INTRODUCTION

Rheumatoid arthritis (RA) is a chronic inflammatory disease mediated by proinflammatory cytokines of the Th1 type leading to the destruction of joints when uncontrolled. There is increased secretion of tumor necrosis factor-alpha (TNF-α), interleukin-1 (IL-1), and interleukin-6 (IL-6), all key players in the pathogenesis of RA. Many studies, both in mice and in humans, have confirmed the importance of a naturally occurring T regulatory (Tr) CD4$^+$ cell subset, comprising approximately 10% of all CD4$^+$ T cells in the pathogenesis of many autoimmune diseases.[1–3] Those CD4$^+$ T cells expressing the interleukin-2 (IL-2) receptor α-chain (CD25) appear to play a pivotal role in the control of T cell homeostasis by suppressing the proliferation of effector T cells, thus maintaining self-tolerance.[4] Experimental *in vivo* studies have demonstrated that absence of regulatory T cells allows organ- and non–organ-specific autoimmune diseases such as thyroiditis, gastritis, and systemic lupus erythematosus (SLE) to occur, whereas the addition of this T cell population can prevent or delay these diseases.[5–7] This observation is consistent with the finding of reduced Tr cell count in active SLE in comparison with values in the peripheral blood of healthy individuals.[8,9]

In a recent study, CD4$^+$CD25^{bright} Tr cells with the potential to suppress the proliferation of autologous CD4$^+$ T cells were relatively enriched in the synovia of patients with active RA compared with their peripheral blood.[10] This local increase was explained by several possibilities, such as their attraction by dendritic cell–derived chemokines, in an attempt to suppress local Th1-induced inflammation. In another recent study,[11] it was shown that CD4$^+$CD25$^+$ cells from the peripheral blood of active RA patients failed to suppress proinflammatory cytokine secretion from activated T cells and monocytes, and that treatment with the anti–TNF-α antibody infliximab restored the capacity of these cells to inhibit cytokine production and suppress CD4$^+$CD25$^-$. Moreover, anti–TNF-α therapy was followed by an increase in the number of peripheral blood Tr cells, in correlation with both clinical and laboratory improvement.

TNF-α, in parallel to its many stimulatory effector functions, is able to stimulate activated cell death (apoptosis) of lymphocytes and monocytes, shown to be mediated through the activation of caspases.[12] In another study, TNF-α induced apoptosis was demonstrated to correlate with overexpression of Bak, a proapoptotic member of the Bcl-2 family, suggesting that TNF-α–induced apoptosis could also occur via a caspase-3–independent pathway.[13]

In consideration of the above, it was elected to investigate the possibility of increased CD4$^+$CD25$^+$ Tr cell apoptosis in RA patients, and to assess whether this alteration correlates with RA activity. In the present study, the tendency of CD4$^+$CD25$^+$ Tr cells to undergo increased spontaneous apoptosis was evaluated. The possibility that the beneficial effect of anti–TNF-α therapy in RA involves the reversal of increased Tr cell apoptosis was evaluated as well.

METHODS

Patients

The study included 17 RA patients, (11 women and 6 men; ages 36 to 68 years, mean 48 years), all with active disease. All satisfied the American College of Rheumatology criteria and were followed at the outpatient rheumatology clinic of the Bnai-Zion Medical Center. All patients had no or only partial response to treatment with methotrexate 10 to 15 mg/week, nonsteroidal anti-inflammatory drugs (NSAIDs), and at least two other disease-modifying drugs. RA disease severity was assessed by two senior rheumatologists using a global physician's score, namely articular swelling/deformity, radiographic erosions, subcutaneous nodules, and serological markers of activity such as rheumatoid factor (RF), C-reactive protein (CRP) and hypergammaglobulinemia.

In an attempt to achieve disease control, infliximab at 3 mg/kg was added, with the methotrexate/NSAID dose held constant. In all patients, the sensitivity of $CD4^+CD25^+$ Tr cells to spontaneous apoptosis was measured at baseline and three months after the initiation of infliximab. In addition to the extent of apoptosis, the absolute number of $CD4^+CD25^+$ cells was also counted. These parameters were compared to those of 15 healthy age- and sex-matched individuals.

Cell Separation

Peripheral blood mononuclear cells (PBMCs) were isolated by Ficoll-Hypaque density gradient centrifugation. Washed PBMCs were cultured in RPMI-1640 supplemented with 10% FCS, L-glutamine 2 mM, penicillin 100 U/mL, streptomycin 5 µg/mL, and IL-2 at 5 µg/mL. Cells were cultured in 24-well plates (Corning Glass Works, Corning, NY) at a final concentration of 1×10^6 cells/well for 48 hours.

Flow Cytometry

Fresh PBMCs were stained with PE-conjugated monoclonal antibodies to CD4 cells and with FITC-conjugated monoclonal antibodies to CD25 (Genzyme Corporation, Cambridge, MA) and counted by flow cytometry. Tr cells were defined when $CD4^+$ cells coexpressed only highly bright CD25, aiming to exclude $CD25^{low}$ cells. Annexin V binding to $CD4^+CD25^+$ Tr cells was assayed by direct (one-step) triple immunostaining using FITC-conjugated monoclonal antibody (mAb) to annexin V (Annexin V kit, MedSystems Diagnostics GmbH, A-1030 Vienna, Austria), PE-conjugated mAb to CD25 (Genzyme Corporation, Cambridge, MA), and APC-conjugated mAb to CD4 T cells (Dako, Glostrup-Denmark, Pharmaceutical Inc., OH). Flow cytometry was carried out with an FACS operating with Cellquest software (Becton Dickinson, Mountain View, CA). The total population of viable cells was gated according to their typical forward and right-angle light scatter. The fluorescence of cells treated with fluorescent isotype mAb was evaluated in each experiment to determine the level of background fluorescence of negative cells. The percentage of stained cells for annexin V, $CD4^+$, and $CD25^+$ cells was determined taking only the positive cells into account.

Association between Tr Cell Apoptosis and Disease Severity

Possible correlation between the degree of spontaneous apoptosis, Tr cell count, and RA disease severity was assessed. The beneficial effect of anti–TNF-α therapy was analyzed in relation to the reversal of Tr cell apoptosis and improvement of both clinical and laboratory parameters.

Statistical Analyses

Comparison of continuous variables of RA patients versus matched controls was performed using the paired Student's t test. The correlation between RA disease severity, CRP values, and annexin V binding was evaluated using the Spearman's Rank correlation coefficient. Two-tailed P values of 0.05 or less were considered to be statistically significant.

RESULTS

Prior to infliximab initiation, spontaneous apoptosis of $CD4^{+}CD25^{+}$ cells was found to be increased in 12 out of 17 of the RA patients as compared with none of

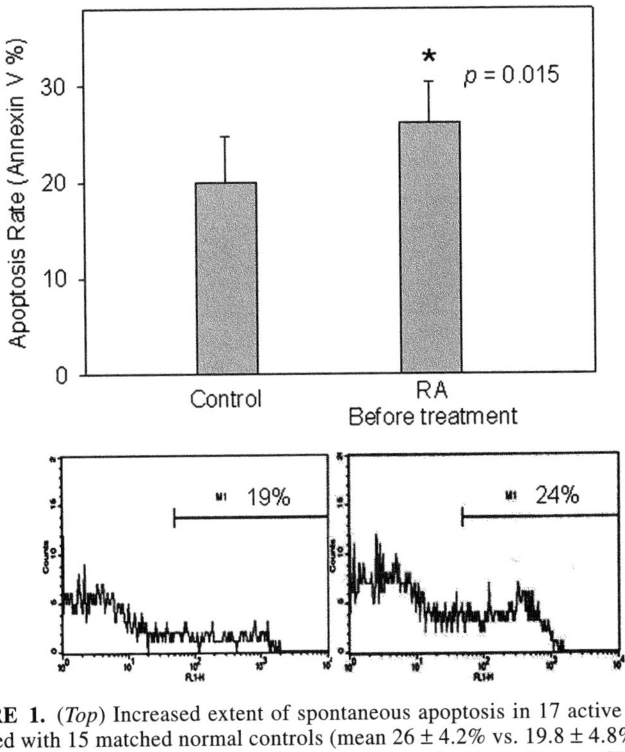

FIGURE 1. (*Top*) Increased extent of spontaneous apoptosis in 17 active RA patients as compared with 15 matched normal controls (mean 26 ± 4.2% vs. 19.8 ± 4.8%, $P = 0.01$). (*Bottom*) A representative experiment of increased annexin V binding on $CD4^{+}CD25^{+}$ T cells from an active RA patient (*right*), as compared with its binding on Tr cells from a normal control (*left*) (24% vs. 19%).

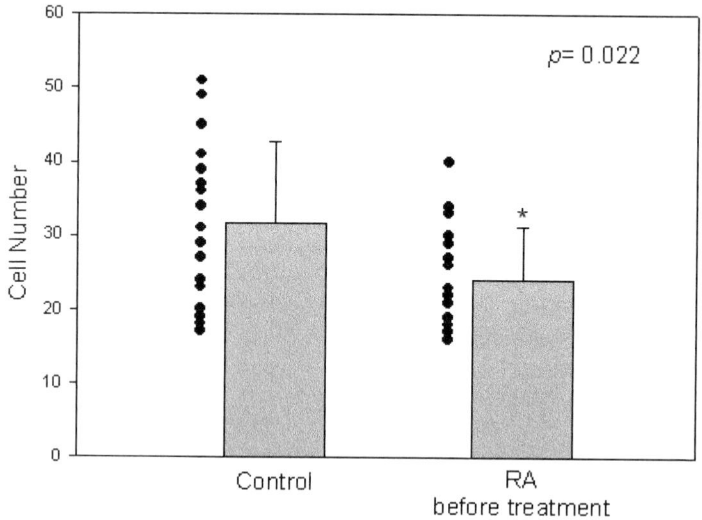

FIGURE 2. Absolute numbers of $CD4^+CD25^{bright}$ T cells were reduced in patients with active RA before infliximab initiation, in comparison with their number in normal individuals.

the normal control group (mean 26 ± 4.2% vs. 19.8 ± 4.8%, respectively; $P = 0.01$) (FIG. 1, top, and a representative experiment, FIG. 1, bottom). Three months later (while still on infliximab), spontaneous apoptosis was comparable in the two groups (remaining increased in only one of the RA patients) (mean 20.7 ± 5.2% vs. 20.8 ± 3.4%; $P = 0.8$). The number of $CD4^+CD25^{bright}$ cells/mL in the peripheral blood at baseline was altered in 11 out of 17 of the RA patients when compared with that of the control group (mean 24 ± 7 vs. 32 ± 10, respectively; $P = 0.02$) (FIG. 2). Following anti–TNF-α therapy, $CD4^+CD25^+$ cell counts were comparable in the two groups (mean 29 ± 8 vs. 31 ± 9; $P = 0.8$).

When spontaneous apoptosis was analyzed (prior to infliximab initiation) in $CD4^+CD25^-$ T cells, it was found to be similar in both active RA patients and normal individuals (32 ± 5.1% vs. 30 ± 4.4%), indicating that increased spontaneous apoptosis in this setting is selective for Tr cells. The deviation in spontaneous apoptosis of $CD4^+CD25^+$ Tr cells was found to be in positive correlation with RA disease severity ($P = 0.01$). The clinical benefit of anti–TNF-α therapy was evident in the RA patients, with achievement of near full remission in 14 of 17 patients, in positive correlation with reversal of increased spontaneous apoptosis of Tr cells in 9 of 12 patients in whom spontaneous apoptosis was increased pretreatment ($P = 0.021$). Similarly, increased spontaneous apoptosis in RA patients pretreatment was demonstrated to be in significant correlation with increased CRP levels; reversal of increased spontaneous apoptosis following anti–TNF-α therapy was also found in correlation with CRP normalization ($r^2 = 0.78$) (FIG. 3).

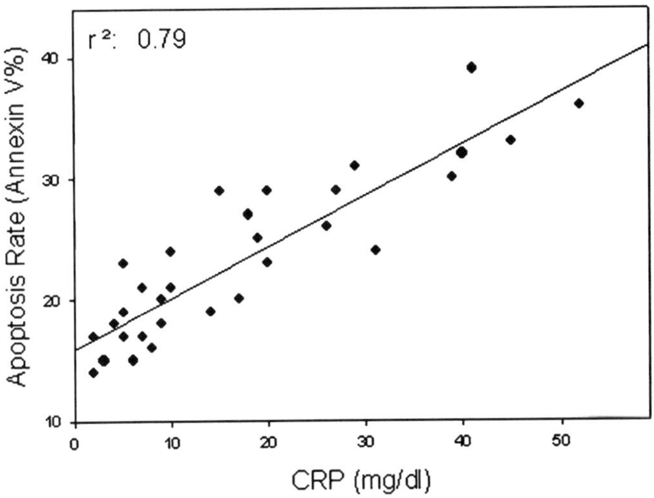

FIGURE 3. Positive correlation between the extent of spontaneous apoptosis and CRP values in RA patients before and after treatment.

DISCUSSION

The investigation of $CD4^+CD25^+$ Tr cell status in active RA is more than relevant, due to the crucial role that this subset of cells plays in maintaining immune homeostasis and self-tolerance.[10,14] Alterations in the apoptotic properties of Tr cells may favor the ratio of responder $CD4^+CD25^-$ T cells to suppressor $CD4^+CD25^+$ T cells, thus leading to the breakdown of self-tolerance, and permitting excessive inflammation and autoimmunity. Immunomodulatory therapies have been shown to restore self-tolerance and to inhibit inflammation in graft rejection or autoimmune diseases by increasing the activation/expansion of Tr cells.[15]

The exact mechanism by which alterations in Tr function could play a role in the development of active human RA is still not clear. In murine models, impaired secretion of TGF-β and IL-10 seem to be essential; however, the role of these cytokines in human RA is yet not well established.[16] The suppressive function of $CD4^+CD25^+$ T cells in autoimmune diseases has been shown to be mediated in part through the expression of the CTLA-4 molecule on their surface. In this regard, the inhibition of CTLA-4 was able to block these suppressive abilities and to increase inflammation in an *in vivo* model of colitis.[17]

This study shows for the first time that $CD4^+CD25^+$ Tr cells are sensitive to the induction of spontaneous apoptosis, and that this is associated with a decrease in the absolute number of peripheral $CD4^+CD25^+$ Tr cells in patients with active RA. This was followed by the demonstration that anti–TNF-α therapy was able to reverse this sensitivity and to restore the absolute number of these cells towards normal. RA disease activity, with its associated increased spontaneous apoptosis of $CD4^+CD25^+$ T cells, may be the result of a quantitative decrease in the absolute number of these cells. In addition, qualitative dysfunction of these cells, with impaired secretion of IL-10 and/or CTLA-4 expression, may allow increases of TNF, other proinflammatory cytokines, and CRP, and, thus, favor RA activity.[18]

Another finding in this study is the reversal of increased spontaneous apoptosis and return to normal of absolute numbers of $CD4^+CD25^+$ T cells following anti–TNF-α therapy. This was found to occur in parallel with its beneficial clinical effect in decreasing RA disease activity, with correlate reduction in CRP levels. This clinical response may be mediated by retained suppressive $CD4^+CD25^+$ cell properties and the inhibition of effector T cell proliferation (i.e., inhibiting Th1 cytokine secretion such as IFN-γ or TNF-α).[19,20]

One possible mechanism by which anti–TNF-α therapy could reverse increased sensitivity of $CD4^+CD25^+$ T cells to spontaneous apoptosis, restoring by this means their absolute number, is by downregulating inflammation and decreasing proinflammatory cytokines, as was elegantly demonstrated in a TNF-induced experimental model of diabetes.[21] In this model, the proportion of pancreatic $CD4^+CD25^+$ regulatory T cells was markedly enhanced when the disease was delayed by TNF withdrawal. Another possible mechanism is for infliximab to act as a growth factor, selectively protecting these cells from apoptosis, by enhancing the expression of CTLA-4 on $CD4^+CD25^+$ Tr cells, similar to that induced by other immunosuppressive drugs, thus selectively protecting Tr cells from increased spontaneous apoptosis.[22]

In contrast to our findings, Ehrenstein *et al.*[11] found the suppressive defects of T regulatory cells in active RA not to correlate with increased apoptosis of these cells, as detected by a nonspecific viability assay, nor to a reduction in T regulatory cell percentage at baseline. Nevertheless, in that study anti–TNF-α therapy was followed by an increase in the $CD4^+CD25^+$ T cell count and decrease in CRP values. The discrepancy with our results may be due to the different cut-off used in $CD25^{high}$ cell detection by FACS analyses in the two studies.

Different gating on CD25 brightness in various studies may lead to the inclusion of $CD4^+CD25^{low}$ cells, which are not true regulatory T cells, and thereby change the total number of regulatory T cells.[23] This is consistent with the concept that $CD4^+CD25^+$ T cells are not a homogeneous subset of cells, and that CD25 brightness in FACS analyses may result in the inclusion of some nonregulatory cells.[24] In the present study we found that absolute $CD4^+CD25^+$ T cell count was decreased in active RA, and that the actual cell count was more representative of this finding than was their relative percentage.

The present finding of reduced absolute $CD4^+CD25^+$ cell count in patients with active RA is consistent with other studies in which a reduced count was demonstrated, such as in SLE. Our ability to demonstrate increased spontaneous apoptosis of $CD4^+CD25^+$ Tr cells in active RA may also be due to the use of a more specific assay for detecting early apoptosis, that is, annexin V binding. Another explanation for our discrepant results in this respect may relate to the DMARD regimen of our RA patients at baseline, including a higher methotrexate dosage, which could affect CD25 expression or contribute somehow to the extent of spontaneous apoptosis.[10,25]

Further studies are underway to better understand how proinflammatory cytokines may promote the induction of spontaneous $CD4^+CD25^+$ Tr cell apoptosis, and how, precisely, anti–TNF-α therapy may attenuate this alteration.

REFERENCES

1. SAKAGUCHI, S., N. SAKAGUCHI, J. SHIMIZU, *et al.* 2001. Immunologic tolerance maintained by CD25+CD4+ regulatory T cells: their common role in controlling autoimmunity, tumor immunity, and transplantation tolerance. Immunol. Rev. **182:** 18–32.
2. CUROTTO DE LAFAILLE, M.A. & J.J. LAFAILLE. 2002. CD4+ regulatory T cells in autoimmunity and allergy. Curr. Opin. Immunol. **14:** 771–778.
3. SHEVACH, E.M. 2000. Regulatory T cells in autoimmunity. Annu. Rev. Immunol. **18:** 423–428.
4. SAKAGUCHI, S., N. SAKAGUCHI, M. ASANO, *et al.* 1995. Immunologic self-tolerance maintained by activated T cells expressing IL-2 receptor alpha-chain (CD25). Breakdown of a single mechanism of self-tolerance causes various autoimmune diseases. J. Immunol. **155:** 1151–1164.
5. SAKAGUCHI, S., K. FUKUMA, K. KURIBAYASHI & T. MASUDA. 1985. Organ-specific autoimmune diseases induced in mice by elimination of T cell subset. I. Evidence for the active participation of T cells in natural self-tolerance; deficit of a T cell subset as a possible cause of autoimmune disease. J. Exp. Med. **161:** 72–87.
6. READ, S., V. MALMSTROM & F. POWRIE. 2000. Cytotoxic T lymphocyte-associated antigen 4 plays an essential role in the function of CD4+CD25+ regulatory cells that control intestinal inflammation. J. Exp. Med. **192:** 295–302.
7. LEVINGS, M.K., R. SANGREGORIO & M.G. RONCAROLO. 2001. Human CD25+CD4+ regulatory cells suppress naive and memory T cell proliferation and can be expanded in vitro without loss of function. J. Exp. Med. **193:** 1295–1302.
8. CRISPIN, J.C., A. MARTINEZ & J. ALCOCER-VARELA. 2003. Quantification of regulatory T cells in patients with SLE. J. Autoimmunity **21:** 273–276.
9. LIU, M.F., C.R.WANG, L.L. FUNG & C.R. WU. 2004. Decreased CD4+ CD25+ T cells in peripheral blood of patients with SLE. Scand. J. Immunol. **59:** 198–202.
10. CAO, D., V. MALMSTROM, C. BAECHER-ALLAN, *et al.* 2003. Isolation and functional characterization of regulatory CD25 bright CD4+ T cells from the target organ of patients with RA. Eur. J. Immunol. **33:** 215–223.
11. EHRENSTEIN, M.R., J.G. EVANS, A. SINGH, *et al.* 2004. Compromised function of regulatory T cells in RA and reversal by anti-TNF alpha therapy. J. Exp. Med. **200:** 277–285.
12. BAI, S., H. LIU, K.H. CHEN, *et al.* 2004. NF-kappa B-regulated expression of cellular FLIP protects rheumatoid arthritis synovial fibroblasts from tumor necrosis factor alpha-mediated apoptosis. Arthritis Rheum. **50:** 3844–3855.
13. SALOMON, B., D.J. LENSCHOW, L. RHEE, *et al.* 2000. B7/CD28 costimulation is essential for the homeostasis of the CD4+CD25+ immunoregulatory T cells that control autoimmune diabetes. Immunity **12:** 431–440.
14. VAN PARIJS, L. & A.K. ABBAS. 1998. Homeostasis and self-tolerance in the immune system: turning lymphocytes off. Science **280:** 243–248.
15. FELDMAN, M. 2002. Development of anti-TNF therapy for rheumatoid arthritis. Nat. Rev. Immunol. **2:** 364–371.
16. ANNACKER, O., R. PIMENTA-ARAUJO, O. BURLEN-DEFRANOUX, *et al.* 2001. CD25+CD4+ T cells regulate the expansion of peripheral CD4 T cells through the production of IL-10. J. Immunol. **166:** 3008–3018.
17. ASSEMAN, C. & M. VON HERRATH. 2002. About CD4+CD25+ regulatory cells. Autoimmun. Rev. **1:** 190–197.
18. SARIN, A., M. CONAN-CIBOTTI & P.A. HENKART. 1995. Cytotoxic effect of TNF and lymphotoxin on T lymphoblasts. J. Immunol. **155:** 3716–3718.
19. SCHUERWEGH, A.J., J.F. VAN OFFEL, W.J. STEVENS, *et al.* 2003. Influence of therapy with chimeric monoclonal tumor necrosis factor-alpha antibodies on intracellular cytokine profiles of T lymphocytes and monocytes in rheumatoid arthritis patients. Rheumatology (Oxford) **42:** 541–548.
20. AKBAR, A.N., L.S. TAAMS, M. SALMON & M. VUKMANOVIC-STEJIC. 2003. The peripheral generation of CD4+CD25+ regulatory T cells. Immunology **109:** 319–325.
21. GREEN, E., Y. CHOI & R. FLAVELL. 2002. Pancreatic lymph node-derived CD4+CD25+ T reg cells: highly potent regulators of diabetes that require TRANCE-RANK signals. Immunity **16:** 183–191.

22. CHEN, X., T. MURAKAMI, J.J. OPPENHEIM & O.M. HOWARD. 2004. Differential response of murine CD4+CD25+ and CD4+CD25– T cells to dexamethasone-induced cell death. Eur. J. Immunol. **34:** 859–869.
23. BAECHER-ALLAN, C., J.A. BROWN, G.J. FREEMAN & D.A. HAFLER. 2001. CD4+CD25+ regulatory cells in human peripheral blood. J. Immunol. **167:** 1245–1253.
24. LEVINGS, M.K., R. SANGREGORIO, C. SARTIRANA, *et al.* 2002. Human CD25+CD4+ T suppressor cell clones produce transforming growth factor beta but not interleukin 10, and are distinct from type I T regulatory cells. J. Exp. Med. **196:** 1335–1346.
25. RUDWALEIT, M., Z. YIN, S. SIEGERT, *et al.* 2000. Response to methotrexate in early rheumatoid arthritis is associated with a decrease of T cell derived tumor necrosis factor alpha, increase of interleukin 10, and predicted by the initial concentration of interleukin 4. Ann. Rheum. Dis. **59:** 311–314.

Synergistic Effect of Avemar on Proinflammatory Cytokine Production and Ras-Mediated Cell Activation

ANDRÁS TELEKES,[a] ENDRE KISS-TÓTH,[b] TÜNDE NAGY,[c] EVA E. QWARNSTROM,[b] ERZSÉBET KÚSZ,[c] TIMEA POLGÁR,[b,c] ÁKOS RESETÁR,[d] STEVEN K. DOWER,[b] AND ERNŐ DUDA[c,e]

[a]*National Institute of Oncology, Budapest, Hungary*

[b]*Functional Genomics Group, Division of Genomic Medicine, University of Sheffield, Royal Halamshire Hospital, Sheffield, United Kingdom*

[c]*Institute of Biochemistry, Biological Research Center, Szeged, Hungary*

[d]*Biromedicina First Hungarian Corporation for Cancer Research and Oncology, Budapest, Hungary*

[e]*Institute of Medical Microbiology and Immunobiology, Szeged University, Szeged, Hungary*

ABSTRACT: Macrophages activated by lipopolysaccharide and/or phorbol esters exhibited high sensitivity to Avemar, a fermented wheat germ extract. Avemar synergized with lipopolysaccharide and PMA in the induction of the transcription of cytokine genes and release of inflammatory cytokines. At higher concentrations the preparation had a significant negative effect on the proliferation and survival of activated myeloid cell types. Avemar treatment induced the synthesis of ICAM-1 and synergized with the ICAM-inducing effect of TNF, but had no effect on VCAM-1 expression on microvascular endothelial cells. The effect of Avemar on signaling pathways, which are involved in cell activation was studied on HeLa cells as a model system. Avemar treatment increased the activity of stress kinases in a concentration-dependent way, resulting in the activation of AP-1 transcription factor. NF-kappa B–sensitive reporters were also activated by Avemar; in contrast, no effect of the preparation was observed on PKA-sensitive signaling pathways.

KEYWORDS: cytokine; synergism; Avemar; TNF; ICAM; NF-κB

INTRODUCTION

Avemar, a standardized wheat germ extract, developed by a Hungarian chemist, Máté Hidvégi, was launched as a dietary supplement in 1998. After extensive

Address for correspondence: András Telekes, M.D., Ph.D., Head, Chemotherapy Day-Ward Unit, National Institute of Oncology, Ráth György u. 7-9, 1122 Budapest, Hungary. Voice: +36-1-224-8600; fax: +36-1-224-8620.
telekes@oncol.hu

Ann. N.Y. Acad. Sci. 1051: 515–528 (2005). © 2005 New York Academy of Sciences.
doi: 10.1196/annals.1361.096

research, it was approved in Hungary (Registration No. 503) and in other European countries as a dietary food for cancer patients. The inhibitory effect of Avemar on tumor progression has been proven in several experimental models.[1–3] Moreover, Avemar significantly inhibited azoxymethane-induced colon carcinogenesis in F-344 rats determined by the number of animals with tumor as well as the average number of colon tumors per animal.[4] Avemar induced apoptosis in human cell lines such as MCF-7 breast cancer,[5] Jurkat acute lymphoid leukemia T cells,[2,6] A2058 melanoma,[1] and HT-29 colon cancer.[3] Avemar induced proteolytic cleavage of poly (ADP-ribose) polymerases (PARPs), which is considered to be a hallmark of activation of caspase-3–like proteases during apoptosis. In fact, incubation of Jurkat cells for 48 h with 0, 0.3, 0.5, and 0.7 mg/ml of Avemar resulted in prominent cleavage of PARP at a concentration of 0.5 mg/ml or greater.[6] Moreover, Avemar can control tumor propagation by a dose-dependent decrease in cell glucose consumption and regulation of glucose carbon redistribution between cell proliferation-related and cell differentiation-related macromolecules.[7] Interestingly, glucose deprivation itself can trigger apoptosis through different mechanisms.[8,9] Avemar showed activity in certain immmunologic processes as well. The rejection time of skin graft in thymectomized mice was significantly shortened with Avemar treatment, indicating an immunity-restoring effect.[10] As a result of Avemar treatment, the amount of cell surface MHC class I proteins was downregulated by 90 and 69% in Jurkat and Raji B cells, respectively, compared to nonstimulated controls.[2] Avemar reduced autoantibody production by inhibiting the Th2 response and it improved clinical manifestations (erythrocyte sedimentation rate [ESR], WBC count, and proteinuria) of the disease in an experimental model of systemic lupus erythematosus.[11] Avemar, by its complex mechanism of action, reduced disease progression and the incidence of metastases and consequently significantly improved the survival of patients with colorectal cancer compared to that of patients treated with conventional regimens alone.[12]

Tumor necrosis factor-alpha (TNF-α), first identified as a serum factor from lipopolysaccharide (LPS)-treated mice, induced hemorrhagic necrosis in tumors. In the human body, TNF is mainly produced by activated macrophages and epithelial cells. In contrast, TNF receptor-1 (TNF-R1) is widely expressed in different cells, which could implicate the manifold effect of TNF in physiologic and/or pathophysiologic processess. In fact, the interaction of TNF with TNF-R1 activates several signal transduction pathways. TNF is a major mediator of apoptosis, inflammation, and immunity; therefore, the role of TNF has been implicated in the pathogenesis of a wide range of human diseases including sepsis, diabetes, inflammatory bowel diseases, osteoporosis, multiple sclerosis, rheumatoid arthritis, and cancer.[13]

Because of the importance of TNF in the natural defense against cancer as well as the fact that Avemar induces apoptosis in malignant hematologic and solid tumor cell lines and exhibits immunomodulatory activities, the effect of Avemar treatment on proinflammatory cytokine production and Ras-mediated cell activation was studied, particularly, TNF-mediated cytotoxicity, TNF production of activated leukocytes, and the proliferation, sensitivity, and survival of TNF-producing and target cells. The molecular mechanisms of Avemar were also studied using signaling pathway-specific transcription reporters.

MATERIAL AND METHODS

Cell Line Culture and Reagents

Tumor necrosis factor was measured by bioassay on WEHI 164 cells (ECACC No. 87022501). A genetically modified clone (WC1) of this cell line, produced in our laboratory, was also used.[14] WC1 cells are several hundred-fold more sensitive to TNF and provide us with a reproducible bioassay. WEHI 164 or WC-1 cells were grown in 96-well plates to a density of 3 × 104 cells/well. After 24 h of incubation at 37°C, serial dilutions of TNF were added to the cells containing 5% fetal calf serum (FCS). In WEHI assays, 0.1 μg/ml actinomycin D was also used. After 16-24 h of incubation cell viability was determined using the MTT assay.[15]

Several human (THP-1, ECACC No. 88081201, MonoMac6, from Dr. D. Wallach, Rehovot) and mouse (P388D and RAW264.7, ECACC Nos. 85011439 and 91062702, respectively) myeloid leukemia cell lines, an Epstein-Barr virus-immortalized human B-cell lymphoma cell line (Raji, ECACC No. 85011429), Sci1, a human B-cell lymphoma (ECACC No. 960905313), and BCL1, a mouse B-cell lymphoma (ECACC No. 90061904) were used to measure TNF production after *in vitro* activation of the cells by different combinations of Avemar, lipopolysaccharide (LPS), and phorbol-myristyl-acetate (PMA). (The human CDC-HMEC microvascular endothelial cell line was a kind gift of Prof. Hunyadi, Debrecen, Hungary.)

WEHI 164, WC/1, and RAW 264.7 cells were grown on DMEM + 5% FCS, Raji was propagated on RPMI-1640 + 10% FCS, and all other cells (including HeLa and CDC-HMEC) were cultured on DMEM + 10% FCS. Media, sera, and reagents were purchased from Sigma Chemical Co. (St. Louis, Mo). Cell viability, proliferation, and cytotoxicity measurements were done using the MTT (3-[4,5-dimethylthiazol-2-yl]-2,5-diphenyltetrazolium bromide) assay.[15]

Human microvascular cells were treated *in vitro* with TNF and/or Avemar in six plates (35 mm) overnight. For flow cytometry the cells were dislodged with EDTA, rubber policeman, and repeated pipetting.

PMA and LPS (*Escherichia coli* serotype O55:B5) were purchased from Sigma-Aldrich (Budapest, Hungary). Avemar (Biromedicina, Budapest) was freshly dissolved, cleared by centrifugation, and filtered through a 0.1-μ filter just before the experiments. When cells were treated for extended periods, Avemar was replaced every other day.

Recombinant human TNF and TNF ELISA were purchased from Genzyme (Wiesbaden-Nordenstadt, Germany). Expression of cell adhesion molecules ICAM-1 and VCAM-1 on the surface of CDC-HMEC cells was followed by flow cytometry using monoclonal antibodies from Beckton Dickinson (Soft-Flow, Pécs, Hungary) and a BD Facscalibur apparatus.

Analysis of RNA

Total cellular RNA was prepared from Avemar-treated macrophages using the guanidium isothyocianate method according to standard protocols, and the integrity of the RNA samples was checked by running 5 μg RNA on formaldehyde gels.

The ribonuclease protection assay (RPA) was carried out with the ML-11 multiple probe set using 10 μg of total cellular RNA, essentially as described earlier.[16] This set detects transcripts of 10 different murine cytokine genes (lymphotoxin α, TNF, interleukin (IL)-4, IL-5, IL-1α, interferon (IFN)-γ, IL-2, IL-6, IL-1β, and IL-3) and the housekeeping L-32 gene used as a control. In each gel, 1/10 part of the total amount of probe and a commonly used mixed spleen sample from LPS-treated mice were always included as a molecular weight marker and a positive contol, respectively. TNF mRNA was also detected on Northern blots using 10 μg total RNA for electrophoresis. For these assays a DNA fragment containing the first 885 base-pair of the coding region of the murine TNF gene from the pGMTNF-MJ plasmid (a kind gift from Dr. J.-F. Arrighi) was used as the probe. After stripping, blots were rehybridized with a GAPDH probe, pHcGAP (from ATCC, Rockville, MD) for blotting control. RPA gels and Northern blots were visualized and quantified by using a Phosphorimager 445SI (Molecular Dynamics).

Plasmids and Transformation

All inducible reporter plasmids were purchased from Stratagene; the control, pTK-RL, containing the HSV promoter was from Promega. The reporter plasmid containing the promoter region of the human IL-8 gene (pIL-8-luc) was previously described.[17]

Constructs coding for the wild-type and mutant Ras proteins, used for the cotransformation experiments, were derivatives of pCDNA3.

Cells were transformed by liposomes according to standand protocols, as suggested by the manufacturers of Lipofectamine (GIBCO) and Superfect (Qiagene), respectively. For transient expression, 1–2 × 10^4 cells were plated into the wells of microtiter plates 1 day before transformation. Next, 500 ng reporter construct and 100 ng control plasmid were mixed with 2.5 μl Superfect or 5 μl Lipofectamine.

Measurement of Reporter Activity

Activity of the individual promoters was measured by luciferase assay in Avemar-treated cells using the Dual Luciferase Assay kit (Promega). Cells were washed in phosphate-buffered saline solution and lysed *in situ* in 25 μl of lysis buffer. Ten microliters of this solution was used for measurement. Because TK promoter was not influenced by Avemar treatment, it was used as an internal control during the experiments. Luciferase activity was expressed, for example, as a ratio of IL8-luc/TK-Rluc. At least two independent transformations were performed in each experiment, and treatments were repeated at least in three parallels.

RESULTS

Effect of Avemar on Proliferation and Survival of Different Cell Lines

Avemar is used by cancer patients as medical nutriment for prolonged periods. Consequently, experiments were planned to be of long duration (6–7 days) so that the proliferation and survival of the investigated cells in the presence of Avemar could be followed. Cells were grown in the presence of Avemar for 72 h before the

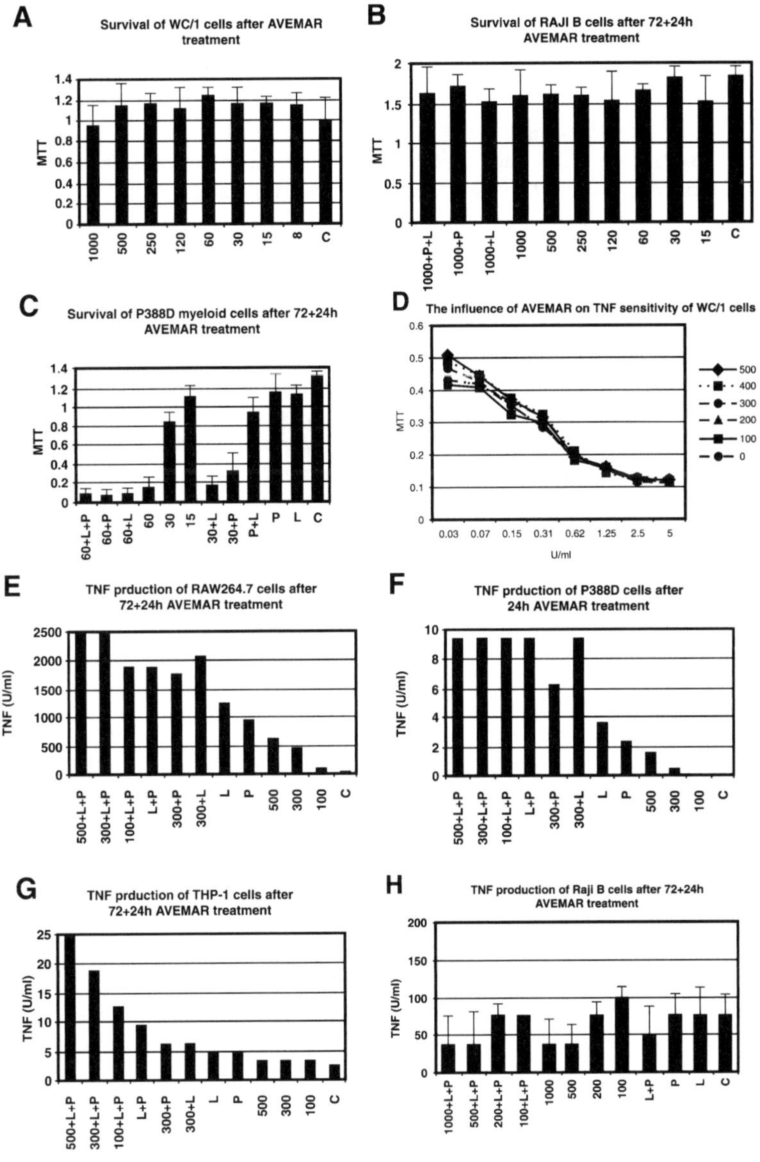

FIGURE 1. Effect of Avemar on proliferation of cells, TNF sensitivity of target cells, and LPS/PMA-induced TNF production of myeloid and lymphoid cells. (**A**) Presence of Avemar (up to 1,000 μg/ml) did not influence the proliferation rate and survival of (highly TNF-sensitive) WC1 cells (MTT measured at the end of the 24-h experiment; control is 100). (**B**) In one type of experiment (here EBV-immortalized B cells [Raji cells] are shown) the cultures were exposed to the same concentrations of Avemar for 72 h before the experiment to follow its long-term effects (MTT values were compared to the untreated control,

experiments, followed by another 24 h during the experiment, and the number of living cells was estimated by MTT methods.

Avemar (at a concentration of 8 μg/ml to 10 mg/ml) did not influence the growth rate and surival of any of the investigated, nonmyeloid cell lines (WEHI 164, WC1, Raji, Sci1, BCL1, CDC-HMEC, and HeLa). However, cells of the monocyte-macrophage lineage (MonoMac6, THP-1, P388D, and RAW264.7) were sensitive to the drug, and some lines exhibited highly inhibited growth and limited survival at higher concentrations (0.5 mg/ml and up). This sensitivity was further increased in the presence of macrophage-activating compounds such as LPS or PMA (FIG. 1A, B, and C).

Avemar Did Not Modify the TNF Sensitivity of Target Tumor Cells

WC1 cells, used for the titration of TNF, were grown in the presence and absence of Avemar. In three parallel experiments, Avemar did not modify the TNF sensitivity of target cells significantly. As in FIGURE 1D, slight changes were observed, but in this assay system only a two- to fourfold increase or decrease in TNF sensitivity was judged as significant. Since WC1 is a genetically modified line of WEHI 164, similar experiments were carried out with the parental WEHI 164 line. As expected, WEHI cells, although they were less sensitive to TNF, exhibited similar TNF sensitivities in both the presence and the absence of Avemar (data not shown).

100, at the beginning of the 24-h experiment.) (**C**) Myeloid cells (here P388D mouse myeloid leukemia cells) showed very strong growth inhibition and decreased survival in the presence of Avemar, especially if TNF-inducing agents were also present. The doses of Avemar applied are as follows: 1,000, 500, 250, 120, 60, 30, 15, and 8 μg/ml. L represents 1 μg/ml lipopolysaccharide, and P corresponds to 0.5 μM PMA. (These compounds were used only during the 24 h of the experiment.) C, untreated control cells. Each figure shows the results of at least three parallel experiments. (**D**) Highly TNF-sensitive WC1 cells were incubated with Avemar for 24 h (pretreatment), and then cells were exposed to a serial dilution of TNF (in the presence of Avemar). TNF sensitivity or survival of WC1 cells was not significantly influenced by Avemar treatment. (Similar results were obtained on WEHI and L929 cells, not shown. 500, 400, 300, 200, 100, and 0 labels Avemar concentrations in μg/ml. L corresponds to 1 μg/ml LPS; P, 0.5 μM PMA; C, control cells.) Three experiments were carried out; SD was within 27%. (**E–G**) Treatment with PMA + LPS induced the production of TNF in different myeloid cell types. They produced very different amounts of TNF in the absence of Avemar; however, all cell types increased TNF production significantly in the presence of Avemar. Cells were exposed to the indicated concentrations of Avemar for 72 h before the experiment. LPS and PMA were added only during the experiment. Avemar concentrations are given in μg/ml (namely, 100, 300, and 500 μg/ml.) L, 1 μg/ml lipopolysaccharide; P, 0.5 μM PMA; C, control cells. Each figure shows the results in three independent experiments; SD was within 11%. (**H**) Raji cells were grown in the absence or presence of the indicated concentrations of Avemar for 72 h, then exposed for 24 h to combinations of Avemar, LPS, and PMA, as labeled. Avemar pretreatment had little influence on the LPS + PMA-induced TNF production of Raji cells, and several other lymphoid lines behaved in a similar way (not shown). (Avemar concentrations are given in μg/ml, such as 1,000, 500, 200, and 100 μg/ml. L, 1 μg/ml lipopolysaccharide; P, 0.5 μM PMA; C, untreated control).

Effect of Avemar on the Induced Cytokine Production of Myeloid and Lymphoid Cells

Most myeloid cell types produce insignificant amounts of TNF in the absence of activation. LPS and/or PMA induce a high increase in TNF production, usually with slight upregulation of mRNA synthesis, influencing mostly translational activity.

Different myeloid cells responded differently, but all increased LPS/PMA-induced TNF production in the presence of Avemar. In the lower concentration range upregulation of TNF synthesis was dependent on the dose of Avemar (FIG. 1E, F, and G).

High concentrations of Avemar proved to be toxic to certain myeloid cells. Net TNF production of some cultures decreased rapidly in the presence of higher concentrations of Avemar. Activated cells of these lines could not survive the simultaneous presence of Avemar, LPS, and PMA. The molecular mechanisms leading to cell death (overstimulation, production of toxic substances, and apoptosis) remains to be investigated (annexin assays yielded ambiguous results).

This effect of Avemar proved to be specific for myeloid cells. Unlike myeloid cells, lymphoid cells (virus-immortalized and leukemic B cells) were not greatly influenced by the presence of Avemar. LPS and PMA increased TNF synthesis in these cells, but the production rate was much the same in the presence or absence of Avemar. Also, Epstein-Barr virus–immortalized Raji B-cells did not seem to be sensitive to relatively high concentrations of Avemar in either the presence or the absence of LPS and/or PMA (FIG. 1H).

Avemar Upregulated the Synthesis of Cell Adhesion Molecules on Endothelial Cells

TNF has a profound effect on the expression of cell adhesion molecules in endothelial cells, an effect that is mediated by the activation of the NF-κB/Rel family of transcription factors. The effect of Avemar on ICAM-1 and VCAM-1 expression on cultured human microvascular endothelial cells was investigated. As demonstrated in FIGURE 2A, Avemar induced the production of ICAM-1 and synergized the effect of TNF. VCAM-1 expression or TNF-mediated induction of VCAM-1, however, was not influenced by the presence of Avemar (FIG. 2B).

Avemar Upregulated the Expression of Cytokine Genes on Myeloid Cells

The effect of Avemar on myeloid cells was not restricted to the increased production of TNF. RNase protection experiments (FIG. 3A) showed the upregulated expression of a number of cytokine genes in Avemar and LPS- and/or PMA-treated myeloid cultures. Avemar treatment upregulated the production of mRNAs of IL-1α, IL-2, IL-5, and IL-6 by 3.7-, 6-, 8.4- and 4.5-fold, respectively, an average of three sets of experiments, with less than 13% SD for the bands of these cytokines. Interestingly, the addition of PMA and/or Avemar to LPS decreased the intensity of IL-1 mRNA synthesis. The pattern of activation was not identical in LPS/PMA- and Avemar-treated cells, suggesting the participation of somewhat different signaling pathways.

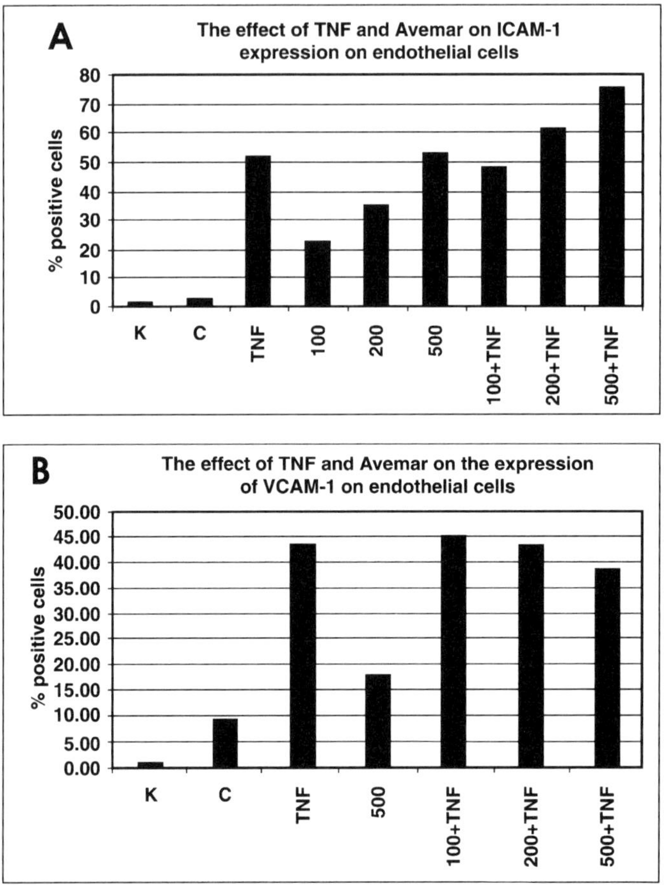

FIGURE 2. Effect of Avemar treatment on the expression of cell adhesion molecules. Human microvascular endothelial cells were exposed to TNF in the presence or absence of Avemar for 24 h, and the expression of cell adhesion molecules was followed by flow cytometry using fluorescent antibodies against CAMs. (**A**) ICAM-1 expression (percentage of fluorescent cells in flow cytometry) after cells were treated with TNF (1,000 U/ml TNF) or Avemar (100, 200, and 500 μg/ml) or their combinations, as labeled. K, untreated cells labeled with isotype control; C, control cells. Results of three independent experiments yielded values with less than 14% SD. (**B**) VCAM-1 expression on human microvascular cells (percentage of fluorescent cells in flow cytometry). Cells were treated with TNF (1,000 U/ml TNF), Avemar (100, 200, and 500 μg/ml), or their combination, as labeled; K, untreated cells labeled with isotype control; C, control cells. Results of three independent experiments yielded values with less than 17% SD.

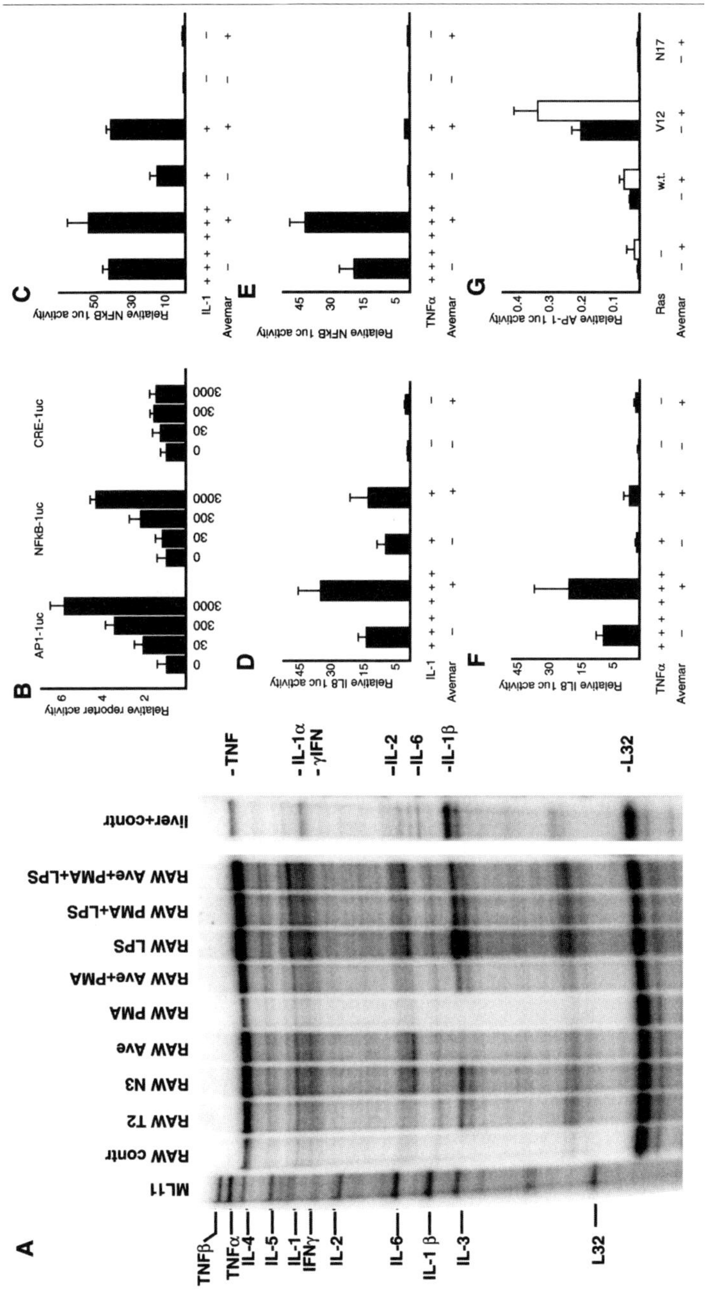

FIGURE 3. *See following page for legend.*

Avemar Upregulated AP-1 and NF-κB but Not CRE-Sensitive Reporters in Cervix Carcinoma (HeLa) Cells Using a Signaling Pathway, Which Involves P21ras

These results indicate that signaling pathways usually triggered by inflammatory cytokines[18] might be involved in the effects of Avemar. To learn more about the molecular events elicited by Avemar, HeLa cells were transiently transfected with signaling pathway-specific reporters and treated with increasing doses of Avemar. As in FIGURE 3B, Avemar activated the stress kinase-sensitive *AP-1 luc* and *NF-κB luc* responsive reporters in a dose-dependent manner, whereas it had no effect on the cAMP-responsive *CRE luc* reporter activity. The possible synergism between Avemar and proinflammatory cytokine-mediated reporter activation was investigated by costimulating HeLa cells with nonsaturating and saturating doses of IL-1 or TNF in the presence or the absence of Avemar. A cytokine–sensitive *IL-8 luc* reporter, which contains binding sites for NF-κB and AP-1 or an *NF-κB luc* reporter was transiently transfected and used as a readout signal (FIG. 3C, D, E, and F). Except for using IL-1 in a saturating dose on *IL-8 luc*, Avemar was able to synergize with the cytokine-mediated stimulation. The ability to superinduce proinflammatory cytokine stimulation even in a saturating dose suggests that Avemar-mediated responses might be coupled with other second messenger pathways. This hypothesis was tested using *AP-1 luc* as a readout and constitutively active or dominant negative *p21ras* mutants as activators. As in FIG. 3G, Avemar-mediated activation was completely blocked upon transfection with the dominant negative *ras* mutant. These data indicate that Avemar activates the AP-1 reporter via a signaling pathway that is controlled by *p21ras*.

DISCUSSION

Apoptosis is a physiologic process critical for organ development, tissue homeostasis, and elimination of defective or potentially dangerous cells in complex organisms. Apoptosis in mammalian cells can be initiated through two major interrelated pathways, one involving engagement of the TNF family of death receptors and the other involving the release of cytochrome *c* from mitochondria. Apoptosis and proliferation are intimately coupled. Some cell cycle regulators can influence both cell

FIGURE 3. RNase protection assay of cytokine mRNAs produced by Avemar treatment and proinflammatory signaling in HeLa cells. (**A**) RAW264.7 cells were exposed to different combinations of Avemar, LPS, and PMA, and the cytokine profiles were analyzed using RNase protection assay. T2 and N3 are extracts that induce TNF synthesis. Raw contr, cells without any treatment (negative control); liver + contr, RNA purified from the liver of LPS-treated mice (positive control); Ave, Avemar, 500 μg/ml, for 24 h. (Protected RNAs run somewhat faster than the probes.) Phosphoimager was used to evaluate the results. Relative band intensities from four experiments differed within 5–22%. (**B**) HeLa cells were transiently transfected with the appropriate reporter plasmid and treated with none, 30 μg/ml, 300 μg/ml, and 3,000 μg/ml freshly dissolved Avemar for 6 h, respectively. (**C–F**) Transfected HeLa cells were stimulated with 1 nM (+++) or 10 pM (+) IL-1 or with 1 ng/ml (+++) or 10 pg/ml (+) TNF in the presence or absence of 3,000 μg/ml Avemar for 6 h. (**G**) HeLa cells were transfected with AP-1 luc reporter and the stated p21 Ras expression construct and treated with 3 μg/ml Avemar for 6 h. Results of three parallel experiments.

division and programmed cell death. The linkage of cell cycle and apoptosis has been recognized for c-Myc, p53, pRb, PKA, PKC, Bcl-2, CDK, cyclins, CKI, Ras, and NF-κB.[19] It is of importance that both NF-κB and Ras can either induce programmed cell death or protect cells from apoptosis depending on the specific cell type and the type of inducer.[20, 21] Experimental data clearly indicate that NF-κB is a major regulator of the inflammatory reaction by controlling the expression of proinflammatory molecules in response to cytokines, oxidative stress, and infectious agents.[22] Moreover, NF-κB pathway activation occurs during transformation induced by a number of classic oncogenes, including Bcr/abl, Ras, and Rac, and it is necessary for full transforming potential.[23] TNF plays a critical role in mediating inflammatory responses by upregulation of genes encoding cell-adhesion molecules required for the recruitment of inflammatory cytokines.[24] Because the promoter regions of many of the TNF-regulated genes contain DNA binding sites for NF-κB, activation of NF-κB by TNF is essential to elicit effective immune and inflammatory responses.[13] Moreover, the link between NF-κB and cancer stems, in part, by the fact that this transcription factor can induce gene products that control proliferative responses and that suppress apoptotic cascades, such as those induced by TNF.[25]

That the regulatory cascades of inflammation, immunity, apoptosis, transformation, and cell cycle seem to entwine, at least partly, the effects of Avemar on TNF-mediated cytotoxicity of sensitive tumor cells is somewhat difficult to interpret. On the one hand, Avemar did not exhibit any significant effect on TNF-mediated killing of tumor cells; it neither protected target cells against TNF nor increased their sensitivity to this cytokine. On the other hand, TNF and IL-6 production of activated macrophages was considerably increased when cells were exposed to Avemar for prolonged periods. IL-6 and TNF are typical examples of multifunctional cytokines involved in the regulation of the immune response, hematopoiesis, and inflammation. Their functions are widely overlapping, but each shows its own characteristic properties.[26] It is noteworthy that nonmyeloid cell lines such as WEHI 164, WCI1, Raji, Sci1, and BCL1 were not sensitive to Avemar, but monocyte-macrophage lineage (MonoMAc6,THP-1, P388D, and RAW264.7) showed growth inhibition and reduced survival to Avemar treatment at higher concentrations (0.5 mg/ml and up). The oncogenic transformation of myeloid cells in CML results from the expression of a constitutively active tyrosine-kinase signaling protein construct generated by the realigment of the breakpoint cluster region and Abelson leukemia virus protooncogene sequences (Bcr/Abl).[27] This construct stimulates glucose transport in multipotent hematopoietic cells.[28] Decreased glucose carbon flow towards nucleic acid synthesis has been observed in cancer cells after treatment with Avemar.[7] It is of interest that Gleevec, one of the most effective agents against CML, has been shown to influence glucose utilization in a similar manner.[29] One of the difference between Gleevec and Avemar is that Gleevec decreases glucose intake and carbon flow through the oxidative pentose cycle, whereas Avemar does the same through the nonoxidative pentose cycle.[30] The efficacy of Avemar on myeloid cell lines can further be explained by the fact that Avemar not only impedes the enzymes regulating carbon flow in the pentose cycle (transketolase and G6PDH), but also is a potent inhibitor of key enzymes regulating glycolytic flux.[6]

In synergy with LPS and PMA, Avemar induced the activity of a number of cytokine genes. The pattern of activated genes was slightly different in LPS/PMA-treated cells in the absence or persence of Avemar, according to the RNase protection experiments shown in FIGURE 3A. These results suggest that the signaling pathways leading to cytokine production were overlapping, but not identical. Further experiments using transcription reporter constructs corroborated this finding and revealed that Avemar activated several intracellular signaling pathways. The MAPK signal transduction cascade plays a pivotal role in cell responses given to extracellular stimuli. Within this system traditionally three subunits are distinguished. The stress kinases activate the AP-1 transcription factor and therefore increase the transcription of several genes including IL-1 and TNF, thus influencing cell growth, survival, differentiation, and apoptosis. The extracellular signal-regulated kinases (ERK) also play an important role in cell growth and differentiation (actvation of ERK leads to expression of SRE). Finally, the p38 kinases regulate cytokine production and other processess leading to apoptosis. The activity of p38 kinases can be measured by a reporter construct containing CRE. All inflammatory processess (induced by cytokines, endotoxins, radiation, etc.) activate NF-κB transcription factor and consequently induce the production of new cytokines, growth factors, adhesion molecules, and immunoreceptors. The signal transduction systems just discussed were measured by reporter constucts containing elements of AP-1, SRE, CRE, and NF-κB. Avemar increased the activity of constructs containing sequences responsive to AP-1 and NF-κB in a dose-dependent manner via a mechanism that involves activation of p21 ras, as shown in FIGURE 3B. SRE showed a dose-dependent increase in activation as well (data not shown).

Endothelial cells in the vasculature of human solid tumors have decreased expression of intercellular adhesion molecule-1 (ICAM-1) compared to normal endothelial cells. Incubation of tumor-derived endothelial cells with TNF resulted in expression levels of only 20%, achieved in similarly treated normal tissue-derived endothelial cells because tumor angiogenesis induces anergy in endothelial cells.[18] This phenomenon may serve as a tumor-protecting mechanism because leukocytes require ICAM-1 to leave the vascular system to infiltrate the tumor tissue. Avemar induced the production of ICAM-1 as well as showing synergy with TNF in this respect. This observation may explain, at least in part, the antitumor activity of Avemar.

In summary, it can be concluded that similar to previous experiments, Avemar showed a wide range of biologic activity. Metabolic pathways triggered by Avemar lead to increased TNF and cytokine production and, if overactivated, to the destruction of the cells. It can be hypothesized that Avemar-treated activated macrophages overproduce proinflammatory cytokines and possibly other mediators (nitric oxide, free oxygen radicals, etc.), so that the cells could not survive ("suicide" mechanism). Alternatively, two signaling pathways, not mutually exclusive, can be envisioned to be set by Avemar in activated myeloid cells, namely, one leading to upregulation of inflammatory mediators and another to apoptosis. Considering the immunologic and anticancer activity of Avemar, further studies are still warranted to elucidate its mechanisms of action.

COMPETING INTEREST: Ákos Resetár is CEO of Biromedicina First Hungarian Corporation for Cancer Research and Oncology, Budapest, Hungary.

REFERENCES

1. Hidvégi, M., E. Rásó, R. Tömösközi-Farkas, *et al.* 1999. MSC, a new benzoquinone-containing natural product with antimetastatic effect. Cancer Biother. Radiopharm. **14:** 277–289.
2. Fajka-Boja, R., M. Hidvégi, Y. Shoenfeld, *et al.* 2002. Fermented wheat germ extract induces apoptosis and downregulation of major histocompatibility complex class I proteins in tumor T and B cell lines. Int. J. Oncol. **20:** 563–570.
3. Illmer, C., S. Madlener, Z. Horvath, *et al.* 2005. Immunologic and biochemical effects of the fermented wheat germ extract Avemar. Exp. Biol. Med. **230:** 144–149.
4. Zalatnai, A., K. Lapis, B. Szende, *et al.* 2001. Wheat germ extract inhibits experimental colon carcinogenesis in F–344 rats. Carcinogenesis **22:** 1649–1652.
5. Marcsek, Z., Zs. Kocsis, M. Jakab, *et al.* 2004. The efficacy of tamoxifen in estrogen receptor-positive breast cancer cells is enhanced by a medical nutriment. Cancer Biother. Radiopharm. **19:** 746–753.
6. Comín-Anduix, B., L.G. Boros, S. Marin, *et al.* 2002. Fermented wheat germ extract inhibits glycolysis/pentose cycle enyzmes and induces apoptosis through poly (ADP-ribose) polymerase activation in Jurkat T-cell leukemia tumor cells. J. Biol. Chem. **277:** 46408–46414.
7. Boros, L.G., K. Lapis, B. Szende, *et al.* 2001. Wheat germ extract decreases glucose uptake and RNA ribose formation but increases fatty acid synthesis in MIA pancreatic adenocarcinoma cells. Pancreas **23:** 141–147.
8. Moley, K.H. & M.M. Mueckler. 2000. Glucose transport and apoptosis. Apoptosis **5:** 99–105.
9. Kansara, M. & M.V. Berridge. 2004. Oncogenes modulate cell sensitivity to apoptosis induced by glucose deprivation. Anticancer Res. **24:** 2503–2510
10. Hidvégi, M., E. Rásó, R. Tömösközi-Farkas, *et al.* 1999. Effect of MSC on immune response of mice. Immunopharmacology **41:** 183–186.
11. Ehrenfeld, M., M. Blank, Y. Shoenfeld, *et al.* 2001. AVEMAR (a new benzoquinone-containing natural product) administration interferes with the Th2 response in experimental SLE and promotes amelioration of the disease. Lupus **10:** 622–627.
12. Jakab, F.,Y. Shoenfeld, Á. Balogh, *et al.* 2003. A medical nutriment has supportive value in the treatment of colorectal cancer. Br. J. Cancer **89:** 465–469.
13. Chen, G. & D.V. Goeddel. 2002. TNF-R1 signaling: a beautiful pathway. Science **296:** 1634–1635.
14. Győrfi, Z., S. Benkő, E. Kúsz, *et al.* 1997. Highly increased TNF sensitivity of tumor cells expressing the yeast delta 9-desaturase gene. Biochem. Biophys. Res. Commun. **2412:** 465–470.
15. Deniyot, F. & R. Lang. 1986. Rapid colorimetric assay for cell growth and survival. Modifications to the tetrazolium dye procedure giving improved sensitivity and reliability. J. Immunol. Methods **892:** 271–277.
16. Hobbs, M.V., W.O. Weigle, D.J. Noonan, *et al.* 1993. Patterns of cytokine gene expression by CD4+ T cells from young and old mice. J. Immunol. **150:** 3602–3614.
17. Kiss-Tóth, E., F.M. Guesdon, D.H. Wyllie, *et al.* 2000. A novel mammalian expression screen exploiting green fluorescent protein-based transcription detection in single cells. J. Immunol. Methods **239:** 125–135.
18. Griffioen, A.W., C.A. Damen, G.H. Blijham, *et al.* 1996. Tumor angiogenesis is accompanied by decreased inflammatory response of tumor-associated endothelium. Blood **882:** 667–673.
19. Vermeulen, K., Z.N. Berneman & D.R. Van Bockstaele. 2003. Cell cycle and apoptosis. Cell Proliferat. **36:** 165–175.
20. Sonensheim, G.E. 1997. Rel/NF-kappa B transcription factors and the control of apoptosis. Semin. Cancer Biol. **8:** 113–119.
21. Downward, J. 1998. Ras signalling and apoptosis. Curr. Opin. Genet. Dev. **8:** 49–54.
22. Bours, V., G. Bonizzi, M. Bentires-Alj, *et al.* 2000. NF-kappa B activation in response to toxical and therapeutical agents: role in inflammation and cancer treatment. Toxicology **153:** 27–38.

23. Joyce, D., C. Albanese, J. Steer, *et al.* 2001. NF-kappa B and cell-cycle regulation: the cyclin connection. Cytokine Growth Factor Rev. **12:** 73–90.
24. Bazzoni, F. & B. Beutler. 1996. The tumor necrosis factor ligand and receptor families. N. Engl. J. Med. **334:** 1717–1725.
25. Mayo, M.W. & A.S. Baldwin. 2000. The transcription factor NF-kappa B: control of oncogenesis and cancer therapy resistance. Biochim. Biophys. Acta **1470:** M55–62.
26. Akira, S., T. Hirano, T. Taga, *et al.* 1990. IL 6 and related molecules (IL 1 and TNF). FASEB J. **4:** 2860–2867.
27. Gyger, M., C. Perrault, R. Belanger, *et al.* 1985. Chronic myeloid leukemia with an unusual simple variant translocation: t(22;22)(q13;q11). Acta Hematol.-Basel **73:** 193–195.
28. Bentley, J., I. Walker, E. McIntosh, *et al.* 2001. Glucose transport regulation by p210 Bcr-Abl in a chronic myeloid leukaemia model. Br. J. Haematol. **112:** 212–215.
29. Boren, J. M. Cascante, S. Marin, *et al.* 2001. Gleevec (ST1571) influences metabolic enzyme activities and glucose carbon flow towards nucleic acid and fatty acid synthesis in myeloid tumor cells. J. Biol. Chem. **276:** 27747–37753.
30. Boros, G.L. M. Cascante & W.-N. P. Lee. 2002. Metabolic profiling of cell growth and death in cancer: applications in drug discovery. Drug Discovery Today **7:** 18–26.

Fermented Wheat Germ Extract (Avemar) in the Treatment of Cancer and Autoimmune Diseases

LASZLO G. BOROS,[a] MICHELE NICHELATTI,[b] AND YEHUDA SHOENFELD[c]

[a]*Los Angeles Biomedical Research Institute at Harbor-UCLA Medical Center, Torrance, California 90502, USA*

[b]*Department of Hematology, Niguarda Ca' Granda Hospital, Milan, 20162 Italy*

[c]*Department of Medicine 'B' and Center for Autoimmune Diseases, Sheba Medical Center, Sackler Faculty of Medicine, Tel-Aviv University, Tel-Hashomer, 52621 Israel*

ABSTRACT: Avemar, the product of industrial fermentation of wheat germ, possesses unique cancer-fighting characteristics. Taken orally, Avemar can inhibit metastatic tumor dissemination and proliferation during and after chemotherapy, surgery, or radiation. Benefits of Avemar treatment have been shown in various human cancers, in cultures of *in vitro* grown cancer cells, in the prevention of chemical carcinogenesis, and also in some autoimmune conditions. This document reviews the clinical and experimental results obtained with this extract so far. Special references are made for its safety, including its coadministration with anticancer drugs, as well as for its immunomodulatory activity, its molecular targets, and its use in cancer clinical trials.

KEYWORDS: fermented wheat germ extract; Avemar; cancer; autoimmune diseases

INTRODUCTION

Wheat germ, if left in flour, has an adverse effect on the functional properties of dough and therefore on breadmaking quality. Therefore, most germ is milled as part of mill feed, and a smaller portion is separated during the milling process. Separated wheat germ is traditionally included in healthy foods, is consumed as is, or serves as raw material for extracts rich in vitamin E.

During the 1990s, a new, fermented wheat germ extract for human consumption was invented by Professor Máté Hidvégi in Hungary.[1] The standardized manufacturing technology included the extraction of wheat germ, the fermentation of the extract, followed by separation of the fermentation liquid, microencapsulation, drying, and granulation. The resulting powder was named Avemar pulvis (or simply Avemar), and the granulate is also known as Avemar. For a 70-kg weight adult, the

Address for correspondence: Prof. Yehuda Shoenfeld, M.D., FRCP (Hon.), Head, Department of Medicine 'B' and Center for Autoimmune Diseases, Sheba Medical Center, Tel-Hashomer 52621, Israel. Voice: +972-3-530-2652; fax: +972-3-535-2855.
shoenfel@post.tau.ac.il

**Ann. N.Y. Acad. Sci. 1051: 529–542 (2005). © 2005 New York Academy of Sciences.
doi: 10.1196/annals.1361.097**

single daily dosage of Avemar contains 8.5 g of Avemar pulvis plus flavoring ingredients, such as fructose and arome. After being dissolved in 150 ml of cold water, Avemar should be drunk preferably before a meal. The product has been approved as a dietary food for special medical purposes in cancer patients by the National Institute of Food Safety and Nutrition of Hungary. Avemar has been consumed by cancer patients for more than 6 years.

Since its invention, a series of *in vitro* and *in vivo* studies and clinical trials have been carried out to determine whether Avemar could help cancer patients struggling with both the effects of their disease and the side effects of standard anticancer therapy (SAT). Subsequently, evidence of the efficacy of the fermented wheat germ extract in some autoimmune diseases has also been found. At this time, sufficient study of this compound has been done and enough data have emerged that some useful and valid conclusions can be made regarding the value of Avemar as a supportive tool in therapy. The benefits observed, mechanisms of action known, and study results are summarized in this review. (In the following text and references, the terms "fermented wheat germ extract," "Avemar," and its code name "MSC" denote the same preparation.)

COMPOSITION

The original composition of wheat germ is substantially modified due to extraction followed by fermentation; therefore, Avemar cannot be replaced by wheat germ, germinated wheat, or any extract or derivative of these. Methoxy-substituted benzoquinones, present originally in the crude wheat germ as glycosides and liberated as aglycones by glycosidases during fermentation, are the indicator compounds for quantitative standardization.[2] Avemar is also characterized by its specific high performance liquid chromatography fingerprint spectra. Avemar is currently manufactured by Biromedicina in Hungary in a Good Manufacturing Practice (GMP)-certified pharmaceutical plant in the Kunfeherto-Kiskunhalas region.

SAFETY

Much evidence is available to demonstrate the safety of Avemar under the conditions of its intended use.[3] Avemar has been investigated in numerous animal and human studies of its efficacy; in none of these studies has any indication of adverse effects been identified. Avemar has been sold in numerous countries for many years with no reports of adverse effects. Finally, Avemar has been subjected to acute toxicity studies in the rat and mouse, a subacute toxicity study in the rat, and subchronic toxicity studies in the rat and mouse in addition to genotoxicity, mutagenicity, and carcinogenicity screening tests, and it has been evaluated for hematologic effects in multi-year studies in human cancer patients.

Based on the absence of adverse effects, the acute oral LD_{50} of Avemar in male and female mice and rats was >2,000 mg/kg, and the no-observable adverse effect level (NOAEL) of the extract in a subacute study with rats was determined to be the tested dose of 2,000 mg/kg/day. The NOAEL of Avemar in a subchronic study with mice and rats was determined also to be the tested dose of 3,000 mg/kg/day.

The effect of long-term administration of Avemar on the hematologic status of carcinoma patients was examined in two hospital centers in Hungary. Hematologic data included white blood cell count, red blood cell count, hemoglobin level, hematocrit, platelet count, erythrocyte sedimentation rate, lymphocyte count, neutrophil granulocyte count, monocyte count, eosinophil granulocyte count, and prothrombin level. After 1, 3, and 5 years of Avemar treatment, all values remained within normal limits.

DRUG INTERACTIONS

Vitamin C

In an early animal study, the effects of Avemar alone and Avemar plus vitamin C on tumor growth and metastasis in laboratory mice and rats were studied.[4] Involved were an aggressive variant of the Lewis lung carcinoma (3LL-HH), B16 melanoma, a rat nephroblastoma (RWT-M), and a human colon carcinoma xenograft (HCR25) in immunosuppressed mice. Effects on metastases were studied both with the primary tumors intact and after their surgical removal. Vitamin C alone had a significant inhibitory effect on metastases in some of these tumor models but not in others. However, combined treatment with Avemar plus vitamin C administered simultaneously profoundly inhibited metastases in all tumor models. Interestingly, in some tumor models, treatment with Avemar alone had a greater inhibitory effect on metastasis formation than did Avemar plus vitamin C. It was therefore recommended that if vitamin C is being administered, Avemar should be consumed at least 2 hours before or after treatment with vitamin C-containing preparations.

Cytostatic Drugs

To determine whether Avemar's beneficial effects might or might not compromise the efficacy of a variety of cytostatic drugs commonly used in cancer treatment, researchers tested Avemar alone and in combination with those drugs in malignant cell lines and in animals with cancer.[5] *In vitro*, Avemar neither increased nor decreased the effect on viability of MCF-7, HepG2, or Vero cells resulting from treatment with dacarbazine (DTIC), 5-fluorouracil (5-FU), or doxorubicin. In mice with transplanted 3LL-HH tumors, the combination of Avemar with cyclophosphamide, vinorelbine, and doxorubicin did not lessen those drugs' inhibition of tumor growth. Avemar produced no toxic effects in the mice, and its addition to the treatment regimen did not increase the toxicity of the drug treatment. Strong synergism in antimetastatic activities was seen with the combined use of Avemar and cytostatic drugs: DTIC plus Avemar in B16 mouse melanoma, muscle/lung metastasis model and 5-FU plus Avemar in C38 mouse colorectal carcinoma, spleen/liver metastasis model resulted in statistically complete eradication of lung and liver metastases, respectively.[6] These results make us confident that Avemar may be administered along with these conventional chemotherapy drugs with little risk of negatively affecting the cytostatic drugs' efficacy, or increasing their undesirable side effects.

Cytokines

Avemar may safely be administered together with the cytokine preparations used in clinical practice. The antineutropenic efficacy of the hematopoietic cytokines plus Avemar in combination is better than that of the cytokines alone.[3]

Tamoxifen

Researchers at the National Institute of Chemical Safety in Budapest conducted an *in vitro* study of the effects of a tamoxifen plus Avemar combination administered to cultures of the MCF-7 (ER+) breast cell line as a preclinical model of human breast cancer.[7] MCF-7 cells were treated with tamoxifen and/or Avemar for 24, 48, and 72 h. Cytotoxicity was measured by MTT assay; the percentages of mitosis and apoptosis were determined by hematoxylin and eosin staining and by immunochemistry, and estrogen receptor activation was studied by semiquantitative determination of the estrogen-responsive pS2 gene mRNA production. The percentage of apoptotic and proliferating cell fraction (S-phase) was determined by flow cytometry. Tamoxifen had no effect on the percentage of apoptotic cell fraction, while significantly reducing the ratio of S-phase cells. After an exposure time of 48 h, Avemar increased apoptosis significantly. Tamoxifen + Avemar increased apoptosis significantly after 24 h, with a negligible effect on mitosis and S phase. Estrogen receptor activity of MCF-7 cells treated for 24, 48, and 72 h was enhanced by Avemar and decreased by tamoxifen as well as by tamoxifen + Avemar. The increase in apoptosis by the combined use of tamoxifen + Avemar suggests that the addition of Avemar to tamoxifen may enhance the efficacy of tamoxifen in ER+ breast cancer. There is no contraindication to their combination in clinical practice.

AVEMAR AND IMMUNITY

Evidence of the immunomodulatory effects of Avemar was first obtained in a study on the effect of the compound on immune function in mice.[8] Results in this study showed that Avemar significantly increased the degree of blastic transformation of peripheral blood T lymphocytes stimulated by concanavalin A.

In other experiments, $C_{57}B1$ mice were given skin transplants from the coisogenic mice strain $B_{10}LP$, which normally could be expected to be tolerated for 16–25 days before rejection. Thymectomized control (untreated) mice rejected the transplants at a gender mean of 52 (male) or 41 (female) days. Thymectomized mice treated with Avemar rejected the grafts at a mean of 29 days (male) or 33 days (female). Control (untreated) mice not thymectomized rejected the transplants at a gender mean of 21 or 29 days. These results, with immune function of mice seriously immunocompromised by thymectomy restored to near that of nonthymectomized mice (untreated), demonstrate the very significant immune restorative effects of Avemar treatment in these animals.[8] Interestingly, other experiments done as part of this group, aimed at determining whether Avemar's immunostimulatory effects could be ascribed to one active molecule, 2,6-dimethoxy-*p*-benzoquinone, showed they could not, as this substance administered alone did not shorten graft rejection time. From a therapeutic point of view, the immunomodulatory and immunorestoring effects of Avemar may be exploited in various clinical manifestations of impaired immune response.

The potential of Avemar treatment on features of experimental systemic lupus erythematosus (SLE) in naive mice, induced by idiotypic manipulation, was also studied.[9] When the product was given in the preimmunization period, downregulation of autoantibody production (anti-dsDNA, mouse 16/6 Id, and antihistones) after treatment with Avemar was noted (e.g., anti-dsDNA decreased from 0.898 OD at 405 nm to 0.519 after treatment). This effect was sustained for at least 4 weeks after discontinuation of therapy. Serologic manifestations were associated with a delay in the Th2 (interleukin [IL]-4 and IL-10) response (e.g., IL-4 decreased from 92 to 60 ng/ml in splenocyte condition media). The mice showed normal erythrocyte sedimentation rate and WBC, and less than 100 mg/dl of protein in the urine in comparison to >300 mg/dl protein in the SLE nontreated mice. It was concluded that oral intake of Avemar could ameliorate the clinical manifestations of experimental SLE by affecting the Th1/Th2 network inhibiting the Th2 response. Based on these results, a double-blind clinical study with Avemar in lupus patients was recently initiated.[10]

In mice, Avemar proved effective in the restoration of hemopoiesis in bone marrow impairment induced by sublethal irradiation and/or cyclophosphamide therapy.[11] Elevation of the platelet count started on postirradiation day 7, and the baseline level was achieved on day 21. At the same time, no substantial increase was detected in the WBC count. As regards cyclophosphamide therapy, restoration of thrombopoiesis as well as of erythropoiesis could be observed as a result of Avemar treatment. These results are in consonance with the 5-year long clinical observation that Avemar has no hematotoxic side effect. A decrease in febrile neutropenia episodes during intensive chemotherapy of Avemar-treated pediatric cancer may help confirm the clinical relevance of bone marrow protection assessed in the experimental setting.

MOLECULAR TARGETS OF AVEMAR

Although the one (or more) molecule of fermented wheat germ extract responsible for the wide variety of biologic effects of this medical food has not yet been identified, molecular targets of Avemar, which could explain the effects, are (at least, partially) known.

PARP

Proliferation, differentiation, and cell death are under similar molecular control in all mammalian cells. Cancer cells develop severe defects in the regulation of homeostasis and cell proliferation, including resistance to apoptosis. Avemar inhibited the growth of leukemia cells in a dose-dependent manner. Laser scanning cytometry and gel electrophoresis with Western immunoblotting of stained cells indicated that the growth-inhibiting effect was consistent with a strong induction of apoptosis by activating the caspase-3–catalyzed cleavage of the poly(ADP-ribose) polymerase (PARP) enzyme.[12] PARP is a key player in DNA repair. The activity of this enzyme is extremely high in cancer cells.[13] Cleavage of PARP results in genomic instability, leading to DNA fragmentation and thus to apoptosis in tumor cells. As the activity of PARP is accelerated in cancer cells, these cells can be selectively sensitized by PARP inhibitors (such as Avemar) to agents (such as 5-fluorouracil [FU] or DTIC), inducing base excisions or lesions in DNA. It has also been indicated that besides apoptosis induction, the mechanism through which Avemar mitigates metastasis involves decreasing cell motility. It was further demonstrated that although Avemar induced apoptosis in different leukemic human cells, it did not trigger programmed cell death in their healthy, resting counterpart, peripheral blood mononuclear cells.

MHC-I

Avemar treatment resulted in a decrease in the MHC class I (MHC-I) protein level on the surface of tumor cells, and hence it may expose them to natural killer (NK) cell activity.[14] As inhibition of tyrosine phosphatase activity also resulted in elevated downregulation of MHC-I molecules, control of protein tyrosine phosphorylation in this process was indicated. Involvement of lymphocyte-specific signaling molecules, the nonreceptor tyrosine kinase $p56^{lck}$, and the receptor tyrosine phosphatase CD45 in the Avemar-triggered cell response has been excluded.

A way for tumors to survive in the host environment is to evade the defense control of the host by mimicking themselves as normal cells for the survey of the immune system. Natural killer cells, which play an important role in antitumor defense, recognize and are blocked by the expression of MHC-I molecules on their target cells.[15] Consequently, tumor cells develop an effective camouflage by expressing high levels of MHC-I to avoid recognition by NK cells. This is a common characteristic of metastatic tumor cells to avoid NK surveillance.[16] As Avemar reduces the MHC-I level on human tumor cells, it may sensitize them against NK killing, thus reducing their metastatic activity.

ICAM-1

Endothelial cells of the vasculature of human solid tumors are known to have decreased expression of ICAM-1 compared to normal endothelial cell tissue, and this phenomenon can be considered a tumor-derived escape mechanism because the development of an efficient leukocyte infiltrate of the tumor is impaired.[17] It has been shown that Avemar upregulates the expression of intercellular adhesion molecule-1 (ICAM-1) on tumor-derived endothelial cells and also potentiates the similar effect of the primary anticancer cytokine, tumor necrosis factor-alpha (TNF-α).[18]

Pentose Phosphate Pathway

Avemar regulates tumor cell proliferation also by altering the rate of glucose intake and the synthesis of nucleic acid ribose through the nonoxidative steps of the pentose phosphate pathway (PPP).[19] This effect of Avemar is most efficiently present in the ribosomal RNA fraction of cancer cells. As ribose is a close metabolite of glucose and ribosomal RNA is essential for *de novo* enzyme protein synthesis and cell proliferation, it is evident that inhibiting the formation of ribose from glucose to build ribosomal structures is one of the important underlying mechanisms by which Avemar regulates tumor cell growth. Avemar also has remarkable effects on lipid synthesis and the oxidation of the first carbon of glucose through the oxidative steps of the PPP. Avemar increases glucose oxidation in the PPP in a dose-dependent fashion and therefore acts as an important agent in controlling oxidative stress and damage to the cells. The oxidative steps of the PPP play a very limited role in the synthesis of ribose to build nucleic acids in tumor cells. Tumor cells broadly use nonoxidative reactions, whereas normal cells heavily depend on oxidative synthesis, and then recycling of ribose back to glycolysis through the nonoxidative steps. The selectivity of Avemar in inhibiting tumor cell proliferation but promoting normal immune cell expansion can be explained by its selective inhibitory action on unique metabolic steps only observed in cancer. The metabolic changes observed in Avemar-treated cancer cells provide explanations for the clinically detected weight gain and slow disease progression in Avemar-treated cancer patients. Increased PPP activity (glucose oxidation and pentose recycling) increases *de novo* fatty acid synthesis, chain elongation, and desaturation. It is also likely that decreased oxidative ribose synthesis is unable to supply tumor cells' metabolic needs for reducing equivalents that would intensively be used for the reduction of ribonucleotides to deoxyribonucleotides during DNA replication. The simultaneous decrease in nucleic acid synthesis from glucose leads to a decrease in cell proliferation, which explains the slow disease progression and the increased survival rate of the patients. Decreased glucose consumption of the tumors also leads to a metabolic harmony with the host and weight gain in patients with even advanced cancers. As a result, Avemar-treated patients also have improved tolerance for surgeries, chemotherapy, or radiation therapy. This effect of redistributing glucose carbon use from nonoxidative nucleic acid ribose synthesis to direct glucose oxidation and lipid synthesis is a novel mechanism of antiproliferative action only described in connection with Avemar treatment.[20] Avemar treatment is likely associated with the phosphorylation or transcriptional regulation of metabolic enzymes that are involved in reverting glucose carbons from cell proliferation-related structural and functional macromolecules (RNA, DNA) to direct oxidative degradation of glucose. It was demonstrated that Avemar treatment was about 50 times less effective in peripheral blood lymphocytes in inducing the aforementioned effects than in cancer (leukemia) cells, which provides a comfortable therapeutic window for Avemar to apply in patients as a supplemental treatment modality with minimal or no toxic side effects.[12]

Ribonucleotide Reductase

Ribonucleotide reductase (RR) is responsible for the conversion of ribonucleotides to deoxyribonucleoside triphosphates, which are precursors of DNA synthesis. Ribonucleotide reductase was demonstrated to be significantly upregulated in tumor cells in order to meet the increased need for dNTPs of these rapidly proliferating cells for DNA synthesis.[21] The enzyme was therefore indicated as being an excellent target for cancer chemotherapy, and various inhibitors of RR have entered clinical practice or are under preclinical or clinical development. The enzyme consists of two subunits, the effector binding and the nonheme iron subunits. The inhibition of the nonheme iron subunit can be caused, for instance, by iron chelation or the free radical scavenging of a free tyrosine radical, which is needed for iron stabilization. To determine whether Avemar's action in HT-29 human colon carcinoma cell line involves such RR inhibition, first an *in situ* enzyme assay was employed. Radiolabeled cytidine had to be reduced by RR in order to be incorporated into DNA. The *in situ* RR activity of HT-29 cells were inhibited by Avemar in a concentration-dependent manner. These results were then confirmed by the determination of dNTP pool sizes after the incubation of HT-29 cells with Avemar. The compound did inhibit RR, the key enzyme of *de novo* DNA synthesis, which might also explain its effect on tumor cells, in particular its antitumor effects in patients with colorectal cancer.[22]

Cyclooxygenases

Cyclooxygenases (COX-1 and COX-2 enzymes) were incubated with increasing concentrations of Avemar. The inhibition of COX-1 and COX-2 in the presence of Avemar was then determined, and IC_{50} values (Avemar concentration resulting in 50% enzyme inhibition) were calculated. For COX-1 activity, the IC_{50} was 100 μg/ml, whereas a concentration of 300 μg/ml inhibited COX-2 activity to 50% of the control.[22] These significant results demonstrate the COX-inhibiting capacity of Avemar, and no selectivity towards one of the COX enzymes could be observed.

The nonselective inhibition of COX enzymes by Avemar may partly explain this extract's anti-inflammatory activities against adjuvant arthritis in rats and rheumatoid arthritis in humans, the results of which are currently in publication.

As inhibition of COX enzymes is also generally considered a preventive tool in colorectal cancer, these results may also shed light on the mechanism of the chemopreventive activity of Avemar against carcinogenic chemically induced experimental colon cancer. It was examined whether Avemar might inhibit colon carcinogenesis in mammals, using as a model F-344 rats.[23] One hundred 4-week-old rats were divided into four groups. *Group 1*: untreated controls; *Group 2*: rats given the carcinogen azoxymethane (AOM) in three subcutaneous injections 1 week apart; *Group 3*: animals that started to receive Avemar via gastric tube 2 weeks prior to the first injection of AOM, daily and continuously thereafter until all animals were killed 32 weeks later; *Group 4*: animals that received the basal diet and Avemar only. At autopsy, no tumors were found in the untreated controls and in *Group 4* (Avemar only) animals. In *Group 2* (AOM only) 83.0% developed colon tumors with a mean of 2.3 tumors per animal; in *Group 3* (Avemar and AOM) 44.8% (P <.001) developed tumors with 1.3 (P <.004) tumors per animal. All the tumors were neoplastic. There were 4.85 aberrant crypt foci per cm^2 in *Group 2* (AOM only) compared to 2.03 in *Group 3* (AOM plus Avemar) (P <.0001). These results showed a powerful anticarcinogenic effect associated with the prophylactic use of Avemar as a cancer preventative in animals.

AVEMAR IN CLINICAL CANCER TRIALS

Oral Cavity Cancer

An open-label, nonrandomized, controlled, phase-II clinical study was performed in the Semmelweis University Clinic of Oral and Maxillofacial Surgery, Budapest. Forty-three patients with a definitive diagnosis of less than 3 months of either locally advanced oral cavity squamous cell carcinoma (OCC) (UICC stage II-III) or locally advanced stage IV (i.e., T4a N0-N1M0) were enrolled. Twenty-one consecutive patients received SAT, consisting of radical surgery + postoperative irradiation and/

or adjuvant chemotherapy, and 22 consecutive patients received SAT + 12 months of Avemar treatment. The objective was to assess whether Avemar has any influence on the outcome of locally advanced OCC when applied concomitantly with SAT. The end-point was disease progression. As regards baseline characteristics (age, clinical stage, chemotherapy, and site of primary tumor), there was no significant difference between the two groups apart from the previous treatment with radiotherapy drawback to the Avemar group (3 of 22 in the Avemar group vs 9 of 21 in the control group) ($P < .05$). At end-point, incidences of local recurrences and disease progression differed significantly between the two groups: 4.5% and 9.09% in the SAT + Avemar, 57.1% and 61.9% in the control group (SAT alone), respectively ($P < .001$). Risk analysis revealed that the 12 months of Avemar treatment significantly reduced the risk of overall progression (death, new loco-regional recurrences, new distant metastases) by 85% (Mantel-Haenszel test, $P < .001$).[24]

Based on these results and taking into consideration the results obtained in a noncomparative quality of life (QOL) study (QLQ-C30 questionnaire of the European Organization for Research and Treatment of Cancer [EORTC], Brussels) of 50 patients with head and neck cancer treated at the Oto-rhino-laryngology Clinic of Semmelweis University, in which patients experienced substantial improvement in cachectic symptoms, and long-term delay of progression in five of six advanced-stage salivary gland tumor patients, supportive use of Avemar in this manner may improve QOL and enhance the antitumor efficacy of SAT.[25]

Colorectal Cancer

Between 1998 and 1999, an open-label, pilot-scale, nonrandomized, controlled, phase II clinical study was carried out in the Uzsoki Hospital of Budapest to document whether or not supportive Avemar treatment adds any benefit to SAT in colorectal cancer.[26] Altogether 30 patients with advanced colorectal cancer (CRC) had been enrolled. All patients underwent curative surgery. The control group (18 patients) received SAT, whereas the Avemar group (12 patients) received SAT plus continuous and uninterrupted Avemar treatment. The end-point was progressive disease. Although, at baseline, patients of the Avemar group had more advanced disease stages, after an average observation period of 9 months, no disease progression had developed in the Avemar group, whereas three patients died and one patient had developed metastatic disease in the control group. Due to the small sample size, this difference had no statistical significance.

Between 1998 and 2003 also an open-label, pilot-scale, nonrandomized, controlled, phase II clinical study was done in the Berettyoujfalu Regional Hospital, including 34 patients with advanced adenocarcinoma of the rectum or the sigma.[27] Following radical surgery, 17 patients received SAT and 17 SAT plus continuous Avemar. The end-point was overall survival. After an average observation period of 46 months, significantly longer survival was found in the Avemar group.

A multicentric, open-label, cohort, phase III clinical study with the participation of 170 CRC patients enrolled from three onco-surgical centers in Hungary (Uzsoki Hospital of Budapest, University Clinics of Szeged and Debrecen) compared SAT vs. SAT + Avemar therapy.[28] Cohort allocation was based on the patient's choice. Sixty-six patients received Avemar as a supportive agent in addition to SAT (radical surgery plus radiotherapy and/or chemotherapy), whereas 104 patients were enrolled as controls without Avemar. The Mayo Clinic chemotherapy regimen and/or postoperative irradiation were regarded as SAT. Major eligibility criteria were: histologically or cytologically confirmed adenocarcinoma, curative surgery (at the time of diagnosis) with complete removal of primary tumor (completed with removal of metastases in selected cases of solitary or localized multifocal liver metastases) + removal of an adequate number of regional lymph nodes, a World Health Organization (WHO) performance status of 0–2, and life expectancy of at least of 6 months. Clinicopathologic stage, date of diagnosis, prior chemotherapy-/radiotherapy were disregarded as selection criteria. The primary end-point for both cohorts was progression-free survival. The mean age of control patients was higher, while distribution according to clinical stages was significantly less favourable in the Avemar group, which had a substantially (and significantly) higher percentage of International Union Against Cancer (UICC) stage IV (Dukes D) patients. There was a substantial difference between cohorts in average time elapsed from diagnosis to onset of therapy (drawback to the prognosis of Avemar cohort), while the interval from diagnosis to evaluation was similar. There was a significant difference between the two groups in number of patients previously treated with radiotherapy ($P < .001$) also drawback to the Avemar cohort. In summary: apart from mean age alone, prognostic variables in Avemar-treated cohort were much less favourable than in the control one.

Results: Progression-related events (new recurrences, new distant metastases, death) occurred with a substantially (and significantly) higher frequency in the control group. The cumulative probabilities of both disease-free (DFS) and overall survival (OS) proved to be more favorable in the Avemar group (DFS: $P = .0184$, OS: $P = .0278$). Cox regression analysis identified UICC staging ($P = .0004$) and Avemar treatment of ≥ 6 months ($P = .0045$) as independent predictors of survival. Side effects were extremely rare, mild and transient: diarrhea (4), nausea/vomiting (2), flatulence, repletion, soft stool and constipation: one instance of each. No serious adverse event (SAE) occurred either related or non-related to the test product.

Although other clinical observations regarding the efficacy of supportive Avemar therapy in CRC have been made, this study is currently the most complete source of data sufficient for drawing conclusions about the role of Avemar in this malignancy. Although there was not optimal homogeneity of previous treatment criteria among patients, it seems clear from this study, run in a more or less adjuvant setting, that Avemar has substantial potential benefit in improving the efficacy of adjuvant therapy (or in lengthening the tumor-free interval following radical surgery) in CRC. Specifically, Avemar may reduce likelihood of CRC recurrence; it may reduce new metastatic disease occurrence; and it may increase chances of survival after diagnosis with CRC.

Malignant Melanoma of the Skin

Being aware that most patients with UICC stage III (high-risk) malignant melanoma of the skin treated with SATs will eventually develop progressive disease, and because delay of progression in this condition is specially of high clinical importance, an open-label, pilot-scale, randomized, controlled, phase II clinical study was carried out in the N.N. Blokhin Cancer Center of the Russian Academy of Sciences in Moscow to test the possible value of supportive therapy with Avemar in this respect.[29] This year-long study compared, in the postsurgical adjuvant setting, DTIC plus 1 year of continuous Avemar administration (Avemar group, 22 patients) to treatment with dacarbazine alone (control group, 24 patients) in stage III melanoma of the skin. These patients were at high risk of recurrence and death from their disease. Interferon-alpha treatment is sometimes given to such patients, but its efficacy is controversial, undesirable side effects can be extreme, so DTIC remains an option. Chemotherapy naive, postoperative patients were randomized to either DTIC plus Avemar or to DTIC on its own (control) groups. In addition to cytostatic monotherapy, patients of the Avemar group took Avemar uninterruptedly up to 12 months. All patients were evaluated at baseline, at the end of each DTIC cycle, and 1, 5, and 9 months after completion of chemotherapy. The end-point was progression-free survival. Primary and/or nodal disease recurrence and new lymphatic and/or distant metastatic disease occurrence were regarded as progression-related events. There was no statistical difference in baseline parameters of the two groups. Eligibility criteria were: histologically confirmed malignant melanoma of the skin, with regional lymph node metastases and without evidence of distant metastases (stage III disease: pT1a-4bN1-3M0); WHO performance status: 0, 1, or 2; life expectation of ≥12 months; radical surgery including complete removal of the primary tumor followed by complete lymph node resection, achieving a macroscopically disease-free state. At end-point analysis, there were significantly more control patients with progressive disease (Avemar: 36% vs control: 75%; $P < .01$). Log-rank analysis (Kaplan-Meier estimate) showed a significant difference in time-to-progression (median, days) in favor of the Avemar group (Avemar: 366 vs control: 231, $P = .0042$). Continuous supplementation of dacarbazine treatment with Avemar is beneficial to stage III (high-risk) melanoma patients in terms of progression-free survival.

Side effects were related to DTIC treatment in both groups. Note that there were generally fewer toxic side effects in patients receiving the combined treatment than in those of the DTIC only group.

QUALITY OF LIFE

Lung Cancer

Downturn of quality of life (QOL) of advanced-stage cancer patients is a significant clinical issue, potentially influencing even patient survival probabilities. Consequently, improvement of QOL is of great importance among these patients. A pilot study was performed with enrolment of 16 lung cancer patients (8 males, 8 females, 7 small-cell and 9 adenocarcinoma cases) in the Korányi National Institute of Pulmonology, Budapest.[30] The patients had been treated with chemotherapy and/or radiotherapy. Avemar was administered for 8 months; the EORTC QLQ-C30 questionnaire was self-administered and the resulting data used for assessing the change in QOL. After 12 weeks of Avemar administration, significant improvement was reported in global state of health ($P < .01$) and in fatigue ($P < .05$). This improvement was maintained throughout the observation period. A modest improvement developed in pain, loss of appetite, and mood parameters. No adverse side effects were reported. Improvement in fatigue syndrome is of special importance.

Breast Cancer

A multicentric clinical study of Avemar in breast cancer is still ongoing. However, a QOL study involving Avemar use in breast cancer patients has been completed.[31] A total of 55 patients were enrolled in the study at Szeged Unversity Clinic of Surgery, and gauging of QOL and changes in it were based on the EORTC QLQ-C30 questionnaire. Main baseline characteristics included: mean age: 55 years; UICC stage: I: 8, II: 19, III: 15, and IV: 13; concurrent therapies: chemoradiotherapy: 10, chemotherapy only: 9, radiotherapy only: 2, and none in 34 cases. The mean observation period was 32 months. Several components of QOL showed significant improvement due to supportive therapy with Avemar. Significant improvements were achieved in physical functions ($P < .05$), emotional functions ($P < .001$), global state of health ($P < .01$), fatigue ($P <.01$), nausea, vomiting ($P < .01$), insomnia ($P < .01$), and constipation ($P < .01$). Effects were manifested after 3 months of treatment and remained stable throughout the entire length of the study.

FEBRILE NEUTROPENIA

There is a very attractive clinical observation concerning the indirect beneficial effect of Avemar—in malignant tumors—in connection with immune-stimulatory and bone marrow protective properties. An open-label, matched pair-based, controlled clinical study was performed in the 2nd Clinic of Pediatrics of the Semmelweis University in Budapest, with the enrolment of 22 (2×11) children with various types of pediatric solid cancers.[32] The matched pair setting was based on diagnosis, histopathology, clinical stage, gender, treatment schedule, and age. Avemar treatment was started simultaneously with cytostatic therapy and continued until the end of treatment and later on. Eleven children were given Avemar, and eleven served as controls. The end points of the study were the number and frequency of febrile neutropenia episodes accompanying intensive chemotherapy in the two groups. In the course of 121 cycles of chemotherapy, altogether 30 episodes of febrile neutropenia (24.8%) were observed in the Avemar group, 106 cycles were completed in the control group, and 46 episodes of febrile neutropenia (43.3%) were registered. The difference is significant in favor of the Avemar group ($P <.01$). It should be emphasized that principles in prophylaxis and therapy of febrile neutropenia were identical in the two groups. The results are convincing in the successful control of a life-threatening complication; the study can be regarded as clinical evidence of the immunostimulatory and bone marrow-protecting effect of Avemar.

OTHER CANCERS

Clinical studies with Avemar in cancer of the urinary tract and in chronic myelogenous leukemia are still ongoing in Europe.[33] In Israel, a multicentric, double-blind clinical trial with Avemar in metastatic CRC is currently under an interim analysis. There is much observational data about the favorable use of Avemar in a variety of other human malignancies, including ovarian cancer, gastric cancer, thyroid cancer, non-Hodgkin's lymphoma, and multiple myeloma.[3] Regression in patients with advanced hepatocellular carcinoma who were taking Avemar on a continuous basis has been observed.[3] Interestingly, regression in skeletal metastatic lesions has also been reported in last-stage breast, prostatic, and non-small-cell lung cancer patients after Avemar administration.[3] The therapeutic spectrum of Avemar is much wider than it had been thought some years ago.

REFERENCES

1. HIDVÉGI, M. 1998. Current results of Avemar research. (In Hungarian). Nogyogyaszati Onkol. **3:** 241–243.
2. TOMOSKOZI-FARKAS, R. & H.G. DAOOD. 2004. Modification of chromatographic method for the determination of benzoquinones in cereal products. Chromatographia **60:** S227–S230.
3. AVEMAR. (In Hungarian). 2004. Pharmindex Handbook of Oncology 2004/2005. :611–617. CMP Medica. Budapest.
4. HIDVEGI, M. *et al.* 1998. Effect of Avemar and Avemar + vitamin C on tumor growth and metastasis in experimental animals. Anticancer Res. **18:** 2353–2358.
5. SZENDE, B. *et al.* 2004. Effect of simultaneous administration of Avemar and cytostatic drugs on viability of cell cultures, growth of experimental tumors, and survival of tumor-bearing mice. Cancer Biother. Radiopharm. **19:** 343–349.
6. HIDVEGI, M. *et al.* 1999. MSC, a new benzoquinone-containing natural product with antimetastatic effect. Cancer Biother. Radiopharm. **14:** 277–289.
7. MARCSEK, Z. *et al.* 2004. The efficacy of tamoxifen in estrogen receptor-positive breast cancer cells is enhanced by a medical nutriment. Cancer Biother. Radiopharm. **19:** 746–753.
8. HIDVEGI, M. *et al.* 1999. Effect of MSC on the immune response of mice. Immunopharmacology **41:** 183–186.
9. EHRENFELD, M. *et al.* 2001. Avemar (a new benzoquinone-containing natural product) administration interferes with the Th2 response in experimental SLE and promotes amelioration of the disease. Lupus **10:** 622–627.
10. SUKKAR, S.G. & E. ROSSI. 2004. Oxidative stress and nutritional prevention in autoimmune rheumatic diseases. Autoimmunity Rev. **3:** 199–206.
11. GIDALI, J. *et al.* 2000. The effect of Avemar treatment on the regeneration of leukocytes, thrombocytes and reticulocytes in sublethally irradiated or cyclophosphamide treated mice. 1st Congress of the Hungarian Society of Clinical Oncology. Budapest, Hungary, November 10–11.
12. COMIN-ANDUIX, B. *et al.* 2002. Fermented wheat germ extract inhibits glycolysis/pentose cycle enzymes and induces apoptosis through poly(ADP-ribose) polymerase activation in Jurkat T-cell leukemia tumor cells. J. Biol. Chem. **277:** 46408–46414.
13. VIRAG, L. & CS. SZABO. 2002. The therapeutic potential of poly(ADP-ribose) polymerase inhibitors. Pharmacol. Rev. **54:** 375–429.
14. FAJKA-BOJA, R. *et al.* 2002. Fermented wheat germ extract induces apoptosis and downregulation of major histocompatibility complex class I proteins in tumor T and B cell lines. Int. J. Oncol. **20:** 563–570.
15. LOPEZ-BOTET, M. & T. BELLON. 1999. Natural killer cell activation and inhibition by receptors for MHC class I. Curr. Opin. Immunol. **11:** 301–307.
16. KUNDU, N. & A.M. FULTON. 1997. Interleukin-10 inhibits tumor metastasis, downregulates MHC class I, and enhances NK lysis. Cell Immunol. **180:** 55–61.
17. GRIFFIOEN, A.W. *et al.* 1996. Endothelial intercellular adhesion molecule-1 expression is suppressed in human malignancies: the role of angiogenic factors. Cancer Res. **56:** 1111–1117.
18. TELEKES, A. *et al.* 2005. Synergistic effect of Avemar on proinflammatory cytokine production and Ras-mediated cell activation. Ann. N.Y. Acad. Sci. **1051:** 515–528.
19. BOROS, L.G. *et al.* 2001. Wheat germ extract decreases glucose uptake and RNA ribose formation but increases fatty acid synthesis in MIA pancreatic adenocarcinoma cells. Pancreas **23:** 141–147.

20. CASCANTE, M. *et al.* 2002. Metabolic control analysis in drug discovery and disease. Nat. Biotechnol. **20:** 243–249.
21. TAKEDA, E. & G. WEBER. 1981. Role of ribonucleotide reductase in expression in the neoplastic program. Life Sci. **28:** 1007–1014.
22. ILLMER, C. *et al.* 2005. Immunologic and biochemical effects of the fermented wheat germ extract Avemar. Exp. Biol. Med. **230:** 144–149.
23. ZALATNAI, A. *et al.* 2001. Wheat germ extract inhibits experimental colon carcinogenesis in F-344 rats. Carcinogenesis **22:** 1649–1652.
24. FULOP, E. *et al.* 2004. Results of the administration of Avemar in oral cavity cancer patients. 7th Congress of the Hungarian Society of Oral and Maxillofacial Surgery. Pecs, Hungary, October 16–18.
25. RIBARI, O. *et al.* 2000. Early results on the supportive treatment of head and neck cancer patients with Avemar. 1st Congress of the Hungarian Society of Clinical Oncology. Budapest, Hungary, November 10–11.
26. JAKAB, F. *et al.* 2000. First clinical data of a natural immunomodulator in colorectal cancer. Hepatogastroenterology **47:** 393–395.
27. KOTI, CS. & L. LENGYEL. 2004. Tumours of the sigma and rectum: the completion of postoperative chemotherapy with Avemar. (In Hungarian). Magy Seb **57:** 168.
28. JAKAB, F. *et al.* 2003. A medical nutriment has supportive value in the treatment of colorectal cancer. Br. J. Cancer **89:** 465–469.
29. DEMIDOV, L.V. *et al.* 2002. Antimetastatic effect of Avemar in high-risk melanoma patients. 18th UICC International Cancer Congress. Oslo, Norway, June 30–July 5.
30. HIDVEGI, M. *et al.* 2003. Fermented wheat germ extract improves quality of life in lung cancer patients. (In Hungarian.) Medicus Anonymus/Pulmono **11:** 13–14.
31. BALOGH, A. 2001. The supportive value of AVEMAR during chemotherapy. New Results of Avemar Research. Symposium. 24th Congress of the Hungarian Cancer Society. Budapest, Hungary, November 22–24.
32. GARAMI, M. *et al.* 2004. Fermented wheat germ extract reduces chemotherapy induced febrile neutropenia in pediatric cancer patients. J. Pediatr. Hematol. Oncol. **26:** 631–635.
33. FARKAS, E. 2004. The role of Avemar in oncology. A review. (In Hungarian). Magy Belorv. Arch. **57:** 4–9.

Open-Label 24-Month Study Evaluating Infliximab Therapy in Patients with Psoriatic Spondyloarthropathy

J. J. SCALI,[a] A. KAMINSKY,[b] J. SALOMÓN,[a] S. VISENTINI,[a] AND E. DANCZIGER[b]

[a]*Department of Rheumatology, Autoimmune and Metabolic Bone Diseases, Durand Hospital, Buenos Aires, Argentina*

[b]*Dermatology Unit, Durand Hospital, Buenos Aires, Argentina*

ABSTRACT: Psoriatic spondyloarthropathy (PsSA) is a common and relatively typical form of spondyloarthropathy, affecting the axial skeleton with peripheral synovitis. Also, extraarticular as well as skin manifestations are sometimes difficult to diagnose and to treat. Recent studies demonstrated that anti-tumor necrosis factor therapies are useful in treating and controlling disease activity. We conducted an open-label 2-year study in 16 patients to evaluate the efficacy and safety of long-term compliance with intravenous infliximab therapy in patients with severe skin and refractory PsSA, with an incomplete response to methotrexate, azathioprine, cyclosporine, and/or sulfasalazine. Patients continued to receive only weekly methotrexate therapy during the study that included 16 patients (9 men, 7 women; mean age 38 ± 12.5 years [SD]) with psoriatic spondyloarthropathy for 16.4 ± 9.2 years. Each patient underwent complete physical examination before treatment and at each visit until the end of the study. Results of patient global pain assessment (VAS scale), investigator opinion on global assessment of disease activity (100 mm VAS), patient body weight and blood pressure, ACR response (20%, 50%, and 70%), laboratory parameters (CRP, ESR, WBC, RBC, liver enzymes, etc.), and PASI (skin score) were recorded. We conclude that infliximab therapy was effective in controlling joint and skin disease, having an acceptable safety profile and very good compliance when considering this type of patient. However, further long-term, double-blind, placebo-controlled trials are necessary to validate these results.

KEYWORDS: psoriatic spondyloarthropathy; infliximab

INTRODUCTION

Psoriatic arthritis (PsA) is a difficult disease to treat. Its symptoms range from mild to severe skin and joint involvement, developing erosions, and deforming arthritis in a significant number of affected patients.[1] DMARDs, such as sulfasalazine, azathioprine, cyclosporine, and methotrexate, do not control the disease manifestations satisfactorily, with no evidence of control of damage progression.[2,3]

Address for correspondence: Juan José Scali, Department of Rheumatology, Autoimmune and Metabolic Bone Diseases, Durand Hospital, Buenos Aires, Argentina.
jjscali@intramed.net.ar

Ann. N.Y. Acad. Sci. 1051: 543–550 (2005).
doi: 10.1196/annals.1361.098

Tumor necrosis factor-alpha (TNF-α), a proinflammatory cytokine, has a role in the pathophysiogenesis of PsA. TNF-α is upregulated in skin lesions and sinovitis. Recent studies show that infliximab can improve both skin lesions and sinovitis of the joints. Some investigators have reported positive results with this anticytokine-neutralizing agent in the treatment of spondyloarthropathies, including PsA.[4–7]

MATERIAL AND METHODS

We conducted an open-label study to evaluate the efficacy, long-term safety, and patient's compliance with infliximab intravenous therapy for 2 years in patients with severe skin and refractory psoriatic spondyloarthropathy with an incomplete response to methotrexate, azathioprine, cyclosporine, and/or sulfasalazine. Patients continued to receive only methotrexate weekly (15 mg/week) throughout the study period.

The primary endpoints were to evaluate arthritis by means of the American College of Rheumatology response score (ACR 20%, 50%, and 70%) and psoriatic arthritis response criteria (PsARC), the skin response by means of the Psoriasis Activity Skin Index (PASI), and the quality of life by the Health Assessment Questionaire Disability Index (HAQ).

The study included 16 patients (9 men, 7 women) with a mean age of 38 ± 12.5 (SD) years. The disease was present for 16.4 ± 9.2 (SD) years, with psoriatic spondyloarthropathy fulfilling the Moll & Wright criteria. Seven of the 16 patients were HLA B27 positive, having active axial and skin disease (refractory for almost 3 months to predetermined methotrexate therapy).

Infliximab 5 mg/kg body weight/infusion was given intravenously over a 2.5 hour period, as follows: baseline, 2 weeks, 6 weeks, and then every 2 months for 24 months.

We chose a dose of 5 mg/kg body weight of infliximab without scientific proof as in other studies. Co-medications such as methotrexate (15 mg/wk) and folic acid supplement (5 mg/day, only 3 days a week) were also administered.

Patients with a history of malignant disease, liver or kidney abnormalities or viral B or C hepatitis, major complicating diseases, blood dyscrasias, positive tuberculin test to PPD 2UT, or other positive test results (radiography, laboratory biopsy, cultures, etc.) suggesting chronic infectious and/or granulomatous diseases were excluded.

Each patient underwent complete physical examination before starting treatment, at 2 weeks, and at each monthly follow-up visit until the end of the study. Primary analyses included ACR scores (ACR response 20%, 50%, and 70%) at 24 months and the HAQ disability index (physical function). Patient global pain assessment on the Visual Analogue Scale of 10 (VAS), physician's opinion on the global assessment of disease activity (VAS), patient's body weight and blood pressure, laboratory parameters (CRP, ESR, WBC, RBC, liver enzymes, etc.), PASI (skin score), number of swollen and tender joints, morning stiffness, night pain, and peripheral joint pain were evaluated.

The disease was defined as active if patients had a PASI (TABLE 3) score of ≥ 16, C-reactive protein (CRP) of 10 mg/L or more, a VAS pain score of more than 6, more than three swollen or tender joints, and a stable methotrexate dose for 3 months equal

TABLE 1. Characteristics of patients at baseline

Number of patients	16
Gender (men/women)	9/7
Age (yr), mean (range)	54 (25–71)
Disease duration (yr)	16.4 (8–38)
TJC (mean, 0–28 joints)	11
SJC (mean, 0–28 joints)	10
HAQ (mean, 0–3)	1.6
CRP (mean, mg/L)	16
Peripheral joint involvement	10
HLA-B 27 positive	7

TABLE 2. PASI: composite index of disease severity

Evaluation
Scale
Erythema
Induration
Weighted
By severity
By body surface area

to 15 mg/week prior to the study without a positive or significant response to treatment. Statistical significance was estimated with Wilcoxon's test (for pairs of data) and the nonparametric Fisher's exact test. Statistical comparisons were performed using an analysis of variance followed by Student's *t* test.

The baseline clinical characteristics of the patients in this study are very similar to those of patients in the infliximab pivotal trials. Patients had long-standing, moderate to severe PsA (TABLE 1).

The enrolled patients represent a broad patient population, including those with no previous biologic experience. The PASI was evaluated in each patient, taking into consideration the scale, erythema, and induration weighted by severity and by body surface area traditional punctuation.

RESULTS

A total of 21 patients having all of these prefixed conditions were recruited for the study. Four patients were excluded because of a positive PPD test, and one had severe arterial hypertension with a positive HBV test, leaving 16 patients. The number of affected joints was reduced from 11 to 3 tender joints and from 10 to 4 swollen joints (TABLE 3).

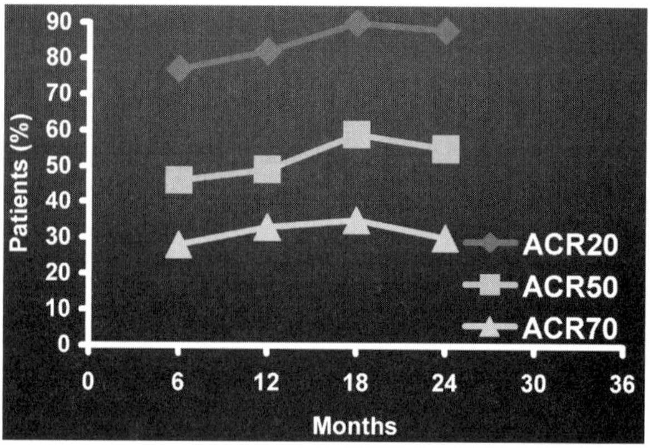

FIGURE 1. American College of Rheumatology(ACR) responses to infliximab.

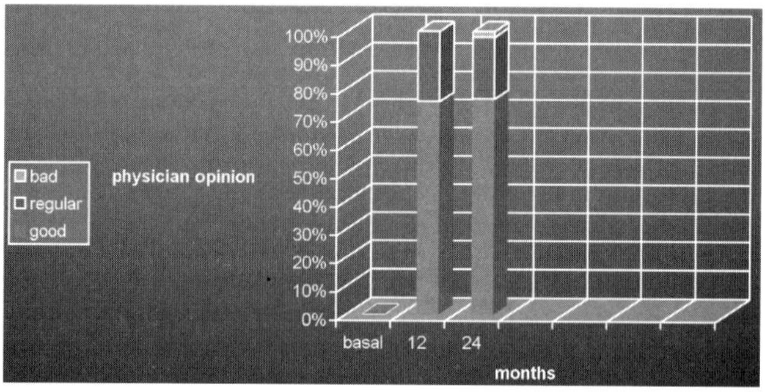

FIGURE 2. Physicians' opinions on overall disease condition.

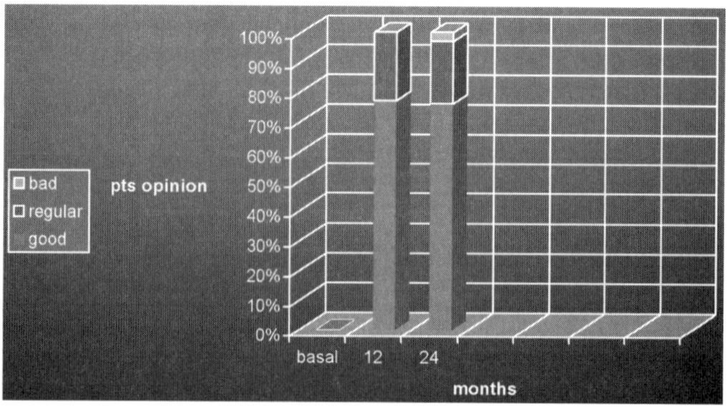

FIGURE 3. Patients' opinions on global assessment of the disease (%).

The ACR response rate (FIG. 1) at the end was ACR 20%: 88%; ACR 50%: 55%; and ACR 70%: 30%. The physicians' opinions on global assessment (FIG. 2) were good, 76%; regular, 22%; and bad, 2%.

The patients' opinions on global assessment were very interesting (FIG. 3), with a very effective percentage of improvement until 18 months, when the percentage of good results diminished.

Night pain assessment indicated good improvement from 15 days to 18 months. From 18–24 months, 4 of 16 patients had night pain again but in a VAS lower intensity scale. The same results were seen with morning stiffness and peripheral joint pain on VAS (FIG. 4).

The secondary endpoint was the change in PASI score. The mean PASI score changed from 25.4 (range 12.5–39.1) to 3.9 (range 0.4–4.7), revealing rapid and complete clearing of psoriasis erythroderma and widespread psoriasis plaque depending on the affected patient (FIG. 5).

Laboratory results were generally normal. CRP, ESR, and hemoglobin showed a better profile at the end of the study than at baseline (FIG. 6). Only two cases had elevated transaminase levels (GOAT and GPT) at 18 and 24 months, respectively, returning to normal after this period without any change in infliximab therapy, decreasing methotrexate only to 7.5 mg/week. Also, one case of mild transient thrombocytopenia at 16 months had a good outcome without any treatment.

Clinical skin scores (PASI: basal, 25.4; end of study, 3.9 [range: basal, 12.5–39.1; end study, 0.4–4.7]) and joints scores were statistically significant ($P < .0002$) compared with baseline data (FIG. 5).

No allergic reactions or systemic infections were present. Treatment was very well tolerated. Adverse events were mild and resolved at the end (neurologic: 1 case of paresthesia of the right arm; infection: the common cold in two cases and reactivation of osteomyelitis in one patient, believed to have resolved 15 years earlier).

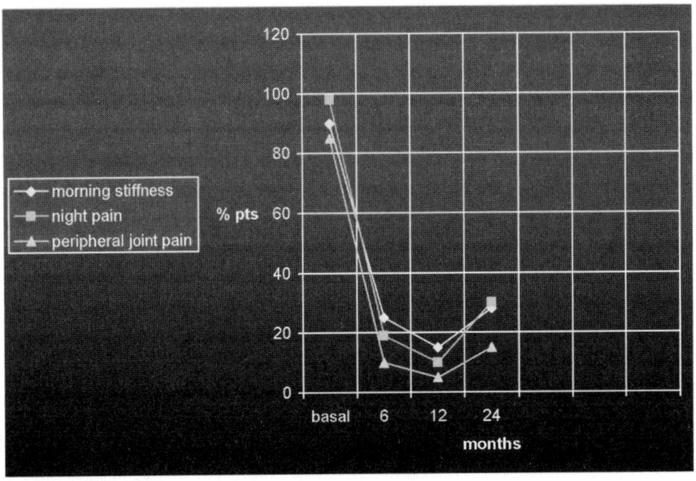

FIGURE 4. Outcome in morning stiffness, night pain, and peripheral pain from baseline to the end of the study.

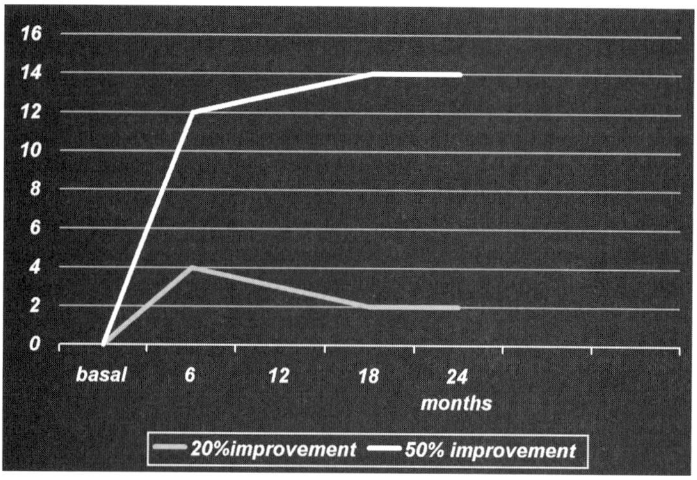

FIGURE 5. Degree of 20% or 50% improvement in PASI from baseline, 6, 12, 18, and 24 months.

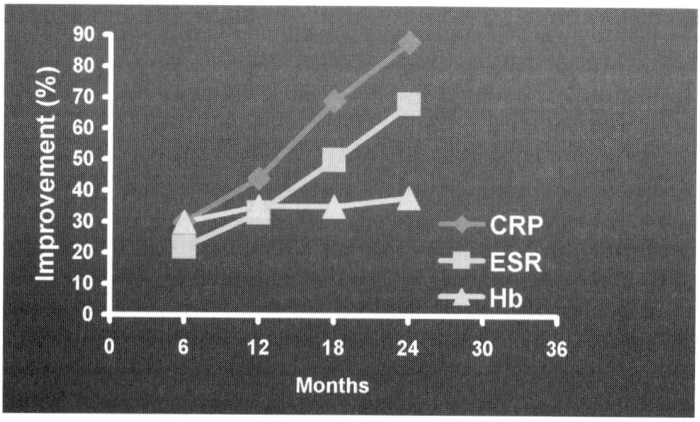

FIGURE 6. Percentage of improvement in hemoglobin, C-reactive protein (CRP), and erythrocyte sedimentation rate (ESR) during the study.

One patient developed an ANA (+) homogeneous pattern at 1/320 titers at the end of the study. No other antibodies were detected during the study.

Infliximab plus methotrexate was efficacious for over 2 years in patients with active PsA, resulting in sustained, marked improvements in the ACR response and the HAQ DI (FIG. 7).

We conclude that infliximab therapy was effective in controlling joint and skin disease, having an acceptable safety profile and very good compliance when considering this type of patient. However, further long-term, double-blind, placebo-controlled trials are necessary to validate these results.

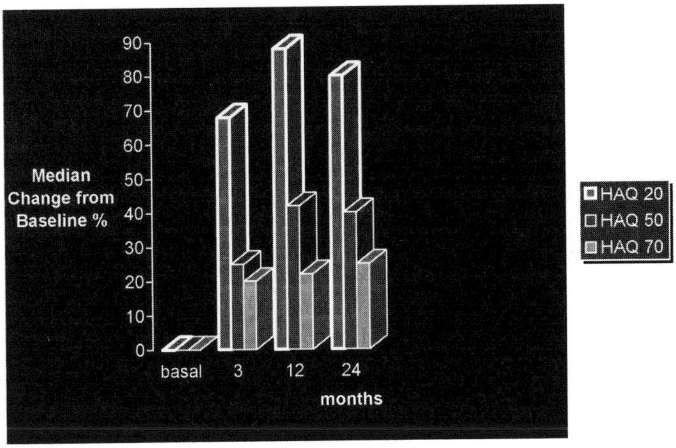

FIGURE 7. Health Assessment Questionaire Disability Index (HAQ DI) values from baseline to 2 years of treatment.

TABLE 3. General changes in parameters during the study and their degree of significance

Parameter	Baseline	24 weeks	Significance
Number of tender joints	11	3	$P < .001$
Number of swollen joints	10	4	$P < .001$
Physicians' global opinion	7.0	2.0	$P < .003$
Patients' global opinion	8.0	2.0	$P < .008$
PAIN (VAS)	8.5	1.9	$P < .001$
Morning stiffness (*min)	105	15	$P < .0001$
Erythrocyte sedimentation rate (mm/1h)	34	18	$P < .0004$
CRP (mg/dl) (*)	16	0.5	$P < .001$

DISCUSSION

Our data show significant efficacy of infliximab, almost similar to data from other studies reporting an almost 50–70% improvement in different scores and response rates.[6,7] Patients must be carefully selected for treatment by rheumatologists, given the high costs and potential risks cited in other trials. However, our results suggest that it may be the preferred treatment in patients resistant to conventional DMARD therapy. The anti–TNF-α treatments offer improvement in disease activity, quality of life, and radiologic progression as determined by a review of some references in the literature.

The efficacy we obtained is slightly less marked than that described in some other reports,[5,6] probably because of certain factors, including selection of affected patients, comorbidity, and therapeutic regimen if thought to be medication asssociated (methotrexate may enhance the therapeutic effects of infliximab). Some psychologic aspects as well as the season are important to consider when treating these kinds of patients. Summer is normally the time that psoriatic patients achieve a good sun response in skin lesions, then ameliorating their psychologic aspects and thus the overall rate of pain perception.

In our study, maximum effect was found between 3 and 18 months of treatment; starting at 18 months, a stable condition or a smaller effect on articular parameters was noted. Psoriatic arthropathy is known to lead to substantial morbidity and mortality. When considering the published trials, numerous studies show that treatment improves the signs, symptoms, and function and leads to improved quality of life for patients with this condition.

Trials considering these kinds of variables must be performed in the future to obtain precise information on the effects of infliximab, even when multiple cost-effectiveness studies have been performed, especially in rheumatoid arthritis, suggesting that anti–TNF-α treatment should be cost effective, and maybe PsA is in the same line.

REFERENCES

1. Mease, P.J. 2002. Tumor necrosis factor (TNF) in psoriatic arthritis pathophysiology and treatment with TNF inhibitors. Ann. Rheum. Dis. **61:** 298–304.
2. Mease, P.J., B.S. Gaffe, J. Metz, *et al.* 2000. Etanercept in the treatment of psoriatic arthritis and psoriasis: a randomized trial. Lancet **356:** 385–390.
3. Gladman, D.D., F. Stafford-Brady, C.H. Chang, *et al.* 1990. Longitudinal study of clinical and radiological progression in psoriatic arthritis. J. Rheumatol. **17:** 809–812.
4. Dougados, M., S. van der Linden, R. Juhlin, *et al.* 1991. The European Spondyloarthropathy Study Group preliminary criteria for the classification of spondyloarthropathy. Arthritis Rheum. **34:** 1218–1227.
5. Kruithof, E. F. van den Bosch, D. Baeten, *et al.* 2002. Repeated infusions of infliximab, a chimeric anti-TNFalpha monoclonal antibody, in patients with active spondyloarthropathy: one year follow up. Ann. Rheum. Dis. **61:** 207–212.
6. Herfarth, H., F. Obermeier, T. Andus, *et al.* 2002. Improvement of arthritis and arthralgia after treatment with infliximab (Remicade) in a German prospective, open-label, multicenter trial in refractory Crohn's disease. Am. J. Gastroenterol. **97:** 2688–2690.
7. Braun, J. & J. Sieper. 2002. Therapy of ankylosing spondylitis and other spondyloarthritides: established medical treatment, anti-TNF-α therapy and other novel approaches. Arthritis Res. **4:** 307–321.

Cyclosporine: From Renal Transplantation to Autoimmune Diseases

CLAUDIO PONTICELLI

IRCCS Istituto Auxologico Italiano, Milan, Italy

ABSTRACT: **Over the last 20 years, cyclosporine (CsA) has been the mainstay of immunosuppression in renal transplantation. Initially, CsA was administered at high doses, which enhanced its potential nephrotoxicity. Better handling of the drug was obtained by lowering the dose, monitoring CsA concentration and renal function, and using graft biopsy in difficult cases. In the early 1990s, a new microemulsion showed better pharmacokinetics and efficacy than did the previous formulation. A few years later, evidence showed that checking blood levels 2 hours after administration was a more reliable indicator of CsA exposure than were trough blood levels. The combination with newer immunosuppressive drugs allowed further reduction in the doses of CsA to maintain stable renal allograft function and to improve long-term graft survival. CsA has largely been used in autoimmune diseases. There is concern about its nephrotoxicity, however, as in some studies control renal biopsies showed that CsA-treated patients developed progressive interstitial fibrosis. The risk of nephrotoxicity was related to the initial doses of CsA and to the increase in serum creatinine. Avoiding CsA in patients with creatinine clearance <60 mL/min and in those with uncontrolled hypertension, starting with CsA microemulsion at doses not higher than 4 mg/kg, and reducing the doses whenever serum creatinine increases to 30% or more over baseline may prevent deterioration of renal function. If these guidelines are followed, CsA may be safely used in autoimmune diseases.**

KEYWORDS: **renal transplantation; autoimmune diseases; cyclosporine; cyclosporine nephrotoxicity**

CYCLOSPORINE IN RENAL TRANSPLANTATION

Before the discovery of cyclosporine (CsA), immunosuppressive therapy in renal transplantation was based on azathioprine (Aza) and corticosteroids, which allowed good graft function to be obtained in some patients. However, acute rejection was frequent and often irreversible, one-year cadaveric graft survival was around 50%, mortality rate was elevated, and quality of life was severely impaired by the need for high-dose corticosteroids. Taken together, the results were far from satisfying, and transplantation was often considered only a temporary respite from dialysis, which remained the basic form of treatment of uremia.[1]

Address for correspondence: Claudio Ponticelli, M.D., FRCP, Via Ampere 126, 20131 Milan, Italy. Voice: +39-0226112952.
claudio.ponticelli@fastwebnet.it

Ann. N.Y. Acad. Sci. 1051: 551–558 (2005). © 2005 New York Academy of Sciences.
doi: 10.1196/annals.1361.099

After the discovery of its immunosuppressive properties, CsA was studied in experimental transplantation by Calne and his group.[2] Its initial use in patients with renal transplantation resulted in good protection from rejection. However, patients had poor renal function and an increased risk of lymphoma because doses of CsA were too high.[3] A few years passed before dose management could be clarified. Eventually, in 1983, two multicenter randomized trials showed that CsA could significantly improve the probability of graft survival at one year over that of standard treatment with Aza and steroids.[4,5] After these results were repeated in other transplant centers, the drug was almost universally adopted for basic immunosuppression in renal transplant recipients. However, the doses of CsA used in the initial experiences were still too high, ranging from 17 mg/kg/day with a gradual reduction to maintenance doses of 5–7 mg/kg/day, much higher doses than those currently used. The administration of such elevated doses strongly enhanced the potential nephrotoxicity of CsA, a complication that is usually dose dependent and that may lead to renal dysfunction and severe histologic lesions.

Cyclosporine can cause strong vasoconstriction from activation of the renin-angiotensin system,[6] reduced synthesis of nitric oxide,[7] increased sympathetic nervous activity,[8] increased production of vasoconstrictive thromboxane A2,[9] and excessive renal synthesis of endothelin.[10] Because of continuous renal vasoconstriction, the glomerular filtration rate reduces the urea and uric acid increases in the blood. Blood pressure may also increase both because of the increase in peripheral vascular resistance[11] and because the vasoconstrictive effect on afferent arterioles enhances the proximal resorption of sodium chloride with consequent volume expansion.[12] When severe or protracted, these pathophysiologic factors can lead to histologic changes that initially can be reversible with adequate adjustment of the CsA dosage, but that can also result in irreversible renal damage.

Histologic changes caused by CsA may involve tubular cells, arterioles, and/or interstitium (TABLE 1). Earlier lesions affect proximal tubuli, with the appearance of giant mitochondria in the convoluted part of the proximal tubule, isometric vacuolization in the straight part of the proximal tubule, and microcalcifications caused by calcification of Tamm-Horsfall protein casts.[13] These lesions, which are frequent but not specific signs of CsA toxicity, may be reversed by reducing the doses of CsA.

TABLE 1. Main histologic features of cyclosporine-related nephrotoxicity

Tubulopathy (fully reversible with dose reduction)	Arteriolopathy (partially reversible with dose adjustement or CsA withdrawal)	Scarring (irreversible)
Giant mitochondria	Circular nodular protein deposits in the arteriolar wall	Stripe interstitial fibrosis
Isometric vacuolization		Diffuse interstitial fibrosis and tubular atrophy Glomerular sclerosis
Calcification	Mucinoid thickening of the intima	

The microvascular changes that predominate in the afferent arterioles may be more severe. Mihatsch *et al.*[14] described two forms of CsA-related arteriolopathy. In one form, circular nodular protein deposits permeate the arteriolar wall and may narrow or occlude the lumen. The second form is characterized by mucinoid thickening of the intima, causing narrowing of the lumen. Early arteriolopathy may be reversible if CsA is stopped or reduced;[15] otherwise, persistent ischemia may lead to scarring. Moreover, continuous activation of the renin-angiotensin system and increased synthesis of osteopontin, a powerful macrophage chemoattractant, may trigger over-expression of TGF-β1, which can eventually lead to interstitial fibrosis and tubular atrophy,[16] with progressive kidney dysfunction.

The wrong doses used in the early experience strongly contributed to the development of CsA nephropathy in some renal transplant recipients. However, in many others, doses could be adjusted by monitoring serum creatinine levels and trough blood levels of CsA. Kidney allograft biopsy in difficult cases helped to diagnose CsA-related nephrotoxicity and to prevent progressive graft dysfunction by adjusting the doses of CsA.

Because of the fear that CsA could predispose the transplant recipient to renal function deterioration in the long term, some transplant centers decided to administer CsA at low doses, whereas others converted from CsA to Aza or mycophenolate mofetil (MMF) treatment a few months after transplantation. However, by analyzing the data of the Collaborative Transplant Study, Opelz[17] demonstrated that mean doses of CsA lower than 3 mg/kg/day in the first year were associated with poor graft survival at 7 years, a result similar to that with doses >6 mg/kg/day. The best 7-year graft survival was observed in patients who received doses between 3 and 6 mg/kg/day in the first year. However, the switch from CsA to Aza-MMF resulted in a better lipid profile and lower blood pressure, but at control biopsy 50% of patients showed histologic deterioration.[18] Only one randomized trial compared CsA and Aza and reported the long-term results.[19] In this trial, begun in 1983, patients were followed up for 10 years. De novo cadaveric renal transplant recipients were allocated to receive Aza (3 mg/kg/day) plus steroids or cyclosporine (15 mg/kg/day progressively tapered) plus steroids. The risk of rejection was significantly lower in Csa-treated patients (0.3 vs. 1.4). According to the intention-to-treat analysis the 10-year graft survival was significantly better in CsA-treated patients than in those given Aza (56 vs. 35%). Mean levels of creatinine clearance were lower in the CsA group at any time point, but levels remained stable over the time. From year 1 to year 10 there was a mean decline in creatinine clearance of 12 mL/min in the Aza group versus 13 mL/min in the CsA group. Thus, despite the initial high doses, CsA-treated patients maintained great advantages over the Aza-treated patients, even over the long term.

Besides the potential nephrotoxicity, other drawbacks of CsA were represented by large inter- and intraindividual variabilities in its bioavailability, which could increase the risk of rejection.[20] Moreover, CsA reached a steady state only after about 3 months, and its absorption was food dependent. The solubility of CsA depends on its dissolution, a process that is influenced by many factors, the most important of which are particle size, gastric mixing/emptying, and absorptive surface. In the early 1990s, a new microemulsion of CsA (Neoral, Novartis Pharma, Basel) was made available. When compared with the old formulation, Neoral showed better bioavailability, more predictable pharmacokinetics, and dose linearity in CsA exposure.[21,22] This improved pharmacologic profile resulted in increased efficacy. A meta-analysis of trials comparing Neoral with the old formulation of CsA showed a significant reduction in the risk of acute rejection in patients treated with Neoral.[23] A review of the U.S. Renal Data Systems (USRDS) showed that Neoral reduced the relative risk of graft failure to 0.6 compared to the old formulation of CsA.[24] The superior performance of Neoral coupled with a progressively better understanding of CsA administration led to improved patient and graft survival in the long term. Analysis of the USRDS showed a mortality rate of 3.8 deaths per 100 patient-years in kidney graft recipients compared with 6.3 deaths in those awaiting transplantation.[25] The graft half-life of living and cadaveric renal transplants performed in the United States almost doubled between 1988 and 1996.[26] By reviewing our own cumulative experience with cyclosporine, we found an estimated graft half-life of 19 years in cadaveric renal transplant patients and 31 years in living transplant recipients treated with CsA.[27] Despite the potential nephrotoxicity of CsA, mean levels of serum creatinine remained stable in our experience, even in the long term.[28] Recent evidence indicates that measuring blood CsA concentration at 2 hours after administration (C2) could be a better guide for adjusting the dosage than trough blood levels.[29] The major risk of long-term graft dysfunction was observed in patients with low C2 levels,[30] supporting the hypothesis that chronic rejection is more important than chronic toxicity as a cause of late kidney allograft failure.

Together with Neoral, MMF and the calcineurin inhibitor tacrolimus were made available almost in the same period. In the last few years, two monoclonal antibodies directed against the alpha chain of the interleukin (IL)-2 receptor, basiliximab and daclizumab, and more recently two mTOR inhibitors, sirolimus and everolimus, were also made available. The combination of different immunosuppressive agents further reduced the risk of rejection, while safely allowing the doses of calcineurin inhibitors to be decreased. Although cyclosporine is still considered a cause of graft dysfunction and interstitial fibrosis in renal transplant recipients,[31] compared with 20 years ago the scenario of kidney transplantation is completely changed. One-year graft survival improved from approximately 50% to over 90%.[32] Acute rejection has become increasingly more rare and is usually reversible. Steroids may be used at low doses or may even be avoided.[33] Currently, the most frequent causes of failure are death, mostly caused by cardiovascular disease, and chronic allograft nephropathy, mainly caused by chronic rejection and the use of marginal donors.[34]

CYCLOSPORINE IN AUTOIMMUNE DISEASES

Cyclosporine is a prodrug that gains pharmacologic activity after binding to its specific cytoplasmic receptor cyclophilin. It is the complex CsA-cyclophilin that interferes with a system of phosphatases called calcineurin. Calcineurin has a key role in the immune response. Contact with the antigen-presenting cell generates a strong influx of calcium ions into the lymphocyte, which results in activation of the calcineurin with consequent dephosphorylation of a family of proteins, called nuclear factor-activating T cells (NFAT). After being dephosphorylated, NFAT enters the nucleus where it participates in the synthesis of IL-2, which triggers lymphocyte proliferation. Thus, CsA may disrupt progression of the activated cascade by dampening T-cell production of proinflammatory lymphokines and arresting the cell cycle between G0 and G1.[35] This mechanism of action makes CsA an attractive drug for autoimmune diseases. CsA has been used with variable success in almost all autoimmune diseases. It is beyond the scope of the current review to analyze in detail the results with CsA in the different autoimmune diseases. Currently, the more frequent indications for CsA are psoriasis,[36] atopic dermatitis,[37] rheumatoid arthritis,[38] uveitis,[39] systemic lupus erythematosus,[40] sympathetic ophtalmia,[41] and the idiopathic nephrotic syndrome.[42] However, anecdotal cases in which CsA was used with success have been reported in many other autoimmune diseases.

Some reports indicate that CsA may cause interstitial fibrosis and tubular atrophy in patients with autoimmune disease.[43,44] These reports raise concern that the use of CsA in this setting could expose to nephrotoxicity with the same frequency and severity observed in renal transplant recipients. In 1992, Feutren and Mihatsch[45] analyzed the main risk factors associated with the development of CsA-induced nephropathy in 192 patients with nonrenal autoimmune diseases who had been subjected to a control renal biopsy. Fifty-one patients had CsA nephropathy, defined as at least moderate focal interstitial fibrosis, with tubular atrophy, arteriolar alterations, or both. Compared with patients who did not develop renal toxicity, patients with CsA nephropathy had received larger initial doses of CsA, had a higher maximal increase in serum creatinine concentration, and were older. After that report, initial doses of CsA were reduced and serum creatinine was monitored more frequently. A study of patients with rheumatoid arthritis showed that none of the patients who started CsA at doses lower than 4 mg/kg/day and did not exceed 5 mg/kg/day during follow-up developed CsA-induced nephropathy at renal biopsy or at any sign of renal function deterioration.[46] Therefore, using lower doses of CsA and monitoring the serum creatinine concentration should help prevent the development of severe renal lesions in patients with autoimmune disease. Another advantage of the use of CsA in autoimmune diseases is the possibility of interrupting treatment after 1–2 years and reassuming CsA after an adequate interval.

There are many important differences in the risk of CsA-related nephrotoxicity between patients with autoimmune diseases and renal transplant recipients. The transplanted kidney is exposed to the risk of alloimmune reactivity, including acute rejection, subclinical rejection, and chronic rejection, as well as the risk of alloantigen-independent injuries such as old age of the donor, ischemia-reperfusion injury, hypertension, diabetes, and viral infections.[47] Instead, with the possible exception of renal diseases, the kidney in patients with autoimmune diseases usually has normal function, and it is not exposed to the risk of alloimmune reactivity, ischemia-reperfusion injury, or comorbidity. Currently, the large doses used in early experiences have been abandoned. In patients with autoimmune disease the starting dose of CsA does not exceed 5 mg/kg/day and the maintenance dosage ranges between 2 and 3 mg/kg/day, whereas in renal transplant recipients the starting dose ranges from 8–10 mg/kg/day and the maintenance dose ranges from 4–5 mg/kg/day when cyclosporine is used as the basic immunosuppressive agent. Moreover, in some patients with autoimmune disease, treatment may be discontinued or CsA may be alternated with other immunosuppressive drugs while it has to be given indefinitely in transplant patients.

Although the risk of renal insufficiency is low in patients with autoimmune diseases, we should not forget that CsA is a potentially nephrotoxic drug. The risk of renal damage is dose-dependent and is particularly increased in patients with

TABLE 2. Factors that may interfere with CsA pharmacokinetics or may enhance nephrotoxicity

Increased CsA blood levels	Decreased CsA blood levels	Enhanced nephrotoxicity
Diltiazem	Barbiturates	Older age
Verapamil	Carbamazepin	Renal failure
Nicardipine	Rifampin	Hypertension
Ketoconazole	Rifabutin	Dehydration
Fluconazole	Isoniazid?	Aminoglycosides
Erythromycin	Nafcillin	Amphotericin B
Clarythromycin		Ciprofloxacin
High-dose methyl-prednisolone		Sulfonamides

elevated serum creatinine concentration and/or already established tubulointerstitial lesions. The respect of some guidelines may minimize the risk of nephrotoxicity and may further improve the therapeutic index of CsA. Patients with a stable creatinine clearance <60 mL/min and/or patients with severe uncontrolled hypertension should not receive CsA. Renal patients with severe interstitial fibrosis and tubular atrophy at renal biopsy should also be excluded by CsA treatment. Caution is recommended in patients with subnormal levels of creatinine clearance (between 60 and 80 mL/min) and/or moderate tubulointerstitial lesions. In hypertensive patients it is advisable to initiate CsA treatment only when blood pressure has returned to the normal range with therapy. It should be kept in mind that drugs such as nondihydropyridinic calcium channel blockers, ketoconazole and derivates, and macrolide antibiotics may increase the blood levels of CsA, while rifampin and derivates, nafcillin, barbiturates, and carbamazepin, reduce blood levels of CsA. Moreover, many factors and drugs may enhance the potential nephrotoxicity of CsA (TABLE 2). In the presence of the latter factors it is advisable to reduce the doses of CsA.

In patients with autoimmune disease, the initial doses of Neoral should not exceed 4 mg/kg/day with slow reduction to a maintenance of 2–3 mg/kg/day. Patients should be checked regularly. The higher the increase in serum creatinine, the higher the risk of severe renal toxicity. The risk is minimal if the increase in creatinine is lower than 20–30%. It ranges from 10–12% for stable increases of 30%, but it is around 50% when serum creatinine levels reach twice the baseline concentration, and it approaches 100% for further increases.[45] To be on the safe side, we feel that when serum creatinine increases >30–50% over baseline, the doses of CsA should be reduced. If serum creatinine does not return to normal, the drug may be stopped for one month. Administration of CsA may be resumed when serum creatinine returns to normal or to values not exceeding 10% over baseline. If serum creatinine increases >75% over baseline, the drug should be stopped and resumed only after serum creatinine returns to baseline levels. With these precautions, CsA can be considered a safe drug that can be added to the available armamentarium for the treatment of several autoimmune diseases.

COMPETING INTERESTS. The author is an external consultant of Novartis Pharma, Italy.

REFERENCES

1. RENNIE, D. 1978. Home dialysis and the costs of uremia N. Engl. J. Med. **298:** 399–400.
2. CALNE, R. 2004. Cyclosporine as a milestone in immunosuppression Transplant. Proc. **36** (Suppl. 2S9)**:** 13S–15S.
3. CALNE, R.Y., K. ROLLES, D.J.G. WHITE, *et al.* 1978. Cyclosporin A initially as the only immunosuppressant in 34 recipients of cadaveric organs: 32 kidneys, 2 pancreas, and 2 livers. Lancet **2:** 1033–1036.
4. EUROPEAN MULTICENTRE TRIAL GROUP. 1983. Cyclosporin in cadaveric renal transplantation: one-year follow-up of a multicentre trial. Lancet **2:** 986–989.
5. CANADIAN MULTICENTER TRANSPLANT STUDY GROUP. 1983. A randomized clinical trial of cyclosporine in cadaveric renal transplantation N. Engl. J. Med. **309:** 809–815.
6. RUIZ-ORTEGA, M. & J. EGIDO. 1997. Angiotensin II modulates cell growth-related events and synthesis of matrix protein in renal interstitial fibroblasts. Kidney Int. **52:** 1497–1510.
7. CHANDER, V. & K. CHOPRA. 2005. Effect of molsidomine and l-arginine in cyclosporine nephrotoxicity: role of nitric oxide. Toxicology **207:** 463–474.
8. SCHERRER, U., S.F. VISSING, B.J. MORGAN, *et al.* 1990. Cyclosporine-induced sympathetic activation and hypertension after heart transplantation. N. Engl. J. Med. **323:** 693–699.
9. SMITH, S.R., E.A. CREECH, A.V. SCHAFFER, *et al.* 1992. Effects of thromboxane synthase inhibition with CGS 13080 in human cyclosporine nephrotoxicity Kidney Int. **41:** 199–205.
10. RAMIREZ, C., A. OLMO, F. O'VALLE, *et al.* 2000. Role of intrarenal endothelin 1, endothelin 3, and angiotensin II expression in chronic cyclosporin A nephrotoxicity in rats. Exp. Nephrol. **8:** 161–172.
11. XUE, H., R.D. BULOSKI, D.A. MC CARRON, *et al.* 1987. Induction of contraction in isolated rat aorta. Transplantation **43:** 715–718.
12. LUKE, R.G. 1991. Mechanism of cyclosporine-induced hypertension. Am. J. Hypertens. **4:** 468–471.
13. MIHATSCH, M.J., B. RYFFEL & F. GUDAT. 1995. The differential diagnosis between rejection and cyclosporine toxicity. Kidney Int. **48** (Suppl. 52)**:** S63–69.
14. MIHATSCH, M.J., K. MOROZUMI, E.H. STROM, *et al.* 1995. Renal transplant morphology after long-term therapy with cyclosporine. Transplant. Proc. **27:** 39–42.
15. MOROZUMI, K., A. TAKEDA, K. UCHIDA, *et al.* 2004. Cyclosporine nephrotoxicity how does it affect renal allograft function and transplant morphology? Transplant. Proc. **36** (Suppl. 2)**:** 216–256.
16. BENNETT, W.M., A. DE MATTOS, M.M. MEYER, *et al.* 1996. Chronic cyclosporine nephropathy: the Achille's heel of immunosuppressive therapy. Kidney Int. **50:** 1089–1100.
17. OPELZ, G. & B. DOHLER. 2001. Cyclosporine and long-term kidney graft survival. Transplantation **72:** 1267–1273.
18. THERVET, E., E. MORELON, D. DUCLOUX, *et al.* 2000. Cyclosporine withdrawal in stable renal transplant recipients after azathioprine-mycophenolate mofetil conversion. Clin. Transplant. **14:** 561–566.
19. PONTICELLI, C., G. CIVATI, A. TARANTINO, *et al.* 1996. Randomized study with cyclosporine in kidney transplantation: 10 year follow-up. J. Am. Soc. Nephrol. **7:** 792–797.
20. LINDHOLM, A. & B.D. KAHAN. 1993. Influence of cyclosporine pharmacokinetics through concentrations and AUC monitoring on outcome after kidney transplantation. Clin. Pharmacol. & Ther. **54:** 205–218.
21. MUELLER, E.A., J.M. KOVARIK, J.B. VAN BREE, *et al.* 1991. Improved dose linearity of cyclosporine pharmacokinetics from a microemulsion formulation. Pharm. Res. **11:** 301–304.
22. KOVARIK, J.M., E.A. MUELLER, J.B. VAN BREE, *et al.* 1994.Reduced inter- and intraindividual variability in cyclosporine pharmacokinetics from a microemulsion formulation J. Pharmacol. Sci. **83:** 444–446

23. SHAH, M.B., J.E. MARTIN, T.J. SCHROEDER, *et al.* 1999. A meta-analysis to assess the safety and tolerability of two formulations of cyclosporine: Sandimmune and Neoral. Transplant. Proc. **8:** 4048–4053.
24. MEIER-KRIESCHE, H.U. & B. KAPLAN. 2002. Cyclosporine microemulsion and tacrolimus are associated with decreased chronic allograft failure and improved long-term graft survival as compared with sandimmune. Am. J. Transplant. **2:** 100–104.
25. WOLFE, R.A., V.B. ASHBY, E.L. MILFORD, *et al.* 1999. Comparison of mortality in all patients on dialysis, patients on dialysis awaiting transplantation, and recipients of a first cadaveric transplant N. Engl. J. Med. **341:** 1725–1730.
26. HARIHARAN, S., C.P. JOHNSON, B.A. BRESNAHAN, *et al.* 2000. Improved graft survival after renal transplantation in the United States. N. Engl. J. Med. **342:** 605–612.
27. PONTICELLI, C., M. VILLA, B. CESANA, *et al.* 2002. Risk factors for late kidney allograft failure. Kidney Int. **62:** 1848–1852.
28. PONTICELLI, C., A. AROLDI, A. ELLI, *et al.* 1999. The clinical status of cadaveric renal transplant patients treated for 10 years with cyclosporine therapy. Clin. Transplant. **4:** 324–329.
29. LEVY, G.A. 2004. Neoral C2 monitoring in solid organ transplantation. Transplant. Proc. **36** (Suppl. 2)**:** 392S–395S.
30. DI PAOLO, S., A. TEUTONICO, A. SCHENA, *et al.* 2004. Conversion to C2 monitoring of cyclosporine A exposure in maintenance kidney transplant recipients: results at 3 years. Am. J. Kidney Dis. **44:** 886–892.
31. NANKIVELL, B.J., R.J. BORROWS, C.L. FUNG, *et al.* 2004. Calcineurin inhibitor nephrotoxicity: longitudinal assessment by protocol histology. Transplantation **78:** 557–565.
32. KEOWN, P. 2004. Composite outcomes in renal transplantation using cyclosporine. Transplant. Proc. **36** (Supp.l 2)**:** 35S–39S.
33. PONTICELLI, C. 2001. Steroid free immunosuppression. Transplant. Proc. **33:** 3259–3260.
34. PASCUAL, M., T. THERUVATH, T. KAWAI, *et al.* 2002. Strategies to improve long-term outcomes after renal transplantation. N. Engl. J. Med. **346:** 580–590.
35. KAHAN, B.D. & C. PONTICELLI. 2000. Immunosuppressive drugs: molecular and cellular mechanisms of action. *In* Principles and Practice of Renal Transplantation. B.D. Kahan and C. Ponticelli, Eds.: 315–345. Martin Dunitz. London.
36. GRIFFITHS, C.E., L. DUBERTRET, C.N. ELLIS, *et al.* 2004. Ciclosporin in psoriasis clinical practice: an international consensus statement. Br. J. Dermatol. **150** (Suppl. 67)**:** 11–23.
37. BUNIKOWSKI, R., D. STAAB, F. KUSSELEI, *et al.* 2004. Low-dose cyclosporine A microemulsion in children with severe atopic dermatitis. Clinical and immunological effects. Pediatr. Allergy Immunol. **4:** 216–223.
38. GREMESE, E. & G.F. FERRACCIOLI. 2004. Benefit/risk of cyclosporine in rheumatoid arthritis. Clin. Exp. Rheumatol. **5** (Suppl. 35)**:** 101–107.
39. SONG, J. Systemic management of posterior uveitis. 2003. J. Ocul. Pharmacol. Ther. **19:** 325–343.
40. WALLACE, D.J. 2002. Management of lupus erythematosus: recent insights. Curr. Opin. Rheumatol. **3:** 212–219.
41. VOTE, B.J., A. HALL, J. CAIRNS, *et al.* 2004. Changing trends in sympathetic ophtalmia. Clin. Exp. Ophtalmol. **32:** 545–545.
42. PONTICELLI, C. & P. PASSERINI. 1999. The place of cyclosporine in the management of primary nephrotic syndrome. Biodrugs **12:** 327–341.
43. PALESTINE, A.G., H.A. AUSTIN, III, J.E. BALOW, *et al.* 1986. Renal histopathologic alterations in patients treated with cyclosporine for uveitis. N. Engl. J. Med. **314:** 1293–1298.
44. ZACHARIE, H., K. KRAGBALLE, H.E. HANSEN, *et al.* 1997. Renal biopsy findings in long-term cyclosporine treatment of psoriasis. Br. J. Dermatol. **136:** 531–535.
45. FEUTREN, G. & M.J. MIHATSCH. 1992. Risk factors for cyclosporine-induced nephropathy in patients with autoimmune diseases. N. Engl. J. Med. **326:** 1654–1660.
46. RODRIGUEZ, F., J.C. KRAYENBUHL, W.B. HARRISON, *et al.* 1996. Renal biopsy findings and followup of renal function in rheumatoid arthritis patients treated with cyclosporine A. An update from the International Kidney Biopsy Registry. Arthritis Rheum. **39:** 1491–1498.
47. PONTICELLI, C. 2004. Renal transplantation. Where do we stand today? Nephrol. Dial. Transplant. **12:** 2937–2947.

Autoimmunity and Anti–TNF-α Agents

FABIOLA ATZENI,[a] MAURIZIO TURIEL,[b] FRANCO CAPSONI,[c] ANDREA DORIA,[d] PIERLUIGI MERONI,[e] AND PIERCARLO SARZI-PUTTINI[a]

[a]*Rheumatology Unit, Department of Rheumatology, L Sacco University Hospital, 20157 Milan, Italy*

[b]*Cardiology Unit, Istituto Galeazzi, Milan, Italy*

[c]*Department of Internal Medicine, Ospedale Maggiore Policlinico, IRCCS, University of Milan, Milan, Italy*

[d]*Chair of Rheumatology, University of Padua, Padua, Italy*

[e]*Allergy, Clinical Immunology and Rheumatology Unit, Department of Internal Medicine, University of Milan, IRCCS Istituto Auxologico Italiano, Milan, Italy*

ABSTRACT: **Treatment of rheumatoid arthritis (RA) patients with anti-tumor necrosis factor-alpha (anti–TNF-α) biologic agents has been associated with a reduction in the levels of specific autoantibodies, such as rheumatoid factor (RF) and anticyclic citrullinated peptide (anti-CCP), and the induction of non-organ-specific autoantibodies (antinuclear antibodies [ANAs], anti-dsDNA, and antiphospholipid antibodies [aPLs]). The mechanisms by which the blockade of anti–TNF-α decreases the generation of specific autoantibodies, such as anti-CCP and RF, are not yet known. However, it has been shown that these agents can downregulate the production of several inflammatory cytokines and mediators and that these anti-inflammatory effects may account for reduced autoantibody generation, particularly in the synovial compartment. Infliximab treatment leads to the induction of ANAs in 63.8% of RA patients and 49.1% of Crohn's disease (CD) patients, and anti-dsDNA antibodies in 13% of RA patients and 21.5% of CD patients, respectively. The development of ANAs and anti-dsDNA antibodies has also been described after etanercept therapy in 11% and 15% of RA patients, respectively. In the controlled trials, increases in ANA and anti-dsDNA titers were observed in 5.3% and in 12.9% of adalimumab-treated RA patients. Only limited data on the induction of aPL antibodies during TNF-α blocking treatment are available.**

KEYWORDS: **infliximab; etanercept; adalimumab; autoantibodies; rheumatoid factor; anticyclic citrullinated peptide antibodies (anti-CCP); autoimmunity**

INTRODUCTION

Treatment with biologic agents directed against anti-tumor necrosis factor-alpha (TNF-α), such as infliximab, etanercept, and adalimumab, has significant clinical

Address for correspondence: Piercarlo Sarzi-Puttini, M.D., Rheumatology Unit-University Hospital L Sacco, Via GB Grassi, 74, 20157 Milan, Italy. Voice: +39-02-39042208; fax: +39-02-39043454.
sarzi@tiscali.it

Ann. N.Y. Acad. Sci. 1051: 559–569 (2005).
doi: 10.1196/annals.1361.100

TABLE 1. Pharmacologic characteristics of TNF-α inhibitors

Pharmacologic characteristic	Infliximab	Etanercept	Adalimumab
Half-life	8–10 days	3–5.5 days	14 days
Binding affinity	1.8×10^9	10^{10}	2.3×10^{10}
Target binding	TNF	TNF, lymphotoxin	TNF
Structure	chimeric mAb	TNF receptor-IgG1 fusion protein	Human mAb
Complement	+	–	+
Cell lysis cytotoxicity	+	–	+
Administration and dose	i.v. 4–8 q wk 3–10 mg/kg	s.c. 2 q wk 25 mg	s.c. 2 q mo 40 mg

benefits in inflammatory diseases such as Crohn's disease (CD), ankylosing spondylitis (AS), rheumatoid arthritis (RA), and a variety of autoimmune and non-autoimmune diseases.[1–3]

Infliximab

Infliximab, a recombinant chimeric antibody produced by mouse myeloma cells (TABLE 1), contains sequences from human IgG1 constant and mouse variable regions, is specific for the membrane-bound or secreted or extracellular space TNF-α of humans and chimpanzees,[3–8] and prevents TNF from binding to its membranous and soluble receptors. After initial parenteral administration, its serum half-life is approximately 8.9 days and is maintained by dosing every 8 weeks thereafter. Its intravenous administration ensures that maximum serum concentrations are reached within 1 hour. Multiple clinical studies have confirmed that 30 weeks of treatment lead to a 20% improvement in the American College of Rheumatology (ACR) score in more than 50% of patients with active RA as against only 20% of patients treated with placebo.[9] The same effect is generally maintained after 54 weeks.[10–13]

Infliximab is registered by the Food and Drug Administration (FDA) and the European Medicines Evaluation Agency (EMEA) as therapy for treatment-resistant RA, treatment-resistant moderate to severe CD, and CD with fistulas.[8,10–14] Recently, its efficacy was demonstrated in seronegative spondyloarthritis (SS).[15,16]

Etanercept

Etanercept , a fusion protein (decoy receptor) secreted by Chinese ovary (CHO) cells, combines the ligand binding portion of human TNF receptor 2 (TNFR2=p75=CD120b) with sequences of human IgG1 (TABLE 1). Unlike TNFR1 (p55=CD120a), TNFR2 is a constitutive membrane receptor that is inducible upon stimulation and can be found on the surface of almost all cells except red blood cells and resting lymphocytes.[4] Because its affinity for TNF-α is greater than that for TNFR1, it can capture the cytokine more easily. Inasmuch as active TNFR2 is a trimer, the recombinant decoy receptor need not be a monomer to reach the required bioactivity in competing with natural receptors.[3,4,17] Etanercept is administered twice weekly in 25-mg subcutaneous injections, its median half-life in serum is 4.8 days, and its maximum concentration is reached within 3 days. A 20% improvement in the ACR score was achieved in 60–75% of RA patients on 12 weeks of etanercept therapy as against 14–33 % of those on placebo.[17–21] Reports suggest that the benefit of etanercept treatment is maintained for years.

Etanercept is approved by the FDA and the EMEA for use in treatment-resistant RA as well as for severe active and progressive RA and treatment-resistant polyarticular juvenile chronic arthritis. It is also approved by the FDA for treatment-resistant psoriatic arthritis,[17–20,22,23] and it has a beneficial effect in AS.[24,25]

Adalimumab

Adalimumab is a recombinant human immunoglobulin G1 monoclonal antibody that is specific for human TNF. It specifically binds to circulating and cell surface TNF-α and blocks its interaction with p55 and p75 cell surface TNF receptors[26] (TABLE 1).

The first fully human anti–TNF-α monoclonal antibody, it was approved for the treatment of moderate to severe RA by the FDA in 2002 and by the EMEA in September 2003.[27,28] The standard dose is 40 mg subcutaneously every other week, and the drug can be used alone or in combination with disease-modifying antirheumatic drugs (DMARDs) such as methotrexate (MTX).[26] After a single 40-mg subcutaneous dose to a healthy adult, it reaches a maximum serum concentration of 4.7 ± 1.6 g/ml within 131 ± 5 hours. The average absolute bioavailability of adalimumab, estimated from three studies, is 64%. Population pharmacokinetic analyses have revealed a trend towards a greater apparent clearance in the presence of anti-adalimumab antibodies and a lower clearance with increasing age in patients 40 to >75 years. A 20% improvement in ACR score was achieved in 67% of RA patients on 12 weeks of adalimumab in the ReaAct Trial and a moderate European League Against Rheumatism (Eular) response in 81%.[29,30]

TOXICITY PROFILE AND AUTOIMMUNITY

The safety issues relating to all current TNF antagonists are infections (including *Mycobacterium tuberculosis* and other opportunistic infections), demyelinating dis-

TABLE 2. Serious adverse events correlate with anti-TNF agents

Adverse events	Refs.
Infections (sepsis, mainly candida, aspergillus, cytomegalovirus, cryptococcus, mycobacterium)	31,32,26
Hematology (anemia, neutropenia, lymphoma)	31,32,26
Neurology (demyelination)	31,32,26
Bone-muscle-connective tissue (lupus-like syndrome)	31,32,26,47–49
Anti-infliximab antibodies and infusion/injection reaction	31,32,26,39

TABLE 3. Effects on immunogenicity of biologic agents: review of the literature

Authors	Year	Anti-TNF agent	Pts (n)	ANA (%)	Anti–ds-DNA (%)	aCl (%)	Refs.
Charles *et al.*	2000	Infliximab	156	–	5-7	–	42
Antivalle *et al.*	2002	Infliximab	91	54.9	20.9	–	45
Ferraccioli *et al.*	2002	Etanercept	8	–	–	62.5 (post-infections)	64
De Richie *et al.*	2003	Infliximab	62	82.3	16.7	–	43
Jonsdottir *et al.*	2004	Infliximab Etanercept	67 57	–	–	28 25	65
Ferrero *et al.*	2004	Infliximab	24			87.5	54
Bobbio-Pallavicini *et al.*	2004	Infliximab	30	80	3.3	6.7	35
Allanore *et al.*	2004	Infliximab	59	63.8	32	–	46
Keystone *et al.*	2004	Adalimumab	–	12.9	5.3	–	26
Atzeni *et al.*	In press	Adalimumab	57	28	3.5	1.7	37

orders, autoimmune syndromes (i.e., systemic lupus erythematosus), congestive heart failure, and administrative reactions[26,31,32] (TABLE 2).

Antibody formation can follow the administration of biologic agents such as the TNF antagonists including the development of neutralizing and non-neutralizing antibodies[4,26,33] (TABLE 3).

Rheumatoid Factor and Anticyclic Citrullinated Peptide

Specific autoantibodies such as rheumatoid factor (RF) and anticyclic citrullinated peptide (CCP) are related to the severity of the rheumatoid process and could be reduced by effective TNF-α–blocking agents.[34]

Bobbio-Pallavicini *et al.*[35] found a significant decrease in the titers of both anti-CCP antibodies and RF after 30 weeks of infliximab therapy, which suggests that serial evaluations of these antibodies may be useful in monitoring the clinical course of RA patients undergoing treatment with infliximab. However, they observed a different evolution of RF and anti-CCP antibody titers during long-term therapy: after 54 and 78 weeks, there was a progressive decrease with the former but not the latter despite the persistence of clinical improvement indicated by DAS 28.[35] Alessandri *et al.*[36] reported that infliximab treatment led to a decrease in the serum titers of RF and anti-CCP antibodies in RA patients showing improvement, suggesting that these measurements may be a useful adjunct in assessing treatment efficacy. In a study of 57 patients with RA,[37] we found that 46 (80.7%) were positive for anti-CCP antibodies at baseline, and 43 (75%) were positive for RF. Although none of these patients became negative after adalimumab treatment, the serum titer of anti-CCP antibodies and RF decreased significantly after 12 months of treatment ($P < .001$ for both). When the patients were grouped on the basis of their clinical response, a significant decrease in serum levels of anti-CCP antibody and RF was observed only in those who showed clinical improvement according to ACR 20 and ACR 50 criteria (both $P < .001$) (data submitted for publication).[9,37]

The mechanisms by which the infliximab-induced blockade of anti–TNF-α decreases the generation of specific autoantibodies such as anti-CCP and RF are not yet known; however, it has been shown that infliximab can downregulate the production of several inflammatory cytokines and mediators and that these anti-inflammatory effects may account for reduced autoantibody generation, particularly in the synovial compartment.[38]

Citrullination represents a post-translational modification of proteins involved in apoptosis. As citrullinated fibrin is one of the major citrullanated proteins in rheumatoid synovium, it is an important antigenic target of anti-fillaggrin antibodies.[38] Anti–TNF-α treatment can modulate apoptotic processes (as in inflammatory bowel disease), so that regulation of apoptosis after TNF-α blockade may at least partially explain this observation.[38]

Neutralizing Antibodies

Infliximab therapy can lead to the formation of anti-infliximab antibodies[32,39] whose presence was associated with infusion reactions in 6.9–19% of patients. Infusion reactions are important immunologic events induced by the presence of substantial serum concentrations of such antibodies.[31,32,39] Thereafter, infliximab rapidly disappears from the serum and becomes undetectable within 4 weeks. Once an infusion reaction has occurred, the duration of the response to subsequent infusions decreases, but, although the relation between the duration of response and infliximab concentrations was clear, it was no stronger than the correlation with antibody concentrations. As antibodies develop soon after the initial infusion in most patients, Baert *et al.*[39] believe that immunosuppressive therapy should be started before the administration of infliximab to prevent antibody formation and improve the duration of the drug response; however, concomitant treatment with immunomodulators in ACCENT I (a Crohn's disease clinical trial evaluating infliximab in a new long-term treatment regimen) did not substantially increase the benefit of the three-dose induction regimen and 8-week maintenance therapy.[40]

It remains to be established whether any of the immunosuppressive agents (azathioprine, mercaptopurine, or MTX) provides greater protection against immunogenicity than the others. A drug interaction between MTX and infliximab has been proposed because, although maximum serum infliximab levels remain the same with or without concomitant MTX therapy, one study found that the rate of disappearance of infliximab was slower among patients taking MTX than among those receiving infliximab alone.[41]

In conclusion, it is clear that immunosuppressive treatment prevents the formation of antibodies against infliximab, thus reducing the incidence of infusion reactions and increasing the duration of response. When necessary, anti-TNF therapy can temporarily be discontinued and restarted without the loss of a clinical response or an increased risk of anaphylaxis or immunologic reaction.

Adalimumab. As might be expected with infusion of any immunoglobulin, a proportion of patients develop human anti-idiotypic antibodies specific for adalimumab that, in clinical trials, have been observed in 12% of patients receiving monotherapy and 1% of those receiving combination therapy with MTX.[26,28] These antibodies probably account for the somewhat lower ACR responses observed in the monotherapy study; a significantly better response was observed with adalimumab 40 mg weekly, and it is estimated that 5–15% of patients may require weekly doses while receiving monotherapy.[26,28] There is no evidence that weekly adalimumab dosing may be beneficial in patients receiving concomitant MTX therapy or that the anti-idiotypic antibodies affect the safety profile of adalimumab.

Antinuclear, Anti-dsDNA Antibodies, and Lupus-Like Syndrome

Infliximab treatment has led to the induction of ANAs in 63.8% of RA patients and 49.1% of CD patients and to anti-dsDNA antibodies in 13% of RA patients and 21.5% of CD patients, respectively.[33,42–46] The development of ANAs and anti-dsDNA antibodies has also been described after etanercept therapy in 11% and 15% of RA patients, respectively.[33] Clinical studies of the effect of adalimumab in RA have reported the appearance of autoantibodies, including ANAs (12.9%) and anti–dsDNA antibodies (5.3%),[26] and one case of a lupus-like syndrome in which serositis and arthritis resolved upon discontinuation of therapy.[26] We[37] found that 4 of 57 adalimumab-treated RA patients (7.2%) and 5 of 55 MTX-treated patients with RA (9%) were ANA positive at baseline; after 12 months of therapy, ANA induction was observed in 12 adalimumab-treated RA patients and 6 MTX-treated RA patients, with the total number of ANA-positive patients being 16 (28%) in the adalimumab group and 8 (14.5%) in the control group. The difference in ANA positivity before and after follow-up was statistically significant only in the adalimumab group ($P <.001$), and the difference in induction between the two treatment groups was also significant ($P <.001$) (data in press). However, despite the development of ANAs and anti-dsDNA antibodies in a fairly high proportion of patients during anti–TNF-α therapy, the incidence of possible lupus-like syndromes was low. Some cases of lupus-like symptoms (with or without autoantibodies) in patients receiving infliximab or etanercept treatment have been reported, but it is difficult to determine whether they were related to anti–TNF-α treatment, the underlying disease, or other concomitant drugs or whether they occurred coincidentally.[47–49] The identification of drug-induced SLE in RA patients is especially difficult because of overlaps between the two diseases. Charles *et al.*[42] described the induction of anti-dsDNA antibodies in 7% of RA patients treated with infliximab (with or without MTX therapy) and noted that their isotypes differed from those of IgG. De Rychie *et al.*[43] confirmed the high prevalence of ANAs and anti-dsDNA antibodies in RA patients after infliximab treatment. Moreover, increased ANA titers and induction of anti-dsDNA antibodies are more pronounced in SA than in RA.[43] However, ANAs may be more likely in untreated RA that in untreated SA, and the absence of associated MTX therapy in SA may contribute to the observed differences. Of interest is the observation by Boehm *et al.*[50] that MTX therapy can lead to a decrease in circulating autoantibodies in patients with cutaneous lupus.The diagnostic and prognostic value of anti-dsDNA antibodies remains controversial, because lupus-associated anti-dsDNA antibodies are classically of the IgG isotype, whereas IgM or IgA anti-dsDNA antibodies may occur in other diseases as well (mixed connective tissue disease, primary Sjögren's syndrome, scleroderma, RA, AS, chronic active hepatitis, and primary biliary cirrhosis).[42,51] Other ANA reactivities have not been systematically studied in relation to infliximab therapy. One study found an increase in the number of patients with antinucleosome antibodies before and after infliximab treatment, but this was not statistically significant.[52,53] Antihistone antibodies are particularly common in SLE and drug-induced lupus (with respective sensitivities of 50–70% and 90–95%), but they may also occur in other diseases (RA, juvenile chronic arthritis, autoimmune chronic hepatitis, and chronic infection) or even in healthy controls.[53] Some infliximab-treated patients with RA or SA have shown the newly developed antihistone antibodies.[43,54]

Mechanism of Antinuclear and Anti-DNA Antibody Induction

Autoantibody induction may be a predictable consequence of anti–TNF-α blockade, which could promote humoral autoimmunity by inhibiting the induction of the cytotoxic T-lymphocyte response that normally suppresses autoreactive B cells.[55] Infliximab may also neutralize the biologic activity of TNF-α by binding the soluble forms and thus preventing its interaction with its p55 and p75 cell receptors. Infliximab also binds the transmembrane form of TNF-α and could induce antibody or complement-dependent cytotoxicity in the cells expressing it. Furthermore, it increases the number of apoptotic T lymphocytes in the lamina propria and apoptotic monocytes in peripheral blood in Crohn's disease.[55,56] In this case, one hypothesis concerning the development of autoimmune diseases such as SLE is that increased apoptosis may promote the release of numerous autoantigens, thus leading to the development of autoantibodies against cytoplasmic and nuclear compounds such as ANA and dsDNA, especially if their production is no longer suppressed by the action of infliximab on the suppressor T-cell population.[56] This process may not occur in organ-specific cells such as thyrocytes, because they do not harbor TNF-α receptors, which may partially explain the absence of organ-specific autoantibodies associated with autoimmune vasculitis, hepatitis, or endocrine diseases. Charles *et al.*[42] and Ferrero *et al.*[54] demonstrated that most of the anti-dsDNA autoantibodies detected during the treatment of RA were of the IgM isotype. Furthermore, Ferrero *et al.*[54] showed that most of the detected aPL autoantibodies were also of IgM isotype. The role of IgM in the development of autoimmune diseases remains to be elucidated, but natural autoreactive IgM autoantibodies may suppress autoimmunity by inducing B-cell tolerance and thus participating in the negative selection of autoreactive B cells. The larger pool of autoantibodies of the IgM isotype observed during infliximab treatment could be due to a higher production of natural autoreactive IgM, but it may also be an induced population that can further switch to IgG with a well-known pathogenic effect.[42,54] The high frequency of IgM may also be caused by TNF blockade, as demonstrated in a murine model of collagen-induced arthritis in which anti–TNF-α monoclonal antibodies reduced isotype switching to IgG in the local draining lymph node.[57]

Antiphospholipid Autoantibodies

Antiphospholipid (but not aCL) autoantibodies are found in 2–6% of healthy blood donors and up to 12% in an aging population.[58] In RA patients, aCLs have been found at even higher frequencies.[59] aCL antibodies associated with recurrent thromboembolic disease and fetal loss, but their clinical significance in RA is uncertain and their presence has been considered a nonspecific marker of activation of the immune system.[60,61] Only limited data on the induction of aPL antibodies during TNF-α blocking treatment have been reported. Elliott *et al.*[62] found aCL antibodies (cA2) in 1 of 20 RA patients treated with anti–TNF-α in an 8-week open trial. Rankin *et al.*[63] measured the serologic effects of repeated doses of the humanized anti–TNF-α antibody CDP 571 in patients with RA and found that some develop positive aCL (IgG). Ferraccioli *et al.*[64] showed variations in aCL titers over time in etanercept-treated patients with concomitant bacterial infection in whom reduced titers were seen after treatment with antibiotics. In a recent paper, Jonsdottir *et al.*[65] described a correlation between treatment with TNF-α antagonists (infliximab and etanercept), the appearance of aCL antibodies, and a worse clinical outcome; however, two other studies did not confirm the association between aCL antibodies and clinical outcome. We[37] found that none of 57 RA patients before adalimumab treatment and none of 55 MTX-treated RA patients was positive for aCL or anti–β-$_2$GPI autoantibodies at baseline, and after 12 months, aCL levels were not significantly different between both groups (2 of 57 vs. 2 of 55) (data in press).

CONCLUSIONS

This review indicates that anti-TNF agents induced a decrease in RF and anti-CCP levels and an increase in the production of neutralizing and non-neutralizing autoantibodies. The possible mechanisms underlying these phenomena and their correlation with clinical manifestations remain to be elucidated. Although the fact that the production of ANAs and anti-dsDNA antibodies does not correlate with clinical features suggestive of autoimmune diseases is reassuring in terms of treatment safety, longer-term observational studies of anti-dsDNA–positive patients are essential and the mechanism of anti-dsDNA antibodies by anti–TNF-α therapy must still be clarified.

REFERENCES

1. Skapenko, A., J.R. Kalden & H. Schulze-Koops. 2001. Treatment of rheumatoid arthritis in the third millennium. Scand. J. Rheumatol. **30:** 249–254.
2. McLain, D.A. 2001. Rheumatoid arthritis: update on new therapies. South Med. J. **94:** 893–895.
3. Calabrese, L.H. 2003. Molecular differences in anticytokine therapies. Clin. Exp. Rheumatol. **21:** 241–248.
4. Bencsath, M., A. Blaskovits & J. Borvendeg. 2003. Biomolecular cytokine therapy. Pathol. Onc. Res. **9:** 25–29.
5. Sharma, P.K., D. Hota & P. Pandhi. 2004. Biologics in rheumatoid arthritis. Japi **52:** 231–236.
6. Feldmann, M., F.M. Brennan & R.N. Maini. 1996. Role of cytokines in rheumatoid arthritis. Ann. Rev. Immunol. **14:** 397–440.
7. Vassalli, P. 1987. The pathophysiology of tumor necrosis factors. N. Engl. J. Med. **316:** 379–385.
8. Elliott, M.J., R.N. Maini & M. Feldmann. 1994. Randomized double-blind comparison of chimeric monoclonal antibody tumor necrosis factor alpha (cA2) versus placebo in rheumatoid arthritis. Lancet **344:** 1105–1110.
9. Felson, D.T., J.J. Anderson, M. Boers, *et al.* 1993. The American College preliminary core set of disease activity measures for rheumatoid arthritis clinical trials. Arthritis Rheum. **36:** 729–740.

10. Kavanaugh, A., E.W. St, Clair, W.J. McCune, *et al.* 2000. Chimeric anti-tumor necrosis factor-alpha monoclonal antibody treatment of patients with rheumatoid arthritis receiving methotrexate therapy. J. Rheumatol. **27:** 841–850.
11. Maini, R., E.W. St. Clair, F. Breedveld, *et al.* 1999. Infliximab versus placebo in rheumatoid arthritis patients receiving concomitant methotrexate: a randomised phase III trial. Lancet **354:** 1932–1939.
12. Lipsky, P.E., D.M. van de Heijde, E.W. St. Clair, *et al.* 2000. 102-week clinical and radiological results from the ATTRACT trial: a 2 year, randomized, controlled, phase 3 trial of infliximab in patients with active RA despite MTX. Arthritis Rheum. **43:** abstr. 269.
13. Lipsky, P.E., D.M. Van der Heijde, E.W. St. Clair, *et al.* 2000. Infliximab and methotrexate in the treatment of rheumatoid arthritis. Anti-Tumor Necrosis Factor Trial in Rheumatoid Arthritis with Concomitant Therapy Study Group. N. Engl. J. Med. **343:** 1594–1602.
14. Present, D.H., P. Rutgeerts, S. Targan, *et al.* 1999. Infliximab for the treatment of fistulas in patients with Crohn's disease. N. Engl. J. Med. **340:** 1398–1405.
15. Brandt, J., H. Haibel, D. Cornely, *et al.* 2000. Successful treatment of active ankylosing spondylitis with the anti-tumor necrosis factor alpha monoclonal antibody infliximab. Arthritis Rheum. **43:** 1346–1352.
16. Braun, J., J. Brandt, J. Listing, *et al.* 2002. Treatment of active ankylosing spondylitis with infliximab: a randomised controlled multicentre trial. Lancet **359:** 1187–1193.
17. Moreland, L.W., G. Margolies, L.W. Heck, *et al.* 1996. Recombinant solubile tumor necrosis factor receptor (p80) fusion protein: toxicity and dose finding trial in refractory rheumatoid arthritis. J. Rheumatol. **23:** 1849–1855.
18. Moreland, L.W., S.B. Cohen, S.W. Baumgartner, *et al.* 2001. Long-term safety and efficacy of etanercept in patients with rheumatoid arthritis. J. Rheumatol. **28:** 1238–1244.
19. Moreland, L.W., M.H. Schiff, S.W. Baumgartner, *et al.* 1999. Etanercept therapy in rheumatoid arthritis. A randomized controlled trial. Ann. Intern. Med. **130:** 478–486.
20. Martin, R., E. Ruderman, R. Fleischmann, *et al.* 2000. A phase III trial of etanercept vs methotrexate (MTX) in early rheumatoid arthritis. Ann. Rheum. Dis. **59:** 48.
21. Genovese, M.C., J.M. Bathon, R.W. Martin, *et al.* 2002. Etanercept vs methotrexate in patients with early rheumatoid arthritis: two-year radiography and clinical outcomes. Arthritis Rheum. **46:** 1443–1450.
22. Kietz, D.A., P.H. Pepmueller & T.L.Moore. 2001. Clinical response to etanercept in polyarticular course juvenil arthritis. J. Rheumatol. **28:** 360–362.
23. Mease, P.J., B.S. Goffe, J. Metz, *et al.* 2000. Etanercept in the treatment of psoriatic arthritis and psoriasis: a randomised trial. Lancet **356:** 385–390.
24. Brandt, J., J. Listing, J. Sieper, *et al.* 2004. Development and presentation of criteria for short term improvement after TNF alpha treatment in ankylosing spondylitis. Ann. Rheum. Dis. **63:** 1438–1444.
25. Mease, P.J. 2003. Disease-modifying anthireumatic drugs therapy for spondyloarthropathies: advances in treatment. Curr. Opin. Rheumatol. **15:** 12–25.
26. Keystone, E. & B. Haraoui. 2004. Adalimumab therapy in rheumatoid arthritis. Rheum. Dis. Clin. N. Am. **30:** 349–364.
27. Weinblatt, M.E., E.C. Keystone, D.E. Furst, *et al.* 2003. Adalimumab, a fully human antitumor necrosis factor–monoclonal antibody, for the treatment of rheumatoid arthritis in patients taking concomitant methotrexate. The ARMADA trial. Arthritis Rheum. **48:** 35–39.
28. Furst, D.E., E. Schiff, R. Fleischman, *et al.* 2002. Safety and efficacy of adalimumab, a fully human anti-TNF-α monoclonal antibody, given in combination with stardard antirheumatic therapy: safety trial of adalimumab in rheumatoid arthritis (STAR). Arthritis Rheum. **46:** S572.
29. Van Gestel, A.M., M.L. Prevoo, T. Van Hofma, *et al.* 1996. Development and validation of the European League Against Rheumatism response criteria for rheumatoid arthritis. Comparison with preliminary American College of Rheumatology and World Health Organization/International League Against Rheumatism criteria. Arthritis Rheum. **39:** 34–40.

30. BOMBARDIERI, S., A.G. TZIOUFAS, F. MCKENNA, *et al.* 2004. Efficacy evaluation of adalimumab (Humira) in patients with a single and multiple prior biologics in the ReAct Trial. Arthritis Rheum. **50** (suppl.9): abstr. 365.
31. DAY, R. 2002. Adverse reactions to TNF-alpha inhibitors in rheumatoid arthritis. Lancet **359:** 540–541.
32. ANTONI, C. & J. BRAUN. 2002. Side effects of anti-TNF therapy: current knowledge. Clin. Exp. Rheumatol. **20:** 152–157.
33. ZIOLKOWSKA, M. & W. MASLINSKI. 2003. Laboratory changes on anti-tumor necrosis factor treatment in rheumatoid arthritis. Curr. Opin. Rheumatol. **15:** 267–273.
34. MEYER, O., C. LABARRE, M. DOUGADOS, *et al.* 2003. Anticitrullinated peptide antibody assays in early rheumatoid arthritis for predicting five years radiographic damage. Ann. Rheum. Dis. **42:** 677–680.
35. BOBBIO-PALLAVICINI, F., C. ALPINI, R. CAPORALI, *et al.* 2004. Autoantibody profile in rheumatoid arthritis during long-term inflimab treatment. Arthritis Res. Ther. **6:** 264–272.
36. ALESSANDRI, C., M. BOMBARDIERI, N. DEL PAPA, *et al.* 2004. Decrease of anti-cyclic citrullinated peptide antibodies and rheumatoid factor following ant-TNF therapy (infliximab) in rheumatoid arthritis is associated with clinical improvement. Ann. Rheum. Dis. **63:** 1218–1221.
37. ATZENI, F., P. SARZI-PUTTINI, D. DELL'ACQUA, *et al.* 2005. Adalimumab clinical efficacy is associated with rheumatoid factor and anti-cyclic citrullinated peptide antibody titre reduction and anti-nuclear antibody appearance: a one year prospective study. Submitted for publication.
38. REPARON-SCHIJT, C.C., W.J. VAN ESCH, C. VAN KOOTEN, *et al.* 1988. Functional analysis of rheumatoid factor-producing B cells from the synovial fluid of rheumatoid arthritis patients. Arthritis Rheum. **41:** 2211–2220.
39. BAERT, F., M. NOMAN, S. VERMEIRE, *et al.* 2003. Influence of immunogenicity on the long-term efficacy of Infliximab in Crohn's disease. N. Engl. J. Med. **348:** 601–608.
40. HANAUER, S.B., B.G. FEAGAN, G.R. LICHTENSTEIN, *et al.* 2002. Maintenance infliximab for Crohn's disease: the ACCENT I randomised trial. Lancet **359:** 1541–1549.
41. MAINI, R.N., F.C. BREEDVELD, J.R. KALDEN, *et al.* 1988. Therapeutic efficacy of multiple intravenous infusions of anti-tumor necrosis factor alpha monoclonal antibody combined with low-dose weekly methotrexate in rheumatoid arthritis. Arthritis Rheum. **41:** 1552–1563.
42. CHARLES, P.J., R.J. SMEENK, J. DE JONG, *et al.* 2000. Assessment of antibodies to double-stranded DNA induced in rheumatoid arthritis patients following treatment with infliximab, a monoclonal antibody to tumor necrosis factor alpha: findings in open-label and randomized placebo-controlled trials. Arthritis Rheum. **43:** 2383–2390.
43. DE RYCKE, L., E. KRUITHOF, N. VAN DAMME, *et al.* 2003. Antinuclear antibodies following infliximab treatment in patients with rheumatoid arthritis or spondylarthropathy. Arthritis Rheum. **48:** 1015–1023.
44. VERMEIRE, S., M. NOMAN, G. VAN ASSCHE, *et al.* 2003. Autoimmunity associated with anti-tumor necrosis factor alpha treatment in Crohn's disease: a prospective cohort study. Gastroenterology **125:** 32–39.
45. ANTIVALLE, M., G. RANDISI, M. MARRAZZA, *et al.* 2002. Clinical relevance of the induction of antibodies to double-stranded DNA during long-term treatment of rheumatoid arthritis with Infliximab. Ann. Rheum. Dis. Abstr. 0166.
46. ALLANORE, Y., J. SELLAM, F. BATTEUX, *et al.* 2004. Induction of autoantibodies in refractory rheumatoid arthritis treated by infliximab. Clin. Exp. Rheum. **22:** 756–758.
47. DE BANDT, M.J., V. DESCAMPS & O. MEYER. 2001. Two cases of etanercept-induced systemic lupus erythematosus in patients with rheumatoid arthritis. Ann. Rheum. Dis. **60:** 175.
48. SHAKOOR, N., M. MICHALSKA, C.A. HARRIS, *et al.* 2002. Drug-induced systemic lupus erythematosus associated with etanercept therapy. Lancet **359:** 579–580.
49. SARZI-PUTTINI, P., S. ARDIZZONE, G. MANZIONNA, *et al.* 2003. Infliximab-induced lupus in Crohn's disease: a case report. Dig. Liver Dis. **35:** 814–817.

50. BOEHM, I.B., G.A. BOEHM & R. BAUER. 1998. Management of cutaneous lupus erythematosus with low-dose methotrexate: indication for modulation of inflammatory mechanisms. Rheumatol. Int. **18:** 59–62.
51. MILTENBURG, A.M.M., A. ROOS, L. SLEGTENHORST, *et al.* 1993. IgA anti-dsDNA antibodies in SLE: occurrence, incidence and association with clinical and laboratory variables of disease activity. J. Rheumatol. **20:** 53–58.
52. AMOURA, Z., S. KOUTOUZOV & J.C. PIETTE. 2000. The role of nucleosomes in lupus. Curr. Opin. Rheumatol. **12:** 369–373.
53. BERNSTEIN, R. 1996. Autoantibodies to histones, Sm and ubiquitins. *In* Manual of Biological Markers of Disease. W.J. Van Venrooij & R.N. Maini, Eds. C2.: 1–7. Kluwer Academic Publishers. Dordrecht, the Netherlands.
54. FERRERO-PEYRET, C., F. COURY, J.G. TEBIB, *et al.* 2004. Infliximab therapy in rheumatoid arthritis and ankylosing spondylitis-induced specific antinuclear autoantibodies without autoimmune clinical manifestations: a two-year prospective study. Arthritis Res. Ther. **6:** 535–543.
55. LUGERING, A., M. SCHMIDT, N. LUGERING, *et al.* 2001. Infliximab induces apoptosis in monocytes from patients with chronic active Crohn's disease by using a caspase-dependent pathway. Gastroenterology **121:** 1145–1157.
56. BELL, D.A. & B. MORRISON. 1991. The spontaneous apoptotic cell death of normal human lymphocytes *in vitro*: the release of, and immunoproliferative response to, nucleosomes *in vitro*. Clin. Immunol. Immunopathol. **60:** 13–26.
57. CAMPBELL, I.K., K. O'DONNELL, K.E. LAWLOR, *et al.* 2001. Severe inflammatory arthritis and lymphadenopathy in the absence of TNF. J. Clin. Invest. **107:** 1519–1527.
58. FIELDS, R.A., H. TOUBBEH, R.P. SEARLES, *et al.* 1989. The prevalence of anticardiolipin antibodies in a healthy elderly population and its association with antinuclear antibodies. J. Rheumatol. **16:** 623–625.
59. KEANE, A., R. WOODS, V. DOWDING, *et al.* 1987. Anticardiolipin antibodies in rheumatoid arthritis. Br. J. Rheumatol. **26:** 346–350.
60. WOLF, P., J. GRETLER, F. AGLAS, *et al.* 1994. Anticardiolipin antibodies in rheumatoid arthritis: their relation to rheumatoid nodules and cutaneous vascular manifestations. Br. J. Dermatol. **131:** 48–51.
61. KAPIOTIS, S., W. SPEISER, I. PABINGER-FASCHING, *et al.* 1991. Anticardiolipin antibodies in patients with venous thrombosis. Haemostasis **21:** 19–24.
62. ELLIOTT, M.J., R.N. MAINI, M. FELDMANN, *et al.* 1993. Treatment of rheumatoid arthritis with chimeric monoclonal antibodies to tumor necrosis factor-α. Arthritis Rheum. **36:** 1681–1690.
63. RANKIN, E.C., E.H. CHOY, D. KASSIMOS, *et al.* 1995. The therapeutic effects of an engineered human anti-tumour necrosis factor alpha antibody (CDP571) in rheumatoid arthritis. Br. J. Rheumatol. **34:** 334–342.
64. FERRACCIOLI, G., M. MECCHIA, E. DI POI, *et al.* 2002. Anticardiolipin antibodies in rheumatoid patients treated with etanercept or conventional combination therapy: direct and indirect evidence for a possible association with infections. Ann. Rheum. Dis. **61:** 358–361.
65. JONSDOTTIR, T., J. FORSLID, M.A. VAN VOLLENHOVEN, *et al.* 2004. Treatment with tumour necrosis factor alpha antagonists in patients with rheumatoid arthritis induces anticardiolipin antibodies. Ann. Rheum. Dis. **63:** 1075–1078.

Combination Treatment of Rat Adjuvant-Induced Arthritis with Methotrexate, Probiotic Bacteria *Enterococcus faecium*, and Selenium

JOZEF ROVENSKÝ,[a] KAROL ŠVÍK,[a] VLADIMÍR MAŤHA,[b] RICHARD IŠTOK,[a] VOJTĚCH KAMARÁD,[b] LIBOR EBRINGER,[c] MIROSLAV FERENČÍK,[d] AND MÁRIA STANČÍKOVÁ[a]

[a]*National Institute of Rheumatic Diseases, 921 12 Piešt'any, Slovak Republic*

[b]*IVAX, Pharmaceuticals s.r.o., Opava, Czech Republic*

[c]*Institute of Cell Biology, Faculty of Science,* [d]*Institute of Immunology, Faculty of Medicine, Comenius University, 811 07 Bratislava, Slovak Republic*

ABSTRACT: The effects of the probiotic bacteria *Enterococcus faecium* (EF) and selenium were studied on methotrexate (MTX) treatment in rats with adjuvant arthritis. Arthritic rats were treated orally with the following substances: lyophilized EF (15 mg/kg/day, 5 days a week), sodium selenite pentahydrate (SSe; 0.050 mg/kg containing 0.015 mg/kg selenium, 5 days a week), MTX (0.6 mg/kg/week), and their combinations for the period of 50 days from adjuvant application. Levels of serum albumin, serum nitrite/nitrate concentrations, hind paw swelling, arthrogram scores, whole-body bone mineral density (BMD), and bone erosions were evaluated as markers of inflammation and destructive changes associated with arthritis. Long-term preventive treatment with low-dose MTX significantly inhibited the markers of both inflammation and arthritis. EF or SSe when administered singly or in combination had no significant effect on the given parameters in arthritic rats. EF, but not SSe, potentiated the beneficial effects of MTX, which resulted in a more significant reduction of hind paw swelling, arthrogram scores, and whole-body BMD decrease. EF also had a tendency to improve the effect of MTX on serum albumin and nitrite/nitrate concentrations. Our results indicate that EF may increase the preventive effect of MTX treatment in rat adjuvant arthritis by improving its anti-inflammatory and antiarthritic effects.

KEYWORDS: **adjuvant arthritis; *Enterococcus faecium;* methotrexate; selenium**

INTRODUCTION

Increasing interest in an influence of intestinal microflora on human and animal health has resulted in attempts to optimally improve its composition by using probi-

Address for correspondence: Professor MUDr. J. Rovenský, DrSc, National Institute of Rheumatic Diseases, Nábrežie I. Krasku 4, 921 12 Piešt'any, Slovak Republic. Voice: +421-33-772-3586; fax: +421-33-772-1192.
rovensky@nurch.sk

**Ann. N.Y. Acad. Sci. 1051: 570–581 (2005). © 2005 New York Academy of Sciences.
doi: 10.1196/annals.1361.101**

otics. Probiotics are defined as live cultures of microorganisms that, if administered in sufficient quantities, beneficially affect the host by improving its intestinal microbial balance.[1] They influence favorably both development and stability of the microflora, inhibit colonization by pathogens, influence the mucosal barrier by their trophic effect on intestinal epithelium, and stimulate both specific and nonspecific components of the immune system.[2,3] The bacteria most frequently used as probiotics are those from *Lactobacillus* and *Bifidobacteria* strains. However, some nonpathogenic strains of *E. coli* proved to be suitable for this purpose as well.

Enterococcus faecium (EF), like many other lactic-acid bacteria in functional foods, can transiently colonize the human intestine and exert beneficial probiotic effect.[4] Significant immunostimulatory effects on both phagocytosis by neutrophils and antibody production by EF have been described in several studies.[5,6] As a food additive, this probiotic agent is available in a selenium-enriched form. Selenium is an essential trace element with antioxidant properties able to modulate the anti-inflammatory and immune responses.[7] Deficiencies in selenium attenuate especially the cellular immune response by oxidative stress and increase the risk of bacterial and viral infections. Inflammatory and arthritic manifestations of adjuvant arthritis (AA) in rats significantly worsened after 6 and 12 weeks of being fed a selenium-deficient diet.[8] Selenium supplementation in rheumatoid arthritis (RA) patients did not decrease the arthritic score but improved some symptoms of the disease.[9] The combination of EF with organic selenium may enhance the immunostimulatory and anti-inflammatory actions of this probiotic agent.

Long-lasting unfavorable composition of intestinal microflora could be associated with occurrence of diseases that may have no relation to the bacteria living in intestines; it may also increase susceptibility to infectious diseases or worsen absorption of some drugs. Certain associations were observed among the gastrointestinal system, arthritis, and the immune system.[10,11] Patients with newly diagnosed RA have an altered intestinal microflora composition (especially in terms of Gram-positive anaerobic bacteria) compared to healthy controls (HCs).[12] It has also been suggested that in arthritis the intestinal defensive barrier is disturbed.[13] In one study, short-term therapy with *Lactobacillus GG* showed a tendency to increase IgA secretion and thus improve the mucosal barrier mechanism.[14] The positive alterations in intestine flora can also be induced by an uncooked, lactobacilli-rich, vegan diet. Decrease of RA activity,[15] or the subjective symptoms of the disease,[16] was observed in RA patients using the vegan diet.

Kano *et al.*[17] showed that oral intake of *Lactobacillus delbrueckii* subsp. *bulgaricus* OLL1073R-1 prevents development of collagen-induced arthritis in mice. On the other hand, it has been suggested that the Gram–positive bacteria belonging to the normal intestinal flora (*e.g., Eubacterium aerofaciens, Lactobacillus casei*) may induce arthritis and the production of proinflammatory cytokines in rats.[18,19] The beneficial and the harmful effects of probiotics are clearly strain dependent; therefore, it is important to test different probiotics and their affect on the development and course of arthritis. This work is continuation of our previous study with selenium-enriched EF.[20] The results of our previous study proved that this probiotic agent had a tendency to improve some inflammatory and arthritic parameters in AA rats and significantly potentiate the preventive effect of methotrexate (MTX). MTX is widely used in RA therapy for its anti-inflammatory and immunosuppressive effects. However, one of its side effects is the damage of intestinal mucosa.

The purpose of the present study is to determine whether the beneficial effect of the probiotic agent selenium-enriched EF on the MTX treatment is a result of EF, selenium, or both of these components.

METHODS

Materials

MTX and sodium selenite pentahydrate (SSe) were purchased as pure substances from Pliva-Lachema Ltd. (Brno, Czech Republic). EF M74—the lyophilized probiotic agent containing 360×10^9/g colony-forming units (CFU)—was prepared by MEDIPHARM (Hustopeče, Czech Republic). Mycobacterium butyricum in lyophilized form was purchased from Difco Laboratories Co., Ltd. (Detroit, MI, USA), and the incomplete Freund's adjuvant was purchased from Sigma-Aldrich Chemie GmbH (Taufkirchen, Germany).

Animals

Male Lewis rats (170 ± 10 g; Charles River Wiga, Sulzfeld, Germany) were maintained during the experiment in standard animal facilities that comply with the European Convention for the Protection of Vertebrae Animals Used for Experimental and Other Scientific Purposes. The animals were fed pelleted food (TOP DOVO, Dobrá Voda, Slovak Republic) and had free access to both food and water. The State Veterinary and Food Committee of the Slovak Republic and the Ethics Committee for Control of Animals Experimentation on the National Institute of Rheumatic Diseases approved the experimental protocol and all procedures.

Induction of Arthritis

The rats were injected with a 0.1-mL suspension of heat-killed *Mycobacterium butyricum* (12 mg/mL) in incomplete Freund's adjuvant intradermally at the base of the tail.

Treatment

Tested substances were administered in corresponding doses from day 0 (day of immunization) to day 50 of the study. Lyophilized *Enterococcus faecium* (15 mg/kg), sodium selenite pentahydrate (0.050 mg/kg containing 0.015 mg/kg selenium), and their combinations were prepared in distilled water to reach the required concentration and were applied *per os* in a once-daily dose, five times a week. MTX was prepared in sterile saline to yield the desired concentration of 0.3 mg/kg in 0.1 mL saline, and applied twice a week *per os* (0.6 mg/kg in total per week). A fresh solution of the tested substances was prepared on each day of the administration. The untreated groups received vehicle (sterile saline) in the same manner daily for 50 days.

Rat Groups

The animals were divided into the following nine groups of 10 animals: group 1—nonarthritic untreated controls; group 2—untreated rats with AA; group 3—AA rats treated with EF; group 4—AA rats treated with SSe; group 5—AA rats treated with the combination of EF + SSe; group 6— AA rats treated with MTX; group 7—AA rats treated with the combination of MTX + EF; group 8—AA rats treated with the combination of MTX + SSe; group 9—AA rats treated with the combination of MTX + EF + SSe.

Evaluated Parameters

Hind Paw Swelling

The volume of hind paws swelling was measured with an electronic water plethysmometer (UGO BASILE, Comerio-Varese, Italy) on days 14, 21, and 28.

Arthrogram Score

The severity of arthritis was quantified by scoring each paw from 1 to 5, based on increasing levels of swelling and periarticular erythema. The sum of the scores for the limbs was calculated as the arthritic index, with a maximum possible score of 20 per rat. Arthrogram scores were evaluated on days 14, 21, and 28.

Serum Albumin

Serum albumin levels were measured on days 14, 21, and 28 in the rat serum by spectrophotometric method, using SYS 1 kit (BM/Hitachi, Boehringer Mannheim, Germany) on a Hitachi 911 automatic biochemical analyzer.

Serum Nitrite/Nitrate

Serum nitrite/nitrate concentration in deproteinized serum was determined by the method of Cortas and Waking[21] on days 14, 21, and 28. Cu-coated cadmium granules in glycine buffer at pH 9.7 reduced nitrate, and the resulting nitrite was evaluated by Griess reaction.

Bone Mineral Density

Bone mineral density (BMD) was measured by dual-energy X-ray absorptiometry (DEXA) using a Hologic QDR®-4500 (Waldham, MA, USA) with the equipment for measuring small laboratory animals. The whole-body BMD of rats was determined on day 50 after immunization.

Bone Erosions

Bone changes, indicated by erosions of tarsal and metatarsal bone structures of the hind paws, were evaluated from radiographic prints. They were taken on a computer-controlled X-ray generator (Philips Super 80CP, Hamburg, Germany) on day 50 after immunization, using the modified arthrogram scoring system.[22] Every hind paw radiograph was checked for matching to one of five degrees of bone erosion: degree 1—osteoporosis of the distal part of the tibia and the tarsal bones; degree 2—hyperostosis with osteophytes in the tibiotarsal joint region; degree 3—as in degree 2 plus hyperostosis with osteophytes in the tarsometatarsal joint region; degree 4—as in degree 3 plus hyperostosis with osteophytes in the tarsometatarsal phalangeal joint region; degree 5—as in degree 4 plus deformation of the joint spaces.

TABLE 1. The effects of MTX, EF, SSe, and their combinations on hind paw swelling (mL) in AA rats

Groups of rats	Day 14	Day 21	Day 28
Healthy controls	1.22 ± 0.02	1.25 ± 0.08	1.35 ± 0.08
AA controls	2.20 ± 0.23	2.31 ± 0.17	2.18 ± 0.22
AA rats treated with			
EF	2.11 ± 0.44	2.20 ± 0.37	2.09 ± 0.28
SSe	2.09 ± 0.26	2.20 ± 0.24	2.12 ± 0.27
EF + SSe	2.15 ± 0.19	2.36 ± 0.21	2.19 ± 0.25
MTX	1.79 ± 0.27**	2.01 ± 0.26*	1.85 ± 0.23**
MTX + EF	1.48 ± 0.22***†	1.69 ± 0.33***†	1.58 ± 0.22***†
MTX + SSe	1.81 ± 0.31**	1.98 ± 0.38*	1.79 ± 0.36*
MTX + EF + SSe	1.39 ± 0.23***†	1.65 ± 0.41***†	1.56 ± 0.27***†

NOTE: Data represent mean values ± SD for 10 rats. Significantly different from arthritic control rats: *, $P < .05$; **, $P < .01$; ***, $P < .001$. Significantly different from arthritic rats treated with MTX alone: †, $P < .05$.

Statistical Analysis of the Results

One-way analysis of variance (ANOVA) was used for statistical analysis of the results, and $P < .05$ was taken as the significance limit for all comparisons.

RESULTS

Hind Paw Swelling

Hind paw swelling reflects both inflammatory and arthritic changes occurring in rats with AA. The volume of the swollen hind paws in arthritic rats on day 21 was about twice of that found in healthy controls (TABLE 1). A statistically significant decrease was observed in rats treated with MTX compared to untreated arthritic controls. The reduction of hind paw volume was more pronounced in rats treated with the combination of MTX + EF than in those treated with MTX alone ($P < .05$). Selenium alone had no effect on MTX treatment. The best preventive effect observed with the three-agent combination of MTX + EF + SSe may be the result of the presence of EF in this treatment regiment. EF or SSe when administered singly or in combination had no significant effect on hind paw swelling.

Arthrogram Score

The arthrogram score is a more comprehensive variable to indicate the severity of arthritis. Only MTX and its combinations were associated with a significant decrease in arthrogram scores (TABLE 2). Similar to hind paw swelling, reductions in arthrogram scores were more pronounced for the groups treated with combinations of MTX with EF (MTX + EF and MTX + EF + SSe).

TABLE 2. The effects of MTX, EF, SSe, and their combinations on the arthrogram score in rats with AA

Groups of rats	Day 14	Day 21	Day 28
AA controls	16.67 ± 1.87	19.13 ± 1.83	19.33 ± 1.87
AA rats treated with			
EF	14.63 ± 5.15	17.13 ± 2.95	18.25 ± 3.20
SSe	15.00 ± 2.78	18.38 ± 2.20	19.38 ± 2.72
EF + SSe	16.25 ± 1.91	17.38 ± 1.50	19.75 ± 2.43
MTX	10.50 ± 2.62***	14.88 ± 3.31**	14.00 ± 4.57**
MTX + EF	7.50 ± 1.20***†	13.50 ± 3.42***	12.38 ± 4.37***
MTX + SSe	10.13 ± 3.40***	15.75 ± 2.31**	14.88 ± 4.73**
MTX + EF + SSe	7.30 ± 2.06***†	11.00 ± 2.40***†	11.25 ± 3.08***

NOTE: Data represent mean values ± SD for 10 rats. Significantly different from arthritic control rats: **, $P < .01$; ***, $P < .001$. Significantly different from arthritic rats treated with MTX alone: †, $P < .05$.

TABLE 3. The effects of MTX, EF, SSe, and their combinations on serum albumin concentrations (g/L) in rats with AA

Groups of rats	Day 14	Day 21	Day 28
Healthy controls	33.18 ± 1.02	34.55 ± 1.86	34.95 ± 1.84
AA controls	25.90 ± 0.99	26.34 ± 1.21	26.40 ± 1.95
AA rats treated with			
EF	26.33 ± 1.37	26.58 ± 0.85	25.66 ± 1.79
SSe	25.61 ± 1.85	26.26 ± 0.82	24.91 ± 1.47
EF + SSe	26.04 ± 0.97	26.34 ± 1.54	25.40 ± 1.66
MTX	27.15 ± 1.10*	29.06 ± 2.78*	28.80 ± 2.11*
MTX + EF	27.81 ± 2.10*	29.14 ± 2.89*	29.21 ± 1.24**
MTX + SSe	27.34 ± 1.56*	28.96 ± 2.74*	28.84 ± 1.48*
MTX + EF + SSe	28.02 ± 2.62*	30.25 ± 3.95*	29.87 ± 2.00**

NOTE: Data represent mean values ± SD for 10 rats. Significantly different from arthritic control rats: *, $P < .05$; **, $P < .01$.

Serum Albumin

Serum albumin behaves as a negative acute-phase reactant in both rat and human arthritis. Lower levels of serum albumin correspond to higher levels of inflammatory activity. The concentration of albumin in the serum of arthritic controls was significantly lower than in healthy controls (HC vs. AA $P < .001$). All treatments containing MTX significantly inhibited the decrease in serum albumin (TABLE 3). EF potentiated the beneficial effect of MTX (on day 28). EF or SSe used singly and in combination (EF + SSe) without MTX did not influence this inflammatory marker.

TABLE 4. The effects of MTX, EF, SSe, and their combinations on serum nitrite/nitrate concentrations (nmol/mL) in rats with AA

Groups of rats	Day 14	Day 21	Day 28
Healthy controls	39.75 ± 4.83	38.76 ± 8.57	40.94 ± 4.71
AA controls	91.14 ± 14.63	84.24 ± 14.70	74.69 ± 7.93
AA rats treated with			
EF	88.21 ± 12.67	79.53 ± 10.22	71.62 ± 10.69
SSe	97.79 ± 14.56	77.89 ± 8.11	78.56 ± 18.87
EF + SSe	89.72 ± 15.61	77.11 ± 16.80	70.65 ± 13.09
MTX	76.82 ± 12.08*	71.34 ± 8.40*	67.53 ± 5.51*
MTX + EF	75.51 ± 8.14*	69.61 ± 7.15*	58.85 ± 10.97**
MTX + SSe	75.81 ± 11.54*	69.77 ± 11.64*	64.51 ± 9.95*
MTX + EF + SSe	74.17 ± 11.74*	65.77 ± 13.69*	57.97 ± 13.16**

NOTE: Data represent mean values ± SD for 10 rats. Significantly different from arthritic control rats: *, $P < .05$; **, $P < .01$.

Serum Nitrite/Nitrate

Serum concentrations of nitrite/nitrate reflect nitric oxide (NO) production in various tissues and inflammatory responses. The clinical onset of AA was associated with a significant rise in nitrite/nitrate concentrations. MTX alone and in combination with EF and SSe significantly decreased nitrite/nitrate concentrations during the whole study compared to arthritic controls (TABLE 4). SSe, EF, or their combination (EF + SSe) had no significant effect on the serum nitrite/nitrate concentrations; but EF potentiated the beneficial effect of MTX on day 28 of the study.

Whole-Body BMD

Development of arthritis in both humans and rats is associated with the development of osteopenia due to the activation of proinflammatory cytokines. At the end of the study (on day 50), AA rats had markedly lower values of the whole-body BMD compared to healthy controls (FIG. 1). Evaluation of different treatments showed that only the combinations MTX + EF and MTX + EF + SSe significantly inhibited the whole-body BMD decrease in AA rats.

Bone Erosions

X-ray scans of AA rats on day 50 revealed destruction of joint structures characteristic of arthritis. The radiographic scores positively correlated with hind paw swelling; bone erosions increased with increased swelling. No changes were detected in healthy controls, whereas arthritis was manifested by pronounced destruction (FIG. 2). MTX and its combinations (MTX + EF and MTX + SSe) significantly reduced the radiographic scores. The most pronounced reduction was observed for the three-agent combination (MTX + EF + SSe). EF or SSe administered singly or in combination did not influence this parameter.

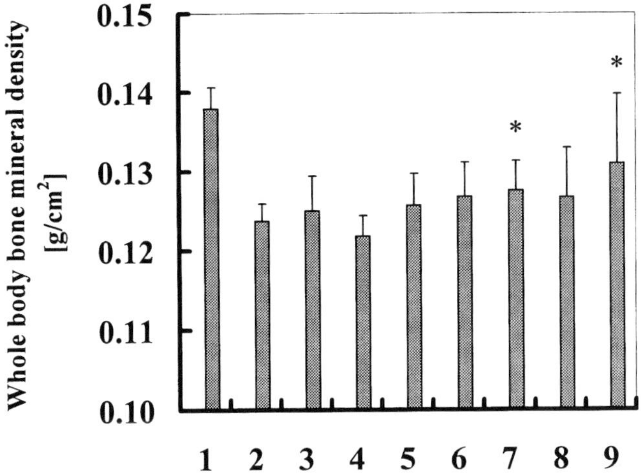

FIGURE 1. The effects of MTX, EF, SSe, and their combinations on whole-body BMD in rats assessed on day 50. The nine groups of animals are described in the text. Data represent mean values ± SD for 10 rats. Significantly different from arthritic control rats: *, $P < .05$.

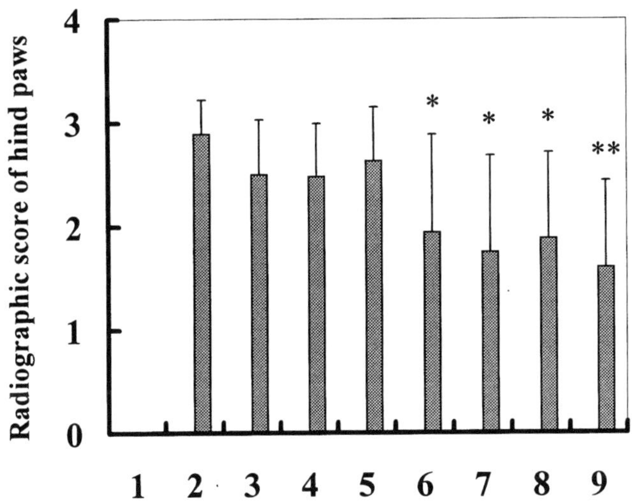

FIGURE 2. The effects of MTX, EF, SSe, and their combinations on radiographic scores in rats assessed on day 50. The nine groups of animals are described in the text. Data represent mean values ± SD for 10 rats. Significantly different from arthritic control rats: *, $P < .05$; **, $P < .01$.

DISCUSSION

The purpose of our study was to evaluate the effect of the probiotic agent EF and selenium on MTX treatment of AA in rats. Because the effects on BMD and radiographic scores were also investigated, the duration of the treatment was longer (50 days) than usually administered for AA (10–14 days) to prevent exacerbation of arthritis after discontinuation of the therapy.

The results of our investigation confirmed the previously reported effect of MTX treatment in rats with AA.[22] MTX at a dose of 0.6 mg/kg/week suppressed, but did not prevent, arthritis development. In our study, MTX significantly suppressed the hind paw swelling and decreased the arthrogram scores. EF but not SSe potentiated the beneficial effect of MTX, which resulted in a more significant reduction of hind paw swelling and arthrogram scores. Parnham *et al.*[23] have observed a weak inhibition of carrageenan paw edema and adjuvant arthritis in rats with the organo-selenium compound ebselen.

Serum albumin acts as a negative acute-phase reactant in rat arthritis, and the decrease of serum albumin levels reflects the changes in synthesis of this protein in the liver secondary to the activation of hepatic cells by inflammatory cytokines, mainly interleukin 1 (IL-1).[24] Our results correlate with the observation that MTX markedly prevents the albumin decrease in rat AA.[24] The administration of EF was positively manifested in both combinations (MTX + EF and MTX + EF + SSe) on day 28. The combination of MTX with SSe had no additional effect compared to MTX alone. In patients with RA, the concentration of selenium containing glutathione peroxidase is decreased in polymorphonuclear leucocytes.[25] Supplementation with selenium increases the concentration of selenium in the serum and erythrocytes but only weakly increases its concentration in polymorphonuclear leucocytes, and that might be the cause of its insufficient anti-inflammatory effect in arthritis.[25]

NO, an unstable free radical produced by the action of the enzyme NO synthase (NOS) on L-arginine, is a mediator of multiple physiologic functions, and may also mediate local inflammation and tissue destruction.[26] Nitric oxide is involved in both initiation and development of AA in rats.[27] Moreover, inhibitors of NOS have been shown to suppress arthritis in several animal models,[28,29] and increased NO levels have been found in patients with RA.[30] Omata *et al.*[31] reported MTX to suppress *ex vivo* production of NO in macrophages of rats with AA. In our study, markedly increased serum nitrite/nitrate concentrations were measured in AA rats. EF or SSe administered singly or in combination did not decrease the concentration of nitrite/nitrate, but EF potentiated the inhibitory effect of MTX on day 28.

AA rats developed marked osteopenia, predominantly in the distal periarticular region of the femur, as a result of the suppression of bone formation and increased bone resorption.[32] Suzuki *et al.*[33] reported short-term low doses of MTX to ameliorate abnormal bone metabolism and decrease the bone loss in adjuvant arthritis. In AA rats, MTX in the dose of 3 mg/kg/week suppressed arthritis and restored the decreased osteogenic activity of bone marrow cells and significantly increased periarticular BMD in the femur. The lower dose of 0.3 mg/kg/week had no effect on femoral BMD. In our study, MTX (0.6 mg/kg/week) had no effect on the whole-body BMD in rats. It was interesting that EF alone, similarly to MTX, was ineffective. But EF in combination with MTX significantly reduced the whole-body BMD loss in

AA rats. This observation needs further study, and BMD should be measured in different sites (*e.g.,* femur or tibia).

Bone erosions of the hind paws are typical sign of chronic arthritis; reduction of radiographic response in AA with MTX is dose dependent. Low doses of MTX (0.1 or 0.2 mg) did not normalize the radiographic findings in AA.[34] Morgan *et al.*[35] found that MTX at 1 mg/kg/week resulted in mean total radiographic scores not different from healthy controls; lower or higher doses of MTX were less effective. In our experiment, MTX 0.6 mg/kg/week significantly decreased the radiographic scores. The more pronounced reduction of radiographic scores with the three-agent combination (MTX + EF + SSe) may be result of the additional effect of the probiotic agent, SSe, or their combination.

Our results demonstrate that administration of the probiotic agent EF alone does not worsen the clinical, inflammatory, or destructive markers of adjuvant arthritis. On the contrary, it potentiates the beneficial effect of MTX treatment on arthritis-associated inflammation and destruction. Our results also show that the beneficial effect of selenium-enriched EF observed in our previous study[20] results mainly from the bacteria and not from selenium. The possible explanation may be the altered intestinal absorption of MTX after colonization of gut by this probiotic agent. During the experiment, no diarrhea was observed in rats. Mao *et al.*[36] showed that administration of lactobacilli, especially *L. plantarum*, is helpful in reducing the severity of the methotrexate-induced enterocolitis in rats. Owing to the fact that EF not only increases the efficacy of MTX treatment but may favorably influence the intestinal flora and may protect against related infectious diseases, we can see the rationale for the use of this probiotic agent for the MTX treatment of arthritis.

The focus of the present study is on the long-term preventive treatment of arthritic rats; further studies are needed to explore the role of EF in the MTX therapy regimen and the possible therapeutical use of this probiotic agent in arthritis.

REFERENCES

1. Reid, G., J. Jass, *et al.* 2003. Potential uses of probiotics in clinical practice. Clin. Microbiol. Rev. **16:** 658–672.
2. Isolauri, E., Y. Sütas, *et al.* 2001. Probiotics: effect on immunity. Am. J. Clin. Nutr. **73:** 444S–450S.
3. Tlaskalova-Hogenova, H., R. Stepankova, *et al.* 2004. Commensal bacteria (normal microflora), mucosal immunity and chronic inflammatory and autoimmune diseases. Immunol. Lett. **93:** 97–107.
4. Belicova, A., J. Krajcovic, *et al.* 1999. Antimutagenicity of milk fermented by *Enterococcus faecium*. Folia Microbiol. **44:** 513–518.
5. Mikes, Z., M. Ferencik, *et al.* 1995. Hypocholesterolemic and immunostimulatory effects of orally applied *Enterococcus faecium M-74* in man. Folia Microbiol. **40:** 639–646.
6. Ferencik, M., Z. Mikes, *et al.* 2000. Immunostimulatory and other beneficial health effects of lactic acid bacteria. Bratisl. Lek. Listy **101:** 51–53.
7. Rayman, M.P. 2000. The importance of selenium to human health. Lancet **356:** 233-41.
8. Parnham, M.J., J. Winkelmann & S. Leyck. 1983. Macrophage, lymphocyte and chronic inflammatory responses in selenium deficient rodents. Association with decreased glutathione peroxidase activity. Int. J. Immunopharmacol. **5:** 455–461.
9. Peretz, A., V. Siderova & J. Néve. 2001. Selenium supplementation in rheumatoid arthritis investigated in a double blind, placebo controlled trial. Scand. J. Rheumatol. **30:** 208–212.

10. SARTOR, R.B. 1997. Review article: role of enteric microflora in the pathogenesis of intestinal inflammation and arthritis. Aliment. Pharmacol. Ther. **11:** 17–32.
11. CEBRA, J.J. 1999. Influences of microbiota on intestinal immune system development. Am. J. Clin. Nutr. **69:** 1046–1051.
12. EEROLA, E., T. MÖTTÖ, *et al.* 1994. Intestinal flora in early rheumatoid arthritis. Br. J. Rheumatol. **33:** 1030–1038.
13. MALIN, M., P. VERRONEN & A. KORHONEN. 1997. Dietary therapy with *Lactobacillus GG*, bovine colostrum or bovine immune colostrum in patients with juvenile chronic arthritis: evaluation of effect on gut defense mechanism. Inflammopharmacology **5:** 219–236.
14. HATAKKA, K., J. MARTIO, *et al.* 2003. Effects of probiotic therapy on the activity and activation of mild rheumatoid arthritis—a pilot study. Scand. J. Rheumatol. **32:** 211–215.
15. PELTONEN, R., M. NENONEN, *et al.* 1997. Faecal microbial flora and disease activity in rheumatoid arthritis during a vegan diet. Br. J. Rheumatol. **36:** 64–68.
16. MCDOUGALL, J., B. BRUCE, *et al.* 2002. Effects of a very low fat, vegan diet in subjects with rheumatoid arthritis. J. Altern. Complement Med. **8:** 71–75.
17. KANO, H., T. KANEKO & S. KAMINOGAWA. 2002. Oral intake of *Lactobacillus delbrueckii* subsp. *bulgaricus* OLL1073R-1 prevents collagen-induced arthritis in mice. J. Food Prot. **65:** 153–160.
18. CHEN, T., P. ISOMÄKI, *et al.* 1999. Human cytokine responses induced by Gram-positive cell walls of normal intestinal microbiota. Clin. Exp. Immunol. **118:** 261–267.
19. SIMELYTE, E., M. RIMPILÄINEN, *et al.* 2000. Bacterial cell wall-induced arthritis chemical composition and tissue distribution of four *Lactobacillus* strains. Infect. Immun. **68:** 3535–3540.
20. ROVENSKY, J., K. SVIK, *et al.* 2002. Treatment of experimental adjuvant arthritis with the combination of methotrexate and lyophilized *Enterococcus faecium* enriched with organic selenium. Folia Microbiol. **47:** 573–578.
21. CORTAS, N.K. & N.W. WAKING. 1990. Determination of inorganic nitrate in serum and urine by a kinetic cadmium-reduction method. Clin. Chem. **36:** 1440–1443.
22. WELLES, W.L., J. SILKWORTH, *et al.* 1985. Studies on the effect of low dose methotrexate in adjuvant arthritis. J. Rheumatol. **12:** 904–906.
23. PARNHAM, M.J., S. LEYCK, *et al.* 1987. Ebselen a new approach to the inhibition of peroxide-dependent inflammation. Int. J. Tissue React. **9:** 45–50.
24. CONNOLLY, K.M., V.J. STECHER, *et al.* 1988. Alteration of interleukin-1 production and the acute phase response following medication of adjuvant arthritic rats with cyclosporin-A or methotrexate. Int. J. Immunopharmacol. **10:** 717–728.
25. TARP, U. 1994. Selenium and selenium-dependent glutathione peroxidase in rheumatoid arthritis. Dan. Med. Bull. **41:** 264–274.
26. STAMLER, J.S., D.J. SINGEL & J. LOSCALZO. 1992. Biochemistry of nitric oxide and its redox-activated forms. Science **258:** 1898–1902.
27. OYANAGUI, Y. 1994. Nitric oxide and superoxide radical are involved in both initiation and development of adjuvant arthritis in rats. Life Sci. **54:** PL285–PL289.
28. CANNON, G.W., S.J. OPENSHAW, *et al.* 1996. Nitric oxide production during adjuvant-induced and collagen-induced arthritis. Arthritis Rheum. **39:** 1677–1684.
29. STEFANOVIC-RACIC, M., K. MEYERS, *et al.* 1995. Comparison of the nitric oxide synthase inhibitors methylarginine and aminoguanidine as prophylactic and therapeutic agents in rat adjuvant arthritis. J. Rheumatol. **22:** 1992–1998.
30. UEKI, Y., S. MIYAKE, *et al.* 1996. Increased nitric oxide levels in patients with rheumatoid arthritis. J. Rheumatol. **23:** 230–236.
31. OMATA, T., Y. SEGAWA, *et al.* 1997. Methotrexate suppresses nitric oxide production *ex vivo* in macrophages from rats with adjuvant-induced arthritis. Res. Exp. Med. **197:** 81–90.
32. BONNET, J., E. ZERATH, *et al.* 1993. Bone morphometric changes in adjuvant-induced polyarthritic osteopenia in rats: evidence for an early bone formation defect. J. Bone Miner. Res. **8:** 659–668.
33. SUZUKI, Y., M. NAKAGAWA, *et al.* 1997. Short-term low dose methotrexate ameliorates abnormal bone metabolism and bone loss in adjuvant-induced arthritis. J. Rheumatol. **24:** 1890–1895.

34. Kawai, S., K. Nagai, *et al.* 1997. Low-dose pulse methotrexate inhibits articular destruction of adjuvant arthritis in rats. J. Pharm. Pharmacol. **49:** 213–215.
35. Morgan, S.L., J.E. Baggott, *et al.* 2001. MTX affects inflammation and tissue destruction differently in the rat AA model. J. Rheumatol. **28:** 1476–1481.
36. Mao, Y., S. Nobaek, *et al.* 1996. The effect of *Lactobacillus* strains and oat fiber on methotrexate-induced enterocolitis in rats. Gastroenterology **111:** 334–344.

Comparative Analysis of Antigen Specificities in the Monomeric and Dimeric Fractions of Intravenous Immunoglobulin

SYLVIA M. MIESCHER,[a,b] ALEXANDER SCHAUB,[b] MARCO GHIELMETTI,[a] MICHAEL BAUMANN,[b] MONIQUE VOGEL,[b] REINHARD BOLLI,[a] AND BEDA STADLER[b]

[a]*ZLB Behring AG, 3000 Bern 22, Switzerland*

[b]*Institute of Immunology, Inselspital, 3010 Bern, Switzerland*

ABSTRACT: Intravenous immunoglobulin (IVIG) preparations are derived from the pooled plasma of thousands of healthy donors and contain a complex mix of antibodies. Depending on the formulation, IVIG preparations contain variable amounts of monomeric and dimeric IgG. The biological and therapeutic significance of these IVIG fractions is still ill defined. Kinetic analysis of monomeric and dimeric IgG isolated by size-exclusion chromatography revealed a stable monomeric versus an unstable dimeric IgG fraction tending to dissociation. Biochemical analysis by 2D gel electrophoresis and isotype analysis showed no significant differences between the fractions. In contrast, comparative analysis by immunodot, ELISA, FACS, and immunohistology of monomeric and dimeric IgG fractions showed a preferential reactivity of the dimeric IgG on a variety of both self-antigens and exoantigens.

KEYWORDS: intravenous immunoglobulin; monomeric IgG; dimeric IgG; size-exclusion chromatography; two-dimensional gel electrophoresis; antigen specificity

INTRODUCTION

Intravenous immunoglobulin (IVIG) preparations are derived from pooled plasma of thousands of healthy donors (current pool sizes range from 1000 to 60,000 donors) and contain both immune and natural antibodies (NAbs), reflecting the cumulative antigen experience of the donor population. IVIG thus contains a large spectrum of so-called immune antibodies with specificities directed against pathogens and foreign antigens as well as NAbs reacting with self/autoantigens.[1–3]

Generally, IVIG consists of intact IgG molecules with an IgG isotype distribution similar to that of normal human serum; and depending on the product, there may be trace amounts of IgA and IgM. Final IVIG products also contain variable amounts of monomeric and dimeric IgG, depending on the formulation (FIG. 1). Monomers represent the monomeric IgG (molecular weight ~150,000), whereas dimers repre-

Address for correspondence: Sylvia M. Miescher, Ph.D., ZLB Behring AG, Wankdorfstrasse 10, 3000 Bern 22, Switzerland. Voice: +41-31-344-5543; fax: +41-31-344-5745. sylvia.miescher@zlb.com

Ann. N.Y. Acad. Sci. 1051: 582–590 (2005). © 2005 New York Academy of Sciences. doi: 10.1196/annals.1361.102

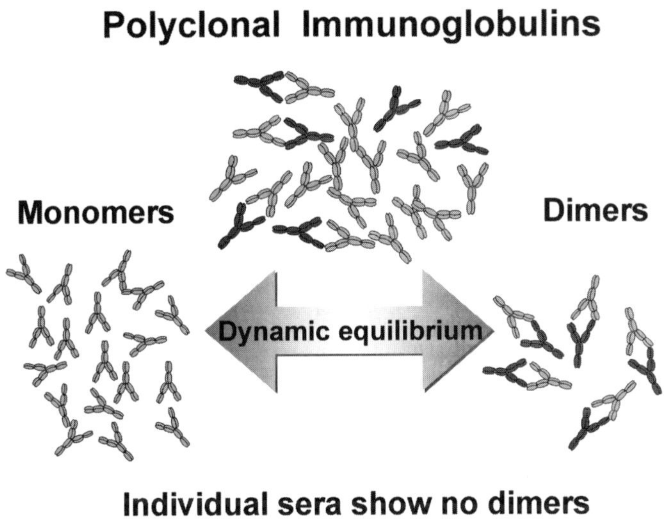

FIGURE 1. IVIG preparations contain both monomeric and dimeric IgG fractions, which are in a state of dynamic equilibrium, depending on various factors, such as IgG concentration, temperature, pH, and the pool size (number of donors in original plasma pool). A dimeric IgG fraction has not been observed in single donors.

sent two IgG molecules, which can be orientated in various forms, including the classical idiotype anti-idiotype pairs.[4–8]

Therapeutic applications of IVIG are diverse and include antibody replacement in immune-deficient patients and immunomodulation in patients with inflammatory and autoimmune diseases.[3,9–19] Tolerability of IVIG preparations during the infusion period is significantly influenced by the content of dimeric IgG in the product and can induce hypotension in the rat model and headache, nausea, and fever in humans.[20–22] For this reason, the plasma fractionation industry formulate their IVIG products to maintain the dimeric IgG content within specified limits.[23–25] However, the biological characteristics and potential significance of the monomeric and dimeric IgG fractions with respect to the mechanism of action of IVIG have only been marginally addressed.[5,26,27]

Therefore, this study aims at separating the monomeric and dimeric IgG fractions of IVIG to provide two dynamically stable fractions that can be used for comparative analyses of their recognition patterns on a variety of self-antigens and exoantigens.

MATERIALS AND METHODS

Isolation of Dimeric and Monomeric IgG Fractions from IVIG

A total of 12 g IVIG (provided by ZLB Behring AG, Bern, Switzerland) was dissolved in 84.6 mL 0.9% NaCl to obtain a 12% IgG solution. Molecular size exclusion (SEC) HPLC analysis on a TSK G3000SWXL column (Tosoh Biosep GmbH, Stuttgart, Germany) gave a profile of 12.54% dimers, 86.9% monomers, and 0.55% polymers. Preparative fractionation of the IVIG solution was performed by size-exclusion chromatography on a ReproSil 300 × 20 mm column (Dr. Maisch GmbH, Ammerbuch-Entringen, Germany). Elution was performed at 1.5 mL/min using PBS containing 0.02% azide as the mobile phase. SEC HPLC analysis of the separated fractions showed typical purities of 98% and 95% for the monomeric and dimeric IgG fractions, respectively.

Dissociation of IgG Dimers

The dimeric IgG fraction was dialyzed for 24 h at 4°C against 10 mM sodium acetate buffer (pH 4) and immediately frozen and stored at –20°C. Control samples of IVIG solution and the separated monomeric IgG fraction were prepared in the same buffer.

Two-Dimensional Gel Electrophoresis; Immunodot Blot, ELISA, and FACS

Two-dimensional (2D) PAGE analysis of the monomer and dimer fractions was performed as described in the supplier's instructions in 2D-Electrophoresis, Principles and Methods (Amersham Biosciences). In brief, 4 µg IgG was applied for electrofocusing (first dimension) on a 7-cm IPG strip (pH 3–10) (Amersham Biosciences) and run on an IPGphor II unit (Amersham Biosciences) according to the strip specifications. The second-dimension electrophoresis was performed under reducing conditions on a 12% polyacrylamide gel (MiniProtean chamber, BioRad). Silver staining was performed using the PlusOne silver staining kit (Amersham Biosciences).

Immunodots

Nitrocellulose strips were dotted with 10 ng of respective antigen and air dried. Blocking was done in PBS/0.15% casein for 1.5 h at RT. The first antibody (IgG of IVIG, monomer or dimer fraction) was incubated at 10, 100, and 500 µg/mL overnight at 4°C. The developing antibody, sheep antihuman IgG peroxidase (The Binding Site, UK) was incubated for 2 h at RT.

ELISA

Antigens were coated at 10 or 1 µg/mL and blocked for 2 h at 37°C in PBS/0.15% casein. The first antibody (IgG of IVIG, monomer or dimer fraction) was incubated at 10, 100, and 500 µg/mL for 4 h at 37°C. The developing antibody was the same as used in the immunodot assays. Commercially available kits were used for tetanus toxoid, *H. influenzae B* (both from The Binding Site), and respiratory syncytial virus (RSV) (Morvell Diagnostics GmbH, Zurich); the results were expressed as units per gram immunoglobulin calculated from a standard curve.

FACS

Immunofluorescence was performed on adherent cell lines that had been previously detached with PBS-EDTA 0.03% (w/v). Cells were analyzed for both membrane and intracellular staining by preparing nonpermeabilized versus permeabilized (saponin-treated) cells, respectively. The developing antibody was an isotype-specific fluorescein isothiocyanate (FITC)-labeled sheep antihuman IgG-FC (PFO04; The Binding Site). Flow cytometric data acquisition was performed on a FACSCalibur machine using *Cell Quest Pro* software (both Becton-Dickinson), and subsequent data analysis used *WinMDI* software (© Joseph Trotter).

Cells Used

Epithelial cells from monkey (COS-7), human (HepG2, HEp-2) and Chinese hamster ovary (CHO) cells were obtained from the American Type Culture Collection (ATTC).

RESULTS

Characterization of the Separated Monomeric and Dimeric IgG Preparations

Stability and kinetic analyses of the two separated fractions confirmed previous reports indicating that the monomeric IgG fraction was stable whereas the dimeric IgG fraction showed a dynamic instability—that is, tended to partially revert to the monomeric form. In contrast, the dissociated dimer fraction at pH 4 remained dynamically stable and did not reconvert to dimers under specified conditions during their use in the assay or in storage. Thus all experiments were performed using the treated (pH 4 buffer) fractions.

There was no significant difference between the monomeric and dimeric fractions as assessed by 2D gel electrophoresis. Isoelectric focusing showed that both fractions were widely distributed over the pH range 3–10 and demonstrated the expected overall patterns for heavy and light chains under reducing conditions. The light chains of the dimeric fraction showed a slight tendency for a wider isoelectric distribution extending more into the acidic region (FIG. 2). Comparative isotype analysis showed equal distribution of all four IgG isotypes and a slight increase of IgA in the dimeric IgG fractions (data not shown), which, however, represented only a small fraction of the actual total protein (3%).

Differential Reactivities of Monomeric and Dissociated Dimer Preparations

Reactivities to both exoantigens and self/autoantigens in a range of different assays were performed and are summarized in TABLE 1. The results are presented as a comparison between pH 4–treated fractions for both the monomeric and dimeric IgG fractions. To allow a convenient comparison, the monomers and dimers have been compared on a simple reactivity scale (++ to –), as explained in the table. Reactivities are clearly seen in the monomers and dimers to both categories of antigens (exoantigens and self/autoantigens). Monomers and dimers showed positive reactions on the same antigens. We have not found an antigen specificity for which the reactivity is present only in the monomeric or in the dimeric IgG fraction. Overall, there was a tendency for the dimeric IgG fraction to show an increased reactivity compared to the monomeric IgG fraction, which was also verified by using different assay systems. In some cases (*e.g.,* tetanus toxoid), we also measured the antibody–

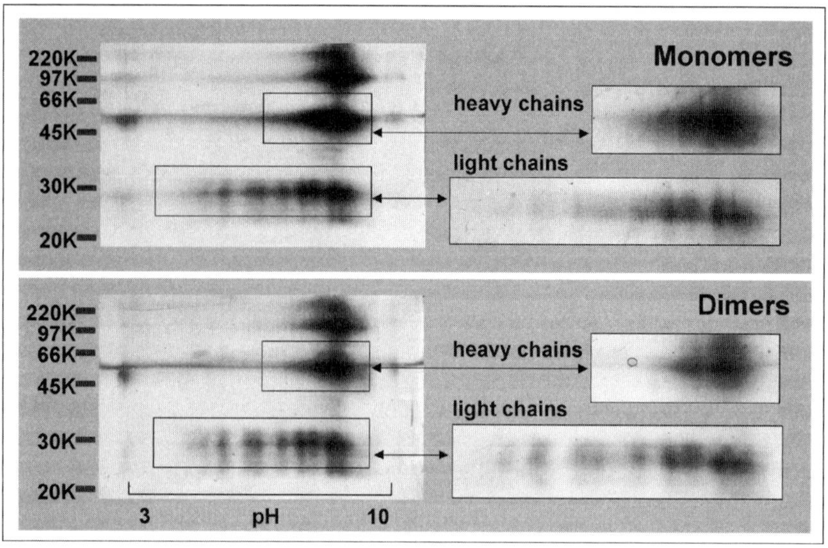

FIGURE 2. Characterization of the monomeric and dissociated dimeric IgG fractions by 2D gel electrophoresis. For the first dimensions, both fractions were focused on IPG strips over a pH range of 3–10; the second dimension involved separation on a reducing SDS-12% polyacrylamide gel. Molecular weight markers are indicated. The expected overall patterns for heavy and light chains were seen for both fractions. The light chains of the dimeric IgG fraction showed a slight tendency for a wider isoelectric distribution extending more into the acidic region (enlarged gel, *at right*).

antigen binding affinity, which was clearly increased in the dimeric IgG fraction (data not shown). FACS analysis on different cell lines showed a marked increase of intracellular staining when using the dimeric IgG fraction on permeabilized cells.

In summary, the dimeric IgG fraction shows an increased reactivity to certain antigens of both self-antigens and exoantigens.

DISCUSSION

IVIG is a heterogeneous and intriguing mix of antibodies representing a cumulative immune repertoire resulting from the thousands of donors that contributed to the original plasma pools. Nevertheless, a precise analysis of all the antibody specificities present is not possible with current state of the art technologies. In contrast, the presence of monomeric and dimeric IgG fractions in IVIG is well documented.[5,8,20,28] In this study, we isolated up to 100% pure fractions of monomeric and dimeric IgG by size-exclusion chromatography. Our results indicate that these fractions cannot be considered as equivalent, although they both contain IgG, show the same distribution of IgG isotypes, and demonstrate a comparable biochemical profile on 2D gel electrophoresis. In agreement with other studies, there was a difference in their dynamic equilibrium, which was influenced by pH, temperature, protein concentration of the solution, and storage time.[5,28] Thus the monomeric IgG

TABLE 1. Differential reactivity of monomeric and dimeric immunoglobulin fractions on selected antigens[a]

	IVIG Fractions			IVIG Fractions	
Exoantigens	Monomers	Dimers	Self-Antigens	Monomers	Dimers
Tetanus toxoid[b,c]	+	++	Myosin[c]	+	++
Diphtheria toxoid[b]	+	+	Phosphorylase B[c]	+	++
RSV[d]	+	++	Fibronectin[b,c]	–	–
H. influenzae B[c]	+	+	α_2-macroglobulin[b,c]	+	+
Campylobacter jejuni[b]	+	+	C-reactive protein[b]	+	+
E. coli[b]	+	±	IgE, IgA, IgM[b,c]	±	±
Bacteriophage[b]	+	+	HSA[b]	-	–
KLH[b,c]	+	+	Erythropoietin[b,c]	-	–
BSA[b]	±	±	FcεRI-α-chain[b,c]	±	±
Streptavidin[b]	–	–	C1q[b]	+	+
Cos 7[d]	+	++	HEp-2[d]	+	++
CHO[d]	+	++	HepG2[d]	+	++
SUS 11[d]	+	++			

ABBREVIATIONS: RSV, respiratory syncytial virus; KLH, keyhole limpet hemocyanin; HSA, human serum albumin; Cos 7, monkey kidney fibroblast; CHO, Chinese hamster ovary; SUS 11, mouse hybridoma; HEp-2, human epithelial cells; HepG2, human hepatoma.

[a]Antigens (10 ng/dot) were incubated with various concentrations (500, 100, and 10 μg/mL) of monomeric and dimeric IgG fractions.

[b]Immunodot blots: scanned on a densitometer and assessed qualitatively on a scale from ++ (strong signal), +, ±, to – (no signal).

[c]ELISA: comparison of reactivity at 10 μg/mL antigen with 100 μg/mL immunoglobulin fractions and assessed as follows: the ++ dimer signal titrates out at least a log-fold more than monomers; + and ±, clear/weak signal over background; –, no signal.

[d]FACS: immunofluorescence was assessed quantitatively based on the mean fluorescence intensity values for monomers and dimers.

fraction remained stable, whereas the dimers in the dimeric IgG fraction tended to dissociate until an equilibrium between the dimeric and the monomeric form was reached.

Therefore, a dynamically stable IgG fraction of highly dissociated dimers was produced that also served to simulate the *in vivo* dissociation of dimers once injected. Thus the antigen-binding activities of the IgG in the monomer and dimer fractions could be directly compared.

The choice of antigens to test was guided by the types of antibodies found in IVIG—that is, both "immune," resulting from an immune response, and NAbs, defined as generated in the absence of deliberate immunization and independently of exposure to foreign antigens.[29] Indeed a long list of antibodies to self-antigens has been detected and even purified by affinity chromatography from IVIG preparations.[30–37] These NAbs are often polyreactive, can bind to pathogens, and, by tagging and clearing senescent or altered molecules from the circulation, are thought to be important in maintaining immunohomeostasis.[1,38] Furthermore, it has been proposed that these NAbs recognize a conserved subset of immunodominant antigens referred to as the "immunological homunculus," which is essential for maintaining tolerance to self.[39–41]

For this preliminary screen, a selection of antigens was chosen to represent the major categories of exoantigens and self/autoantigens. A heterogeneous reactivity pattern, ranging from strongly positive to negative, was observed in both antigen categories. Monomer and dimer fractions differed in that the intensity of the positive reactions, with a few exceptions, was stronger in the dimer fraction, which was confirmed by affinity measurements. This may represent a graded response to an antigen that is preferentially found in either the monomeric or the dimeric IgG fraction but not exclusively in one or the other. Indeed, previous data based on a computer simulation analysis suggested the presence of two major IgG populations in IVIG differing in their apparent association rate constants.[28] Our analysis of the self-antigen category revealed an increased activity with the dimer fraction, in agreement with previous reports.[27] It is interesting that this increased activity was particularly marked on self-antigens located in the intracellular compartment.

It is tempting to try to link the reactivity pattern of IVIG and its subfractions to the potential therapeutic mechanisms of action of IVIG. In particular, reactivity to self-antigens has been linked to the existence of a highly conserved immune repertoire represented by the NAb repertoire and with the immunoregulatory action of IVIG.[3,16,42,43] Many of the current therapeutic indications for IVIG are based on counterbalancing, neutralizing, or blocking pathological autoimmune antibodies and thus restoring a healthy idiotype network.[27,44,45] Recent reports have also shown direct effects on neutrophils, dendritic cells, endothelial, and both T and B lymphocytes.[46–50] This complexity reflects the essential functions of circulating antibodies in maintaining homeostasis in healthy individuals.

There is still insufficient information to attribute the various functional activities of IVIG to particular subfractions. However, these preliminary results indicate that further experiments, aimed at delineating the differential specificities and functional activities of monomeric and dimeric IgG fractions found in IVIG, are warranted.

ACKNOWLEDGMENTS

We thank Roland Zehnder for his excellent technical assistance and Martin Spycher for critical input and scientific discussions (ZLB Behring AG). This work was supported by the KTI/CTI The Innovation Promotion Agency, Grant No. 6369.1 MTS-LS.

REFERENCES

1. HUREZ, V. *et al.* 1993. Polyreactivity is a property of natural and disease-associated human autoantibodies. Scand. J. Immunol. **38:** 190–196.
2. KAZATCHKINE, M.D. 1994. Natural IgG autoantibodies in the sera of healthy individuals. J. Interferon. Res. **14:** 165–168.
3. KAZATCHKINE, M.D. & S.V. KAVERI. 2001. Immunomodulation of autoimmune and inflammatory diseases with intravenous immune globulin. N. Engl. J. Med. **345:** 747–755.
4. TANKERSLEY, D.L., M.S. PRESTON & J.S. FINLAYSON. 1988. Immunoglobulin G dimer: an idiotype-anti-idiotype complex. Mol. Immunol. **25:** 41–48.

5. Tankersley, D.L. 1994. Dimer formation in immunoglobulin preparations and speculations on the mechanism of action of intravenous immune globulin in autoimmune diseases. Immunol. Rev. **139:** 159–172.
6. Roux, K.H. & D.W. Metzger. 1982. Immunoelectron microscopic localization of idiotypes and allotypes on immunoglobulin molecules. J. Immunol. **129:** 2548–2553.
7. Roux, K.H. & D.L. Tankersley. 1990. A view of the human idiotypic repertoire. Electron microscopic and immunologic analyses of spontaneous idiotype-anti-idiotype dimers in pooled human IgG. J. Immunol. **144:** 1387–1395.
8. Gronski, P. *et al.* 1988. On the nature of IgG dimers. II. Idiotype—anti-idiotype complexes of polyclonal and monoclonal origin: size distribution patterns and molecular geometries. Behring Inst. Mitt. 144–153.
9. So, A. *et al.* 1984. Intravenous gammaglobulin treatment in patients with hypogammaglobulinaemia. Br. Med. J. Clin. Res. Ed. **289:** 1177–1178.
10. Ryan, A., B.J. Thomson & A.D. Webster. 1988. Home intravenous immunoglobulin therapy for patients with primary hypogammaglobulinaemia. Lancet **2:** 793.
11. Webster, A.D. *et al.* 1988. Critical dependence on antibody for defence against mycoplasmas. Clin. Exp. Immunol. **71:** 383–387.
12. Webster, A.D. 1991. Intravenous immunoglobulins. Br. Med. J. **303:** 375–376.
13. Imbach, P. *et al.* 1981. High-dose intravenous gammaglobulin for idiopathic thrombocytopenic purpura in childhood. Lancet **1:** 1228–1231.
14. Viard, I. *et al.* 1998. Inhibition of toxic epidermal necrolysis by blockade of CD95 with human intravenous immunoglobulin. Science **282:** 490–493.
15. Lutz, H.U. *et al.* 2004. Intravenously applied IgG stimulates complement attenuation in a complement-dependent autoimmune disease at the amplifying C3 convertase level. Blood. **103:** 465–472.
16. Sewell, W.A. & S. Jolles. 2002. Immunomodulatory action of intravenous immunoglobulin. Immunology **107:** 387–393.
17. Gold, R., M.C. Dalakas & K.V. Toyka. 2003. Immunotherapy in autoimmune neuromuscular disorders. Lancet Neurol. **2:** 22–32.
18. Ahmed, A.R. & M.V. Dahl. 2003. Consensus statement on the use of intravenous immunoglobulin therapy in the treatment of autoimmune mucocutaneous blistering diseases. Arch. Dermatol. **139:** 1051–1059.
19. Dalakas, M.C. 2004. Intravenous immunoglobulin in autoimmune neuromuscular diseases. JAMA **291:** 2367–2375.
20. Bleeker, W.K. *et al.* 2000. Vasoactive side effects of intravenous immunoglobulin preparations in a rat model and their treatment with recombinant platelet-activating factor acetylhydrolase. Blood **95:** 1856–1861.
21. Spycher, M. 1999. Second International Congress on Autoimmunity. Tel Aviv, Israel, March 7–11, 1999. Abstracts J. Autoimmun. (Suppl.): 1–126, 1–9.
22. Kroez, M. *et al.* 2003. Hypotension with intravenous immunoglobulin therapy: importance of pH and dimer formation. Biologicals **31:** 277–286.
23. Andresen, I. *et al.* 2000. Product equivalence study comparing the tolerability, pharmacokinetics, and pharmacodynamics of various human immunoglobulin-G formulations. J. Clin. Pharmacol. **40:** 722–730.
24. Knezevic-Maramica, I. & M.S. Kruskall. 2003. Intravenous immune globulins: an update for clinicians. Transfusion **43:** 1460–1480.
25. Morell, A. 2004. Manufacturing of intravenous immunoglobulin: challenges, achievements and opportunities. *In* Intravenous Immunoglobulins in the Third Millennium. M.C. Dalakas & P.J. Späth, Eds.: 3–8. Parthenon Publishing Group. London.
26. Dietrich, G., S.V. Kaveri & M.D. Kazatchkine. 1992. A V region-connected autoreactive subfraction of normal human serum immunoglobulin G. Eur. J. Immunol. **22:** 1701–1706.
27. Vassilev, T.L. *et al.* 1995. Variable region-connected, dimeric fraction of intravenous immunoglobulin enriched in natural autoantibodies. J. Autoimmun. **8:** 405–413.
28. Gronski, P. *et al.* 1988. On the nature of IgG dimers. I. Dimers in human polyclonal IgG preparations: kinetic studies. Behring Inst. Mitt. 127–143.
29. Coutinho, A., M.D. Kazatchkine & S. Avrameas. 1995. Natural autoantibodies. Curr. Opin. Immunol. **7:** 812–818.

30. KAVERI, S. *et al.* 1996. Antibodies to a conserved region of HLA class I molecules, capable of modulating CD8 T cell-mediated function, are present in pooled normal immunoglobulin for therapeutic use. J. Clin. Invest. **97:** 865–869.
31. BOUHLAL, H. *et al.* 2001. Antibodies to C-C chemokine receptor 5 in normal human IgG block infection of macrophages and lymphocytes with primary R5-tropic strains of HIV-1. J. Immunol. **166:** 7606–7611.
32. VASSILEV, T. *et al.* 1993. Antibodies to the CD5 molecule in normal human immunoglobulins for therapeutic use (intravenous immunoglobulins, IVIg). Clin. Exp. Immunol. **92:** 369–372.
33. HUREZ, V. *et al.* 1994. Anti-CD4 activity of normal human immunoglobulin G for therapeutic use. (Intravenous immunoglobulin, IVIg). Ther. Immunol. **1:** 269–277.
34. BENDTZEN, K. *et al.* 1998. High-avidity autoantibodies to cytokines. Immunol. Today **19:** 209–211.
35. PASHOV, A. *et al.* 2002. Autoantibodies to heat shock protein 90 in the human natural antibody repertoire. Int. Immunol. **14:** 453–461.
36. ALTZNAUER, F. *et al.* 2003. Concurrent presence of agonistic and antagonistic anti-CD95 autoantibodies in intravenous Ig preparations. J. Allergy Clin. Immunol. **112:** 1185–1190.
37. LACROIX-DESMAZES, S. *et al.* 2000. Natural antibodies to factor VIII. Semin. Thromb. Hemost. **26:** 157–165.
38. LUTZ, H.U. *et al.* 1987. Naturally occurring anti-band-3 antibodies and complement together mediate phagocytosis of oxidatively stressed human erythrocytes. Proc. Natl. Acad. Sci. USA **84:** 7368–7372.
39. STOLLAR, B.D. 1991. Autoantibodies and autoantigens: a conserved system that may shape a primary immunoglobulin gene pool. Mol. Immunol. **28:** 1399–1412.
40. COHEN, I.R. 1992. The cognitive paradigm and the immunological homunculus. Immunol. Today **13:** 490–494.
41. NOBREGA, A. *et al.* 1993. Global analysis of antibody repertoires. II. Evidence for specificity, self-selection and the immunological "homunculus" of antibodies in normal serum. Eur. J. Immunol. **23:** 2851–2859.
42. MARCHALONIS, J.J. *et al.* 2002. Natural recognition repertoire and the evolutionary emergence of the combinatorial immune system. FASEB J. **16:** 842–848.
43. SIMON, H.U. & P.J. SPATH. 2003. IVIG—mechanisms of action. Allergy **58:** 543–552.
44. ROSSI, F., G. DIETRICH & M.D. KAZATCHKINE. 1989. Anti-idiotypes against autoantibodies in normal immunoglobulins: evidence for network regulation of human autoimmune responses. Immunol. Rev. **110:** 135–149.
45. SCHUSSLER, O. *et al.* 1998. Intravenous immunoglobulins for therapeutic use contain anti-idiotypes against xenophile antibodies and prolong discordant graft survival. Clin. Immunol. Immunopathol. **86:** 183–891.
46. TEELING, J.L. *et al.* 2001. Intravenous immunoglobulin preparations induce mild activation of neutrophils in vivo via triggering of macrophages—studies in a rat model. Br. J. Haematol. **112:** 1031–1040.
47. BAYRY, J. *et al.* 2003. Inhibition of maturation and function of dendritic cells by intravenous immunoglobulin. Blood **101:** 758–765.
48. XU, C. *et al.* 1998. Modulation of endothelial cell function by normal polyspecific human intravenous immunoglobulins: a possible mechanism of action in vascular diseases. Am. J. Pathol. **153:** 1257–1266.
49. ICHIYAMA, T. *et al.* 2004. An immunoglobulin agent (IVIG) inhibits NF-kappaB activation in cultured endothelial cells of coronary arteries in vitro. Inflamm. Res. **53:** 253–256.
50. DE GRANDMONT, M.J. *et al.* 2003. Intravenous immunoglobulins induce the in vitro differentiation of human B lymphocytes and the secretion of IgG. Blood **101:** 3065–3073.

Treatment of Pemphigus Vulgaris with Protein A Immunoadsorption

Case Report of Long-Term History Showing Favorable Outcome

NINA FROST,[a] GERALD MESSER,[b] GERHARD FIERLBECK,[c] TEUT RISLER,[a] AND SIMON D. LYTTON[d]

[a]*Universitätsklinikum Tübingen, Abteilung Innere Medizin IV, Sektion Nieren und Hochdruckkrankheiten, 72076 Tübingen, Germany*

[b]*Klinik und Poliklinik für Dermatologie und Allerlogie der Ludwig-Maximillians Universität, 80337 München, Germany*

[c]*Universitätsklinikum Tübingen, Universitäts-Hautklinik, 72076 Tübingen, Germany*

[d]*SeraDiaLogistics, 81545 München, Germany*

ABSTRACT: A pemphigus vulgaris (PV) patient with a 14-year history of severe and painful blistering of skin and mucous membranes as well as side effects from corticosteroids and concomitant immunosuppressive drug treatment was managed successfully by protein A immunoadsorption (IA). After 19 sessions of protein A IA, the patient showed remission of PV and healing of mucocutaneous lesions and the skin. The level of the pathogenic autoantibodies to the adhesion proteins desmoglein 1 (Dsg-1) and desmoglein 3 (Dsg-3) measured by ELISA and immunofluorescence microscopy revealed a significant removal of autoantibodies after each IA therapy. There was a weak rebound of anti–Dsg-1 and anti–Dsg-3 antibodies between IA sessions but an overall decrease over the period of IA therapy. This case demonstrates the effective use of protein A IA as an adjuvant and corticosteroid-sparing therapy in severe pemphigus refractory to standard immunosuppressive therapy and underscores the need for careful monitoring of autoantibodies.

KEYWORDS: pemphigus; protein A immunoadsorption; anti-Dsg autoantibodies

INTRODUCTION

The mainstay treatments of the chronic autoimmune blistering diseases pemphigus vulgaris (PV) and pemphigus foliaceus (PF), associated with formation of autoantibodies to the adhesion molecules desmoglein 1 (Dsg-1) and desmoglein 3 (Dsg-3), are systemic steroids and immunosuppressive drugs such as azathioprine, mycophenolate mofetil, cyclophosphamide, and cyclosporine A. Immunoglobulin infu-

Address for correspondence: Dr. Simon D. Lytton, SeraDiaLogistics Hertlingstrasse 1, 81545 München, Germany. Voice: +49-0-1724911169; fax: +49-89-642-54137.
simon.lytton@t-online.de

Ann. N.Y. Acad. Sci. 1051: 591–596 (2005). © **2005 New York Academy of Sciences.**
doi: 10.1196/annals.1361.103

sion,[1–3] plasma exchange,[4] and recently B lymphocyte depletion with anti-CD20 monoclonal antibody[5] have been used to remove immunoglobulins from the circulation and to alleviate symptoms caused by pathogenic autoantibodies. In a few patients who display only a partial response to these treatments, severe illness ensues; for this reason, there is a need to consider alternative therapeutic modalities. In cases of therapy-refractory PV with acute or long-term side effects, immunoadsorption (IA) can be an effective adjuvant treatment, as previously demonstrated.[6,7] In contrast with plasmapheresis, protein A IA specifically removes IgG and immune complexes without requiring plasma substitution and allows treatment of large plasma volumes.[8] In the patient presented here, we show controlled and successful management of severe PV with 19 successive protein A IA treatments adjuvant to standard immunosuppressive medication.

CASE REPORT

A 56-year-old female, 155 cm and 50 kg, was first diagnosed with PV in December 1987, presenting with widespread intraepidermal blisters and erosive lesions on her breasts, trunk, and buttocks. The initial treatment was oral prednisolone (8 mg/day) and azathioprine (30 mg/day). Because of the appearance of mucocutaneous erosions and ulcers in the oral cavity, the dosages of corticosteroids were increased to 30 mg/day for 6 months and then for 10 months combined with 1.5 g/day mycophenolate mofetil. This treatment was only partially effective, and the skin condition worsened. For 14 years of 5–30 mg/day prednisolone, the blistering continued in cycles, with the exception of one 1–2-month period in which no new blisters emerged.

In 2001, the patient presented with Cushing syndrome osteoporosis and had 100–150 lesions on her trunk, chest, and arms and complained of painful erosions with sores in the mouth. To manage these conditions, we reduced the corticosteroid dose to 5 mg/day, and the patient received analgesic medication (rofecoxib 25 mg/day). In addition, 26 high-dose intravenous infusions of 25 g bolus IgG (iv-IG) and 5 mg cyclophosphamide in pulse were given for 6 months. This treatment was only partially effective and the high Dsg-1 and Dsg-3 autoantibody levels and the PV lesions persisted.

From September 2002 to July 2003 and from April 2004 to February 2005, protein A IA was performed as an adjuvant therapy. During each of these periods, the patient received 19 sessions of protein A IA with prednisolone (100 mg/day) and azathioprine (100 mg/day). Each IA session involved extracorporeal separation of the patient's plasma and cells on Fresenius Citem10 and passage of two to three plasma volumes over two tandem Immunosorba Protein A columns. Sera samples were collected immediately before and after each IA, and the IgG fraction obtained from the column elution wash cycle was saved for the analysis of antibody reactivity. Anti–Dsg-1- and anti–Dsg-3 autoantibodies were monitored by ELISA (FIG. 1A).

The response to IA was an immediate anti-inflammatory effect. Lesions started to heal at the palate and the skin, with a subsequent absence of mucous membrane involvement. Serological findings indicated a significant removal of pathogenic Dsg-1 and Dsg-3 autoantibodies. At the onset of IA therapy, the patient's Dsg-1 and

Dsg-3 ELISA reactivities were in the range of 600–1000 U/mL. After each protein A IA, the ELISA reactivity decreased by 10-fold (results not shown).

To prepare the patient for hip surgery in August 2003, we discontinued IA, and the corticosteroid dosage was reduced to prednisolone (8 mg/day) and azathioprine (50 mg/day). The patient was maintained on this dose until March 2004. After cessation of protein A IA, there was mild recurrence of the disease in the form of approximately five new blisters every 2 weeks (FIG. 1B).

Between April 2004 and August 2004, the patient had another 13 sessions of protein A IA therapy with prednisolone (50 mg/day) and azathioprine (50 mg/day) (FIG. 1A). During this second cycle of protein A IA therapy, the anti–Dsg-1 and anti–Dsg-3 antibodies were eliminated after each IA (anti–Dsg-1 = mean, 1.7 U/mL;

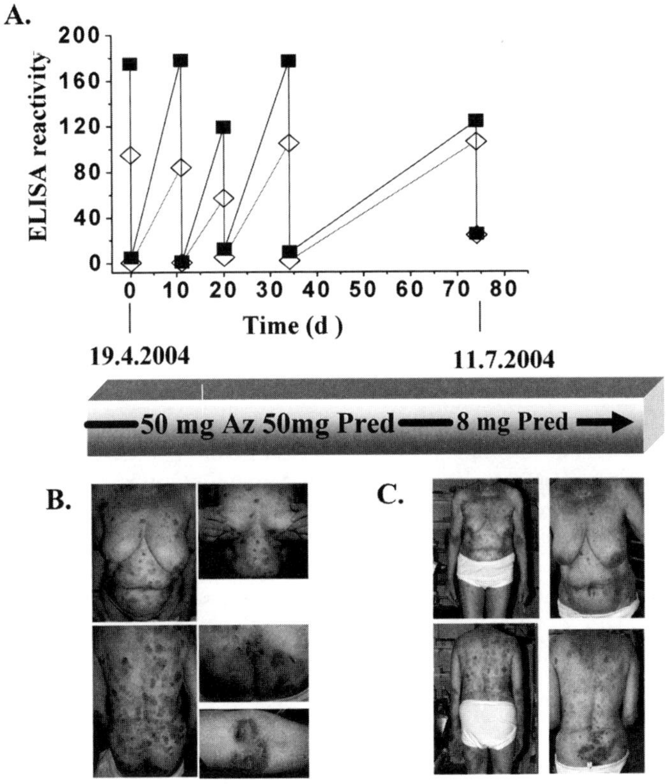

FIGURE 1. Anti-Dsg autoantibodies and skin lesions in a pemphigus vulgaris patient (RF) during protein A IA and corticosteroid therapy. (**A**) ELISA reactivity in the patient's sera taken before and immediately after protein A IA. The values of anti–Dsg-3 (*filled squares*) and anti–Dsg-1 (*open diamonds*) represent the mean of duplicate samples in the second series of protein A IA measured, using MESACUP Desmoglein Test (MBL, Nagoya, Japan). (**B, C**) Clinical presentation of the pemphigus lesions. Lesions on chest and buttocks of the patient (**B**) in September 2003 before the second series of protein A IA and (**C**) in August 2004 after the 13th treatment.

range, 0.4–5 U/mL; and anti–Dsg-3 = mean, 5.6 U/mL; range, 1–12 U/mL). A rebound to positive anti–Dsg-1 and anti–Dsg-3 reactivity in the range of 50–150 U/mL and 100–175 U/mL, respectively, was consistently detected between each IA session (FIG. 1A).

From September 2004 to the present, the patient was treated with maintenance therapy of prednisolone (8–15 mg/day) and protein A IA (once a month). The skin condition is currently stable with mild non-mucous-membrane blisters and erythema with features of PF (FIG. 1C).

RECOVERY OF AUTOANTIBODY REACTIVITY IN PROTEIN A–PURIFIED IGG

To better monitor the pathogenic autoantibodies in this case of PV, we analyzed the ELISA reactivities and immunofluorescence of the eluted wash fraction of the protein A columns during the course of IA therapy. The normalized (per milligram IgG) ELISA reactivity in the pre-IA plasma was as follows: anti–Dsg-1 = mean, 2000 U/mg IgG; range, 1500–2500 U/mg IgG; and anti–Dsg-3 = mean, 3800 U/mg IgG; range, 3500–6000 U/mg IgG. The autoantibody reactivity in the protein A–purified IgG fraction was as follows: anti–Dsg-1 = mean, 1160 U/mg IgG; range, 750–1500 U/mg IgG; and anti–Dsg-3 = mean, 2350 U/mg IgG; range, 1500–3800 U/mg IgG. This indicates a 50% lower level of specific reactivity compared with the plasma. The plasma IgG levels before and after protein A IA were in the range of 0.5–0.96 g/dL and 0.05–0.07 g/dL, respectively.

In two of seven measured IA sessions in 2004, anti–Dsg-3 reactivity was detected in the plasma circulation after protein A IA. The residual reactivity after protein A IA suggests that IgG isotypes emerge during protein A IA therapy that do not bind to protein A. Technical problems—such as insufficient plasma flows, incomplete washing cycles, or regeneration of the protein A columns—were unlikely to explain the residual autoantibody reactivity during these sessions. Autoantibody reactivity was recovered from the protein A column, and the amount of total IgG depletion was similar to IA sessions in which anti-Dsg reactivity was abolished. Although flareup in circulatory autoantibodies continued between IA sessions, further increase in residual anti–Dsg-3 ELISA reactivity was not detected after subsequent IA.

Because indirect immunofluorescence microscopy tests (IFTs) are routine for pemphigus diagnostics, we monitored the IFT titers of patient plasma on esophagus tissue sections of monkey (FIG. 2A) and rabbit (FIG. 2B) before and after IA. The patient's autoantibody reactivities in the IFTs revealed a similar pattern to that of ELISA. After each IA session, there was a 10- to 20-fold decrease in plasma IFT titer and a subsequent rebound between sessions. It is interesting that confocal immunofluorescence of the protein A–purified IgG showed typical cell membrane localization characteristic of desmosomal staining and no cytoplasmic staining. No colocalization was seen for nuclear fluorescence of the DNA-binding dye TOPRO-3 and the fluorescein isothiocyanate–labeled antihuman IgG (FIG. 2C, panel a). A similar immunofluorescence was found in the plasma before IA (data not shown), but no specific staining was detected from the patient's plasma obtained immediately after IA (FIG. 2C, panel b).

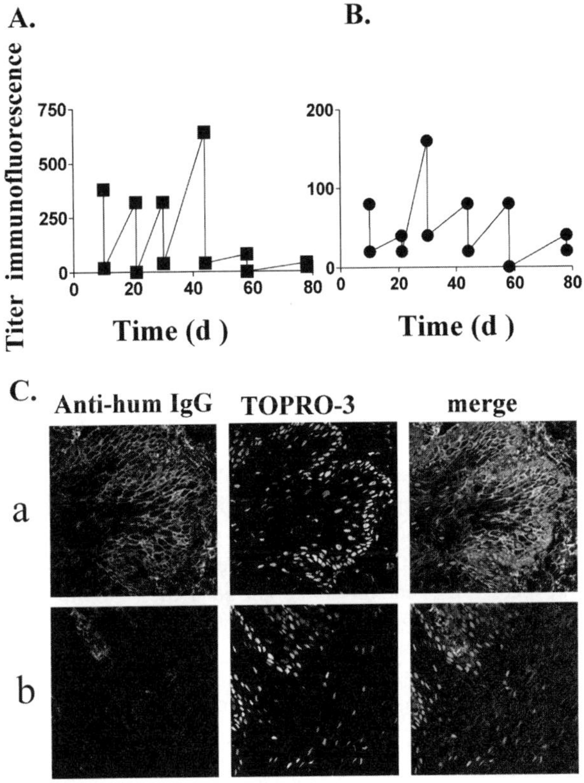

FIGURE 2. Serum autoantibodies show positive immunofluorescence reactivity. Titers of serum IMTs on tissue sections prepared from the esophagus of (**A**) monkey and (**B**) rabbit. (**C**) Confocal immunofluorescence of monkey esophagus. Immunofluorescence reactivity of DNA-binding dye TOPR-3 and fluorescein isothiocyanate–labeled antihuman IgG in the presence of 1:40 diluted protein A–purified IgG of the patient (RF) (panel **a**) and 1:40 diluted serum of the patient after protein A IA (panel **b**). Sera samples were taken on February 6, 2004.

DISCUSSION

The use of protein A IA as an adjuvant and corticosteroid-sparing therapy in PV is demonstrated in this case report. The removal of pathogenic autoantibodies by protein A IA alleviated the blister severity and had a positive impact on the patient's skin condition and overall well-being. Clonal expansion of autoreactive pathogenic B cells is driven by antigen-specific T cells,[9] and the underlying T cell defect is not corrected by IA. For this reason, the B cell factory remains intact, and rebound in circulating autoantibodies is predicted. The development of T cell–targeting therapies that interfere with the autoimmune process and deliver long-lasting effects in PV and other related autoimmune diseases is needed. For the present, extracorporal protein A IA remains a safe, efficient, and noninvasive treatment to complement the available therapeutic regimens with corticosteroids and further immunosuppressive drugs.

In our patient, with long-term PV of 16 years, the use of azathioprine, mycophenolate, and iv-IgG as well as rofecoxib had no major effect on the painful erosions, blistering, and serious corticosteroid side effects and did not lead to stable remission of the disease. No further therapeutic options were available. Protein A IA reduced the circulating IgG and provided the patient with a window of relief from tissue-destructive anti-Dsg autoantibodies. This regimen was well tolerated, and, under renewed corticosteroid dosing, partial intraepidermal healing has been achieved. Up until now, the use of repeated protein A IA for PV was restricted to a last-resort therapy. The results of this case suggest that use of protein A IA should be considered as an intervention earlier in the course of disease to prevent PV with painful erosions and severe corticosteroid side effects, which can be life threatening.

Future studies are needed to assess in more detail the pathogenicity of autoantibodies that persist between protein A IA sessions. The isotype of the anti-Dsg antibodies that show residual reactivity immediately after protein A IA has to be characterized. The ability to recover large quantities of IgG with autoantibody reactivity from protein A IA columns, as shown here, will allow investigations of pathogenic antibodies in experimental animals to determine the specificity of these antibodies with respect to Dsg and other autoantigens, their binding to keratinocytes, and the effects on cell-signaling cascades in apoptotic pathways.

ACKNOWLEDGMENTS

The authors are grateful to Karin Woischwill and Andrea Hess for their technical assistance and expertise in ELISA and immunofluorescence measurements.

REFERENCES

1. MESSER, G. *et al.* 1995. High-dosage intravenous immunoglobulins for immediate control of severe pemphigus vulgaris. Br. J. Dermatol. **133:** 1014–1015.
2. HUMBERT, P. *et al.* 1990. Effects of intravenous γ-globulin in pemphigus. J. Am. Acad. Dermatol. **22:** 326–330.
3. SHEEHAN, D. *et al.* 2004. Deep venous thrombosis after high-dose intravenous immunoglobulin in the treatment of pemphigus vulgaris. Curtis **73:** 403–406.
4. MAZZI, G. *et al.* 2003. Plasmapheresis therapy in pemphigus vulgaris and bullous pemphigoid. Transf. Apher. Sci. **28:** 13–18.
5. ESPANA, A. *et al.* 2004. Long-term complete remission of severe pemphigus vulgaris with monoclonal anti-CD20 antibody therapy and immunophenotype correlations. J. Am. Acad. Dermatol. **150:** 1018–1024.
6. SCHMIDT, E. *et al.* 2003. Protein A immunoadsorption: a novel and effective adjuvant treatment of severe pemphigus. Br. J. Dermatol. **148:** 1222–1229.
7. LÜFTL, M. *et al.* 2003. Successful removal of pathogenic autoantibodies in pemphigus by immunoadsorption with a tryptophan-linked polyvinylalcohol adsorber. Br. J. Dermatol. **149:** 598–605.
8. BRAUN, N. *et al.* 2000. Immunoadsorption onto protein A induces remission in severe systemic lupus erythematosus. Nephrol. Dial. Transplant. **15:** 1367–1372.
9. LIN, M. *et al.* 1997. Development and characterization of desmoglein-3 specific T cells from patients with pemphigus vulgaris. J. Clin. Invest. **99:** 31–40.

Immunosuppressive Therapy and Clinical Evolution in Forty-nine Patients with Antineutrophil Cytoplasmic Antibody–Associated Glomerulonephritis

E. KOKOLINA, E. ALEXOPOULOS, C. DIMITRIADIS, A. VAINAS, P. GIAMALIS, A. PAPAGIANNI, D. EKONOMIDOU, AND D. MEMMOS

Department of Nephrology, Aristotle University, Hippokration General Hospital, Thessaloniki, Greece

ABSTRACT: **Immunosuppressive therapy and clinical evolution were studied in 49 patients (29 females) with antineutrophil cytoplasmic antibody (ANCA)–associated glomerulonephritis. The mean age of patients at presentation was 55 years, and the mean (±SD) follow-up was 43 months (±33) (range, 3–140). Among the 49 patients, 10 had biopsy-proven Wegener's granulomatosis, 33 microscopic polyangiitis, 2 Churg-Strauss syndrome, and 4 idiopathic crescentic glomerulonephritis. IgG ANCA autoantibodies were detected in all patients. Induction therapy included pulses and oral administration of methylprednisolone (MP) with oral administration of cyclophosphamide (CP) and plasma exchange in patients with alveolar hemorrhage and serum creatinine (SCr) levels ≥6 mg/dL. CP was converted to azathioprine (AZA) or mycophenolate mofetil (MMF) after 3–6 months of therapy. Low doses of MP with or without AZA or MMF were administered until the end of follow-up. Therapy institution resulted in remission of disease in all patients. The mean SCr levels decreased from 4.9 mg/dL (±2.5) at the onset of the disease to 2.8 mg/dL (±1.7) ($P > 0.0001$), and 3.2 mg/dL (±2.3) ($P > 0.0001$) after 3 and 6 months, respectively. At the end of follow-up, 17 (35%) patients progressed to end-stage renal disease after 34 months (±29) (range, 3–98), and 30 (61%) patients maintained sufficient renal function. Two patient deaths were attributed to immunosuppression. Patients with high SCr levels at diagnosis and severe interstitial fibrosis found in renal biopsy had poor renal outcome ($P > 0.01$ and $P > 0.02$, respectively). Induction therapy with MP and CP seems to be the regimen of choice in patients with ANCA-associated glomerulonephritis. Early diagnosis and therapy institution as well as long-term treatment lead to acceptable renal survival.**

KEYWORDS: **ANCA-associated glomerulonephritis; immunosuppressive therapy; renal survival; renal pathology**

Address for correspondence: Dr. Elisabeth Kokolina, 13, Kath Rossidou Str., 54655-Thessaloniki, Greece. Voice: +30-2310-892328; fax: +30-2310-992855.
kokolina@med.auth.gr

Ann. N.Y. Acad. Sci. 1051: 597–605 (2005). © 2005 New York Academy of Sciences.
doi: 10.1196/annals.1361.104

INTRODUCTION

Antineutrophil cytoplasmic antibody (ANCA)–associated glomerulonephritis is a pauci-immune necrotizing crescentic glomerulonephritis (NCGN) and occurs as part of small-vessel vasculitides or as idiopathic NCGN without extrarenal manifestations.[1–5] Wegener granulomatosis (WG), microscopic polyangiitis (MPA), Churg-Strauss syndrome (CSS), and the renal-limited form of rapidly progressive glomerulonephritis are described as small-vessel vasculitides and are commonly associated with ANCAs.[1–5] ANCAs are directed against antigens in the azurophilic granules of neutrophils and the peroxidase-positive lysosomes of monocytes.[2–4] The two major antigenic targets recognized by ANCAs are proteinase 3 (PR3) and myeloperoxidase (MPO).[2–4] ANCAs are now considered a useful tool for diagnosis and, by some authors, a sensitive marker of disease activity and remission.[6,7] In addition, recent data suggest that ANCAs are involved in the pathogenesis of vasculitis.[8,9]

The prognosis of untreated ANCA-associated vasculitis (AASV) is poor. Immunosuppressive therapy is usually effective in controlling disease progression in most patients, leading to better patient and kidney survival. Induction therapy with the combination of corticosteroids and cyclophosphamide is now considered as the gold standard treatment for this group of diseases. However, immunosuppressive therapy is toxic and contributes to morbidity and mortality of the disease. A successful treatment of AASV must include early diagnosis and institution of therapy before permanent scarring occurs and must reduce the potentially life-threatening side effects of immunosuppression. On the other hand many patients progressed to chronic renal failure despite an initially favorable response to treatment. Probably, the time to convert the initial aggressive therapy to a milder maintenance immunosuppression, such as azathioprine (AZA) or mycophenolate mofetil (MMF), and the time to stop the immunosuppression are of particular importance for patient and renal survival.

The aim of this study is to determine the results of the immunosuppressive therapy in patients with AASV using aggressive induction therapy with methylprednisolone (MP) and cyclophosphamide (CP) and low doses of MP with or without AZA or MMF as maintenance therapy until the end of follow-up.

PATIENTS AND METHODS

Patients

From January 1994 until January 2004, 89 patients with AASV were diagnosed in our nephrology department. Of these patients, 49 (29 women) were followed up adequately in our center. The mean age of patients at presentation was 55 years and the mean follow-up was at 43 (±33) months (range, 3–140). Among the 49 patients, 10 had biopsy-proven WG, 33 had MPA, 2 had CSS, and 4 had the limited form of idiopathic NCGN. All patients had an ANCA-positive test by indirect immunofluorescence (IIF) and ELISA and renal involvement by means of the pauci-immune NCGN. WG was considered to be present in any patient with NCGN and granulomatous inflammation in any organ, and MPA was considered to be present in patients with NCGN and systemic clinical manifestations. The diagnosis of CSS was based on the findings of NCGN with or without giant-cell granuloma formation in combination with asthma and eosinophilia. The idiopathic NCGN was considered to be present in patients with NCGN without systemic disease manifestations.

All patients were followed up every 15 days for the first 3 months, every month until the first year, and every 2–3 months thereafter. At every visit, a complete clinical and laboratory workup was performed.

METHODS

The inclusion criteria for the study were as follows: (1) a renal biopsy showing a pauci-immune focal or diffuse segmental NCGN; (2) detection of ANCA in the patient's sera by IIF, followed by ELISA for further characterization of the antigenic target; and (3) adequate follow-up, consecutive clinical and laboratory examinations, and serial ANCA testing until the end of the study.

The age of the patients; the clinical extrarenal manifestations; the presence of hypertension; and laboratory findings such as proteinuria, hematuria, and serum creatinine (SCr) levels and the type and titer of ANCA were estimated in all patients. The severity of histologic findings at initial biopsy were assessed by two pathologists, as has been described previously.[10] A paucity of the immune deposits was defined as <2+ (of 0 to 4+) immunoglobulin deposits on immunofluorescence microscopy. The starting day of the study was considered to be the date of renal biopsy, and the end point for renal survival was the start of renal replacement therapy. The patients who died during the study were excluded from the study.

The patients were divided in two groups. Group A included patients who maintained an adequate renal function during follow-up, and group B included patients who progressed to end-stage renal disease (ESRD). A subgroup in group A included patients who maintained normal renal function until the end of the study. Statistical analysis was done using the Kruscal-Wallis one-way analysis of variance and the Mann-Whitney U test.

ANCA Detection

IIF

The serum of all patients, diluted 1:20, was subjected to an IIF assay on ethanol-fixed granulocytes using commercially available slides (INOVA Diagnostics, San Diego, CA). The preparations were considered to be positive for c-ANCA if the neutrophils showed a diffuse fluorescence in the cytoplasm; for p-ANCA, if the neutrophils showed a perinuclear staining; and atypical ANCA, if the type of fluorescence was not distinguishable.

ELISA

When ANCA detection was positive by using IIF, serum was tested by ELISA for both antimyeloperoxidase and antiproteinase activities using standard commercial kits: PR3-ANCA (Varelisa, Freiburg, Germany) ELISA and MPO-ANCA (Varelisa) ELISA. In addition, over the last 5 years, positive serum by IIF was tested not only for PR3 and MPO ANCA but also for other antigenic targets of the primary granules (ANCA Panel-kit; Wieslab, Lund, Sweden). The results for MPO and PR3 ANCA were graded positive or negative according to a scale from 0 to 100 U/mL provided from the manufacturer. ELISA results were categorized as positive when the result was > 7 U or exactly 7 U, and negative when the result was < 7 U. At presentation all patients had an ANCA titer of more than 40 U. An ANCA titer of less or more than 7 U or exactly 7 U was noted during follow-up in both groups.

Patients with an atypical fluorescence of ANCA or with an antigenic target other than PR3 or MPO were excluded from this study.

Treatment and Follow-up

The induction therapy of patients with NCGN with or without extrarenal manifestations consisted of MP and oral administration of CP. Intravenous MP was administered, at a dose of 1 g for 3 days consecutively, followed by oral administration of MP at a maximum dose of 48 mg/day for 2 months with progressive tapering to the dose of 6 mg/day. CP was given orally from the first day of treatment (1–1.5 mg/kg/day), depending on the white blood cell count. Once remission was achieved, the daily dose of CP was tapered by 25 mg every 1–2 months. Plasma exchange was added to the induction therapy in case of either alveolar hemorrhage and SCr levels >6 mg/dL or persistence of active disease. In one patient, cyclosporine, instead of CP, in combination with MP was used successfully as induction therapy.

After 3–6 months of therapy, CP was converted to AZA (1–2 mg/kg/day) or MMF (15–25 mg/kg/day). Low doses of MP (6 mg/day) were maintained alone or in combination with AZA or MMF until the end of follow-up.

The patients were considered to have relapses when a rapid SCr level accompanied by an active urine sediment occurred. Recurrence of clinical manifestations of AASV, increase of ANCA levels, and a new renal biopsy showing new necrotizing lesions contributed to the diagnosis of relapses. Patients with a relapse were treated according to the same protocol of induction therapy.

RESULTS

By definition, all patients had ANCA-associated pauci-immune NCGN. A total of 10 patients (20.4%) had WG, and in 9 of these patients the granulomas were found from extrarenal manifestations. MPA was diagnosed in 33 (67.3%) patients, and idiopathic NCGN and CSS were diagnosed in 2 (4%) and 4 (8.2%) patients, respectively.

At presentation, the mean (±SD) SCr levels were 4.9 mg/dL (±2.5). Clinical and laboratory findings at presentation are shown in TABLE 1. A total of 11 patients (22%) required hemodialysis (HD) at presentation. Microscopic hematuria and proteinuria were observed in all patients. Low-grade proteinuria (<1.5 g/day) was found in 33 (67%) patients, and high-grade proteinuria (>1.5 g/day) was found in 16 (33%) patients. Two female patients, who maintained a satisfactory renal function (2 mg/dL), had a nephrotic syndrome rate proteinuria before treatment, which decreases to a rate of 1.5–2 g/day after treatment. Hypertension was present in 38 (77%) patients, but 13 of them were hypertensive before this diagnosis. Anti-MPO ANCAs were detected in 30 (61%) patients, and anti-PR3 ANCAs were detected in 19 (39%) patients. The mean ANCA level at diagnosis was 54 U (±34). Initial renal biopsy

TABLE 1. Clinical and laboratory findings at diagnosis

Measure	Patients	
	Number	Percentage
Microscopic hematuria	49	100
Proteinuria <1.5 g/day	33	67
Proteinuria >1.5 g/day	16	33
Hypertension	38	77
ANCA positivity	49	100
IgG anti-MPO	30	61
IgG anti-PR3	19	39
Pauci-immune NCGN	49	100

NOTE: SCr: mean = 4.9 mg/dL (±2.5); range, 0.80–10.40 mg/dL.

showed NCGN in 47 patients and necrotizing glomerulonephritis without crescents in two patients. The latter two patients had normal SCr levels at presentation, no clinical manifestations of vasculitis, an abnormal urine sediment, and high IgG anti-MPO titers. On immunofluorescence, all patients had a pauci-immune glomerulonephritis.

Induction therapy resulted in remission of disease activity in all patients. Most patients responded immediately to treatment, and, within a week, symptoms and signs of extrarenal manifestations improved. ANCA levels measured by ELISA decreased during the first 10 days of treatment. Renal disease responded slowly in most patients, and the maximal improvement occurred 1–2 months after induction therapy. At 3 months after immunosuppressive treatment, the mean value of initial ANCA levels decreased from 54 U (±34) to 9.5 U (±12) ($P < 0.001$). The mean SCr levels also decreased from 4.9 mg/dL (±2.5) to 2.8 mg/dL (±1.7) ($P < 0.0001$) and then to 3.2 mg/dL (±2.3) ($P < 0.0001$) after 3 and 6 months of therapy, respectively. As noted, 11 patients initially required HD. During follow-up, seven of these patients progressed to ESRD and four remained off dialysis.

The outcome of renal function at the end of follow-up is shown in TABLE 2. A total of 30 (61%) patients (group A) remained off dialysis, with a mean SCr level of 2.1 mg/dL (±1.2) (range, 0.8–5.5). Of these, 10 (33.3%) patients maintained normal renal function at the end of the observation period. At presentation, they showed a lower SCr value (3.5 mg/dL [±2.45]) than the other patients, with a mean follow-up period of 57.8 months (±18.60). The remaining 20 (66.6%) patients in group A had an initial SCr of 4.8 mg/dL (±2.2) and for a mean period of 60 months (±140) maintained a SCr value of 2.59 mg/dL (±1.2).

The remaining 17 (35%) patients (group B) progressed to ESRD in a mean period of 34 months (±29) (range, 3–98). Of these, 2 patients progressed to ESRD in 3 months, 4 in 6 months after induction therapy, and the remaining 11 in a mean period of 45 months (±7) (range, 24–98). The seven patients who progressed to ESRD in the first 6 months had severe histologic changes by means of glomerular sclerosis and interstitial fibrosis, and, in five of them the duration of the disease was 2–6 months before treatment was initiated. It is likely that they came to the hospital too late and their disease was untreated for too long a time before admission. Two

TABLE 2. Comparative clinical and laboratory data at presentation according to the outcome of the patients

	Renal function at end of study		
	Group A		Group B
Patients' data at diagnosis	Normal RF	Impaired RF (2.59 ±1.2)	ESRD
No. of patients	10	20	17
Mean age (yr)	53.80 (±18.67)	49.85 (±19.10)	58.82 (±17.33)
Mean follow-up (mo)	57.8 (±18.60)	60.00 (±40.00)	34 (±29)
Mean SCr (mg/dL)	3.5 (±2.45)	4.8 (±2.2)	6.59 (±2.16) ($P < 0.01$)
Proteinuria (no. of patients; g/day)	4; >1.5 6; <1.5	9; 1.5 11; <1.5	3; >1.5 14; <1.5
Hypertension (no. of patients)	6	17	15
ANCA (no. patients; type)	5; anti-PR3 5; anti-MPO	17; anti-MPO 3; anti-PR3	8; anti-MPO 9; anti-PR3

NOTE: Renal pathology: more severe and extent lesions in group B—glomerular sclerosis ($P < 0.03$), fibrocellular crescents ($P < 0.01$), interstitial inflammation ($P < 0.05$), and interstitial fibrosis ($P < 0.01$).

patients' deaths were related to immunosuppressive therapy. Both patients were older (75 and 80 years), and they died of severe lung infection (cytomegalovirus and pseudomonas), after 8 and 10 months of therapy and while their SCr levels were 0.8 mg/dL and 2.0 mg/dL, respectively.

Relapses were noted in 12 (24%) patients in a mean period of 15 months (±5) after treatment initiation. All patients showed an increase in SCr levels, and 8 (67%) of them had a threefold increase in ANCA titers; four of these patients were in group B, progressing to ESRD.

The possible prognostic parameters for renal survival (e.g., age, extrarenal clinical manifestations, entry SCr level, proteinuria, hypertension, and type of ANCA) were evaluated at the end of the observation period between the two groups of patients. We did not find any significant influence of these parameters on renal survival, except for SCr level and the age of the patient at diagnosis. Patients with higher proteinuria had a slightly worse outcome of renal disease, but the difference was not statistically significant. In contrast, a high SCr value at presentation was a poor predictor of renal survival ($P < 0.01$). In addition, the entry SCr level correlated significantly with the extent of tubular atrophy found in the initial biopsy ($P < 0.01$).

Clinicopathologic correlations revealed that poor renal outcome correlated with the severity of glomerular sclerosis ($P < 0.03$), the percentage of fibrocellular crescents ($P < 0.01$), and tubulointerstitial changes such as interstitial inflammation ($P < 0.05$) and interstitial fibrosis ($P < 0.02$). All these changes predicted a poor renal outcome in our study. The immunofluorescence findings did not affect prognosis in our patients. The estimated duration of the disease before histologic diagnosis was similar in both groups (*P* value not significant).

DISCUSSION

Early immunosuppressive treatment and better understanding of the pathogenesis of AASV have led to marked improvement in both patient and kidney survival.[2,4,11,12] However, patients with AASV are still prone to ESRD and to severe side effects of immunosuppression. In this study, 30 (61%) patients (group A) remained off dialysis, maintaining a sufficient renal function until the end of the follow-up, and 17 (35%) progressed to ESRD (group B). Of the 17 patients of group B, 6 lost renal function in a small period of 3–6 months, despite a transient remission after induction therapy. The remaining 11 patients maintained sufficient renal function for a mean period of 45 months (±7) (range, 24–98). It is now well known that up to 20% of patients with AASV reach ESRD and need renal replacement therapy over a mean period of follow-up of 32 months.[13,14] Renal failure is the result of either treatment resistance and repeated inflammatory insult to the kidneys or slowly progressive fibrosis and glomerulosclerosis.

Our results showed that the mean SCr level at presentation was significantly higher in group B of patients, reflecting a sign of poor renal outcome. The predictive value of SCr level at presentation in ASSV is controversial. Some authors believe that the SCr level at diagnosis is the strongest predictor of renal oucome,[15] but others found that the SCr level at diagnosis does not differ between patients with a favorable renal outcome and those who developed chronic renal failure.[16] From our data, four (13%) patients of group A and seven (41%) patients of group B presented with advanced renal failure requiring dialysis. In other words, patients in both groups had both low SCr levels and high SCr levels requiring dialysis. Although our statistical analysis revealed that the initial SCr level predicts renal outcome, we believe that high SCr levels only in combination with chronic renal lesions and renal scarring or active lesions at presentation accurately predict long-term renal survival.

Of the 30 patients in group A, 10 who had normal renal function at the end of follow-up had an initial SCr level of 3.5 mg/dL (±2.4). In contrast, the remaining 20 of this group who progressed had much higher SCr levels at presentation (4.8 mg/dL [±2.2]). During follow-up, these 10 patients maintained normal renal function with mild proteinuria and negative ANCA testing. One of them experienced a relapse, which was treated successfully. We believe that for these patients there was no delay in diagnosis and institution of therapy. In this subgroup, two patients had abnormal urine sediment on admission, and only the high titer of ANCA led us to perform a renal biopsy, which revealed necrotizing glomerulonephritis without crescents. Another two patients were admitted with high fever and alveolar hemorrhage in combination with high ANCA titer, and the remaining six patients had mild signs and symptoms of the disease. In all 10 patients, there was no suspicion of subclinical disease before admission. The remaining 20 patients in group A maintained sufficient renal function at the end of follow-up (SCr, 2.59 mg/dL ±1.2). All patients who relapsed were off CCP at the time of relapse, but they were receiving AZA plus MP.

In all, 12 relapses (24%) were observed in our patients. Only two patients of group B lost renal function after a relapse: one during the 8th month and the other in the 24th month of treatment. All other relapses manifested in both groups were treated successfully. The remaining patients progressed slowly to ESRD without signs of relapse or acute deterioration of renal function due to another cause. Franssen *et al.* found that most patients with anti-MPO AASV progressed to ESRD without signs of relapse.[16] An elevation of SCr levels in all patients and threefold ANCA titers in 8/12 (66.6%) patients were observed. In patients without an elevation of the ANCA titer, the diagnosis was difficult, especially in patients with lung infection.

Statistical analysis, concerning renal outcome between the two groups, revealed that the chronic renal lesions, such as glomerulosclerosis, fibrocellular crescents, and interstitial fibrosis, are associated with the poor renal outcome in group B. In addition, the only active lesion predictive of renal function was the amount of diffuse interstitial infiltration. These chronic and active interstitial lesions at initial biopsy probably account for the high SCr levels at admission of the patients in group B.

One study suggests that the more chronic lesions found in renal biopsy, the higher the SCr level will be 1 year later.[17] In another study, the authors believe that chronic lesions at biopsy are not of predictive value of poor renal outcome and suggest that the mechanism underlying renal function loss may be the hyperfiltration of remnant glomeruli. The same authors found a significant correlation between the grade of proteinuria and loss of renal function, and they suggest that proteinuria is a consequence of glomerulosclerosis and interstitial scarring.[16] In this study, we did not note a statistical significance between the loss of renal function and the grade of proteinuria.

We continued treatment of our patients with low doses of immunosuppression until the end of follow-up. Although the combination of MP and CP is effective as an induction therapy, long-term maintenance treatment with AZA and MMF is associated with unacceptable morbidity and mortality. Less toxic and more effective therapeutic agents are needed for more effective long-term treatment.

In conclusion, patients with AASV and NCGN are still prone to ESRD. Although treatment with corticosteroids and cyclophosphamide has improved patient and renal survival, a high percentage of patients progressed to ESRD. Disease-related morbidity usually arises from delays in therapy institution and progression of subclinical disease. Important predictors of poor renal outcome at diagnosis are the high entry SCr levels in combination with sclerosing renal lesions and active interstitial infiltration at initial biopsy. Early diagnosis and therapy institution and individualization of induction and long-term therapy in these patients should be the first step toward long-term control of the disease.

REFERENCES

1. Davies, D.J., J.E. Moran, J.F. Niall & G.B. Ryan. 1982. Segmental necrotising glomerulonephritis with antineutrophil antibody: possible arbovirus aetiology? Br. Med. J. **285:** 606.
2. van der Woude, F.J., N. Rasmussen, S. Lobatto, *et al.* 1985. Autoantibodies against neutrophils and monocytes: tool for diagnosis and marker of disease activity in Wegener's granulomatosis. Lancet **1:** 425–429.
3. Falk, R.J. & J.C. Jenette. 1988. Antineutrophil cytoplasmic antibodies with specificity for myeloperoxidase in patients with systemic vasculitis and idiopathic crescentic glomerulonephritis. N. Engl. J. Med. **318:** 1651–1657.

4. Kallenberg, C.G., E. Brouwer, J.J. Weening & J.W. Tervaert. 1994. Antineutrophil cytoplasmic antibodies: current diagnostic and pathophysiological potential. Kidney Int. **46:** 1–15.
5. Savage, C.O.S., L. Harper, P. Cockwell, *et al.* 2000. Vasculitis. Br. Med. J. **320:** 1325–1328.
6. Cohen Tervaert, J., R. Goldschmeding, J.D. Elema, *et al.* 1990. Association of autoantibodies to myeloperoxidase with different forms of vasculitis. Arthritis Rheum. **33:** 1264–1272.
7. Girard, T., A. Mahr, L.H. Noel, *et al.* 2001. Are antineutrophil cytoplasmic antibodies a marker of predictive of relapse in Wegener's granulomatosis? A prospective study. Arthritis Rheum **40:** 147–151.
8. Xiao, H., P. Heeringa, P. Hu, *et al.* 2002. Antineutrophil cytoplasmic autoantibodies specific for myeloperoxidase cause glomerulonephritis and vasculitis in mice. J. Clin. Invest. **110:** 955–963.
9. Heeringa, P. & J.W. Cohen Tervaert. 2004. Pathophysiology of ANCA-associated vasculitides: are ANCA really pathogenic? Kidney Int. **65:** 1564–1567.
10. Bajema, I.M., E.C. Hagen, B. Hansen, *et al.* 1996. Scoring renal histopathology in systemic vasculitis: an international survey study of inter and intra observer agreement. Nephrol. Dial. Transplant. **11:** 1989–1995.
11. Hoffman, G.S., G.S. Kerr, R.Y. Leavitt, *et al.* 1992. Wegener's granulomatosis an analysis of 158 patients. Ann. Intern. Med. **116:** 488–498.
12. Kamesh, L., L. Harper & C.O.S. Savage. 2002. ANCA-positive vasculitis. J. Am. Soc. Nephrol. **13:** 1953–1960.
13. Westman, K.W.A., P.G. Bygren, H. Olsson, *et al.* 1998. Relapse rate, renal survival and cancer morbidity in patients with Wegener's granulomatosis or microscopic polyangiitis with renal involvement. J. Am. Soc. Nephrol. **7:** 842–852.
14. Nachman, P.H., S. Hogan, J.C. Jennette & R.J. Falk. 1996. Treatment response and relapse in ANCA-associated microscopic polyangiitis and glomerulonephritis. J. Am. Soc. Nephrol. **7:** 33–39.
15. Hogan, S., P.H. Nachman, A.S. Wilkman, *et al.* 1996. Prognostic markers in patients with antineutrophil cytoplasmic antibody-associated microscopic polyangiitis and glomerulonephritis. J. Am. Soc. Nephrol. **7:** 23–32.
16. Franssen, C.F.M., C.A. Stegeman, W.W. Oost-Kort, *et al.* 1998. Determinants of renal outcome in anti-myeloperoxidase-associated necrotizing crescentic glomerulonephritis. J. Am. Soc. Nephrol. **9:** 1915–1923.
17. Bajema, I.M., E.C. Hagen, J. Hermans, *et al.* 1999. Kidney biopsy as a predictor for renal outcome in ANCA-associated necrotizing glomerulonephritis. Kidney Int. **56:** 1751–1758.

Management of Thrombosis in Antiphospholipid Syndrome and Systemic Lupus Erythematosus in Pregnancy

GUILLERMO RUIZ-IRASTORZA[a] AND MUNTHER A. KHAMASHTA[b]

[a]*Service and Department of Internal Medicine, Hospital de Cruces, University of the Basque Country, Bizkaia, Spain*

[b]*Lupus Research Unit, Guy's, King's and St. Thomas' Medical School, The Rayne Institute, St. Thomas' Hospital, London, United Kingdom*

ABSTRACT: Pregnancy is a high risk period for thrombosis in women with antiphospholipid syndrome (APS) and systemic lupus erythematosus (SLE) with antiphospholipid antibodies (aPL). Thrombosis may affect the mother, both in the venous and arterial beds, and also have a role in pregnancy loss. Thromboprophylaxis thus is warranted in most of these women. However, specific regimens containing low-dose aspirin, unfractionated heparin (UH), low molecular weight heparin (LMWH), and even dicumarinics in some circumstances after the first trimester are still a matter of controversy. Women with previous thrombosis should receive full antithrombotic doses of UH or LMWH during the whole pregnancy. Treatment of pregnancy losses is more debated, consisting of low-dose aspirin with or without associated heparin. The choice of treatment for a given patient must always take into account the woman's opinion after a careful discussion with the treating physician. Peripartum thromboprophylaxis with LMWH in women receiving aspirin-only regimens and prevention of osteoporosis in those treated with heparin are considered essential in the medical management of these patients.

KEYWORDS: pregnancy; thrombosis; antiphospholipid syndrome; systemic lupus erythematosus

INTRODUCTION

Pregnancy is characterized by the combination of a procoagulant state, meant to avoid massive maternal bleeding during delivery, and venous stasis caused by venous dilation and compression by the gravid uterus.[1] Thus, pregnant women are at an increased risk for thromboembolic complications, a risk that is obviously higher among women suffering any prothrombotic condition.

Thrombosis is a major risk factor in patients with systemic lupus erythematosus (SLE), particularly in those with antiphospholipid (aPL) antibodies. Likewise, the clinical course of patients with the primary antiphospholipid syndrome (APS) is mainly defined by the occurrence of recurrent thrombotic events. Either primary or

Address for correspondence: Munther A. Khamashta, Lupus Research Unit, The Rayne Institute, St. Thomas' Hospital, London SE1 7EH, UK. Voice: +20-76202567; fax: +20-76202658. munther.khamashta@kcl.ac.uk

Ann. N.Y. Acad. Sci. 1051: 606–612 (2005). © 2005 New York Academy of Sciences. doi: 10.1196/annals.1361.105

secondary to SLE, APS is unique among common thrombophilias in producing arterial and venous thrombosis with similar frequency.[2] Furthermore, recurrent miscarriage is a major manifestation of APS, and placental thrombosis seems to play a relevant, albeit not unique, role.[3]

Thromboprophylaxis thus is mandatory for many woman with SLE and APS. However, clinical management in this setting is often challenging owing to the lack of prospective data coming from well-designed studies, the potential fetal and maternal toxicity of antithrombotic drugs, their impact on delivery and use of epidural anesthesia, and the wide spectrum of APS-related manifestations.

INDICATION OF THROMBOPROPHYLAXIS IN PREGNANT WOMAN WITH SLE AND/OR APS

Long-term anticoagulation is indicated in patients with APS suffering any thrombotic complication.[4] Several studies have shown the high risk of thrombotic recurrences when secondary prophylaxis is not initiated or withdrawn.[5–8] Therefore, women with APS and previous thrombosis should maintain antithrombotic treatment throughout their whole pregnancy and, more important, during the postpartum period.[9] The same principle applies to those women with aPL antibodies whose first thrombotic event occurs during pregnancy.

It is far less clear how to treat women with SLE and aPL antibodies but no thrombosis and those with persistently positive aPL antibodies at significant levels discovered by chance. It is common practice to offer these patients low-dose aspirin and recommend stronger thromboprophylaxis during the postpartum period. However, this approach is largely empirical, and the pros and cons of antiaggregant/antithrombotic therapy must be discussed with each woman on an individualized basis.

Women with purely obstetric APS, that is, recurrent miscarriage, fetal loss, or severe preeclampsia leading to premature delivery in the absence of thrombosis, are also a subject of controversy. First, this group has been shown to be at high risk of subsequent thromboses, which are partially prevented by aspirin.[10] One randomized study showed that the combination of heparin and low-dose aspirin is superior to aspirin alone in achieving successful pregnancies in women with nonthrombotic APS with recurrent early pregnancy losses;[11] however, such increased efficacy of the combination treatment was not seen in a later randomized controlled trial of similar design.[12] In addition, data from several uncontrolled series show that a subset of women with APS and poor obstetric history do well with low-dose aspirin in monotherapy.[13–19] Although routine use of heparin, unfractionated heparin (UH), or low molecular weight heparin (LMWH) is generally advocated for pregnant women with APS and adverse obstetric history, particularly late fetal losses,[4,9] this approach is not supported by unquestionable data; therefore, such an option must be discussed too on an individual basis.

SPECIFIC REGIMENS

Management of women with APS and previous thrombosis is largely empirical, because this group of patients has been systematically excluded from clinical trials analyzing the effects of heparin and aspirin in the prevention of pregnancy losses.[19] In 1999, Sanson *et al.*[20] published a systematic review focused on the safety of LMWH during pregnancy. They analyzed 486 pregnant woman who received antithrombotic prophylaxis with LMWH because of several conditions (including previous thromboembolism, miscarriage, mechanical heart valves, or presence of autoantibodies). Three groups of LMWH regimens were examined: low dose (< 75 anti-Xa U/kg/day), intermediate dose (75–150 anti-Xa U/kg/day), and high dose (>150 anti-Xa U/kg/day). Only three thromboembolic complications were reported, one of them in a woman with APS. Yet, because of the heterogeneity of both patients and therapies, it is difficult to draw specific recommendations for women with APS from these data.

More recent guidelines recommend that women with APS and previous thrombotic events, most of whom would already be fully anticoagulated before pregnancy, should receive antithrombotic therapy with UH or LMWH throughout the whole pregnancy, with oral anticoagulants being reinstituted as soon as possible after delivery.[21,22] Specific doses are still open to discussion,[9,21,22] with proposed schedules ranging from adjusted doses of calcium heparin according to activated partial thromboplastin time (aPTT) or anti-Xa activity to full therapeutic doses of LMWH (dalteparin, 200 U/kg/day; or enoxaparin, 1 mg/kg/12 h or 1.5 mg/kg/day; or nadroparin, 171 U/kg/day) to prophylactic doses of LMWH (dalteparin, 5000 U; or enoxaparin 40 mg/once daily to 16 weeks of gestation, doubling the dose every 12 h onward). Concomitant treatment with low-dose aspirin is generally recommended whatever heparin regimen is prescribed.

There is more debate regarding management of women with APS with poor obstetric history but no previous thrombosis. It has already been discussed that monotherapy with aspirin may suffice for a subgroup of these patients in terms of achieving a successful pregnancy.[19] However, recent guidelines advocate combined therapy with aspirin (75–150 mg/day) and heparin in prophylactic doses.[9,21] Although this approach can be argued, thromboprophylaxis with LMWH is mandatory in all women with APS (and is also recommended in asymptomatic women with aPL antibodies, especially in those with SLE) during the postpartum period.

Thromboprophylaxis may represent a risk during labor and, particularly, with the use of epidural anesthesia. Stopping heparin during the 12 h before and 12 h after any interventional procedure is generally considered safe. Many anesthesiologists also require a minimum of 7 days without aspirin to perform a spinal tap.[23] Even under these circumstances, some anesthesiologists feel more comfortable using general anesthesia in this group of patients.

POTENTIAL SIDE EFFECTS

Antithrombotic and anticoagulant drugs have the potential for some serious side effects. Regarding the fetus, neither UH nor LMWH cross the placenta, thus any form of heparin is safe for the baby.[22] Conversely, vitamin K antagonists can cross the placenta and thus increase the risk of bleeding and malformations. The so-called warfarin embryopathy, consisting of nasal hypoplasia and/or stippled epiphysis, has been reported in as many as 6.4% of fetus exposed to vitamin K antagonists.[22] The risk is highest between the 6th and 12th weeks of pregnancy. Fetal bleeding can take place at any time during pregnancy.

Pautzner *et al.*[24] reported 11 women with primary APS treated with warfarin to a target international normalized ratio (INR) of 2.0–2.5 between gestational weeks 14 and 34. No episode of fetal bleeding or malformation was seen, and the treatment was effective in preventing thrombosis and fetal loss in these high-risk women. The authors thus advocated the efficacy and safety of warfarin in pregnant women with APS. Nevertheless, because of the risk of fetal morbidity, vitamin K antagonists are absolutely contraindicated during the early phases of pregnancy (between weeks 6 and 12), although in selected cases their use in later phases of pregnancy may be justified. In these cases, strict control of the INR is critical. Note that both heparin and vitamin K antagonists are safe in nursing mothers.[25]

Maternal bleeding is also a matter of concern with the use of antithrombotic or anticoagulant drugs. Experience with heparin is extensive and favorable, with a low risk of serious bleeding.[20,26,27] LMWH probably offers a better safety profile than UH, including a lower incidence of heparin-induced thrombocytopenia.[1] Risk of bleeding in any patient treated with vitamin K antagonists is directly related to the intensity of anticoagulation as measured by INR.[28]

Finally, pregnant women treated with heparin for prolonged periods may be exposed to an increased risk of osteoporosis (recently reviewed in Refs. 29 and 30). Pregnancy and, especially, lactation may result in a net negative calcium balance. Yet, the frequency of symptomatic osteoporosis (i.e., fractures) in women treated with heparin during the whole pregnancy is low. Women with a previously reduced bone mass (e.g., those receiving long courses of corticosteroids) are more susceptible to the potential deleterious effects of heparin on bone. It is now accepted that LMWH is safer than UH with regard to osteoporosis. Prophylaxis with calcium (1000 mg/day) plus vitamin D (400–800 IU/day) is generally recommended during the full course of pregnancy and the postpartum period. Nonpharmacological measures include exposure to sunlight (which can be contraindicated in woman with photosensitive SLE) and regular exercise.

RECURRENT THROMBOSIS DURING PREGNANCY

Despite optimal thromboprophylaxis, recurrent thrombotic events do occur in some patients with APS.[31] Pregnant women are not an exception. In fact, the protection against arterial thrombosis given by heparin may not be enough for some patients. Women with previous arterial events, particularly stroke, must be considered as high risk.[32,33] Warfarin may be needed in cases in which recurrent thrombosis despite therapeutic doses of heparin occurred.[33]

FUTURE DIRECTIONS

The relationship between complement activation and clinical expression of APS is currently the subject of major research in this field. Studies in mouse models suggest that complement activation is necessary for aPL antibody–induced

TABLE 1. Take-home messages

- Women with any form of APS are subject to an increased risk of thromboembolic complications during pregnancy. Patients with SLE and aPL antibodies without previous thrombosis also must be considered as high risk.
- Thromboprophylaxis during the whole pregnancy and early puerperium is mandatory in these patients.
- Women with previous thrombosis should receive full antithrombotic doses of UH or LMWH.
- Women with previous miscarriage or fetal losses but no thrombosis must be treated with low-dose aspirin with or without heparin at prophylactic doses. Whether all women in this group should receive heparin is not well defined, although it is recommended by most authors.
- Women with SLE and aPL antibodies but no previous thrombosis or pregnancy complications can be offered low-dose aspirin on an empirical basis.
- Warfarin must never be used between weeks 6 and 12 of pregnancy owing to the risk of embryopathy. Later use is generally disregarded, although selected patients with insufficient response to heparin could be candidates to treatment with vitamin K antagonist.
- Women treated with heparin during pregnancy should be given calcium plus vitamin D to prevent bone mass loss. LMWH is less deleterious for bone than UH.
- The pathogenetic role of complement activation in APS manifestations is being investigated. This, in return, might lead to more targeted therapies.

thrombosis[34] and miscarriage.[3] Moreover, interventions toward inhibition of complement activation can prevent both types of APS manifestations.

Data from Girardi *et al.*[3] show that low-dose heparin, without anti–factor X activity but retaining the capacity of complement inactivation, prevented miscarriage. On the contrary, full antithrombotic doses of fondaparinux and hirudin, both of which have no any effect on complement activation, were unable to avoid miscarriage in this murine model.

Although data in humans are still lacking, this line of research may help us understand the complex and wide range of APS manifestations and design more targeted therapies. It is possible that women with recurrent early miscarriage, fetal losses, or thrombosis belong to different pathogenetic subgroups of APS, and thus treatment may differ for these different manifestations of APS. TABLE 1 lists some current recommendations.

REFERENCES

1. BAZAAN, M. & V. DONVITO. 2001. Low-molecular-weight heparin during pregnancy. Throm. Res. **101:** V175–V186.
2. RUIZ-IRASTORZA, G., M.A. KHAMASHTA & G.R.V. HUGHES. 2002. Hughes syndrome crosses boundaries. Autoimmun. Rev. **1:** 43–48.
3. GIRARDI, G., P. REDECHA & J.E. SALMON. 2004. Heparin prevents antiphospholid antibody-induced fetal loss by inhibiting complement activation. Nat. Med. **10:** 1222–1226.
4. LEVINE, J.S., D.W. BRANCH & J. RAUCH. 2002. The antiphospholipid syndrome. N. Engl. J. Med. **346:** 752–763.

5. KHAMASHTA, M.A., M.J. CUADRADO, F. MUJIC, *et al.* 1995. The management of thrombosis in the antiphospholipid-antibody syndrome. N. Engl. J. Med. **332:** 993–997.
6. ROSOVE, M.H. & P.M.C. BREWER. 1992. Antiphospholipid thrombosis: clinical course after the first thrombotic event in 70 patients. Ann. Intern. Med. **117:** 303–308.
7. SCHULMAN, S., E. SVENUNGSSON, S. GRANQVIST, *et al.* 1998. Anticardiolipin antibodies predict early recurrence in thromboembolism and death among patients with venous thromboembolism following anticoagulant therapy. Am. J. Med. **104:** 332–338.
8. KEARON, C., M. GENT, J. HIRSH, *et al.* 1999. A comparison of three months of anticoagulation with extended anticoagulation for a first episode of idiopathic venous thromboembolism. N. Engl. J. Med. **340:** 901–907.
9. DERKSEN, R.H.W.M., M.A. KHAMASHTA & D.W. BRANCH. 2004. Management of the obstetric antiphospholipid syndrome. Arthritis Rheum. **50:** 1028–1039.
10. ERKAN, D., J.T. MERRILL, Y. YAZICI, *et al.* 2001. High thrombosis rate after fetal loss in antiphospholipid syndrome: effective prophylaxis with aspirin. Arthritis Rheum. **44:** 1466–1467.
11. RAI, R., H. COHEN, M. DAVE & L. REGAN. 1997. Randomised controlled trial of aspirin and aspirin plus heparin in pregnant women with recurrent miscarriage associated with phospholipid antibodies (or antiphospholipid antibodies). Br. Med. J. **314:** 253–257.
12. FARQUHARSON, R.G., S. QUENBY & M. GREAVES. 2002. Antiphospholipid syndrome in pregnancy: a randomized, controlled trial of treatment. Obstet. Gynecol. **100:** 408–413.
13. SILVER, R.K., S.N. MACGREGOR, J.S. SHOLL, *et al.* 1993. Comparative trial of prednisone plus aspirin versus aspirin alone in the treatment of anticardiolipin antibody-positive obstetric patients. Am. J. Obstet. Gynecol. **169:** 1411–1417.
14. LIMA, F., M.A. KHAMASHTA, N.M.M. BUCHANAN, *et al.* 1996. A study of sixty pregnancies in patients with the antiphospholipid syndrome. Clin. Exp. Rheumatol. **14:** 131–136.
15. GRANGER, K.A. & R.G. FARQUHARSON. 1997. Obstetric outcome in antiphospholipid syndrome. Lupus **6:** 509–513.
16. PATTISON, N.S., L.W. CHAMLEY, M. BIRDSALL, *et al.* 2000. Does aspirin have a role in improving pregnancy outcome for women with the antiphospholipid syndrome? A randomized controlled trial. Am. J. Obstet. Gynecol. **183:** 1008–1012.
17. HUONG, D.L.T., B. WECHSLER, O. BLETRY, *et al.* 2001. A study of 75 pregnancies in patients with antiphospholipid syndrome. J. Rheumatol. **28:** 2025–2030.
18. MUÑOZ-RODRIGUEZ, F.J., J. FONT, R. CERVERA, *et al.* 1999. Clinical study of 100 patients with the antiphospholipid syndrome. Semin. Arthritis Rheum. **29:** 182–190.
19. RUIZ-IRASTORZA, G., M.A. KHAMASHTA & G.R.V. HUGHES. 2002. Treatment of pregnancy loss in Hughes syndrome: a critical update. Autoimmun. Rev. **1:** 298–304.
20. SANSON, B.J., A.W.A. LENSING, M.H. PRINS, *et al.* 1999. Safety of low-molecular-weight heparin in pregnancy: a systematic review. Thromb. Haemost. **81:** 668–672.
21. BRANCH, D.W. & M.A. KHAMASHTA. 2003. Antiphospholipid syndrome: obstetric diagnosis, management and controversies. Obstet. Gynecol. **101:** 1333–1344.
22. BATES, S., I.A. GREER, J. HIRSH & J.S. GINSBERG. 2004. Use of antithrombotic agents during pregnancy. The seventh ACCP conference on antithrombotic and thrombolytic therapy. Chest **126:** 627S–644S.
23. Wetzl, R.G. 2004. Anestesiological aspects of pregnancy in patients with rheumatic diseases. Lupus **13:** 699–702.
24. PAUZNER, R., M. DULITZKI, P. LANEVITZ & M.A. KENETT. 2001. Low molecular weight heparin and warfarin in the treatment of patients with antiphospholipid syndrome during pregnancy. Thromb. Haemost. **86:** 1379–1384.
25. JILMA, B., S. KAMATH & G.Y.H. LIP. 2003. Antithrombotic therapy in special circumstances. I—pregnancy and cancer. Br. Med. J. **326:** 37–40.
26. NELSON-PIERCY, C., E. LETSKY & M. DE SWIET. 1997. Low-molecular-weight heparin for obstetric thromboprophylaxis: experience of sixty-nine pregnancies in sixty-one women at high risk. Am. J. Obstet. Gynecol. **176:** 1062–1068.
27. HUNT, B.J., H.A. DOUGHTY, G. MAJUMDAR, *et al.* 1997. Thromboprophylaxis with low molecular weight heparin (Fragmin) in high risk pregnancies. Thromb. Haemost. **77:** 39–43.

28. BRITISH COMMITTEE FOR STANDARDS IN HAEMATOLOGY. 1998. Guidelines on oral anticoagulation, 3rd ed. Br. J. Haematol. **101:** 374–387.
29. RUIZ-IRASTORZA, C. NELSON-PIERCY & G.R. HUGHES. 2001. Lupus pregnancy: is heparin a risk factor for osteoporosis? Lupus **10:** 597–600.
30. RUIZ-IRASTORZA, G., M.A. KHAMASHTA & G.R. HUGHES. 2002. Heparin and osteoporosis during pregnancy: 2002 update. Lupus **11:** 680–682.
31. RUIZ-IRASTORZA, G., M.A. KHAMASHTA, B.J. HUNT, *et al.* 2002. Bleeding and recurrent thrombosis in definite antiphospholipid syndrome: analysis of a series of 66 patients treated with oral anticoagulation to a target international normalized ratio of 3.5. Arch. Intern. Med. **162:** 1164–1169.
32. CUADRADO, M.J., L.L.F. MENDONÇA, M.A. KHAMASHTA, *et al.* 1999. Maternal and fetal outcome in antiphospholipid syndrome pregnancies with a history of previous cerebral ischemia [Abstract]. Arthritis Rheum. **42:** S265.
33. HUNT, B.J., M.A. KHAMASHTA, L. LAKASING, *et al.* 1998. Thromboprophylaxis in antiphospholipid syndrome pregnancies with previous cerebral arterial thrombotic events: is warfarin preferable? Thromb. Haemost. **79:** 1060–1061.
34. PIERANGELI, S.S., M. VEGA-OSTERTAG, X. LIU, *et al.* 2004. An anti C5 monoclonal antibody reverses antiphospholipid-induced thrombosis [abstract]. Arthritis Rheum. **50:** S639–S640.

Gene-Gun Biolistic Immunization Encoding Glutamic Acid Decarboxylase

A Model for Studying Langerhans Cell Abnormalities and Mimicry in the Nonobese Diabetic Mouse

BÉATRICE JOUSSEMET, ANH-TUAN VU, PIERRE SAI, AND JEAN-MARIE BACH

IECM Unit, ENVN/INRA/University, Nantes, France

ABSTRACT: Plasmid-DNA gene-gun immunization may be an efficient approach for investigating the role of skin dendritic cells (DCs) in type 1 diabetes (T1D) pathogenesis and the significance of the presentation of peptides that mimic autoantigenic epitopes in aggravating or modulating the autoimmune reaction. Gene-gun immunization has been described as producing long-lasting immune responses elicited by skin DCs, especially Langerhans cells (LCs). Therefore, we tested the immune response and diabetes modulation in nonobese diabetic (NOD) mice and in control BALB/c mice, by gene-gun administration of plasmid-DNA encoding (1) human 65 kDa glutamic acid decarboxylase (hGAD65) mimicking the crucial mouse autoantigen GAD65 (similarity of 95.7%) or (2) β-galactosidase (βGAL) as a negative control. Expression of GAD and βGAL in skin of pc-GAD– and pc-LacZ–injected mice, respectively, was confirmed. It was surprising that both pc-LacZ–injected BALB/c and NOD mice exhibited a βGAL-specific Th1 immune response: spleen cells of pc-LacZ mice proliferated specifically to βGAL ($P < 10^{-4}$) and secreted significant amounts of IFNγ ($P < 10^{-4}$). pc-LacZ mice also developed a βGAL-specific Th1-related (IgG2a/2c) and Th2-related (IgG1) humoral response. Although pc-GAD BALB/c mice showed Th2-related GAD-specific IgG1 production and a significant secretion of IL4 ($P < .03$), pc-GAD NOD mice did not generate either an antibody response or a T cell response specific to GAD. Moreover, gene-gun immunization encoding hGAD65 did not clearly modulate diabetes onset in NOD mice. This absence of detectable GAD-specific response may implicate skin DC deficiencies in NOD mice. The gene-gun technique could thus provide an interesting model for studying skin DC abnormalities in NOD mice and their potential implication of presenting mimetic peptides that modulate the autoimmune response in T1D.

KEYWORDS: DNA immunization; gene-gun; type 1 diabetes; autoimmunity; T cell; glutamic acid decarboxylase; NOD mouse mimicry

Address for correspondence: Jean-Marie Bach, Immuno-Endocrinology Unit, ENVN/INRA/University, ENVN, Atlanpôle-La Chantrerie, BP 40706, 44307 Nantes cedex 03, France. Voice: +33-24-0687804; fax: +33-24-0687805.
bach@vet-nantes.fr

**Ann. N.Y. Acad. Sci. 1051: 613–625 (2005). © 2005 New York Academy of Sciences.
doi: 10.1196/annals.1361.106**

INTRODUCTION

Type 1 diabetes (T1D) results from the autoimmune destruction of pancreatic islet β cells. In the nonobese diabetic (NOD) mouse model of human T1D, this β cell injury is known to involve autoreactive $CD4^+$ T helper type 1 (Th1) cells secreting large amounts of IFNγ and IL2, and $CD8^+$ T lymphocytes (reviewed in Ref. 1). On the other hand, diabetes development in NOD mice could be controlled by regulatory T cells such as Th2 or Th2/3 $CD4^+$ T cells,[1,2] $CD4^+CD62L^+$,[3,4] $CD4^+CD25^+Foxp3^+$,[5] $CD4^+CD45RB^{lo}$,[6] and natural-killer (NK) T cells.[7] Environmental factors, such as microbes, are actually suspected to participate in the initiation, aggravation, or modulation of the autoimmune process leading to T1D, presumably by influencing the balance between β cell–specific aggressive and suppressive responses. One mechanism put forward to explain autoreactive T cell stimulation by microbial compounds is the attractive concept of mimicry between a self and a microbial peptide antigen (discussed in Refs. 8 and 9). Mimetic peptides are likely able to activate $CD4^+$ or $CD8^+$ T cells, recognizing self-peptides, or to induce regulatory cells when they act as weak or partial agonists, antagonist peptides, or altered-peptide ligands (APLs).[10] However, although several sets of observations support this concept, it is not clearly understood whether mimicry plays a significant role in aggravating or attenuating T1D. New experimental approaches are required to clarify the role of antigen mimicry in autoimmune diabetes.

The skin constitutes a functional defense barrier from contact with microbes. Skin is a specialized immune organ that contains numerous specialized antigen-presenting cells (APCs): skin-specific immature dendritic cells in the epidermis (termed Langerhans cells [LCs]) and dendritic cells (DCs) in the dermis. Skin APCs are specialized for initiating primary immune naive T and B cells and play a key role in orientating microbial-specific immune responses.[11,12] These APCs process foreign antigens and may present peptides derived from microbial proteins to β cell–specific immune cells, activating or modulating them.

To test this hypothesis and to establish an experimental animal model for targeting APC in skin, we used gene-gun biolistic immunization consisting of the cutaneous delivery of gold microscopic beads coated with plasmid DNA encoding for a recombinant antigen. Although the majority of skin cells transfected by this gene-gun immunization are not APCs, such as fibroblasts and keratinocytes, approximately 5% of the cells transfected are LCs.[13] Antigen-specific immune responses evoked by gene-gun immunization are essentially initiated by the presentation of the recombinant antigen expressed by direct transfected LCs.[14,15] In a limited action, cross-presentation by cutaneous untransfected DCs of antigen released by transfected cells could also participate in the initiation of immune responses.[14,16] After migration to draining lymph nodes,[14,17,18] DCs can elicit humoral responses and both $CD4^+$ and $CD8^+$ T cell responses, depending on class II– and class I–mediated antigen presentation, respectively (reviewed in Ref. 19).

In the present study, human 65 kDa glutamic acid decarboxylase (hGAD65) was chosen as a model of strong mimetic antigen of a crucial β cell autoantigen in NOD mouse diabetes pathogenesis, the mouse GAD65.[1,20,21] Human and mouse GAD65 share strong amino acid sequence similarities (95.7%). β-Galactosidase (βGAL) was used as a negative control because it is not known to share amino acid sequence similarities with the known β cell autoantigens. To target the skin environmental barrier,

NOD and BALB/c mice were injected twice by gene-gun with plasmid-DNA encoding hGAD65 (pc-GAD mice) or βGAL (pc-LacZ mice).

MATERIAL AND METHODS

Mice and Diabetes

Female BALB/c (Janvier, Le Genest-St-Isle, France) and NODLtj mice (Jackson Laboratory, Bar Harbor, MA, USA) were maintained in controlled and clean conventional conditions at the Veterinary School of Nantes (France). Diabetes incidences at 280 days in female and male NOD mice were 80% and 60%, respectively, in these house-breeding conditions. Diabetes was diagnosed when glycemia was ≥16.7 mmol/L for 2 weeks consecutively.

Plasmid Construction and Production

Details of the construction of pc-GAD were described previously.[22] Briefly, pc-GAD was obtained by cloning EcoRI-XbaI PCR amplicons containing the full-length hGAD65 cDNA into pcDNA3.1/B (Invitrogen, Groningen, the Netherlands). pc-LacZ (pcDNA3.1/LacZ) encoding βGAL (Invitrogen) was used as control. Plasmids were amplified in Top10 competent *E. coli* (Invitrogen), and endotoxin-free large volumes of plasmids were produced by the alkaline lysis method (Giga kit, Qiagen, Hiden, Germany).

Gene-Gun Biolistic Immunization

Before plasmid immunization by particle bombardment with Helios Gene-Gun System (Bio-Rad, Hercules, CA, USA), cartridges containing 1 μg of plasmid DNA precipitated onto 0.5 mg of 1.6 mm gold beads were prepared, according to manufacturer instructions, using CaCl2 and spermidine (Sigma, St. Louis, MO, USA). To control the efficiency of plasmid DNA precipitation onto gold beads, plasmids were solubilized by water from coated beads. Plasmid DNA quality and quantity were then controlled after migration in agarose gel and by spectrophotometry (U-2001 Spectrophotometer, Hitachi Instruments), respectively. Then 3-week-old female mice were randomly allocated and received two shots, at 7-week intervals, of one cartridge of pc-GAD, pc-LacZ, or empty gold beads under a 300-psi helium pulse in the abdominal skin. Both BALB/c and NOD mice were included in each experiment and injected with the same cartridge batch.

Detection of GAD or βGAL Expression in Injected Skin

The 3-week-old female BALB/c and NOD mice were injected with pc-GAD or pc-LacZ using a Helios gene-gun, as indicated above. Injected and noninjected skin samples were removed 24 h after DNA immunization. Nonspecific staining of 5-μm cryosections was inhibited using the Dako ARK kit (Dako, Glostrup, Denmark). GAD and βGAL expression was detected by direct immunostaining with 4 μg/section biotinylated primary monoclonal antibodies (MAbs) specific to GAD (Clone GAD6, mouse IgG2a, BD Biosciences) or to βGAL (clone GAL-13, mouse IgG1, Sigma) in combination with peroxidase-conjugated streptavidin (Sigma). Sections were then incubated with substrate (DAB, 3,3′-Diaminobenzidine, Sigma), which produced a brown color when activated, and stained with hematoxylin. As controls, adjacent sections from immunized mice were stained identically but without primary MAbs, and uninjected skin sections were stained with the primary MAbs.

Quantification of GAD- or βGAL-Specific Antibodies

Titers of GAD- and βGAL-specific IgG1, IgG2a/2c, and IgG2b antibodies in the serum of immunized mice were measured at regular time points using a sandwich ELISA technique, described previously.[22] Briefly, 96-well Maxisorb plates (Nunc, Roskilde, Denmark) were coated with recombinant hGAD65 (Diamyd, Stockholm, Sweden) or βGAL (Sigma). Diluted sera were then added in duplicates and incubated for 2 h at RT. Diluted horseradish peroxidase (HRP)-conjugated goat antimouse IgG1, IgG2a/2c, or IgG2b (CALTAG, Burlingham, CA, USA) were added for 2 h at RT. Specific OD_{450nm} (OD with antigen minus OD without antigen) samples were evaluated by following incubation with *o*-phenylenediamine dihydrochloride (OPD, Sigma). Antibody titers (μg/mL) were calculated based on calibration curves obtained with various dilutions of a standard serum included in each plate and previously quantified for antibody to GAD or to βGAL, respectively.

T Cell–Proliferation Assay

Spleens were removed from DNA-immunized mice. After incubation with NH4Cl (0.17 M) for 10 min at 4°C, cells were washed and resuspended in AIMV® serum-free medium (Life technologies, Paisley, Scotland, UK), then distributed in triplicates into flat-bottom 96-well culture plates (Nunc) at a density of 5×10^5/well and cultured in the presence or absence of 15 μg/mL of recombinant hGAD65 or βGAL at 37°C and 5% CO_2. After 72 h of culture, cells were pulsed with methyl-^{3}H[thymidine] (Amersham, Saclay, France), 1 μCi/well. Cells were harvested 16 h later, and thymidine uptake was measured using a β scintillation counter (LS 7500, Beckman, France). Proliferative responses were calculated for each triplicate as stimulation indexes (SIs): mean counts per minute (cpm) in the presence of antigen divided by mean cpm in the absence of antigen.

Detection of Cytokines in Culture Supernatants

Spleen cells from vaccinated mice were cultured in AIMV® serum-free medium, in flat-bottom 24-well plates in the presence or absence of 15 μg/mL of recombinant hGAD65 or βGAL. After 72 h, IFNγ, IL2, and IL4 secretions were determined in culture supernatants using the BD Cytometric Bead Array (CBA) according to the manufacturer's instructions (BD Biosciences). Analysis was performed on a FACS-Calibur™ (BD Biosciences). IL10 secretions were measured by ELISA (Duoset, R&D Systems, MN, USA).

Pancreatic Histopathology

The 15-μm frozen pancreas sections were stained with hematoxylin-eosin to analyze Langerhans islet infiltrations. At least 30 islets were graded as follows: grade 0, noninvaded normal islet; grade 1, peri-insulitis or insulitis occupying up to 25% of islet; grade 2, infiltration of 25–50% of the islet; and grade 3, severe insulitis with significant destruction of β islet cells. The percentage of islets affected by each degree of insulitis was calculated for each mouse.

Statistical Analysis

Statistical significance was evaluated using the Mann-Withney *U* test. The time course of diabetes was analyzed using Kaplan-Meier curves, and significance differences among curves were evaluated by log-rank and Chi^2 tests.

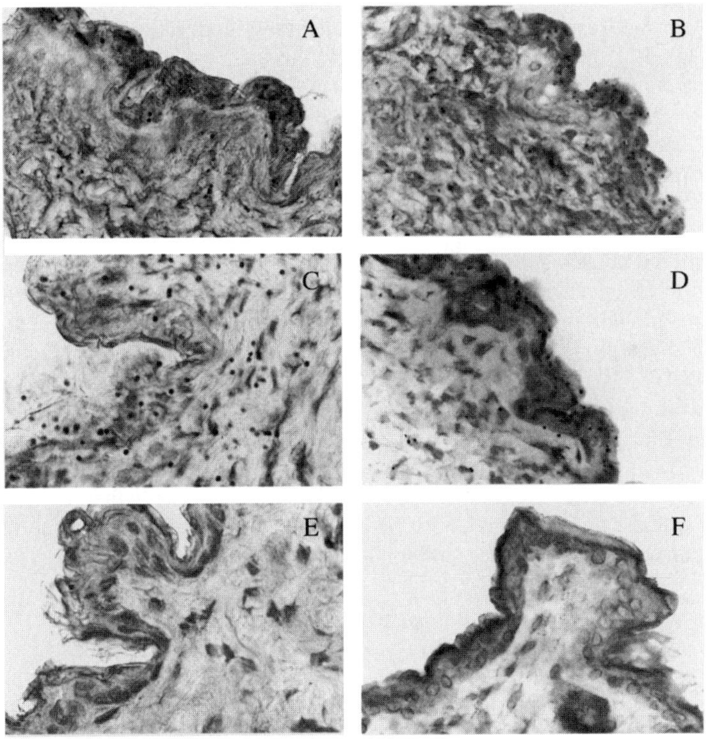

FIGURE 1. GAD expression in injected skin. Abdominal skin patches from BALB/c and NOD mice were obtained 24 h after one gene-gun administration of pc-GAD. (**A**) injected skin of pc-GAD BALB/c mice incubated with anti-GAD primary MAbs. (**C**) Injected skin from pc-GAD BALB/c mice in the absence of anti-GAD primary MAbs. (**E**) Uninjected skin from BALB/c mice incubated with anti-GAD primary MAbs. (**B**) Injected skin from pc-GAD NOD mice incubated with anti-GAD primary MAbs. (**D**) Injected skin from pc-GAD NOD mice without anti-GAD primary MAbs. (**F**) Uninjected skin from NOD mice incubated with anti-GAD primary MAbs. Original magnification 250×, reduced to 60%.

RESULTS

βGAL and GAD Expression in Skin of Gene-Gun Immunized Mice

βGAL and GAD expressions were clearly detected in both the epidermis and dermis of pc-LacZ mice (data not shown) and pc-GAD mice (FIG. 1A and B). Histologic examination of the injected-tissue revealed little cell damage or inflammation (data not shown). Most of the beads and GAD- or βGAL-expressing cells were present in the different layers of the epidermis, few of them were found in the dermis. Adjacent sections, treated identically but without anti-GAD primary MAb, were not stained positively (FIG. 1C and D). Finally, uninjected skin sections from pc-GAD mice (FIG. 1E and F) or pc-LacZ mice (data not shown), incubated with anti-GAD or anti-βGAL primary Mabs, respectively, did not exhibit brown coloration in the skin cells.

Humoral Responses to βGAL and GAD in Sera of Injected Mice

In both mouse strains, two pc-LacZ injections induced strong and significant βGAL-specific IgG1, IgG2a/2c and IgG2b productions comparative to pc-GAD mice and control mice (who received empty gold-beads; gold mice) (FIG. 2A and C). After two pc-LacZ injections, BALB/c mice exhibited a greater secretion of IgG1 and IgG2a/2c to βGAL than IgG2b ($P < .02$ and $P < 10^{-3}$, respectively) (FIG. 2A). IgG1 response to βGAL was already observed between the two plasmid-DNA immunizations, whereas anti-βGAL IgG2a/2c production seemed to be especially stimulated after the second gene-gun injection (FIG. 2B). Furthermore, pc-LacZ NOD mice produced predominantly anti-βGAL IgG1 even 1 month after the first plasmid DNA injection ($P < 10^{-2}$) (FIG. 2D), which persisted 4 weeks after the second gene-gun administration ($P < 10^{-4}$) (FIG. 2C and D). pc-LacZ NOD mice also developed a slight IgG2a/2c humoral response to βGAL after two gene-gun immunizations ($P < 10^{-3}$) (FIG. 2C and D).

Concerning pc-GAD immunization, pc-GAD BALB/c mice showed a GAD-specific IgG1 response comparative to anti-GAD IgG2a/2c and IgG2b productions ($P < 10^{-4}$) (FIG. 2E). This IgG1 secretion against GAD strongly increased after the second plasmid DNA immunization (FIG. 2F). It was surprising that no humoral response specific to GAD was observed in the NOD mice after either one (data not shown) or two pc-GAD gene-gun immunizations (FIG. 2G).

Spleen T Cell–Proliferative Responses to βGAL and GAD in Spleen of Injected Mice

At 4 weeks after the second immunization, spleen T cells from both pc-LacZ BALB/c mice (FIG. 3A) and NOD mice (FIG. 3B) showed specific and significantly higher proliferations of βGAL than pc-GAD ($P < .01$) or gold mice ($P < .01$). Moreover, proliferations of spleen T cells from pc-LacZ BALB/c and NOD mice were higher in the presence of βGAL than in the presence of GAD ($P < 10^{-4}$ and $P < 10^{-3}$, respectively) (FIG. 3A, B). Spleen T cell–proliferations to GAD were also significantly increased for pc-GAD BALB/c mice compared to pc-LacZ BALB/c mice ($P < .01$) or gold mice ($P < .01$) (FIG. 3A). Contrasting with pc-GAD BALB/c mice, gene-gun vaccination encoding hGAD65 did not induce any specific T cell–

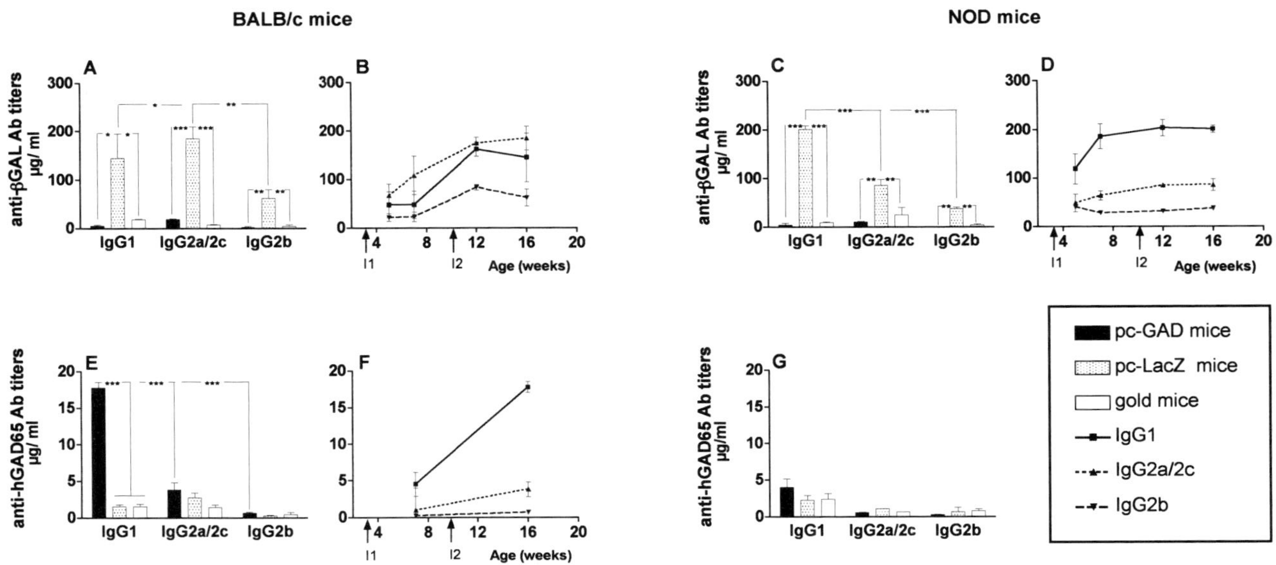

FIGURE 2. (**A**) βGAL-specific antibody titers in serum of pc-GAD ($n = 7$), pc-LacZ ($n = 9$), and gold ($n = 8$) BALB/c mice and (**C**) pc-GAD ($n = 4$), pc-LacZ ($n = 10$), and gold ($n = 7$) NOD mice 4 weeks after the second plasmid-DNA injection. (**B**) βGAL-specific antibody titers in serum of pc-LacZ BALB/c mice ($n = 9$) and (**D**) pc-LacZ NOD mice ($n = 10$) 2 and 4 weeks after the first (I1) and the second (I2) pc-LacZ administrations. (**E**) GAD-specific antibody titers in serum of pc-GAD ($n = 16$), pc-LacZ ($n = 11$), and gold ($n = 10$) BALB/c mice and (**G**) pc-GAD ($n = 10$), pc-LacZ ($n = 5$), and gold ($n = 4$) NOD mice 4 weeks after the second plasmid-DNA injection. (**F**) GAD-specific antibody titers in serum of pc-GAD BALB/c mice ($n = 16$) 4 weeks after the first (I1) and the second (I2) pc-GAD administrations. Results are given as mean titers ± SEM; ∗, $P < .04$; ∗∗, $P < 10^{-3}$; ∗∗∗, $P < 10^{-4}$.

proliferative responses in NOD mice (FIG. 3B), whereas T cells from both treated mouse strains showed similar proliferations to concanavalin A (data not shown).

Cytokine Secretion Patterns of Spleen T Cells from Injected Mice

Spleen T cells from pc-LacZ BALB/c and NOD mice obtained 4 weeks after the second plasmid-DNA injection exhibited significantly higher βGAL-specific IFNγ secretions than pc-GAD and gold mice spleen T cells ($P < .01$) (FIG. 3C,D). Spleen cells from pc-LacZ NOD mice also secreted βGAL-specific quantities of IL10 as compared to pc-GAD and gold NOD mice ($P < .05$) (FIG. 3D). On the other hand,

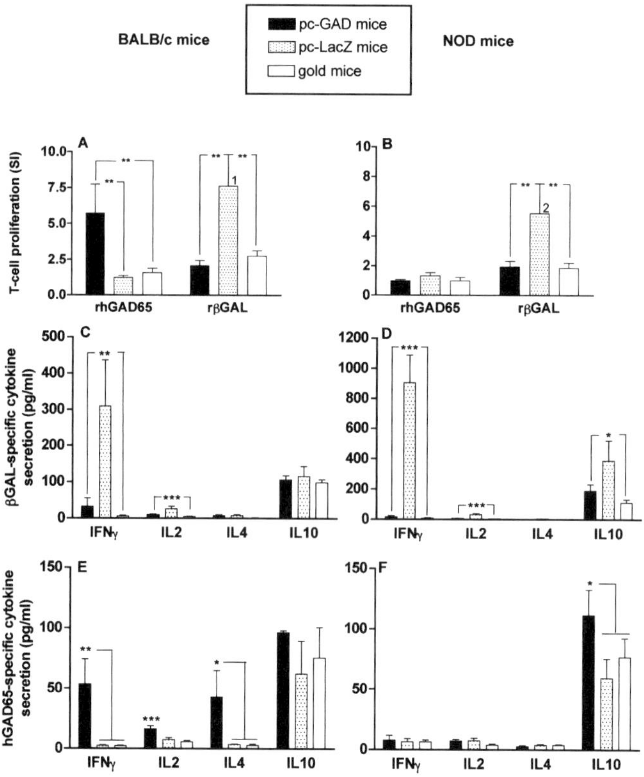

FIGURE 3. βGAL- and GAD-specific proliferations and cytokine secretions of T cells from plasmid-DNA–immunized BALB/c and NOD mice 4 weeks after the second injection. (**A**) Proliferations of spleen T cells from pc-GAD (n = 12), pc-LacZ (n = 11), and gold (n = 9) BALB/c mice and (**B**) from pc-GAD (n = 11), pc-LacZ (n = 14), and gold (n = 11) NOD mice. (**C**) βGAL-specific cytokine production by spleen T cells from pc-GAD (n = 12), pc-LacZ (n = 10), and gold (n = 7) BALB/c mice and (**D**) from pc-GAD (n = 8), pc-LacZ (n = 13), and gold (n = 6) NOD mice. (**E**) GAD-specific cytokine production by spleen T cells from pc-GAD (n = 12), pc-LacZ (n = 10), and gold (n = 7) BALB/c mice and (**F**) from pc-GAD (n = 8), pc-LacZ (n = 13), and gold (n = 6) NOD mice. Results are expressed as mean stimulatory indices ± SEM or mean cytokine quantities in culture supernatants ± SEM; *, $P < .05$; **, $P < .01$; ***, $P < 10^{-4}$.

pc-GAD BALB/c spleen cells secreted lower levels of IFNγ in response to GAD than spleen cells from pc-LacZ BALB/c mice in response to βGAL ($P < 10^{-3}$) (FIG. 3E). Spleen cells from pc-GAD BALB/c mice also exhibited a GAD-specific secretion of IL4 ($P < .05$) (FIG. 3E). Analysis of cytokine expression patterns in pc-GAD mice showed marked differences between BALB/c and NOD mice. No GAD-specific IFNγ IL2 and IL4 productions were observed in pc-GAD NOD mice (FIG. 3F). Spleen T cells from pc-GAD NOD mice showed only a slight increase of GAD-specific IL10 production compared to spleen cells from pc-LacZ and gold NOD mice ($P < .05$) (FIG. 3F).

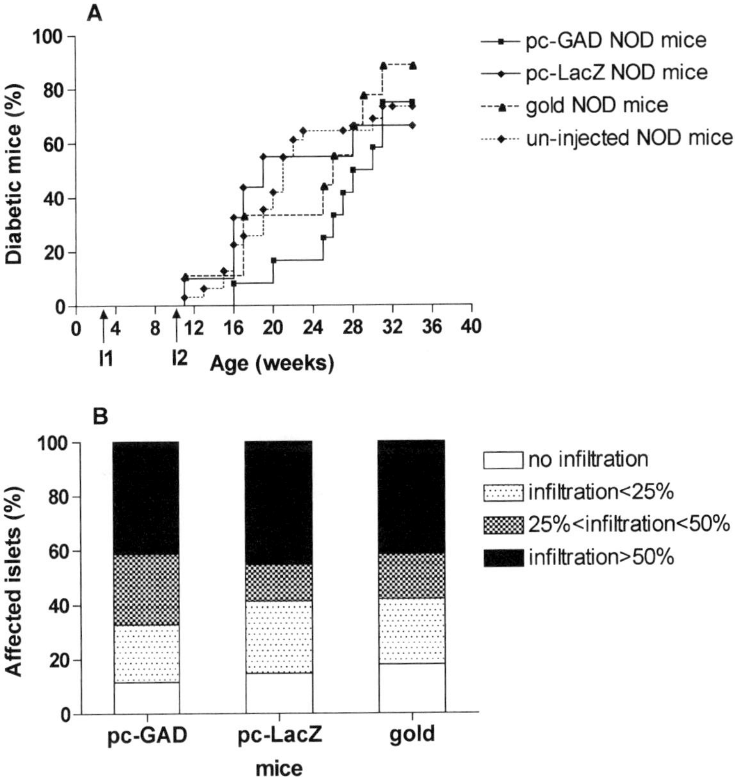

FIGURE 4. (**A**) Diabetes severity in DNA-vaccinated NOD mice. The cumulative incidence of diabetes is indicated for female NOD mice ($n = 31$), uninjected and injected at 3 (I1) and 10 (I2) weeks of age with pc-GAD ($n = 12$), pc-LacZ ($n = 10$), or gold beads ($n = 9$). (**B**) Insulitis in plasmid-DNA–injected NOD mice. Female NOD mice were injected at 3 and 10 weeks of age with pc-GAD ($n = 4$), pc-LacZ ($n = 4$), or gold beads ($n = 4$). Pancreata were removed 4 weeks after the second injection, before diabetes onset. Insulitis was evaluated using scores as indicated in the text. Results are expressed as mean percentage of islets affected by each degree of insulitis.

Diabetes Incidence

No significant change of diabetes incidence was observed for NOD mice receiving gene-gun immunization with pc-GAD compared to pc-LacZ, gold, or uninjected NOD mice (FIG. 4A). At the end of our observation (34 weeks of age), 75% and 73% of pc-GAD and uninjected female NOD mice, respectively, became diabetic. However, a slight delay of diabetes was observed between 16 and 20 weeks of age in the pc-GAD NOD group compared to the other ones ($P < .01$) (FIG. 4A). At 4 weeks after the second plasmid-DNA gene-gun administration, pancreatic islet infiltrations were almost identical among pc-GAD, pc-LacZ, and gold NOD mice (FIG. 4B).

DISCUSSION

The gene-gun technique allows direct intracellular synthesis, processing, and presentation by epidermal LCs of antigen-derived peptides and is thus an attractive approach to study the potential role of exogenous peptides mimicking β cell–derived autoantigenic epitopes in T1D pathogenesis. Using the hGAD65 model as a strong mimetic antigen, we have shown that two pc-GAD gene-gun administrations seemed to slightly delay diabetes in NOD mice. This result suggests that gene-gun immunization may procure an interesting approach to investigate the mimicry concept. However, we do not know by what way GAD expression in skin LCs influences progression to T1D in NOD mice. Mimetic peptides may influence organ-specific autoimmunity by favoring or inhibiting the avidity maturation of autoreactive T lymphocytes or by inducing a regulatory autoantigenic T cell response.[8,9]

It was surprising that no immune reaction was clearly detected in the pc-GAD NOD mice included in our study, neither GAD-specific IgG1, IgG2a/2c and IgG2b Ab responses nor spleen cell proliferations or clear cytokine secretion in response to GAD were noted. Only a moderate GAD-specific IL10 production was observed after two pc-GAD immunizations in NOD mice compared to control mice. In contrast, pc-GAD BALB/c mice developed a clearly polarized Th2 immune response characterized by a GAD-specific IL4 secretion by spleen cells and an exclusive production of Th2-related anti-GAD IgG1. Thus gene-gun immunization suggests a probable dysfunction of NOD LCs known to induce a strong and durable specific immune response in control mice after gene-gun immunization.[14,15] This absence of detectable immune response to GAD is not attributable to a lack of the protein expression in the skin of NOD-treated mice as shown by the immune detection of the antigen in targeted tissue. Moreover, the same cartridge batch was used in each experiment for BALB/c and NOD mice. GAD-unresponsiveness described in our study may involve antigen processing or presentation as well as maturation and migration of LCs.

As previously described, NOD mice were known to present several DC abnormalities. NOD bone marrow– and spleen-derived progenitors were unable to differentiate into tolerogenic semimature DCs that express MHC class II and costimulatory molecules but secrete low levels of IL12.[23–25] Semimature DCs were shown to be able to efficiently stimulate regulatory CD4 T cells,[26,27] which were implicated in suppression of autoimmune processes,[28] or to prevent the autoimmune aggression of islet allograft in NOD mice.[29] A deficient maturation of DCs to a tolerogenic state may contribute to the dysfunctional immune regulation and then to the autoimmune process. A low number of regulatory T cells exist in NOD mice, and their development requires expression of co-stimulatory molecules.[30] DCs and particularly epidermal LCs are positioned at the interface with environmental factors. Such factors as microbial infections can prevent autoimmune diabetes, probably by controlling the balance between the Th1 or Tc1 aggressive T cell responses and the regulatory T cells.[31] In our study, a maturation defect of epidermal LCs and a decreased expression of co-stimulatory molecules may explain the lack of strong Th2 T cell activation after gene-gun administration of a plasmid encoding hGAD65 in NOD mice.

The absence of a GAD-specific immune response elicited by pc-GAD gene-gun immunization in NOD mice may also reflect a defect of LC migration to draining lymph nodes. We are presently testing this hypothesis. After transfection by gene-gun administration, LCs were known to maturate into fully competent DCs during their migration to the dermis and further when they reached the draining lymph nodes.[14,17,18] It is interesting that a specific humoral and cellular response to another antigen (βGAL) could be induced by the same protocol of gene-gun immunization in NOD mice, suggesting strongly that the antigen-specific immune response observed in NOD mice receiving a gene-gun shot is intimately associated with the encoded antigen. In both NOD and BALB/c mice, pc-LacZ administration induced a βGAL-specific Th1 immune response characterized by IFNγ and IL2 secretion by spleen cells and an important Th1-related βGAL-specific IgG2a/2c production. A significant Th2-related βGAL-specific IgG1 secretion could be also detected after pc-LacZ immunization in both mouse strains.

The nature of the antigen itself, particularly its immunogenicity, could strongly influence the quantity and quality of the type of immune response elicited.[32–34] βGAL is a Th1-biased antigen and constitutes a strong stimulus that may drive the response down the Th1 path. βGAL immunogenicity was probably sufficient to prime a humoral and cellular immune response in NOD mice, whereas intracellular GAD65 did not constitute a sufficiently strong immunogenic protein. Differences observed between GAD- and βGAL-specific immune responses could also implicate affinity differences between the T cell receptor (TCR) to GAD or to βGAL. High-affinity lymphocytes become Th1 relatively easily, whereas the GAD-specific $CD4^+$ T cells may exhibit low-affinity TCR that tends to express a Th2 phenotype in the control mouse strain,[33,35] as observed in our study for pc-GAD BALB/c mice.

The gene-gun technique is usually described as producing a typical antigen-specific Th2 T-cell activation,[36,37] but is also an efficient method that primes a Th1-like or a balanced Th1/Th2 response, depending on the antigen encoded and the delay between the two particle shots.[38–40] Sudowe *et al.*[41] recently demonstrated that, after gene-gun immunization encoding βGAL, T cells exhibit a more Th1 phenotype in the spleen, whereas they exhibit a more polarized Th2 immune response in lymph nodes draining the injection site. These observations are consistent with our data. Indeed, pc-LacZ BALB/c and pc-LacZ NOD mice developed a humoral balanced Th1- and Th2-related immune response to βGAL, whereas spleen T cells from pc-LacZ NOD and BALB/c mice showed a βGAL-specific secretion of IFNγ.

In conclusion, our study shows for the first time that NOD LCs probably exhibit functional abnormalities. Furthermore, we show that the gene-gun technique could provide an interesting model for studying skin DC dysfunctions in NOD mice and their potential implication in presenting mimetic peptides for modulating the autoimmune response in T1D.

REFERENCES

1. DELOVITCH, T.L. & B. SINGH. 1997. The nonobese diabetic mouse as a model of autoimmune diabetes: immune dysregulation gets the NOD. Immunity **7:** 727–7238.
2. PICCIRILLO, C.A., Y. CHANG & G.J. PRUD'HOMME. 1998. TGF-beta1 somatic gene therapy prevents autoimmune disease in nonobese diabetic mice. J. Immunol. **161:** 3950–3956.
3. YOU, S. *et al.* 2004. Unique role of CD4+CD62L+ regulatory T cells in the control of autoimmune diabetes in T cell receptor transgenic mice. Proc. Natl. Acad. Sci. USA **101** (Suppl. 2): 14580–14585.
4. LEPAULT, F. & M.C. GAGNERAULT. 2000. Characterization of peripheral regulatory CD4+ T cells that prevent diabetes onset in nonobese diabetic mice. J. Immunol. **164:** 240–247.
5. PENG, Y. *et al.* 2004. TGF-beta regulates in vivo expansion of Foxp3-expressing CD4+CD25+ regulatory T cells responsible for protection against diabetes. Proc. Natl. Acad. Sci. USA **101:** 4572–4577.
6. MARTINS, T.C. & A.P. AGUAS. 1999. A role for CD45RBlow CD38+ T cells and costimulatory pathways of T-cell activation in protection of non-obese diabetic (NOD) mice from diabetes. Immunology **96:** 600–605.
7. SHARIF, S. *et al.* 2001. Activation of natural killer T cells by alpha-galactosylceramide treatment prevents the onset and recurrence of autoimmune Type 1 diabetes. Nat. Med. **7:** 1057–1062.
8. FOURNEAU, J.M. *et al.* 2004. The elusive case for a role of mimicry in autoimmune diseases. Mol. Immunol. **40:** 1095–1102.
9. CHRISTEN, U. & M.G. VON HERRATH. 2004. Induction, acceleration or prevention of autoimmunity by molecular mimicry. Mol. Immunol. **40:** 1113–1120.
10. KERSH, G.J. & P.M. ALLEN. 1996. Essential flexibility in the T-cell recognition of antigen. Nature **380:** 495–498.
11. STINGL, G. 1990. Dendritic cells of the skin. Dermatol. Clin. **8:** 673–679.
12. TUTING, T. 1999. The immunology of cutaneous DNA immunization. Curr. Opin. Mol. Ther. **1:** 216–225.
13. BOYLE, C.M. & H.L. ROBINSON. 2000. Basic mechanisms of DNA-raised antibody responses to intramuscular and gene gun immunizations. DNA Cell Biol. **19:** 157–165.
14. PORGADOR, A. *et al.* 1998. Predominant role for directly transfected dendritic cells in antigen presentation to CD8+ T cells after gene gun immunization. J. Exp. Med. **188:** 1075–1082.
15. TIMARES, L. *et al.* 2003. Drug-inducible, dendritic cell-based genetic immunization. J. Immunol. **170:** 5483–5490.
16. RAZ, E. *et al.* 1994. Intradermal gene immunization: the possible role of DNA uptake in the induction of cellular immunity to viruses. Proc. Natl. Acad. Sci. USA **91:** 9519–9523.
17. CONDON, C. *et al.* 1996. DNA-based immunization by in vivo transfection of dendritic cells. Nat. Med. **2:** 1122–1128.
18. GARG, S. *et al.* 2003. Genetic tagging shows increased frequency and longevity of antigen-presenting, skin-derived dendritic cells in vivo. Nat. Immunol. **4:** 907–912.
19. GURUNATHAN, S., D.M. KLINMAN & R.A. SEDER. 2000. DNA vaccines: immunology, application, and optimization. Annu. Rev. Immunol. **18:** 927–974.
20. KATZ, J.D., C. BENOIST & D. MATHIS. 1995. T helper cell subsets in insulin-dependent diabetes. Science **268:** 1185–1188.
21. YOON, J.W. *et al.* 1999. Control of autoimmune diabetes in NOD mice by GAD expression or suppression in beta cells. Science **284:** 1183–1187.
22. GAUVRIT, A. *et al.* 2004. DNA vaccination encoding glutamic acid decarboxylase can enhance insulitis and diabetes in correlation with a specific Th2/3 CD4 T cell response in non-obese diabetic mice. Clin. Exp. Immunol. **137:** 253–262.

23. Feili-Hariri, M. & P.A. Morel. 2001. Phenotypic and functional characteristics of BM-derived DC from NOD and non-diabetes-prone strains. Clin. Immunol. **98:** 133–142.
24. Peng, R. *et al.* 2003. Defective maturation of myeloid dendritic cell (DC) in NOD mice is controlled by IDD10/17/18. Ann. N. Y. Acad. Sci. **1005:** 184–186.
25. Boudaly, S. *et al.* 2002. Altered dendritic cells (DC) might be responsible for regulatory T cell imbalance and autoimmunity in nonobese diabetic (NOD) mice. Eur. Cytokine Netw. **13:** 29–37.
26. Lutz, M.B. & G. Schuler. 2002. Immature, semi-mature and fully mature dendritic cells: which signals induce tolerance or immunity? Trends Immunol. **23:** 445–449.
27. Wakkach, A. *et al.* 2003. Characterization of dendritic cells that induce tolerance and T regulatory 1 cell differentiation in vivo. Immunity **18:** 605–617.
28. Menges, M. *et al.* 2002. Repetitive injections of dendritic cells matured with tumor necrosis factor alpha induce antigen-specific protection of mice from autoimmunity. J. Exp. Med. **195:** 15–21.
29. Adorini, L. 2003. Tolerogenic dendritic cells induced by vitamin D receptor ligands enhance regulatory T cells inhibiting autoimmune diabetes. Ann. N. Y. Acad. Sci. **987:** 258–261.
30. Salomon, B. *et al.* 2000. B7/CD28 costimulation is essential for the homeostasis of the CD4+CD25+ immunoregulatory T cells that control autoimmune diabetes. Immunity. **12:** 431–440.
31. Lund, T. & J. Strid. 2000. Is lack of peripheral tolerance induction a cause for diabetes in the non-obese diabetic mouse? Arch. Immunol. Ther. Exp. (Warsz). **48:** 405–416.
32. Lee, S.W. & Y.C. Sung. 1998. Immuno-stimulatory effects of bacterial-derived plasmids depend on the nature of the antigen in intramuscular DNA inoculations. Immunology **94:** 285–289.
33. von Herrath, M.G. & J.L. Whitton. 2000. DNA vaccination to treat autoimmune diabetes. Ann. Med. **32:** 285–292.
34. Boyle, J.S., C. Koniaras & A.M. Lew. 1997. Influence of cellular location of expressed antigen on the efficacy of DNA vaccination: cytotoxic T lymphocyte and antibody responses are suboptimal when antigen is cytoplasmic after intramuscular DNA immunization. Int. Immunol. **9:** 1897–1906.
35. Coon, B. *et al.* 1999. DNA immunization to prevent autoimmune diabetes. J. Clin. Invest. **104:** 189–194.
36. Feltquate, D.M. *et al.* 1997. Different T helper cell types and antibody isotypes generated by saline and gene gun DNA immunization. J. Immunol. **158:** 2278–2284.
37. Weiss, R. *et al.* 2002. Gene gun bombardment with gold particles displays a particular Th2-promoting signal that over-rules the Th1-inducing effect of immunostimulatory CpG motifs in DNA vaccines. Vaccine **20:** 3148–3154.
38. Prayaga, S.K., M.J. Ford & J.R. Haynes. 1997. Manipulation of HIV-1 gp120-specific immune responses elicited via gene gun-based DNA immunization. Vaccine **15:** 1349–1352.
39. Haynes, J.R. *et al.* 1996. Particle-mediated nucleic acid immunization. J. Biotechnol. **44:** 37–42.
40. Leitner, W.W. *et al.* 1997. Immune responses induced by intramuscular or gene gun injection of protective deoxyribonucleic acid vaccines that express the circumsporozoite protein from Plasmodium berghei malaria parasites. J. Immunol. **159:** 6112–6119.
41. Sudowe, S., *et al.* 2003. Transcriptional targeting of dendritic cells in gene gun-mediated DNA immunization favors the induction of type 1 immune responses. Mol. Ther. **8:** 567–575.

Intra-bone Marrow–Bone Marrow Transplantation

A New Strategy for Treatment of Stem Cell Disorders

SUSUMU IKEHARA

First Department of Pathology, Transplantation Center, Regeneration Research Center for Intractable Diseases, Center for Cancer Therapy, Kansai Medical University, Osaka, Japan

ABSTRACT: We have established new bone marrow transplantation (BMT) methods for the treatment of stem cell disorders such as autoimmune diseases. The methods include the perfusion method (PM) and intra-bone marrow (IBM)–BMT. PM, in comparison with the conventional aspiration method, can minimize the contamination of bone marrow cells (BMCs) with T cells from the peripheral blood. Therefore, without removing T cells, no graft-versus-host disease develops in the case of PM. Because BMCs collected using the PM contain not only hemopoietic stem cells (HSCs) but also mesenchymal stem cells (MSCs), the injection of both cells directly into the bone marrow cavity (IBM-BMT) facilitates the engraftment of donor hemopoietic cells. With IBM-BMT, no graft failure therefore occurs even if the radiation dose is reduced. IBM-BMT is applicable to regeneration therapy and various age-associated diseases such as osteoporosis, because it can efficiently recruit donor-derived normal MSCs into the bone marrow. We believe that this strategy heralds a revolution in the field of transplantation and regenerative therapy.

KEYWORDS: bone marrow transplantation; intra-bone marrow injection; perfusion method; regeneration medicine

INTRODUCTION

Bone marrow transplantation (BMT) is becoming a powerful strategy for the treatment of hematologic disorders (leukemia, aplastic anemia, etc.), congenital immunodeficiencies, metabolic disorders, and autoimmune diseases. Using various animal models for autoimmune diseases, we have recently shown that BMT can be used to treat autoimmune diseases such as systemic lupus erythematosus (SLE), rheumatoid arthritis (RA), immune thrombocytic purpura (ITP), insulin-dependent diabetes mellitus (IDDM), chronic glomerulonephritis, and a certain type of non-insulin-dependent diabetes mellitus (NIDDM).[1–8]

Address for correspondence: Susumu Ikehara, M.D., Ph.D., First Department of Pathology, Kansai Medical University, 10-15 Fumizono-cho, Moriguchi City, Osaka 570-8506, Japan. Voice: +81-6-6993-9429; fax: +81-6-6-994-8283.
ikehara@takii.kmu.ac.jp

Ann. N.Y. Acad. Sci. 1051: 626–634 (2005). © 2005 New York Academy of Sciences.
doi: 10.1196/annals.1361.107

In addition, we have found that autoimmune diseases are stem cell disorders.[9,10] However, in MRL/lpr mice, which are radiosensitive (<8.5 Gy), we found that conventional intravenous BMT (iv-BMT) had a transient effect on autoimmune diseases, which were found to recur.[5] Therefore, we concentrated on how we could prevent and treat autoimmune diseases in radiosensitive and chimeric-resistant MRL/lpr mice. We found that three types of cells are essential for successful allogeneic BMT: pluripotent hemopoietic stem cells (P-HSCs),[11] natural suppressor cells,[12] and stromal cells (including mesenchymal stem cells [MSCs]).[13,14] Particularly, we recently found that stromal cells play a crucial role in preventing graft failure,[15] because there is an MHC restriction between HSCs and stromal cells.[16] To recruit donor-derived stromal cells, we found that intra-bone marrow–BMT (IBM-BMT)—injection of whole bone marrow cells (BMCs), containing P-HSCs and MSCs, into the bone marrow cavity—is the best strategy for allogeneic BMT.[15] We here show that the perfusion method (PM) plus IBM-BMT will become a valuable strategy for the treatment of various intractable diseases, including autoimmune diseases.

PERFUSION METHOD VERSUS ASPIRATION METHOD

To study the application of IBM-BMT to humans, we used cynomolgus monkeys to establish a method, termed the perfusion method, that can minimize the contamination of BMCs with T cells. As shown in FIGURE 1, two needles were inserted into a long bone, such as the humerus, femur, or tibia, to the shaft. The end of the extension tube was connected to a needle. The other end was placed in a culture flask containing 20 mL PBS with heparin. The other needle was connected to a syringe containing 30 mL PBS, and the PBS was then pushed gently from the syringe into the medullary cavity to flush out the bone marrow (BM). The medium containing the BM fluid was collected in the culture flask.

There is significantly less contamination with T cells when using the PM (<6%) than with the conventional aspiration method (>20%), which consists of multiple bone marrow aspirations from the iliac crest.[17] Therefore, T cell depletion is unnecessary with the PM, and whole BMCs can be used. In contrast, with the conventional aspiration method, T cell depletion is necessary, and the loss of some important cells, such as MSCs, during the process of T cell depletion is inevitable. Furthermore, the number and progenitor activities of the cells harvested using this PM are greater than when using the conventional aspiration method.[17]

It has been generally accepted that more than 1×10^8 BMCs/kg are necessary for BMT. Therefore, multiple bone marrow aspirations are essential for collecting BMCs; this results in a large burden on donors owing to the duration of the operation. In contrast, the PM is completed within 15 min of anesthetization. Consequently, using the PM, a large number of BMCs can rapidly be harvested without any complications, such as pulmonary infarction or paralysis (when tested more than 100 times using more than 50 cynomolgus monkeys), thus reducing the burden on the donors.

In humans, because there has been a rapid increase in the number of patients for whom BMT is indispensable in recent years, HLA-one-locus-mismatched BMT and unrelated BMT have been performed, but graft-versus-host disease (GvHD), graft rejection, and incomplete T cell recovery have been reported.[18–21] The PM, which

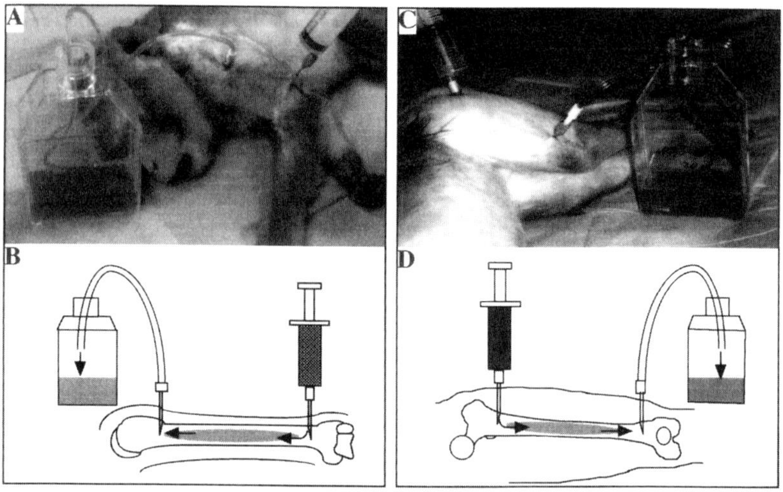

FIGURE 1. Perfusion method. Two needles are inserted into the humerus (**A, B**) or femur (**C, D**). One needle is connected to an extension tube, and the end of the tube is inserted into a culture flask to collect the bone marrow fluid. The other needle is connected to a syringe containing 30 mL PBS. The solution is pushed gently from the syringe into the bone marrow cavity. The medium containing the bone marrow fluid is collected into the flask.

minimizes the contamination of the BMCs with T cells from the peripheral blood, may prevent these problems, particularly GvHD (unpublished data). In addition, since the red bone marrow is detected in the long bones to age 20,[22] it may be possible to harvest BMCs using the PM from adolescent donors who are brain dead. We have also found that the PM could contribute to gene therapy[23] and organ allografts in conjunction with BMT (unpublished data).

NECESSITY FOR RECRUITMENT OF DONOR STROMAL CELLS

Using radiosensitive and chimeric-resistant MRL/lpr mice, we found that the recruitment of donor stromal cells is essential for successful allogeneic BMT. We carried out three experiments to recruit donor stromal cells including MSCs: (1) conventional iv-BMT plus bone grafts (as described in Ref. 24), (2) BMT from the portal vein (PV-BMT; as described in Ref. 25) because it is well known that tolerance can easily be induced when the antigen is injected into the liver via the portal vein, and (3) IBM-BMT.[15]

First, we compared the effects of the various BMT methods on the survival rates of MRL/lpr mice. As shown in FIGURE 2, all recipients treated with 5.5 Gy × 2 plus iv-BMT died within 200 days after the treatment owing to the recurrence of autoimmune diseases. However, the survival rate of recipients treated with 5.5 Gy × 2 plus PV-BMT was 70%, and all recipients treated with 5.5 Gy × 2 plus PV-BMT + iv-BMT survived for more than 350 days, indicating that additional iv-BMT is helpful for successful engraftment.[25]

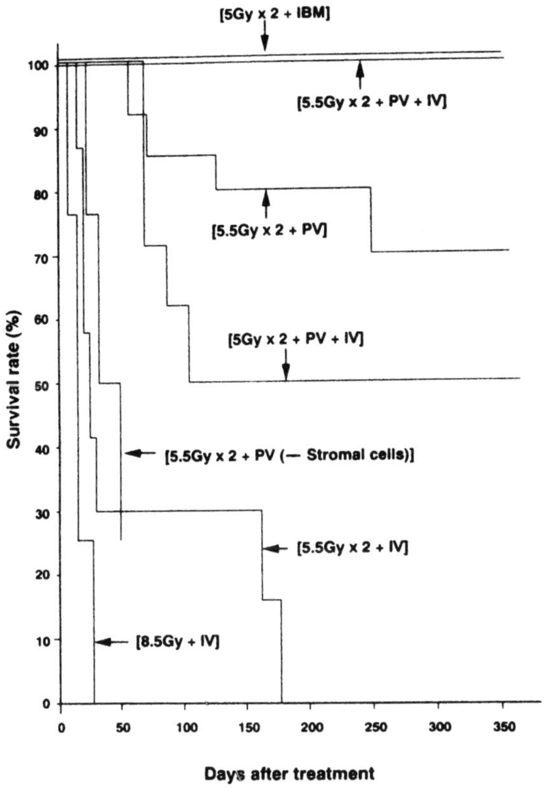

FIGURE 2. Treatment of autoimmune diseases in MRL/lpr mice by IBM-BMT (5 Gy × 2). IBM-BMT can be used to treat autoimmune diseases in MRL/lpr mice even when the radiation dose is reduced to 5 Gy × 2. When stromal cell–depleted BMCs were injected via the PV, the recipients died of graft failure.

When BMCs from which the stromal cells had been removed were injected from the PV, the survival rate of the recipients was markedly reduced (FIG. 2), indicating the crucial role of stromal cells in the successful engraftment. Donor-derived stromal cells are trapped in the liver when whole BMCs are injected from the PV, and the stromal cells not only support the proliferation and differentiation of donor-derived P-HSCs trapped in the liver but also protect those P-HSCs from being attacked by the host's immunocompetent cells by directly embracing the P-HSCs[13] and/or by producing immunosuppressive cytokines such as hepatocyte growth factor (HGF) and transforming growth factor–β (TGF-β).[26]

We next injected whole BMCs (including MSCs) directly into the bone marrow cavity (IBM-BMT), because we have found that the hemopoietic site moves from the liver to the bone marrow, even when the whole BMCs are PV-injected. As shown in FIGURE 2, IBM-BMT–treated recipients showed excellent survival rates, even when the radiation dose was reduced to 5 Gy × 2.[15] These findings indicate that IBM-BMT is the best strategy for allogeneic BMT.

SEVERE COMBINED IMMUNODEFICIENCY/ HUMAN (hu) BY IBM-BMT

The xenotransplant assay system using severe combined immunodeficiency (SCID) mice provides a powerful tool for characterizing the frequency, cell surface markers, cell cycle status, homing, and response to cytokine stimulation of human HSCs.[27–29] However, all HSC repopulation assays are based on intravenous injection, a complex process that requires circulation through blood, recognition and extravasation through bone marrow vasculature, and migration to a supportive microenviroment.[30–32] Recently, several groups have reported that nonobese diabetic (NOD-)–SCID xenograft models using IBM-BMT provide powerful tools for the detection of new classes of HSCs that are rare, poorly detected using traditional intravenous-based assays, or from atypical sources (such as embryonic stem cells or nonhematopoietic tissues).[33–35] Indeed, we found using IBM-BMT that $Lin^-CD34^-CD38^-$ cells have high SCID-repopulating cell (SRC) activity.[33] Thus the SCID/hu system using IBM-BMT would become a valuable strategy not only for producing animal models of various intractable diseases but also for analyzing real HSCs in mice and humans.

IBM-BMT FOR REGENERATION THERAPY

Because we found that donor stromal cells could be effectively recruited by IBM-BMT, we next attempted to prevent osteoporosis in SAMP6 mice. The SAMP6 mouse (a substrain of senescence-accelerated mice) spontaneously develops osteoporosis early in life and is therefore a useful model for examining the mechanisms underlying osteoporosis. After IBM-BMT, the hematolymphoid system was completely reconstituted with donor-type cells. Thus-treated SAMP6 mice showed marked increases in trabecular bone even at 12 months of age, and the bone mineral density (BMD) remained similar to that of normal B6 mice. Bone marrow stromal cells in IBM-BMT–treated SAMP6 mice were replaced by donor stromal cells.[36] Thus we succeeded in preventing osteoporosis in SAMP6 mice by IBM-BMT, which can recruit not only donor P-HSCs but also MSCs. Therefore, we believe that IBM-BMT should become a powerful strategy in regeneration therapy.

TRANSLATIONAL RESEARCH FOR IBM-BMT

Because IBM-BMT was found to be the most effective strategy for allogeneic stem cell transplantation in mice, rats, and rabbits, we carried out monkey experiments as a preclinical step for human application. It is well known that there are three main problems concerning allogeneic BMT in humans: GvHD, graft failure, and incomplete restoration of T cell functions.

First, to prevent the development of GvHD, we established a new method (PM) for BMC harvesting using cynomolgus monkeys, as already mentioned. If bone marrow needles are inserted into the iliac crest more than 100 times and BMCs are collected using an aspiration method, as in conventional BMT (FIG. 3A), peripheral blood contamination is inevitable. In contrast, if the PM is carried out using long bones (FIG. 3B), not only HSCs but also MSCs can be collected without contamination from the peripheral blood. If thus-collected BMCs are directly injected into the bone marrow cavity (IBM-BMT) (FIG. 3B), donor-derived HSCs and MSCs can be retained at the bone marrow site and can proliferate and differentiate. However, if BMCs are intravenously injected, most BMCs are trapped in the lung and only a few cells migrate into the bone marrow (FIG. 3A).

Second, as already discussed, donor stromal cells play a crucial role in the prevention of graft failure, because they can protect HSCs from the attack of host-

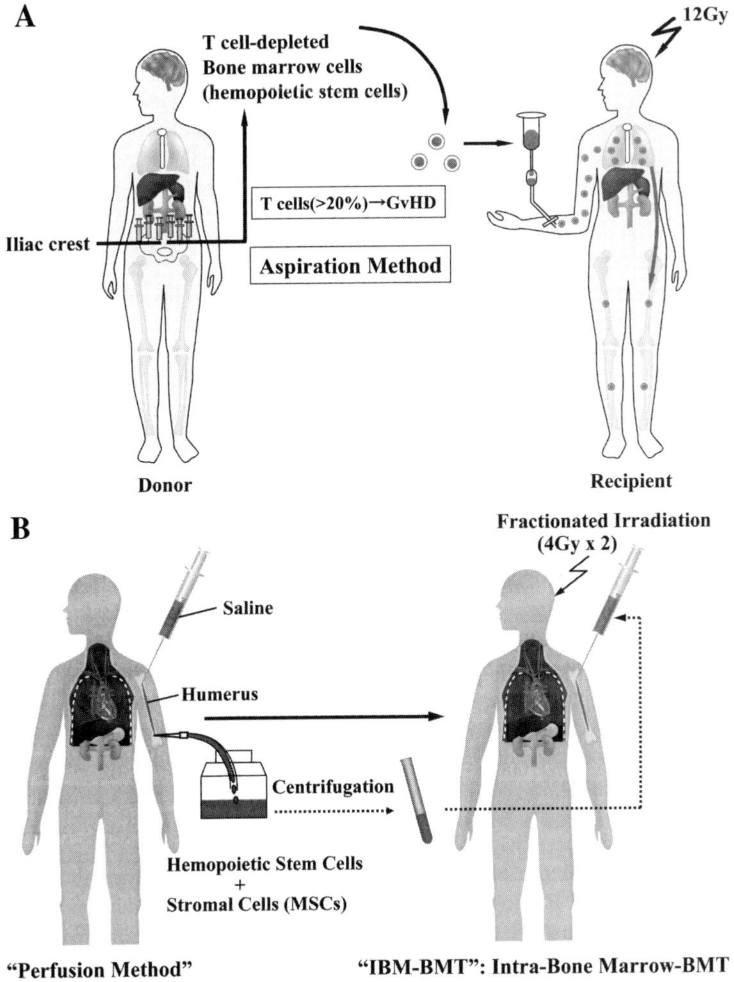

FIGURE 3. Conventional (**A**) BMT vs. new methods (**B**) for allo-BMT. Conventional BMT is carried out using an aspiration method, followed by the intravenous injection of BMCs. In contrast, new methods consist of the PM + IBM-BMT using long bones.

derived cells such as T cells and natural-killer (NK) cells, and IBM-BMT efficiently recruits donor stromal cells into the bone marrow of recipients.

Third, concerning impaired T cell functions in BMT across MHC barriers, we recently found that, in the case of IBM-BMT, donor stromal cells migrate into the thymus, where they are engaged in positive selection.[37] Thus IBM-BMT can overcome all three problems in allogeneic BMT.

DISEASES CURABLE BY PM + IBM-BMT

We believe that PM + IBM-BMT will become a valuable strategy not only for the treatment of intractable diseases such as autoimmune diseases but also for regeneration therapy for injured organs and tissues such as myocardial infarction, cerebral infarction, and Alzheimer disease because this strategy can efficiently reconstitute recipients with both donor-derived P-HSCs and MSCs, which can differentiate into all cells, including hepatocytes,[38] epithelial cells,[38] nerve cells,[39] and retinal cells.[40]

Finally, I would like to propose a new concept of stem cell disorders. On the one hand, there are *hemopoietic stem cell disorders,* which include:

- Monoclonal or oligoclonal abnormal HSC proliferative syndromes (leukemias and myelodysplastic syndrome).
- Polyclonal abnormal HSC proliferative syndromes (autoimmune diseases).
- Aplasia of HSCs (aplastic anemia).

On the other hand, there are *mesenchymal stem cell disorders*, which include age-associated diseases such as osteoporosis, Alzheimer disease, and arteriosclerosis.

We think it may be possible for most diseases to be cured by the transplantation of both P-HSCs and MSCs from young normal donors because all cells are derived from the bone marrow.

In conclusion, because most intractable diseases are stem cell disorders (not only HSC disorders but also MSC disorders), we believe that our new BMT method (PM + IBM-BMT), which can efficiently collect both HSCs and MSCs and transplant both, will become a valuable strategy for the treatment of various intractable diseases. We also believe that the development of this strategy heralds a revolution in the field of transplantation and regeneration therapy.

ACKNOWLEDGMENTS

This work was supported by a grant from Haiteku Research Center of the Ministry of Education; a grant from the Millennium program of the Ministry of Education, Culture, Sports, Science and Technology; a grant from the Science Frontier program of the Ministry of Education, Culture, Sports, Science and Technology; a grant from the The 21st Century Center of Excellence (COE) program of the Ministry of Education, Culture, Sports, Science and Technology; a grant-in-aid for scientific research (B) 11470062; grants-in-aid for scientific research on priority areas (A)10181225 and (A)11162221; Health and Labour Sciences research grants (Research on Human Genome, Tissue Engineering Food Biotechnology); a grant from the Department of Transplantation for Regeneration Therapy (Sponsored by Otsuka Pharmaceutical Company, Ltd.); a grant from Molecular Medical Science Institute,

Otsuka Pharmaceutical Co., Ltd.; and a grant from Japan Immunoresearch Laboratories Co., Ltd. (JIMRO).

We thank Mr. Hilary Eastwick-Field and Ms. K. Ando for their help in the preparation of the manuscript.

REFERENCES

1. Ikehara, S., R.A. Good, T. Nakamura, *et al.* 1985. Rationale for bone marrow transplantation in the treatment of autoimmune diseases. Proc. Natl. Acad. Sci. USA **82:** 2483–2487.
2. Ikehara, S., H. Ohtsuki, R.A. Good, *et al.* 1985. Prevention of type I diabetes in non-obese diabetic mice by allogeneic bone marrow transplantation. Proc. Natl. Acad. Sci. USA **82:** 7743–7747.
3. Yasumizu, R., K. Sugiura, H. Iwai, *et al.* 1987. Treatment of type I diabetes mellitus in non-obese diabetic mice by transplantation of allogeneic bone marrow and pancreatic tissue. Proc. Natl. Acad. Sci. USA **84:** 6555–6557.
4. Oyaizu, N., R. Yasumizu, M. Inaba-Miyama, *et al.* 1988. (NZW × BXSB) F1 mouse. A new model of idiopathic thrombocytopenic purpura. J. Exp. Med. **167:** 2017–2022.
5. Ikehara, S., R. Yasumizu, M. Inaba, *et al.* 1989. Long-term observations of autoimmune-prone mice treated for autoimmune disease by allogeneic bone marrow transplantation. Proc. Natl. Acad Sci. USA **86:** 3306–3310.
6. Adachi, Y., M. Inaba, Y. Amoh, *et al.* 1995. Effects of bone marrow transplantation on antiphospholipid syndrome in murine lupus mice. Immunobiology **192:** 218–230.
7. Soe T., H. Ishida, M. Inaba, *et al.* 1992. Bone marrow transplantation as a strategy for treatment of non-insulin-dependent diabetes mellitus in KK-Ay mice. J. Exp. Med. **176:** 1233–1238.
8. Nishimura, M., J. Toki, K. Sugiura, *et al.* 1994. Focal glomerulonephritis is a stem cell disorder. J. Exp. Med. **179:** 1053–1058.
9. Ikehara, S., M. Kawamura, F. Takao, *et al.* 1990. Organ-specific and systemic autoimmune diseases originate from defects in hematopoietic stem cells. Proc. Natl. Acad. Sci. USA **87:** 8341–8344.
10. Kawamura, M., H. Hisha, Y. Li, *et al.* 1997. Distinct qualitative differences between normal and abnormal hemopoietic stem cells in vivo and in vitro. Stem Cells **15:** 56–62.
11. Doi, H., M. Inaba, Y. Yamamoto, *et al.* 1997. Pluripotent hemopoietic stem cells are c-kit$^{<\text{low}}$. Proc. Natl. Acad. Sci. USA **94:** 2513–2517.
12. Sugiura, K., M. Inaba, H. Ogata, *et al.* 1988. Wheat germ agglutinin-positive cells in a stem cell-enriched fraction of mouse bone marrow have potent natural suppressor activity. Proc. Natl. Acad. Sci. USA. **85:** 4824–4826.
13. Ikehara, S. 1998. Autoimmune diseases as stem cell disorders: normal stem cell transplant for their treatment. Int. J. Molec. Med. **1:** 5–16.
14. Ikehara, S. 2001. Treatment of autoimmune diseases by hematopoietic stem cell transplantation. Exp. Hematol. **29:** 661–669.
15. Kushida, T., M. Inaba, H. Hisha. et al. 2001. Intra-bone marrow injection of allogeneic bone marrow cells: a powerful new strategy for treatment of intractable autoimmune diseases in MRL/lpr mice. Blood **97:** 3292–3299.
16. Hashimoto, F., K. Sugiura, K. Inoue, *et al.* 1997. Major histocompatibility complex restriction between hematopoietic stem cells and stromal cells in vivo. Blood **89:** 49–54.
17. Kushida, T., M. Inaba, K. Ikebukuro, *et al.* 2000. A new method for bone marrow cell harvesting. Stem Cells **18:** 453–456.
18. Beatty, P.G., C. Anasetti, J.A. Hansen, *et al.* 1993. Marrow transplantation from unrelated donors for treatment of hematologic malignancies: effect of mismatching for one HLA locus. Blood **81:** 249–253.
19. Ferrara, J.L.M. & H.J. Deeq. 1991. Graft-versus-host disease. N. Engl. J. Med. **324:** 667–674.
20. Kerhan, N.A., G. Bartsch, R.C. Ash, *et al.* 1993. Analysis of 462 transplantations from unrelated donors facilitated by the national marrow donor program. N. Engl. J. Med. **328:** 593–602.

21. SULLIVAN, K.M., H.M. SHULMAN, R. STORB, *et al.* 1981. Chronic graft-versus-host disease in 52 patients: adverse natural course and successful treatment with combination immunosuppression. Blood **57:** 267–276.
22. BLOCK, M.H. 1976. Atlas of Hematology. Lea & Febiger. Philadelphia.
23. UEDA, K., Y. HANAZONO, H. SHIBATA, *et al.* 2004. High-level in vivo gene marking after gene-modified autologous hematopoietic stem cell transplantation without marrow conditioning in nonhuman primates. Mol. Ther. **10:** 469–477.
24. ISHIDA, T., M. INABA, H. HISHA, *et al.* 1994. Requirement of donor-derived stromal cells in the bone marrow for successful allogeneic bone marrow transplantation: complete prevention of recurrence of autoimmune diseases in MRL/MP-lpr/lpr mice by transplantation of bone marrow plus bone (stromal cells) from the same donor. J. Immunol. **152:** 3119–3127.
25. KUSHIDA, T., M. INABA, K. TAKEUCHI, *et al.* 2000. Treatment of intractable autoimmune diseases in MRL/lpr mice using a new strategy for allogeneic bone marrow transplantation. Blood **95:** 1862–1868.
26. NICOLA, M.D., C. STELLA-CARLO, M. MAGNI, *et al.* 2002. Human bone marrow stromal cells suppress T-lymphocyte proliferation induced by cellular or nonspecific mitogenic stimuli. Blood **99:** 3838–3843.
27. WANG, J.C., *et al.* 2001. Normal and leukemic human stem cells assayed in immune-deficient mice. *In* Hematopoiesis: A developmental Approach. L. I. Zon, Ed.: 99–118. Oxford University Press. New York.
28. LAPIDOT, T., I. PETIT. 2002. Current understanding of stem cell mobilization: the roles of chemokines, proteolytic enzymes, adhesion molecules, and stromal cells. Exp. Hematol. **30:** 973–981.
29. PELED, A., *et al.* 2000. The chemokine SDF-1 activates the integrins LFA-1, VLA-4, and VLA-5 on immature human CD34(+) cells: role in transendothelial/stromal migration and engraftment of NOD-SCID mice. Blood **95:** 3289–3296.
30. VAN HENNIK, P.B., A.E. DE KONING, R.E. PLOEMACHER. 1999. Seeding efficiency of primitive human hematopoietic cells in nonobese diabetic/severe combined immune deficiency mice: implications for stem cell frequency assessment. Blood **94:** 3055–3061.
31. QUESENBERRY, P.J. & P.S. BECKER. 1998. Stem cell homing: rolling, crawing, and nesting. Proc. Natl. Acad. Sci. USA **95:** 15155–15157.
32. CASHMAN, J. & C. EAVES. 2000. High marrow seeding efficiency of human lymphomyeloid repopulating cells in irradiated NOD-SCID mice. Blood **96:** 3979–3981.
33. WANG, J., T. KIMURA, R. ASADA, *et al.* 2003. SCID-repopulating cell activity of human cord blood-derived $CD34^-$ cells assured by intra-bone marrow injection. Blood **101:** 2924–2931.
34. YAHATA, T., K. ANDO, T. SATO, *et al.* 2003. A highly sensitive strategy for SCID-repopulating cell assay by direct injection of primitive human hematopoietic cells into NOD/SCID mice bone marrow. Blood **101:** 2905–2913.
35. MAZURIER, F., M. DOEDENS, O.I. GAN, *et al.* 2003. Rapid myeloerythroid repopulation after intrafemoral transplantation of NOD-SCID mice reveals a new class of human stem cells. Nat. Med. **9:** 959–963.
36. ICHIOKA, N., M. INABA, T. KUSHIDA, *et al.* 2003. Prevention of senile osteoporosis in SAMP6 mice by intrabone marrow injection of allogeneic bone marrow cells. Stem Cells **20:** 542–551.
37. LI Y, HISHA H, INABA, *et al.* 2000. Evidence for migration of donor bone marrow stromal cells into recipient thymus after bone marrow transplantation plus bone grafts: a role of stromal cells in positive selection. Exp. Hematol. **28:** 950–960.
38. WANG, X., S. GE, G. MCNAMARA, *et al.* 2003. Albumin-expressing hepatocyte-like cells develop in the livers of immune-deficient mice transmitted with highly purified human hematopoietic stem cells. Blood **101:** 4201–4208.
39. MEZEY, E., S. KEY, G. VOGELSANG, *et al.* 2003. Transplanted bone marrow generates new neurons in human brains. Proc. Natl. Acad. Sci. USA **100:** 1364–1369.
40. TOMITA, M., Y. ADACHI, H. YAMADA, *et al.* 2002. Bone marrow-derived stem cells can differentiate into retinal cells in injured rat retina. Stem Cells **320:** 279–283.

Removal of Pathogenic Autoantibodies by Immunoadsorption

ALON Y. HERSHKO AND YAAKOV NAPARSTEK

Department of Medicine, Hadassah University Hospital, Jerusalem, Israel

ABSTRACT: Autoimmune diseases result from disrupted tolerance to self-antigens and subsequent damage to tissues and organs. In several diseases, specific autoantibodies have been either proved or suspected to play a role in this process. Consequently, several strategies have been devised in an attempt to discard the destructive immunoglobulins. Currently, both nonselective and epitope-specific methods are applied in several diseases. In this review, we provide a summary of the available data on elimination of pathogenic autoantibodies and discuss the advantages and pitfalls of the different approaches.

KEYWORDS: autoantibodies; immunoadsorption; apheresis; myasthenia gravis; dilated cardiomyopathy; systemic lupus erythematosus

INTRODUCTION

The presence of antibodies that recognize self-antigens is the hallmark of many autoimmune diseases, and these autoantibodies are regarded as pathogenic if they contribute directly to disease formation. Alternatively, they may not be the causative factors but rather a consequence of tissue damage or merely represent markers of a pathogenic process.[1] Several criteria have been suggested to indicate that an autoantibody is harmful: the titers should roughly correlate with disease activity, the antibody must cause the relevant lesion in experimental systems, and the antibody should be detected along with a plausible target antigen at the site of tissue damage. Pathogenicity is convincingly established when passive transfer of serum induces experimental autoimmune disease or when elimination of the autoantibody from the serum alleviates disease manifestations. Obviously, the latter is the more difficult to fulfill because it requires both isolation of the culprit antibody and the technical means for its removal.

Until two decades ago, therapeutic plasma exchange was the only procedure used for antibody removal from the plasma, allowing reduction of immunoglobulins to approximately 50%. The most significant disadvantages were depletion of essential plasma components such as albumin and clotting factors, and the adverse effects re-

Address for correspondence: Alon Y. Hershko, Department of Medicine, Hadassah University Hospital, P.O.B. 12000, IL-91120, Jerualem, Israel. Voice: +972-2-6777644; fax: +972-2-6423216.

alonh@md.huji.ac.il

Ann. N.Y. Acad. Sci. 1051: 635–646 (2005). © 2005 New York Academy of Sciences. doi: 10.1196/annals.1361.108

sulting from administration of their substitutions, including allergic reactions and viral contamination. To overcome these problems, several types of immunoadsorption devices have been developed to remove immunoglobulins only. More recently, attempts have been made to eliminate pathogenic antibodies in an antigen-specific manner with sparing of irrelevant immunoglobulins and other plasma proteins.

In this review, we chose to present and discuss therapeutic approaches based on removal of antibodies from the blood, with a special emphasis on treatment modalities designed to reduce titers of specific pathogenic autoantibodies. For this purpose we focus on three diseases that represent promising candidates for these novel treatments: myasthenia gravis (MG), idiopathic dilated cardiomyopathy (DCM), and systemic lupus erythematosus (SLE).

NONSPECIFIC ELIMINATION OF ANTIBODIES

Several immunoadsorption columns are currently available for clinical use in conjunction with apheresis systems (TABLE 1).[2] Each column is characterized by an adsorbent, consisting of a matrix and a ligand. Immusorba columns (Ashahi Medical, Tokyo, Japan) contain cross-linked polyvinyl alcohol gel beads as the matrix, to which the hydrophobic amino acids tryptophan (TR) and phenylalanine (PH) are immobilized.[3] In small clinical trials, efficacy was demonstrated in a variety of neurologic disorders, including MG.[4] In the Selesorb system (Kaneka, Osaka, Japan), cellulose beads are linked to the negatively charged dextran sulfate. This ligand enables electrostatic bonding with anti-DNA and anticardiolipin antibodies[5] but may also be effective in the treatment of hepatitis C virus (HCV-)–related cryoglobulinemia.[6]

Both Immusorba and Selesorb possess nonselective physical features and are, therefore, applicable in more than one disease, depending on their capacity to interact with the pathogen. However, they may cause reduction of plasma levels of various substances other than immunoglobulins, such as fibrinogen, albumin, and lipids.[7] A larger spectrum of antibodies can be extracted by the Ig-Therasorb column (Therasorb Medical Systems, Unterschleissheim, Germany), which is made of cellulose beads with sheep polyclonal anti-human immunoglobulin as the ligand.[8] The efficacy of Ig-Therasob was demonstrated in several diseases, one of which is DCM (discussed below).

Protein A is the ligand of two widely used extracorporeal immunoadsorption systems that have earned the approval of the U.S. Food and Drug Administration (FDA) for treatment in indicated diseases. Protein A of the staphylococcus bacterium (SPA) is a cell wall component that was found in *S. aureus* isolates, more than 40 years ago.[9] Its capacity to react with the constant regions of antibodies renders it useful as a means for extraction of immunoglobulins. The SPA-based products that are mostly used are Immunosorba, in which SPA is coupled to agarose beads, and Prosorba (Fresenius Hemocare, USA) which is silica-based.

Immunosorba is a double-column system with a nearly unlimited adsorption capacity and is efficacious where rapid and effective antibody removal is required. For this reason, Immunosorba was approved by the FDA for treatment of patients with hemophilia who develop inhibitors,[10–12] which are allo-antibodies stimulated by, and directed against, factor concentrates. In this specific disease, Immunosorba has

TABLE 1. Nonspecific immunoadsorption system

Apparatus	Base material	Ligand	Selected applications	Comments
Immusorba	Polyvinyl-alcohol gel	Tryptophan (TR) Phenylalanine (PH)	MG	
Selesorb	Cellulose	Dextran-sulfate	Anti-DNA ab Anti-cardiolipin HCV cryoglobulin	
Ig Therasorb	Cellulose	Sheep anti-human Ig	DCM	
Immunosorba	Agarose	SPA	Hemophilia inhbitors	FDA approved
Prosorba	Silica	SPA ITP	Rheumatoid arthritis	FDA approved

unequivocal superior cost-efficiency over excess administration of factor concentrates.[9]

Unlike Immunosorba, the capacity of Prosorba is restricted to a maximum of 2000 mL of plasma.[13,14] Despite the limited volume of processed plasma, which does not allow significant removal of immunoglobulins or circulating immune complexes, this device has been shown to exert immune modulating effects. Its mode of action remains, however, somewhat obscure.[15–17] The Prosorba system is approved by the FDA for treatment of rheumatoid arthritis refractory to therapy with conventional drug regimens. This decision was largely based on the results of a prospective, controlled, randomized, and double-blinded study on 99 patients.[13,18] Prosorba is also an FDA-approved treatment for resistant idiopathic thrombocytopenic purpura unresponsive to conventional therapy. The major analysis in this respect cites 72 treated patients with platelet counts < 50,000/mL.[14]

Apart from these FDA-approved indications, SPA-based immunoadsorption has been tried in several other autoimmune entities. There are data supporting a possible beneficial effect in patients with diseases such as Goodpasture syndrome,[19] Wegener's granulomatosis,[9] thrombotic thrombocytopenic purpura/hemolytic uremic syndrome,[20] and myasthenia gravis.[21–23] In SLE, Immunosorba has induced complete elimination of circulating immune complexes and normalization of antibodies against double-stranded DNA (dsDNA), with concomitant amelioration of inflammation.[7,24] Acute vascular rejection of transplanted kidneys, which is mediated by anti-HLA antibodies also appears to respond well to SPA-based extracorporeal immunoadsorption.[25]

Because many of the diseases mentioned in this section have not been recognized as indications for SPA immunoadsorption, a prudent conservative approach is to consider this treatment modality only in exceptionally refractory cases. Alternatively, it may be used in individuals who should avoid cytotoxic drugs—for example, SLE patients with bone marrow depression caused by cyclophosphamide. We should also note, that it seems that most adverse effects are attributed to the apheresis procedure per se, rather than to the column.[18]

TABLE 2. Epitope-specific elimination of autoantibodies

Disease and pathogenic autoantibody	Method of removal	Comments
Myasthenia gravis Anti-AChR (α-domain)	Immunoadsorption	Successful removal of blocking antibodies only
Dilated cardiomyopathy Anti–β1-AR	Immunoadsorption	Antibodies not specific for DCM
Systemic lupus erythematosus Anti-dsDNA	LJP394 (drug)	LJP394 removes pathogenic antibodies and suppresses antibody-producing cells
Anti-laminin	Immunoadsorption	Specific marker of lupus nephritis

ANTIGEN-SPECIFIC REMOVAL OF PATHOGENIC AUTOANTIBODIES

During the past few years, a novel strategy has emerged for treatment of autoimmune diseases, aimed at specific removal of identified pathogenic autoantibodies (TABLE 2). The concept underlying this approach assumes that elimination of these antibodies is sufficient to suppress or reverse the autoimmune process. The validity of this assumption can now be tested in three model systems: MG, DCM and SLE.

Myasthenia Gravis

The major clinical manifestations in MG are the result of a postsynaptic dysfunction of the neuromuscular junction that causes muscle weakness. The functional disturbances are accompanied by structural changes, such as widening of the synaptic cleft and reduced folding of the postsynaptic membrane. In most cases, antibodies to various sites on the extracellular portion of the acetylcholine receptor (AChR) can be detected. However, in nearly 15–20% of MG patients, these antibodies are absent (seronegative myasthenia gravis) and the pathogenic agents are probably circulating antibodies against other muscle antigens, such as muscle-specific kinase (MuSK). The AChR is a transmembrane protein consisting of five subunits: α, β, γ, δ, and ε.[26] The MG autoantibodies are predominantly of the IgG class and mostly directed against the α unit. Antibodies against the α domain can be divided into two subclasses, according to the role they play in the pathogenetic process. One subclass includes antibodies recognizing residues 183–200[27] and prevents the binding of ACh to its receptor (blocking antibodies). The other subclass is directed against segments α67–76[28] and 125–147,[29] which are implicated in enhancement of AChR degradation and destruction of postsynaptic membrane through complement activation (binding or modulating antibodies).

Immunization of Lewis rats with the *Torpedo californica* and human segments of α183–200 induces myasthenic features, as evidenced by elevated antipeptide antibodies and reduced endplate potential amplitudes.[27] In contrast, α67–76 fails to induce disease, unless artificially linked to a putative T cell stimulatory site, α106–116. The data obtained from animal models combined with subsequent detection of anti-Torpedo α183–200 antibodies in the sera MG patients led directly to clinical trials of antigen-specific immunoadsorption therapy using the corresponding peptide.

After a successful pilot study in two patients whose sera were positive for anti-Torpedo α183–200 peptide and anti-native AChR blocking antibodies, the study was expanded to include 22 randomly selected patients. Consequently, both significant reduction of blocking antibodies and clinical improvement were demonstrated in one-half to two-thirds of the subjects.[30] It was disappointing that attempts for selective removal of the antibodies involved in accelerated receptor degradation and membrane destruction were apparently not feasible. This is due to the low affinity of peptides containing the sequence of α67–76 to anti-native AChR binding antibodies, even when subjected to conformational modifications (model peptides) that are designed to enhance their antigenicity.[30]

It therefore seems that patients may benefit from short-term stabilizing therapy by specific removal of pathogenic blocking antibodies using plasma perfusion treatment based on the synthetic peptide (α183–200)-bound adsorbent. Nevertheless, the specificity of this technique, which is its major advantage, proved to be a significant drawback because the anti-AChR blocking antibody is merely one subpopulation among several others implicated in the pathogenesis of MG.

Dilated Cardiomyopathy

The cause of cardiomyopathy can be attributed to mutations in genes encoding for myocyte structural proteins[31,32] and cardiotoxic substances in only 30–40% of cases. The remaining 60–70% are thought to result from either chronic viral myocarditis[33] or from primary abnormalities in the immune system. Heart-specific autoantibodies have been detected in such patients,[34] and those directed against β1-adrenergic receptor (β1-AR) are presently implicated in the pathogenesis of DCM. Their prevalence in patients with idiopathic DCM is approximately 80%.[35] A subset of these antibodies—those that bind to the second extracellular receptor loop (β1-ECII)—is capable of activating the receptor[36] and is associated with poor left ventricular function.[37] It should be noted, however, that IgG antibodies with agonist activity for the β1-AR are definitively not specific for DCM, and their presence has been detected in sera of patients with Chagas disease and ischemic heart disease.

A large body of data regarding the cardiotoxic effects of β1-AR overstimulation lends support to the concept that agonist anti-β1-AR IgGs are pathogenic rather than markers of myocardial inflammation or result of myocardial damage. Genetic and pharmacologic manipulations indicate that excessive β1-AR activation yields cardiomyocyte toxicity. For example, excessive isoproterenol stimulation–induced damage is mediated primarily by its effect on β1-AR,[38] and transgenic mice overexpressing β1-AR develop cardiomyopathy.[39]

Recently, direct and convincing data were introduced indicating that antibodies against the cardiac β1-AR are indeed pathogenic.[40] After inducing left ventricular dilatation and dysfunction by immunization of inbred rats against β1-ECII, sera were transferred to healthy isogenic rats, and the recipient animals developed similar cardiac abnormalities. This experiment established the role of the antibodies as pathogenic agents.

Preliminary data suggest a similar conclusion in humans. In a limited study, 8 patients were subjected to specific immunoadsorption with peptide columns mimicking the autoantibody-binding epitope of the β1-AR.[41] Consequently, long-term improvement in cardiac function was detected, manifested by increased ejection fraction and decreased left ventricular dimension. However, a clinical trial in which nonselective immunoadsorption was employed in 22 DCM patients added complexity to the proposed model of DCM pathogenesis. In this study, immunoglobulins were extracted from the plasma using the Ig-Therasorb device.[2] It is interesting that both β1-AR-antibody-positive and -negative groups showed similar hemodynamic improvements as well as augmentation of left ventricular ejection fraction.[42] This implies that the mechanism of improvement after immunoadsorption therapy involves multiple factors, such as elimination of antibodies directed at several cardiac proteins. Even though anti-β1-AR antibodies are clearly pathogenic, their relative impact in the pathogenesis of DCM *in vivo,* compared to other putative pathogenic autoantibodies, has yet to be determined.

Systemic Lupus Erythematosus

When discussing novel treatments for SLE, one should keep in mind that although the disease involves multiple organ systems, it is the renal disease that primarily determines the prognostic outcome. Therefore, prevention of renal function deterioration is usually a major end-point in clinical trials.

Anti-double-stranded DNA antibodies have so far attracted much of the attention as the likely pathogenic agent in lupus nephritis. This hypothesis is supported by several observations: Elevated titers of serum antibodies to dsDNA were often correlated with glomerulonephritis,[43] sustained reductions in antibody levels are associated with improved treatment outcomes, and antibodies to DNA can be eluted from diseased glomeruli. The mechanism of damage seems to consist of two arms. Some antibodies cause glomerulonephritis by direct attachment to glomerular structures, whereas others form complexes with DNA that are passively trapped in the glomeruli. We should remark, however, that in recent years doubts have been raised concerning the significance of circulating immune complexes (CICs) in SLE owing to lack of direct evidence demonstrating their pathogenetic role and the fact that DNA and DNA-anti-DNA complexes are rapidly cleared from the serum in experimental models of the disease.[44,45]

Suppression of disease activity and reduction of dsDNA production can be effectively achieved by the use of corticosteroids and cytotoxic drugs, which also exert a favorable effect on the prognosis of SLE patients. Nevertheless, these agents are nonselective and do not discriminate between normal and pathogenic immune cells. Thus far, experimental approaches to specifically reduce dsDNA antibody levels in SLE patients have included immunoadsorbent extracorporeal perfusion,[7,24] intravenous administration of immunoglobulins enriched with anti-idiotypes that bind to dsDNA antibodies,[46] and administration of recombinant human DNase.[47]

The investigational drug LJP394 represents another novel strategy. LJP394 is a selective B lymphocyte immunomodulator that consists of four double-stranded 20-mer oligodeoxynucleotides attached to an inert scaffold composed of a triethylene glycol core.[48] The administration of LJP394 to mice reduces serum dsDNA antibodies and dsDNA antibody–producing cells.[49] In humans, several clinical trials have been conducted thus far, establishing the safety and tolerability of LJP394 and its dsDNA antibody–lowering effect.[50] This drug was shown to improve health-related quality of life in SLE patients in a randomized prospective trial.[51] Significant improvement in renal manifestations is apparently restricted to a subpopulation of patients with high-affinity antibodies.[52] This result is in line with a previous observation that not all anti-dsDNA antibody subsets contribute equally to kidney disease.

The manner by which LJP394 reduces dsDNA antibody titers is thought to involve two mechanisms. Binding of the drug to circulating antibody and subsequent clearance of these complexes probably account for the immediate decline in dsDNA antibody levels in SLE patients after a single intravenous dose.[50] Antigen-specific tolerance is another proposed explanation, supported by drug-induced decline in dsDNA antibody–producing cells in mice[49] and a sustained suppression of anti-dsDNA antibody levels, exceeding the calculated period required for antibody synthesis.[48] The precise mode of action underlying tolerance induction has yet to be elucidated.

Apart from the anti-dsDNA antibodies, a different type of antibodies, which bind to the extracellular matrix, has been implicated in the pathogenesis of lupus glomerulonephritis. Initially, the existence of such antibodies was hypothesized owing to the fact that DNA and other intracellular antigens are artificially exposed *in vitro* after fixation of cells but are not accessible to antibodies *in vivo*. Indeed, direct immunofluorescence demonstrates binding of antibodies from nephritic patients to the kidney at the subepithelial and subendothelial basement membrane.[53] Rigorous analysis of the target epitope disclosed a 21-mer peptide located in the globular part of the α-chain of laminin. Treatment of mice with competitive peptides prevents antibody deposition in the kidneys, suppresses renal disease, and prolongs survival (unpublished data). In humans, significant correlation seems to exist between levels of antipeptide antibodies and disease activity. Furthermore, antibodies were found in high titers even in active SLE patients who were anti-DNA-negative (unpublished data). Peptide-bound columns allow specific removal of the pathogenic antibodies, implying that extracorporeal specific immunoadsorption on the laminin-epitope columns may serve as a new therapeutic alternative for SLE.

CONCLUSION

In autoimmune diseases, the immune system attacks constituents of self-tissues and causes damage or impairs organ function. Such pathologic processes can be mediated by either the cellular or humoral arms of the immune system. In several diseases, the pathogenic roles of autoantibodies have been established. Having realized that autoantibodies cause disease, they have been regarded as toxic agents that should be eliminated from the circulation. In this review, we assessed the advantages and drawbacks of this approach, based on data provided by application of antibody removal in autoimmune diseases. For this purpose, we focused on nonselective immunoadsorption and on specific antibody removal in three distinct clinical entities: myasthenia gravis, dilated cardiomyopathy, and systemic lupus erythematosus.

A striking feature that is common to all three diseases is that more than one type of autoantibody is implicated in the pathogenetic process, such as anti-dsDNA and anti-laminin in SLE and the blocking and modulating antibodies in MG. In DCM, the comparable improvement in both anti β1-AR–positive and –negative groups[42] after treatment with Therasorb suggests that other cardiac epitopes are involved as well. These observations raise an intriguing conceptual dilemma regarding the preferable strategy for elimination of pathogenic autoantibodies.

The nonspecific extracorporeal immunoadsorption may remove all of the putative harmful antibodies, rendering the characterization of each individual pathogen redundant. The disadvantage of this approach derives from the unwanted global loss of antibodies against viral and bacterial epitopes as well as protective antibodies that counter-regulate inflammatory processes. These systems may require polyclonal immunoglobulin substitution to reduce the risk of infection and to prevent rebound of autoantibody production.[42] Alternatively, the use of a low-adsorption-capacity system (Prosorba) does not permit substantial removal of immunoglobulins or circulating immune complexes, and its immunomodulatory effects are not yet clearly understood. Specific removal of autoantibodies has the advantage of a potentially high capacity for elimination of the pathogenic agent while sparing immunoglobulins that are irrelevant to the disease process. However, this approach may be hampered by several pitfalls. The identification and isolation of a specific antibody and its target epitope do not guarantee the feasibility of an efficient column. Such is the case in the modulating antibodies of MG implicated in receptor and membrane destruction, which could not be removed due to low affinity to their corresponding peptide. Furthermore, epitope-specific strategies ignore the possible existence of several pathogenic antibodies in a certain disease, and it is of interest to compare the efficacy and side effects of nonspecific immunoadsorption with specific removal of pathogenic antibodies.

We should note that in many cases, a specific pathogenic antibody has not been defined (e.g., in rheumatoid arthritis) and that identification of autoantibodies in different diseases is not uniformly convincing. For example, in lupus, many of the pathophysiologic aspects of anti-dsDNA antibodies, remain obscure. Attempts to induce immunogenic responses by introduction of DNA in adjuvant to animals were disappointing, thus curtailing attempts to devise an experimental model of the primary immunogenic epitope. Similarly, it is difficult to define the target proteins that are recognized by anti-dsDNA antibodies or to determine to which cellular compartment they bind: nuclear, cell surface, or perhaps extracellular. The fact that only a subset of seropositive patients demonstrate renal function improvement upon treatment with LJP394[52] indicates that anti-dsDNA antibodies are heterogenous and make up different subclasses that are not equally pathogenic.

In short, we cannot confidently delineate the mechanism underlying the generation of anti-dsDNA antibodies, nor can we define their target epitope and mode of action. However, data are much less elusive in myasthenia gravis and DCM, in which anti-AChR and anti-β1-AR antibodies, respectively, are implicated in pathogenesis. These antibodies provide a plausible explanation for clinical manifestations, and they can be used to induce passive-transfer experimental autoimmune disease when injected in animals.[40,54,55] Moreover, their specific removal from the serum of patients seems to be beneficial. Even though these manipulations establish the pathogenic effects of both autoantibodies, observations *in vivo* indicate that other critical factors may participate in the disease process as well. For example, in MG, the anti-AChR antibody titers correlate poorly with the severity of neuromuscular dysfunction,[56] implying a role for AChR gene polymorphism[57] or a possible effect of the immunoglobulin subclass on antibody pathogenicity.

Past experience shows that epitope-directed strategies may yield treatments that are eventually applied in diseases other than those for which they were originally tailored. This diversion is exemplified in glatiramer acetate (GLAT), which is a myelin basic protein analog that was shown to reduce severity of multiple sclerosis.[58,59] GLAT was also found to effectively suppress experimental autoimmune uveitis[60] as well as graft-versus-host reaction *in vivo*.[61] Another example is provided by the rat model of adjuvant arthritis, which is induced by immunization with heat-killed *Mycobacterium tuberculosis*. In the late stages of disease, the animals recover and acquire immunity to arthritis by producing monoclonal antibodies against a specific epitope of the 65kDa mycobacterial heat shock protein (HSP65). These antibodies have also been successfully used to suppress autoimmune diabetes mellitus in mice (unpublished data). Both GLAT and the monoclonal anti-HSP65 antibodies seem to possess anti-inflammatory features beyond the context of the disease from which they were derived. At least part of this effect can be explained by nonspecific induction of IL10 secretion.[62,63] Therefore, it should not be surprising if some of the treatment modalities described in this review (e.g., LJP394) will eventually be used in more than one autoimmune disease.

In conclusion, removal of epitope-specific pathogenic antibodies is a relatively novel and rapidly evolving strategy for treatment of autoimmune disease, with promising prospects. However, owing to the paucity of data, large-scale prospective clinical studies are required to accurately define the effect of nonselective and antibody-specific immunoadsorption and to allow optimal incorporation of these techniques into traditional therapeutic regimens. We hypothesize that specific ligands may eventually also be used for recognition of immunoglobulins on the surface of B lymphocytes and thus allow removal of pathogenic antibody–producing cells.

REFERENCES

1. Naparstek, Y. & P. H. Plotz. 1993. The role of autoantibodies in autoimmune disease. Annu. Rev. Immunol. **11:** 79–104.
2. Nakaji, S. 2001. Current topics on immunoadsorption therapy. Therap. Apher. **5:** 301–305.
3. Hirata N., T. Kuriyama & N. Yamawaki. 2003. Immusorba TR and PH. Therap. Apher. Dial. **7:** 85–90.
4. Shibuya, N., T. Sato, M. Osame, *et al.* 1994. Immunoadsorption therapy for myasthenia gravis. J. Neurol. Neurosurg. Psychiatry **57:** 578–581.
5. Kutsuki, H., S. Takata, K. Yamamoto, *et al.* 1998. Therapeutic selective adsorption of anti-DNA antibody using dextran sulfate cellulose columns (Selesorb) for the treatment of systemic lupus erythematosus. Therap. Apher. **2:** 18–24.
6. Stefanutti, C., S. Di Giacomo, M. Mareri *et al.* 2003. Immunoadsorption apheresis (Selesorb) in the treatment of chronic hepatitis C virus–related type 2 mixed cryoglobulinemia. Transfus. Apheresis. Sci. **28:** 207–214.
7. Braun, N., S. Gutenberger, C. M. Erley, *et al.* 1999. Immunoglobulin and circulating autoimmune complex kinetics during immunoadsorption onto protein A sepharose. Transfus. Sci. **19** (Suppl)**:** 25–31.
8. Sueoka, A. 1997. Present status of apheresis technologies, part 3: adsorbent. Therap. Apher. **1:** 271–283.
9. Matic, G., T. Bosch & W. Ramlow. 2001. Background and indications for protein A-based extracorporeal immunoadsorption. Therap. Apher. **5:** 3 94–403.
10. Uehlinger, J., G.R. Button, J. McCarthy, *et al.* 1991. Immunoadsorption for coagulation factor inhibitors. Transfusion **31:** 265–269.

11. FREIBURGHAUS, C., E. BERNTORP, M. EKMAN, *et al.* 1998. Immunoadsorption for removal of inhibitors: update on treatments in Malmo-Lund between 1980 and 1995. Haemophilia **4:** 16–20.
12. WATT, R.M., K. BUNITSKY, E.B. FAULKNER, *et al.* Treatment of congenital and acquired hemophilia patients by extracorporeal removal of antibodies to coagulation factors: a review of US clinical studies 1987–1990. Hemophilia Study Group. Transfus. Sci. **13:** 233–253.
13. FELSON, D.T., M.P. LAVALLEY, A.R. BALDASSARE, *et al.* 1999. The Prosorba column for treatment of refractory rheumatoid arthritis: a randomized, double-blinded, sham-controlled trial. Arthritis. Rheum. **42:** 2153–2159.
14. SNYDER, H.W. JR., S.K. CHOCHRAN, J.P. BALINT JR., *et al.* 1992. Experience with protein A-immunoadsorption in treatment-resistant adult immune thrombocytopenic purpura. Blood **79:** 2237–2245.
15. BALINT, J.P. JR., M. A. HUSSEIN, F. QUAGLIATA, *et al.* 1996. Modulation of idiotypic and antiidiotypic immunoglobulin G responses in an alloimmune thrombocytopenic patient associated with extracorporeal protein A immunoadsorption. Artif. Organs. **20:** 266–270.
16. BOSCH, T. 1996. Current status in extracorporeal immunomodulation: immune disorders. Artif. Organs. **20:** 902–905.
17. SNYDER, H.W. JR., B.W. SEAWELL, S.K. COCHRAN, *et al.* 1992. Specificity of antibody responses affected by extracorporeal immunoadsorption of plasma over columns of protein A silica. J. Clin. Apheresis. **7:** 110–118.
18. GENDREAU, R.M. 2001. Randomized double-blinded sham-controlled trial of the Prosorba column for treatment of refractory rheumatoid arthritis. Therap. Apher. **5:** 79–83.
19. STEGMAYR, B.G., G. ALMORTH, G. BERLIN, *et al.* 1999. Plasma exchange or immunoadsorption in patients with rapidly progressive crescentic glomerulonephritis. A Swedish multi-center study. Int. J. Artif. Organs. **22:** 81–87.
20. BUENO, D. JR., J. SEVIGNY & A.A. KAPLAN. 1999. Extracorporeal treatment of thrombotic microangiopathy: a ten year experience. Therap. Apher. **3:** 294–297.
21. SCHNEIDEWIND, J.M., U.K. ZETTL, R.E. WINKLER, *et al.* 1999. Therapeutic apheresis in myasthenia gravis patients: a six year follow-up. Therap. Apher. **3:** 298–302.
22. BENNY, W.B., D.M. SUTTON, J. OGER, *et al.* 1999. Clinical evaluation of a staphylococcal protein A immunoadsorption system in the treatment of myasthenia gravis patients. Transfusion **39:** 682–687.
23. BERTA, E., P. CONFALONIERI, O. SIMONCINI, *et al.* 1994. Removal of anti-acetylcholine receptor antibodies by protein–A immunoadsorption in myasthenia gravis. Int. J. Artif. Organs. **17:** 603–608.
24. BRAUN, N., C. ERLEY, R. KLEIN, *et al.* 2000. Immunoadsorption onto protein A induces remission in severe systemic lupus erythematosus. Nephrol. Dial. Transplant. **15:** 1367–1372.
25. PRETAGOSTINI, R., P. BERLOCO, L. POLI, *et al.* 1996. Immunoadsorption with protein A in humoral rejection of kidney transplants. ASAIO J. **42:** M645–M648.
26. PROTTI, M.P., A.A. MANFREDI, R.M. HORTON, *et al.* 1993. Myasthenia gravis: Recognition of a human autoantigen at the molecular level. Immunol. Today **14:** 363–368.
27. TAKAMORI, M., S. OKUMURA, N. NAGATA, *et al.* 1988. Myasthenogenic significance of synthetic alpha-subunit peptide 183–100 of *Torpedo californica* and human acetylcholine receptor. J. Neurol. Sci. **85:** 121–129.
28. TZARTOS, S.J., A. KOKLA, S.L. WALGRAVE, *et al.* 1988. Localization of the main immunogenic region of human muscle acetylcholine receptor to residues 67–76 of the alpha subunit. Proc. Natl. Acad. Sci. USA **85:** 2899–2903.
29. LENNON, V.A., D.J. MCCORMICK, E.H. LAMBERT, *et al.* 1985. Region of peptide 125–147 of acetylcholine receptor alpha-subunit is exposed at neuromuscular junction and induces experimental autoimmune myasthenia gravis, T-cell immunity and modulating antibodies. Proc. Natl. Acad. Sci. USA **82:** 8805–8809.
30. TAKAMORI, M. & M. TAKAHIRO. 2001. Immunoadsorption in myasthenia gravis based on specific ligands mimicking the immunogenic sites of the acetylcholine receptor. Therap. Apher. **5:** 340–350.

31. GRAHAM, R.M. & W.A. OWENS. 1999. Pathogenesis of inherited forms of dilated cardiomyopathy. N. Engl. J. Med. **341:** 1759–1762.
32. SEIDMAN, J.G. & C. SEIDMAN. 2001. The genetic basis for cardiomyopathy: from mutation identification to mechanistic paradigms. Cell *104*: 557–567.
33. KUHL, U., M. NOUTSIAS, B. SEEBERG, *et al.* 1996. Immunohistological evidence for a chronic intramyocardial inflammatory process in dilated cardiomyopathy. Heart **75:** 295–300.
34. LIMAS, C.J. 1997. Cardiac autoantibodies in dilated cardiomyopathy. Circulation **95:** 1979–1980.
35. MULLER, J., G. WALLUKAT, M. DANDEL, *et al.* 2000. Immunoglobulin adsorption in patients with idiopathic dilated cardiomyopathy. Circulation **101:** 385–391.
36. JAHNS, R., V. BOIVIN, T. KRAPF, *et al.* 2000. Modulation of b1-adrenoreceptor activity by domain-specific antibodies and heart failure-associated auto-antibodies. J. Am. Coll. Cardiol. **36:** 1280–1287.
37. JAHNS, R., V. BOIVIN, C. SIEGMUND, *et al.* 1999. Autoantibodies activating human b1-adrenergic receptors are associated with reduced cardiac function in chronic heart failure. Circulation **99:** 649–654.
38. ROHRER, D.K., K.H. DESAI, J.R. JASPER, *et al.* 1996. Targeted disruption of the mouse beta1-adrenergic receptor gene: developmental and cardiovascular effects. Proc. Natl. Acad. Sci. USA **93:** 7375–7380.
39. LIGGETT, S.B., N.M. TEPE, J.N. LORENZ, *et al.* 2000. Early and delayed consequences of beta2-adrenergic receptor overexpression in mouse hearts: critical role for expression level. Circulation **101:** 1707–1714.
40. JAHNS, R., V. BOIVIN, L. HEIN, *et al.* 2004. Direct evidence for a beta1-adrenergic receptor-directed autoimmune attack as a cause of idiopathic dilated cardiomyopathy. J. Clin. Invest. **113:** 1419–1429.
41. WALLUKAT, G., J. MULLER & R. HETZER. 2002. Specific removal of beta1-adrenergic autoantibodies from patients with idiopathic dilated cardiomyopathy. N. Engl. J. Med. **347:** 1806.
42. MOBINI, R., A. STAUDT, S. B. FELIX, *et al.* 2003. Hemodynamic improvement and removal of autoantibodies against beta1-adrenergic receptor by immunoadsorption therapy in dilated cardiomyopathy. J. Autoimmun. **20:** 345–350.
43. HAHN, B. H. 1998. Antibodies to DNA. N. Engl. J. Med. **338:** 1359–1368.
44. BEN-CHETRIT, E., E.H. DUNSKY, S. WOLLNER, *et al.* 1985. In vivo clearance and tissue uptake of an anti-DNA monoclonal antibody and its complexes with DNA. Clin. Exp. Immunol. **60:** 159–68.
45. FINBLOOM, D S. & P.H. PLOTZ. 1979. Studies of the reticuloendothelial function in the course with model immune complexes. II. Serum clearance, tissue uptake and reticuloendothelial saturation in NZB/W mice. J. Immunol. **23:** 1600–1603.
46. SILVESTRIS, F., O. D'AMORE, P. CAFFORIO, *et al.* 1996. Intravenous immune globulin therapy of lupus nephritis: use of pathogenic anti-DNA-reactive IgG. Clin. Exp. Immunol. **104:** 91–97.
47. DAVIS, J.C., S. MANZI, C. YARBORO, *et al.* 1999. Recombinant human DNase I (rhDNase) in patients with lupus nephritis. Lupus **8:** 68–76.
48. FURIE, R.A., J. M. CASH, M.E. CRONIN, *et al.* 2001. Treatment of systemic lupus erythematosus with LJP 394. J. Rheumatol. **28:** 257–265.
49. JONES, D.S., P.A. BARSTAD, M.J. FIELD, *et al.* 1995. Immunospecific reduction of antioligonucleotide antibody-forming cells with a tetrakis-oligonucleotide conjugate (LJP394), a therapeutic candidate for the treatment of lupus nephritis. J. Med. Chem. **38:** 2138–2144.
50. WEISMAN, M.H., H.G. BLEUSTEIN, C.M. BERNER, *et al.* 1997, Reduction in circulating dsDNA antibody titer after administration of LJP394. J. Rheumatol. **24:** 314–318.
51. STRAND, V., C. ARANOW, M.H. CARDIEL, *et al.* 2003. Improvement in health-related quality of life in systemic lupus erythematosus patients enrolled in a randomized clinical trial comparing LJP394 treatment with placebo. Lupus **12:** 677–686.
52. ALARCON-SEGOVIA, D., J.A. TUMLIN, R.A. FURIE, *et al.* LJP394 for the prevention of renal flare in patients with systemic lupus erythematosus: results from a randomized, double-blinded, placebo-controlled study. Arthritis. Rheum. **48:** 442–454.

53. Ben-Yehuda, A., L. Rasooly, R. Bar-Tana, *et al.* 1995. The urine of SLE patients contains antibodies that bind to the laminin component of the extracellular matrix. J. Autoimmun. **8:** 279–291.
54. Toyka, K.V., D.B. Drachman, A. Pestronk, *et al.* 1975. Myasthenia gravis: passive transfer from man to mouse. Science **190:** 397–399.
55. Tzartos, S., S. Hochschwender, P. Vasquez, *et al.* 1987. Passive transfer of experimental autoimmune myasthenia gravis by monoclonal antibodies to the main immunogenic region of the acetylcholine receptor. J. Neuroimmunol. **15:** 185–194.
56. Roses, A., W. Olanow, M. McAdams, *et al.* 1981. No direct correlation between serum antiacetylcholine receptor antibody levels and clinical state of individual patients with myasthenia gravis. Neurology **31:** 220–224.
57. Hoedemaekers, A., J.L. Besseraeu, Y. Graus, *et al.* 1998. Role of the target organ in determining susceptibility to experimental autoimmune myasthenia gravis. J. Neuroimmunol. **89:** 131–141.
58. Bornstein, M.B., A. Miller, S. Slagle, *et al.* 1987. A pilot trial of Cop 1 in exacerbating-remitting multiple sclerosis. N. Engl. J. Med. **317:** 408–414.
59. Johnson, K.P., B.R. Brooks, J.A. Cohen, *et al.* 1995, Copolymer I reduces relapse rate and improves disability in relapsing-remitting multiple sclerosis: results in phase III multicenter, double blind placebo-controlled trial. The copolymer I multiple sclerosis study group. Neurology **45:** 1268–1276.
60. Zhang, M., C.C. Chan, B. Vistica, *et al.* 2000. Copolymer I inhibits experimental autoimmune uveoretinitis. J. Neruoimmunol. **103:** 189–194.
61. Schlegel, P.G., R. Aharoni, Y. Chen, *et al.* 1996. A synthetic random basic copolymer with promiscuous binding to class II major histocompatibility complex molecules inhibits T-cell proliferative responses to major and minor histocompatibility antigens in vitro and confers the capacity to prevent murine graft-versus-host disease in vivo. Proc. Natl. Acad. Sci. USA **93:** 5061–5066.
62. Jung, S., I. Siglienti, O. Grauer, *et al.* 2004. Induction of IL-10 in rat peritoneal macrophages and dendritic cells by glatiramer acetate. J. Neuroimmunol. **148:** 63–73.
63. Ulmansky, R., C.J. Cohen, F. Szafer, *et al.* 2002. Resistance to adjuvant arthritis is due to protective antibodies against heat shock protein surface epitopes and the induction of IL-10 secretion. J. Immunol. **168:** 6463–6469.

Chemokine Receptors

Attractive Targets for Drug Discovery

NURIA GODESSART

Department of Biology, Almirall Research Center, Barcelona, Spain

ABSTRACT: Studies of two antibodies, efalizumab and natalizumab, have recently demonstrated that the blockade of leukocyte migration is of therapeutic benefit for the treatment of diseases such as psoriasis and multiple sclerosis. The role of chemokines in the control of cell traffic led to their receptors being considered one of the most promising family of targets aimed at disrupting cell recruitment in chronic inflammatory processes. Choosing the appropriate chemokine receptor for each disease was not easy, and the interpretation of target validation studies proved to be extremely difficult. Despite an intense effort in the search for chemokine receptor antagonists in the last decade, no compounds in advanced clinical trials exist as such. The inherent complexity of the family, the differences between the chemokine system in mice and men, and the species selectivity of small-molecule compounds could account for this fact. Pharmaceutical companies still believe in chemokine receptors as therapeutic targets, as demonstrated by the number of compounds reported to be in development. In the next years, the developmental progression of these compounds will reveal which target within the chemokine family is of real therapeutic value.

KEYWORDS: chemokines; leukocyte recruitment; G protein–coupled receptors; chronic inflammation; autoimmune diseases; drug discovery; target validation

INTRODUCTION TO CHEMOKINES: STRUCTURAL AND FUNCTIONAL CLASSIFICATION

Chemokines are a large family of small secreted proteins of 8–14 kDa that control cell trafficking. They are structurally divided into four classes—C, CC, CXC, and CX_3C—depending on the number and the relative position of their amino terminal cysteine residues (FIG. 1).[1] Individual chemokines are named using the acronyms of the structural class they belong to, followed by an L (for ligand) and their gene number.[2]

In the last decade, it has been clearly established that these mediators play a significant role in processes such as embryonic development, host defense, immune surveillance, inflammation, angiogenesis, autoimmunity, and cancer.[2–4] The biologic effects of chemokines are mediated by receptors expressed on the cell surface. Chemokine receptors are themselves classified according to the chemokine family

Address for correspondence: Nuria Godessart, Department of Biology, Almirall Research Center, Cardener 68–74, 08024 Barcelona, Spain. Voice: +34-932-913-540; fax: +34-932-912-827. ngodessa@almirall.es

Ann. N.Y. Acad. Sci. 1051: 647–657 (2005). © 2005 New York Academy of Sciences.
doi: 10.1196/annals.1361.109

they bind (FIG. 1). The nomenclature of the receptors is analogous to that of chemokines, using the family acronym followed by an R (for receptor) and a number that corresponds to the order of its discovery.[5] Chemokine receptors belong to class A of the G protein–coupled receptor (GPCR) superfamily. They are rhodopsin-like receptors that span the membrane seven times and are coupled to heterotrimeric $G\alpha\beta\gamma$ proteins.[6] Upon ligand–receptor interaction, different intracellular signaling pathways are activated, ultimately leading to cell mobilization and activation.[7]

From a functional point of view, chemokines can be divided into inflammatory, homeostatic, and dual function.[8] Inflammatory chemokines are induced by pathogens, cytokines, or growth factors and recruit effector leukocytes to sites of infection, inflammation, tissue injury, and tumor. CCR1, CCR2, CCR3, CCR5, CXCR2, XCR1, and CX_3CR1 are some examples of receptors that bind inflammatory chemokines. Homeostatic chemokines are expressed in bone marrow and lymphoid tissues and are involved in hematopoiesis, immune surveillance, and adaptive immune responses. The receptors for homeostatic chemokines (CCR7, CXCR4, and CXCR5) are expressed on B cells, follicular-helper T cells, central-memory T cells, and mature dendritic cells, among others. Chemokines that share properties of these two groups are classified as dual function. These chemokines are involved in adaptive immunity, T lymphopoiesis, dendritic cell development, and homing to particular anatomic compartments. Regulatory T cells, CLA4$^+$ cells (homing to skin), and

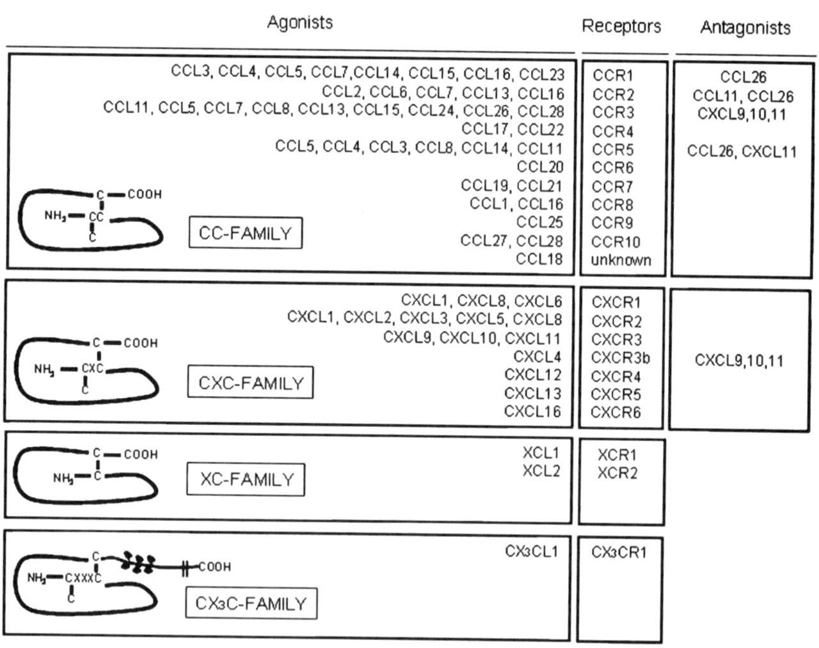

FIGURE 1. Structural classification of the chemokine superfamily. For each receptor, chemokines acting as agonists and antagonists are depicted. The systematic nomenclature of chemokines was used.[2]

$\alpha 4\beta 7^+$ cells (homing to intestinal mucosa) express receptors for these chemokines (CCR4, CCR6, CCR8, CCR9, CXCR3, and/or CXCR6). See Ref. 8 for a detailed description of the functional classification of chemokines.

A feature of the chemokine system is the complexity of the ligand–receptor interactions, especially evident in the inflammatory and dual-function chemokine groups. Thus, a particular chemokine (i.e., CCL5) may bind several receptors (CCR1, CCR3, and CCR5), and different chemokines (i.e., CXCL9, CXCL10, and CXCL11) may bind a single receptor (CXCR3). Some evidence suggest that in some cases ligand redundancy does not mean duplicity of functions. *In vitro* studies comparing the behavior of the two CCR7 ligands, CCL19 and CCL21, revealed differences in their affinity, their ability to desensitize the receptor,[9] and the signaling pathways evoked.[10] These results indicate that the roles of the two ligands were not merely redundant. Similar findings have been recently reported for the two ligands of human CCR4[11] and those of mouse CXCR2.[12] These results suggest that different ligands for the same receptor act in different compartments; one ligand would act at the endothelial surface to promote vascular recognition, and the other chemokine would engage the receptor within the tissue microenvironment to guide cellular localization. As expected, the ligand acting in the vascular compartment always exhibits a low capacity to desensitize the receptor, to allow cells to respond to the second stimulus.[9,11,12]

A series of discoveries made in the past 5 years have added a new degree of complexity. As FIGURE 1 shows, a chemokine may act either as an agonist or an antagonist, depending on the receptor it binds.[13–19] The antagonistic effect of some chemokines were revealed in *in vitro* studies, but it has also been reported to occur *in vivo*.[20,21] It has been postulated that the meaning of this effect is to increase the selectivity of cell recruitment.[20] A chemokine such as CXCL11, agonist of a receptor mainly expressed on T helper type 1 (Th1) cells (CXCR3), is at the same time an antagonist of the responses mediated by CCR3, a receptor expressed on Th2 cells. The opposite is also true: a chemokine such as CCL26 attracts Th2 cells *via* CCR3 cells while blocking CCR1- and CCR5-mediated responses on Th1 cells. In this scenario, the consequences of blocking a particular chemokine or a receptor *in vivo* could be unpredictable.

CHEMOKINES AND CELL MIGRATION

Leukocyte migration is a multistep process that takes place in homeostasis as well as in pathological conditions. In the last decade, the role of chemokines in the regulation of cell traffic has been clearly established. Proinflammatory stimuli induce the synthesis of chemokines by stromal cells, endothelial cells, and leukocytes. Chemokines may bind to heparin sulfate proteoglycans on the luminal surface of vascular endothelial cells, are exposed to the lumen of blood vessels (or high endothelial venules), and capture rolling leukocytes expressing the appropriate receptor. Chemokine binding activates the heterotrimeric G proteins coupled to the receptor. The α and the $\beta\gamma$ subunits dissociate and may activate several signaling pathways involving small GTPases (RAP1, RhoA, Rac) and/or kinases (PI_3K, atypical PKC, Pyk2), depending on the chemokine and the cell type.[22,23] This process results in a change in the conformation and avidity of the leukocyte integrins, together with the formation of a polarity complex and the focal recruitment of integrins, culminating in transendothelial migration. Leukocytes are then guided to the target tissue, probably following the concentration gradient of chemokines bound to proteoglycans (haptotaxis). Once there, the high local concentration of chemokines would induce the phosphorylation and internalization of the receptor, making cells unresponsive to the same or other ligands of that receptor. Different chemokines may participate in different parts of the process, in a sequential manner, as it has been hypothesized to occur in the transmigration of lymphocytes from high endothelial venules.[22]

BLOCKADE OF LEUKOCYTE MIGRATION AS A THERAPEUTIC STRATEGY

The excessive infiltration of leukocytes is a hallmark of many autoimmune and chronic inflammatory diseases. Several approaches can be exploited to prevent cell recruitment to inflamed tissues, such as blocking adhesion molecules (selectins, integrins), or preventing the effect of chemotactic mediators such as peptidic (chemokines) or lipidic (eicosanoids, sphingolipids) mediators. TABLE 1 lists some agents, in different stages of development or in the market, that target cell migration.

TABLE 1. Therapies directed at blocking cell migration

Target family	Strategy	Drug name and company	Disease	Status
Integrins	Anti-α4 antibody	Tysabri® (natalizumab) Biogen and Elan	Multiple sclerosis	Launched
	Anti-CD11a antibody	Raptiva® (efalizumab) Xoma, Genetech, Serono	Psoriasis	Launched
Selectins	Selectin antagonist	Bimosiamose Revotar Pharm	Asthma, psoriasis	Phase II
	Anti-L-selectin antibody	Aselizumab Scil Biomedicals	Atherosclerosis, vascular injury	Phase II
Sphingosine	S1P receptor agonist	FTY-720 Novartis	Transplant rejection	Phase II
PGD_2	DP antagonist	L-888839 Merck Frosst	Seasonal allergic rhinitis	Phase I
	CRTh2 antagonist	Astra-Zeneca Pfizer	Allergic asthma, allergic rhinitis	Preclinical

Two biologicals that block lymphocyte integrins have validated cell traffic blockade as a therapeutic strategy. In November 2004, Tysabri® (natalizumab; Biogen Idec and Elan Corporation) was approved for the treatment of relapsing forms of multiple sclerosis.[24] This monoclonal antibody blocks the α4 integrin subunit, preventing T cells from transendothelial migration and probably from crossing the blood–brain barrier. Natalizumab has also demonstrated activity in a phase III clinical trial for Crohn disease.[25] Another monoclonal antibody, Raptiva® (efalizumab; Genentech and Xoma), was approved one year before for the treatment of chronic plaque psoriasis.[26] Raptiva is a humanized monoclonal antibody that binds human CD11a (a subunit of the LFA-1 integrin) and prevents the recruitment of T cells to the skin as well as their activation.

Treatment with both natalizumab and efalizumab is associated with an increase in the number of blood lymphocytes owing to the inhibition of their migration out of the vascular space. A different strategy is represented by FTY-720, a compound derived from the fungus *Isaria sinclairii*.[27] The compound is phosphorylated *in vivo* by the enzyme sphingosine kinase, forming FTY-720-P, a high-affinity nonselective agonist of sphingosine 1-phosphate receptor 1 ($S1P_1$), necessary for lymphocytes to exit lymphoid tissues. The compound induces the internalization of the receptor, preventing lymphocytes from responding to egress signals from circulating sphingosine 1-P (S1P), the natural ligand of $S1P_1$. The drug induces accumulation of naive and activated CD4 and CD8 T cells and B cells in lymph nodes and Peyer patches, preventing lymphocytes from being recruited at the graft. FTY720 (Novartis) is currently in phase III clinical trials for renal transplantation[27] and is also in development for multiple sclerosis. It is interesting that S1P has been described as inducing chemokine and/or chemokine receptor expression in several cell subsets, such as eosinophils and T cells.[28,29] Thus targeting S1P receptors represents an alternative strategy for modulating chemokine receptor expression.

Other agents in development include Bimosiamose®, a pan-selectin blocker in clinical trials of psoriasis and asthma, and low molecular weight antagonists of the prostaglandin D_2 (PGD_2) receptors, DP and CRTh2, in clinical trials of allergy and/or asthma (TABLE 1).

CHEMOKINE RECEPTORS AS THERAPEUTIC TARGETS

Proinflammatory cytokines induce the synthesis of chemokines,[1,8] and blocking the biological effects of cytokines could be a nonselective way of inhibiting cell recruitment. This has been demonstrated to be the case for the anti-TNFα antibody Remicade® in psoriasis.[30] The only therapies, either in the market or in advanced clinical trials, that inhibit cytokine effects are biologicals—for example, anti-TNFα antibodies such as Remicade® and Humira®, soluble TNFα receptors such as Enbrel®, the IL-1 receptor antagonist Kineret®, the anti-IL-6 receptor MRA®, and the anti-IL-15 antibody HuMax-IL-15®. Probably the nature of cytokine receptors and the complex interactions established between cytokines and their receptors make this interaction difficult to be inhibited by small organic compounds.

The interest in chemokines as therapeutic targets increased with the discovery that their receptors, unlikely those of cytokines, are GPCRs. About half of the drugs currently in the market are either agonists or antagonists of GPCR, demonstrating that at least some members of the family are "druggable" targets.[6] In 1996, just 5 years after the discovery of the first chemokine receptor, it was confirmed that chemokine receptor antagonists could be obtained.[31] The discovery of the role of CCR5 and CXCR4 as co-receptors in HIV infection gave researchers an impetus to search for antagonists of those receptors.

According to the information in the public domain, after a decade of drug discovery on chemokines, there are no compounds in advanced phases of development. The analysis of the difficulties found in drug discovery on chemokines have been reviewed[6,12] and is out of the scope of this chapter. Instead, we focus on the difficulty in interpreting results from target validation studies within the chemokine family.

TARGET VALIDATION ON CHEMOKINES: FROM MICE TO MEN

Evidence for the role of chemokines in disease states comes essentially from studies of animal models of disease and the analysis of human pathological samples.[7,32] These studies provided a list of potential targets for the treatment of diseases such as multiple sclerosis, atherosclerosis, psoriasis, asthma, arthritis, diabetes, and cancer.[3,6,7,32] Most of these targets correspond to receptors for inflammatory chemokines, characterized by redundancy and promiscuity. Would inhibition of a single receptor be enough to achieve efficacy? Which was the best target for each pathology? Choosing the target was difficult, especially for diseases like rheumatoid arthritis (RA), in which more than six potential targets have been suggested.[33]

Validation of the candidate compound in animal models was desirable for reducing failures in the clinic. However, target validation with small molecule receptor antagonists soon proved to be difficult. As occurs for antagonists of other GPCRs with peptidic ligands,[6] compounds often exhibit species selectivity, thus cannot be used in mouse or rat models. This explains why only limited information about the *in vivo* effects of receptor antagonists exists.[34–38]

Biological reagents (antibodies or modified natural ligands) and knockout mice are also good validation tools. However, results obtained using different validation strategies sometimes led to contradictory conclusions. The receptors CCR2 and CCR5, previously validated for arthritis by two independent groups using modified chemokines,[39,40] have since been devalidated using knockout mice.[41] These studies showed that the lack of CCR5 had no impact on the progression of arthritis, whereas CCR2 knockout mice developed more severe disease than did controls.[41]

Independent groups working with the same chemokine receptor knockout mice have also obtained contradictory results. This is the case for CCR2 and multiple sclerosis.[42,43] Factors such as the use of different experimental protocols and/or the mouse strain have been argued to explain these differences.

The true target validation occurs in the clinic, but these data are still missing. Several compounds have progressed to clinical trials and failed,[31] and the reasons are not always known. Toxicity issues, a deficient ADME profile, and an inadequate target can account for this fact. However, there is still an intense activity in the field, as illustrated by the number of agents targeting chemokine receptors currently in development (TABLE 2). As an update of previous reviews,[12,31,44,45] a more detailed explanation of the situation of the antagonists of CCR1, CCR2, and CXCR3 receptors is given below.

TABLE 2. Chemokine receptor antagonists reported to be in clinical development

Target	Compound name and company	Development status	Disease
CCR1	BX-471 (ZK-811752) (Berlex Biosciences/Schering AG)	Phase II	MS, Pso, eczema
	BX-471 (ZK-811752) (Berlex Biosciences/Schering AG)	Phase I	Alzheimer disease
	MLN-3897 (Millennium Pharmaceuticals/ Aventis)	Phase II	RA, MS, Pso
	MLN-3701 (Millennium Pharmaceuticals)	Phase I	RA
CCR2	MLN-1202 (antibody) (Millenium Pharmaceuticals)	Phase II	RA
	Unknown (Incyte Pharmaceuticals)	Phase I	RA
CCR3	CAT-213 (antibody, bertilimumab) (Cambridge AT)	Phase II	Rhinitis, conjunctivitis
	GW-766994 (GlaxoSmithKline)	Phase II	Asthma, allergic rhinitis
	DPC-168 (Bristol-Myers Squibb)	Phase I	Asthma
CCR5	UK-427857 (Pfizer)	Phase II	HIV infection,
	ONO-4128 (Ono Pharmaceutical /GlaxoSmith-Kline)	Phase II	HIV infection
	Sch-351125/Sch-417690 (Schering-Plough)	Phase I	HIV infection
CXCR1/2	SB-332235 (GlaxoSmithKline)	Phase I	COPD, RA, Pso
CXCR4	AMD-3100 (AnorMED)	Phase II Phase I	Stem cell transplantation Repair of cardiac tissue after heart attack
	AMD-070 (AnorMED)	Phase I	HIV infection
	CTCE-0214 (Chemokine Therapeutics)	Phase II	Stem cell transplantation

NOTE: Data from Refs. 12 and 44–46.

ABBREVIATIONS: COPD, chronic obstructive pulmonary disease; MS, multiple sclerosis; Pso, psoriasis; RA, rheumatoid arthritis.

CCR1

The most advanced CCR1 antagonist in development is apparently compound BX-741, also named ZK-811752 (Banyu/Schering). It is a potent and selective antagonist of the human receptor[34,47] but 100–200 times less potent against the rat and the mouse receptor. However, the compound has proven to be effective in several animal models when administered at high doses.[34,47] The phase I studies gave positive results, and phase II trials for multiple sclerosis patients were reported to be planned for March 2002.[47] A total of 94 patients were supposed to be treated three times a day for 16 weeks, but results from this trial have not been released yet. The compound is also in development for psoriasis and Alzheimer disease.

The compound CP-481,715, a potent human CCR1 antagonist (Pfizer) provided the first proof of concept for a chemokine receptor antagonist in RA.[48] In this trial, 12 patients received 300 mg of the compound every 8 h and 4 patients received placebo by oral route for 15 days. Biopsy specimens taken on days 1 and 15 showed that patients treated with the compound had a reduced number of $CCR1^+$ cells in their joints. A trend toward a clinical improvement was also observed.[48] The compound progressed into a 6-week phase II clinical trial, and development was canceled.[45]

Millenium Pharmaceuticals recently reported the completion of phase I with its candidate, MLN-3897, a CCR1 antagonist. Another candidate targeting the same receptor is MLN3701, which has recently advanced to a phase I trial.

CCR2

Incyte Pharmaceuticals has a small-molecule CCR2 antagonist in phase I trials for RA. Millennium Pharmaceuticals is developing an anti-CCR2 antibody (MLN-1202), which is currently in phase II for the same indication. It will be interesting to know whether CCR2 blockade shows a beneficial effect on patients with RA, given the results obtained with CCR2 knockout mice.[41]

CXCR3

Compound T0906487 (originally from Tularik) was being developed by Amgen and Chemocentryx. The compound was evaluated in a phase IIa clinical trial in 40 patients with moderate to severe psoriasis who received 50 and 200 mg of the compound once a day for 28 days. Results indicated that the treatment had no effect on the psoriatic area severity index (PASI) or on the patient's global assessment (PGA) scores. The development of the compound for psoriasis was canceled.[49] The compound was also in development for RA, but no results for this disease have been reported yet.

CONCLUSIONS

The discovery of chemokines exerted a profound effect on our understanding of cell trafficking in health and disease. The potential of chemokines as therapeutic targets soon become evident, but initial optimism has been moderated by failures of compounds in the clinic. In the future, chemokine receptor antagonists will compete with other agents currently in development that also target cell migration. Time will tell whether chemokines are useful therapeutic targets or just a fascinating family of mediators.

[NOTE ADDED IN PROOF:] After less than four months on the market, Tysabri was withdrawn because one person died and another one contracted a rare disease of the cental nervous system called "progressive multifocal leukoencephalopathy." It is believed that both cases were caused by adverse side effects from the combination therapy of Tyrsabri and Avonex (interferon). Source: Press Release. Available at: <http://ms.about.com/b/a/150342.htm>

REFERENCES

1. LUSTER, A.D. 1998. Chemokines-chemotactic cytokines that mediate inflammation. N. Engl. J. Med. **338:** 436–445.
2. ZLOTNIK, A. & O. YOSHIE. 2000. Chemokines: a new classification system and their role in immunity. Immunity **12:** 121–127.
3. GERARD, C. & B.J. ROLLINS. 2001. Chemokines and disease. Nat. Immunol. **2:** 108–115.
4. GODESSART, N. & S.L. KUNKEL. 2001. Chemokine in autoimmune disease. Curr. Opin. Immunol. **13:** 670–675.
5. MURPHY, P.M., *et al.* 2000. International Union of Pharmacology. XXII. Nomenclature for chemokine receptors. Pharmacol. Rev. **52:** 145–176.
6. ONUFFER, J. & R. HORUCK. 2002. Chemokines, chemokine receptors and small-molecule antagonists: recent developments. Trends Pharm. Sci. **23:** 459–467.
7. JOHNSON, Z. *et al.* 2004. Chemokine inhibition—why, when where, which and how? Biochem. Soc. Trans. **32:** 366–377.
8. MOSER, B. *et al.* 2004. Chemokines: multiple levels of leukocyte migration control. Trends Immunol. **25:** 75–84.
9. BARDI, G. *et al.* 2001. The T cell chemokine receptor CCR7 is internalized on stimulation with ELC, but not with SLC. Eur. J. Immunol. **31:** 3291–3297.
10. KOHOUT, T.A. *et al.* 2004. Differential desensitization, receptor phosphorylation, beta-arrestin recruitment, and ERK1/2 activation by the two endogenous ligands for the CC chemokine receptor 7. J. Biol Chem. **279:** 23214–23222.
11. MARIANI, M. *et al.* 2004. Dominance of CCL22 over CCL17 in induction of chemokine receptor CCR4 desensitization and internalization on human Th2 cells. Eur. J. Immunol. **34:** 231–240.
12. TERRICABRAS, E., C. BENJAMIN & N. GODESSART. 2004. Drug discovery and chemokine receptor antagonists: eppur si muove! Autoimmunity Rev. **3:** 550–556.
13. PETKOVIC, V. *et al.* 2004. Eotaxin-3/CCL26 is a natural antagonist for CC chemokine receptors 1 and 5. A human chemokine with a regulatory role. J. Biol. Chem. **279:** 23357–23363.
14. OGILVIE, P. *et al.* 2003. Eotaxin-3 is a natural antagonist for CCR2 and exerts a repulsive effect on human monocytes. Blood **102:** 789–794.
15. OGILVIE, P. *et al.* 2004. Unusual chemokine receptor antagonism involving a mitogen-activated protein kinase pathway. J. Immunol.**172:** 6715–6722
16. LOETSCHER, P. *et al.* 2001. The ligands of CXC chemokine receptor 3, I-TAC, Mig, and IP10, are natural antagonists for CCR3. J. Biol. Chem. **276:** 2986–2991.
17. XANTHOU, G. *et al.* 2003. CCR3 functional responses are regulated by both CXCR3 and its ligands CXCL9, CXCL10 and CXCL11. Eur. J. Immunol. **33:** 2241–2250.
18. PETKOVIC, V. *et al.* 2004. I-TAC/CXCL11 is a natural antagonist for CCR5. J. Leukoc. Biol. **76:** 701–708.
19. LASAGNI, L. *et al.* 2003. An alternatively spliced variant of CXCR3 mediates the inhibition of endothelial cell growth induced by IP-10, Mig, and I-TAC, and acts as functional receptor for platelet factor 4. J. Exp. Med. **197:** 1537–1549.
20. FULKERSON, P.C. *et al.* 2004. Negative regulation of eosinophil recruitment to the lung by the chemokine monokine induced by IFN-gamma (Mig, CXCL9). Proc. Natl. Acad. Sci. USA **101:** 1987–1992.
21. THOMAS, M.S. *et al.* 2004. Regulation of cockroach antigen-induced allergic airway hyperreactivity. J. Immunol. **173:** 615–623.

22. MIYASAKA, M. & T. TANAKA. 2004. T lymphocyte trafficking across high endothelial venules: dogmas end enigmas. Nat. Rev. Immunol. **4:** 360–370.
23. IMHOF, B.A. & M. AURRAND-LIONS. 2004. Adhesion mechanisms regulating the migration of monocytes. Nat. Rev. Immunol. **4:** 432–444.
24. O'CONNOR, P.W. *et al.* 2004. Natalizumab Multiple Sclerosis Trial Group. Randomized multicenter trial of natalizumab in acute MS relapses: clinical and MRI effects. Neurology **62:** 2038–2043.
25. SANDBORN, W. *et al.* 2004. A phase III, double-blind, placebo-controlled study of the efficacy, safety, and tolerability of antegren (Natalizumab) in maintaining clinical response and remission in Crohn's disease (ENACT-2). Gastroenterology **127:** 332–339.
26. LEBWOHL, M. *et al.* 2003. Efalizumab Study Group. A novel targeted T-cell modulator, efalizumab, for plaque psoriasis. N. Engl. J. Med. **349:** 2004–2013.
27. BRINKMANN, V. 2004. FTY720: Mechanism of action and potential benefit in organ transplantation. Yonsei Med. J. **45:** 991–997.
28. ROVIEZZO, F. *et al.* 2004. Human eosinophil chemotaxis and selective in vivo recruitment by sphingosine 1-phosphate. Proc. Natl. Acad. Sci. USA **101:** 11170–11175.
29. YOPP, A.C. *et al.* 2004. FTY720-enhanced T cell homing is dependent on CCR2, CCR5, CCR7, and CXCR4: evidence for distinct chemokine compartments. J. Immunol. **173:** 855–865.
30. BENOIT, S., A. TOKSOY, E.B. BROCKER, *et al.* 2004. Treatment of recalcitrant pustular psoriasis with infliximab: effective reduction of chemokine expression. Br. J. Dermatol. **150:** 1009–1012
31. SCHWARZ, M.K. & T.N.C. WELLS. 2002. New therapies that modulate chemokine networks. Nat. Rev. Drug Discov. **1:** 347–358.
32. KUNKEL, S.L. & N. GODESSART. 2002. Chemokines in autoimmunity: from pathology to therapeutics. Autoimmunity Rev. **1:** 313–320.
33. SZEKANECZ, Z. *et al.* 2003. Chemokines and chemokine receptors in rheumatoid arthritis. Semen. Immunol. **15:** 15–21.
34. HORUK, R. 2003. Development and evaluation of pharmacological agents targeting chemokine receptors. Methods **29:** 369–375.
35. MATTHYS, P. *et al.* 2001. AMD3100, a potent and specific antagonist of the stromal cell-derived factor chemokine receptor CXCR4, inhibits autoimmune joint inflammation in IFN-gamma receptor-deficient mice. J. Immunol. **167:** 4686–4692.
36. NAYA, A. *et al.* 2001. Design, synthesis, and discovery of a novel CCR1 antagonist. J. Med. Chem. **44:** 1429–1435
37. GARCIA-RAMALLO, E. *et al.* 2002. Resident cell chemokine expression serves as the major mechanism for leukocyte recruitment during local inflammation. J. Immunol. **169:** 6467–6473.
38. YANG, Y.F. *et al.* 2002. A non-peptide CCR5 antagonist inhibits collagen-induced arthritis by modulating T cell migration without affecting anti-collagen T cell responses. Eur. J. Immunol. **32:** 2124–2132.
39. GONG, J.H. *et al.* 2004. Post-onset inhibition of murine arthritis using combined chemokine antagonist therapy. Rheumatology (Oxford) **43:** 39–42.
40. PLATER-ZYBERK, C. *et al.* 1997. Effect of a CC chemokine receptor antagonist on collagen induced arthritis in DBA/1 mice. Immunol. Lett. **57:** 117–220.
41. QUINONES, M.P. *et al.* 2004. Experimental arthritis in CC chemokine receptor 2-null mice closely mimics severe human rheumatoid arthritis. J. Clin. Invest. **113:** 856–866.
42. IZIKSON, L. *et al.* 2000. Resistance to experimental autoimmune encephalomyelitis in mice lacking the CC chemokine receptor (CCR)2. J. Exp. Med. **192:** 1075–1080.
43. GAUPP, S. *et al.* 2003. Experimental autoimmune encephalomyelitis (EAE) in CCR2–/– mice. Am. J. Pathol. **162:** 139–150.
44. BHALAY, G. & A. DUNSTAN. 2004. Chemokine receptors and drug discovery-SMR meeting. I. Drugs **7:** 441–443.
45. GLADUE, R.P., S.H. ZWILLICH, A.T. CLUCAS & M.F. BROWN. 2004. CCR1 antagonists for the treatment of autoimmune diseases. Curr. Opin. Investig. Drugs **5:** 499–504.
46. PROUS SCIENCE PUBLISHERS. 2005. Prous Science Integrity database. Barcelona.

47. Elices, M.J. 2002. BX-471 Berlex. Curr. Opin. Investig. Drugs **3:** 865–869 .
48. Haringman, J.J. *et al.* 2003. Chemokine blockade and chronic inflammatory disease: proof of concept in patients with rheumatoid arthritis. Ann. Rheum. Dis. **62:** 715–721.
49. Berry, K. *et al.* 2004. Evaluation of T0906487, a CXCR3 antagonist, in a phase 2a psoriasis trial [Abstract]. Inflammation Res. Suppl. **53:** pS222.

Rationale for T Cell Inhibition by Cyclosporin A in Major Autoimmune Diseases

G. F. FERRACCIOLI, P. TOMIETTO, AND M. DE SANTIS

Division of Rheumatology, Department of Internal Medicine and Geriatrics, Catholic University of the Sacred Heart, Rome, Italy

ABSTRACT: T cells exert a fundamental role in different autoimmune chronic inflammatory diseases. The low-affinity autoreactive T cell clones provide the first amplification loop after the antigen (AgX) presentation, and if not counterregulated by the T regulatory cells (Treg), they maintain the inflammation and predispose to organ damage. Interrupting the T cell amplification loop through calcineurin antagonists leads to maintenance of the whole process under the autoimmune threshold.

KEYWORDS: T cell; autoimmune chronic inflammatory diseases; cyclosporin A

INTRODUCTION

Autoimmune chronic inflammatory diseases (ACIDs), mostly affecting the musculoskeletal and connective tissues, are all characterized by the presentation of an autoantigen (AgX) by the antigen-presenting cells (APCs) to the autoreactive T cells.[1] After these early events, the cascade of activation of co-stimulatory receptors leads to gene activation and synthesis of proinflammatory cytokines.[2,3] The APCs may belong to different lineages (macrophages, B cells, dendritic cells, etc.)[4,5] in different tissues, yet the *sine qua non* is that without them no inflammatory reaction can occur. This means the activation of genes leading to expression and synthesis of several cytokines crucial for the maintenance of the inflammation and for the appearance of autoimmunity. Experimental evidence strongly supports the hypothesis that cytokines released in this context have a definite role in the development of autoimmunity.[6]

The debate governing autoimmune diseases relies on whether the initial AgX (the "original antigen sin")[7] governs the whole course of the disease or not. *In vivo* evidence has shown that as a patient progresses to a disease state (e.g., multiple sclerosis), the T cells lose reactivity to the initial epitope (myelin) recognized during the early immune response, yet they develop immune reactivity to other epitopes.[8] This means that in autoimmune diseases the autoimmune response can be spread to intermolecular as well as to intramolecular epitopes. The key points are the loss of toler-

Address for correspondence: G. F. Ferraccioli, M.D., Professor of Rheumatology, Catholic University of the Sacred Heart, Division of Rheumatology, Complesso Integrato Columbus Via Moscati 31, 00168 Rome, Italy. Voice: +39-06-3503-654; fax: +39-06-3503-523.
gf.ferraccioli@rm.unicatt.it

**Ann. N.Y. Acad. Sci. 1051: 658–665 (2005). © 2005 New York Academy of Sciences.
doi: 10.1196/annals.1361.110**

ance owing to the presence of autoreactive T cells and the lack of governance of the whole process.

CYTOKINES AND T CELL TOLERANCE IN AUTOIMMUNE DISEASES

The general view is that the low-affinity autoreactive T cell clones present in humans, escaping central deletion, need a strong antigenic stimulation to expand and proliferate up to a biological disease state. This requires AgX presentation and at least one of two possible events: (1) intense co-stimulation by signals from APCs, in the form of either membrane expression of co-stimulatory molecules or synthesis of cytokines capable of increasing the reactivity of the T cells and (2) activation of a subset of T cells capable of regulating the autoreactive T cells. These are T regulatory cells (Tregs), which act as bystander suppressors and mediate localized or systemic immune deviation. Tregs can be divided into three subsets: Tr1, which includes cells producing IL10; Th3, which produces transforming growth factor β (TGFβ); and true Treg $CD4^+CD25^+$, which constitutes 5–10% of the circulating pool in humans.[9] This means also that some cytokines, such as IL10 and TGFβ may be considered regulatory and, as such, autoimmunity regulatory molecules. Among the cytokines involved in this process of the control of tolerance, some appear crucial; for example, IL2 is necessary for the repletion of T cells carrying the functional Treg $CD4^+CD25^+$ population;[10] and IL10 and TGFβ, released after cell–cell contact, exert an immunosuppressive function.[11]

In human diseases, Tregs should be capable of suppressing the production of two major proinflammatory cytokines, TNFα and IFNγ, released by AgX-activated responder $CD4^+$Th1 cells,[12] but it has been shown that TNFα might impair the ability of regulatory T cells to suppress disease in the nonobese diabetic model of autoimmune diabetes.[13]

A switch in the immune response toward a Th2-driven biology is even more difficult to reverse because $CD4^+$Th2 cells are less susceptible to the suppressive activity of Treg $CD4^+CD25^+$ cells.[14]

Since in all immune inflammatory reactions IL2, TNFα, and IFNγ are locally produced in tissues infiltrated by the immune cells, the fate of the reaction is tightly regulated by the balance between Tregs and the milieu created by the cytokines.

CYTOKINES AND CO-STIMULATORY MOLECULES IN AUTOIMMUNE INFLAMMATION

The first molecule shown to function as a co-stimulator on the membrane of T cells is CD28, which interacts with its ligand B7.1/B7.2 on the membrane of APCs. The activation of T cells is regulated by two other receptors, CTLA-4 and PD-1, which also bind the B7 family. The second molecule on the T cell membrane that is recruited during the stimulation is CD40 ligand (CD40L), which interacts with CD40 present on the membrane of APCs and, enhancing the B7.1/B7.2 expression, reinforces the CD28 loop. These co-stimulatory molecules are crucial for low-avidity autoreactive T cells to become activated and start an autoimmune response to the AgX.[15] Besides the intrinsic control for such activation mediated by the CTLA-4–

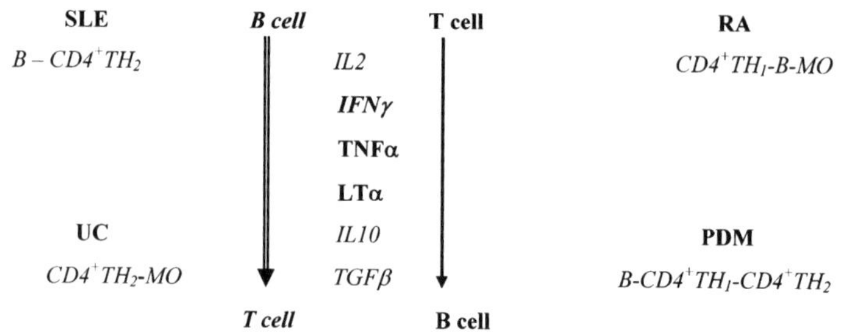

FIGURE 1. Prevalent cell function and role of various cytokines in the pathobiology of four major autoimmune chronic inflammatory diseases. Different cytokines play major roles in the various diseases, but all are important in defining the severity and chronicity of the disease.

PD-1 complex, the local inflammatory milieu is also crucial. In fact TNFα downregulates CD28 expression,[16] and IFNγ seems to play a fundamental role in the activation of B cells by $CD4^+$ T cells.[17]

Following from this background, in ACIDs a resetting of the biology of the disease should be envisioned based on the type of imbalance: cellular or cytokine-related. FIGURE 1 summarizes the type of imbalances in the cytokine milieu that have been described for systemic lupus erythematosus (SLE), ulcerative colitis (UC), rheumatoid arthritis (RA), and polydermatomyositis (PDM). This chapter focuses on why a T cell–oriented therapy may provide biological benefits.

Systemic Lupus Erythematosus

The biology of SLE is mainly driven by a strong cooperation between dendritic cells that present apoptotic bodies to the T cells and by B cells that present nucleoproteins to the T cells. In this setting, the co-stimulatory role of the CD40L–CD40 loop is especially relevant.[4] Of special interest is the biology of the tissue at the kidney level, where $CD4^+$Th1 cytokines clearly overcome the Th2 cytokines and the expression of TGFβ is much lower than expected.[18] If we consider the role played by some growth factors in the mesangial cell proliferation in class IV SLE nephritis, a resetting of the tissue biology would immediately become clear (FIG. 2).[19] All these data clearly suggest that blocking T cell activation might result in a downregulation of the whole inflammatory process.

Ulcerative Colitis

UC is thought to be a $CD4^+$Th2-driven disease in which IL13, a Th2 cytokine could play the major role. T cells obtained from the mucosal lesions in patients with UC also produce increased amounts of IL4 and macrophage-derived cytokines (e.g., TNFα, IL1β, IL6). Most important, however, the B cells produce IgG1 and G4 isotypes (as driven by $CD4^+$Th2 cells) and antineutrophil cytoplasmic (ANCA) and antitropomyosin autoantibodies.[20] Substantial evidence of T cell activation through co-stimulatory molecules has been provided.[21]

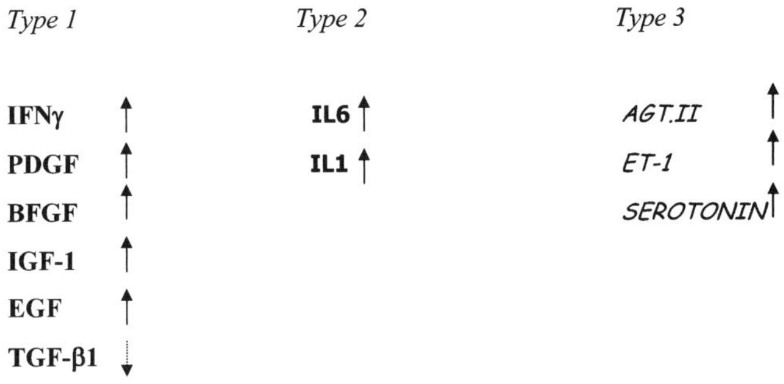

FIGURE 2. Mesangial growth factors implicated in human nephritides. Types 1, 2, and 3 are classified according to the relevance of their role in several models of nephritides. Up arrows show increased protein; down arrows show descreased protein expression and synthesis in the kidneys.

Rheumatoid Arthritis

RA is a classic $CD4^+$Th1-driven disease in which a fundamental role is played by monocyte/macrophage–driven cytokines such as TNFα and IL1β.[22] These are the key mediators of tissue destruction. T cells are thought to control the whole inflammatory process because it has been shown that in severe combined immunodeficiency (SCID) mice, the cartilage-damaging effects of transplants of long-standing synovial tissue could be shut down by the depletion of invading T cells.[23]

More important, the few B cells present in the tissue were demonstrated to be even more critical when it was shown that B cell depletion of the synovial tissue led to a profound functional downregulation not only of the monocytes-macrophages (MOs) but also of the functional T cells.[24]

The demonstration that blocking TNFα leads to an increase in the number and function of Tregs[25] and to a decrease, in some patients, of the production of rheumatoid factor (RF)[26] lends credit to the hypothesis that the interrelationship of B cells–T cells and MOs is very tight. Disrupting this loop is crucial for putting the whole process under adequate control. Leaving one pathway unchecked means more severe and chronic disease.

In RA, functional CD40L is expressed by T cells; it is functional because it stimulates immunoglobulin production by B cells and IL12 by dendritic cells, therefore demonstrating that the co-stimulatory molecules are clearly upregulated. Via the CD40–CD40L interaction, T cells can contribute to the activation of B cells, in particular, to the synthesis of RF.[27] If we consider that sCD40L can induce MOs to synthesize Blys (B cell activating factor), thus recruiting B cells and activating them, we may foresee a loop in which T cells–B cells and monocytes amplify each other's activation.[28] When examining a group of RA patients (n = 15) in their first years of disease (range of disease duration = 6–48 months) and all with active disease (range of CRP levels = 20–106 mg/L), we observed that plasma levels of TNFα and IL1β were increased in some patients and that a substantial number of patients had high levels of IL10 but low levels of TGFβ1. This demonstrates an imbalance in the counterregulatory molecules during the active phase (FIG. 3).

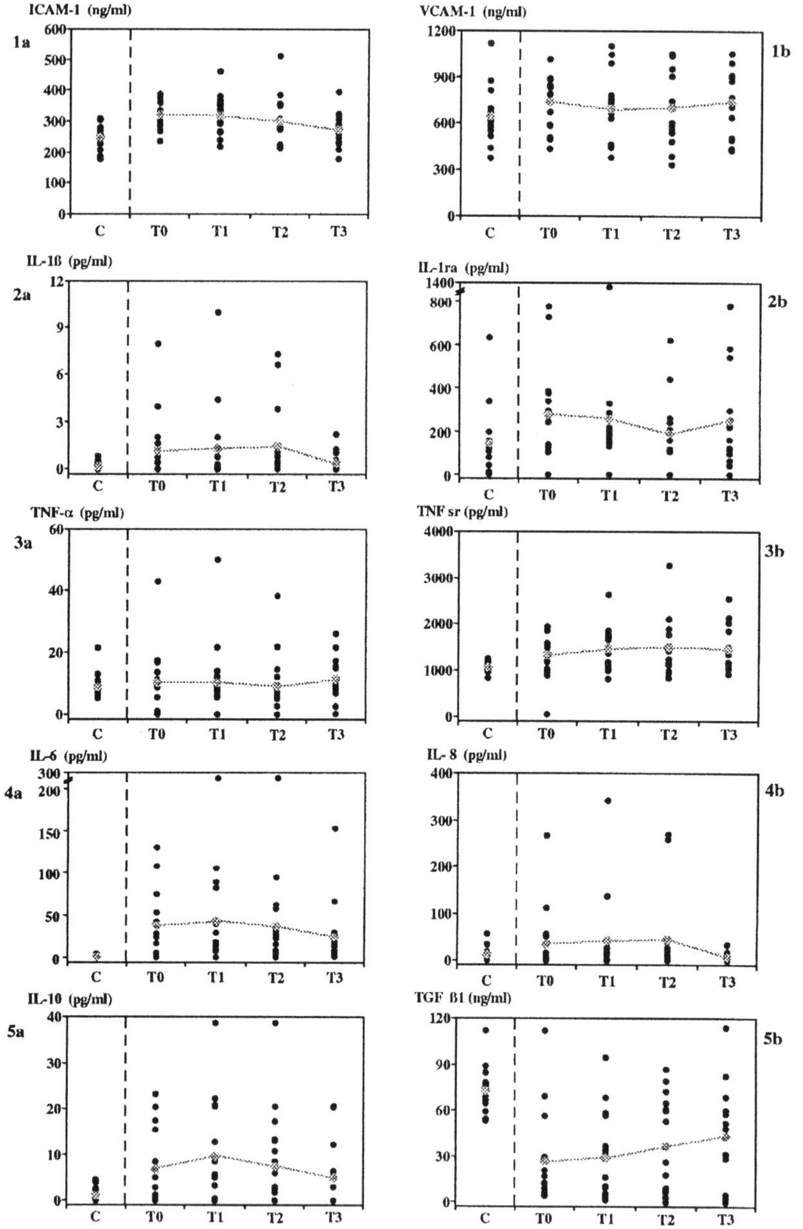

FIGURE 3. Fifteeen patients with active rheumatoid arthritis (CRP levels range from 20–105 mg/L) of short duration (6–48 months) never treated with DMARDs (disease-modifying antirheumatic drugs) and 20 healthy controls (C) were tested at entry (T0 = baseline), and after 15 days (T1 = 15 days), 30 days (T2 = 1 month), and 6 months (T3 = 6 months)

Polydermatomyositis

In polymyositis, the role of $CD8^+$ T cells in the pathogenesis of muscle damage is fairly well established[29]; and in dermatomyositis, the only definite biological process is the endothelial muscle damage caused by antibody binding complement and giving rise to the membrane attack complex (MAC), the true effector of muscle damage. The role played by $CD4^+$ T cells and B cells infiltrating the muscles of dermatomyositis patients is still ill defined.[30] What we know is that co-stimulatory molecules, in particular, CD40, are clearly expressed at the muscle tissue level and contribute to the local chronic inflammatory process by increasing the production of several cytokines.[31]

T CELLS AS TARGETS OF CYCLOSPORINE A IN ACIDS

Cyclosporine A (CsA) represents the mainstay of immunosuppressive therapy in transplantation. The mechanism of action is the inactivation of the Ca/calmodulin-dependent serine–threonine phosphatase calcineurin by the drug-immunophilin complex. This leads to the inactivation of the nuclear factor of activated T cells (NFAT), a transcription factor that is required for the expression of the IL2, IFNγ, and granulocyte-macrophage colony–stimulating factor (GM-CSF) genes.[32] Furthermore, CsA is capable of activating the gene for TGFβ1[33] and of shutting down the expression of CD40L in T cells.[34] In addition, CsA inhibits the maturation of dendritic cells from monocytes when stimulated by TNFα.[35] All these effects explain the clinical and biological results obtained for SLE,[36] in which an adequate control of nephritis was demonstrated; for UC, in which intravenous infusion, as an induction therapy, has been shown to almost fully control the acute phases of the disease[37]; for RA, for which, in combination with methotrexate, CsA has proved to control the progression of the erosive structural damage much more efficiently than methotrexate alone[3,8]; and for polydermatomyositis, in which 81% of patients demonstrated reduction of creatine kinase (CK) levels and clinical improvement.[39]

CONCLUSIONS

IL2 and IFNγ synthesis by activated T cells is crucial in all autoimmune diseases, whether T or B cell dependent. CsA may shut down the autoreactivity through the inhibition of IL2 and IFNγ and the downregulation of CD40L on T cells and may reset the immunologic milieu by inducing the synthesis of TGFβ1. Through these effects, it helps keep ACIDs under the autoimmune threshold.[40]

---

while receiving CsA 3–5 mg/kg/day. As shown, some patients presented increased levels of adhesion molecules at entry; very few patients has increased levels of TNFα, IL1β, and IL8; several patients had increased levels of TNFsRI (soluble TNF receptor I p55) or IL6 and IL10; and several had decreased levels of TGFβ1. During treatement there was a progressive trend toward a normalization of the whole immunologic setting. CsA seems to reset the immune derangement observed in early RA.

REFERENCES

1. Sykulev, Y., M. Joo, I. Vlturina, *et al.* 1996. Evidence that a single peptide-MHC complex on a target cell can elicit a cytolytic T cell response. Immunity **4:** 565–571.
2. Lenschow, D.J., T.L. Walunas & J.A. Bluestone. 1996. CD28/B7 system of T cell costimulation. Annu. Rev. Immunol. **14:** 233–258.
3. Chambers, C.A., T.J. Sullivan & J.P. Allison. 1997. Lymphoproliferation in CTLA-4-deficient mice is mediated by co-stimulation-dependent activation of $CD4^+$ T cells. Immunity **7:** 885–895.
4. Shlomchik, M.J., J.E. Craft & M.J. Mamula. 2001. From T to B and back again: positive feedback in systemic autoimmune disease. Nat. Rev. Immunol. **1:** 147–153.
5. Banchereau, J. & R.M. Steinman. 1998. Dendritic cells and the control of immunity. Nature **392:** 245–252.
6. O'Shea J.J., A. Ma & P.E. Lipsky. 2002. Cytokines and autoimmunity. Nat. Rev. Immunol. **2:** 37–45.
7. Fazekas de St. Groth, B. & R. Webster. 1966. Disquisition on original antigenic sin. J. Exp. Med. **124:** 331–345.
8. Tuohy, V.K., M. Yu, Y. Ling, *et al.* 1999. Spontaneous regression of primary autoreactivity during chronic progression of experimental autoimmune encephalomyelitis and multiple sclerosis. J. Exp. Med. **189:** 1033–1042.
9. Nelson, B.H. 2004. IL2, regulatory T cells and tolerance. J. Immunol. **172:** 3983–3988.
10. Almeida, A.R., N. Legrand, M. Papiernik & A.A. Freitas. 2002. Homeostasis of peripheral $CD4^+$ T cells: IL2Ra and IL2 shape a population of regulatory cells that controls $CD4^+$ T cell numbers. J. Immunol. **169:** 4850–4855.
11. Bach, J.F. & J. Francois Bach. 2003. Regulatory T cells under scrutiny. Nat. Rev. Immunol. **3:** 189–190.
12. Shevach, E.M. 2002. $CD4^+CD25^+$ suppressor T cells: more questions than answers. Nat. Rev. Immunol. **2:** 389–400.
13. Wu A.J., H. Hua, S.H. Munson & H.O. McDevitt. 2002. Tumor necrosis factor alpha regulation of $CD4^+CD25^+$ T cells in NOD mice. Proc. Natl. Acad. Sci. USA **99:** 12287–12292.
14. Cosmi, L., F. Liotta, R. Angeli, *et al.* 2004. Th2 cells are less susceptible than Th1 cells to the suppressive activity of CD25+ regulatory thymocytes because of their responsiveness to different cytokines. Blood **103:** 3117–3121.
15. Frauwirth, K.A. & C.B. Thompson. 2002. Activation and inhibition of lymphocytes by costimulation. J. Clin. Invest. **109:** 295–299.
16. Bryl, E., A.N. Vallejo, C.M. Weyand & J.J. Goronzy. 2001. Down-regulation of CD28 expression by TNFa. J. Immunol. **167:** 3231–3238.
17. Johnson-Leger, C., J. Hasbold, M. Holan & G.G. Klaus. 1997. The effects of IFNγ on CD40-mediated activation of B cells from X-linked immunodeficient or normal mice. J. Immunol. **159:** 1150–1159.
18. Murata, H., R. Matsumura, A. Koyama, *et al.* 2002. T cell receptor repertoire of T cells in the kidneys of patients with lupus nephritis. Arthritis Rheum. **46:** 2141–2147.
19. Uhm, W.S., K. Na, G.W. Song, *et al.* 2003. Cytokine balance in kidney tissue from lupus nephritis patients. Rheumatology **42:** 935–938.
20. Bouma, G. & W. Strober. 2003. The immunological and genetic basis of inflammatory bowel disease. Nat. Rev. Immunol. **3:** 521–533.
21. Liu, Z., S. Colpaert, G.R. D'Haens, *et al.* 1999. Hyperexpression of CD40 ligand (CD154) in inflammatory bowel disease and its contribution to pathogenic cytokine production. J. Immunol. **163:** 4049–4057.
22. Firestein, G.S.. 2003. Evolving concepts of rheumatoid arthritis. Nature **423:** 356–361.
23. Klimiuk, P.A., H. Yang, J.J. Goronzy & C.M. Weyand. 1999. Production of cytokines and metalloproteinases in rheumatoid synovitis is T cell dependent. Clin. Immunol. **90:** 65–70.
24. Takemura, S., P.A. Klimiuk, A. Braun, *et al.* 2001. T cell activation in rheumatoid synovium is B cell dependent. J. Immunol. **167:** 4710–4718.

25. EHRENSTEIN, M.R., J.G. EVANS, A. SINGH, *et al.* 2004. Compromized function of regulatory T cells in rheumatoid arthritis and reversal by anti-TNFα therapy. J. Exp. Med. **200:** 277–285.
26. FERRACCIOLI, G. & E. GREMESE. 2004. Thrombogenicity of TNFa in rheumatoid arthritis defined through biological probes: TNFα blockers. Autoimmunity Rev. **3:** 261–266.
27. KYBURZ, D., M. CORR, D.C. BRINSON, *et al.* 1999. Human rheumatoid factor production is dependent on CD40 signaling and autoantigen. J. Immunol. **163:** 3116–3122.
28. OHATA, J., N.J. ZVAIFLER, M. NISHIO, *et al.* 2005. Fibroblast-like synoviocytes of mesenchymal origin express functional B cell-activating factor of the TNF family in response to proinflammatory cytokines. J. Immunol. **174:** 864–870.
29. DALAKAS, M.C. & R. HOHLFELD. 2003. Polymyositis and dermatomyositis. Lancet **362:** 971–982.
30. GREENBERG, S.A. & A.A. AMATO. 2004. Uncertainties in the pathogenesis of adult dermatomyositis. Curr. Opin. Neurol. **17:** 359–364.
31. SUGIURA, T., Y. KAWAGUCHI, M. HARIGAI, *et al.* 2000. Increased CD40 expression on muscle cells of polymyositis and dermatomyositis: role of CD40-CD40 ligand interaction in IL6, IL8, IL15 and monocyte chemoattractant protein 1 production. J. Immunol. **164:** 6593–6600.
32. GIESE, T., M. ZEIER, P. SCHEMMER, *et al.* 2004. Monitoring of NFAT-regulated gene expression in the peripheral blood of allograft recipients: a novel perspective toward individually optimized drug doses of cyclosporine A. Transplantation **77:** 339–344.
33. SAGGI, S.J., T.F. ANDOH, R. SAFIRSTEIN & W.M. BENNETT. 2004. Cyclosporin induces renal proto-oncogene RNA message and increased transforming growth factor beta prior to renal fibrosis: modification by calcium channel blockade in the salt repleted rat. Nephrology **9:** 58–64.
34. FULEIHAN, R., N. RAMESH, A. HORNER, *et al.* 1994. Cyclosporin A inhibits CD40L expression in T lymphocytes. J. Clin. Invest. **93:** 1315–1320.
35. DUPERRIER, K., A. FARRE, J. BIENVENU, *et al.* 2002. Cyclosporin A inhibits dendritic cell maturation promoted by TNFα or LPS but not by double-stranded RNA or CD40L. J. Leukoc. Biol. **72:** 953–961.
36. TAM, L.S., E.K. LI, C.B. LEUNG, *et al.* 1998. Long term treatment of lupus nephritis with cyclosporin A. Q. J. Med. **91:** 573–580.
37. HANAUER, S.B. 2004. Medical therapy for ulcerative colitis. Gastroenterology **126:** 1582–1592.
38. MARCHESONI, A., N. BATTAFARANO, M. ARREGHINI, *et al.* 2003. Radiographic progression in early RA: a 12 month randomized controlled study comparing the combination of cyclosporin and methotrexate with methotrexate alone. Rheumatology **42:** 1545–1549.
39. QUSHMAQ, K.A., A. CHALMERS & J.M. ESDAILE. 2000. Cyclosporine A in the treatment of refractory adult polymyositis/dermatomyositis population based experience in 6 patients and literature review. J. Rheumatol. **27:** 2855–2859.
40. VON HERRATH, M.G. & L.C. HARRISON. 2003. Antigen-induced regulatory T cells in autoimmunity. Nat. Rev. Immunol. **3:** 223–232.

Partial Response to Anti-CD20 Monoclonal Antibody Treatment of Severe Immune Thrombocytopenic Purpura in a Patient with Common Variable Immunodeficiency

J. CARBONE,[a] A. ESCUDERO,[b] M. MAYAYO,[b] M. BALLESTEROS,[b] A. PEREZ-CORRAL,[b] S. SANCHEZ-RAMON,[a] E. SARMIENTO, D. MICHELOUD,[a] AND E. FERNANDEZ-CRUZ[a]

[a]*Immunology Division, University Hospital Gregorio Marañón, Madrid, Spain*

[b]*Hematology Division, University Hospital Gregorio Marañón, Madrid, Spain*

ABSTRACT: Immune thrombocytopenic purpura (ITP), alone or in combination with autoimmune hemolytic anemia (Evans syndrome) and/or autoimmune neutropenia, is frequent in patients with common variable immunodeficiency (CVID). A 34-year-old man with CVID had long-standing unresponsive ITP. The patient had a 9-year history of CVID on substitutive therapy with intravenous immunoglobulin (IVIG). The clinical course of CVID was complicated with refractory fistulizing inflammatory bowel disease, nodular regenerative hyperplasia of the liver, splenomegaly, severe portal hypertension, and hypercatabolism of IgG. ITP was refractory to medical therapy, including different combinations of corticosteroids, high-dose IVIG, azathioprine, and vincristine. Splenectomy was not performed because of severe portal hypertension. He received a total five doses of rituximab, a monoclonal antibody directed against CD20 antigen, at a dose of 375 mg/m^2. After an initially slow response, his platelet count increased to more than 50,000/μL by the fourth week of infusion. Therapy was well tolerated, and B lymphocytes were effectively depleted from the peripheral blood. The patient was completely tapered off glucocorticoids and maintained platelets at above 40,000/μL. The patient has not taken immunosuppressive agents for 11 months. Early treatment with rituximab might be an option for patients with CVID and ITP that do not respond to other treatments or for patients for whom a splenectomy is contraindicated.

KEYWORDS: common variable immunodeficiency; immune thrombocytopenic purpura; rituximab; anti-CD20

Address for correspondence: Dr. Javier Carbone, Immunology Division, University General Hospital Gregorio Marañón, Dr. Esquerdo, 46, 28007 Madrid, Spain. Voice: +34-91-5868423; fax: +34-91-5866698.
carbone@teleline.es

**Ann. N.Y. Acad. Sci. 1051: 666–671 (2005). © 2005 New York Academy of Sciences.
doi: 10.1196/annals.1361.111**

INTRODUCTION

Common variable immunodeficiency (CVID) is a primary immunodeficiency characterized by deficient antibody production.[1] It is the most frequent clinically significant primary antibody deficiency in humans. Most patients are recognized to have immunodeficiency in the second to the fourth decade of life, after they have had recurrent infections. Even though serum immunoglobulins may be quite reduced in CVID, 20–25% of patients develop clinical features suggesting an autoimmune disease; immune thrombocytopenic purpura (ITP) and autoimmune hemolytic anemia (AHA) are among the most prevalent.[2,3] ITP occurs in 7–10% of patients with CVID. Although this association is well established, the immunodeficiency background of CVID patients manifesting autoimmune disorders is often overlooked. Patients with CVID who develop ITP generally respond well to standard treatment regimens, including corticosteroids and intravenous immunoglobulin (IVIG).[2] However, not infrequently, clinicians see patients who have CVID and ITP that are more difficult to resolve. We report one CVID patient with severe ITP refractory to multiple courses of high-dose IVIG, high-dose steroid treatment, azathioprine, and vincristine who partially responded after adding rituximab (a monoclonal antibody directed against CD20 antigen) while continuing IVIG substitution therapy.

CASE REPORT

A 34-year-old man with CVID had long-standing unresponsive ITP. The patient had a 9-year history of CVID on substitutive therapy with IVIG. He had suffered from recurrent pneumonia, otitis, sinusitis, and diarrhea. At the time of diagnosis of CVID, low levels of all three classes of serum immunoglobulins (IgG = 35 mg/dL; IgA = 6 mg/dL; IgM = 12 mg/dL) and absence of specific antibody activity in the serum were demonstrated. The clinical course of CVID was complicated with intestinal tuberculosis, refractory fistulizing inflammatory bowel disease, splenomegaly, and hypercatabolism of IgG. One month before the onset of ITP, his platelet count was 215,000/μL, with IgG levels of 755 mg/dL. In March 2003, his platelet count decreased to 14,000/μL; his thrombocytopenia was severe, with platelet counts between 1000 and 36,000/μL, accompanied by recurrent bouts of epistaxis and intestinal hemorrhage. Hematologic malignancies were ruled out by normal bone marrow biopsy. Increased numbers of megakaryocytes were observed on bone marrow examination. There was no evidence of disseminated intravascular coagulation or active viral infections.

Treatment with multiple courses of prednisone (1–1.5 mg/kg) and high-dose IVIG (1–2 g/kg) (March–April 2003); prednisone, azathioprine, and high-dose IVIG (April 2003); prednisone, azathioprine, vincristine, and high-dose IVIG (May 2003); and the prednisone and high-dose IVIG (August 2003) all were without prolonged response (TABLE 1). The patient required repeated platelet transfusions to maintain his platelet count above 10,000/μL. In May 2003, granulocyte-colony stimulating factor was introduced because of the development of neutropenia. The number of blood neutrophils was maintained above 1000/μL. In August 2003, he developed interstitial pneumonia. Cytomegalovirus antigenemia was subsequently positive; the CD4 count was 48 cells/μL, and IgG levels were 755 mg/dL.

TABLE 1. Clinical characteristics of a patient with refractory ITP and CVID

Date	Clinical data	Treatments	Pretreatment (platelets/μL)	Posttreatment (highest platelets/μL)
3-7-03	ITP, hematochezia	PS(1.0) + Hd-IVIG	14,000	>70,000
3-28-03	Epistaxis	PS(1.5) + Hd-IVIG	28,000	62,000
4-24-03	Epistaxis	PS(1.5) + AZA + Hd-IVIG	36,000	34,000
5-30-03	Epistaxis, neutropenia	PS(1.0) + AZA + VNC + Hd-IVIG; G-CSF started	17,000	>70,000
8-14-03	GI bleeding, CMV disease, CD4 48/μL	PS(1.0) + Hd-IVIG; ganciclovir	8,000	<30,000
1-23-04	GI bleeding, PHT, RNH	5 doses rituximab (375 mg/m^2)	1,000	>100,000

ABBREVIATIONS: AZA, azathioprine (100 mg/day); CMV, cytomegalovirus; GI, gastrointestinal; Hd-IVIG, high-dose intravenous immunoglobulin; PS(1.0), prednisone (1.0 mg/kg/day); PS(1.5), prednisone (1.5 mg/kg/day); PTH, severe portal hypertension; RNH, regenerative nodular hyperplasia of the liver; VNC, vincristine.

Cytomegalovirus culture in bronchoalveolar lavage (BAL) fluid was positive. The patient started treatment with intravenous ganciclovir. Prednisone was tapered and discontinued in October 2003. A transjugular biopsy of the liver, performed at this time because of MRI findings of hepatic nodules, disclosed nodular regenerative hyperplasia of the liver. Imaging studies showed splenomegaly and severe portal hypertension. In January 2004, the patient's platelet count decreased to 1000/μL; the B cell count was 11%, and IgG levels were 635 mg/dL. Hemorrhagic bullae of the buccal mucosa and purpura developed. Splenectomy was deemed too risky because of the severe portal hypertension.

The patient was then treated with five weekly doses of rituximab at 375 mg/m^2 intravenously. One cycle of 40 mg dexamethasone once daily for 4 days was also administered. After an initially slow response, the patient's platelet count increased to >50,000/μL by the fourth week of infusion (FIG. 1). Then 2 weeks later, after the last dose of rituximab, his platelet count had increased to 110,000/μL. Two months later, his platelet count was 78,000/μL and had remained >40,000/μL thereafter.

Therapy was well tolerated, and B lymphocytes were effectively depleted from the peripheral blood (<1% B cell count). The patient was completely tapered off glucocorticoids. He has not taken immunosuppressive agents for 11 months, despite the return of B lymphocytes to the peripheral circulation. His most recent platelet count (January 2005) was 105,000/μL. CMV antigenemia was cleared on March 2004. IVIG substitution therapy was continuously administered to maintain levels of IgG > 700 mg/dL. The patient received valganciclovir prophylaxis for the development of CMV disease.

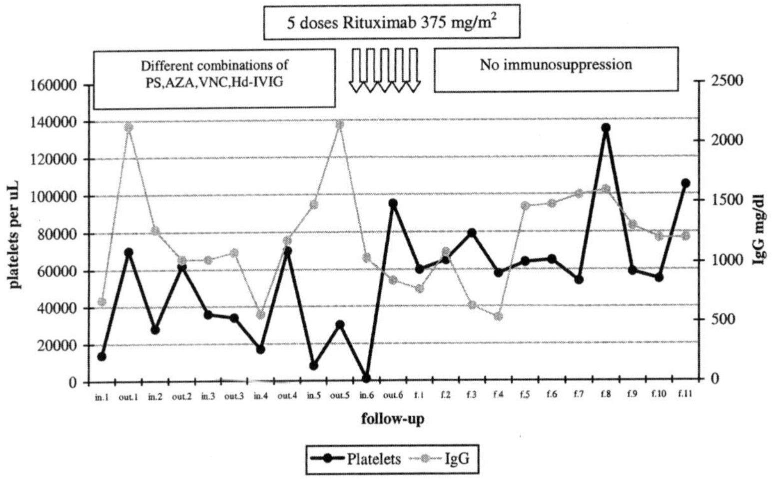

FIGURE 1. Response to anti-CD20 monoclonal antibody treatment in a patient with refractory immune thrombocytopenic purpura and CVID. ABBREVIATIONS: AZA, azathioprine; f., months of follow-up after treatment with rituximab; Hd-IVIG, high-dose intravenous immunoglobulin; in., patient was hospitalized; out., patient was discharged from the hospital; PS, prednisone; VNC, vincristine.

DISCUSSION

There is a paradoxical relationship between immunodeficiency diseases and autoimmunity.[3] In many cases, immunodeficiencies are associated with troublesome and sometimes life-threatening autoimmune complications. Persistent antigen stimulation, owing to an inherent defect in the immune system's ability to eradicate pathogens, is the primary cause leading to autoimmunity in patients with PID. Defects in T cell regulation, cytokine defects, abnormal apoptosis, and abnormal production of immunoglobulins with autoimmune features are other potential mechanisms.[2]

Steroids and other immunosuppressive agents frequently used to treat autoimmune diseases should be used with caution in patients with CVID because such drugs will further increase the risk of infection.[4] As a general rule, unless prolonged medical management fails, splenectomy should be avoided if at all possible in patients with CVID, because these patients are susceptible to overwhelming postsplenectomy infection.[2]

Michel *et al.*[4] described the outcome of ITP in 21 patients with CVID. ITP was not prevented by IVIG substitution therapy. With a median follow-up after ITP onset of 12 years, 62% of patients were in treatment-free remission; 23% were in remission while taking prednisone, with or without azathioprine; and only 1 patient still had a platelet count <50,000/μL. Severe infections, including three fatal bacterial infections and two opportunistic infections, occurred in six patients during or after treatment of ITP.[4]

A few case reports of successful treatment with danazol[5] or anti-D immunoglobulin[6] for ITP in patients with primary antibody deficiency have been published. In the case presented here, ITP was refractory to conventional medical therapy. The clinical course in our patient was complicated by the existence of a severe portal hypertension and CMV disease. Some believe that splenectomy is contraindicated in patients with portal hypertension because the perioperative risks are considerably greater than normal.

Recently, a novel approach using rituximab has shown promising results in patients with refractory ITP.[7,8] Rituximab is a genetically engineered, humanized, mouse monoclonal antibody directed against the CD20 antigen found on the surface of normal and malignant B cells.[9] Rituximab is used in the treatment of recurrent or refractory low-grade non-Hodgkin lymphoma.[10] To the best of our knowledge, this is the first case of refractory ITP in a patient with CVID for which a partial but durable response has been obtained by rituximab therapy. Improved platelet counts were sustained for at least 11 months. There has been one previous report of successful treatment with rituximab in a child with CVID and severe autoimmune hemolytic anemia owing to warm reactive IgM autoantibody.[11] Previous studies have demonstrated that although rituximab treatment induces prolonged B cell depletion, it does not lead to a decrease in immunoglobulin levels. However, a significantly decreased response to recall antigens after rituximab treatment has been suggested.[12] IVIG substitutive therapy in patients with CVID can solve this possible adverse effect.

Rituximab might have clinical advantages in this group of patients who have antibody deficiencies and for whom treatments resulting in further immunosuppression are relatively contraindicated.

REFERENCES

1. Cunningham-Rundles, C. & C. Bodian. 1999. Common variable immunodeficiency: clinical and immunological features of 248 patients. Clin. Immunol. **92:** 34–48.
2. Cunningham-Rundles, C. 2002. Hematologic complications of primary immune deficiencies. Blood Rev. **16:** 61–64.
3. Arkwright, P.D., M. Abinun & A.J. Cant. 2002. Autoimmunity in human primary immunodeficiency diseases. Blood **99:** 2694–2702.
4. Michel, M. *et al.* 2004. Autoimmune thrombocytopenic purpura and common variable immunodeficiency: analysis of 21 cases and review of the literature. Medicine (Baltimore) **83:** 254–263.
5. Saulsbury, F.T. & K.A. Bringelsen. 1991. Danazol therapy for chronic immune-mediated thrombocytopenic purpura in a patient with common variable immunodeficiency. Am. J. Pediatr. Hematol. Oncol. **13:** 326–329.
6. Longhurst, H.J. 2002. Anti-D immunoglobulin treatment for thrombocytopenia associated with primary antibody deficiency. J. Clin. Pathol. **55:** 64–66
7. Shanafelt, T.D. 2003. Rituximab for immune cytopenia in adults: idiopathic thrombocytopenic purpura, autoimmune hemolytic anemia, and Evans syndrome. Mayo Clin. Proc. **78:** 1340–1346.
8. Cooper, N. *et al.* 2004. The efficacy and safety of B-cell depletion with anti-CD20 monoclonal antibody in adults with chronic immune thrombocytopenic purpura. Br. J. Haematol. **125:** 232–239.
9. Cragg, M.S. 2005. The biology of CD20 and its potential as a target for mAb therapy. Curr. Dir. Autoimmun. **8:** 140–174.
10. Czuczman, M.S. 1999. Treatment of patients with low-grade B-cell lymphoma with the combination of chimeric anti-CD20 monoclonal antibody and CHOP chemotherapy. J. Clin. Oncol. **17:** 268–276.

11. WAKIM, M. *et al.* 2004. Successful anti-CD20 monoclonal antibody treatment of severe autoimmune hemolytic anemia due to warm reactive IgM autoantibody in a child with common variable immunodeficiency. Am. J. Hematol. **76:** 152–155.
12. VAN DER KOLK, L.E. *et al.* 2002. Rituximab treatment results in impaired secondary humoral immune responsiveness. Blood **100:** 2257–2259.

CD20 Mimicry by a mAb Rituximab-Specific Linear Peptide

A Potential Tool for Active Immunotherapy of Autoimmune Diseases

FEDERICO PEROSA, ELVIRA FAVOINO, MARIA ANTONIETTA CARAGNANO, AND FRANCO DAMMACCO

Department of Internal Medicine and Clinical Oncology (DIMO), University of Bari Medical School, Bari, Italy

ABSTRACT: An attractive, whether alternative or complementary, approach to passive immunotherapy (IT) with the anti-CD20 mAb rituximab for the treatment of autoimmune diseases is to stimulate the host to produce an anti-CD20 immune response by using peptides that mimic CD20 (mimotopes). The only mimotope reported to target CD20 antigen is a 43-mer polypeptide corresponding to the exposed domain of the molecule (from amino acid 142 to 184). Owing to its length, however, it failed to efficiently induce a CD20-specific response. A search has now been made for a smaller mimotope by biopanning a phage-display peptide library with rituximab. A total of 10 positive phage clones expressing six distinct sequences were isolated. Their alignment produced a motif that did not match any portion of the CD20 extracellular loop, whereas the motif bearing the 12-mer linear peptide Rp10-L specifically reacted with rituximab and inhibited its binding to CD20. Furthermore, in BALB/c mice Rp10-L-induced antibodies that reacted with the CD20$^+$ B lymphoid cell line Raji but not with the C20$^-$ T lymphoid cell line CEM. This peptide is currently being investigated to determine the effectiveness of CD20-based active IT for the treatment of autoimmune diseases.

KEYWORDS: autoimmune disease; CD20 antigen; immunotherapy; mimotopes; molecular mimicry; peptide, vaccine

INTRODUCTION

CD20 antigen is a 33–35-kDa phosphoprotein expressed at high density on B lymphocytes from the early pre-B to the late-B stage. Its expression is lost after differentiation of B cells into plasma cells. CD20 sequence analysis predicts a four-transmembrane domain with intracellular termini and only one extracellular 43–amino acid loop (from 142 to 184), which is the contact site of most anti-CD20 mAbs, including rituximab, which is effective in the immunotherapy (IT) of lymphoma.[1,2]

Address for correspondence: Franco Dammacco, M.D., DIMO, University of Bari Medical School, Piazza G. Cesare 11, 70124, Bari, Italy. Voice: +39-80-547-88-62; fax: +39-80-547-88-20.

f.dammacco@dimo.uniba.it

Ann. N.Y. Acad. Sci. 1051: 672–683 (2005). © 2005 New York Academy of Sciences. doi: 10.1196/annals.1361.112

The lack of CD20 downregulation on mAb binding, rituximab-induced antibody-dependent cell-mediated cytotoxicity (ADCC), and complement-dependent cytotoxicity (CDC)[3] have all been postulated as explanations of rituximab-induced B cell ablation *in vivo*. Furthermore, the expression of CD20 on autoreactive B cells, along with recent evidence indicating an important role played by B cells in the maintenance of the autoimmune T cell–mediated response,[4] has lead to the use of rituximab to treat autoimmune or immune-mediated diseases.[5–9]

Passive IT, however, is hampered by the fact that the mAb employed is effective only during its administration, whereas autoimmune diseases are chronic and hence require repeating large doses at short intervals, with a greater risk of toxicity and tachyphylaxis.[10,11] These limitations could be overcome by stimulating the immune system against the target molecule.[12] This would achieve the same biological effects as passive IT and allow the use of smaller amounts of immunogen, the use of longer intervals between administrations, and long-lasting efficacy.

In the case of CD20, a conjugate vaccine containing a peptide mimicking an epitope of its extracellular domain would induce an active response and generate biological effects similar to those obtained by passive anti-CD20 mAb IT. Furthermore, a polyclonal response would result in more effective recruitment of effector cells.[13]

We have, therefore, biopanned a phage-display peptide library (PDPL) with rituximab to look for a peptide that is able to mimic the CD20 epitope recognized by this mAb. The characterization of six rituximab-specific phage clones and a 12-mer linear peptide synthesized with the insert sequence of one clone are described.

MATERIALS AND METHODS

Animals

Female BALB/c mice (8–12 weeks old) were purchased from Charles River Breeding Laboratory (Milan, Italy).

Cells

The Raji ($CD20^+$) human B lymphoid cell line and the CEM ($CD20^-$) T cell line were grown in RPMI 1640 medium supplemented with 10% fetal calf serum (complete medium; Hyclone, South Logan, UT) and 5 mM L-glutamine.

Conventional Reagents, mAbs, and Peptides

Electrophoresis reagents were purchased from Bio-Rad Laboratories (Hercules, CA). Unless otherwise specified, all chemicals were purchased from BDH Chemicals (Poole, UK). Rituximab (chimeric IgG1) and its isotype-matched TNF-α–specific mAb, infliximab, were purchased from Genentech, Inc. (South San Francisco, CA) and Centocor (Malvern, PA), respectively. The anti-HLA class I mAb TP25.99[14] and the anti-CD4 mAb HP2/6[15] have been previously characterized. The anti-HLA class I mAb HC-10–specific phagotope and its insert-derived peptide, HC-Qp1a, have also been described.[16] The anti-CD4 mAb HP2/6-specific phage clone HP-41 is available in our laboratory.

Horseradish peroxidase (HRP)–conjugated avidin and xenoantibodies to human IgG (Fc portion) were purchased from Jackson Immunoresearch Laboratories (Avondale, PA). HRP-conjugated anti-M13 antibodies were purchased from Pharmacia-LKB Biotech AB (Uppsala, Sweden).

Monoclonal antibodies were purified from ascites by sequential precipitation with caprylic acid and ammonium sulfate[17] or by affinity chromatography on protein G (or protein A)–Sepharose (Pharmacia-LKB). Purity was assessed by sodium dodecyl sulfate–polyacrylamide gel electrophoresis (SDS-PAGE), as previously described.[18] Concentrations of mAb were determined in a bicinchoninic acid assay (BCA; Pierce, Rockford, IL). Purified mAb was coupled to biotin using the biotin-*N*-hydroxysuccinimide ester (Sigma-Aldrich, St. Louis, MO), as previously described.[19]

Linear peptides were synthesized at the Sigma (Sigma-Genosys Ltd., Cambridge, UK) and the Primm (San Raffaele, Milan, Italy) peptide synthesis service. Their quality was assessed by analytical reverse-phase chromatography and mass spectral analysis. Their purity was >80%.

Phage-Display Peptide Library

The 12-mer PDPL was purchased from New England Bio Lab (Beverly, MA). It is a filamentous phage-display system containing a repertoire of 1.2×10^9 sequences of random 12–amino acid peptides fused to the N-terminal sequence of the M13 synthetic minor coat protein PIII (five for each virion), via the flexible linker GGGs, with an overall sequence of PFYSHS-X-GGGSA.

Biopanning of PDPL with mAb Rituximab

Biopanning was performed as described previously,[16] except that infliximab was used as a rituximab isotype–matched mAb to remove allotype and isotype-specific phage particles.

Immunoscreening of Phage Clones

ELISA screening of phage clones was performed as previously reported.[16] The procedure for western blot was also performed as previously described,[20] with minor modifications. In brief, purified phage particles (1×10^{10} pfu/lane) were electrophoresed onto a 10% polyacrylamide gel under nonreducing conditions, with the mini-Protean II apparatus (Bio-Rad) at constant 200 V for 30 min. Resolved proteins were transferred to a polyvinylidene-diflouride (PVDF) filter (Millipore Corporation, Billerica, MA), with a semidry electrophoresis transfer cell (Bio Rad) by applying a current of 0.2 A for 30 min. After blockade of its free protein active-binding site with PBS containing 0.5% Tween-20 (PBS-T20), the filter was incubated for 2 h at 25°C with an appropriate dilution of biotinylated mAb (dissolved in PBS-T20), rinsed in PBS for 5 min, incubated with HRP-avidin, and developed with a diaminobenzidine substrate.

Nucleotide Sequence Analysis of Phage Inserts and Motif Identification

The nucleotide sequence analyses were performed as previously described.[16]

Keyhole Limpet Hemocyanin Conjugation of Peptides

Keyhole limpet hemocyanin (KLH) conjugation was performed by mixing 2 mg of each peptide with an equal amount of KLH in PBS (final volume, 1 mL) in the presence of glutaraldehyde (final concentration, 0.025%). After a 1-h incubation at 25°C, the reaction was stopped by extensively dialyzing the mixture against PBS at 4°C. KLH-conjugated peptides (KLH peptides) were stored at –80°C until used.

Immunochemical Assay

The indirect binding assay to test the reactivity of mAbs to peptides and the cross-blocking assay to determine the ability of a synthetic peptide to inhibit the binding of rituximab to it were performed in 96-well poly(vinyl chloride) microtiter plates (Falcon; Becton Dickinson, Mountain View, CA) as described previously[16] but with minor modifications.

In the indirect binding assay, plates were coated with peptide by overnight incubation at 4°C of 50 μL/well of a PBS solution containing 5 μg/mL of KLH peptide. After two washings with PBS-T20 and the blockade of the free protein–binding site with PBS containing 0.5% BSA (PBS-BSA), 50 μL of PBS-T20 solution containing mAb (2.5 μg/mL) was added to each well.

After a 4-h incubation at 25°C and three washings, binding of mAb to peptide was detected by the sequential addition of an appropriate dilution of HRP-conjugated, affinity-purified xenoantibodies to human IgG (Fc portion; 90 min incubation at 25°C) and a freshly prepared *o*-phenylenediamine (OPD)–H_2O_2 substrate solution. Color reaction was stopped with 100 μL/well of 2 N H_2SO_4. Absorbance was read at 492 nm in a Multiscan plate reader (Benchmark; Bio-Rad).

The cross-blocking assay was performed by mixing 50 μL of PBS solution containing a twofold dilution of peptide (starting concentration 400 μg/mL) with an equal volume of PBS-T20 containing the highest dilution of rituximab, giving 90% of the maximal binding (3 μg/mL). After a 1-h incubation at 25°C, the mixture was added to plates, which had been previously coated with KLH peptide. After a 4-h incubation at 25°C, the wells were washed and mAb binding to peptide was detected with an appropriate dilution of HRP-conjugated affinity-purified xenoantibodies to human IgG (Fc portion). The assay was then continued as described above for the indirect binding assay. Results were expressed as percentage of inhibition calculated from the following formula: % inhibition = [(A_{492} in the absence of inhibitor-A_{492} in the presence of inhibitor)/A_{492} in the absence of inhibitor] × 100.

Cell Assays

The inhibition assay to determine the ability of synthetic peptides to inhibit the binding of mAbs to $CD20^+$ Raji cells was performed by mixing 50 μL PBS-BSA solution containing a twofold serial dilution of inhibitor (starting concentration 400 μg/mL) with an equal volume of an appropriate dilution of biotinylated rituximab. After a 2-h incubation at 4°C, the mixture was added to target cells (7×10^5), and incubation was prolonged for 2 h. Next, cells were washed twice with PBS, and the binding of biotinylated mAbs to the corresponding antigen was detected by sequential addition of HRP-conjugated avidin and OPD substrate solution. Color reaction was stopped with 100 μL/well of 2 N H_2SO_4. Absorbance was read at 492 nm in a Multiscan plate reader. Results were expressed as a percentage of inhibition compared with the binding in absence of the inhibitor.

The indirect binding assay was performed by incubating mouse sera or mAbs with human B or T lymphoid cells (5×10^5 cells/well) for 2 h at 4°C. Cells then were washed twice with PBS and incubated with an appropriate dilution of HRP-conjugated xenoantibodies to mouse IgG (Fc portion) for 90 min at 4°C. After three washings with PBS, antibody binding to cells was detected by the addition of OPD solution. A solution of 2 N H_2SO_4 (100 µL/well) was used to stop the reaction. Absorbance was read at 492 nm. Background binding was determined by measuring absorbance with cells incubated with plain PBS.

BALB/c Mice Immunization

BALB/c mice were primed with an intraperitoneal injection of 100 µg of purified KLH peptide mixed with complete Freund's adjuvant (Invitrogen Co-Gibco-BRL, Carlsbad, CA). They were then boosted with 100 µg of the same immunogen in incomplete Freund's adjuvant on day 14. Sera were harvested on day 28 and every week thereafter up to the eighth week. Sera drawn on day 28 displayed the highest binding titer with the corresponding immunogen and were used for the assay.

RESULTS

Selection of Rituximab-Specific Phage Clones

To identify linear peptides recognized by rituximab, we isolated phage clones by panning the 12-mer PDPL with rituximab. Immunoscreening of 20 randomly selected colonies at the end of the third round of panning showed that 10 clones reacted with rituximab in ELISA. The binding was specific, because no reactivity with infliximab was detected (FIG. 1A,B), and this was confirmed by Western blot. Biotinylated rituximab reacted with minor coat protein III (PIII) fused peptide of the selected phagotopes (FIG. 1C). The reactivity was specific because rituximab did not react with the anti-CD4 mAb HP2/6-specific phagotope HP41-C, nor did rituximab-specific phage clones react with anti-CD4 mAb HP2/6 (FIG. 1D).

Nucleotide Sequence of Phage Clones and Synthesis of Peptides

Nucleotide sequence analysis of phage clones identified five sequences in the peptides expressed by 10 clones. Alignment of the deduced amino acid sequence of the inserts from 12-mer PDPL-derived phage positive clones resulted in a motif that could not be aligned with any portion of human protein sequences in the nonredundant (NR) database.

TABLE 1 lists the peptides synthesized. Linear peptide Rp10-L was synthesized on the basis of the insert sequence expressed by the 12-mer PDPL-derived positive clones R10-L, and an additional three peptides were synthesized using as template the CD20 amino acid stretch containing the amino acids A^{170} and P^{172}, which were found to be critical for extracellular CD20 epitope expression[21]: the cyclic 7-mer $RpCD20^{168-174}$-C, the linear 9-mer $RpCD20^{168-176}$-L and the linear 20-mer

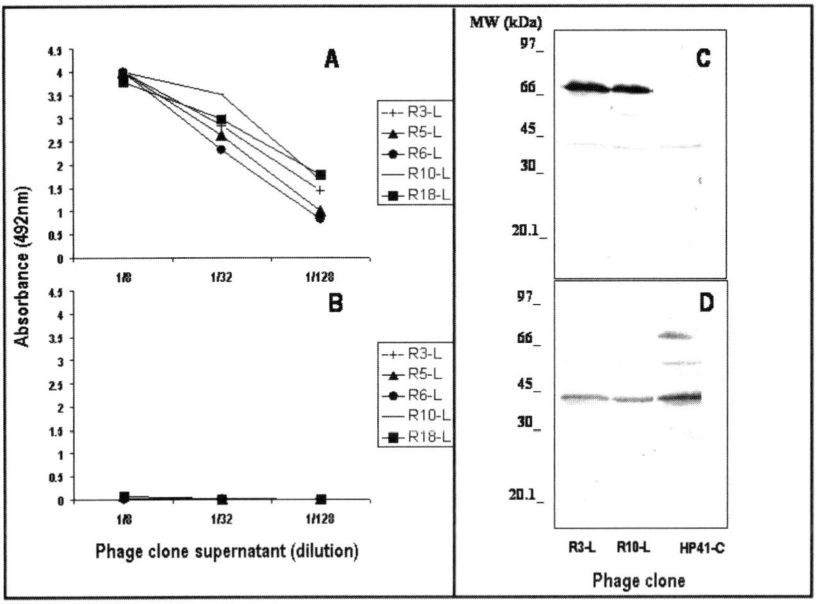

FIGURE 1. Specificity of the reactivity of phage clones isolated by biopanning of a 12-mer PDPL with mAb rituximab. (**A, B**) For this analysis, 96-well poly(vinyl chloride) microtiter plates were incubated with 50 μL of PBS solution containing rituximab (**A**) and infliximab (**B**) (5 μg/mL) for 12 h at 4°C. After two washings and blockade of free protein-binding sites, 50 μL of a fourfold dilution of phage clone supernatants was added to wells and incubation was prolonged for 2 h at 25°C. After four washings, the wells were incubated for 90 min with an appropriate dilution of HRP-conjugated, affinity-purified anti-M13 antibodies. Plates were then washed and developed by the addition of 100 μL of freshly prepared OPD. Color reaction was stopped with 100 μL 2 N H_2SO_4. Absorbance was read at 492 nm in a Multiscan plate reader. Background binding was determined by absorbance generated in wells with blocking solution alone. (**C, D**) Purified rituximab-specific phage particles (1×10^{10} pfu/lane) were run on a 10% polyacrylamide gel under nonreducing conditions and transferred to a PVDF filter. After blocking of free protein-binding sites, the filter was incubated for 2 h at 25°C with an appropriate dilution of biotinylated rituximab (**C**) and anti-CD4 mAb HP2/6 (**D**), rinsed in PBS for 5 min, incubated with HRP-avidin, and developed with a diaminobenzidine substrate. Binding of rituximab to anti-CD4 mAb HP2/6-specific phage clone HP41-C was included as negative control.

$RpCD20^{165-184}$-L (RpCD20-L). Only the last of these displayed detectable binding with rituximab in preliminary assay and was, therefore, always used as the control.

Reactivity of Peptides with Rituximab

A preliminary set of experiments showed that rituximab did not bind Rp10-L and RpCD20-L coated to the plates (data not shown), probably because they were unable to bind to the plates. Therefore, peptides were conjugated to a protein carrier, KLH, and used to sensitize the plate. FIGURE 2A shows that rituximab reacted with KLH peptides. Binding was specific because rituximab did not react with KLH alone, nor

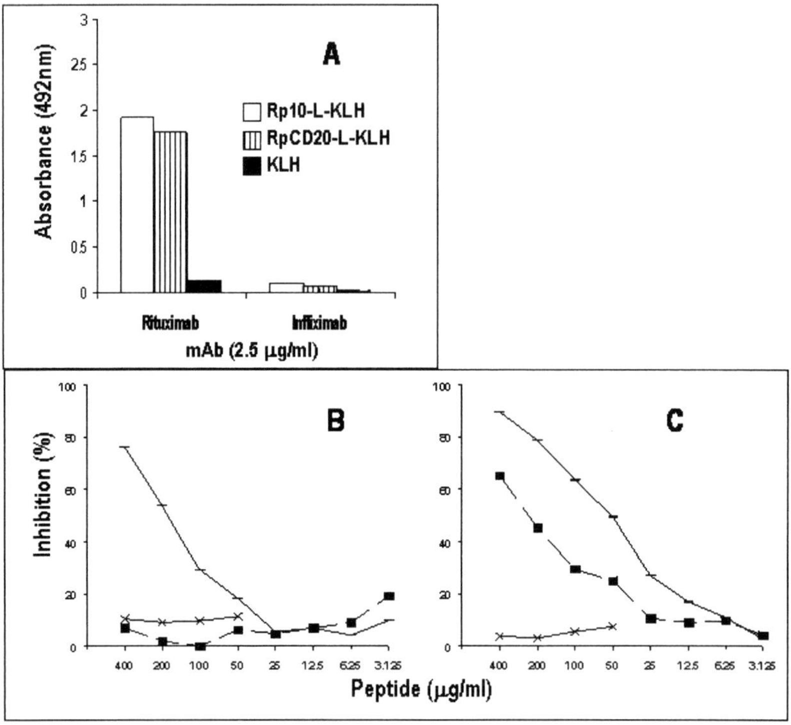

FIGURE 2. Peptides Rp10-L and RpCD20-L specifically react with rituximab and recognize the same (or spatially related) rituximab-associated epitope. (**A**) A total of 50 μL of PBS solution containing rituximab (2.5 μg/mL) was added to wells of a 96-well microtiter plate previously coated with KLH peptide. After a 4-h incubation at 25°C, the wells were washed and mAb–peptide interaction was detected by the addition of HRP-conjugated xenoantibodies to the Fc portion of human IgG, followed by an OPD-substrate solution. Binding of rituximab to KLH and of infliximab to rituximab-specific peptides were included as negative controls. (**B, C**) A total of 50 μL of a PBS solution containing different concentrations of Rp10-L (-) and RpCD20-L (■) were mixed with an equal volume of an appropriate dilution of purified rituximab (3 μg/mL). After a 1-h incubation at 25°C, the mixture was added to wells of a 96-well microtiter plate previously sensitized with peptide Rp10-L (**B**) and RpCD20-L (**C**). After a 4-h incubation at 25°C, rituximab binding to peptide was detected by sequential addition of xenoantibodies to human IgG (Fc portion) and an OPD-substrate solution. Binding of rituximab to peptide in the presence of peptide HC-Qp1a (X) was included as negative control. Results are expressed as the percentage of binding compared with binding in the absence of inhibitor.

TABLE 1. Peptides synthesized for immunochemical assay

Sequence origin	Deduced amino acid sequence of phagotope insert	Peptide	
		Denomination[a]	Sequence[b]
Ph.D.12-phagotope insert	ITPWPHWLERSS	Rp10-L	ITPWPHWLERSSg
CD20		RpCD20$^{168-174}$-C	cEPANPSEc
		RpCD20$^{168-176}$-L	EPANPSEKN
		RpCD20$^{165-184}$-L	YNCEPANPSEKNSPSTQYCY

[a]Cyclic (C) and linear (L) peptides.
[b]Flanking sequences are shown in lowercase letters.

did rituximab-specific peptides react with infliximab. The data indicate that conjugation to KLH of peptides did not change their antigenic profiles.

To define whether the epitopes recognized by two linear peptides are distant or spatially related to each other, a cross-blocking assay was performed whereby the binding of mAb rituximab to linear KLH-Rp10-L and KLH-RpCD20-L in the presence of different concentrations of free peptide was evaluated. FIGURE 2B,C shows that the two peptides inhibited rituximab-binding to the homologous peptide to a similar extent. The inhibition was dose dependent and dose specific, because peptide HC-Qp1a displayed no inhibitory effect. Although Rp10-L affected rituximab-RpCD20-L interaction, RpCD20-L failed to interfere with Rp-10-L-rituximab binding, indicating that Rp-10-L and RpCD20-L recognize the same rituximab epitope, though the binding avidity for rituximab of Rp10-L is higher than that of RpCD20-L.

To determine whether the synthesized peptides recognized the rituximab Ag-combining site, we evaluated their ability to inhibit biotinylated rituximab binding to CD20$^+$ Raji cells. As shown in FIGURE 3, Rp10-L inhibited rituximab binding with an inhibition profile similar to that of unlabeled rituximab. The inhibition was dose dependent and dose specific, because HC-Qp1a did not affect the binding. RpCD20-L, on the other hand, barely inhibited rituximab binding at high concentrations. The data suggest that the epitope recognized by Rp-10-L was within or spatially related to the rituximab Ag-combining site and that Rp10-L was a more efficient inhibitor than RpCD20-L.

Induction of CD20$^+$ Cell-Specific Antibodies after Immunization of Mice with Peptide

Sera drawn on day 28 from BALB/c mice immunized with Rp10-L were tested in a binding assay with the CD20$^+$ Raji cell line. As depicted in FIGURE 4, a 1:20 dilution of anti–Rp10-L serum displayed a detectable binding with this line. The reactivity was specific because anti–Rp10-L serum did not react with the CD20$^-$ CEM line. On the other hand, RpCD20-L-immune sera reacted with neither cell line. The lack of reactivity was not the result of peptide immunogenicity because RpCD20-L induced antibodies to the corresponding immunizing peptide (data not shown). The data strongly suggest that anti–Rp10-L immune sera contained anti-CD20 antibodies.

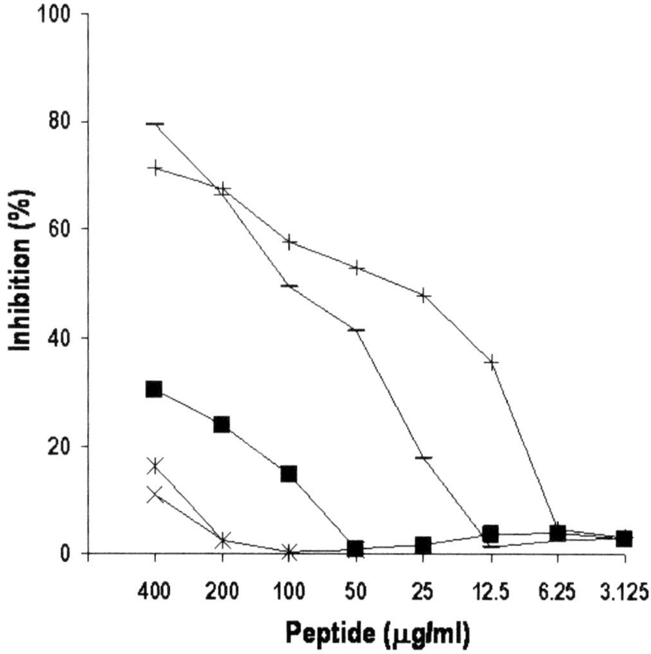

FIGURE 3. Inhibition assay to define the spatial relationship between the peptide-specific epitopes and the rituximab antigen-combining site. A total of 50 µL of a PBS solution containing twofold serial dilutions of Rp10-L (-) and RpCD20-L (■) (starting concentration, 400 µg/mL) were mixed with an equal volume of an appropriate dilution of biotinylated rituximab. After a 2-h incubation at 4°C, the mixture was added to target Raji cells (7×10^5/well), and incubation was prolonged for 2 h at 4°C. Then cells were washed with PBS-BSA, incubated with HRP-conjugated avidin, and developed by OPD-solution. Binding of rituximab in the presence of unlabeled rituximab (+) and mAb HC-10–specific peptide HC-Qp1a (**X**) were included as positive and negative controls, respectively. Results are expressed as the percentage of inhibition of binding compared with binding in the absence of inhibitor.

DISCUSSION

Induction of an active immune response to self-antigens successfully used as targets for passive IT has represented a major challenge because it is based on the assumption that active IT is a more feasible way to control or even cure autoimmune or immune-mediated disorders.[22–26] Because CD20 is regarded as a successful target in rituximab-based passive IT for the treatment of B cell neoplasms and, more recently, autoimmune diseases, we looked for a peptide able to mimic the CD20 epitope recognized by rituximab and assessed its ability to break tolerance to this widely expressed antigen. Biopanning of a PDPL to isolate phage clones specifically reacting with rituximab disclosed a peptide that behaves as CD20 mimotope.

Alignment of rituximab-specific phage clone insert sequences identified a motif that did not display any homology with the CD20 sequence. Even so, the motif-bearing the 12-mer linear peptide Rp10-L, synthesized with the sequence of the insert of

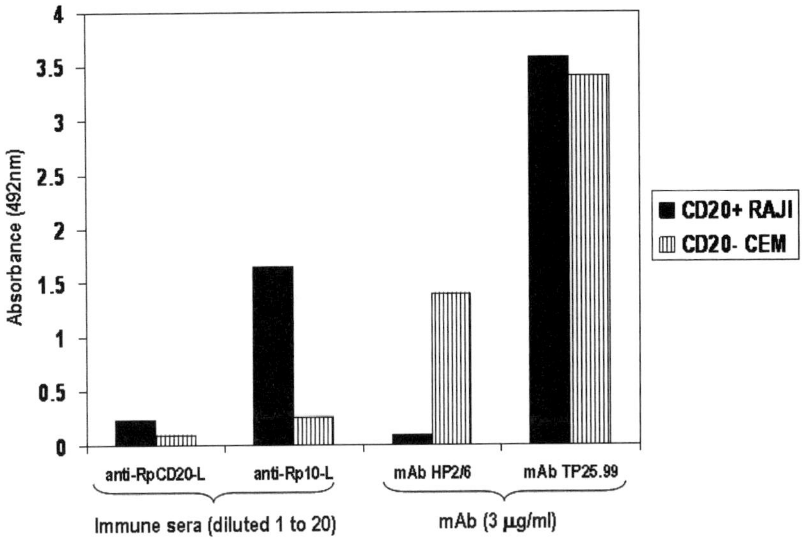

FIGURE 4. Rp10-L–induced antibodies react with Raji $CD20^+$ human B lymphoid cells. A total of 50 µL of sera drawn on day 28 from BALB/c mice immunized with Rp10-L and RpCD20-L were incubated with Raji human B lymphoid cells (*closed bar*) and CEM human T cells (*hatched bar*) (5×10^5 cells/well) for 2 h at 4°C. Cells were then washed twice with PBS and incubated with 50 µL of an appropriate dilution of HRP-conjugated xeno-antisera to mouse IgG (Fc portion). After a 90-min incubation at 4°C and three washings with PBS, sera reactivity with cells was detected by addition of OPD solution. Background binding was determined by absorbance generated in wells incubated with plain PBS. Bindings of the anti-HLA class I mAb TP25.99 and of anti-CD4 mAb HP2/6 were included as specificity controls.

phage clone R10-L, reacted specifically with rituximab and inhibited its binding to CD20. It is unlikely that this inhibition was the result of steric hindrance because this is not a common phenomenon with low molecular weight molecules. It was more probably the result of recognition by Rp10-L of the rituximab antigen-combining site, which means that it mimics the CD20 epitope. The ability of Rp10-L-immunized mouse serum to specifically react with CD20+ B cells supports this conclusion.

The lack of sequence homology between the peptide and the rituximab-specific CD20 epitope can be explained by the fact that the Rp10-L mimics a conformational epitope and does not need to share such homology.[27] The results of previous efforts to develop peptide-based vaccines to induce protection against infectious diseases[28] or tumor growth support this conclusion.[26,29] In the first case, Westerink *et al.*[28] showed that the peptide mimic of the CDR3 region of anti-idiotype that induced protection against *Neisseria* meningitides infection in mice had no homology with the CDR3 region. In the second, the peptide H98 mimic of the HER-2–epitope recognized by trastuzumab shared no homology with HER-2, although it induced anti–HER-2–specific antibodies.[26] Finally, peptide mimics of carbohydrate antigens,[30] and hence of molecules with a completely different structure that bind the antigen ligand[31] or induce tumor protection,[29] have also been reported.

There is only one previous description of a CD20 mimotope.[12] Here, however, the reagent used to induce a CD20-specific response was an abnormally long 43-mer polypeptide corresponding to the whole extracellular loop of CD20, which was likely to assume different conformations not necessarily resembling that on naive CD20.

The 12-mer peptide described here is less susceptible to the assumption of conformations other than that resembling the CD20 epitope recognized by rituximab, and its lack of sequence homology with CD20 make it more likely to bypass the established immune tolerance against CD20 in syngeneic settings in humans. The potential usefulness of this reagent for active IT of autoimmune diseases remains to be ascertained.

ACKNOWLEDGMENTS

This work was supported by grants from the Associazione Italiana per la Ricerca sul Cancro, Milan; the foundation Cassa di Risparmio di Puglia, Bari; and University of Bari Medical School, Bari. The authors are grateful to Mr. Vito Iacovizzi for his excellent secretarial assistance.

REFERENCES

1. COIFFIER, B. 2004. New treatment strategies in lymphomas: aggressive lymphomas. Ann. Hematol. **83:** S73–S74.
2. HENNESSY, B.T., E.O. HANRAHAN & P.A. DALY. 2004. Non-Hodgkin lymphoma: an update. Lancet Oncol. **5:** 341–353.
3. DI GAETANO, N., E. CITTERA, R. NOTA, *et al.* 2003. Complement activation determines the therapeutic activity of rituximab in vivo. J. Immunol. **171:** 1581–1587.
4. LIPSKY, P.E. 2001. Systemic lupus erythematosus: an autoimmune disease of B cell hyperactivity. Nat. Immunol. **2:** 764–766.
5. LOONEY, R.J. 2002. Treating human autoimmune disease by depleting B cells. Ann. Rheum. Dis. **61:** 863–866.
6. KNEITZ, C., M. WILHELM & H.P. TONY. 2002. Effective B cell depletion with rituximab in the treatment of autoimmune diseases. Immunobiology **206:** 519–527.
7. LEANDRO, M.J., J.C. EDWARDS, G. CAMBRIDGE, *et al.* 2002. An open study of B lymphocyte depletion in systemic lupus erythematosus. Arthritis Rheum. **46:** 2673–2677.
8. WAKIM, M., A. SHAH, P.A. ARNDT, *et al.* 2004. Successful anti-CD20 monoclonal antibody treatment of severe autoimmune hemolytic anemia due to warm reactive IgM autoantibody in a child with common variable immunodeficiency. Am. J. Hematol. **76:** 152–155.
9. EDWARDS, J.C., L. SZCZEPANSKI, J. SZECHINSKI, *et al.* 2004. Efficacy of B-cell-targeted therapy with rituximab in patients with rheumatoid arthritis. N. Engl. J. Med. **350:** 2572–2581.
10. D'ARCY, C.A. & M. MANNIK. 2001. Serum sickness secondary to treatment with the murine-human chimeric antibody IDEC-C2B8 (rituximab). Arthritis Rheum. **44:** 1717–1718.
11. HERISHANU, Y. 2002. Rituximab-induced serum sickness. Am. J. Hematol. **70:** 329.
12. ROBERTS, W.K., P.O. LIVINGSTON, D.B. AGUS, *et al.* 2002. Vaccination with CD20 peptides induces a biologically active, specific immune response in mice. Blood **99:** 3748–3755.

13. UCHIDA, J., Y. HAMAGUCHI, J.A. OLIVER, *et al.* 2004. The innate mononuclear phagocyte network depletes B lymphocytes through Fc receptor-dependent mechanisms during anti-CD20 antibody immunotherapy. J. Exp. Med. **199:** 1659–1669.
14. DESAI, S.A., X. WANG, E.J. NORONHA, *et al.* 2000. Structural relatedness of distinct determinants recognized by monoclonal antibody TP25.99 on beta 2-microglobulin-associated and beta 2-microglobulin-free HLA class I heavy chains. J. Immunol. **165:** 3275–3283.
15. CARRERA, A.C., F. SANCHEZ-MADRID, M. LOPEZ-BOTET, *et al.* 1987. Involvement of the CD4 molecule in a post-activation event on T cell proliferation. Eur. J. Immunol. **17:** 179–186.
16. PEROSA, F., G. LUCCARELLI, M. PRETE, *et al.* 2003. Beta 2-microglobulin-free HLA class I heavy chain epitope mimicry by monoclonal antibody HC-10-specific peptide. J. Immunol. **171:** 1918–1926.
17. PEROSA, F., R. CARBONE, S. FERRONE, *et al.* 1990. Purification of human immunoglobulins by sequential precipitation with caprylic acid and ammonium sulphate. J. Immunol. Methods **128:** 9–16.
18. LAEMMLI, U.K. 1970. Cleavage of structural proteins during the assembly of the head of bacteriophage T4. Nature **227:** 680–685.
19. STREICHER, H.Z., F. CUTTITTA, G.K. BUCKENMEYER, *et al.* 1986. Mapping the idiotopes of a monoclonal anti-myoglobin antibody with syngeneic monoclonal anti-idiotypic antibodies: detection of a common idiotope. J. Immunol. **136:** 1007–1014.
20. PEROSA, F., S. FERRONE & F. DAMMACCO. 1991. Anti-idiotypic monoclonal antibodies reacting with idiotope on isolated-denatured chains of an anti-CD4 monoclonal antibody. Immunology **74:** 748–750.
21. POLYAK, M.J. & J.P. DEANS. 2002. Alanine-170 and proline-172 are critical determinants for extracellular CD20 epitopes; heterogeneity in the fine specificity of CD20 monoclonal antibodies is defined by additional requirements imposed by both amino acid sequence and quaternary structure. Blood **99:** 3256–3262.
22. MORELAND, L.W., E.E. MORGAN, T.C. ADAMSON III, *et al.* 1998. T cell receptor peptide vaccination in rheumatoid arthritis: a placebo-controlled trial using a combination of Vbeta3, Vbeta14, and Vbeta17 peptides. Arthritis Rheum. **41:** 1919–1929.
23. ST. CLAIR, E.W., S.B. COHEN, M.L. LEE, *et al.* 2000. Treatment of rheumatoid arthritis with a DR4/1 peptide. J. Rheumatol. **27:** 1855–1863.
24. PEROSA, F., G. LUCCARELLI, M. SCUDELETTI, *et al.* 2002. Assessment of safety and the immune response to the CD4 "internal antigen" mouse anti-idiotypic Mab 16D7 in four patients with SLE. J. Clin. Immunol. **22:** 13–22.
25. BYNOE, M.S., J.T. EVANS, C. VIRET, *et al.* 2003. Epicutaneous immunization with autoantigenic peptides induces T suppressor cells that prevent experimental allergic encephalomyelitis. Immunity **19:** 317–328.
26. RIEMER, A.B., M. KLINGER, S. WAGNER, *et al.* 2004. Generation of peptide mimics of the epitope recognized by trastuzumab on the oncogenic protein Her-2/neu. J. Immunol. **173:** 394–401.
27. VAN REGENMORTEL, M.H. 2002. Reductionism and the search for structure-function relationships in antibody molecules. J. Mol. Recognit. **15:** 240–247.
28. WESTERINK, M.A., P.C. GIARDINA, M.A. APICELLA, *et al.* 1995. Peptide mimicry of the meningococcal group C capsular polysaccharide. Proc. Natl. Acad. Sci. USA **92:** 4021–4025.
29. KIEBER-EMMONS, T., P. LUO, J. QIU, *et al.* 1999. Vaccination with carbohydrate peptide mimotopes promotes anti-tumor responses. Nat. Biotechnol. **17:** 660–665.
30. VALADON, P., G. NUSSBAUM, L.F. BOYD, *et al.* 1996. Peptide libraries define the fine specificity of anti-polysaccharide antibodies to *Cryptococcus neoformans*. J. Mol. Biol. **261:** 11–22.
31. OLDENBURG, K.R., D. LOGANATHAN, I.J. GOLDSTEIN, *et al.* 1992. Peptide ligands for a sugar-binding protein isolated from a random peptide library. Proc. Natl. Acad. Sci. USA **89:** 5393–5397.

Anticytokine Therapy, Especially Anti–Interferon-γ, as a Pathogenetic Treatment in TH-1 Autoimmune Diseases

SIMON SKURKOVICH[a] AND BORIS SKURKOVICH[a,b]

[a]*Advanced Biotherapy, Inc., Rockville, Maryland 20852, USA*

[b]*Brown Medical School, Providence, Rhode Island, USA*

ABSTRACT: We pioneered anticytokine therapy (ACT) in 1974 and 1989, proposing to remove interferon (IFN) and tumor necrosis factor (TNF)–α together with IFNs to treat various autoimmune diseases, including AIDS. This hypothesis was confirmed in different laboratories and opened a new line to produce and test different anticytokines. We have had good, sometimes striking results treating various Th1-mediated autoimmune diseases, including inflammatory skin diseases, using anti–IFN-γ and sometimes anti–TNF-α. Anti–IFN-γ may be a universal treatment for these conditions. Because TNF-α inhibitors, now successfully used in certain autoimmune disorders, have many severe side effects, there are opportunities for the development of other ACT and TNF-α antagonists with fewer side effects.

KEYWORDS: anticytokine therapy; autoimmune diseases; inflammatory skin diseases; AIDS; Th1 cytokines; interferon-γ; interferon-α; tumor necrosis factor–α inhibitors

INTRODUCTION

Anticytokine therapy (ACT) was pioneered by S. Skurkovich, who in 1974 proposed in *Nature* that a disturbance of interferon (IFN) (cytokine) synthesis can bring autoimmune disease and that neutralization of IFN could be therapeutic.[1] In 1975, IFN was found in the blood of autoimmune patients, and the first ACT was tested.[2] Later, in 1989, because IFN-γ induces TNF-α and these cytokines sometimes work in the same way, we first proposed to remove TNF-α (presently various TNF-α blockers are used, such as Enbrel, Remicade, and Humira) together with antibodies to certain IFNs in treating autoimmune diseases and AIDS, which has an autoimmune component.[3] After our early work, a number of researchers conducted experimental and later clinical studies on the pathogenetic role of cytokines and the therapeutic benefit of blocking various cytokines in different autoimmune diseases.

We first proposed (1973–2002) ACT to treat such autoimmune conditions as skin allograft rejection, collagenosis, rheumatoid arthritis, systemic lupus erythematosus, rheumatism, hemolytic anemia, immune form of idiopathic thrombocytopenic pur-

Address for correspondence: Simon Skurkovich, 802 Rollins Avenue, Rockville, MD 20852. Voice: 301-770-7285; fax: 301-770-4833.
sskurkovich@erols.com

**Ann. N.Y. Acad. Sci. 1051: 684–700 (2005). © 2005 New York Academy of Sciences.
doi: 10.1196/annals.1361.113**

TABLE 1. IFN-γ or IFN-γ–producing T cells are found at the site of pathology in various autoimmune diseases

Autoimmune disease	Site of pathology	Reference(s)
Rheumatoid arthritis	Synovial fluid	16
Multiple sclerosis	Cerebrospinal fluid and plaques	17,18
Corneal transplant rejection	Aqueous humor and corneal infiltrating cells	19
Type I diabetes	Islet β-cells	20
Uveitis	Ocular cells	21
Psoriasis, alopecia, vitiligo, acne	Skin lesions	22–24

pura, eczemas, nephritis, myasthenia gravis, Hashimoto disease, autoimmune diseases of the organs of sight and hearing, multiple sclerosis, Ménière disease, Parkinson disease, pemphigus, schizophrenia and possibly some mental derangements, psoriasis, Crohn disease, and others.[1,4]

Studies in experimental rodent models of autoimmune disease confirm our hypothesis that IFNs can trigger or exacerbate disease, as in animal models of thyroiditis,[5] anterior uveitis,[6] autoimmune neuritis,[7] and neonatal autoimmune ovarian disease,[8] and that anti–IFN-γ can bring beneficial results, such as preventing type I diabetes[9,10] and treating experimental autoimmune thyroiditis,[11] neuritis,[12] and orchitis.[13] Mice lacking the IFN-γ receptor were also found less susceptible to collagen-induced arthritis.[14] In addition, giving IFN-α or IFN-γ to patients to treat cancer and other diseases has led to the triggering or exacerbation of a variety of underlying autoimmune diseases.[15]

We would like to emphasize that various autoimmune diseases have several features in common, including disturbed cytokine synthesis as a mechanism of pathology. The different clinical manifestations of these diseases may depend on the site of disturbed T helper type 1 (Th1) cytokine production. High levels of IFN-γ and other Th1 cytokines, T cells producing IFN-γ and other cytokines, or Th1 cytokine mRNA compared with controls have been found at the disease site of many Th1 autoimmune diseases (TABLE 1).

We conducted the first anti–IFN-γ therapy in Th1-mediated diseases together with several clinics using a polyclonal anti–IFN-γ antibody (both IgG and F[ab′]2 antibody fragments) and in some cases, for comparison, a polyclonal anti–TNF-α. The antibodies were given intramuscularly or topically once or twice daily for 5–7 days. Side effects have been limited mainly to local dermatitis at the injection site, which disappeared within 2–3 days. TABLE 2 provides a summary of the results of these studies.

Our investigations suggest that anti–IFN-γ may have clinical effects that are as good as and sometimes superior to anti–TNF-α. Rapid responses to anti–IFN-γ and anti–TNF-α were observed in most autoimmune diseases treated. For example, in rheumatoid arthritis, a reduction in pain and edema was observed after a short course of five to six injections. In some conditions, such as multiple sclerosis (MS), anti–TNF-α was ineffective, confirming other studies.[25] This may be connected with the

TABLE 2. Th1-mediated autoimmune diseases treated with anti–IFN-γ and in some cases anti–TNF-α

Disease	Treatment	Results	Reference(s)
Rheumatoid arthritis	Open-label and randomized, double-blind, placebo-controlled studies with anti–IFN-γ and anti–TNF-α	• Open-label (23 patients), randomized (55 patients: 20 receiving anti–IFN-γ; 20 receiving anti–TNF-α; 15 receiving placebo) • 5 of 17 anti–IFN-γ patients, 5 of 16 anti–TNF-α patients completing trial achieved ACR 50% response rate by day 28 • 6 anti–IFN-γ patients achieved ACR 70% response by day 28 compared to none receiving anti–TNF-α or placebo • Clinical remission longer in those receiving anti–IFN-γ than anti–TNF-α in open-label and randomized trials • Comparison by ultrasound of joint swelling found significant decrease only in anti–IFN-γ group	27–29
Secondary progressive multiple sclerosis	Open-label and randomized, double-blind, placebo-controlled studies with anti–IFN-γ and anti–TNF-α	• Open-label (22 patients), randomized (45 patients: 15 receiving anti–IFN-γ; 15 receiving anti–TNF-α; 15 receiving placebo) • After 12-month observation, anti–IFN-γ group had significant increase in number of patients free of sustained EDSS progression, in mean time without sustained EDSS progression and without gadolinium-enhancing lesions (using MRI) • No significant response in anti–TNF-α or placebo group	30
Corneal transplant rejection	Anti–IFN-γ and anti–TNF-α as eye drops	• By 2–3 days after start of treatment, transplant transparency improved and edema decreased in 10 of 13 patients • By 1 week, transplant almost fully transparent, no eye inflammation, improved visual acuity • Other 3 patients improved with additional treatment courses • Comparable response in 4 anti–TNF-α patients	31

TABLE 2. (*continued*) Thl-mediated autoimmune diseases treated with anti–IFN-γ and in some cases anti–TNF-α

Disease	Treatment	Results	Reference(s)
Type I diabetes	Anti–IFN-γ, anti–TNF-α in separate groups	• 3 patients received anti–IFN-γ • Treatments associated with increase in C-peptide levels, decrease in blood glucose, and reduction in insulin dose • Note: Skin ulcers, a complication of diabetes, may also be connected with disturbed cytokine production and treatment could be local or systemic injection of anti–IFN-γ, anti–TNF-α, or an IL-1 receptor antagonist	32
Psoriatic arthritis	Anti–IFN-γ intramuscularly	• 5 patients • Clinical response of lesions same as in psoriasis vulgaris	33
Psoriasis vulgaris	Anti–IFN-γ intradermally around lesion and intramuscularly	• 7 patients • Rapid reduction of erythema intensity and disappearance of papular infiltrates 3–4 days after treatment • Clearing of psoriatic plaques and complete remission in 4 patients after several weeks (see FIG. 1, bottom)	34
Alopecia areata	Anti–IFN-γ intradermally around lesion and intramuscularly	• 16 patients (aged 6–15 years) • 8 of 9 patients with patchy, progressive hair loss stabilized by day 4 with no additional hair loss • After 4–6 months, partial but ongoing (4 patients), or full (4 patients) terminal: fully restored hair growth was observed, including eyebrows and/or eyelashes (see FIG. 1, top) • No response in 9th patient • Little or no response in 5 patients who were 100% bald • Of 2 patients with stable, but patchy hair loss, one had eyelash and eyebrow hair restoration, but neither had hair growth in scalp	35
Vitiligo	Anti–IFN-γ intradermally around lesion and intramuscularly	• 4 patients • 2 responded with repigmentation in treated area • An additional course of intramuscular injections led to gradual diminishment of border between depigmented area and normal skin in other 2 patients	36

TABLE 2. (*continued*) **Th1-mediated autoimmune diseases treated with anti–IFN-γ and in some cases anti–TNF-α**

Disease	Treatment	Results	Reference(s)
Uveitis associated with juvenile rheumatoid arthritis	Anti–IFN-γ with NSAIDs vs. NSAIDs alone	• In 4 of 6 patients, anti–IFN-γ + NSAID therapy halved duration of acute period, decreased severity of symptoms during acute period, and substantially increased length of remission compared to NSAIDs alone	37
Acne vulgaris	Anti–IFN-γ compress applied to lesion	• Pustular elements dried with no fresh elements appearing by day 2 of treatment • By day 4, infiltrated elements remained but had paled in color	38
Seborrheic dermatitis	Anti–IFN-γ compress applied to lesion every 2 h for 1–2 min	• By day 2 of treatment, itching decreased, large area of peeling shrank to small scaly area • By day 3, skin paled	38
Herpes simplex virus type 1	Anti–IFN-γ-compress applied to lesions every 2 h for 1–2 min.	• After 3–3.5 h, patients noted rapid reduction of burning and pain in lesion • After 2 days, scabs formed, which faded in 5 days	38

EDSS, Expanded Disability Status Scale.

reported demyelinating effect of anti–TNF-α.[26] This suggests it would be rational to treat MS with standard therapy (IFN-β) together with anti–IFN-γ and IL-10.

TABLE 2 presents results of treating various Th1-mediated skin diseases, but a Th1-mediated immune response appears to be involved in many other skin diseases, including rosacea, oral lichen planus, and dermatophytosis. T cell subsets are found in the dermal infiltrates of rosacea lesions frequently associated with the parasite *Demodex folliculorum*.[39] Although there is little research on this parasite as an inducer of proinflammatory cytokines, chronic dermatitis was found associated with large numbers of *Demodex* ectoparasites, and pronounced CD4 and CD8 T cell infiltrates in the dermis and lymphadenopathy associated with increased IFN-γ and IL-12 expression were observed.[40] IFN-γ–producing cells are found in the skin lesions of dermatophytosis.[41] In oral lichen planus, mononuclear cells express IFN-γ in the superficial lamina propria.[42] Our near-term goal is to test ACT in these conditions. TABLE 3 shows the Th1 cytokines, particularly IFN-γ and TNF-α, found in the lesions of these skin diseases as well as in psoriasis vulgaris and alopecia areata. Thus, IFN-γ and/or Th1 cells found the lesions of these skin diseases appear to be induced by various viruses, bacteria, fungi, and other factors.

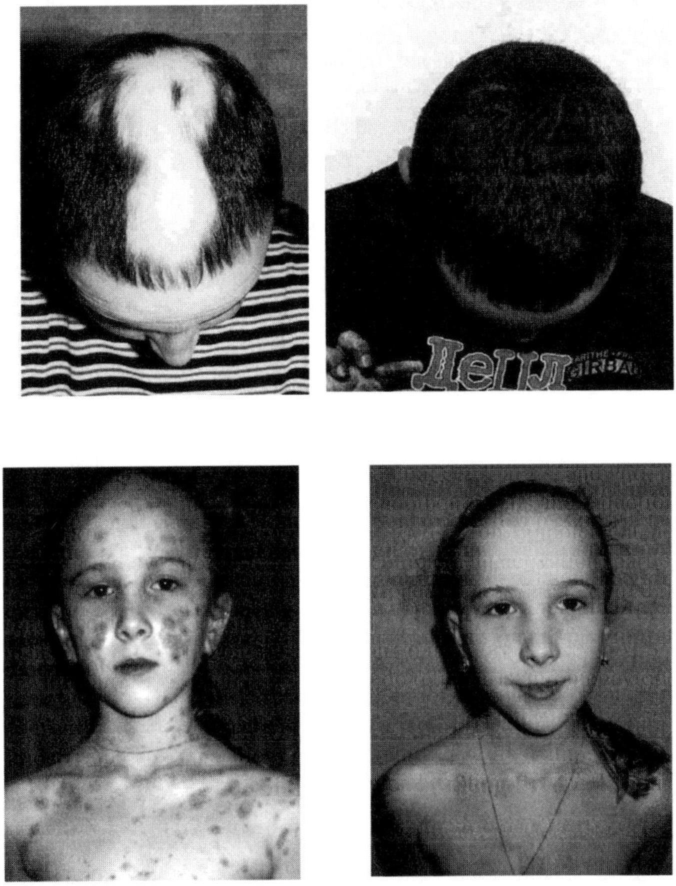

FIGURE 1. Alopecia areata and psoriasis vulgaris treated with anti–IFN-γ antibodies. (*Top left*) Fourteen-year-old patient with alopecia areata lasting 4.5 months before intradermal treatment with anti–IFN-γ antibodies. (*Top right*) Patient 12 weeks after start of treatment. (*Bottom left*) Eleven-year-old patient before treatment with anti–IFN-γ antibodies. (*Bottom right*) Patient 15 days after start of treatment.

Crohn Disease

We first proposed to treat Crohn disease with ACT in 1991. A humanized monoclonal antibody to IFN-γ HuZAF® (fontolizumab) was later developed and is now in clinical testing for the treatment of Crohn disease (Protein Design Labs, California). Remicade® (infliximab; TNF-α antibody) is approved for treatment of Crohn disease. Because the colon is involved, we have proposed that Crohn disease be treated with ACT (anti–IFN-γ or anti–TNF-α) together with vitamin B_{12} in tablet form, as an injection, or as a chemical compound with an anticytokine.

TABLE 3. Th1-mediated inflammatory skin diseases and implicated or possibly associated infectious agents

Disease	Implicated or possible factors or cofactors	Th1 cytokines detected in lesions	Reference(s)
Psoriasis vulgaris	Group A β-hemolytic streptococci	IFN-γ	43
Alopecia areata	Human endogenous retrovirus as found in other autoimmune diseases	T-cell clones that release large amounts of IFN-γ and/or TNF-α	44
Acne vulgaris	*P. acnes* (bacteria) estrogen	IFN-γ, IL-1, TNF-α	24,45
Seborrheic dermatitis	*Pityrosporum ovale* (fungus)	IFN-γ, TNF-α	46
Rosacea	*Demodex follicularium* (parasite)	T cell infiltrates: source of IFN-γ production	39,40
Dermatophytosis	Fungi	IFN-γ	41
Oral lichen planus	Unknown	IFN-γ, TNF-α	42

AIDS

We first proposed that HIV belongs to a category of viruses in which hyperproduced IFN increases rather than stops viral replication. We first suggested that IFN-α plays a pathological role in AIDS and removal of IFN-α could be therapeutic.[47] Later, we suggested removal of TNF-α together with IFN-α in AIDS.[3] These cytokines are closely connected.[48] Many of the clinical manifestations of HIV-infected individuals are related to the immune dysfunction of HIV disease, often caused by the overproduction of proinflammatory cytokines, including excessive production of TNF-α and IFN-α. Laboratory studies have concluded that TNF-α contributes significantly to HIV-1–induced pathology in transgenic mice; anti–TNF-α has prevented the development of pathology by suppressing the level of TNF-α.[49] TNF-α inhibitors have also shown promising results in small trials with AIDS patients.[50,51] It is possible in AIDS, use of three anticytokines, anti–IFN-γ, anti–IFN-α, and anti–TNF-α, could be beneficial.

IFN-α has been found to be highly correlated with disease progression in AIDS.[52] Anti–IFN-α was tested in four patients with advanced AIDS with encouraging results.[53,54] After our work, a vaccine against IFN-α was developed and demonstrated good effects in HIV infection in placebo-controlled, double-blind studies.[55] This work was supported by research showing that anti–IFN-α prevents generation of HIV-1–induced suppressor cells.[56]

SOME GENETIC SKIN DISEASES IN WHICH TH1 CYTOKINES MAY BE INVOLVED

Dystrophic epidermolysis bullosa (DEB) is a genetic disease involving a defect in the gene for type VII collagen.[57] However, it may also involve autoimmune mechanisms. IFN-γ could also be involved by altering gene expression.[58] Based on evidence in the literature of immune system involvement and signs of inflammation in a patient suffering severely from DEB, we treated two cases with striking results, including normalization of temperature; disappearance of pain, swelling, and hyperemia around ulcerative lesions at the back of the neck; and signs of infectious damage to the skin on the back. By day 7 after start of treatment, active epithelialization of the ulcerative skin lesions was observed along with improvement in a general sense of well-being and sleep.[59] Observation continues. Anti–TNF-α was ineffective in one patient.

Very low levels of IFN-γ, IL-1, and IL-2 have been found to be produced *in vitro* by peripheral blood mononuclear cells (PBMCs), common in autoimmune disease, from patients with severe forms of epidermolysis bullosa (EB; recessive dystrophic and dominant dystrophic) as compared with sex- and age-matched controls.[60] Individuals with more severe forms of EB have demonstrated significant reductions in natural-killer (NK) cell activity.[61] Deficiencies in NK cells have been shown to be associated with certain autoimmune diseases.[62] This case brought us strong emotional satisfaction. We plan to test the treatment using humanized monoclonal antibodies to IFN-γ or other depressors of the production of certain other cytokines.

BENEFICIAL EFFECT OF ANTI–IFN-γ IN POSSIBLY NON–TH1-MEDIATED SKIN DISEASES

Herpes Simplex Virus Type 2

IFN is generally known to stop viral replication in herpes simplex virus type 2 (HSV2). Recurrent HSV2 genital lesions, however, appear to be a special case in which dysregulated production of IFN-γ exerts a pathological effect on the organism by paradoxically helping the virus survive or replicate.[63] We have proposed that certain viruses may belong to a special category in which dysregulated production of IFNs may help sustain the virus.[47] In this category may belong oncogenic viruses, HIV, rubella virus, papillomavirus, and possibly certain other bacteria and viruses, including some human endogenous retroviruses (HERVs). In the case of HERVs, for example, which are associated with various autoimmune diseases, these viruses may induce IFN-γ, which, in turn, increases release of the virus.[64] HSV2 may also belong to this category. IFN-γ may directly damage cells in this disease. Thus, removal of IFN-γ, TNF-α, or IL-1 could help destroy the viruses or other agents sustained by these cytokines and ameliorate the condition. We have very preliminary positive data from the topical application of anti–IFN-γ in three patients with recurrent HSV2 genital lesions. Pain was immediately relieved on application of the antibody, and the skin began to quickly epithelialize. Further studies using anti–IFN-γ need to be undertaken to confirm this preliminary finding. In addition, topical use of antagonists of TNF-α and IL-1 in different combinations should be tested in this condition.

Parenteral injection and oral administration of a special form of ACT should also be tested.

OTHER ANTICYTOKINE THERAPIES

In this section, we discuss some of the major ACTs. This is not a comprehensive list. Many of these have been extensively reviewed elsewhere.

Anti–TNF-α

As mentioned, we first proposed use of anti–TNF-α together with certain anti–IFN antibodies to treat AIDS and other autoimmune diseases.[3] Now, inhibitors of TNF-α (infliximab/Remicade®; etanercept/Enbrel®; and adalimumab/Humira®) have been approved by the U.S. FDA as therapies for patients with various autoimmune diseases, including rheumatoid arthritis, ankylosing spondylitis (AS), psoriasis and psoriatic arthritis, and inflammatory bowel disease (Crohn disease). These TNF-α blockers have been quite successful. In patients with rheumatoid arthritis, when used repeatedly for a long time, these drugs (etanercept or adalimumab) produce a generally good clinical response and reduce radiographic disease progress.[65,66] In psoriasis, TNF-α antagonists are reported to be dramatically effective in moderate to severe psoriasis and to produce long-lasting remission.[67] In patients with AS, improvement has been observed in several clinical, function, and quality-of-life parameters.[68] However, these therapies have many risks, including those of increased infections, reactivation of latent tuberculosis, malignancies (e.g., lymphoma), worsening of congestive heart failure, and inflammatory demyelinating disease of the central nervous system.[69] Most of these conditions were not observed until after the drugs were used for several years in the broad patient population. Additional adverse effects of these therapies continue to appear in the literature, such as the triggering of alopecia areata.[70] This experience is important and must be considered in using anti–TNF-α in treating any autoimmune disease in the future. The cause of the complications must also be understood to develop safer TNF-α blockers.

IL-1 Receptor Antagonist

An IL-1 receptor antagonist (anakinra/Kineret) to treat rheumatoid arthritis has not been used as long as the TNF-α antagonists, so its long-term efficacy and safety are still unknown.

Anti–IL-6

An anti–IL-6 receptor antibody (atlizumab) has been tested at two dose levels in a double-blind, placebo-controlled trial in patients with rheumatoid arthritis with good results.[71]

Anti–IFN-α

Anti–IFN-α was first used in rheumatoid arthritis and later in AIDS with promising results.[2,53,54] Anti–IFN-α has also been used with good effect in preventing type I diabetes in a mouse model.[72] In very preliminary studies, patients with arthroses and rheumatic fever were given a short course of donkey anti–IFN-α affinity-purified antibodies with dramatic results. In the patients with arthroses, pain was reduced and joint mobility was increased. In the rheumatic fever cases, heart edema disappeared in a short time, and the patients noted an increased sense of well-being (unpublished data).

Other Anticytokine Drugs and Vitamins

Certain natural factors may also help stabilize IFN-γ production, such as vitamins A and D. Vitamin A (retinoids) inhibits IFN-γ release by PBMCs.[73] Vitamin D, which, among other effects, inhibits IFN-γ synthesis,[74] may be an important factor in MS, in which a correlation of increasing prevalence with increasing latitude has been observed, attributed to an ultraviolet radiation–induced increase in serum vitamin D levels, which may have a protective effect.[75]

ACT in Th1/Th2 Diseases

Although Th1/Th2 autoimmune disease is not in the purview of this chapter, we would like to make some observations on the treatment of some of these diseases. Atopic dermatitis is a disease in which hyperproduced Th1 and Th2 cytokines are involved, depending on the phase of the disease. In the initiation phase, IL-4 production by Th2 and Th0 cells is predominant over IFN-γ production by Th1 cells, whereas in the late and chronic phases, the situation is reversed with IFN-γ production dominant over IL-4, IL-5, and IL-13 production by Th2 and Th0 cells.[76] Use of anti-Th1 cytokines or anti-Th2 cytokines thus may be effective, depending on the phase of the disease.

In diseases that involve hyperproduction of both Th1 and Th2 cytokines, such as systemic lupus erythematosus (SLE), use of inhibitors of Th1 cytokines alone may not be effective. As an example, ACT tested in four patients with SLE (two with anti–IFN-γ alone, two with both anti–IFN-γ and anti–TNF-α) at first gave some positive response but later was found ineffective, with the condition worsening in three of four patients (two who received anti–IFN-γ and one who received the combination).[29]

PRE-AUTOIMMUNE DISEASE

High-Risk Relatives

Many autoimmune diseases may be preceded by a period of hyperproduction of Th1 or Th2 cytokines before clinical manifestations. Symptoms may appear with damage from autoantibody action or the direct action of the cytokines. Before symptoms of autoimmune disease begin, it is possible that checking the PBMCs, cell surface, and spinal fluid for cytokines from high-risk relatives of people with autoimmune diseases could give a strong indication of coming disease. A study investigating high-risk first-degree relatives of type 1 diabetic patients found a high production of IFN-γ in the PBMCs,[77] which may explain why in many fully developed autoimmune diseases, *in vitro* stimulation of PBMCs results in low IFN-γ production—that is, it may be the result of exhaustion of IFN-γ or other cytokine production in a pre-autoimmune phase.

Viruses and Autoimmune Disease

Viruses are long known to be associated with autoimmunity. This may be through the induction of Th1 cytokines, particularly IFN-γ. Mumps, measles, coxsackie B viruses,[78] and possibly others appear to induce IFN-γ or other Th1 cytokines *in vivo*. IFN-γ has been found to be elevated in measles, rubella, and parvovirus infection[79] and in PBMCs of infected autologous or allogenic mumps virus–infected target cells.[80] Also, IFN-γ levels in the serum are increased in patients in the acute phase of measles.[81] Mumps virus, a virus often associated with type 1 diabetes, also brings autoimmune complications, such as orchitis. It may be that orchitis associated with mumps viruses is actually triggered by the IFN-γ induced by the virus. IFN-γ may also directly destroy the cells at the same time. Thus anti–IFN-γ may prevent complications after infection with mumps. Anti–IFN-γ as a downregulator of testicular autoimmunity has been confirmed in a mouse model.[13]

As was pointed out by Deng *et al.*,[82] in cases in which an autoimmune disease is associated with a virus, autoimmunity may not always result from a response to a specific pathogen, as in cases of molecular mimicry, but rather from a generic immune response triggered by certain types of viruses. In some autoimmune diseases, as in many inflammatory skin diseases associated with infectious agents, this may involve the induction of a Th1 cytokine pathway and Th1 cytokine hyperproduction. Testing for high levels of IFN-γ may be useful after infection with certain viruses associated with autoimmune disease, such as those mentioned above; removing this IFN-γ may help prevent onset of certain viral-induced autoimmune diseases or prevent autoimmune complications, such as orchitis in mumps infection.

DISCUSSION

Many cytokines, including IFN-γ, play a fundamental role in the regulation of the metabolism and immunologic status of cells in a healthy state, which begins in the embryonic period.

The function of IFN-γ is broad, thus we cannot dismiss, as mentioned, the idea that IFN-γ participates in normal metabolism and the function of the normal physiologic action of cells. IFN-γ plays a significant role in the establishment of immunity and the realization of cell-mediated and humoral immunity. Every change or disturbance in the production of IFN-γ, in addition to other pathological actions, may, as we have hypothesized,[1,27,83] also play a key role in the development of autoantigen and autoantigen complexes, which in some cases may have mimicry with antigens of normal organs. There may be more than one type of IFN-γ. Moreover, every antigen and autoantigen may induce (have) a specific IFN-γ that helps commit lymphocytes to a specific immune response. We have proposed that possibly, besides IFN-γ, IFN-α may play a similar role as IFN-γ.[83] As is known, IFN-α has 12 subtypes[84] and some of them may also play a role in the formation of autoantigens alone or together with IFN-γ. Some types of autoimmune diseases may be connected with a special or defective type of IFN-γ or IFN-α or an altered IFN-γ or IFN-α pathway.

The main goal for rational treatment of Th1, Th2, and combined Th1/Th2-mediated autoimmune diseases is to return the organism to homeostasis or a Th1/Th2 balance. Suppressing or removing the hyperproduced cytokines with the help of antibodies or other repressors, soluble receptors, vitamins, minerals and microelements, or various agents that suppress cytokine synthesis may effectively do this.

In regard to immunologic methods to treat autoimmune and allergic diseases, besides passive immunization, active immunization with various cytokines (e.g., IFN-α, IFN-γ, TNF-α, IL-6, IL-4, IL-5, IL-13, and others) could also be used, as we have described, to treat autoimmune and allergic conditions. Such vaccines can be used alone, in combination, independently, or after passive immunization and other methods.

As is apparent, the role of cytokines in human physiology and pathology is enormous. The level and quality of cytokine production, especially in different brain cells, may directly or indirectly influence a wider range of behavior than is now appreciated. It has been argued that syphilis may have played a role in the achievements of some of history's most creative artists, including Beethoven, Schubert, and van Gogh.[85] Syphilis has been called the Great Imitator because its later stages can mimic measles, system lupus erythematosus, manic depression, epilepsy, and schizophrenia, all cytokine-disturbance diseases. The general T cell response to *T. pallidum* antigens in syphilis infection has been shown to be biased toward the Th1 phenotype.[86] We speculate that genius may involve the heightened sensitivity of certain brain cells to unusually high levels of cytokines or other changes in cytokine production.[83] At the same time, syphilis may have had darker effects by somehow exacerbating extreme obsessions or hatred. Thus, cytokine production could be what separates genius and psychosis.

The kind of production of cytokines in the brain may determine certain aspects of character. Besides depression and schizophrenia, many other neuropsychiatric illnesses such as Parkinson disease, Alzheimer disease, obsessive-compulsive disorder, anorexia nervosa, autism, and post-traumatic stress disorder are associated with disturbed cytokine production. In other words, cytokines may be key to understanding a connection between certain extreme or abnormal behaviors, including great creativity and dementia. Brain trauma may also have this effect as in the example of Mozart, who suffered a long-lasting brain hematoma after a fall. In all these cases, persistent hyperproduction of inflammatory cytokines and the neurotoxic effects of nitric oxide induced by inflammatory cytokines may be at the basis.

In conclusion, Th1-mediated autoimmune diseases share certain characteristics. First, anti–IFN-γ or anti–TNF-α may generally be universal treatments for Th1 autoimmune diseases, particularly skin diseases. Second, every Th1 autoimmune disease develops through a pathological immune cascade such that removal of one member of the cascade can have some therapeutic effect. Third, all autoimmune diseases develop with a reduced ability of the mononuclear cells to induce *in vitro* IFN-γ in response to stimulation. Fourth, deficiencies in NK cells are associated with autoimmune disease.[62] Fifth, autoimmune diseases are generally chronic but in some cases can be temporary.

Research on the use of ACT, first introduced in 1974[1] and 1989,[3] will continue to stimulate the development of other cytokine repressors and contribute to the understanding and treatment of these diseases.

REFERENCES

1. SKURKOVICH, S.V., E.G. KLINOVA, E.I. EREMKINA & N.V LEVINA. 1974. Immunosuppressive effect of an anti-interferon serum. Nature **247:** 551–552.
2. SKURKOVICH, S.V. & E.I. EREMKINA. 1975. The probable role of interferon in allergy. Ann. Allergy **35:** 356–360.
3. SKURKOVICH, S.V. & B. SKURKOVICH. 1989. Development of autoimmune diseases is connected with the initial disturbance of IFN synthesis in the cells. J. IFN Res. **9** (Suppl. 2): S305.
4. SKURKOVICH, S.V., A.S. SKORIKOVA, N.A. DUBROVINA, *et al.* 1977. Lymphocytes' cytotoxicity towards cells of human lymphoblastoid lines in patients with rheumatoid arthritis and systemic lupus erythematosus. Ann. Allergy **39:** 344–350.
5. KAWAKAMI, Y., N. KUZUYA, T. WATANABE, *et al.* 1990. Induction of experimental thyroiditis in mice by recombinant interferon gamma administration. Acta Endocrinol. (Copenh.) **122:** 41–48.
6. EGWUAGU, C.E., R.M. MAHDI, C.C. CHAN, *et al.* 1999. Expression of interferon-gamma in the lens exacerbates anterior uveitis and induces retinal degenerative changes in transgenic Lewis rats. Clin. Immunol. **91:** 196–205.
7. HARTUNG, H.P., B. SCHAFER, P.H. VAN DER MEIDE, *et al.* 1990. The role of interferon-gamma in the pathogenesis of experimental autoimmune disease of the peripheral nervous system. Ann. Neurol. **27:** 247–257.
8. SETIADY, Y.Y., P. PRAMOONJAGO & K.S. TUNG. 2004. Requirements of NK cells and proinflammatory cytokines in T cell-dependent neonatal autoimmune ovarian disease triggered by immune complex. J. Immunol. **173:** 1051–1058.
9. DEBRAY-SACHS, M., C. CARNAUD, C. BOITARD, *et al.* 1991. Prevention of diabetes in NOD mice treated with antibody to murine IFN gamma. J. Autoimmun. **4:** 237–248.
10. NICOLETTI, F., P. ZACCONE, R. DI MARCO, *et al.* 1997. Prevention of spontaneous autoimmune diabetes in diabetes-prone BB rats by prophylactic treatment with anti-rat interferon-gamma antibody. Endocrinology **13:** 281–288.
11. TANG, H., K. MIGNON-GODEFROY, P.L. MERONI, *et al.* 1993. The effects of a monoclonal antibody to interferon-gamma on experimental autoimmune thyroiditis (EAT): prevention of disease and decrease of EAT-specific T cells. Eur. J. Immunol. **23:** 275–278.
12. TSAI, C.P., J.D. POLLARD & P.J. ARMATI. 1991. Interferon-gamma inhibition suppresses experimental allergic neuritis: modulation of major histocompatibility complex expression of Schwann cells in vitro. J. Neuroimmunol. **31:** 133–145.
13. ITOH, M., A. YANO, Q. XIE, *et al.* 1998. Essential pathogenic role for endogenous interferon-gamma (IFN-gamma) during disease onset phase of murine experimental autoimmune orchitis. I. In vivo studies. Clin. Exp. Immunol. **111:** 513–520.
14. KAGEYAMA, Y., Y. KOIDE, A. YOSHIDA, *et al.* 1998. Reduced susceptibility to collagen-induced arthritis in mice deficient in IFN-gamma receptor. J. Immunol. **161:** 1542–1548.
15. MIOSSEC, P. 1997. Cytokine-induced autoimmune disorders. Drug Saf. **17:** 93–104.
16. CANETE, J.D., S.E. MARTINEZ & J. FARRES. 2000. Differential Th-1/Th-2 cytokine patterns in chronic arthritis: interferon gamma is highly expressed in synovium of rheumatoid arthritis compared with seronegative spondyloarthropathies. Ann. Rheum. Dis. **59:** 263–268.
17. WOODROOFE, M.N. & M.L. CUZNER. 1993. Cytokine mRNA expression in inflammatory multiple sclerosis lesions: detection by non-radioactive in situ hybridization. Cytokine **5:** 583–588.
18. TRAUGOTT, U. & P. LEBON. 1988. Interferon-gamma and Ia antigen are present on astrocytes in active chronic multiple sclerosis lesions. J. Neurol. Sci. **84:** 257–264.
19. YAMAGAMI, S., H. KAWASHIMA & H. ENDO. 1998. Cytokine profiles of aqueous humor and graft in orthotopic mouse corneal transplantation. Transplantation **66:** 1504–1510.
20. VON HERRATH, M.G. & M.B. OLDSTONE. 1997. Interferon-gamma is essential for destruction of beta cells and development of insulin-dependent diabetes mellitus. J. Exp. Med. **185:** 531–539.

21. Whitcup, S.M., C.C. Chan, Q. Li &R.B. Nussenblatt. 1992. Expression of cell adhesion molecules in posterior uveitis. Arch. Ophthalmol. **110:** 662–666.
22. Barker, J.N., G.D. Karabin, T.J. Stoof, *et al.* 1991. Detection of interferon-gamma mRNA in psoriatic epidermis by polymerase chain reaction. J. Dermatol. Sci. **2:** 106–111.
23. Grimes P.E. & R. Morris. 2004. Topical tacrolimus therapy for vitiligo: therapeutic responses and skin messenger RNA expression of proinflammatory cytokines. J. Am. Acad. Dermatol. **51:** 52–61.
24. Mouser, P.E., B.S. Baker, E.D. Seaton & A.C. Chu. 2003. Propionibacterium acnes-reactive T helper-1 cells in the skin of patients with acne vulgaris. J. Invest. Dermatol. **121:** 1226–1228.
25. Lenercept Multiple Sclerosis Study Group and the University of British Columbia MS/MRI Analysis Group. 1999. TNF neutralization in MS: results of a randomized, placebo-controlled multicenter study. Neurology **53:** 457–465.
26. Thomas, C.W., Jr., B.G. Weinshenker & W.J. Sandborn. 2004. Demyelination during anti-tumor necrosis factor alpha therapy with infliximab for Crohn's disease. Inflamm. Bowel Dis. **10:** 28–31.
27. Skurkovich, S.V., G.V. Loukina, Y.A. Sigidin & B.S. Skurkovich. 1998. Successful first-time use of antibodies to interferon-gamma alone and combined with antibodies to tumor necrosis factor-alfa to treat rheumatic diseases (rheumatoid arthritis, systemic lupus erythematosus, psoriatic arthritis, Behcet's syndrome). Int. J. Immunotherapy **14:** 23–32.
28. Sigidin, A.Y., G.V. Loukina, B. Skurkovich & S.V. Skurkovich. 2001. Randomized double-blind trial of anti-interferon-γ antibodies in rheumatoid arthritis. Scan. J. Rheumatol. **30:** 203–207.
29. Loukina, G., Y. Sigidin, O. Pashkova, *et al.* 2004. Clinical response to anti-interferon (IFN)-gamma and anti-tumor necrosis factor (TNF)-alpha compared in Th1-mediated autoimmune disease—rheumatoid arthritis(RA)—and Th1/Th2 disease (systemic lupus erythematosus (SLE)) [Abstract W51.46]. Twelfth International Congress of Immunology, Montreal.
30. Skurkovich, S.V., A. Boiko, I. Beliaeva, *et al.* 2001. Randomized study of antibodies to IFN-γ and TNF-α in secondary progressive multiple sclerosis. Mult. Scler. **7:** 277–284.
31. Skurkovich, S., A. Kasparov, N. Narbut & B. Skurkovich. 2002. Treatment of corneal transplant rejection in humans with anti-interferon-gamma antibodies. Am. J. Ophthalmol. **133:** 829–830.
32. Skurkovich, S.V., I.E. Volkov, V.M. Delyagin, *et al.* 2003. First use of anti-interferon (IFN)-γ in the treatment of type I diabetes in children [Abstract]. Eighth International Workshop on Autoantibodies and Autoimmunity, Berlin.
33. Skurkovich, S., Y. Sigidin, G. Loukina, *et al.* 1998. Successful anti-cytokine therapy using antibodies to IFN-γ, IFN-α, and TNF-α in patients with acute rheumatoid arthritis (RA), psoriatic arthritis (PA) and schizophrenia. Eur. Cytok. Network **9:** 451.
34. Skurkovich, S., N. Korotky, N.M. Sharova & B. Skurkovich. 2004. Successful anticytokine therapy in psoriasis [Abstract]. Ninth International Congress of Dermatology, Beijing.
35. Skurkovich, S., N. Korotky, N.M. Sharova & B. Skurkovich. 2004. Successful treatment with anti-IFN-γ of alopecia areata (AA) [Abstract]. Ninth International Congress of Dermatology, Beijing.
36. Skurkovich, S., N. Korotky, N. Sharova & B. Skurkovich. 2002. Anti-interferon-γ to treat alopecia areata, psoriasis vulgaris, vitiligo, pemphigus vulgaris, and epidermolysis bullosa. In Proceedings of the 5th Asia Pacific Congress of Allergology and Clinical Immunology. Y.-Y. Kim, *et al.*, Eds.: 121–125. Monduzzi Editore. Bologna.
37. Skurkovich, S., V.M. Delyagin, A.G. Rumyantsev, *et al.* 2003. Anti-IFN-γ in the treatment of rheumatoid arthritis-associated uveitis in children [Abstract]. Eighth International Workshop on Autoantibodies and Autoimmunity, Berlin.
38. Skurkovich, S., B. Skurkovich, N. Korotky, *et al.* 2005. Anti-IFN-gamma As a Universal Treatment for Th1 Mediated Skin Diseases [Abstract]. Federation of Clinical Immunology Societies, Boston.

39. RUFLI, T. & S.A. BUCHNER. 1984. T-cell subsets in acne rosacea lesions and the possible role of Demadex folliculorum. Dermatologica **169:** 1–5.
40. LIU, Q., C. ARSECULERATNE, Z. LIU, *et al.* 2004. Simultaneous deficiency in CD28 and STAT6 results in chronic ectoparasite-induced inflammatory skin disease. Infect. Immun. **72:** 3706–3715.
41. KOGA, T., H. DUAN, K. URABE & M. FURUE. 2001. Immunohistochemical detection of interferon-gamma-producing cells in dermatophytosis. Eur. J. Dermatol. **11:** 105–107.
42. KHAN, A., C.S. FARAH, N.W. SAVAGE, *et al.* 2003. Th-1 cytokines in oral lichen planus. J. Oral. Pathol. Med. **32:** 77–83.
43. BROWN, D.W., B.S. BAKER, J.M. OVIGNE, *et al.* 2000. Skin CD4+ T cells produce interferon-gamma in vitro in response to streptococcal antigens in chronic plaque psoriasis. J. Invest. Dermatol. **114:** 576–580.
44. LA PLACA, M., F. VITONE, T. BIANCHI, *et al.* 2004. Serum antibodies against human intracisternal A-type particle (HIAP) endogenous retrovirus in alopecia areata patients: a hallmark of autoimmune disease? J. Invest. Dermatol. **123:** 407–409.
45. KARPUZOGLU-SAHIN, E., B.D. HISSONG & S. ANSAR AHMED. 2001. Interferon-gamma levels are upregulated by 17-beta-estradiol and diethylstilbestrol. J. Reprod. Immunol. **52:** 113–27.
46. FAERGEMANN, J., J.C. JONES, O. HETTLER & Y. LORIA. 1996. Pityrosporum ovale (*Malassezia furfur*) as the causative agent of seborrhoeic dermatitis: new treatment options. Br. J. Dermatol. **134** (Suppl. 46): 12–15 (discussion, 38).
47. SKURKOVICH, S., B. SKURKOVICH & J.A. BELLANTI. 1987. A unifying model of the immunoregulatory role of the interferon system: can interferon produce disease in humans? Clin. Immunol. Immunopathol. **43:** 362–373.
48. LAU, A.S., S.D. DER, S.E. READ & B.R. WILLIAMS. 1991. Regulation of tumor necrosis factor receptor expression by acid-labile interferon-alpha from AIDS sera. AIDS Res. Hum. Retroviruses **7:** 545–552.
49. DE, S.K., K. DEVADAS & A.L. NOTKINS. 2002. Elevated levels of tumor necrosis factor alpha (TNF-alpha) in human immunodeficiency virus type 1-transgenic mice: prevention of death by antibody to TNF-alpha. J. Virol. **76:** 11710–11714.
50. GAYLIS, N. 2003. Infliximab in the treatment of an HIV positive patient with Reiter's syndrome. J. Rheumatol. **30:** 407–411.
51. WALLIS, R.S., P. KYAMBADDE, J.L. JOHNSON, *et al.* 2004. A study of the safety, immunology, virology, and microbiology of adjunctive etanercept in HIV-1-associated tuberculosis. AIDS **18:** 257–264.
52. VADHAN-RAJ, S., G. WONG, C. GNECCO, *et al.* 1986. Immunological variables as predictors of prognosis in patients with Kaposi's sarcoma and the acquired immunodeficiency syndrome. Cancer Res. **46:** 417–425.
53. BELLANTI, J.A., S.V. SKURKOVICH, S.M. PETERS & G. ARIAS. 1987. Treatment of AIDS patients with anti-alpha IFN: an alternative approach. Second Annual Conference on Clinical Immunology of the Clinical Immunology Society, Washington, DC.
54. SKURKOVICH, S., B. SKURKOVICH & J. BELLANTI. 1994. A disturbance of interferon synthesis with the hyperproduction of unusual kinds of interferon can trigger autoimmune disease and play a pathogenetic role in AIDS: the removal of these interferons can be therapeutic. Med. Hypotheses **42:** 27–35.
55. GRINGERI, A., M. MUSICCO, P. HERMANS, *et al.* 1999. Active anti-interferon-alpha immunization: a European-Israeli, randomized, double-blind, placebo-controlled clinical trial in 242 HIV-1—infected patients (the EURIS study). J. AIDS Hum. Retrovirol. **20:** 358–370.
56. GALLO, R.C., A. BURNY & D. ZAGURY. 2002. Targeting Tat and IFN (alpha) as a therapeutic AIDS vaccine. DNA Cell Biol. **21:** 611–618.
57. GARDELLA, R., L. BELLETTI, N. ZOPPI, *et al.* 1996. Identification of two splicing mutations in the collagen type VII gene (COL7A1) of a patient affected by the localisata variant of recessive dystrophic epidermolysis bullosa. Am. J. Hum. Genet. **59:** 292–300.
58. BUNTINX, M., E. GIELEN, P. VAN HUMMELEN, *et al.* 2004. Cytokine-induced cell death in human oligodendroglial cell lines. II: alterations in gene expression induced by interferon-gamma and tumor necrosis factor-alpha. J. Neurosci. Res. **76:** 846–861.

59. KOROTKY, N.G., N.M. SHAROVA, B. SKURKOVICH & S. SKURKOVICH. 2004. Striking therapeutic effects in a patient with dysplastic epidermolysis bullosa using anti-IFN-γ (case report). Ninth International Congress of Dermatology, Beijing.
60. CHOPRA, V., S.K. TYRING, L. JOHNSON & J.D. FINE. 1992. Peripheral blood mononuclear cell subsets in patients with severe inherited forms of epidermolysis bullosa. Arch. Dermatol. **128:** 201–209.
61. TYRING, S.K., V. CHOPRA, L. JOHNSON & J.D. FINE. 1989. Natural killer cell activity is reduced in patients with severe forms of inherited epidermolysis bullosa. Arch. Dermatol. **125:** 797–800.
62. BAXTER, A.G. & M.J. SMYTH. 2002. The role of NK cells in autoimmune disease. Autoimmunity **35:** 1–14.
63. SINGH, R., A. KUMAR, W.D. CREERY, *et al.* 2003. Dysregulated expression of IFN-gamma and IL-10 and impaired IFN-gamma-mediated responses at different disease stages in patients with genital herpes simplex virus-2 infection. Clin. Exp. Immunol. **133:** 97–107.
64. SERRA, C., G. MAMELI, G. ARRU, *et al.* 2003. In vitro modulation of the multiple sclerosis (MS)-associated retrovirus by cytokines: implications for MS pathogenesis. J. Neurovirol. **9:** 637–643.
65. MORELAND, L.W. 2004. Drugs that block tumour necrosis factor: experience in patients with rheumatoid arthritis. Pharmacoeconomics. **22** (2 Suppl): 39–53.
66. SCOTT, D.L. 2004. Pursuit of optimal outcomes in rheumatoid arthritis. Pharmacoecomics **22** (2 suppl): 13–26.
67. GISONDI, P., E. GUBINELLI, B. COCUROCCIA & G. GIROLOMONI. 2004. Targeting tumor necrosis factor-alpha in the therapy of psoriasis. Curr. Drug Targets Inflamm. Allergy **3:** 175–183.
68. WENDLING, D. & E. TOUSSIROT. 2004. Anti-TNF-alpha therapy in ankylosing spondylitis. Expert Opin. Pharmacother. **5:** 1497–1507.
69. SCHEINFELD, N. 2004. A comprehensive review and evaluation of the side effects of the tumor necrosis factor alpha blockers etanercept, infliximab and adalimumab. J. Dermatolog. Treat. **15:** 280–294.
70. ETEFAGH, L., S. NEDOROST & P. MIRMIRANI. 2004. Alopecia areata in a patient using infliximab: new insights into the role of tumor necrosis factor on human hair follicles. Arch. Dermatol. **140:** 1012.
71. NISHIMOTO, N., K. YOSHIZAKI, N. MIYASAKA, *et al.* 2004. Treatment of rheumatoid arthritis with humanized anti-interleukin-6 receptor antibody: a multicenter, double-blind, placebo-controlled trial. Arthritis Rheum. **50:** 1761–1769.
72. STEWART, T.A., B. HULTGREN, X. HUANG, *et al.* 1993. Induction of type I diabetes by interferon-alpha in transgenic mice. Science **260:** 1942–1946.
73. WAUBEN-PENRIS, P.J., D.P. CERNEUS, W.E. VAN DEN HOVEN, *et al.* 1998. Immunomodulatory effects of tretinoin in combination with clindamycin. J. Eur. Acad. Dermatol. Venereol. **11** (Suppl 1): S2–S7.
74. CIPPITELLI M. & A. SANTONI. 1998. Vitamin D3: a transcriptional modulator of the interferon-gamma gene. Eur. J. Immunol. **28:** 3017–3030.
75. PONSONBY, A.L., A. MCMICHAEL & I. VAN DER MEI. 2002. Ultraviolet radiation and autoimmune disease: insights from epidemiological research. Toxicology **181–182:** 71–78.
76. THEPEN, T., E.G. LANGEVELD-WILDSCHUT, I.C. BIHARI, *et al.* 1996. Biphasic response against aeroallergen in atopic dermatitis showing a switch from an initial TH2 response to a TH1 response in situ: an immunocytochemical study. Allergy Clin. Immunol. **97:** 828–837.
77. KARLSSON, M.G., S.S. LAWESSON & J. LUDVIGSSON. 2000. Th1-like dominance in high-risk first-degree relatives of type I diabetic patients. Diabetologia **43:** 742–749.
78. VREUGDENHIL, G.R., P.G. WIJNANDS, M.G. NETEA, *et al.* 2000. Enterovirus-induced production of pro-inflammatory and T-helper cytokines by human leukocytes. Cytokine **12:** 1793–1796.
79. HARI, Y., A. URWYLER, M. HURNI, *et al.* 1999. Distinct serum cytokine levels in drug- and measles-induces exanthema. Int. Arch. Allergy Immunol. **120:** 225–229.

80. Martin, R., A. Vallbracht & H.W. Kreth. 1991. Interferon-gamma secretion by in vivo activated cytotoxic T lymphocytes from the blood and cerebrospinal fluid during mumps meningitis. J. Neuroimmunol. **33:** 191–198.
81. Ohga, S., C. Miyazaki, K. Okada, *et al.* 1992. The inflammatory cytokines in measles: correlation between serum interferon-gamma levels and lymphocyte subpopulations. Eur. J. Pediatr. **252:** 492–496.
82. Deng, C., C. Radu, A. Diab, *et al.* 2003. IL-1 receptor-associated kinase 1 regulates susceptibility to organ-specific autoimmunity. J. Immunol. **170:** 2833–2842.
83. Skurkovich, S.V., B. Skurkovich & J.A. Kelly. 2002. Anticytokine therapy—new approach to the treatment of autoimmune and cytokine-disturbance diseases. Med. Hypotheses **59:** 770–780.
84. Foster, G.R. & N.B. Finter. 1998. Are all type I human interferons equivalent? J. Viral Hepatitis **5:** 142–152.
85. Hayden, D. 2003. Pox: Genius, Madness, and the Mysteries of Syphilis. Basic Books. New York.
86. Arroll, T.W., A. Centurion-Lara, S.A. Lukehart & W.C. Van Voorhis. 1999. T-cell responses to *Treponema pallidum* subsp. *pallidum* antigens during the course of experimental syphilis infection. Infect. Immun. **67:** 4757–4763.

Therapeutic T Cell–Based Vaccination for Neurodegenerative Disorders

The Role of CD4$^+$CD25$^+$ Regulatory T Cells

MICHAL SCHWARTZ AND JONATHAN KIPNIS

Department of Neurobiology, The Weizmann Institute of Science, Rehovot, Israel

ABSTRACT: A well-controlled local immune response is needed for recovery from CNS injury, and autoimmune T cells play a key role in mediating this response. Autoimmunity, at least in the context of the CNS, is the body's fighting force against self-derived destructive compounds, and "tolerance to self" (traditionally though mistakenly equated with nonresponsiveness) should be viewed as the ability to tolerate autoimmune responses without developing an autoimmune disease. This physiological repair mechanism is controlled by naturally occurring CD4$^+$CD25$^+$ regulatory T cells (Treg cells), with an on/off switch regulated by brain-derived compounds. We suggest that ongoing neurodegeneration after acute injuries results from insufficiency of the endogenous fighting force, and chronic neurodegenerative diseases reflect age-related deterioration of the body's two principal regulators: the central nervous system (CNS) and the immune system. If so, then the restoration or boosting of immune function might bridge the gap between such manifestations of CNS-related risk factors and the defensive capacity of the immune system. Boosting of peripheral immunity by the use of weak agonists of CNS self-antigens, might offer a promising potential therapy for different neurodegenerative conditions. This could be accomplished either by vaccination with a universal weak T cell–reactive antigen or with altered peptide ligands of self-antigens, or by weakening the suppressive effect of autoimmunity (e.g., by eliminating Treg cells). T cells that home to the damaged CNS might then help restore local homeostasis by controlling the local microglial response. Because neurodegenerative diseases possess common features (deriving from the local chaos), the same vaccine might protect against several different disorders associated with impaired motor, sensory, cognitive, or mental functions of the brain.

KEYWORDS: neurodegenerative disease; T cell vaccines; central nervous system injury; peripheral neuropathy; microglia; CD4$^+$ cells; neuroprotection

INTRODUCTION

Injury to myelinated axons in the central nervous system (CNS) often has a devastating outcome in terms of neuronal loss, with accompanying loss of function. Part of the damage occurs immediately, and another part is delayed and leads to a

Addresses for correspondence: Michal Schwartz, Ph.D., Department of Neurobiology, Weizmann Institute of Science, 76100 Rehovot, Israel. Voice: +972-8-934-2467; fax: +972-8-934-6018.
michal.schwartz@weizmann.ac.il

Ann. N.Y. Acad. Sci. 1051: 701–708 (2005).
doi: 10.1196/annals.1361.114

loss of neurons that escaped the direct insult. The latter loss is termed *secondary degeneration* or self-perpetuating degeneration.

Autoimmunity has long been viewed as a destructive process. However, our research group recently provided evidence that autoimmunity is the body's endogenous response to CNS injury, and that its purpose is meant to be beneficial. This notion was based on the observation that in rodents, passive transfer of encephalitogenic (disease-inducing) T cells that are reactive to myelin basic protein (MBP) reduces postinjury neuronal losses.

During the last two decades, it has become increasingly clear that degenerative diseases of the CNS share a number of primary and secondary features.[1–4] In many such diseases, the local microglial response is often viewed as an unwelcome contributor to disease pathology.[5–7] Recent data suggest, however, that such a view is oversimplified, and that a well-controlled glial response can be beneficial in protecting the affected tissues,[7,8] whereas malfunctioning glia contribute to the ongoing neurodegenerative process.[9]

The spread of neuronal damage is caused, at least in part, by compounds that are normally essential for the survival and function of neurons; however, these compounds become toxic when their physiological concentrations are exceeded. Among the injury-related mechanisms that might underlie the posttraumatic spread of damage are biochemical and metabolic changes in oxygen and glucose utilization, energy state, lipid-dependent enzymes, free radicals, eicosanoids, tissue ions, biogenic amines, endogenous opioids, and excitatory amino acids. These changes cause alterations in cellular homeostasis, excitotoxicity, local production of agents harmful to nerve cells, and a loss of trophic support from targets—all of which result in secondary neuronal loss.

In the CNS, immune responses are relatively restricted, resulting in the status of the CNS as an immune-privileged site.[10] The unique nature of the communication between the CNS and the immune system can be observed, for example, in the dialogue between the CNS and T cells. In the healthy CNS, memory T cells (but not naive T cells) can cross the blood-brain barrier and enter the CNS parenchyma. However, only T cells capable of reacting with CNS antigens seem to persist there and only to a limited extent.[11] Comparative studies were undertaken of the T cell response at sites of axotomy in the CNS and the peripheral nervous system (PNS), using T cell immunocytochemistry. These studies revealed a significantly greater accumulation of endogenous T cells in injured PNS axons than in injured CNS axons.[12] Moreover, in cases of inflammation, the CNS showed a marked potential for eliminating T cells via apoptosis; such elimination was less effective in the PNS, and was almost absent in other tissues such as muscle and skin.[13]

RESPONSES TO CNS INJURY

Adaptive Immunity in CNS Repair

The first line of defense in any injured tissue is the innate immune response, characterized by activity of the phagocytic immune cells.[14] In the CNS, this defensive activity of the microglia (CNS-resident macrophages) is hardly tolerated unless it is tightly controlled. We have suggested that the local innate response to CNS injury

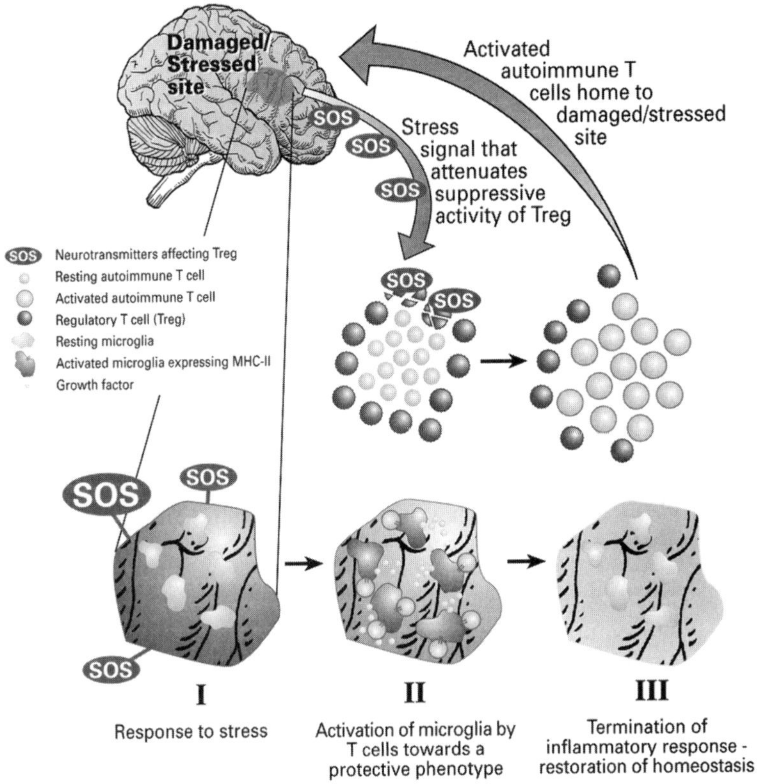

FIGURE 1. An autoimmune response regulated by brain-derived compounds protects damaged or stressed sites in the brain. Brain tissue subjected to damage or stress responds by producing various neurotransmitters and by activating resident glial cells to create a cytotoxic phenotype **(I)**. Compounds (such as dopamine[31]) originating from the damaged or stressed brain, and released to the periphery, apparently weaken the normally suppressive effect of Treg on circulating autoimmune effector T cells. On alleviation of the suppression, the autoimmune T cells home in on sites of CNS damage or stress,[12] where they become activated, upon being presented with their specific antigens by antigen-presenting cells. The autoimmune T cells in turn activate local glial cells to produce growth factors[40] and buffer toxic extracellular compounds such as glutamate **(II)**. Once brain-tissue homeostasis is restored, immune activity at the site diminishes **(III)**, and the autoimmune T cells return to their former state of suppression by Treg cells in the periphery.

can be controlled, at least in part, by the adaptive arm of the immune response in the form of CD4+ T cells (T helper [Th] cells).

There are different subpopulations of CD4+ T cells, and each is responsible for a certain type of immune response. Th1 cells, for example, reinforce cellular immunity, whereas Th2 cells induce humoral (antibody-mediated) immunity. These cells, in order to do their job, must first home in on sites of stress and be locally activated by their specific antigens that reside there. Thus, antigenic specificity apparently dictates the homing of T cells to the site at which their local activation can occur (Fig. 1).

Protective Autoimmunity in CNS Injury

Our group has suggested that neuroprotective T cells are likely to be those T cells that exhibit antigenic specificity to self-proteins that are abundantly expressed and presented at the site of injury, such as MBP. Studies from several laboratories have shown that T cells patrol the healthy CNS but do not accumulate there.[15,16] Autoimmune T cells reactive to MBP, when injected into rats or mice after CNS injury, confer significant protection on neurons; the result is a long-lasting, dramatic increase in neuronal survival accompanied by functional activity. CNS injury triggers a succession of complex processes, and therefore it is not surprising that multiple mechanisms participate in its repair. Any treatment based on a single molecule is likely to fail. It seems reasonable to assume that treatment aimed at multiple targets, such as administration of cells that can reach the site of injury and interact there with resident antigen-presenting cells, microglia, and astrocytes, would become the therapy of choice.

Our studies have also shown that a population of autoimmune ($CD4^+$) T cells locally boosts and controls resident microglia and infiltrating blood-borne monocytes, thereby helping these innate immune cells to acquire activity that allows them to fight off degenerative conditions. The autoimmune T cells allow the innate immune cells to buffer toxic compounds without producing excessive amounts of inflammation-associated cytotoxic compounds such tumor-necrosis factor (TNF)-α, nitric oxide, or cyclo-oxygenase (COX)–2.[17–21] T cells also allow the innate immune cells to produce growth factors, such as insulin-like growth factor-I (IGF-I), which are critical for neuronal survival and renewal.[22]

Thus, according to our results, the role of $CD4^+$ T cells directed against self-antigens is to activate the innate response in a well-controlled way, enabling it to recognize the threat to the tissue, not as a harmful organism that it must kill, but as a toxic substance that it must neutralize or eliminate. In addition, the T cells themselves, if locally activated, can produce protective compounds such as growth factors and neurotrophins.[23–25] All of these tasks can be accomplished by a well-controlled response by Th cells. T cells and factors derived from them can also facilitate the uptake of toxic neurotransmitters (such as glutamate) by astrocytes.[21] The ability of autoimmune T cells to target multiple deficits is probably what enables them to exert such a significant positive effect on neuronal survival. Their multipotency, moreover, allows them to be employed to treat various neurodegenerative conditions, because the therapy is based on a concept applicable to neurodegenerative diseases in general, and not on the over- or underproduction of a single disease-specific molecule.

Spontaneous Protective Autoimmune Response to CNS Injury

A spontaneous autoimmune T cell–based neuroprotective response is not a universal phenomenon. For example, strains of mice and rats differ in their ability to manifest a beneficial T cell–based response after injury, and hence in the extent to which their neurons can withstand an identical insult. In strains endowed with this spontaneous neuroprotection, local immune response of the injured CNS occurs early and is transient.[26] The response is caused by T cells that arrive at the injured site, where they activate resident microglia and astrocytes to express class II major histocompatibility complex (MHC-II).

In strains in which a spontaneous protective response cannot be evoked, the local immune response is delayed and poorly controlled.[26] In rats endowed with the ability to spontaneously manifest a protective autoimmune response to injury, neonatal tolerance to myelin-associated self-antigens (induced by neonatal immunization of neonatal rats with an emulsion of spinal cord homogenate) significantly reduces postinjury neuronal survival.[27] However, the induction of tolerance does not affect neuronal survival in rats that lack this spontaneous response.[27]

These and other results have led our group to propose that not all strains can spontaneously mount a protective T cell response against self-antigens; all strains, however, can benefit from the boosting of T cells directed to relevant self-antigens.[28,29]

Regulation of the T Cell–Mediated Neuroprotective Response by Naturally Occurring CD4+CD25+ Regulatory T Cells

Our group has discovered that autoimmunity is the body's defense mechanism against its own self-compounds, and that, in principle, T cells are spontaneously recruited in individuals with a genetic tendency toward autoimmune disease development. This discovery has led to the conclusion that a constitutively operating mechanism maintains the balance between the need for autoimmunity on the one hand and its attendant risks on the other.[30] This regulatory mechanism was shown to be displayed by a subpopulation of T cells, known as naturally occurring $CD4^+CD25^+$ regulatory T cells, or Treg cells.[31] Moreover, one of the molecular signals responsible for these cells' activity was found to be the stress-related compound dopamine.[32] The interaction between dopamine and Treg cells via the dopamine type 1 (D_1) receptor family downregulates Treg-cell activity.[32] Thus, the elimination or downregulation of Treg cells can be viewed as a means of boosting the physiological protective autoimmune response.[32,33]

THE ROLE OF T CELLS IN NORMAL BRAIN FUNCTIONING

Having discovered that T cells play a key role in brain repair,[36] we suspected that this role might be an extension of the physiological role these cells play in healthy individuals. The recent finding by our group that immune-deficient mice suffer from cognitive impairment[34] substantiated our contention that neurodegenerative diseases and age-related dementias, in addition to their local manifestations, are systemic diseases. This contention was supported by the finding that copolymer-1 (Cop-1) vaccination showed benefit in rodent models whose abnormal behavior reflected mental stress or cognitive impairment. Deviations from normal activity, whether caused by peripheral immune deficiency or local transmitter imbalance or brain damage, require systemic intervention by boosting T cells. Thus, T cell–based vaccination might be viewed as a means of "recharging" the immune system to meet the demands imposed by age and other risk factors.[27,34]

WAYS TO BOOST A PROTECTIVE IMMUNE RESPONSE

Any manipulation that activates the immune system to increase, in a well-controlled way, the chances of relevant T cells homing to a site of injury can be expected to be beneficial. We have examined two ways of obtaining the desired effect:

by inducing lymphopenia and by depleting, or functionally inactivating, naturally occurring regulatory $CD4^+CD25^+$ T cells.

Inducing Lymphopenia

Inducing lymphopenia significantly increases immunoreactivity toward cancer-specific proteins and efficiently suppresses cancer.[35] A sudden drop in the pool of peripheral T lymphocytes stimulates their homeostasis-driven proliferation in order to restore the pool. If the proliferative stimulus coincides with exposure to a relevant specific antigen, the T cell response to this antigen will be boosted. In response to the stimulus of lymphopenia, naive peripheral T cells proliferate and acquire a phenotype that resembles memory T cells.[36] The induced proliferation predisposes the individual to develop an autoimmune response because, under lymphopenic conditions, T cells can proliferate upon interaction with MHC-II molecules alone, with no need for a costimulatory signal.[37–39] If the body undergoes stress during lymphopenia induction, and consequently certain self-antigens are exposed (e.g., antigens related to tissue injury or cancer), an autoimmune response to those antigens will occur, resulting in a high overall proliferation of the relevant T lymphocytes.[40]

Our group has shown that, in rodents with acute or chronic neurodegenerative conditions, inducing lymphopenia significantly benefits postinjury neuronal survival.[33] Lymphopenia and the subsequent homeostatic proliferation can be induced in a number of ways; the most clinically relevant is low-dose irradiation of the lymphoid organs. Owing to lymphopenia, T cells proliferate and become activated. They patrol the body, and their patrol route includes the CNS. On reaching the lesion site, and after being activated by the resident cells that present self-antigens in the MHC-II groove, these lymphopenia-derived T cells perform their effector functions. In doing so, they resemble T cells obtained from immunization with self- or altered self-proteins.[32]

Weakening the Naturally Occurring Treg Cells

Because the aim of neurodegenerative disease therapy is to activate T cells that cross-react with self-antigens at the site of injury, this can also be done by weakening the naturally occurring Treg cells. In an experimental context, nude mice (devoid of mature T cells) repopulated with a T cell population that did not contain the Treg-cell subpopulation[27,41] demonstrated better recovery from a CNS insult than did wild-type mice of the same strain.

For clinical use, however, what is needed is a reagent that will weaken Treg cells. As mentioned earlier, dopamine was found to both weaken the activity and reduce the trafficking of Treg cells.[32] It is possible that dopamine comprises a family of physiological compounds (neurotransmitters and neuropeptides) capable of controlling Treg-cell activity and thereby allowing speedy recruitment of the relevant autoimmune T cells.

The development of synthetic compounds to reproduce the dopamine effect is another feasible approach toward a common immune-based therapy that could be used to fight off neurodegenerative diseases, regardless of their etiology. Although such compounds might weaken Treg cells nonselectively (disregarding their antigenic specificity), the evoked autoimmunity would be specific, and hence restricted to effector cells that encountered their relevant antigens, and would consequently be associated with the site under stress.

REFERENCES

1. Carri, M.T., A. Ferri, M. Cozzolino, *et al.* 2003. Neurodegeneration in amyotrophic lateral sclerosis: the role of oxidative stress and altered homeostasis of metals. Brain Res. Bull. **61:** 365–374.
2. Hur, K., J.I. Kim, S.I. Choi, *et al.* 2002. The pathogenic mechanisms of prion diseases. Mech. Ageing Dev. **123:** 1637–1647.
3. Evert, B.O., U. Wullner & T. Klockgether. 2000. Cell death in polyglutamine diseases. Cell Tissue Res. **301:** 189–204.
4. Rehman, H.U. 2000. Progressive supranuclear palsy. Postgrad. Med. J. **76:** 333–336.
5. Koutsilieri, E., C. Scheller, F. Tribl & P. Riederer. 2002. Degeneration of neuronal cells due to oxidative stress—microglial contribution. Parkinsonism Relat. Disord. **8:** 401–406.
6. Liu, B., H.M. Gao, J.Y. Wang, *et al.* 2002. Role of nitric oxide in inflammation-mediated neurodegeneration. Ann. N. Y. Acad. Sci. **962:** 318–331.
7. Aschner, M., U. Sonnewald & K.H. Tan. 2002. Astrocyte modulation of neurotoxic injury. Brain Pathol. **12:** 475–481.
8. Banati, R.B. & M.B. Graeber. 1994. Surveillance, intervention and cytotoxicity: is there a protective role of microglia? Dev. Neurosci. **16:** 114–127.
9. Teismann, P., K. Tieu, O. Cohen, *et al.* 2003. Pathogenic role of glial cells in Parkinson's disease. Mov. Disord. **18:** 121–129.
10. Streilein, J.W. 1995. Unraveling immune privilege. Science **270:** 1158–1159.
11. Hickey, W.F., B.L. Hsu & H. Kimura. 1991. T-lymphocyte entry into the central nervous system. J. Neurosci. Res. **28:** 254–260.
12. Moalem, G., A. Monsonego, Y. Shani, *et al.* 1999. Differential T cell response in central and peripheral nerve injury: connection with immune privilege. FASEB J. **13:** 1207–1217.
13. Gold, R., H.P. Hartung & H. Lassmann. 1997. T-cell apoptosis in autoimmune diseases: termination of inflammation in the nervous system and other sites with specialized immune-defense mechanisms. Trends Neurosci. **20:** 399–404.
14. Paape, M.J., K. Shafer-Weaver, A.V. Capuco, *et al.* 2000. Immune surveillance of mammary tissue by phagocytic cells. Adv. Exp. Med. Biol. **480:** 259–277.
15. Hickey, W.F. 1999. Leukocyte traffic in the central nervous system: the participants and their roles. Semin. Immunol. **11:** 125–137.
16. Flugel, A., T. Berkowicz, T. Ritter, *et al.* 2001. Migratory activity and functional changes of green fluorescent effector cells before and during experimental autoimmune encephalomyelitis. Immunity. **14:** 547–560.
17. Basu, A., J.K. Krady, J.R. Enterline & S.W. Levison. 2002. Transforming growth factor beta1 prevents IL-1beta-induced microglial activation, whereas TNFalpha- and IL-6-stimulated activation are not antagonized. Glia. **40:** 109–120.
18. Janabi, N. 2002. Selective inhibition of cyclooxygenase-2 expression by 15-deoxy-Delta(12,14)(12,14)-prostaglandin J(2) in activated human astrocytes, but not in human brain macrophages. J. Immunol. **168:** 4747–4755.
19. Levi, G., L. Minghetti & F. Aloisi. 1998. Regulation of prostanoid synthesis in microglial cells and effects of prostaglandin E2 on microglial functions. Biochimie. **80:** 899–904.
20. Schwartz, M., I. Shaked, J. Fisher, *et al.* 2003. Protective autoimmunity against the enemy within: fighting glutamate toxicity. Trends Neurosci. **26:** 297–302.
21. Shaked, I., D. Tchoresh, R. Gersner, *et al.* 2005. Protective autoimmunity: interferon-gamma enables microglia to remove glutamate without evoking inflammatory mediators. J. Neurochem. **92:** 997–1009.
22. Butovsky, O., A.E. Talpalar, K. Ben-Yaakov & M. Schwartz. 2005. Activation of microglia by aggregated beta-amyloid or lipopolysaccharide impairs MHC-II expres-

sion and renders them cytotoxic whereas IFN-gamma and IL-4 render them protective. Mol. Cell. Neurosci. **29:** 381–393.
23. Moalem, G. *et al.* 2000. Production of neurotrophins by activated T cells: implications for neuroprotective autoimmunity. J. Autoimmun. **15:** 331–345.
24. Gielen, A., M. Khademi, S. Muhallab, *et al.* 2003. Increased brain-derived neurotrophic factor expression in white blood cells of relapsing-remitting multiple sclerosis patients. Scand. J. Immunol. **57:** 493–497.
25. Hammarberg, H., O. Lidman, C. Ludnberg, *et al.* 2000. Neuroprotection by encephalomyelitis: rescue of mechanically injured neurons and neurotrophin production by CNS-infiltrating T and natural killer cells. J. Neurosci. **20:** 5283–5291.
26. Shaked, I., Z. Porat, R. Gersner, *et al.* 2004. Early activation of microglia as antigen-presenting cells correlates with T cell–mediated protection and repair of the injured central nervous system. J. Neuroimmunol. **146:** 84–93.
27. Kipnis, J., T. Mizrahi, E. Hauben, *et al.* 2002. Neuroprotective autoimmunity: naturally occurring $CD4^+CD25^+$ regulatory T cells suppress the ability to withstand injury to the central nervous system. Proc. Natl. Acad. Sci. USA. **99:** 15620–15625.
28. Kipnis, J., E. Yoles, H. Schori, *et al.* 2001. Neuronal survival after CNS insult is determined by a genetically encoded autoimmune response. J. Neurosci. **21:** 4564–4571.
29. Schwartz, M. & G. Moalem. 2001. Beneficial immune activity after CNS injury: prospects for vaccination. J. Neuroimmunol. **113:** 185–192.
30. Shevach, E.M. 2000. Regulatory T cells in autoimmunity. Annu. Rev. Immunol. **18:** 423–449.
31. Thornton, A.M. & E.M. Shevach. 1998. $CD4^+CD25^+$ immunoregulatory T cells suppress polyclonal T cell activation in vitro by inhibiting interleukin 2 production. J. Exp. Med. **188:** 287–296.
32. Kipnis, J., M. Cardon, H. Avidan, *et al.* 2004. Dopamine, through the extracellular signal-regulated kinase pathway, downregulates $CD4^+CD25^+$ regulatory T-cell activity: implications for neurodegeneration. J. Neurosci. **24:** 6133–6143.
33. Kipnis, J., H. Avidan, Y. Markovich, *et al.* 2004. Low-dose gamma-irradiation promotes survival of injured neurons in the central nervous system via homeostasis-driven proliferation of T cells. Eur. J. Neurosci. **19:** 1191–1198.
34. Kipnis, J., H. Cohen, M. Cardon, *et al.* 2004. T cell deficiency leads to cognitive dysfunction: implications for therapeutic vaccination for schizophrenia and other psychiatric conditions. Proc. Natl. Acad. Sci. USA. **101:** 8180–8185.
35. Dummer, W., A.G. Niethammer, R. Baccala, *et al.* 2002. T cell homeostatic proliferation elicits effective antitumor autoimmunity. J. Clin. Invest. **110:** 185–192.
36. Ma, J., W.J. Urba, L. Si, *et al.* 2003. Anti-tumor T cell response and protective immunity in mice that received sublethal irradiation and immune reconstitution. Eur. J. Immunol. **33:** 2123–2132.
37. Elflein, K., M. Rodriguez-Palmero, T. Kerkau & T. Hunig. 2003. Rapid recovery from T lymphopenia by CD28 superagonist therapy. Blood. **102:** 1764–1770.
38. Gudmundsdottir, H. & L.A. Turka. 2001. A closer look at homeostatic proliferation of $CD4^+$ T cells: costimulatory requirements and role in memory formation. J. Immunol. **167:** 3699–3707.
39. Sara, E., A. Kotsakis, J. Souklakos, *et al.* 1999. Post-chemotherapy lymphopoiesis in patients with solid tumors is characterized by $CD4^+$ cell proliferation. Anticancer Res. **19:** 471–476.
40. Gelinas, S. & M.G. Martinoli. 2002. Neuroprotective effect of estradiol and phytoestrogens on MPP^+-induced cytotoxicity in neuronal PC12 cells. J. Neurosci. Res. **70:** 90–96.
41. Kipnis, J., H. Avidan, R.R. Caspi & M. Schwartz. 2004. Dual effect of $CD4^+CD25^+$ regulatory T cells in neurodegeneration: a dialogue with microglia. Proc. Natl. Acad. Sci. USA **101** (Suppl 2): 14663–14669.

Tumor Necrosis Factor Inhibitor Therapy for Rheumatoid Arthritis

STANLEY M. NAGUWA

Division of Rheumatology, Allergy, and Clinical Immunology, Department of Internal Medicine, University of California, Davis, Davis, California 95616, USA

ABSTRACT: The immunopathology of rheumatoid arthritis (RA) is now better understood, and this knowledge has been translated into more effective therapy with biologic response modifiers. The first group of biologic response modifiers are the tumor necrosis factor inhibitors. There efficacy in controlling RA has been such that remission is now the goal of RA management. As with any patient treatment, safety is an issue; patients will need ongoing monitoring for infections, tumors, and other rare complications.

KEYWORDS: rheumatoid arthritis; biologic response modifiers; disease-modifying antirheumatic drugs; DMARDs; TNF-α inhibitors; corticosteroids

INTRODUCTION

With the rapid advances in immunology over the past three decades has come the promise that more effective treatment for rheumatoid arthritis (RA) would follow. The development of biologic response modifiers has fulfilled that promise; and rheumatologists, the primary caregivers for RA patients, have experienced a rebirth. Until the late 1990s, therapeutic options to slow the destructive effects of RA were limited to, for example, acetylsalicylic acid (ASA), nonsteroidal anti-inflammatory drugs (NSAIDs), corticosteroids, gold, and D-penicillamine (DPA). At that time, managed care organizations in the United States considered rheumatologists to be superfluous. However, the picture has changed radically since then: the biologic response modifiers, tumor necrosis factor (TNF) inhibitors, are so effective in the management of RA that remission is the new goal of RA treatment.

PATHOPHYSIOLOGY OF RHEUMATOID ARTHRITIS

In the past two decades, intense research into RA, coupled with the rapid advance in immunology, has significantly elucidated the pathophysiology of RA. Even so, the exact cause remains undefined.[1,2]

Address for correspondence: Stanley M. Naguwa, Division of Rheumatology, Allergy and Clinical Immunology, University of California, Davis, 451 E. Health Sciences Drive, Genome and Biomedical Science Facility, Suite 6510, Davis, CA 95616. Voice: 530-752-2884; fax: 530-754-6047.

smnaguwa@ucdavis.edu

Ann. N.Y. Acad. Sci. 1051: 709–715 (2005). © 2005 New York Academy of Sciences.
doi: 10.1196/annals.1361.115

The primary cellular elements in the RA inflammatory process that cause synovitis and other systemic manifestations are the $CD4^+$ lymphocyte, macrophage, and synovial fibroblasts. These cells work in concert to initiate, promote, amplify, and perpetuate inflammation in and around the joints. This inflammation leads to the symptoms of joint pain and stiffness. It also causes joint swelling, erosion of joint structures, joint-space narrowing, and, if prolonged, ankylosis; all of these phenomena result in joint dysfunction.

The cells produce numerous cytokines, of which interleukin (IL)–1, IL-6, and TNF are arguably the most important in the RA inflammatory cascade.[3] Agents have been developed to block cytokine expression and have shown significant clinical benefit.[4] Of interest is the fact that blocking a single cytokine can significantly interrupt the inflammatory process in RA, despite the complexity of numerous cytokines interacting with several cells in this disease. However, the key cytokine that would interfere with the inflammatory cascade is different for each patient.

As part of the inflammatory cascade, matrix metalloproteinases (MMPs) are produced. This effect, in concert with the activation of osteoclasts, may permanently damage the joint structures, as manifested by erosions and cartilage loss. Chemokines attract cells to the inflammation site; these cells include polymorphonuclear leukocytes, which are seen in increased numbers in RA joint fluid. Chondrocytes, which also participate in the inflammatory process, are also targets, leading to alteration in cartilage homeostasis. Although B cells play a part in the production of rheumatoid factor (RF), until recently, the importance of B cells' role in RA inflammation was debated. However, the clinical trials of the anti-CD20 monoclonal antibody (MAb) in RA have identified the B cell as a key player.[5]

The important role of TNF-α has also been verified in clinical trials of TNF inhibitors. TNF-α, a homodimer produced primarily by macrophages/monocytes, is an excellent promoter of RA inflammation. Acting through a p55 or p75 receptor, it stimulates other cells to produce various inflammatory cytokines, for example, IL-2, IL-6, IL-8, IL-12, IL-18, and interferon (IFN)–γ. In experimental models of arthritis and RA, TNF blockade results in decreased levels of important inflammatory cytokines.[6,7]

EVALUATION OF RA TREATMENT WITH TNF INHIBITORS

Through the 1970s, rheumatologists were frustrated at the inability to control RA, until methotrexate (MTX) was introduced as a disease-modifying antirheumatic drug (DMARD). MTX demonstrated an ability to slow joint damage and improve joint functioning while maintaining an acceptable risk profile—far better than available agents: gold, D-penicillamine (DPA), or hydroxychloroquinine (HCQ). By the 1990s, it had become the first-line DMARD prescribed by rheumatologists in the United States; however, not all patients responded, and responses were occasionally modest.[8] Following the lead of oncologists, rheumatologists have experimented with combination therapy regimens, such as MTX + sulfasalazine + hydroxychloroquine.[9] In RA, debate is ongoing as to whether prednisone is disease modifying.

In the late 1990s, biologic response modifiers, therapeutic agents directed against specific targets of the immunologic inflammatory cascade in RA, left the laboratory and underwent human clinical trials. Inhibitors of TNF were the first to successfully complete these trials and become part of the RA treatment armamentarium. Three TNF inhibitors are commercially available, and they utilize two different strategies to block TNF from participating in the inflammatory cascade.

Etanercept was the first available biologic response modifier for RA; the drug is a cleverly engineered coupling of a human p75 TNF receptor with the Fc portion of immunoglobulin G1 (IgG1). Administered as a subcutaneous injection either once or twice weekly, it binds to TNF, preventing it from binding to naturally occurring receptors and thus activating the target cell. The second and third approved TNF inhibitors were infliximab, a chimeric MAb coupled to the Fc portion of IgG1, and adalimumab, a humanized MAb also coupled to the Fc portion of IgG1. Infliximab is administered intravenously every 4 to 8 weeks, and adalimumab is given subcutaneously from every other week to once weekly.

In clinical trials, the three agents have yielded similar results. When added to MTX therapy in patients who had an incomplete treatment response, etanercept plus MTX achieved an American College of Rheumatology definition of improvement in RA in 20% (ACR20) of 70%, ACR50 score of 39%, and ACR70 score of 15%, compared with placebo-plus-MTX patients (whose scores were ACR20 27%, ACR 50 3% and ACR70 0%, respectively).[10] Infliximab can be administered at different doses and different intervals. For infliximab given at 3 mg/kg every 8 weeks (low dose), responses were as follows: ACR20 of 50%, ACR50 of 27%, and ACR70 of 8%; at 10 mg/kg every 4 weeks (high dose), ACR20 was 58%, ACR50 was 26%, and ACR70 was 11%.[11] Patients taking 40 mg adalimumab every other week plus MTX had response rates of ACR20 67%, ACR50 55%, and ACR70 27%.[12]

The TNF inhibitors have also been studied in early RA. As monotherapy in patients with RA of less than three years' duration, etanercept achieved the following results: ACR20 score of 72%, ACR50 score of 48%, and ACR70 score of 29%.[13] In a trial of infliximab, patients with disease of less than one year's duration were given 3 mg/kg at weeks 0, 2, 6, and every eight weeks subsequently, plus MTX; their response was an ACR20 of 80%, an ACR50 of 80%, and an ACR70 of 70%.[14] A subsequent subset analysis of a larger adalimumab study demonstrated this drug's efficacy in early RA.

Unlike for earlier DMARDs, the clinical response to TNF inhibitors is rapid, and results are noted in a few weeks. With regard to durability of the clinical response, TNF inhibitors show sustained benefit, and responses to etanercept have been noted at 7 years,[15] infliximab at 2 years,[16] and adalimumab at 4 years.[17]

Although the ACR20 response was the primary goal of initial TNF inhibitor therapeutic trials, the significant percentage of ACR50 and ACR70 responses (which are more rigorous) have prompted researchers and clinicians to propose *remission* as a goal in the management of RA. To that end, the ACR-N and Disease Activity Score (DAS) are being used to document response to treatment in a continuous versus a discrete fashion, that is, ACR20, ACR50, and ACR70. In the case of DAS28, a score of less than 2.6 is being proposed as indicating remission.[18]

Paralleling the remarkable clinical response to the new drugs has been the prevention of joint damage (joint-space narrowing and erosions) by the use of TNF inhibitors. Joint damage, as quantified by the Sharp/van der Heijde radiographic score, has shown little or no change after treatment with etanercept plus MTX when measured at 52 weeks,[19] infliximab at 54 weeks,[20] and adalimumab at 54 weeks.[21] This finding has stimulated the investigation of more sensitive imaging techniques

(Sharp/van der Heijde uses plain X rays) to document the changes in the joint as a result of inflammation. Magnetic resonance imaging (MRI), computed tomography (CT), and sonography have all been studied. These imaging techniques are more sensitive for showing changes, especially early in the disease process, albeit at a higher cost.[22,23] A study of the cost–benefit ratios of the more sophisticated techniques is needed.

Safety

What then are the potential drawbacks of TNF inhibitor therapy? TNF functions in human homeostasis to control infection and tumors. Thus, its blockade would put a patient at further risk of infection and/or tumors, because RA patients are at increased risk for both owing to their disease and the effects of traditional therapy.[24,25] TNF inhibitor use would be expected to increase the risk for granulomatous infections, given the role of TNF in granuloma formation. This heightened risk has been observed, and recommendations for the evaluation and prophylaxis of tuberculosis (TB) have been advanced.[26] In certain at-risk populations, the standard TB skin test may not be sufficient, and more sophisticated tests may be required.[27] TNF inhibitor–treated patients are at increased risk from other infections including bacterial, fungal, and intracellular pathogenic organisms such as *Pneumocystis carinii* pneumonia.[28]

A concern has been the use of TNF inhibitors in hepatitis C infections. A conservative estimate of hepatitis C prevalence places it above that of the 1% for RA; the concomitant occurrence of both would not be unexpected. Further confusing the issue is the occurrence of RF and joint disease in patients with hepatitis C infections. Fortunately, preliminary data suggest that TNF inhibitor use does not worsen hepatitis C.[29]

Tumors, particularly non-Hodgkin's lymphoma, are more prevalent in RA, but whether TNF inhibitor use would increase their prevalence has not been clearly established.[25] Whether the relative risk for cancer will increase with the duration of TNF inhibitor use is still unknown.

The blocking of TNF, which is a T-helper cell type 1 (Th1) cytokine, may alter the Th1/Th2 immunologic balance. As such, increased autoantibody production would not be unexpected, which has been shown.[30] Although the mechanisms of autoantibody production have not been fully elucidated, clinical correlates have arisen with reports of SLE, vasculitis, and multiple sclerosis–like demyelinating diseases.[28,31,32]

Although TNF levels are elevated in heart failure, a study investigating the use of TNF inhibitors in congestive heart failure (CHF) had adverse results that led to study termination. These results, plus reports of *de novo* CHF, have prompted experts to warn physicians about the use of TNF inhibitors in patients who are at risk for CHF.

Treatment Strategy

Overall, the positive effects of TNF inhibitors in the management of RA have been better than expected.[33] In the Cochrane Reviews, the numbers needed to treat for an ACR20 effect were two patients for etanercept and three patients for infliximab.[34,35] Compare these figures with those for the treatment of hyperlipidemia to prevent death or myocardial infarction: in the latter, the numbers needed to treat are at least tenfold higher.

Because approximately 70% of TNF inhibitor-treated patients respond, there is a 30% nonresponse rate. Thus, research is under way to identify responders and non-responders *before* expensive TNF inhibitor treatment is initiated. With the advent of microarray testing for genomic and proteonomic factors, researchers expect that prognostic signs will be identified.[36–38]

Because of the high cost of TNF inhibitors, guidelines have been proposed recommending their use in patients who have had an inadequate response to MTX.[39,40] But if a patient fails to respond to a selected TNF inhibitor, would switching to another help? In fact, several reports do support such a maneuver.[41–43]

SUMMARY

The treatment of RA with TNF inhibitors has revitalized the specialty of rheumatology. The crucial role that TNF plays in RA pathogenesis has been experimentally documented and clinically confirmed. Remarkable response rates to TNF inhibitor treatment have been observed, even in patients who failed to respond to "older" DMARDs, such as methotrexate, azathroprine, and sulfasalasine. The extent of the response to TNF inhibitors has prompted rheumatologists to consider remission as a realistic goal of RA management.

TNF inhibitor treatment with etanercept, infliximab, or adalimumab may not benefit all patients. Thus, a second generation of agents that interfere with the TNF-promoted inflammatory cascade is being developed. These agents include a TNF-α–converting enzyme inhibitor, which prevents TNF from being released from the cells producing it, and a p38 MAP kinase inhibitor, which would interrupt the downstream signaling in a cell after TNF–TNF receptor coupling.

REFERENCES

1. Choy, E.H. & G.S. Panayi. 2001. Cytokine pathways and joint inflammation in rheumatoid arthritis. N. Engl. J. Med. **344:** 907–916.
2. Smith, J.B. & M.K. Haynes. 2002. Rheumatoid arthritis—a molecular understanding. Ann. Intern. Med. **136:** 908–922.
3. Hata, H., N. Sakaguchi, H. Yoshitomi, *et al.* 2004. Distinct contribution of IL-6, TNF-alpha, IL-1, and IL-10 to T cell-mediated spontaneous autoimmune arthritis in mice. J. Clin. Invest. **114:** 582–588.
4. Olsen, N.J. & C.M. Stein. 2004. New drugs for rheumatoid arthritis. N. Engl. J. Med. **350:** 2167–2179.
5. Edwards, J.C., L. Szczepanski, J. Szechinski, *et al.* 2004. Efficacy of B-cell-targeted therapy with rituximab in patients with rheumatoid arthritis. N. Engl. J. Med. **350:** 2572–2581.
6. Brennan, F.M., K.A. Browne, P.A. Green, *et al.* 1997. Reduction of serum matrix metalloproteinase 1 and matrix metalloproteinase 3 in rheumatoid arthritis patients following anti-tumour necrosis factor-alpha (cA2) therapy. Br. J. Rheumatol. **36:** 643–650.
7. Charles, P., M.J. Elliott, D. Davis, *et al.* 1999. Regulation of cytokines, cytokine inhibitors, and acute-phase proteins following anti-TNF-alpha therapy in rheumatoid arthritis. J. Immunol. **163:** 1521–1528.
8. Borchers, A.T., C.L. Keen, G.S. Cheema & M.E. Gershwin. 2004. The use of methotrexate in rheumatoid arthritis. Semin. Arthritis Rheum. **34:** 465–483.
9. O'Dell, J.R., C.E. Haire, N. Erikson, *et al.* 1996. Treatment of rheumatoid arthritis with methotrexate alone, sulfasalazine and hydroxychloroquine, or a combination of all three medications. N. Engl. J. Med. **334:** 1287–1291.

10. WEINBLATT, M.E., J.M. KREMER, A.D. BANKHURST, *et al.* 1999. A trial of etanercept, a recombinant tumor necrosis factor receptor:Fc fusion protein, in patients with rheumatoid arthritis receiving methotrexate. N. Engl. J. Med. **340:** 253–259.
11. MAINI, R., E.W. ST. CLAIR, F. BREEDVELD, *et al.* 1999. Infliximab (chimeric anti-tumour necrosis factor alpha monoclonal antibody) versus placebo in rheumatoid arthritis patients receiving concomitant methotrexate: a randomised phase III trial. ATTRACT Study Group. Lancet **354:** 1932–1939.
12. WEINBLATT, M.E., E.C. KEYSTONE, D.E. FURST, *et al.* 2003. Adalimumab, a fully human anti-tumor necrosis factor alpha monoclonal antibody, for the treatment of rheumatoid arthritis in patients taking concomitant methotrexate: the ARMADA trial. Arthritis Rheum. **48:** 35–45.
13. BATHON, J.M., R.W. MARTIN, R.M. FLEISCHMANN, *et al.* 2000. A comparison of etanercept and methotrexate in patients with early rheumatoid arthritis. N. Engl. J. Med. **343:** 1586–1593.
14. QUINN, M.A., P.G. CONAGHAN, P.J. O'CONNOR, *et al.* 2005. Very early treatment with infliximab in addition to methotrexate in early, poor-prognosis rheumatoid arthritis reduces magnetic resonance imaging evidence of synovitis and damage, with sustained benefit after infliximab withdrawal: results from a twelve-month randomized, double-blind, placebo-controlled trial. Arthritis Rheum. **52:** 27–35.
15. WEINBLATT, M.E., *et al.* 2004. Efficacy and safety of over 7 years of etanercept therapy in North American patients with early and long standing rheumatoid arthritis. Arthritis Rheum. **50:** 5184.
16. MAINI, R.N., F.C. BREEDVELD, J.R. KALDEN, *et al.* 2004. Sustained improvement over two years in physical function, structural damage, and signs and symptoms among patients with rheumatoid arthritis treated with infliximab and methotrexate. Arthritis Rheum. **50:** 1051–1065.
17. SCHIFF, M.H. *et al.* 2004. Significant clinical improvement at 6 months are sustained over 4 years in patients with rheumatoid arthritis treated with adalimumab plus methotrexate. Arthritis Rheum. **50:** 5182.
18. FRANSEN, J., M.C. CREEMERS & P.L. VAN RIEL. 2004. Remission in rheumatoid arthritis: agreement of the disease activity score (DAS28) with the ARA preliminary remission criteria. Rheumatology (Oxford) **43:** 1252–1255.
19. KLARESKOG, L., D. VAN DER HEIJDE, J.P. DE JAGER, *et al.* 2004. Therapeutic effect of the combination of etanercept and methotrexate compared with each treatment alone in patients with rheumatoid arthritis: double-blind randomised controlled trial. Lancet **363:** 675–681.
20. LIPSKY, P.E., D.M. VAN DER HEIJDE, E.W. ST. CLAIR, *et al.* 2000. Infliximab and methotrexate in the treatment of rheumatoid arthritis. Anti-Tumor Necrosis Factor Trial in Rheumatoid Arthritis with Concomitant Therapy Study Group. N. Engl. J. Med. **343:** 1594–1602.
21. KEYSTONE, E.C., A.F. KAVANAUGH, J.T. SHARP, *et al.* 2004. Radiographic, clinical, and functional outcomes of treatment with adalimumab (a human anti-tumor necrosis factor monoclonal antibody) in patients with active rheumatoid arthritis receiving concomitant methotrexate therapy: a randomized, placebo-controlled, 52-week trial. Arthritis Rheum. **50:** 1400–1411.
22. HOVING, J.L., R. BUCHBINDER, S. HALL, *et al.* 2004. A comparison of magnetic resonance imaging, sonography, and radiography of the hand in patients with early rheumatoid arthritis. J. Rheumatol. **31:** 663–675.
23. GHOZLAN, R. & H. VACHER. 2000. Where is imaging going in rheumatology? Bailliere's Best Pract. Res. Clin. Rheumatol. **14:** 617–633.
24. DORAN, M.F., C.S. CROWSON, G.R. POND, *et al.* 2002. Frequency of infection in patients with rheumatoid arthritis compared with controls: a population-based study. Arthritis Rheum. **46:** 2287–2293.
25. WOLFE, F. & K. MICHAUD. 2004. Lymphoma in rheumatoid arthritis: the effect of methotrexate and anti-tumor necrosis factor therapy in 18,572 patients. Arthritis Rheum. **50:** 1740–1751.
26. HAMILTON, C.D. 2003. Tuberculosis in the cytokine era: what rheumatologists need to know. Arthritis Rheum. **48:** 2085–2091.

27. MEDINA, F., V. RIVERA, J. FUENTES, *et al.* 2004. Is there a role for PPD and chest radiography in identification of asymptomatic tuberculosis in rheumatic diseases? Arthritis Rheum. **50:** 5126.
28. IMPERATO, A.K., S. SMILES & S.B. ABRAMSON. 2004. Long-term risks associated with biologic response modifiers used in rheumatic diseases. Curr. Opin. Rheumatol. **16:** 199–205.
29. CALABRESE, L.H., N. ZEIN & D. VASSILOPOULOS. 2004. Safety of antitumour necrosis factor (anti-TNF) therapy in patients with chronic viral infections: hepatitis C, hepatitis B, and HIV infection. Ann. Rheum. Dis. **63** (Suppl. 2): ii18–ii24.
30. ERIKSSON, C., S. ENGSTRAND, K.G. SUNDQVIST & S. RANTAPAA-DAHLQVIST. 2004. Autoantibody formation in patients with rheumatoid arthritis treated with anti-TNF-alpha. Ann. Rheum. Dis. **64:** 403–407.
31. HYRICH, K.L., A.J. SILMAN, K.D. WATSON & D.P. SYMMONS. 2004. Anti-tumour necrosis factor alpha therapy in rheumatoid arthritis: an update on safety. Ann. Rheum. Dis. **63:** 1538–1543.
32. MOHAN, N., E.T. EDWARDS, T.R. CUPPS, *et al.* 2001. Demyelination occurring during anti-tumor necrosis factor alpha therapy for inflammatory arthritides. Arthritis Rheum. **44:** 2862–2869.
33. JOIS, R., M. SOMERVILLE, A. BROOKSBY, *et al.* 2004. Biologics in clinical practice—better than expected? EULAR 2004 abstr. online FRI 0067.
34. BLUMENAUER, B., M. JUDD, A. CRANNEY, *et al.* 2003. Etanercept for the treatment of rheumatoid arthritis. Cochrane Database Syst. Rev. **4:** CD004525.
35. BLUMENAUER, B., M. JUDD, G. WELLS, *et al.* 2002. Infliximab for the treatment of rheumatoid arthritis. Cochrane Database Syst. Rev. **3:** CD003785.
36. CRISWELL, L.A., R.F. LUM, K.N. TURNER, *et al.* 2004. The influence of genetic variation in the HLA-DRB1 and LTA-TNF regions on the response to treatment of early rheumatoid arthritis with methotrexate or etanercept. Arthritis Rheum. **50:** 2750–2756.
37. SCHOTTE, H., B. SCHLUTER, S. DRYNDA, *et al.* 2004. Interleukin 10 promoter microsatellite polymorphisms are associated with response to long term treatment with etanercept in patients with rheumatoid arthritis. Ann. Rheum. Dis. **64:** 575–581.
38. DRYNDA, S., B. RINGEL, M. KEKOW, *et al.* 2004. Proteome analysis reveals disease-associated marker proteins to differentiate RA patients from other inflammatory joint diseases with the potential to monitor anti-TNFalpha therapy. Pathol. Res. Pract. **200:** 165–171.
39. FURST, D.E., F.C. BREEDVELD, J.R. KALDEN, *et al.* 2002. Updated consensus statement on biological agents for the treatment of rheumatoid arthritis and other rheumatic diseases (May 2002). Ann. Rheum. Dis. **61** (Suppl. 2): ii2–ii7.
40. YOCUM, D. 2004. Effective use of TNF antagonists. Arthritis Res. Ther. **6** (Suppl. 2): S24–S30.
41. HARAOUI, B., E.C. KEYSTONE, J.C. THORNE, *et al.* 2004. Clinical outcomes of patients with rheumatoid arthritis after switching from infliximab to etanercept. J. Rheumatol. **31:** 2356–2359.
42. VAN DER BIJL, A.E., F.C. BREEDVELD, C. ANTONI, *et al.* 2004. Infliximab failures in rheumatoid arthritis can be successfully treated with adalimumab. EULAR 2004 abstr. online FRI 0055.
43. HANSEN, K.E., J.P. HILDEBRAND, M.C. GENOVESE, *et al.* 2004. The efficacy of switching from etanercept to infliximab in patients with rheumatoid arthritis. J. Rheumatol. **31:** 1098–1102.

Pathogenesis of Rheumatoid Arthritis: Targeting Cytokines

JOCHEN ZWERINA, KURT REDLICH, GEORG SCHETT, AND JOSEF S. SMOLEN

Division of Rheumatology, Internal Medicine III,
Medical University of Vienna, Vienna, Austria

ABSTRACT: Although considerable progress has been made by adequate treatment with traditional disease-modifying antirheumatic drugs (DMARDs), therapy of rheumatoid arthritis (RA) still remains difficult. The discovery of the importance of cytokines such as tumor necrosis factor (TNF), interleukin-1 (IL-1), interleukin-6 (IL-6), and interleukin-15 (IL-15), which are also stimulated by consequences of autoimmune responses, has led to the development of anticytokine therapies ("biologicals"). Blocking TNF or also, to some extent, IL-1 has proved beneficial in DMARD-resistant RA patients in multiple clinical trials. Along with clinical improvement, TNF blockade has been shown to halt radiographic disease progression, a major risk factor for disability. Recently, clinical trials have shown a significant therapeutic benefit of biological inhibitors of IL-6, and also of IL-15, with an efficacy comparable to that of TNF blockers. All these agents are particularly efficacious when combined with methotrexate. Although clinical remission is difficult to achieve even with anticytokine treatment, these drugs offer the potential to decrease disease activity and improve quality of life in a majority of RA patients, and it is conceivable that combinations of biological therapies may pave the path to even better success, which ultimately is remission or even cure.

KEYWORDS: rheumatoid arthritis; cytokines; TNF; IL-1; IL-6; IL-15; disease activity; joint damage; osteoclasts; therapy; anti-TNF; IL-1ra; anti–IL-6R (MRA)

INTRODUCTION

Rheumatoid arthritis (RA) is a chronic and symmetric polyarthritis most commonly involving the joints of the hands, feet, and knees. RA is two to three times more frequent in women than in men, and the peak incidence is between the fourth and sixth decade, although it may start at any time. Its prevalence is 0.5% to 1%, and it often leads to disablement and, subsequently, reduced quality of life. Clinically, RA is characterized by joint swelling, pain, and morning stiffness. In addition, extra-articular involvement ranging from rheumatoid nodules to life-threatening vasculitis indicates the systemic nature of the disease. The inflamed synovial tissue transforms into a tumor-like tissue ("pannus") that invades bone and degrades cartilage. This

Address for correspondence: Josef S. Smolen, M.D., Division of Rheumatology, Waehringer Guertel 18-20, A-1090 Vienna, Austria. Voice: +43-1-40400-4300; fax: +43-1-40400-4306. josef.smolen@wienkav.at

Ann. N.Y. Acad. Sci. 1051: 716–729 (2005). © 2005 New York Academy of Sciences.
doi: 10.1196/annals.1361.116

was first described over 120 years ago and was termed "caries of the joint ends;"[1] the invading synovial tissue was called "tumor albus" or "fungoid synovitis." The radiologic occurrence of bone erosions inversely correlates to quality of life and in the long term leads to severe loss of functional capacity of RA patients.

PATHOGENETIC ASPECTS OF RA

The etiology of RA is unclear, although a genetic basis involving the MHC II complex has been proposed. Subjects with the HLA-DR4 haplotype are more susceptible to development of RA, and patients with a "shared epitope" allele more often have extra-articular involvement and a more severe course of the disease.[2] Furthermore, a link between bacterial and viral infections leading to polyarthritis in susceptible subjects has been proposed.[3] Indeed, viral infections (parvovirus, rubella) are able to trigger an RA-like arthritis. Chronic bacterial infection can also lead to arthritis, as in lyme disease, and bacterial cell wall fragments can induce chronic arthritis in animal models. However, no causative infectious agent has ever been isolated from RA patients. Although the ultimate link between the immune system and synovial inflammation has not been found, significant progress has been made in identifying pathogenetic aspects by studying animal models of RA.

After the initiating event of RA, an injury to the synovial vasculature is seen, followed by an influx of T cells, mainly of the CD4 memory type.[4] These cells infiltrate the synovium and are activated further by antigen-presenting cells in connection with (unknown) (auto)antigens. These $CD4^+$ cells are clearly of the Th1 subtype, produce interferon-γ (IFN-γ), interleukin-2 (IL-2), tumor necrosis factor (TNF), interleukin-17 (IL-17), and, in turn, through cell–cell contact and the production of these cytokines, activate monocytes, macrophages, and fibroblasts. The latter cells attract and activate neutrophil granulocytes through production of IL-8. Neutrophils are seen at the site of the cartilage junction zone, but far more cells accumulate in the synovial exudate and produce various cartilage-degrading enzymes such as metalloproteases. B cells, dendritic cells, T cells, and macrophages form lymphoid follicle–like structures within the synovial membrane and produce various autoantibodies,[5] such as rheumatoid factor, autoantibodies directed against the Fc fragment of IgG. These autoantibodies may form immune complexes, and are deposited in the cartilage of RA patients.[6] Whether development of autoimmunity is a sole primary, a coprimary, or a secondary event is enigmatic, but it is at least thought to influence the perpetuation of the inflammatory cascade, because immune complexes can induce secretion of proinflammatory cytokines by macrophages.[7]

In the course of the disease, the normal relatively avascular synovium then becomes heavily infiltrated by a wide variety of cells, including B cells, macrophages, fibroblasts, neutrophil granulocytes, dendritic cells, and many other cells.[8] The synovial lining increases to a thickness of up to 30 cell layers, presumably through influx of macrophages, and by expansion of synovial fibroblasts. The latter produce high amounts of proinflammatory cytokines, mainly TNF, IL-1, and IL-6. Furthermore, many other cytokines—such as IL-17, IL-18, and IL-15—chemokines, and angiogenic molecules are present in the inflamed synovial membrane and drive the disease. Subsequently, these proinflammatory cytokines activate signal transduction pathways and transcription factors, which, in turn, control the transcription of cytokines.[9]

The hallmark of RA is the production of a tumor-like inflammatory tissue that invades bone. Early after the clinical onset of RA, mostly within the first year, synoviocytes become hyperplastic and, in a tumor-like manner, invade the subchondral bone at the cartilage junction zone ("pannus"). In contrast with enzyme-mediated cartilage degradation, bone destruction ultimately depends on the presence of bone-resorbing cells, the osteoclasts.[10] These cells are not present in the inflamed synovial membrane of nondestructive arthritides. Osteoclasts are formed, upon various stimuli, by fusion of monocytes, ultimately depending on the recently discovered cytokine, receptor activator of NFκB ligand (RANKL). TNF, IL-1, and IL-6 are known to play significant roles in osteoclast development and function, cartilage destruction, and synovial hyperplasia. Inhibition of each of the three latter cytokines by so-called biologicals has been found to be beneficial in clinical trials and in clinical practice.

THE ROLE OF CYTOKINES IN RA

TNF

TNF, discovered in the 1970s, binds to two receptors, the type 1 TNF receptor (p55) and the type 2 TNF receptor (p75).[11,12] TNF can be produced by mesenchymal cells (fibroblasts, osteoblasts), monocytes, and T and B cells, whereas both receptors are commonly expressed in many cells. TNF expression is induced by cytokines, endotoxin, heat stress, neoplastic transformation, viral agents, and other stimuli. TNF itself induces proinflammatory cytokines, activates polymorphnuclear leukocytes, natural killer cells, and cytotoxic T cells, drives osteoclastogenesis, inhibits collagen synthesis, and enhances cartilage breakdown.[13] The proinflammatory effects of TNF are mostly mediated via the p55 receptor (TNF-RI), whereas its proapoptotic effects are exerted mainly via the p75 receptor (TNF-RII). In RA, TNF is highly expressed in the rheumatoid synovium and synovial fluid.[14–17] It is highly efficient in inducing the differentiation of monocytes to osteoclasts in the presence of RANKL, a critical factor in osteoclastogenesis.[18] Furthermore, TNF increases the synthesis of proinflammatory cytokines and metalloproteases by synovial fibroblasts and decreases the synthesis of proteoglycans by chondrocytes.[19,20] Animal studies have shown the importance of TNF in joint inflammation. Mice that overexpress TNF systemically develop an erosive polyarticular symmetric arthritis.[21] Moreover, these mice develop systemic bone loss similar to that seen in RA patients.[22] Consistent with these findings, TNF blockade is highly effective in animals and inhibits synovial inflammation, cartilage degradation, and bone erosion.[23–25]

Currently, three TNF blockers are approved for treatment of RA: infliximab (a chimeric monoclonal antibody to TNF), adalimumab (a human monoclonal antibody to TNF), and etanercept (a fusion protein of the p75 TNF receptor). All three agents are efficacious in patients who have previously failed methotrexate (MTX) treatment. Typically, American College of Rheumatology 20% improvement criteria (ACR20) responses between ~50% to 70% and ACR50 responses between ~30% to 50% have been achieved.[26–31] In terms of radiographic progression of RA, the Trial of Etanercept and Methotrexate with Radiographic Patient Outcomes (TEMPO) showed superiority of etanercept plus MTX versus etanercept or MTX alone.[32] Patients who received etanercept alone showed some progression, whereas patients

TABLE 1. Biologicals approved or in clinical development for the treatment of rheumatoid arthritis

Agent	Description	Status	Company
Anti-TNF therapy			
Infliximab	Chimeric monoclonal antibody to TNF	Approved (1999)	
Etanercept	Construct of TNF-RII and Fc portion of IgG1	Approved (1998)	Centocor
Adalimumab	Human monoclonal antibody to TNF	Approved (2002)	Amgen/Wyeth
CDP870	PEGylated humanized anti-TNF antibody Fab′ fragment	Phase II	Abbott
Pegsunercept	PEGylated TNF-RI	Phase II	Celltech
Anti–IL-1 therapy			
Anakinra	Recombinant human (rh)IL-1ra	Approved (2001)	Amgen
Pralnacasan	Interleukin-converting enzyme (ICE) inhibitor	Phase II	Aventis
IL-1 trap	Construct of two IL-1 receptor chains with an IgG-Fc domain	Phase II	Novartis
Anti–IL-1	Monoclonal antibody	Phase I/II	
Anti–IL-6 therapy			
MRA	Humanized anti–IL-6 receptor antibody	Phase III	Chugai/Roche
Anti–IL-15 therapy			
HuMax IL-15	Human monoclonal anti–IL-15 antibody	Phase II	Genmab/Amgen

who received combination therapy showed a slight reduction in total Sharp scores. Interestingly, anti-TNF treatment appears to halt radiographic progression even in patients not achieving clinically significant reduction of disease activity.[33] Moreover, a trial in patients with early RA (disease duration ≤ 3 years) showed that combined treatment with infliximab plus MTX or etanercept plus MTX reduced disease activity and halted bone damage.[34] Recently, a small 1-year trial with very early RA patients (disease duration ≤ 1 year) investigated the combination of infliximab plus MTX versus MTX alone, followed by another year of therapy with MTX only.[35] After 1 year, the combination therapy showed better ACR20 responses and radiographs. Even after discontinuation of infliximab after 12 months, a sustained benefit in quality of life and functional capacity was observed; however, ACR responses, radiologic progression, and DAS28 scores were similar in both groups. Currently, forms of humanized anti-TNF antibodies that have been PEGylated to obtain a prolonged plasma half-life are in clinical development (see TABLE 1). Another question is whether patients who did not respond to one TNF blocker respond to another. Data from a registry in Sweden suggest that a switch from etanercept to infliximab or vice versa could be of benefit.[36]

IL-1

Originally discovered as a fever-inducing humoral factor, two forms of IL-1 are now known: IL-1α is a nonsecreted locally acting form, whereas IL-1β is secreted and is measurable in the serum of patients with an activated immune system.[37] IL-1 acts via the type I IL-1 receptor (IL-1R1), whereas binding of IL-1 to the type II IL-1 receptor (IL-1R2) does not transduce signaling. Interleukin-converting enzyme (ICE) sheds IL-1 from the membranes of cells. IL-1 receptor antagonist (IL-1ra) is a naturally occurring counterregulatory cytokine.[38] Binding of IL-1ra to IL-1 receptor blocks activation and signal transduction. Intracytoplasmically, IL-1RI engagement by IL-1 activates Myd88, then TRAF-6, and subsequently leads to phosphorylation of IκB and to release of NFκB, a proinflammatory transcription factor. IL-1, like TNF, is produced by many cells, although monocytes and macrophages produce the highest amounts of it under inflammatory conditions.[39] IL-1 induces production of TNF, IL-1, IL-6, and other cytokines, stimulates osteoclastogenesis, drives the expression of cartilage- and matrix-degrading metalloproteases, enhances chemokine production, and plays a role in neoangiogenesis.[40–44] Animal models of joint inflammation suggested the importance of IL-1. Injection of IL-1 in knee joints induces joint inflammation,[45] and inhibition of IL-1 by administration of either IL-1ra or antibodies against IL-1 leads to significant reduction of joint inflammation, cartilage destruction, and bone erosion in the collagen-induced arthritis (CIA) model.[46–49] Furthermore, IL-1ra knockout mice develop an RA-like disease with an erosive polyarthritis.[50] However, in TNF-driven RA models such as adjuvant-induced arthritis (AIA) and the TNF transgenic mice, inhibition of IL-1 is much less efficacious.[23,51] In RA patients, IL-1 is detectable in synovial fluid specimens and occasionally in serum, and its levels correlate with disease activity.[52] Increased expression of IL-1 and decreased production of IL-1ra has been detected in RA synovial tissues, suggesting a disturbed IL-1/IL-1ra balance.[53] *Ex vivo* studies with synovial fibroblasts demonstrated the cartilage-degrading potency of IL-1.[54]

Anakinra, a recombinant nonglycosylated form of human IL-1ra produced in *Escherichia coli*, is successful in preventing joint inflammation in animal models of RA. After a dose-finding and frequency study,[55] a large, randomized, placebo-controlled trial with 472 patients was conducted.[56] Active RA patients, who had failed no more than two DMARDs and had stopped treatment for 6 weeks, received either placebo or one of three doses of anakinra (30 mg, 75 mg, 150 mg) by daily subcutaneous injections. The primary end point was the ACR20 response. After 24 weeks, 27% of the placebo-treated patients and 43% of the patients in the 150-mg-dose group reached an ACR20 response ($P < 0.014$); the lower two anakinra doses did not result in significant efficacy. Anakinra at the 150-mg dose also reduced swollen and tender joint counts, HAQ score, pain, erythrocyte sedimentation rate, and serum C-reactive protein statistically more than placebo. A combined analysis of all three doses showed a 45% reduction in the progression of bone erosions as determined by the Larsen score method. A second trial compared MTX plus placebo versus MTX plus anakinra at five different doses (0.04, 0.1, 0.4, 1.0, and 2.0 mg/kg/day s.c.).[57] Patients had to be active despite stable MTX treatment. After 12 weeks, increasing anakinra doses led to improvement of patients, with 46% of patients receiving 1 mg/kg and 38% of patients receiving 2 mg/kg reaching an ACR20 response, compared with 19% of placebo-treated patients. This effect was sustained after 24 weeks of treatment. Also, more treated patients reached an ACR50 and ACR70 response. This was accompanied by significant reduction in secondary end points, as in the above-described study. Radiographic data of these patients showed a 36% lower joint damage progression as determined by the Sharp score method.[58] A third study compared the currently approved dose of daily subcutaneous 100 mg anakinra plus MTX with placebo plus MTX.[59] Confirming the former two studies, significantly more patients reached ACR responses when treated with anakinra in addition to MTX versus placebo plus MTX (ACR20: 38% vs. 22%; ACR50: 17% vs. 8%; ACR70: 6% vs. 2%, respectively). A large, placebo-controlled trial evaluated the safety of adding anakinra to traditionally used DMARDs. Although serious adverse events were slightly higher in the anakinra-treated group (2.1% vs. 0.4%), mortality was similar, suggesting an acceptable safety profile. Thus, IL-1 antagonism by IL-1ra is safe and effective and slows joint damage, although to a lesser degree than observed in clinical trials of TNF blockers. Another IL-1 inhibitor developed is IL-1 trap, which binds to IL-1 and inhibits ligation of the latter to IL-1RI. Although a phase Ib study showed positive results, a phase II study revealed no superiority to placebo.[60] Pralnacasan, an orally available ICE inhibitor, also did not achieve significant ACR20 responses compared with placebo, and serious liver enzyme elevations in mice led to discontinuation of another phase II trial.[61]

IL-6

IL-6 was originally described in 1982 as a B cell differentiation marker.[62,63] It belongs to a family of cytokines with a helical structure, such as leukemia inhibitory factor, IL-11, oncostatin M, cardiotrophin-1, and ciliary neurotrophic factor.[64] IL-6 binds the membrane-bound IL-6 receptor (gp80) and then subsequently binds to gp130, the common signal transducer for the IL-6 family cytokines. Alternatively, IL-6 can bind to soluble IL-6R and then generate signal transduction by binding of membrane-bound gp130. IL-6 is produced by a wide variety of cells, including T cells, B cells, macrophages, fibroblasts, endothelial cells, and tumor cells. It also induces terminal differentiation of macrophages, and acts as a growth factor for both T and B cells.[65,66] Furthermore, it enhances differentiation of megakaryocytes to produce platelets,[67] and is a stem cell growth factor.[68] More evidence of the physiological importance of IL-6 *in vivo* comes from IL-6 transgenic mice. These mice develop multiple complications: (1) polyclonal plasmocytosis with autoantibody production, (2) increased levels of fibrinogen and a reduction of serum albumin, (3) increased megakaryopoeisis, and (4) eventual development of mesangial proliferative glomerulonephritis and lymphocytic interstitial lung disease.[69–72] Treatment of these mice with anti–IL-6R antibodies ameliorates disease.[73]

Because RA is characterized at least partially by events also induced by IL-6, synovial fluid (SF) IL-6 levels of RA patients were first assessed. Indeed, high levels of IL-6 in SF were observed.[74] Moreover, serum IL-6 levels were increased and correlated with levels of acute-phase proteins. IL-6 may contribute to autoantibody production by enhancing B cell proliferation,[75] Locally, IL-6 can be produced by many cells in the inflamed synovium but predominantly is found in mononuclear leukocytes. Its production by synovial fibroblasts is driven by TNF, IL-1, and IL-17 *in vitro*, and it may induce pannus formation itself.[76] With respect to bone turnover, IL-6 inhibits bone formation and stimulates bone resorption. IL-6 knockout mice are protected from estrogen- or androgen-deficiency–driven bone loss,[77,78] and IL-6 administration enhances osteoclastogenesis and bone resorption *in vitro*.[79,80]

Animal studies with CIA in mice[81] and cynomolgus monkeys[82] showed a benefit of inhibition of IL-6 by murine-derived and by humanized anti–IL-6R antibodies (the latter termed MRA), respectively. Additionally, IL-6 receptor knockout mice challenged with collagen develop arthritis less often and with less severity;[83] in another report, CIA development ultimately depends on IL-6.[84]

The first evidence of the beneficial effects of IL-6 inhibition in humans came from an open trial of a murine monoclonal antibody to IL-6 in patients with RA.[85] Subsequently, application of MRA was shown to be efficacious in the treatment of Castleman's disease, which is based on IL-6 overproduction.[86] MRA administration led to improvement in clinical signs as well as acute-phase parameters.[87] In 2002, a phase I/II study of MRA in 45 active RA patients showed significant ACR20 responses compared with placebo after 8 weeks.[88] Moreover, erythrocyte sedimentation rate and C-reactive protein levels were significantly reduced. Consequently, phase II dose-finding trials, with or without methotrexate, were initiated. In the Charisma trial, treatment with MRA plus MTX was superior over MTX plus placebo, with the highest efficacy shown by combining MTX and the highest MRA dose (ACR20 response 74%). A second trial of MRA without MTX was published in 2004,[89] in which patients received placebo, 4 mg/kg MRA, or 8 mg/kg MRA. Again, MRA (8 mg/kg) was superior to placebo, with an ACR20 response of 78%. The ACR20, 50, and 70 response rates were comparable to other available biological drugs, such as TNF blockers. Adverse events included elevated lipid and liver enzyme levels, likely caused by withdrawal of IL-6 action on hepatocytes. Few serious infections occurred, but no cases of tuberculosis were observed. Overall, IL-6 inhibition seems to be safe and effective. Phase III trials are now needed to determine long-term safety and efficacy, as well as the effects of MRA on bone erosion and cartilage damage.

IL-15

IL-15 was first described in 1994, with functional similarities to IL-2.[90] IL-15 uses components of the IL-2 receptor but also requires its own α receptor chain. IL-15 is primarily produced by macrophages.[91] Infectious agents (BCG), TNF, IL-1, and cell–cell contacts (T cell–macrophage) induce IL-15 production. IL-15 is tightly regulated, because many human tissues express IL15 mRNA but not protein. The regulation is on both a transcriptional and a post-transcriptional level. IL-15 stimulates T cell proliferation and migration *in vitro* and *in vivo*.[92] IL-15 drives naive T cells in the Th1-type direction by inducing IFN-γ production. Additionally, a single intradermal injection of recombinant human (rh)IL-15 is sufficient to induce a local inflammatory infiltrate. These cell aggregates mainly consist of $CD3^+$ T cells.[93] Moreover, IL-15 induces natural killer cell toxicity.[94] IL-15 also binds to macrophages and induces TNF, IL-1, and IL-6 production.[95] IL-15 induces the differentiation of bone marrow mononuclear cells into osteoclast precursors and enhances the expression of calcitonin receptor and TRAP, two osteoclast lineage markers.[96]

The proinflammatory actions of IL-15 led to the investigation of the expression of this cytokine in RA. It was first noted in 1996 that IL-15 is present in RA synovial tissue but is detectable far less often in synovial samples from reactive arthritis or osteoarthritis (OA).[93] IL-15–positive cells were detected in the synovial lining layer, sublining layer, and perivascular aggregates, and the majority of these cells were macrophages and fibroblasts.[97] Furthermore, soluble (s)IL-15 was detected in RA synovial fluid specimens, but not in specimens from OA patients, and levels of sIL-15 correlated with synovial fluid TNF levels.

Synovial T cells produced significant amounts of TNF upon incubation with IL-15, but not with IL-2.[98] IL-15–stimulated T cells also elicit TNF production of synovial fluid macrophages in a cell–cell contact–dependent fashion. In turn, TNF and IL-1 are able to induce IL-15 production in synovial fibroblasts and therefore might perpetuate local T cell proliferation.[99] As it has been shown for many other cytokines, IL-15 potently synergizes with other cytokines to enhance T cell growth as well as proliferation and macrophage activation. IL-12 and IL-18 in combination with IL-15 promote macrophage activation at low concentrations.[100] Hence, IL-15 is likely to play a role in RA.

Consequently, therapeutic inhibition of IL-15 has been investigated in animal models of RA. Administration of a soluble fragment of the IL-15R α-chain was tested in the collagen-induced arthritis model in mice.[101] Daily treatment after collagen challenge diminished incidence and severity of disease. Histologically, infiltration of polymorphonuclear cells, cartilage destruction, and bone erosion were prevented. Serologically, antibody levels raised against collagen were significantly reduced. Moreover, levels of IFN-γ and IL-6 in sera of treated CIA mice were lower compared with levels in untreated mice. Discontinuation of treatment, however, exacerbated disease immediately. Another study evaluated the efficacy of a mutant fusion protein (CRB-15) that binds to the IL-15 receptor but does not trigger intracellular signal transduction in CIA mice.[102] Again, incidence and severity of disease were reduced when CRB-15 was administered after collagen challenge, and CRB-15 also alleviated disease when given after clinical onset.

In 2003, a first report of an anti–IL-15–targeted therapy in RA patients was presented.[103] In a phase I study, 30 active RA patients received either a human monoclonal anti–IL-15 antibody (HuMax-IL15) at various doses (0.15 mg/kg up to 8 mg/kg) or placebo. Administration was safe, and patients did not have an increase of antibodies against HuMax-IL15. A combined analysis of the anti–IL-15–treated patients showed an ACR20 response in 63%, an ACR50 response in 38%, and 25% achieved an ACR70 response. Recently, these data were confirmed by a phase II study with comparable ACR responses.[104] This suggests that targeting IL-15 in RA may be beneficial.

CONCLUSION

Although many proinflammatory cytokines are expressed in RA synovium, and many of their actions appear to be additive or even synergistic, or in any case redundant, inhibition of each of them is efficient in preventing signs and symptoms of RA, at least to a certain (and sometimes greater) degree. Why some patients benefit from TNF blockade whereas others do not is unclear but points to different dominance of cytokine pathways in different patients. We have proposed an "inflammatory house of cards model," where more than one molecule has to be targeted for optimal treatment of RA.[105] This is underlined by the fact that combining biologicals with traditional DMARDs such as MTX is superior to treatment with a single agent, especially in terms of radiological and clinical response. Furthermore, animal studies suggest a synergistic action of cytokines, and combined inhibition of TNF and IL-1 is highly efficacious in treating TNF-mediated arthritis and the AIA model.[23] Moreover, some combination therapies lead to healing phenomena in mice.[106]

In summary, the novel and expanding insights into cellular and molecular events governing the evolution of RA, in conjunction with results of therapeutic trials, suggest that multiple cell systems and cytokines are involved in the generation of the joint damage characteristic of the disease. Targeting these events has already improved the fate of patients refractory to other treatment modalities and has led to shifts in treatment paradigms. Further progress is to be expected, with the ultimate aim of remission and cure of the disease.

REFERENCES

1. WEICHSELBAUM, A. 1878. Die feineren Veränderungen des Gelenkknoperpels bei fungöser Synovitis und Caries der Gelenkenden. Arch. Pathol. Anat. Physiol. Klin. Med. 461–475.
2. WINCHESTER, R.J. 1981. Genetic aspects of rheumatoid arthritis. Springer Semin. Immunopathol. **4:** 89–102.
3. HYRICH, K.L. & R.D. INMAN. 2001. Infectious agents in chronic rheumatic diseases. Curr. Opin. Rheumatol. **13:** 300–304.
4. GORONZY, J.J. & C.M. WEYAND. 1995. T cells in rheumatoid arthritis. Paradigms and facts. Rheum. Dis. Clin. North Am. **21:** 655–674.
5. STEINER, G. & J. SMOLEN. 2002. Autoantibodies in rheumatoid arthritis and their clinical significance. Arthritis Res. **4** (Suppl 2)**:** S1–S5.
6. COOKE, T.D., E.R. HURD, H.E. JASIN, *et al.* 1975. Identification of immunoglobulins and complement in rheumatoid articular collagenous tissues. Arthritis Rheum. **18:** 541–551.
7. DEBETS, J.M., C.J. VAN DER LINDEN, I.E. DIETEREN, *et al.* 1988. Fc-receptor cross-linking induces rapid secretion of tumor necrosis factor (cachectin) by human peripheral blood monocytes. J. Immunol. **141:** 1197–1201.
8. HARAOUI, B., J.P. PELLETIER, J.M. CLOUTIER, *et al.* 1991. Synovial membrane histology and immunopathology in rheumatoid arthritis and osteoarthritis. In vivo effects of antirheumatic drugs. Arthritis Rheum. **34:** 153–163.
9. SWEENEY, S.E. & G.S. FIRESTEIN. 2004. Rheumatoid arthritis: regulation of synovial inflammation. Int. J. Biochem. Cell Biol. **36:** 372–378.
10. GRAVALLESE, E.M. 2002. Bone destruction in arthritis. Ann. Rheum. Dis. **61** (Suppl 2)**:** ii84–ii86.
11. PERLMUTTER, D.H., C.A. DINARELLO, P.I. PUNSAL & H.R. COLTEN. 1986. Cachectin/tumor necrosis factor regulates hepatic acute-phase gene expression. J. Clin. Invest. **78:** 1349–1354.
12. TARTAGLIA, L.A. & D.V. GOEDDEL. 1992. Two TNF receptors. Immunol. Today **13:** 151–153.
13. DINARELLO, C.A., J.G. CANNON, S.M. WOLFF, *et al.* 1986. Tumor necrosis factor (cachectin) is an endogenous pyrogen and induces production of interleukin 1. J. Exp. Med. **163:** 1433–1450.

14. CHU, C.Q., M. FIELD, S. ALLARD, *et al.* 1992. Detection of cytokines at the cartilage/pannus junction in patients with rheumatoid arthritis: implications for the role of cytokines in cartilage destruction and repair. Br. J. Rheumatol. **31:** 653–661.
15. STEINER, G., M. TOHIDAST-AKRAD, G. WITZMANN, *et al.* 1999. Cytokine production by synovial T cells in rheumatoid arthritis. Rheumatology (Oxford) **38:** 202–213.
16. PARTSCH, G., G. STEINER, B.F. LEEB, *et al.* 1997. Highly increased levels of tumor necrosis factor-alpha and other proinflammatory cytokines in psoriatic arthritis synovial fluid. J. Rheumatol. **24:** 518–523.
17. CHU, C.Q., M. FIELD, M. FELDMANN & R.N. MAINI. 1991. Localization of tumor necrosis factor alpha in synovial tissues and at the cartilage-pannus junction in patients with rheumatoid arthritis. Arthritis Rheum. **34:** 1125–1132.
18. LAM, J., S. TAKESHITA, J.E. BARKER, *et al.* 2000. TNF-alpha induces osteoclastogenesis by direct stimulation of macrophages exposed to permissive levels of RANK ligand. J. Clin. Invest. **106:** 1481–1488.
19. JORGENSEN, C., I. COURET, F. CANOVAS, *et al.* 1996. Mononuclear cell retention in rheumatoid synovial tissue engrafted in severe combined immunodeficient (SCID) mice is up-regulated by tumour necrosis factor-alpha (TNF-alpha) and mediated through intercellular adhesion molecule-1 (ICAM-1). Clin. Exp. Immunol. **106:** 20–25.
20. FIRESTEIN, G.S. & M.M. PAINE. 1992. Stromelysin and tissue inhibitor of metalloproteinases gene expression in rheumatoid arthritis synovium. Am. J. Pathol. **140:** 1309–1314.
21. KEFFER, J., L. PROBERT, H. CAZLARIS, *et al.* 1991. Transgenic mice expressing human tumour necrosis factor: a predictive genetic model of arthritis. EMBO J. **10:** 4025–4031.
22. SCHETT, G., K. REDLICH, S. HAYER, *et al.* 2003. Osteoprotegerin protects against generalized bone loss in tumor necrosis factor-transgenic mice. Arthritis Rheum. **48:** 2042–2051.
23. ZWERINA, J., S. HAYER, M. TOHIDAST-AKRAD, *et al.* 2004. Single and combined inhibition of tumor necrosis factor, interleukin-1, and RANKL pathways in tumor necrosis factor-induced arthritis: effects on synovial inflammation, bone erosion, and cartilage destruction. Arthritis Rheum. **50:** 277–290.
24. LEWTHWAITE, J., S. BLAKE, T. HARDINGHAM, *et al.* 1995. Role of TNF alpha in the induction of antigen induced arthritis in the rabbit and the anti-arthritic effect of species specific TNF alpha neutralising monoclonal antibodies. Ann. Rheum. Dis. **54:** 366–374.
25. THORBECKE, G.J., R. SHAH, C.H. LEU, *et al.* 1992. Involvement of endogenous tumor necrosis factor alpha and transforming growth factor beta during induction of collagen type II arthritis in mice. Proc. Natl. Acad. Sci. USA **89:** 7375–7379.
26. LIPSKY, P.E., D.M. VAN DER HEIJDE, E.W. ST. CLAIR, *et al.* 2000. Infliximab and methotrexate in the treatment of rheumatoid arthritis. Anti-Tumor Necrosis Factor Trial in Rheumatoid Arthritis with Concomitant Therapy Study Group. N. Engl. J. Med. **343:** 1594–1602.
27. MAINI, R., E.W. ST. CLAIR, F. BREEDVELD, *et al.* 1999. Infliximab (chimeric anti-tumour necrosis factor alpha monoclonal antibody) versus placebo in rheumatoid arthritis patients receiving concomitant methotrexate: a randomised phase III trial. ATTRACT Study Group. Lancet **354:** 1932–1939.
28. MAINI, R.N., F.C. BREEDVELD, J.R. KALDEN, *et al.* 1998. Therapeutic efficacy of multiple intravenous infusions of anti-tumor necrosis factor alpha monoclonal antibody combined with low-dose weekly methotrexate in rheumatoid arthritis. Arthritis Rheum. **41:** 1552–1563.
29. MORELAND, L.W., M.H. SCHIFF, S.W. BAUMGARTNER, *et al.* 1999. Etanercept therapy in rheumatoid arthritis. A randomized, controlled trial. Ann. Intern. Med. **130:** 478–486.
30. VAN DE PUTTE, L.B., C. ATKINS, M. MALAISE, *et al.* 2004. Efficacy and safety of adalimumab as monotherapy in patients with rheumatoid arthritis for whom previous disease modifying antirheumatic drug treatment has failed. Ann. Rheum. Dis. **63:** 508–516.

31. WEINBLATT, M.E., E.C. KEYSTONE, D.E. FURST, *et al.* 2003. Adalimumab, a fully human anti-tumor necrosis factor alpha monoclonal antibody, for the treatment of rheumatoid arthritis in patients taking concomitant methotrexate: the ARMADA trial. Arthritis Rheum. **48:** 35–45.
32. GENOVESE, M.C., J.M. BATHON, R.W. MARTIN, *et al.* 2002. Etanercept versus methotrexate in patients with early rheumatoid arthritis: two-year radiographic and clinical outcomes. Arthritis Rheum. **46:** 1443–1450.
33. SMOLEN, J.S., C. HAN, M. BALA, *et al.* 2005. Evidence of radiographic benefit of infliximab plus methotrexate in rheumatoid arthritis patients who had no clinical improvement: a detailed subanalysis of the ATTRACT trial. Arthritis Rheum. **52:** 1020–1030.
34. ST. CLAIR, E.W., D.M. VAN DER HEIJDE, J.S. SMOLEN, *et al.* 2004. Combination of infliximab and methotrexate therapy for early rheumatoid arthritis: a randomized, controlled trial. Arthritis Rheum. **50:** 3432–3443.
35. QUINN, M.A., P.G. CONAGHAN, P.J. O'CONNOR, *et al.* 2005. Very early treatment with infliximab in addition to methotrexate in early, poor-prognosis rheumatoid arthritis reduces magnetic resonance imaging evidence of synovitis and damage, with sustained benefit after infliximab withdrawal: results from a twelve-month randomized, double-blind, placebo-controlled trial. Arthritis Rheum. **52:** 27–35.
36. VAN VOLLENHOVEN, R., A. HARJU, S. BRANNEMARK & L. KLARESKOG. 2003. Treatment with infliximab (Remicade) when etanercept (Enbrel) has failed or vice versa: data from the STURE registry showing that switching tumour necrosis factor alpha blockers can make sense. Ann. Rheum. Dis. **62:** 1195–1198.
37. DINARELLO, C.A. 1991. Interleukin-1 and interleukin-1 antagonism. Blood **77:** 1627–1652.
38. AREND, W.P., H.G. WELGUS, R.C. THOMPSON & S.P. EISENBERG. 1990. Biological properties of recombinant human monocyte-derived interleukin 1 receptor antagonist. J. Clin. Invest. **85:** 1694–1697.
39. DINARELLO, C.A. 2002. The IL-1 family and inflammatory diseases. Clin. Exp. Rheumatol. **20:** S1–S13.
40. FOX, S.W., K. FULLER & T.J. CHAMBERS. 2000. Activation of osteoclasts by interleukin-1: divergent responsiveness in osteoclasts formed in vivo and in vitro. J. Cell Physiol. **184:** 334–340.
41. LORENZO, J.A., A. NAPRTA, Y. RAO, *et al.* 1998. Mice lacking the type I interleukin-1 receptor do not lose bone mass after ovariectomy. Endocrinology **139:** 3022–3025.
42. KOBAYASHI, M., G.R. SQUIRES, A. MOUSA, *et al.* 2005. Role of interleukin-1 and tumor necrosis factor alpha in matrix degradation of human osteoarthritic cartilage. Arthritis Rheum. **52:** 128–135.
43. RATHANASWAMI, P., M. HACHICHA, W.L. WONG, *et al.* 1993. Synergistic effect of interleukin-1 beta and tumor necrosis factor alpha on interleukin-8 gene expression in synovial fibroblasts. Evidence that interleukin-8 is the major neutrophil-activating chemokine released in response to monokine activation. Arthritis Rheum. **36:** 1295–1304.
44. COXON, A., B. BOLON, J. ESTRADA, *et al.* 2002. Inhibition of interleukin-1 but not tumor necrosis factor suppresses neovascularization in rat models of corneal angiogenesis and adjuvant arthritis. Arthritis Rheum. **46:** 2604–2612.
45. PETTIPHER, E.R., G.A. HIGGS & B. HENDERSON. 1986. Interleukin 1 induces leukocyte infiltration and cartilage proteoglycan degradation in the synovial joint. Proc. Natl. Acad. Sci. USA **83:** 8749–8753.
46. KIM, J.M., J.G. JEONG, S.H. HO, *et al.* 2003. Protection against collagen-induced arthritis by intramuscular gene therapy with an expression plasmid for the interleukin-1 receptor antagonist. Gene Ther. **10:** 1543–1550.
47. PALMER, G., D. TALABOT-AYER, L. SZALAY-QUINODOZ, *et al.* 2003. Mice transgenic for intracellular interleukin-1 receptor antagonist type 1 are protected from collagen-induced arthritis. Eur. J. Immunol. **33:** 434–440.
48. JOOSTEN, L.A., M.M. HELSEN, T. SAXNE, *et al.* 1999. IL-1 alpha beta blockade prevents cartilage and bone destruction in murine type II collagen-induced arthritis, whereas TNF-alpha blockade only ameliorates joint inflammation. J. Immunol. **163:** 5049–5055.

49. van den Berg, W.B., L.A. Joosten, M. Helsen & F.A. van de Loo. 1994. Amelioration of established murine collagen-induced arthritis with anti-IL-1 treatment. Clin. Exp. Immunol. **95:** 237–243.
50. Horai, R., S. Saijo, H. Tanioka, *et al.* 2000. Development of chronic inflammatory arthropathy resembling rheumatoid arthritis in interleukin 1 receptor antagonist-deficient mice. J. Exp. Med. **191:** 313–320.
51. Wooley, P.H., J.D. Whalen, D.L. Chapman, *et al.* 1993. The effect of an interleukin-1 receptor antagonist protein on type II collagen-induced arthritis and antigen-induced arthritis in mice. Arthritis Rheum. **36:** 1305–1314.
52. Fontana, A., H. Hengartner, E. Weber, *et al.* 1982. Interleukin 1 activity in the synovial fluid of patients with rheumatoid arthritis. Rheumatol. Int. **2:** 49–53.
53. Deleuran, B.W., C.Q. Chu, M. Field, *et al.* 1992. Localization of interleukin-1 alpha, type 1 interleukin-1 receptor and interleukin-1 receptor antagonist in the synovial membrane and cartilage/pannus junction in rheumatoid arthritis. Br. J. Rheumatol. **31:** 801–809.
54. Muller-Ladner, U., C.R. Roberts, B.N. Franklin, *et al.* 1997. Human IL-1Ra gene transfer into human synovial fibroblasts is chondroprotective. J. Immunol. **158:** 3492–3498.
55. Campion, G.V., M.E. Lebsack, J. Lookabaugh, *et al.* 1996. Dose-range and dose-frequency study of recombinant human interleukin-1 receptor antagonist in patients with rheumatoid arthritis. The IL-1Ra Arthritis Study Group. Arthritis Rheum. **39:** 1092–1101.
56. Bresnihan, B., J.M. Alvaro-Gracia, M. Cobby, *et al.* 1998. Treatment of rheumatoid arthritis with recombinant human interleukin-1 receptor antagonist. Arthritis Rheum. **41:** 2196–2204.
57. Cohen, S., E. Hurd, J. Cush, *et al.* 2002. Treatment of rheumatoid arthritis with anakinra, a recombinant human interleukin-1 receptor antagonist, in combination with methotrexate: results of a twenty-four-week, multicenter, randomized, double-blind, placebo-controlled trial. Arthritis Rheum. **46:** 614–624.
58. Shergy, W.J., S. Cohen, M.W. Greenwald, *et al.* 2003. Anakinra (Kineret) inhibits the progression of radiographically measured joint destruction in rheumatoid arthritis. Ann. Rheum. Dis. **62:** 273.
59. Cohen, S.B., L.W. Moreland, J.J. Cush, *et al.* 2004. A multicentre, double blind, randomised, placebo controlled trial of anakinra (Kineret), a recombinant interleukin 1 receptor antagonist, in patients with rheumatoid arthritis treated with background methotrexate. Ann. Rheum. Dis. **63:** 1062–1068.
60. Guler, H.P. *et al.* 2001. A phase I, single dose escalation study of IL-1 trap in patients with rheumatoid arthritis. Arthritis Rheum. **44:** 370.
61. Pavelka, K. *et al.* 2002. Clinical effects of pralnacasan (PRAL), an orally active interleukin-1beta converting enzyme (ICE) inhibitor in a 285-patient phase II trial in rheumatoid arthritis (RA). Arthritis Rheum. **48:** 281.
62. Tosato, G., K.B. Seamon, N.D. Goldman, *et al.* 1988. Monocyte-derived human B-cell growth factor identified as interferon-beta 2 (BSF-2, IL-6). Science **239:** 502–504.
63. Okada, M., N. Sakaguchi, N. Yoshimura, *et al.* 1983. B cell growth factors and B cell differentiation factor from human T hybridomas. Two distinct kinds of B cell growth factor and their synergism in B cell proliferation. J. Exp. Med. **157:** 583–590.
64. Hibi, M., K. Nakajima & T. Hirano. 1996. IL-6 cytokine family and signal transduction: a model of the cytokine system. J. Mol. Med. **74:** 1–12.
65. Yoshizaki, K., T. Nakagawa, T. Kaieda, *et al.* 1982. Induction of proliferation and Ig production in human B leukemic cells by anti-immunoglobulins and T cell factors. J. Immunol **128:** 1296–1301.
66. Nishimoto, N., A. Ogata, Y. Shima, *et al.* 1994. Oncostatin M, leukemia inhibitory factor, and interleukin 6 induce the proliferation of human plasmacytoma cells via the common signal transducer, gp130. J. Exp. Med. **179:** 1343–1347.
67. Ishibashi, T., H. Kimura, T. Uchida, *et al.* 1989. Human interleukin 6 is a direct promoter of maturation of megakaryocytes in vitro. Proc. Natl. Acad. Sci. USA **86:** 5953–5957.

68. IKEBUCHI, K., G.G. WONG, S.C. CLARK, *et al.* 1987. Interleukin 6 enhancement of interleukin 3-dependent proliferation of multipotential hemopoietic progenitors. Proc. Natl. Acad. Sci. USA **84:** 9035–9039.
69. GOYA, S., H. MATSUOKA, M. MORI, *et al.* 2003. Sustained interleukin-6 signalling leads to the development of lymphoid organ-like structures in the lung. J. Pathol. **200:** 82–87.
70. HILL, R.J., M.K. WARREN, P. STENBERG, *et al.* 1991. Stimulation of megakaryocytopoiesis in mice by human recombinant interleukin-6. Blood **77:** 42–48.
71. SUEMATSU, S., T. MATSUDA, K. AOZASA, *et al.* 1989. IgG1 plasmacytosis in interleukin 6 transgenic mice. Proc. Natl. Acad. Sci. USA **86:** 7547–7551.
72. FATTORI, E., R.C. DELLA, P. COSTA, *et al.* 1994. Development of progressive kidney damage and myeloma kidney in interleukin-6 transgenic mice. Blood **83:** 2570–2579.
73. KATSUME, A., H. SAITO, Y. YAMADA, *et al.* 2002. Anti-interleukin 6 (IL-6) receptor antibody suppresses Castleman's disease like symptoms emerged in IL-6 transgenic mice. Cytokine **20:** 304–311.
74. HOUSSIAU, F.A., J.P. DEVOGELAER, J. VAN DAMME, *et al.* 1988. Interleukin-6 in synovial fluid and serum of patients with rheumatoid arthritis and other inflammatory arthritides. Arthritis Rheum. **31:** 784–788.
75. GUERNE, P.A., B.L. ZURAW, J.H. VAUGHAN, *et al.* 1989. Synovium as a source of interleukin 6 in vitro. Contribution to local and systemic manifestations of arthritis. J. Clin. Invest. **83:** 585–592.
76. OKAMOTO, H., M. YAMAMURA, Y. MORITA, *et al.* 1997. The synovial expression and serum levels of interleukin-6, interleukin-11, leukemia inhibitory factor, and oncostatin M in rheumatoid arthritis. Arthritis Rheum. **40:** 1096–1105.
77. POLI, V., R. BALENA, E. FATTORI, *et al.* 1994. Interleukin-6 deficient mice are protected from bone loss caused by estrogen depletion. EMBO J. **13:** 1189–1196.
78. BELLIDO, T., R.L. JILKA, B.F. BOYCE, *et al.* 1995. Regulation of interleukin-6, osteoclastogenesis, and bone mass by androgens. The role of the androgen receptor. J. Clin. Invest. **95:** 2886–2895.
79. KUDO, O., A. SABOKBAR, A. POCOCK, *et al.* 2003. Interleukin-6 and interleukin-11 support human osteoclast formation by a RANKL-independent mechanism. Bone **32:** 1–7.
80. KURIHARA, N., D. BERTOLINI, T. SUDA, *et al.* 1990. IL-6 stimulates osteoclast-like multinucleated cell formation in long term human marrow cultures by inducing IL-1 release. J. Immunol. **144:** 4226–4230.
81. TAKAGI, N., M. MIHARA, Y. MORIYA, *et al.* 1998. Blockage of interleukin-6 receptor ameliorates joint disease in murine collagen-induced arthritis. Arthritis Rheum. **41:** 2117–2121.
82. MIHARA, M., M. KOTOH, N. NISHIMOTO, *et al.* 2001. Humanized antibody to human interleukin-6 receptor inhibits the development of collagen arthritis in cynomolgus monkeys. Clin. Immunol. **98:** 319–326.
83. SASAI, M., Y. SAEKI, S. OHSHIMA, *et al.* 1999. Delayed onset and reduced severity of collagen-induced arthritis in interleukin-6-deficient mice. Arthritis Rheum. **42:** 1635–1643.
84. ALONZI, T., E. FATTORI, D. LAZZARO, *et al.* 1998. Interleukin 6 is required for the development of collagen-induced arthritis. J. Exp. Med. **187:** 461–468.
85. WENDLING, D., E. RACADOT & J. WIJDENES. 1993. Treatment of severe rheumatoid arthritis by anti-interleukin 6 monoclonal antibody. J. Rheumatol. **20:** 259–262.
86. YOSHIZAKI, K., T. MATSUDA, N. NISHIMOTO, *et al.* 1989. Pathogenic significance of interleukin-6 (IL-6/BSF-2) in Castleman's disease. Blood **74:** 1360–1367.
87. NISHIMOTO, N., M. SASAI, Y. SHIMA, *et al.* 2000. Improvement in Castleman's disease by humanized anti-interleukin-6 receptor antibody therapy. Blood **95:** 56–61.
88. CHOY, E.H., D.A. ISENBERG, T. GARROOD, *et al.* 2002. Therapeutic benefit of blocking interleukin-6 activity with an anti-interleukin-6 receptor monoclonal antibody in rheumatoid arthritis: a randomized, double-blind, placebo-controlled, dose-escalation trial. Arthritis Rheum. **46:** 3143–3150.
89. NISHIMOTO, N., K. YOSHIZAKI, N. MIYASAKA, *et al.* 2004. Treatment of rheumatoid arthritis with humanized anti-interleukin-6 receptor antibody: a multicenter, double-blind, placebo-controlled trial. Arthritis Rheum. **50:** 1761–1769.

90. Grabstein, K.H., J. Eisenman, K. Shanebeck, *et al.* 1994. Cloning of a T cell growth factor that interacts with the beta chain of the interleukin-2 receptor. Science **264:** 965–968.
91. Doherty, T.M., R.A. Seder & A. Sher. 1996. Induction and regulation of IL-15 expression in murine macrophages. J. Immunol. **156:** 735–741.
92. Kanegane, H. & G. Tosato. 1996. Activation of naive and memory T cells by interleukin-15. Blood **88:** 230–235.
93. McInnes, I.B., J. Al Mughales, M. Field, *et al.* 1996. The role of interleukin-15 in T-cell migration and activation in rheumatoid arthritis. Nat. Med. **2:** 175–182.
94. Carson, W.E., J.G. Giri, M.J. Lindemann, *et al.* 1994. Interleukin (IL) 15 is a novel cytokine that activates human natural killer cells via components of the IL-2 receptor. J. Exp. Med. **180:** 1395–1403.
95. Alleva, D.G., S.B. Kaser, M.A. Monroy, *et al.* 1997. IL-15 functions as a potent autocrine regulator of macrophage proinflammatory cytokine production: evidence for differential receptor subunit utilization associated with stimulation or inhibition. J. Immunol. **159:** 2941–2951.
96. Ogata, Y., A. Kukita, T. Kukita, *et al.* 1999. A novel role of IL-15 in the development of osteoclasts: inability to replace its activity with IL-2. J. Immunol. **162:** 2754–2760.
97. Thurkow, E.W., I.M. van der Heijden, F.C. Breedveld, *et al.* 1997. Increased expression of IL-15 in the synovium of patients with rheumatoid arthritis compared with patients with Yersinia-induced arthritis and osteoarthritis. J. Pathol. **181:** 444–450.
98. McInnes, I.B., B.P. Leung, R.D. Sturrock, *et al.* 1997. Interleukin-15 mediates T cell-dependent regulation of tumor necrosis factor-alpha production in rheumatoid arthritis. Nat. Med. **3:** 189–195.
99. Miranda-Carus, M.E., A. Balsa, M. Benito-Miguel, *et al.* 2004. IL-15 and the initiation of cell contact-dependent synovial fibroblast-T lymphocyte cross-talk in rheumatoid arthritis: effect of methotrexate. J. Immunol. **173:** 1463–1476.
100. Gracie, J.A., R.J. Forsey, W.L. Chan, *et al.* 1999. A proinflammatory role for IL-18 in rheumatoid arthritis. J. Clin. Invest. **104:** 1393–1401.
101. Ruchatz, H., B.P. Leung, X.Q. Wei, *et al.* 1998. Soluble IL-15 receptor alpha-chain administration prevents murine collagen-induced arthritis: a role for IL-15 in development of antigen-induced immunopathology. J. Immunol. **160:** 5654–5660.
102. Ferrari-Lacraz, S., E. Zanelli, M. Neuberg, *et al.* 2004. Targeting IL-15 receptor-bearing cells with an antagonist mutant IL-15/Fc protein prevents disease development and progression in murine collagen-induced arthritis. J. Immunol. **173:** 5818–5826.
103. McInnes, I.B. & J.A. Gracie. 2004. Interleukin-15: a new cytokine target for the treatment of inflammatory diseases. Curr. Opin. Pharmacol. **4:** 392–397.
104. McInnes, I., R. Martin, I. Zimmerman-Gorska, *et al.* 2004. Safety and efficacy of a human monoclonal antibody to IL-15 (AMG 714) in patients with rheumatoid arthritis (RA): results from a multicenter, randomized, double-blind, placebo-controlled trial. Presented at the Annual Meeting of the American College of Rheumatology. San Antonio, TX, Oct 18.
105. Smolen, J.S. & G. Steiner. 2003. Therapeutic strategies for rheumatoid arthritis. Nat. Rev. Drug Discov. **2:** 473–488.
106. Redlich, K., B. Gortz, S. Hayer, *et al.* 2004. Repair of local bone erosions and reversal of systemic bone loss upon therapy with anti-tumor necrosis factor in combination with osteoprotegerin or parathyroid hormone in tumor necrosis factor-mediated arthritis. Am. J. Pathol. **164:** 543–555.

Anti-inflammatory and Immune Regulatory Properties of 5-Androsten-3β, 17β-Diol (HE2100), and Synthetic Analogue HE3204

Implications for Treatment of Autoimmune Diseases

D. AUCI,[a] F. NICOLETTI,[b] K. MANGANO,[b] R. PIETERS,[c] S. NIERKENS,[c] L. MORGAN,[a] H. OFFNER,[d] J. FRINCKE,[a] AND C. READING[a]

[a]*Hollis-Eden Pharmaceuticals, San Diego, California, USA*

[b]*Department of Biomedical Sciences, School of Medicine, University of Catania, Catania, Italy*

[c]*Institute for Risk Assessment Sciences, Utrecht University, Utrecht, the Netherlands*

[d]*Department of Neurology, Oregon Health and Science University, Portland, Oregon, USA*

ABSTRACT: 5-Androsten-3β, 17β-diol (HE2100), and a synthetic analogue HE3204 are regarded as immune-regulating hormones, because both induce changes in the reporter antigen–popliteal lymph node assay (RA-PLNA). Mice were injected in the footpad with either HE2100 or HE3204 (0.01–3 mg), and a nonsensitizing dose of trinitrophenyl ovalbumin (TNP-OVA) was used as bystander reporter antigen. Seven days later, nodes were removed and numbers of cells (CD3, CD4, CD8, CD19; flow cytometry), TNP-specific IgM, IgG1, and IgG2a antibody-forming cells (AFCs; ELISPOT assay), and cytokines (interleukin-4 [IL-4], interferon-γ [IFN-γ]; ELISA) were measured. HE2100 and HE3204 increased cell numbers in a dose-dependent fashion. T (helper and suppressor) cells and B cells were increased (>5-fold). HE3204 was apparently twice as potent as HE2100. Both increased the B/T ratio (fivefold), increased TNP-specific IgM and IgG1 (~50-fold), and induced IgG2a AFCs. Both increased IL-4 and IFN-γ secretion (up to threefold). Both displayed anti-inflammatory activity in the murine model of carrageenan-induced pleurisy, as evidenced by reduced neutrophil numbers and exudate volumes. Our observations suggest that both HE2100 and HE3204 are immune-regulating steroid hormones that exhibit anti-inflammatory properties. HE2100 (1 mg/mouse per day) provided significant benefit when given at disease onset in the SJL/J female mouse model of experimental autoimmune encephalomyelitis. These compounds and their analogues are candidates for further testing in autoimmune diseases.

KEYWORDS: steroids; DHEA; autoimmune disease; immune-regulating hormones

Address for correspondence: Dominick L. Auci, 4435 Eastgate Mall, Suite 400, San Diego, CA 92121. Voice: 858-320-2582; fax: 858-558-6470.
Dauci@holliseden.com

**Ann. N.Y. Acad. Sci. 1051: 730–742 (2005). © 2005 New York Academy of Sciences.
doi: 10.1196/annals.1361.117**

INTRODUCTION

More than 30 steroids are made by the adrenal cortex. Collectively called corticoids, they can be grouped into three main classes: the *mineralocorticoids,* which are involved in ion regulation; the immune suppressive anti-inflammatory *glucocorticoids* (GCs); and a third class of compounds with powerful immune regulatory functions. This third class of immune active steroids, which includes dehydroepiandrosterone (DHEA; 3β-hydroxy-5-androstene-17-one), a precursor of both androgens and estrogens, has well-documented antiglucocorticoid[1] and immunoregulatory properties in several preclinical models.[2–9] DHEA also serves as a precursor for many less well understood immune-active steroids, and a decline in serum levels is associated with aging and the loss of several aspects of immunity and health.[10] Its replacement in immune-suppressed or aged immune-senescent animals restores immunity.[11] DHEA has not proved efficacious in humans. This may be caused by poor oral bioavailability,[12] differential metabolic potential in humans versus rodents, and ready conversion to sex hormones, which causes androgenic and estrogenic effects, rather than the desired clinical benefit. Recently, Lardy and colleagues have characterized an array of DHEA metabolites.[13] In all, 19 metabolites, each with potentially different activities, were identified in that study.

Because of poor potency, high metabolic potential, and androgenic and estrogenic side effects, DHEA does not appear to be suited for use as a pharmaceutical in humans. Instead, an entire family of potential immune-regulating hormones (IRHs) are now under development that are congeners of the androstene steroid series. In many human and animal model systems, these molecules appear to potently reduce inflammation, correct immune system dysregulation, normalize immune function, and preserve or restore effective immunity. Initial studies determined that lead candidates include 5-androsten-3β, 17β-diol (HE2100), 16α-bromoepiandrosterone (HE2000), and 16α-fluroandrosten-17-one (HE2500). Medicinal chemistry approaches have afforded second-generation analogues with improved properties. HE2100 and HE3204 serve as examples of a first-generation metabolite and a metabolically inert second-generation synthetic analogue, respectively. Both are regarded as immune-regulating hormones, because both produce changes in the reporter antigen–popliteal lymph node assay (RA-PLNA). In this communication, we report their potential as candidates to treat autoimmune conditions.

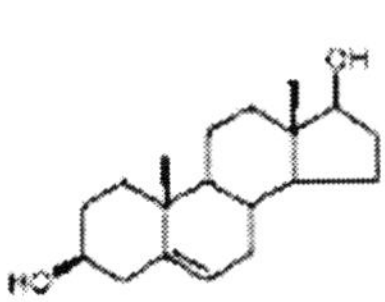

5-androsten-3ß,17ß-diol
(HE2100)

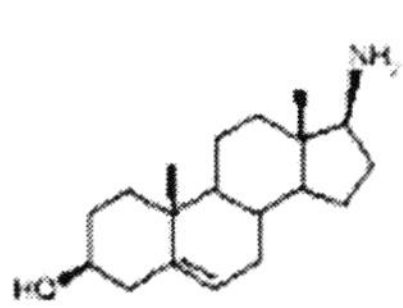

5-androsten-17β-amino-3-ol
(HE3204)

SCHEME 1.

METHODS

Pleurisy Model

Animals

Five- to eight-week-old CD1 male mice (Charles River, Calco, Italy) were used for the study. The animals were housed in a controlled environment and provided with standard rodent chow and water. Animal care was in compliance with Italian regulations on the protection of animals used for experimental and other scientific purposes and with the European Economic Community regulations.

Experimental groups

Mice were allocated into one of the following groups: (1) administration of carrageenan (CAR) only (CAR group); (2) mice treated with HE compound (HE 2100 or HE 3204) subcutaneously (s.c.) 24 h and 1 h before CAR; (3) mice treated with vehicle s.c. 24 h and 1 h before CAR; and (4) mice treated with a rabbit anti-mouse polyclonal anti–TNF-α antibody (200 μg) given by intraperitoneal (i.p.) bolus 24 h and 1 h before CAR. Each group consisted of 10 mice. All treatments were given in a final volume of 100 μL.

Carrageenan-induced pleurisy

Mice were anesthetized with isoflurane and underwent a a skin incision at the level of the left sixth intercostal space. The underlying muscle was dissected and saline (0.1 mL) or saline containing 2% λ-CAR (0.1 mL) was injected into the pleural cavity. The skin incision was closed with a suture and the animals were allowed to recover. At 4 h after the injection of CAR, the animals were killed by inhalation of CO_2. The chest was carefully opened and the pleural cavity rinsed with 1 mL saline solution containing heparin 5 U/mL and indomethacin 10 μg/mL. The exudate and washing solution were removed by aspiration and the total volume was measured. Any exudate that was contaminated with blood was discarded. The amount of exudate was calculated by subtracting the volume used to wash the pleural cavity (1 mL) from the total volume recovered. The leukocytes in the exudate were suspended in phosphate-buffered saline (PBS) and counted with an optical microscope in a Burker's chamber after vital trypan blue staining.

Data analysis

All values in the figures are expressed as mean ± standard deviation (SD).

The results were analyzed by one-way ANOVA, followed by a Bonferroni *post hoc* test for multiple comparisons. For statistical analysis each group was compared with the control group of mice that were challenged with CAR and received no treatment.

Lipopolysaccharide-Induced Shock Model

Mice

Six-week-old female CD1 mice were kept under standard laboratory conditions with free access to food and water.

Induction of septic shock and experimental treatment

To induce lethal endotoxemia, we injected the mice intraperitoneally with 1 mg lipopolysaccharide (LPS; Sigma Chimica, Milan, Italy). Groups of mice were treated with HE2100 (1.0 or 0.1 mg) or vehicle (HERF 405; 0.1% carboxymethylcellulose, 0.9% saline, 2% Tween 80, 0.05% phenol; Hollis-Eden Pharmaceuticals, San Diego, CA).

Data analysis

Statistical analysis was performed on data acquired for cumulative incidence of lethality up to 72 h after LPS administration by the chi-square test. Data from each experimental group were compared with data from vehicle-treated controls.

Reporter Antigen–Popliteal Lymph Node Assay

Mice

Specific pathogen-free female BALB/C mice (6–12 weeks old) were obtained from the Utrecht University breeding facility (Gemeenschappelijk Dier Laboratorium, Utrecht, The Netherlands) and randomly assigned to specific treatments. Mice were allowed to acclimate for 1 week and were maintained under barrier conditions in filter-topped Macrolon cages with wood chip bedding at a mean temperature of 23 ± 2°C, 50% to 55% relative humidity, and a 12-hour light/dark cycle. Drinking water and standard laboratory food pellets were provided *ad libitum*. The experiments were conducted according to the guidelines of the animal care experiments committee of the Veterinary Faculty of the Utrecht University.

Chemicals and reagents

Chemicals were obtained from Sigma-Aldrich (Zwijndrect, The Netherlands) unless stated otherwise. Saline 0.9% (B. Braun Melsungen, Melsungen, Germany) and citrate buffer (0.1 M citric acid, 0.1 M disodium hydrogen phosphate, pH 6.0) were used to dilute test chemicals. Trinitrophenyl ovalbumin (TNP-OVA) and blocking agent trinitrophenyl bovine serum albumin (TNP-BSA) were prepared as previously described by Pieters and Albers.[14] For ELISPOT analyses, alkaline phosphatase (AP)–conjugated goat anti-mouse IgG1 and IgM were obtained from Southern Biotechnology Associates (Birmingham, AL). For development of spots, fresh stock solutions of para-nitroblue tetrazolium and 5-bromo-4 chloro-3 indolylphosphate toluidine salt in dimethylformamide (BDH Laboratory Supplies, Poole, UK) were prepared and diluted in Tris buffer (100 mM Trizma base, 100 mM NaCl, 5 mM $MgCl_2$*6H2O, pH 9.5). For cytokine measurements, interleukin-4 (IL-4) and interferon-γ (IFN-γ) capture and detection antibodies were obtained from BD PharMingen (Hamburg, Germany). Streptavidin coupled to HRP was obtained from CLB (Amsterdam, the Netherlands) and casein was purchased from BDH Laboratory Supplies. The following antibodies used for surface marker staining in tricolor flow cytometry were purchased from BD PharMingen: CD3e CyChrome (CY; 145-2C11), CD4 FITC (RM4-5), CD8a PE (53-6.7), and CD19 PE (1D33).

RA-PLNA

Naive mice (five mice per group) were injected subcutaneously into the right hind footpad with 50 mL of a freshly prepared mixture of the drug together with a subsensitizing dose (10 mg) of TNP-OVA. Seven days after drug injection, mice were killed by cervical dislocation, blood was drawn by orbital puncture, and the popliteal lymph node (PLN) was excised and separated from adherent fatty tissue. PLNs were isolated in ice-cold PBS/1% BSA, and single-cell suspensions were prepared, washed (1000 rpm at 4°C), resuspended in 1 mL PBS/1% BSA, counted using a Coulter counter (Coulter Electronics, Luton UK), and adjusted to 1×10^6 cells/mL.

ELISPOT assay

The ELISPOT assay was performed based on the operating procedure described by Schielen *et al.*[15] Immobilon-P membranes (immobilon PVDF Transfer; Millipore, Etten-Leur, The Netherlands) were coated overnight with PBS/0.05%Tween/TNP-BSA (10 mg/mL) and blocked for 1 h with PBS/Tween/1% BSA. These membranes were clamped in spot blocks (made in-house), and 5 × 105 cells were centrifuged onto the membranes and incubated for 4 h at 37°C. Membranes were removed from the spot block, washed with PBS and PBS/Tween, and incubated overnight at 4°C with AP-conjugated antibodies in PBS/Tween. Membranes were washed and incubated with para-nitroblue tetrazolium/5-bromo-4-chloro-3-indolylphosphate toluidine salt reagent to accomplish color development of TNP-specific antibody spots. These spots were counted by two independent observers using a stereomicroscope.

Cell culture and cytokine measurements

Cell suspensions at 1×10^5 cells in 100 mL complete RPMI 1640 (Life Technologies) supplemented with 10% FCS, 50 mM B-ME, and 200 mM L-glutamine were incubated with 50 mL concavalin A (Con A, 15 mg/mL) or medium in 96-well plates (Highbond 3590; Costar, Cambridge, MA) overnight in 5% CO2. After centrifugation for 10 min at 1000 rpm, supernatant was collected and stored at –70°C until analysis. IFN-γ and IL-4 were determined by sandwich ELISA. Plates were coated overnight at 4°C with 1 mg/mL rat anti-mouse IFN-γ or 1 mg/mL rat anti-mouse IL-4 in 0.05 M carbonate buffer (pH 9.6), washed with PBS/Tween, and blocked with PBS/Tween/casein for 4 h at room temperature. Samples and IL-4 and IFN-γ standards (100 mL) were added in several dilutions and incubated overnight at 4°C. After washing, plates were incubated with 0.25 mg/mL biotinylated rat anti-mouse IFN-γ or IL-4 conjugate diluted in PBS/Tween/casein for 1 h at room temperature. Plates were washed and incubated with streptavidin-HRP (0.3 mg/mL) and diluted in PBS/Tween/casein for 45 min at room temperature. After final washes, tetramethylbenzidine (TMB) substrate (0.1 mg/mL) was added, and after 10 min the color reaction was stopped with 2 M H_2SO_4. Absorbance was measured at 450 nm using an ELISA plate reader (ELX800; Bio-Tek Instruments, Winooski, VT).

Flow cytometry

Flow cytometric analysis using 1×10^5 cells suspended in PBS/BSA were centrifuged, resuspended, and incubated with predetermined dilutions of FITC-, PE-, or CY-conjugated monoclonal antibodies in 96-well plates (30 min in darkness at 4°C).

Cells were washed, resuspended, stored in formalin 0.1%, and analyzed within 18 h using a FACscan with standard FACsflow CellQuest software (BD Biosciences, Franklin Lakes, NJ).

EAE Model

Mice

Female SJL/J mice were used for *in vivo* EAE studies. The mice were housed in the Animal Resource Facility at the Portland Veterans Affairs Medical Center in accordance with institutional guidelines.

Antigens

Mouse proteolipid protein (PLP) 139-151 (HCLGKWLGHPDKF) was used for active immunization. Antigens were synthesized using solid-phase techniques and purified by high-performance liquid chromatography at the Beckman Institute, Stanford University (Palo Alto, CA).

Induction of active EAE

On day 0, SJL/J mice were immunized with 150 μg PLP 139-151 in complete Freund's adjuvant (CFA) containing 200 μg of *Mycobacterium tuberculosis* (MTB) by subcutaneous injection over four sites on the hind flank. The mice were assessed daily for clinical signs of EAE according to the following scale: 0 = no signs; 1 = limp tail or mild hind limb weakness; 2 = moderate hind limb weakness or mild ataxia; 3 = moderately severe hind limb weakness; 4 = severe hind limb weakness or mild forearm weakness or moderate ataxia; 5 = paraplegia with no more than moderate forelimb weakness; 6 = paraplegia with severe forelimb weakness or severe ataxia or moribund condition.

Treatment with DHEA derivative

SJL/J mice were given subcutaneous injections of HE2100 (1 mg in 0.1 mL vehicle) or vehicle alone (control), beginning at onset of disease (approximately 11 days after immunization).

RESULTS

CAR-Induced Pleurisy

All mice challenged with CAR and left untreated, or treated with vehicle alone, developed an acute pleurisy that produced turbid exudates and increased numbers of polymorphonuclear leukocytes (PMNs) in the pleural cavity (FIG. 1; exudate data not shown). Relative to vehicle control mice, prophylactic treatment with HE2100 or HE3204 markedly reduced both the degree of lung inflammatory cell infiltration and the volume of pleural exudates in a dose-dependent fashion. The effect achieved by the higher dose of HE3204 was comparable to that of the polyclonal anti-mouse TNF-α antibody (positive control). Neutrophils observed in the CAR-challenged

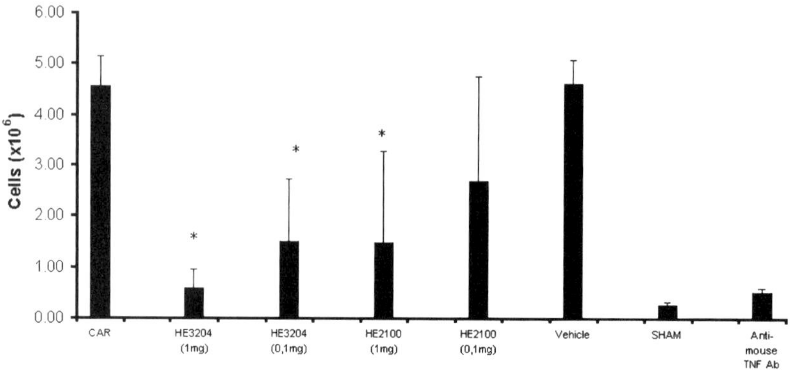

FIGURE 1. Effect of HE2100 and HE3204 on PMN numbers in murine model of carrageenan-induced pleurisy. Mice were anesthetized with isoflurane, and saline (0.1 mL) or saline containing 2% λ-CAR (0.1 mL) was injected into the pleural cavity. Mice were treated with HE2100 or HE3204 (1.0 or 0.1 mg s.c.) 24 h and 1 h before CAR challenge. At 4 h after injection of CAR, the animals were killed, the chests were carefully opened, and the pleural cavities were rinsed with 1 mL saline solution containing heparin 5 U/mL and indomethacin 10 μg/mL. The leukocytes in the exudate were suspended in PBS and counted with an optical microscope in a Burker's chamber, after vital trypan blue staining. Data are the combined results of two separate studies and are expressed as PMNs per mouse ± standard deviation. *Significant difference between vehicle control and experimental treatment ($P < 0.05$). CAR, carrageenan; PBS, phosphate-buffered saline; PMN, polymorphonuclear leukocyte; s.c., subcutaneous.

mice treated with high-dose HE2100 were 13% of those observed in untreated CAR-challenged animals as compared with 11% for the CAR-challenged mice treated with anti-mouse TNF-α antibody. Exudate volumes in the treated CAR-challenged animals were 40% of those observed in the untreated CAR-challenged group as compared with 36% for CAR-challenged animals treated with anti-mouse TNF-α antibody.

LPS-Induced Shock

All vehicle-treated control mice died within 3 days after LPS challenge (FIG. 2). A 40% reduction in the cumulative incidence of lethality was observed in mice that had been treated with 0.1 mg HE2100.

RA-PLN Assay

Neither HE2100 nor HE3204 appeared immune suppressive, even at the highest dose (3 mg) tested. Both appeared to increase B cells and the B/T cell ratio. These effects were dose dependent (FIG. 3). Both compounds increased numbers of antigen-presenting and dendritic cells (up to fivefold; data not shown). Both HE2100 and HE3204 increased numbers of hapten-specific IgM and IgG1 AFCs, and HE3204 appeared more potent than HE2100 (FIG. 4). ConA-induced IFN-γ production by PLN cells was increased by both compounds (FIG. 5), even at the lowest dose

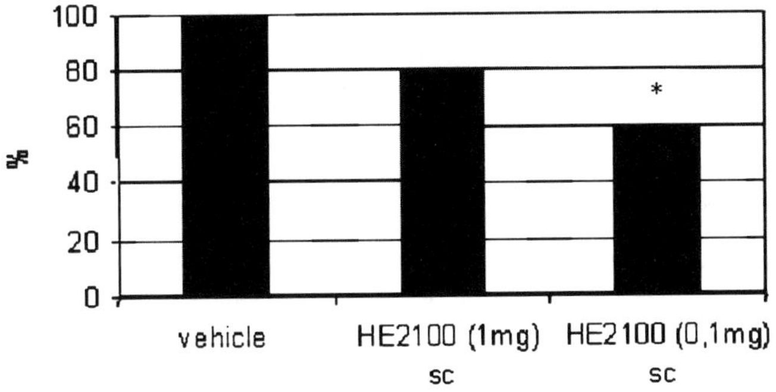

FIGURE 2. Effect of HE2100 on survival of LPS-challenged mice. Mice were challenged with i.p. LPS (1 mg in 100 μL). Mice were treated with HE2100 (1 mg or 0.1 mg s.c.) or vehicle control (100 μL). Percent lethality was determined 72 h later. *Significant difference between vehicle control and experimental treatment ($P < 0.05$). LPS, lipopolysaccharide; i.p., intraperioneal; s.c., subcutaneous.

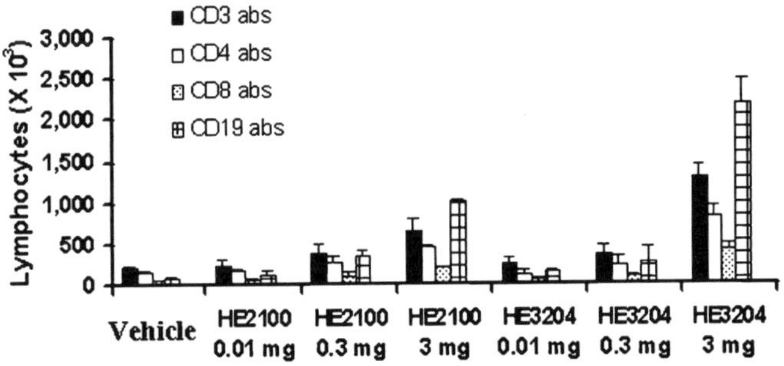

FIGURE 3. Effect of HE2100 or HE3204 on T and B cells in RA-PLN assay. HE2100 or HE3204 (0.01, 0.3, or 3 mg) was injected into the right footpad along with a nonsensitizing dose of TNP-OVA conjugate (total volume, 50 μL). On day 7, PLNs were harvested. Numbers of T or B lymphocytes ($CD3^+$, $CD4^+$, $CD8^+$, or $CD19^+$) were determined by flow cytometry of living cells in suspension. Data are expressed as total cells. Each *bar* represents mean values ± SEM of five mice per group. RA-PLN, reporter antigen–popliteal lymph node; TNP-OVA, trinitrophenyl-ovalbumin.

tested (0.01 mg), and this effect was dose dependent. Both compounds also increased ConA-induced IL-4 production. Both compounds increased TNP-induced IFN-γ production at the high dose. Both compounds increased TNP-OVA–specific IL-4 production in a dose-dependent fashion.

EAE

When female SJL/J mice were injected with PLP 139-151 peptide in CFA, a severe form of relapsing-remitting EAE was observed (FIG. 6 and TABLE 1). Symptoms of EAE first developed on days 10 to 11 and peaked on day 14 (4.81 ± 0.46). Symptoms of EAE remitted and relapsed in certain animals between days 14 to 34 in both

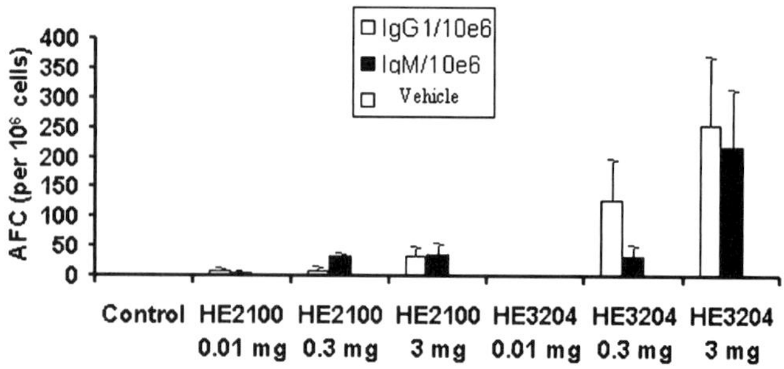

FIGURE 4. Effect of HE2100 or HE3204 on numbers of TNP-specific AFCs in RA-PLN assay. HE2100 or HE3204 (0.01, 0.3, or 3 mg) was injected into the right footpad along with a nonsensitizing dose of TNP-OVA conjugate (total volume, 50 μL). On day 7, PLNs were harvested. Numbers of TNP-specific IgM or IgG1 AFCs were determined by the ELISPOT assay. Data are expressed as AFCs/million cells. Each bar represents mean values ± SEM of five mice per group. AFC, antibody-forming cell; RA-PLN, reporter antigen–popliteal lymph node; TNP-OVA, trinitrophenyl-ovalbumin.

untreated (three of eight mice) and treated (two of eight mice) groups. Cumulative disease index (CDI) for these animals was 81.88 ± 11.55.

In contrast, when mice were treated with HE2100 (1 mg/mouse per day beginning at EAE onset) a lower peak (3.63 ± 1.3) was observed on day 14. Symptoms of EAE followed a relapsing-remitting course. CDI for the HE2100-treated animals was 58.6 ± 22.9, which was significantly less than in the vehicle-treated animals ($P < 0.05$).

DISCUSSION

Several findings stand out from the results reported here. Both HE2100 and HE3204 appear to have potent anti-inflammatory effects, as judged by the ability of both compounds to reduce neutrophil infiltration and exudate volumes in the murine model of carrageenan-induced pleurisy. This model is widely used to assess the anti-inflammatory potential of candidate compounds. HE2100 provided survival benefit in the mouse model of septic shock. Neither compound was found to be immune suppressive in the RA-PLN assay. Both HE2100 and HE3204 are considered to be immune-regulating hormones, based on their ability to increase lymphocytes and to stimulate immune parameters associated with the so-called Th2 responses. These parameters include greater increases in B cells (as opposed to T cells), increases in antibody-forming cells, and increases in IL-4 and IFN-γ.

FIGURE 5. Effect of HE2100 or HE3204 on IFN-γ and IL-4 secretion in RA-PLN assay. HE2100 or HE3204 (0.01, 0.3, or 3 mg) was injected into the right footpad along with a nonsensitizing dose of TNP-OVA conjugate (total volume, 50 μL). On day 7, PLNs were harvested. IFN-γ (*top*) or IL-4 (*bottom*) levels in overnight cell culture supernatants were determined by ELISA. Data are expressed as picograms per milliliters. Each *bar* represents mean values ± SEM of five mice per group. IFN-γ, interferon-γ; IL-4, interleukin-4; RA-PLN, reporter antigen–popliteal lymph node; TNP-OVA, trinitrophenyl-ovalbumin.

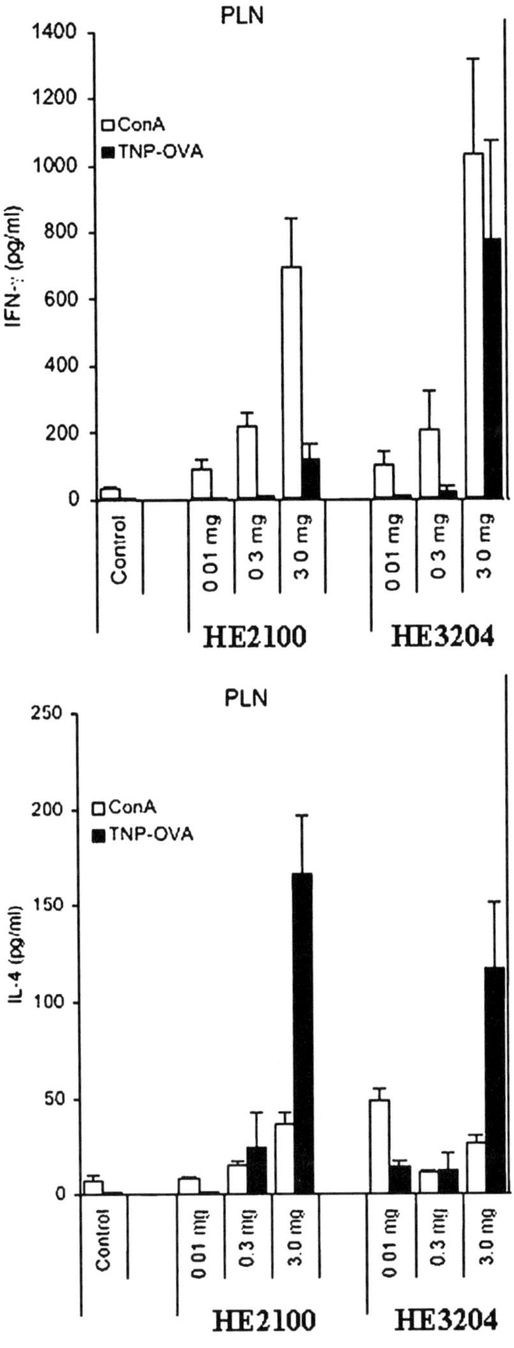

FIGURE 5. *See preceding page for legend.*

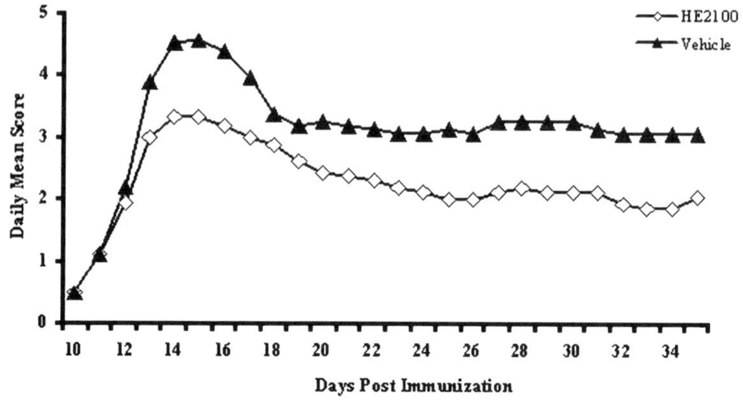

FIGURE 6. Effect of HE2100 treatment on disease scores in the female SJL mouse model of EAE. Female SJL mice were injected subcutaneously with 1 mg HE2100/mouse/day in 100 μL of vehicle, or with vehicle alone, starting at onset of EAE (day 10 to 11 after immunization with 150 mg PLP/200 mg CFA to induce EAE). Data are from 10 mice per group and expressed as daily mean clinical score. CFA, complete Freund's adjuvant; EAE, experimental autoimmune encephalomyelitis; PLP, proteolipid protein; s.c., subcutaneous.

TABLE 1. Amelioration of EAE in female SJL mice treated with HE2100 beginning at onset of disease

Group	Onset	Peak	Mortality	Relapse	CDI
HE2100	11.38 ± 0.52	3.63 ± 1.30	0/8	2/8	58.75 ± 22.89[a]
Vehicle	11.38 ± 0.52	4.81 ± 0.46	0/8	3/8	81.88 ± 11.55

NOTE: Female SJL mice were treated with HE2100 1 mg s.c. per mouse per day beginning at onset of EAE (day 10 to 11 after immunization with PLP 139-151 peptide in CFA). CDI, cumulative disease index.

[a]Significant difference between vehicle control and experimental treatment ($P < 0.05$).

A general "gender gap" in autoimmunity has long been recognized. Attempts to understand the molecular basis for this gender dimorphism with respect to incidence and severity of autoimmune disease, with a view to uncover new therapeutic modalities, has been the focus of much effort over the past two decades. Such work has led to the demonstration of powerful immunoregulatory properties of sex hormones such as 17-beta estradiol in several autoimmune disease models, including EAE.[16] Voskuhl and colleagues, in a recent review of the literature, concluded that the gender difference in EAE susceptibility in mice is caused primarily by a protective effect of testosterone in male animals.[17] The idea that the ratio between male and female sex hormones could modulate demyelinating disease was recently strengthened by Du and colleagues, who showed that subcutaneous treatment with DHEA could ameliorate EAE in female SJL/L mice.[18] However, the inability of humans to produce potent metabolites of DHEA, as found in rodents, and the estrogenic and/or androgenic side effects associated with these compounds make neither estradiol nor DHEA ideal candidates for use in humans. Neither HE2500 (see below) nor HE3204 interact with androgen or estrogen receptors (Hollis-Eden Pharmaceuticals, unpublished observations) and are not expected to produce such unwanted side effects.

In EAE, in this same SJL/J female mouse model, we recently showed that HE2500 could provide significant benefit when given to animals at disease onset.[19] However, benefit was observed only at doses (6 mg per day) not easily achievable in humans. Therefore, analogues were screened as described in this communication to elucidate relationships that could lead to more potent and pharmaceutically relevant compounds. HE2100 provided an ideal opportunity to benchmark our screening process. H2100 is a potent anti-inflammatory steroid that appears to preferentially stimulate Th2 responses. These properties were indicative of possible benefit in EAE, benefits confirmed by these studies. HE3204, a synthetic analogue, is metabolically resistant and appears to be more potent in Th2 immune response stimulation (as judged by the PLN assay) than HE2100. These results suggest that studies of several additional related analogues with a variety of pharmaceutical properties are warranted.

REFERENCES

1. Blauer, K.L., M. Poth, W.M. Rogers & E.W. Bernton. 1991. Dehydroepiandrosterone antagonizes the suppressive effects of dexamethasone on lymphocyte proliferation. Endocrinology **129:** 3174–3179.
2. Daynes, R.A., D.J. Dudley & B.A. Araneo. 1990. Regulation of murine lymphokine production in vivo. II. Dehydroepiandrosterone is a natural enhancer of interleukin 2 synthesis by helper T cells. Eur. J. Immunol. **20:** 793–802.
3. Suzuki, T., N. Suzuki, R.A. Daynes & E.G. Engleman. 1991. Dehydroepiandrosterone enhances IL2 production and cytotoxic effector function of human T cells. Clin. Immunol. Immunopathol. **61:** 202–211.
4. Daynes, R.A. & B.A. Araneo. 1994. The development of effective vaccine adjuvants employing natural regulators of T-cell lymphokine production in vivo. Ann. NY Acad. Sci. **730:** 144–161.
5. Loria, R.M., D.A. Padgett & P.N. Huynh. 1996. Regulation of the immune response by dehydroepiandrosterone and its metabolites. J. Endocrinol. **150** (Suppl): S209–S220.
6. Padgett, D.A., R.M. Loria & J.F. Sheridan. 1997. Endocrine regulation of the immune response to influenza virus infection with a metabolite of DHEA-androstenediol. J. Neuroimmunol. **78:** 203–211.
7. Ben-Nathan, D., D.A. Padgett & R.M. Loria. 1999. Androstenediol and dehydroepiandrosterone protect mice against lethal bacterial infections and lipopolysaccharide toxicity. J. Med. Microbiol. **48:** 25–31.
8. Canning, M.O., K. Grotenhuis, H.J. de Wit & H.A. Drexhage. 2000. Opposing effects of dehydroepiandrosterone and dexamethasone on the generation of monocyte-derived dendritic cells. Eur. J. Endocrinol. **143:** 687–695.
9. Clerici, M., D. Trabattoni, S. Piconi, *et al.* 1997. A possible role for the cortisol/anticortisols imbalance in the progression of human immunodeficiency virus. Psychoneuroendocrinology **22:** S27–S31.
10. Spencer, N.F., S.D. Norton, L.L. Harrison, *et al.* 1996. Dysregulation of IL-10 production with aging: possible linkage to the age-associated decline in DHEA and its sulfated derivative. Exp. Gerontol. **31:** 393–408.
11. Daynes, R.A. & B.A. Araneo. 1992. Prevention and reversal of some age-associated changes in immunologic responses by supplemental dehydroepiandrosterone sulfate therapy. Aging: Immunol. Infect. Dis. **3:** 135–153.

12. DIAMOND, P., L. CUSAN, J.L. GOMEZ, *et al.* 1996. Metabolic effects of 12-month percutaneous dehydroepiandrosterone replacement therapy in postmenopausal women. J. Endocrinol. **150** (Suppl): S43–S50.
13. MARWAH, A., P. MARWAH & H. LARDY. 2002. Ergosteroids. VI. Metabolism of dehydroepiandrosterone by rat liver in vitro: a liquid chromatographic-mass spectrometric study. J. Chromatogr. B. Analyt. Technol. Biomed. Life Sci. **767:** 285–299.
14. PIETERS, R. & R. ALBERS. 1999. Assessment of autoimmunogenic potential of xenobiotics using the popliteal lymph node assay. Methods **19:** 71–77.
15. SCHIELEN, P., W. VAN RODIJNEN, J. TEKSTRA, *et al.* 1995. Quantification of natural antibody producing B cells in rats by an improved ELISPOT technique using the polyvinylidene difluoride membrane as the solid support. J. Immunol. Methods **188:** 33–41.
16. BEBO, B.F., JR., A. FYFE-JOHNSON, K. ADLARD, *et al.* 2001. Low-dose estrogen therapy ameliorates experimental autoimmune encephalomyelitis in two different inbred mouse strains. J. Immunol. **166:** 2080–2089.
17. VOSKUHL, R.R. & K. PALASZYNSKI. 2001. Sex hormones in experimental autoimmune encephalomyelitis: implications for multiple sclerosis. Neuroscientist **7:** 258–270.
18. DU, C., M.W. KHALIL & S. SRIRAM. 2001. Administration of dehydroepiandrosterone suppresses experimental allergic encephalomyelitis in SJL/J mice. J. Immunol. **167:** 7094–7101.
19. OFFNER, H., A. ZAMORA, H. DROUGHT, *et al.* 2002. A synthetic androstene derivative and a natural androstene metabolite inhibit relapsing-remitting EAE. J. Neuroimmunol. **130:** 128.

Immunomodulatory Effects of Intravenous Immunoglobulins as a Treatment for Autoimmune Diseases, Cancer, and Recurrent Pregnancy Loss

TAL SAPIR,[a,b] MIRI BLANK,[a,c] AND YEHUDA SHOENFELD[a,c,d]

[a]*Department of Internal Medicine B and Research Center for Autoimmune Diseases, Sheba Medical Center, Tel Hashomer, Israel*

[b]*Faculty of Life Sciences, Bar-Ilan University, Ramat Gan, Israel*

[c]*Sackler Faculty of Medicine, Tel Aviv University, Tel Aviv, Israel*

ABSTRACT: **Intravenous immunoglobulin (IVIG) is a safe preparation, made of human plasma of thousands of healthy donors. The fascinating history of gamma globulin therapy begins in 1930 when Finland treated pneumococcal pneumonia patients with equine serum, which prolonged their survival from pneumonia. Since then, significant breakthroughs were achieved by Cohn, Bruton, Imbach, and others, whose clinical contribution to the world of medicine was of great importance. Originally IVIG was used to treat immunodeficiencies. Later on the use of IVIG extended to autoimmune diseases as well. The efficacy of IVIG has been established only in several autoimmune diseases; clinical reports of trials, series, and case reports indicate significant improvement in many more autoimmune diseases. IVIG have also showed antimetastatic effects in a variety of cancer cell lines, as well as in a few case reports. The efficiency of IVIG has also been observed in recurrent pregnancy loss (RPL), either as a result of an autoimmune disease or spontaneous. Several attempts were made to discover the immunomodulatory effects of IVIG, but it is still not fully understood. Clearly IVIG has multiple mechanisms of actions, which are thought to cooperate synergistically. One of the main mechanisms of actions of IVIG is its ability to neutralize pathogenic autoantibodies via anti-idiotypic antibodies within IVIG preparation. The ability of IVIG to neutralize pathogenic autoantibodies is of great importance in many autoimmune diseases, as well as in RPL. In cancer cell lines, IVIG modulates the immune system in a few ways, including the induction of IL-12 secretion, which consequently activates natural killer cells, and the induction of expression of proapoptotic genes only in cancer cells. Side effects from IVIG are rare and mostly mild and transient. More importantly adverse effects can be minimized by administration to a selective patient population in a proper way: slow infusion rate of 0.4 g/Kg body weight IVIG for 5 consecutive days, given in monthly cycles. The only**

Address for correspondence: Yehuda Shoenfeld, M.D., F.R.C.P. (Hon.), Department of Medicine B, Sheba Medical Center, Tel Hashomer 52621, Israel. Voice: +972-5302652; fax: 972-3-5352855.

[d]Incumbent of the Laura Schwarz-Kipp Chair for Research of Autoimmunity Diseases, Tel Aviv University, Tel Aviv, Israel.

shoenfel@post.tau.ac.il

Ann. N.Y. Acad. Sci. 1051: 743–778 (2005). © 2005 New York Academy of Sciences.
doi: 10.1196/annals.1361.118

downside of IVIG therapy is its high price. Therefore, clinicians should balance efficiency versus cost in deciding whether or not to treat certain conditions with IVIG.

KEYWORDS: **IVIG; autoimmune disease; cancer therapy; recurrent pregnancy loss**

WHAT IS IVIG?

Intravenous immunoglobulin (IVIG) is a safe preparation made from sterilized purified human plasma from thousands of healthy donors per batch. Therefore, IVIG most likely contains the entire wide spectrum of variable regions present in normal plasma.[1–3] IVIG contains more than 95% intact immunoglobulin G (IgG) molecules, with traces of immunoglobulin A (IgA) (<2.5%) and immunoglobulin M (IgM) (negligible). The IgG subclasses distribution corresponds to that of normal human plasma.[1–4] Petaglobin, an IVIG preparation, is IgM enriched.[5]

The therapeutic immunomodulatory effect of IVIG lies within its content. A standard IVIG preparation contains natural antibodies that are more polyreactive than are immune antibodies, including IgG antibodies against endogenous antibodies. These IgG antibodies are known to be anti-idiotypic and are able to neutralize and immunomodulate autoantibodies.[3,4] IVIG also contains natural autoantibodies against DNA, phospholipids, gangliosides, and glycolipid-sulfatide,[6,7] as well as IgG antibodies against exogenous antigens (bacteria, viruses, etc.), $F(ab')_2$ fragments of IgG, immunomodulating peptides (CD4, CD8, CD95, etc.), and various cytokines (interleukin [IL]–2, IL-4, IL-10, transforming growth factor–β, etc.).[4,8–11] Importantly, the natural autoantibodies (i.e., antiphospholipid and anti-DNA autoantibodies) within IVIG are nonpathogenic *in vivo*, most likely because of low affinity toward the autoantigenic target.[6]

IVIG, when administered properly to a selected patient population, was shown to be an effective treatment in autoimmune and cancer diseases, as well as for recurrent pregnancy loss, with side effects that are mostly mild and transient.[5,12]

THE HISTORY OF IVIG

The origin of IVIG use dates back to 1930 at Boston City Hospital, where a clinical experiment was conducted from 1919 to 1929 by M. Finland, in which equine serum was given to treat pneumococcal pneumonia. Although the treatment had side effects, namely, acute febrile reactions and serum sickness, it seemed that the therapy improved survival from pneumonia.[13] In 1940, Edwin J. Cohn from Harvard University used human albumin from 19 donors to treat combat shock in soldiers wounded on the battlefield in World War II. In 1941, Cohn developed a process to produce human albumin (using ethanol as a precipitant) and recognized fractions containing gamma globulin, as well as prothrombin, lipoproteins, and other proteins.[14] Cohn acknowledged the importance of the globulins as a potent substitute "for convalescent serum." Cohn's collaborator, Oncley, separated (by molecular weight) the gamma globulins from prothrombin, plasminogen, and isohemagglutinins.[15] After World War II, in the mid-1940s, injections of separated gamma globulins became common as a substitute for earlier placental extract preparations of globulin, mainly to prevent or attenuate viral diseases.[16]

The first use of gamma globulin that was not related to infections or immunodeficiencies was attempted in the 1940s by Diamond, who worked with Cohn's fractions and tried to develop an anti-Rh globulin to prevent erythroblastosis fetalis.[14] However, the use of intravenous administration of gamma globulins was discontinued after Janeway[17] found it to be the frequent cause of immediate vasomotor reactions, chills, and fever. A significant case report was detailed in 1952 when an immunodeficiency patient was successfully treated with gamma globulin injections.[18]

A valuable contribution to the use of IVIG as a treatment for autoimmune diseases was made by Imbach *et al.*, who reported in 1981 on its beneficial effect in children with chronic thrombocytopenia and immunodeficiency. Imbach was the first to observe that the IVIG treatment improved the condition of the children with immunodeficiency and ameliorated the thrombocytopenia. Imbach immediately implemented this treatment for idiopathic thrombocytopenia purpura (ITP), indicating the efficacy of IVIG in other autoimmune conditions.[19]

To date, IVIG has been given for a variety of autoimmune, inflammatory, and neurologic diseases and many other conditions. In some diseases, a beneficial effect was proved, such as in ITP and Kawasaki syndrome, whereas in others it is still debatable, for example, multiple sclerosis.[16,20]

IVIG FOR IMMUNODEFICIENCY

The original purpose for using gamma globulin injections in the early to mid-1940s was mainly to prevent or attenuate viral diseases. Back then, immunodeficiency diseases had not yet been discovered.[16] As summarized by Berger,[16] it was Bruton who made a seminal contribution. In 1952, Bruton reported an 8-year-old boy who had recurrent infections associated with agammaglobulinemia. The boy was treated monthly with subcutaneous injections of gamma globulins, and consequently sepsis and serious infections were healed.

In the 1950s and early 1960s, the Medical Research Council in England conducted a clinical trial comprising 176 patients with primary hypogammaglobulinemia who were treated with intramuscular injections of 25 or 50 mg/kg/week gamma globulin. The high-dose treatment was more effective in reducing C-reactive protein levels, febrile episodes, number of death reports, pneumoniae, and otitis media. The Medical Research Council approved the high-dose IVIG only for patients in whom the low-dose treatment failed to prevent severe infections.[21]

Today, IVIG is widely used in immunodeficiencies; that is, IVIG is given as prophylaxis against severe infections or as an adjunctive measure for sepsis. Treatment with IVIG against severe infections led to a reduction in infection occurrence, infection-related mortality, and duration of hospitalization. Treatment of sepsis with IVIG led to a significant reduction in mortality from sepsis and septic shock, as reported in the Cochrane database.[22,23]

Another important use of IVIG is for allogeneic stem cell transplantation. Patients undergoing transplantations are given immunosuppressive treatment to minimize the probability of organ rejection. The value of IVIG in transplantations lies in both preventing infections and reducing the occurrence and severity of acute graft-versus-host disease.[22] In 1982, the U.S. Food and Drug Administration approved the use of IVIG as part of the treatment regimen for chemoblasted recipients of allogeneic bone marrow stem cell transplantation.[22] The experience gained with IVIG in bone marrow transplantation has been controversial. A beneficial effect of IVIG in bone marrow transplantation has yet to be established, although it is clear that IVIG is efficient against some viral (cytomegalovirus, herpes virus, Epstein-Barr virus, parvovirus B19, and others) and bacterial infections (*Mycoplasma pneumoniae, Chlamydia pneumoniae, Helicobacter pylori*, etc.).[24]

IVIG FOR AUTOIMMUNE DISEASES

The first major contribution to the use of IVIG in autoimmunity was made by Imbach in 1981. Using the Swiss Red Cross IV preparation to treat children with Wiskott-Aldrich syndrome and thrombocytopenia, he noticed an improvement in both their immune deficiency and their thrombocytopenia. Thereafter, Imbach used IVIG to treat children with ITP who did not have an immune deficiency and were refractory to conventional treatments. The idea was that IVIG might interfere with the immune responses of the platelet-targeted autoantibody. A drastic increase in platelet count was observed and all the children were cured.[19] In 1990, the National Institutes of Health consensus approved the use of IVIG in ITP.[25]

In the early 1980s, IVIG was used successfully to treat hemophilic patients, as well as patients with Kawasaki syndrome.[26,27] Because Kawasaki syndrome is an inflammatory autoimmune disease, the findings led to IVIG being implemented as a treatment for inflammatory conditions, independent of an autoimmune background. During the 1980s, beneficial effects of IVIG were observed when it was given as a treatment for autoimmune neurological diseases, such as myasthenia gravis,[28,29] Guillain-Barré syndrome,[30] and chronic idiopathic demyelinating polyneuropathy.[31] From the 1990s, IVIG was also shown to be beneficial in polymyositis, dermatomyositis,[32,33] and stiff-person syndrome.[34]

Today, the therapeutic effects of IVIG have been well established for several autoimmune diseases, including ITP, Guillain-Barré syndrome, Kawasaki disease, polymyositis, and dermatomyositis.[20] Moreover, there are indications for the efficacy of IVIG in other autoimmune conditions as well (TABLES 1A-1D). Several beneficial effects of IVIG have been reported with regard to systemic lupus erythematosus (SLE),[127] vasculitides,[104] factor VIII inhibitor,[35] recurrent pregnancy loss as a result of antiphospholipid syndrome (APS),[36,37] fibrosis,[21,132,133] heparin-induced thrombocytopenia,[153,154] and others.[133,136]

TABLE 1A presents diseases in which the therapeutic effect of IVIG has been established in controlled trials.[3] TABLE 1B lists diseases treated with IVIG in uncontrolled trials; that is, the beneficial response of IVIG has yet to be established. TABLE 1C summarizes diseases treated with IVIG in case series. TABLE 1D presents several case reports of diseases treated with IVIG.

Mechanisms of Action of IVIG in Autoimmunity

IVIG exerts its immunomodulatory effects in a multiple mechanistic way that is not fully defined. Some of the mechanisms of action of IVIG involve (1) Fc receptor

TABLE 1A. IVIG treatment for patients with autoimmune diseases, in which the beneficial effect was established in controlled clinical trials

Autoimmune disease	IVIG treatment in human	Results	Ref.
Idiopathic thrombocytopenic purpura	A. 22 children were treated with 2 g/kg IVIG. The treatment succeeded in 19 (86%). B. 34 children were treated with 2 g/kg/d or 0.6 g/kg IVIG. The treatment succeeded in 15/17 (88%) of children who received 2 g/kg IVIG, and 13/17 (76.5%) of children who received 0.6 g/kg IVIG. C. 17 children were treated with 1 g/kg IVIG. The treatment succeeded in 13 (76%). D. 14 patients were treated monthly with 2 g/kg IVIG for 1-4 cycles. The treatment succeeded in 12 (86%).	A. Platelet count increased above 20,000/l in a mean time of 2.9 days and above 50,000/l in a mean time of 5.2 days. No significant difference was observed in the mean platelet counts on treatment days 30, 60, 90, 120 and 180. Chronic disease developed in 4 children (18%). B. Platelet count increased above 20,000/l on the 3rd day of treatment. Chronic disease occurred in 3 patients receiving 2 g/kg IVIG and in 5 patients receiving 0.6 g/kg IVIG. C. Platelet count recovered rapidly from below 20,000/l to above 50,000/l on the 4th day. Four children needed a second dose. In 5 children platelet counts returned to normal without recurrence. In 10 children platelet count declined again after 2-3 weeks, 6 of whom needed re-treatment. All but 1 child had a complete recovery of the platelet count by 6 months. D. Platelet count increased from below 50,000/l to above 150,000/l. Of 12 patients, 6 had a temporary response (a relapse accord in 6 months), 5 had a sustained response (the beneficial effect lasted for at least 6 months) and 1 patient responded well to the treatment but was lost to follow-up.	A. 76 B. 80 C. 81 D. 54
Guillain-Barré syndrome	A. 15 bedridden children were treated with 2 g/kg IVIG. The treatment succeeded in all (100%). B. 22 patients were treated with IVIG. The treatment succeeded in all (100%).	A. Improvement by 1 grade on the motor disability grading scale after IVIG therapy was achieved after a mean of 10.17 days, and the children started walking independently after a mean of 30.35 days. B. Serum tumor necrosis factor-alpha (TNF) concentrations declined from 9.75 to 65.5pg/ml. At the time of discharge from the hospital there was a positive correlation between neurological recovery and decreasing TNF concentration.	A. 82 B. 83

TABLE 1A. (*continued*) **IVIG treatment for patients with autoimmune diseases, in which the beneficial effect was established in controlled clinical trials**

Autoimmune disease	IVIG treatment in human	Results	Ref.
Chronic inflammatory demyelinating polyneuropathy	A. 2 patients with orthotopic liver transplantation were treated with IVIG. Both patients had immunosuppressive therapy, with cyclosporine and prednisolone in one patient and tacrolimus in the other. The treatment succeeded in both (100%). B. 29 patients were treated with 2 g/kg IVIG every 3 weeks. The treatment succeeded in 11 (38%). C. 30 patients were treated with 2 g/kg IVIG. The treatment succeeded in 19 (63%), including 9/16 patients with chronic progressive disease, and 10/14 patients with relapsing disease. D. 15 patients were treated with high-dose IVIG. The treatment succeeded in 4 (27%). E. 7 patients were treated with high-dose IVIG. The treatment succeeded in all (100%).	A. IVIG significantly improved the neuropathy. B. IVIG improved mean average muscle score at day 42 and improved strength by day 10 with continued benefit through day 42. The patients' functional disability scale improved; none worsened. IVIG improved ulnar motor distal latency, tibial distal compound muscle amplitude, and peroneal nerve conduction velocity. C. An improvement in neurological disability score, clinical grade and grip strength was observed. IVIG significantly improved the summed motor conduction velocities and the summed compound muscle action potentials evoked with proximal stimulation of median, ulnar, peroneal and tibial nerves. 8/9 IVIG responders with chronic progressive disease improved gradually to normal function with a single 5 day course of IVIG, of whom 5 received small doses of prednisone during follow-up. In 10 IVIG responders with relapsing disease, improvement lasted a median of 6 weeks and was reproducible with open label treatments. All 10 patients have been maintained and stabilized on 1 g/kg IVIG pulse or less, given as a single infusion prior to the expected relapse. A good response to IVIG was most effective in patients with acute relapse or with disease of one year or less. D. The degree of improvement in patients in the IVIG group was not different from that of the placebo group. Electrophysiological studies did not show significant differences between the groups. E. All patients deteriorated after discontinuation of the treatment in a mean time lapse of 6.4 weeks.	A. 84 B. 85 C. 86 D. 87 E. 88

TABLE 1A. (*continued*) IVIG treatment for patients with autoimmune diseases, in which the beneficial effect was established in controlled clinical trials

Autoimmune disease	IVIG treatment in human	Results	Ref.
Myasthenia gravis	A. 34 patients were treated with 2 g/kg IVIG, of whom 26 patients were in a long-standing, drug-refractory stationary phase of the illness and 11 patients were in an acute phase. The treatment succeeded in the short-term in 70% (26/37) and in the long-term in 59% (22/37). B. 6 patients were treated monthly with 2 g/kg IVIG, followed by maintenance therapy of 0.4 g/kg every 3-4 months for 2 years. All other medications, including prednisone and cholingeric drugs such as Mestinon, were gradually weaned. The treatment succeeded for the long-term in all (100%). C. 10 patients in an acute deterioration unresponsive to conventional therapy including high-dose corticosteroids, cyclosporine, and azathioprine were treated with 2 g/kg IVIG with maintenance IVIG treatment at a dose of 0.4 g/kg, once every 6 weeks. The treatment succeeded in all (100%).	A. A one-degree improvement in OGCCMS (Oosterhuis global clinical classification of myasthenic severity), the disappearance of bulbar involvement or both, were recorded 12 days after beginning the treatment in 70% of patients and persisted up to 60 days in 59%. A two-degree improvement in OGCCMS was recorded in 54% (20/37) and was maintained up to 60 days in 38% (14/37). There was no significant difference between patients entering the treatment in a long-standing, drug-refractory stationary phase and patients who were in an acute phase of the disease. B. For the last 2 years, each of the patients maintained better than functional class 2 on an average of 1.5-2.2 ± 0.5 grades on the University of Virginia modification of Ossermann's classification scale for myasthenia gravis. They were solely treated with IVIG every 3-4 months. C. The severity of the disease decreased by 2.5 ± 0.8 grades of the Osserman scale over a period of one year, parallel to a reduction of immunosuppressive therapy as well as a decrease in acetylcholine receptor antibody titers.	A. 89 B. 90 C. 91
Multifocal neuropathy	A. 10 patients were treated with IVIG for 5-12 years. The treatment succeeded for a mean of 4.8 years in all (100%) and for a mean of 8.2 years in 2 (20%). B. 18 patients were treated with 1.2-2 g/kg IVIG for 9-48 months. 4 patients were initially treated with prednisone, without any clear improvement. The treatment succeeded for the long-term in 12 (67%). 5 unresponsive patients to IVIG or IVIG-dependent were treated with cyclophosphamide, but only one improved. C. 6 patients were treated with 2 g/kg IVIG. The treatment succeeded in 5 (83%).	A. 2/10 patients maintained the maximal improvement achieved during therapy while 8 worsened despite increasing IVIG dosage. This decline started after 3-7 years of therapy and correlated with a reduction of distal compound muscle action potential amplitudes. B. A clinical improvement was observed. Isometric strength increased from 32% to 97%. Often, patients needed repeated courses of IVIG to maintain the improvement. In 2 patients IVIG infusions were stopped without signs of relapse after one year. C. IVIG treatment led to improvement of muscle strength.	A. 92 B. 93 C. 94

TABLE 1A. (*continued*) IVIG treatment for patients with autoimmune diseases, in which the beneficial effect was established in controlled clinical trials

Autoimmune disease	IVIG treatment in human	Results	Ref.
Dermato-myositis	A. 12 treatment-resistant patients were treated monthly with 2 g/kg IVIG for 3 or 6 months. The patients also received concomitant prednisone therapy. The treatment succeeded in 92% (9/12) and partly succeeded in 67% (2/3) of the other patients. B. 19 patients, of whom 4 had paraneoplastic dermatomyositis, were treated with high-dose IVIG. The treatment succeeded in 7 (37%).	A. 9/12 patients with severe disabilities had a major improvement to nearly normal function. Their mean muscle strength scores increased from 74.5 to 84.7 and their neuromuscular symptoms improved. Two of the other 3 patients had mild improvement. B. The patients had severe skin but only moderate muscle involvement, no autoantibodies, and no malignancy. sIL-2R levels reverted to normal. CK levels and other parameters did not correlate with disease activity and/or treatment response.	A. 95 B. 96
Kawasaki disease	A. 22 patients were treated with 2 g/kg Thai Red-Cross IVIG. The treatment succeeded in all (100%). B. 41 patients were treated with a single dose of 1 g/kg IVIG. A second dose of 1 g/kg of IVIG was required in 7 patients due to persistent fever more than 48 hours after the initial treatment. Three patients required 3 doses of 1 g/kg of IVIG due to persistent fever after the second dose. The treatment succeeded in 31 (76%).	A. A good response to a single treatment was observed. During the convalescent phase there were only 2 cases with coronary artery abnormalities (CAA) in the first month and one case at the 3-month follow-up. This only case with CAA had multiple aneurysms at the left main and left anterior descending coronary arteries. One patient had a severe reaction to IVIG and required discontinuation and intervention. B. Patients who received a single treatment responded completely. During the convalescent phase, CAA developed in 19%, 29% and 100% patients treated with 1, 2 or 3 doses of IVIG, respectively. After a 1 year follow-up, the prevalence of CAA decreased to 3%, 0% and 67% in patients treated with 1, 2 or 3 doses of IVIG, respectively. Only one patient treated with 3 doses of IVIG developed a giant aneurysm of the right coronary artery.	A. 97 B. 98

TABLE 1A. (*continued*) **IVIG treatment for patients with autoimmune diseases, in which the beneficial effect was established in controlled clinical trials**

Autoimmune disease	IVIG treatment in human	Results	Ref.
Antineutrophil cytoplasmic autoantibody positive systemic vasculitis *	A. 6 patients were treated with high-dose IVIG as a sole therapy. The treatment succeeded in all (100%). B. 10 patients were treated monthly with 2 g/kg IVIG for 1-6 courses. In all the patients, other therapeutic measures failed to control disease progression prior to IVIG treatment. The treatment succeeded in 6 (60%). C. 16 patients were treated with IVIG. The treatment succeeded in 15 (94%). D. One steroid-resistant Churg-Strauss vasculitis patient was successfully treated monthly with 2 g/kg IVIG for 3 courses.	A. Early reductions in the disease activity were observed. 4/6 patients entered a full, clinical remission, which lasted for at least one year, while in 2 patients the response was partial and transient and they subsequently required conventional treatment. After 16-48 months of follow-up, 2/4 patients in full remission relapsed, but the other 2 have remained well. B. A beneficial clinical response was observed. Anti-myeloperoxidase antibodies and antineutrophil cytoplasmic antibodies (ANCA) levels decreased concomitantly with the clinical improvement observed in the patients with Churg-Strauss vasculitis and Wegener's granulomatosis, respectively. C. A clinical benefit was observed. 8/15 patients sustained remission, which was associated with a decrease in ANCA levels and stimulation of endogenous immunoglobulin production. D. Significant improvement of the dyspnea and pulmonary function were observed, as well as a reduction in ANCA levels, eosinophil levels and erythrocyte sedimentation rate.	A. 99 B. 100 C. 101 D. 102
Graft versus host disease	A. 123 patients who had marrow transplantation were treated monthly with 0.5 g/kg IVIG from day 90 to 360 post-transplantation. Not only did the treatment not reduce late complications, it also impaired the long-term humoral immune recovery after the marrow transplantation.	A. The treatment had no effect on survival, the incidence of obliterative bronchiolitis, severity of airflow obstruction, or the incidence or mortality of chronic GVHD.	A. 103

TABLE 1A. (*continued*) **IVIG treatment for patients with autoimmune diseases, in which the beneficial effect was established in controlled clinical trials**

Autoimmune disease	IVIG treatment in human	Results	Ref.
Multiple sclerosis	A. 42 patients, at the first demyelinating event suggestive of multiple sclerosis (MS), were treated with 2 g/kg IVIG with boosters (0.4 g/kg) given once every 6 weeks for one year. 28/42 patients were treated with corticosteroids during the first neurological event. The treatment succeeded in 31 (74%). B. 159 patients were treated monthly with 1 g/kg IVIG for 27 months. The treatment success was similar to that of the control group. C. 18 patients, previously treated with immunomodulatory or immunosuppressive drugs, were treated monthly with 2 g/kg IVIG. The treatment succeeded in 11 (61%). D. 10 patients were treated with 2 g/kg IVIG. The treatment success was similar to that of the control group.	A. At trial completion, the cumulative probability of fulfilling the criteria for the diagnosis of MS was 26% in IVIG recipients. IVIG reduced the probability of developing clinically definite MS by 48%. IVIG recipients had a significant reduction in the volume and number of T2-weighted lesions and in the volume of gadolinium-enhancing lesions. The corticosteroid treatment did not affect the probability of developing a second neurological event. B. IVIG did not show any clinically beneficial effect on time to confirmed expanded disability status scale (EDSS) progression. The annual relapse rate was 0.46 in both groups. No significant differences between the groups were found in any of the other clinical outcome measures or in the change of T2-lesion load over time. C. The EDSS decreased from 6.77 to less than 1 and 0.75 for secondary and primary progressive diseases, respectively. No worsening was reported. Surprisingly, some patients had partial improvement of neurological functions, which were considered as sequelae. D. IVIG did not affect central motor conduction times measured. Clinically there was no significant difference between IVIG and placebo groups.	A. 104 B. 105 C. 106 D. 107
Uveitis*	A. 10 patients, unresponsive to immunosuppressive medication, were treated monthly with 1.5 g/kg IVIG for 7.5 cycles and continued to receive immunosuppressive medication. The treatment succeeded in 7 (70%). B. A patient with severe reaction to high-dose steroid therapy was successfully treated with high-dose IVIG.	A. 5/7 responders had a clinically important and sustained improvement in visual acuity, and 2/7 responders markedly reduced their immunosuppressive medication. B. Retinal exudation and phlebitis subsided and visual acuity increased dramatically.	A. 108 B. 109

* The results of preliminary trials have been published, and major controlled trials are underway.

TABLE 1B. IVIG treatment for patients with autoimmune diseases: uncontrolled clinical trials

Autoimmune Disease	IVIG treatment in humans	Results	Ref.
Autoimmune hemolytic anemia	A. Combined pilot study and case reports: 73 patients were treated with IVIG. The treatment succeeded in 29 (40%). B. 4 patients were treated with 1 g/kg IVIG for 5-7 days. The treatment succeeded in 3 (75%). C. A corticosteroid-resistant patient after remission of Hodgkin's disease was successfully treated with high-dose IVIG.	A. A good response was strongly observed in patients with hepatomegaly and low pretreatment hemoglobin. A trend towards a better response was observed in children. B. The response was excellent in 1 patient and good in 2 patients. The average response occurred with a dose of 5 g/kg. C. The treatment produced a rapid and long-lasting response.	A. 110 B. 111 C. 112
Anti-factor VIII autoimmune disease	A. 2 patients were treated with high-dose IVIG. The treatment succeeded in both (100%). B. 19 patients were treated with 2 g/kg IVIG, followed by maintenance doses at intervals. The treatment succeeded in 25%-37.5% patients. 6/19 patients received concomitant prednisone therapy.	A. A rapid and prolonged, although not total, suppression of autoantibodies was achieved. B. A reduction of at least 25% in inhibitor titer was observed in 8 patients. A rapid decline in inhibitor titer over 3-4 days was observed in 2 patients, but in 4 additional responding patients the decline was more gradual, with final nadirs being reached several weeks to months after treatment. The inhibitor disappeared in 3 patients with low-level inhibitors. Concomitant prednisone therapy may have contributed to the response in 2 of the patients but was not a factor in 4 patients.	A. 27 B. 113
Polymyositis	A. 35 chronic patients, refractory to traditional treatments (prednisone, methotrexate, azathioprine, cyclophosphamide, cyclosporine, chlorambucil, plasmapheresis, lymphopheresis and total body irradiation), were treated monthly with 2 g/kg IVIG for a mean course of 4-6 months. The treatment succeeded in the short-term in 25 (71.5%). A. 2 treatment-resistant patients were treated monthly with 1.6 g/kg IVIG. The treatment succeeded in both (100%).	A. A significant clinical improvement was observed. The mean muscle power significantly improved. All patients had a significant biochemical response, mean creatine kinase (CK) levels decreased significantly. This benefit allowed the initial prednisone dose to be reduced by >50% in all patients. 12/25 patients remained in full remission following their initial course of IVIG, resulting in complete cessation of medication in 5 patients or low doses of steroids in 7 patients. The condition of 6/25 patients remained improved and no other drugs were prescribed, but the patients remained dependent on IVIG infusions. 7/25 patients relapsed at an average of 17.1 months after the discontinuation of IVIG. B. Serum CK activity decreased to normal and a clear improvement in muscle strength was observed. One patient showed neither clinical relapses nor increase in serum CK activity after 20 months. The other showed a mild increase in serum CK activity after 24 months and was successfully retreated with IVIG.	A. 114 B. 115

TABLE 1B. *(continued)* **IVIG treatment for patients with autoimmune diseases: uncontrolled clinical trials**

Autoimmune Disease	IVIG treatment in humans	Results	Ref.
Antiphospholipid syndrome	A. 15 women (19 pregnancies) were treated monthly with IVIG, beginning in the first or early second trimester in 17/19 pregnancies. Additional therapy consisted of low-dose aspirin and subcutaneous heparin. 6/15 women also received steroid therapy. The live-birth percentage was 84% (16/19). B. 5 women with a history of 17 unsuccessful previous pregnancies were treated monthly with 2 g/kg IVIG, beginning the first or early second trimester. 4/5 women with previous thromboembolic events were treated with concomitant heparin prophylaxis. 4/5 women received aspirin daily. 80% (4/5) of the women delivered healthy infants at term. C. 3 women (4 pregnancies) with a history of 2 pulmonary embolies related to pregnancy and estrogen containing pills, 13 miscarriages and only 1 live born after preeclamptic pregnancy were treated with 1 g/kg IVIG. During the 4 pregnancies the women were treated with concomitant daily heparin. One had SLE secondary to APS. The live-birth percentage was 100% (4/4). D. 14 women with a history of recurrent spontaneous abortion were treated monthly with 1 g/kg IVIG, from the 5th to the 33rd week of gestation. 13 (93%) delivered healthy infants. E. 38 women with history of 3 or more consecutive first trimester spontaneous abortions were treated monthly with 0.3 g/kg IVIG every 3 weeks, beginning as soon as pregnancy had been confirmed, until the 16th-17th week of pregnancy. 31 (81%) delivered healthy infants at 37th-42nd week of gestation.	A. 75% of the women delivered in the 34th week of gestation or later. There were no cases of fetal growth restriction. Preeclampsia and non-reassuring fetal status were each diagnosed in 25% of the pregnancies. Anticardiolipin IgG decreased throughout the course of therapy in 7/19 pregnancies. Placental pathology was minimal. B. One infant was delivered in the 32nd week of gestation with a diagnosis of fetal distress. Short and long-term decreases of anticardiolipin IgG were noted in 3/5 women. Neither preeclampsia nor fetal intrauterine growth retardation was observed. Significant placental histological anomalies were not identified. C. 3/4 pregnancies resulted in the delivery of a healthy infant after 36-38 weeks of gestation and one was born preterm (34 weeks) with slight respiratory distress syndrome. A progressive decrease of anticardiolipin IgG was observed. The effects on lupus anticoagulant were variable. D. One woman developed gestational hypertension and abruptio placentae. No other pregnancy complications were seen. No proteinuria was found. No fetal or neonatal growth retardation was seen. E. Pregnancy proceeded beyond the first trimester in 34/38 (89.4%) women.	A. 116 B. 117 C. 118 D. 119 E. 120

TABLE 1B. ***(continued)*** **IVIG treatment for patients with autoimmune diseases: uncontrolled clinical trials**

Autoimmune Disease	IVIG treatment in humans	Results	Ref.
Rheumatoid arthritis	A. 4 refractory patients who failed at least 4 second-line drugs, including methotrexate, and who were receiving nonsteroidal anti-inflammatory drugs and prednisone only, were treated monthly with 2 g/kg IVIG for 3 months. The treatment did not succeed in any of the patients (0/4). B. 9 patients unresponsive to first and second-line agents were treated monthly with high-dose IVIG for 6 months. The treatment succeeded in all (100%).	A. None of the patients met the Paulus criteria for either improvement or worsening. Furthermore, increased TNF production in lipopolysaccharide-stimulated whole blood assays was consistently noted in 3/4 patients during the course of IVIG. There was no evidence for efficacy of IVIG. B. There was a significant improvement in both subjective and objective parameters of disease activity. This improvement occurred after the second infusion of IVIG. The reduction in clinical activity paralleled a decrease in the CD4+CDw29+:CD4+CD45RA+ cell ratio.	A. 121 B. 122
Juvenile rheumatoid arthritis	A. 22 refractory children were treated with 1.5 g/kg IVIG every 2 weeks for 2 months, and then monthly for 4 months. The treatment succeeded in 11 (50%). B. 25 patients were treated monthly with IVIG for 3-54 months. The treatment succeeded for the short-term (6 months) in 20 (80%) and for the long-term (37.6 ± 18 months) in 14 (70%) of the responder patients.	A. IVIG was not more effective than placebo in reducing the number of days with fever or other systemic manifestations. Changes from baseline in the joint count, hemoglobin, albumin, platelet count, and erythrocyte sedimentation rate did not differ between IVIG and placebo groups. B. Six months after the therapy, a decrease of at least 50% in at least one of the following was observed: the number of days of fever, prednisone dose, and the number of active joints. After a mean of 37.6 ± 18 months 11/20 patients were in remission, and 3/20 patients significantly improved but still had active arthritis.	A. 123 B. 124

TABLE 1B. (*continued*) **IVIG treatment for patients with autoimmune diseases: uncontrolled clinical trials**

Autoimmune Disease	IVIG treatment in humans	Results	Ref.
Systemic lupus erythematosus	A. 20 patients were treated monthly with 2 g/kg IVIG for 1-8 courses. The treatment succeeded in 17 (85%).	A. Some clinical manifestations responded to the treatment: arthritis, fever, thrombocytopenia, and neuropsychiatric lupus. In 9 patients the mean systemic lupus activity measure score decreased from 19. 3 ± 4.7 to 4 ± 2.9.	A. 125
	B. 12 patients refractory to conventional treatments were treated monthly with 2 g/kg IVIG for 6-24 months. The treatment succeeded in 11 (92%).	B. Progressive clinical improvement was observed. This improvement was associated with an increase in hemoglobin, total serum hemolytic complement activity and C3 and C4 components. 2 thrombocytopenic patients showed an increase in platelet count, as well as a progressive reduction in erythrocyte sedimentation rate, serum immunocomplexes and antinuclear antibodies. A marked improvement in serum urea, creatinine clearance and proteinuria was also observed in patients with renal involvement.	B. 126
	C. 2 patients unresponsive to corticosteroid and immunosuppressive therapy were treated monthly with high-dose IVIG for 20 months and continued to receive corticosteroids. The treatment succeeded in both (100%).	C. Lupus pneumonitis and encephalitis in the first patient, and lupus nephritis in the second, resolved. IVIG induced a prolonged clinical and laboratory remission. Treatment with cytotoxic agents was stopped and the dosage of corticosteroids lowered. Exacerbation of lupus nephritis occurred in the second patient after 10 months of IVIG therapy.	C. 127
	D. 2 refractory patients were treated with 2.25 or 0.6-0.8 g/kg IVIG for 1 or 3 courses, respectively. The treatment succeeded in both (100%).	D. 1 patient had immediate recovery from severe pancytopenia and amelioration of proteinuria, and the other showed a significant reduction of massive proteinuria. In both cases there was improvement in immunological variables.	D. 128
	E. 12 patients were treated with 3.75 g/kg sulfonated IVIG on days 1-4 and 21-24. The treatment succeeded in 9 (75%).	E. In 6 weeks the mean disease activity score, the Systemic Lupus Activity Measure (SLAM), declined from 7.33 to 5.25. In 3/12 patients the improvement lasted 5-12 months. At 1 week after the initiation of therapy most patients showed a decline in dsDNA antibodies, whereas titers of antinuclear antibodies and complement proteins were not affected. Transient hypotension was observed in one patient	E. 129

TABLE 1B. (*continued*) IVIG treatment for patients with autoimmune diseases: uncontrolled clinical trials

Autoimmune Disease	IVIG treatment in humans	Results	Ref.
Systemic sclerosis	A. 8 patients were treated with IVIG for 1.5 months to almost 8 years. The treatment succeeded in all (100%). B. 15 patients were treated monthly with 2 g/kg IVIG for 3 cycles to 6 months. The treatment succeeded in 14 (93%). C. 3 patients were treated monthly with 2 g/kg IVIG for 6 courses. The treatment succeeded in all (100%).	A. Fibrotic excess was reduced. 5/8 patients benefited. B. Based on the Rodnan scores, the mean degree of skin involvement decreased by 35%. A significant improvement in the patients' well-being and quality of life was reflected by a decrease in the health assessment questionnaire score. C. A large decrease in the skin score was observed. No modification of PM-Scl antibody titers was noted in any patient. The third patient received 3 courses, after which he developed renal failure and later died of sepsis.	A. 130 B. 131 C. 132
Graves' ophthalmopathy	A. 21 patients were treated with 2 g/kg IVIG every 3 weeks for 6 courses. The treatment succeeded in 13 (62%). B. 34 patients were treated with high-dose IVIG. The treatment succeeded in 26 (76%). C. One steroid-resistant patient, who underwent radioisotopic ablation of the thyroid, was unsuccessfully treated with L-thyroxin for hypothyroidism. The patient's vision was impaired and she suffered from orbital pain. The patient was successfully treated with 2 g/kg IVIG for 6 courses.	A. An improvement in proptosis, visual acuity, intraocular pressure and lid aperture was observed, as well as a decrease in eye muscle area and thyroid antibody titers. B. Soft tissue involvement improved or disappeared in 91% (32/35), and diplopia improved or disappeared in 76% (22/29), and proptosis improved or disappeared in 65% (20/31). A significant reduction of extraocular muscle thickness was observed. One patient discontinued the therapy, not because of side effects. C. The patient's symptoms and exophthalmos reversed.	A. 133 B. 134 C. 135
Birdshot retinochoroidopathy	A. 18 patients (36 eyes) were treated monthly with 1.6 g/kg IVIG as a sole treatment for 6 months, followed by injections of 1.2-1.6 g/kg at 6-8 week intervals. The treatment succeeded in 50% of eyes (18/36).	A. The final visual acuity increased in 50% of eyes (18/36), remained stable in 42% (15/36) and deteriorated in 8% (3/36). When present, macular edema was improved in half the eyes on fluorescein angiography.	A. 136
Insulin-dependent diabetes mellitus	A. 10 children were treated with 2 g/kg IVIG and subsequently, after 15 days, every month for 6 months, and continued to receive Insulin. The treatment success for the long- term was similar to that of the control group.	A. Serum post-prandial C-peptide level was significantly higher after 6 months in IVIG recipients. This difference was no longer significant at 18 and 24 months. Insulin requirement in the IVIG group was significantly lower at 6 months. This difference was no longer significant at 12 months.	A. 137

TABLE 1C. IVIG treatment for patients with autoimmune diseases: case series

Autoimmune Disease	IVIG treatment in humans	Results	Ref.
Pemphigus vulgaris	A. 4 therapy-resistant patients were treated monthly with 2 g/kg IVIG and continued to receive corticosteroids. The treatment succeeded in all (100%). B. 15 corticosteroid-dependent patients were treated with 1-2 g/kg IVIG per cycle. The patients also received concomitant prednisone therapy. The use of other systemic conventional immunosuppressive agents was contraindicated. The treatment succeeded in all (100%). C. 21 patients who did not respond to prolonged use of oral prednisone and multiple immunosuppressive agents were treated with 2 g/kg IVIG per cycle. The treatment succeeded in all (100%).	A. A clinical improvement and a decrease in circulating autoantibodies to desmoglein 3 were observed. Corticosteroids and immunosuppression were reduced and in one patient discontinued. In 3 patients, IVIG was discontinued after 12 cycles; subsequently, new blisters developed and autoantibody levels rose after re-initiation of IVIG; in 2 patients the condition quickly improved, along with a decrease in autoantibody serum levels. B. A satisfactory clinical response was observed. The use of systemic prednisone was gradually discontinued over a mean period of 4.3 months. A statistically significant difference was noted in the total dose of prednisone, total duration of prednisone therapy, and number of relapses before and after the initiation of IVIG. C. Use of IVIG as a monotherapy resulted in effective control of the disease and a sustained remission. The patients became free of lesions and remained so after discontinuation of IVIG therapy. IVIG had a steroid-sparing effect and led to a better quality of life.	A. 138 B. 139 C. 140
Pemphigus foliaceus	A. 7 steroid-dependent patients were treated with IVIG. The treatment succeeded in all (100%). B. 11 patients refractory to prednisone and other immunosuppressive therapies were treated with IVIG according to a defined protocol. The treatment succeeded in all (100%).	A. After the initiation of IVIg, doses of systemic corticosteroids were gradually reduced and eventually discontinued over a mean period of 2.8 months. Thereafter, IVIg was used as monotherapy. A statistically significant difference was noted between pre- and post-IVIG in the total dose, total duration of prednisone, and number of relapses. IVIG induced and maintained a prolonged clinical remission. B. An effective clinical response and a maintained clinical remission for a mean period of 18.6 months after discontinuation of IVIG therapy were observed. IVIg was effective as monotherapy.	A. 141 B. 142

TABLE 1C. (*continued*) IVIG treatment for patients with autoimmune diseases: case

Autoimmune Disease	IVIG treatment in humans	Results	Ref.
Steroid-dependent asthma	A. 10 patients were treated monthly with 2 g/kg IVIG for 6 months, and continued to receive systemic and inhaled corticosteroids as well as beta 2-mimetic. The treatment succeeded in all (100%). B. 7 patients were treated monthly with 1 g/kg IVIG for 6 months, and continued to receive prednisolone. The treatment succeeded in all (100%). C. 11 patients were treated monthly with 2 g/kg IVIG for a total of 7 infusions, and continued to receive steroids and methacholine. The treatment succeeded in all (100%).	A. A reduction of systemic corticosteroids doses and simultaneous improvement of asthma score and forced expiratory volume in one second (FEV1) were observed, as well as a decrease of asthma aggravation and emergency need. In some patients the recovery persisted for 6 months after discontinuing IVIG. B. IVIG significantly reduced daily prednisolone dose, and a decreased rate of hospital admissions was observed. IVIG did not improve lung function. C. Despite substantial steroid reduction, an improvement in pulmonary function and symptom scores was observed. The responses to methacholine were unaffected by IVIG.	A. 143 B. 144 C. 145
Toxic epidermal necrolysis syndrome	A. 16 patients were treated with 0.5-0.9 g/kg/day IVIG for 3-5 days. The treatment success was similar to that of the control group. B. 10 patients were treated with IVIG. The treatment succeeded in all (100%).	A. There were no significant differences with respect to length of stay, duration of mechanical ventilation, severity of systemic inflammatory response syndrome, and multiple organ dysfunction syndrome, the incidence of sepsis or mortality rate. Although there may have been a trend towards less severe wound progression in IVIG recipients, it was not associated with any substantial improvement in the patients' outcome. B. The progression rapidly reversed and the outcome was favorable.	A. 146 B. 147
Inclusion body myositis	A. 19 patients were treated monthly with 2 g/kg IVIG for 3 months. The treatment succeeded in 6 (28%). B. 19 patients were treated monthly with IVIG and prednisone for 3 months. Before IVIG infusions, all patients received high-dose prednisone for 3 months. The treatment success was similar to that of the control group.	A. A functionally important improvement by more than 10 medical research council (MRC) points was observed. During IVIG modest gains were noted in certain muscle groups. The duration of swallowing functions also improved statistically in the IVIG group. B. No significant change was noted in muscle strength, from baseline to the 2nd, 3rd, or 4th month after IVIG. The number of necrotic fibers was reduced in the IVIG group, and the mean number of CD2+ cells decreased significantly in both groups, denoting a steroid effect.	A. 148 B. 149

TABLE 1D. IVIG treatment for patients with autoimmune diseases: case-reports

Autoimmune Disease	IVIG treatment in humans	Results	Ref.
Heparin-induced thrombocytopenia	A. 5 patients were treated with high-dose IVIG. The treatment succeeded in all (100%). B. A patient with thrombosis was successfully treated 7 times with 5 g/kg IVIG. In addition, thrombolysis treatment with streptokinase combined with phenprocoumon was undertaken, until satisfactory anticoagulation was achieved after 4 days.	A. Platelet count was rapidly restored. B. Platelet count increased from 33,000/l to 136,000/l in 20 hours of the first IVIG dose and complete clinical normality was restored. Scintigraphy showed no perfusion deficit in the lungs.	A. 150 B. 151
Autoimmune neutropenia	A. 6 children were treated with 1 g/kg IVIG. The treatment succeeded in all (100%). B. 2 infants were treated with IVIG. The treatment succeeded in both (100%). C. A corticosteroid-resistant patient in the setting of renal carcinoma was successfully treated with high-dose IVIG.	A. Neutrophil count increased from below 300/mm^3 to above 1,000/mm^3. The average response occurred with a dose of 3 g/kg during 5-7 days and lasted an average of 14 days before counts decreased to baseline levels. B. Neutrophil count increased significantly with the initial IVIG therapy. One infant went into remission and the other had a neutrophil count above baseline for 3 weeks and then required a subsequent booster infusion to increase the neutrophil count. The infants remained clinically well. C. A rapid and long-lasting response was observed.	A. 112 B. 113 C. 152
Parvovirus B19-associated red cell aplasia	A. 8 AIDS patients were treated with 1-2 g/kg IVIG. Relapses were treated with 2 g/kg IVIG. Maintenance therapy with 0.4-1g/kg IVIG for 4 weeks was given to those who developed a second or subsequent relapse. The treatment succeeded in all (100%). B. 3 renal transplant recipients with erythroid hypoplasia were treated with IVIG. The treatment succeeded in 2 (67%). C. Combined case reports: 14 patients were treated with high-dose IVIG, of whom 2 were transplant recipients (1 heart and 1 lung) who developed severe anemia with reticulocytopenia and were heavily immunosuppressed. The treatment succeeded in 12 (86%).	A. A response to initial therapy was observed. 6/8 patients with CD4 count <80 cells/mm^3 relapsed and maintained therapy. 4/8 patients were given regular maintenance IVIG following a subsequent relapse and remained in remission. 2/8 patients whose CD4 count was >300 cells/mm^3 remained in continuous un-maintained remission for over 8 and 11 months. B. Anemia responded promptly in 2/3 patients of whom 1 had recurrence of the anemia, which responded to a second course of IVIG. In the third patient, who had received the most intense immunosuppression, despite IVIG treatment a persistent infection with PV B19, recurrent anemia, and *de novo* collapsing glomerulopathy leading to allograft failure, were developed. C. One patient recovered spontaneously and another recovered only after treatment with recombinant human erythropoietin.	A. 153 B. 154 C. 155

TABLE 1D. (*continued*) **IVIG treatment for patients with autoimmune diseases: case-**

Autoimmune Disease	IVIG treatment in humans	Results	Ref.
Acquired von Willebrand disease	A. A patient with monoclonal gammopathy of undetermined significance (MGUS), refractory to a high dose of corticosteroids, had a very transient response to desmopressin acetate, but was successfully treated with high-dose IVIG. B. 2 patients were treated with high-dose IVIG. The treatment succeeded in both (100%). C. 2 patients with acquired von Willebrand disease associated with SLE were treated with IVIG, and continued to receive corticosteroids. The treatment succeeded in 1 (50%). D. A patient was successfully treated with IVIG after replacement therapy was ineffective.	A. The patient remained very responsive to IVIG 2 years later. His underlying MGUS has not progressed during the past 4 years. B. Two days after initiation of therapy, von Willebrand factor (VWF) and factor VIII rose to normal levels. One patient underwent dental surgery, and the 2nd patient underwent a splenectomy without increased bleeding and without additional factor coverage or desmopressin acetate therapy. C. IVIG corrected the patient's plasma VWF level. The severity of the cutaneous lesions in that patient led to the use of cyclophosphamide, which resulted in total correction of VWF levels. Therapy with corticosteroids was partially beneficial in both patients. D. IVIG not only caused symptomatic improvement, but also transiently restored the depleted VWF intermediate and high molecular weight multimers. Subsequently, periodic IVIG infusions were used successfully to treat bleeding complications in this patient over the past 3 years.	A. 156 B. 157 C. 158 D. 159
Felty's syndrome	A. 5 patients were treated with high-dose IVIG. The treatment did not succeed in any of the patients.	A. The neutrophil count did not change.	A. 160
Severe steroid-dependent atopic dermatitis	A. 3 patients, who had steroid-related side effects, were treated monthly with 2 g/kg IVIG, and continued to receive steroids. The treatment succeeded in all (100%). B. 6 treatment-resistant patients were treated monthly with 2 g/kg IVIG for 6 cycles. The treatment succeeded in 4 (67%). C. Combined case reports: 32 treatment-resistant patients were treated with high-dose IVIG. The treatment succeeded in 20 (61%).	A. An improvement in skin scores was observed and the steroid dose was reduced. Total IgE decreased in 1/3 patients. B. Major improvements in skin scores and a significant overall reduction were observed. CD4+ T cell titers decreased following IVIG, and recovered by the next cycle. T cell CD69 expression decreased to 60% of baseline values. Reductions in interferon gamma (IFN) and TNFα were non-significant. C. Adults appeared less likely to respond than children and the duration of response was also more prolonged in children. Adjunctive therapy in adults was more effective than monotherapy, whereas monotherapy was effective in children.	A. 161 B. 162 C. 163

TABLE 1D. (*continued*) **IVIG treatment for patients with autoimmune diseases: case-**

Autoimmune Disease	IVIG treatment in humans	Results	Ref.
A. Crohn's disease	A. A patient was successfully treated with IVIG, after the disease could not be controlled with conventional anti-inflammatory therapy. B. A patient was successfully treated with IVIG, after earlier treatment with various therapeutic regimens had been unsuccessful. C. 3 medically refractory patients, who were reluctant to receive immunosuppressive therapy or have surgical intervention, were treated with 2 g/kg IVIG followed by a maintenance phase: 0.2-0.5 g/kg every 2 weeks for 12 or 24 weeks. Tapering of systemic corticosteroid therapy was attempted, whereas other medications for idiopathic colitis were continued. The treatment succeeded in all (100%).	A. Her condition improved markedly, CD8 T cell levels returned to normal and IgM decreased. B. A complete remission was achieved. During the next 2 relapses the same prompt positive response was obtained, although in the third the dose of IVIG had to be doubled. C. Statistically significant reductions were achieved in the colitis activity score and in daily prednisone dose.	A. 164 B. 165 C. 166
Hemolytic uremic syndrome (HUS)	A. A refractory patient, with a 2 year history of metastatic carcinoid tumor, underwent a multi-visceral transplant and received induction immunosuppression with humanized anti-CD52 panlymphocytic monoclonal antibody. Her maintenance immunosuppression consisted of steroids and tacrolimus. She developed anuric acute renal failure after the transplant, and was unsuccessfully treated with plasmapheresis, platelet transfusion, and discontinuation of tacrolimus. Subsequently, she was successfully treated with plasmapheresis and 20 g bolus IVIG, followed by 10 g/kg IVIG for 5 days, and received red blood cell transfusions. B. A patient, who underwent combined liver-kidney transplantation for hepatorenal polycystic disease, was initially unsuccessfully treated with withdrawal of cyclosporine, introduction of low-dose tacrolimus, and administration of fresh frozen plasma (FFP) transfusion and heparin. Subsequently the FFP treatment was replaced by plasmapheresis, followed by 0.4 mg/kg/day IVIG, and that treatment succeeded. C. 9 children with acute typical post-diarrhea hemolytic uremic syndrome were treated with IVIG. The treatment succeeded in 1 (11%).	A. Platelet count rose promptly and serum lactate dehydrogenase hormone (LDH) decreased. Four weeks later she was discharged home with normal renal function on rapamycin and steroids without recurrence of HUS. She continues to do well 9 months post-transplant. B. Rapid improvements in renal function, platelet count, and hemolytic anemia were observed. C. One child demonstrated both an increase in platelet count and a decrease in white blood cell (WBC) count within 24 hours of receiving the first dose of IVIG, but there were no significant differences found in 8/9 of the treated children in the duration of hemorrhagic colitis, thrombocytopenia, elevation of the WBC, anuria, dialysis, hospitalization, or the presence of a central nervous system complication or pancreatitis.	A. 167 B. 168 C. 169

TABLE 1D. (*continued*) IVIG treatment for patients with autoimmune diseases: case-

Autoimmune Disease	IVIG treatment in humans	Results	Ref.
Behcet's disease	A. 4 patients (6 eyes) refractory to steroids and cyclosporin A were treated with 0.4 g/kg/day IVIG for one year. The treatment succeeded in 100% of the eyes (6/6).	A. IVIG brought the acute inflammation under control and preserved the remission for a period of at least 1 year. In patient 1, the inflammatory process improved and resolved to the degree of no cells and +1 flare in 10 days. After 3 months of treatment the right eye underwent cataract surgery, after which the protocol was continued. During 1 year of treatment the eye remained in remission, with 6/10 vision. In patient 2, ocular inflammation improved in 5 days and full resolution was noted in 10 days. Over 1 year on the treatment, and an additional year follow-up after completion of treatment, vitreal remission was retained, with 6/6 vision in each eye. In patient 3, after 3 weeks of treatment the eye improved. After 6 weeks, no sign of active inflammation, with visual acuity of 6/6, was achieved, and the eye was kept in remission for up to 1 year. In patient 4, After 5 weeks of treatment, the inflammation abated and visual acuity improved to 6/7 in the right eye and 6/9 in the left eye. After 6 months of stabilization, the patient was lost to follow-up and treatment. Three months later she returned with a relapse, and was put back on IVIG therapy. The inflammation abated in 2 weeks, with stabilization. There were no recurrences in the 1 year follow up.	A. 170

blockade[3]; (2) inhibition of complement-mediated damage[3]; (4) modulation of cytokines[11]; (4) neutralization of pathogenic autoantibodies via anti-idiotypic antibodies or by their downregulation[1,38,39]; and (5) neutralization of toxins that trigger autoantibody production.[40]

The primary mechanism of action of IVIG in some autoantibody-mediated cytopenias, like ITP, is considered to be a blockade of macrophage Fc receptors.[41–43] Because Fc receptor blockade may also inhibit antibody-dependent cell-mediated cytotoxicity, it can explain the protective effect of IVIG against demyelination in inflammatory neurological diseases.[4]

IVIG exerts its anti-inflammatory activity in several ways in some autoimmune inflammatory diseases. In Kawasaki disease, IVIG is considered to (1) decrease proinflammatory cytokines levels, such as IL-1[44]; (2) increase plasma levels of IL-1 receptor antagonist[45]; and (3) neutralize the staphylococcal toxin by blocking blastic T cell apoptosis.[46,47] In dermatomyositis, IVIG is assumed to prevent the activated components C3b and C4b from being deposited on target surfaces by binding them, thereby inhibiting the generation of membrane attack complexes (C5b-C9) and subsequent complement-mediated tissue damage.[48] The anti-inflammatory effect of IVIG in Guillain-Barré syndrome is by reduction of IL-1 levels.[49] The mechanism of action of IVIG in toxic epidermal necrolysis is via blocking Fas-mediated keratinocyte death by inhibiting Fas–Fas ligand interactions.[151] IVIG modulates hemolytic uremic syndrome patients by neutralizing antibodies against toxins (Shiga toxin and SLT-1 toxin).[50]

IVIG contains high levels of anti-idiotypic antibodies that are able to bind and neutralize pathogenic autoantibodies in several autoimmune diseases, for example, (1) acquired hemophilia, in which IVIG neutralizes autoantibodies against factor VIII[51]; (2) vasculitides, in which IVIG neutralizes autoantibodies against antineutrophil cytoplasmic autoantibodies[52]; (3) SLE, in which IVIG neutralizes autoantibodies against DNA[53]; (4) ITP, in which IVIG neutralizes autoantibodies against the platelets' glycoprotein[54]; and (5) APS, in which IVIG neutralizes autoantibodies against phospholipids, for example, anticardiolipin.[53] Note that the anti-idiotypic immunomodulatory effects are extended also to T cells.[55,56]

Conclusion

IVIG is an efficient and safe therapy for many autoimmune diseases. The beneficial immunomodulatory effects of IVIG have been established in only a few autoimmune diseases. IVIG provides a good solution for patients with autoimmune diseases refractory to conventional therapy.

IVIG FOR CANCER

Patients with hematological malignancies, such as leukemia, are exposed to recurrent infections. Therefore, IVIG can reduce the frequency of infections in these patients. IVIG might also be an appropriate treatment for cancer patients undergoing chemotherapy.[5]

Cancer and autoimmune diseases share several significant features: (1) an autoimmune disease is often detected in cancer patients, and vice versa, for example, Eaton-Lambert's syndrome in patients with small cell carcinoma of the lung, or thymoma in patients with myasthenia gravis[57–59]; (2) the variety of autoantibodies seen in cancer patients, such as anti-DNA, RNP, and Sm antibodies in patients with lymphoma[60,61]; (3) a possible common genetic background; (4) a common immunodeficiency course, such as IgA deficiency[38,57,62]; (5) etiology due to common viruses (i.e., Epstein-Barr virus and cytomegalovirus) and bacteria (e.g., *Helicobacter pylori*)[38,57,62]; and (6) common treatment, such as immunosuppressive and cytotoxic drugs.[63]

Given the bidirectional relationship between cancer and autoimmunity and the fact that cancer patients are often immunosuppressed, it was logical to treat cancer patients with IVIG. The clinical experience with IVIG in cancer patients is limited, but beneficial effects have been described in several reports. TABLE 2 presents case reports, experimental studies, and trials in which cancer patients received IVIG. Clearly, prospective controlled trials are needed to establish the clinically improving effects of IVIG. Animal experimental models of cancer treated with IVIG have been reported, showing antimetastatic effects.[64]

Mechanisms of Action of IVIG in Cancer

Similar to the effects of IVIG in autoimmune diseases, IVIG exerts its antimetastatic effects in diverse, complicated mechanisms that are not fully defined. Some of the antimetastatic effects of IVIG are (1) elevation of IL-12 secretion and a subsequent enhancement of natural killer cell activity[64]; (2) inhibition of matrix metalloproteinase–9 activity[65]; and (3) inhibition of some malignant cell line growth, including lymphoma and colon carcinoma cell lines, by increasing both the expression of proapoptotic genes and Fas expression.[63]

Conclusion

IVIG significantly reduces metastases in a broad spectrum of cancer cell lines, does not affect normal cell lines (bone marrow progenitors), and is considered an effective and safe agent. It can be a potent anticancer drug, suitable for cancer patients with disease in early and advanced stages.[63,66–68,177]

IVIG FOR RECURRENT PREGNANCY LOSS

There are several reasons why recurrent pregnancy loss (RPL) occurs. One of the causes of RPL is an autoimmune disease, such as APS. Frequently, however, the reason cannot be found and these cases are referred to as spontaneous or idiopathic RPL.

RPL Caused by an Autoimmune Disease

One of the diseases associated with RPL is antiphospholipid syndrome. APS is an autoimmune disease in which RPL might occur as a result of several mechanisms, such as autoantibodies against placental membrane phospholipids, increased platelet aggregation, decreased endogenous anticoagulant activity, and complement activation.[12,69] Interestingly, it was found that women with a history of RPL have higher levels of autoantibodies to a variety of cell and tissue components, especially

TABLE 2. VIG treatment in patients with cancer

Cancer disease	IVIG treatment in humans	Results	Ref.
Multiple melanoma	A patient with unresponsive widespread metastases was treated monthly with 2 g/kg IVIG as a sole treatment; the treatment succeeded initially, but after 9 months of treatment, new metastases appeared and the patient was unsuccessfully treated with combination chemotherapy of interferon and IVIG.	In 6 months of IVIG as a sole treatment, IVIG led to stability and non-progression of the metastases in several organs, and to regression of metastases in other organs. IVIG also led to prolonged survival time. In 5 months of combined treatment, the metastases did not regress and the patient died of septic condition after 14 months of treatment.	171
Malignant peripheral nerve sheath tumor	A patient, unresponsive to doxorubicin-based chemotherapy, surgery and radiation therapy, was diagnosed with progressive multiple sclerosis. She was successfully treated with 0.4 g/kg IVIG once every 6 weeks. After 2.5 years a sacral mass was diagnosed and stabilized by irradiation. When pulmonary metastases appeared she was treated with supportive oncological care and IVIG.	The malignant peripheral nerve sheath tumor course was remarkably longer and more indolent than expected. The patient achieved a disease-free interval of 2.5 years. Stabilization of the multiple sclerosis was observed for 11 months. Three months after discontinuation of the supportive oncological care and IVIG treatment the patient succumbed to her disease.	172
Kaposi's sarcoma	An HIV patient with polymyositis was given immunosuppressive therapy and developed Kaposi's sarcoma. The patient was successfully treated with high-dose IVIG.	IVIG treatment was given for the polymyositis, and the Kaposi's sarcoma regressed abruptly.	173
Chronic lymphocytic leukemia	5 patients, in clinical stage III and IV, were treated with a 5 day infusion of high-dose IVIG for either autoimmune hemolytic anemia or ITP, or by a dose of IgG every 3-4 weeks for prevention and control of infections associated with hypogammaglobulinemia. The treatment succeeded in all (100%).	The IgG treatment succeeded for the autoimmune hemolytic anemia when combined with steroids, chemotherapy, plasmapheresis, and splenectomy, and for the ITP when combined with chemotherapy. Lymphocytopenic effects were observed in all patients during IVIG for 5 days. Furthermore, the maintenance IgG given every 3 weeks controlled both infections and lymphocyte counts with the chemotherapy. Changing the schedule to every 4 weeks resulted in poor control of the lymphocyte counts with chemotherapy. The lymphocytopenic effect suggests immunomodulating effects of IgG, which may alter the response of chronic lymphocytic leukemia cells to chemotherapy.	174

TABLE 2. (*continued*) VIG treatment in patients with cancer

Cancer disease	IVIG treatment in humans	Results	Ref.
Malignant rheumatoid arthritis	A patient, unresponsive to methylprednisolone, prednisolone and cyclophosphamide, successfully underwent an operation because of perforation of an ileum ulcer proven to be caused by vasculitis, was successfully treated with IVIG. The patient responded transiently to plasmapheresis with immunosuppressive treatment. Eventually the patient was successfully treated with 2 g/kg IVIG, and continued to receive immunosuppressive drugs at the same level during and after IVIG.	Clinical improvement emerged 3 days after IVIG, followed by improvement in laboratory variables including C-reactive protein and C-ANCA; both finally became normal. Without any adverse effects, she went into remission after 1 month. Her disease has been inactive for 4 months to date with daily 5 mg oral prednisolone.	175
Malignant epilepsy	15 children, unresponsive to conventional anti-epileptic drugs or hormone therapy, were treated with 0.4 g/kg/day on the 1st and 15th day and subsequently every 3 weeks for 6 months. The treatment succeeded in 10 (67%).	A significant reduction in attacks, or even absence of attacks was observed after 6 months. Apart from one patient with ring chromosomopathy, all 7 patients with IgG2 subclass deficiency responded. The reduction of attacks after IVIG therapy correlates with the improvement or normalization of the EEG findings.	176

anticardiolipin antibodies, but also anticoagulant, antithyroglobulin, antiphosphatidylserine, antiphosphatidylethanolamine, antiphosphatidylinositol, antiphosphatidylglycerol, and antiphosphatidic acid.[12,20,70,71] Moreover, an inverse correlation has been reported between anticardiolipin antibodies levels and the probability of a successful pregnancy.[12]

Although RPL includes several autoimmune characteristics and might occur as a result of an autoimmune disease that has yet to be found, it is still unclear whether the presence of the above-mentioned autoantibodies is the cause or the result of the reproductive failure, or an artifact of prior reproductive losses.[12]

Improved responses to IVIG have been seen in RPL that occur as a result of an autoimmune background (such as APS in TABLE 1B). For example, IVIG therapy (with or without aspirin/heparin) for APS patients with RPL has led to successful pregnancy outcomes.[36,37] Moreover, IVIG was also effective in *in vitro* fertilization for antibody-positive APS patients.[70]

Idiopathic RPL

Encouraging responses to IVIG have been seen for spontaneous RPL as well.[72] Several trials and series testing the therapeutic effect of IVIG in idiopathic RPL have been reported. TABLE 3 presents some of the reports of IVIG therapy for women with spontaneous RPL.

TABLE 3. IVIG treatment in woman with recurrent spontaneous abortions

IVIG treatment in women	Results	Ref.
10 women, with a history of 3-5 spontaneous abortions, were treated monthly with 0.4 g/kg IVIG, beginning in the 5th-6th week of gestation, until the 28th week of gestation in 5-, 3- and 1-day protocols. In 2/10 women therapy followed active immunotherapy with paternal lymphocytes. The treatment succeeded in 8 (80%).	Healthy infants were delivered, 3 preterm.	177
26 women with secondary recurrent abortions and a history of at least 4 unexplained abortions were treated with 0.8 g/kg IVIG, beginning as soon as the pregnancy test was positive, until the 20th week of gestation, and 1 g/kg IVIG was given from gestational weeks 20-26. The treatment succeeded in 15 (58%).	Successful outcomes, in which the pregnancy progressed at least until the 26th gestational week.	178
29 women, experiencing 2 or more consecutive spontaneous abortions, were treated monthly with 0.5 g/kg IVIG. The treatment succeeded in 18 (62%).	Live infants were delivered.	179
72 women with a history of 5 or more abortions were treated with 0.4 g/kg IVIG in one day in the follicular phase of a cycle in which pregnancy was planned. A booster dose was administered when pregnancy was diagnosed. The treatment succeeded in 35 (49%).	Live infants were delivered, or the previous stage of abortion was passed.	180
12 women, with a history of at least 5 abortions, were treated with 0.4 g/kg IVIG, in the follicular phase of a cycle in which pregnancy was planned. A booster dose was administered as soon as pregnancy was diagnosed. Repeat infusions were given to women who had second-trimester losses. One woman received a third dose in the 33rd week, due to growth retardation. The treatment succeeded in 5 (42%).	10 women conceived. 5 live infants were delivered, 2 preterm.	181

Mechanisms of Action of IVIG in RPL

IVIG is believed to exert its immunomodulatory effects via several mechanisms of action that cooperate in different combinations to achieve a synergistic effect in RPL. The mechanisms of action include the following: (1) anti-idiotypic antibodies neutralize cytotoxic antibodies and thereby prevent them from binding to the fetoplacental unit[73]; (2) downregulation of natural killer cell activity [73]; and (3) polarization of Th1/Th2 ratio from Th1 (hostile endometrial environment) toward Th2 (trophoblast-friendly environment) by cytokine immunomodulation.[74,75]

In Conclusion

The reports of IVIG as a treatment for RPL are encouraging, but the efficacy of IVIG has yet to be established.[12,72] Better results can be expected when a population of women is selected with a higher probability to respond to IVIG. In the meantime, one should not exclude IVIG as a potent therapy for RPL.

SIDE EFFECTS OF IVIG

When patients are well selected and when IVIG is given properly, side effects are rarely encountered (occurring in 10–30% of patients). When they do occur, they are mainly mild and transient.[2,5,72] Mild side effects include fatigue, fever, chills, myalgia, and headache. Possible serious side effects (very rare) are myocardial infarction, renal failure, alopecia, aseptic meningitis, and retinal necrosis.[2,4,5,72] Side effects depend, among other factors, on the patient's age, the dose of IVIG, and the infusion rate.[5]

To minimize the side effects, it is recommended that IVIG be administered in a dose not higher than 0.4 g/kg body weight in a 5-day schedule for 1 month (because the half-life of IgG is 3 weeks, except for IgG3, which has a half-life of 1 week).[20,76] It is also recommended to administer IVIG in low-rate infusions, especially in patients with a compromised cardiovascular system or congestive heart failure, to avoid rapid fluid overload.[4,72] Another important way to minimize IVIG side effects is to carefully select the patients receiving the therapy. For example, anaphylactic shock may occur in IgA-deficient patients after IVIG therapy; therefore, it is important to identify these patients to give them an IVIG preparation that is IgA-free. Patients with a history of side effects in general have a higher probability of developing adverse reactions to IVIG. These patients could be treated with corticosteroids intravenously half an hour before the administration of IVIG.[12] Additional risk factors to consider before administering IVIG include serum viscosity and prior thromboembolic events, tendency for migraines, and history of a renal disease or volume depletion in older patients.[4] Acute renal failure was reported to occur mainly when a sucrose-containing IVIG preparation was administered. Today, however, IVIG preparations no longer contain sucrose.[77,78]

COST OF IVIG

IVIG is an expensive therapy, costing close to U.S. $3,000 for one course of 2 g/kg IVIG for a patient weighing 70 kg.[79] The price range depends on several factors, such as where IVIG is administered (hospital, outpatient clinic, or home infusion program) and the number of days IVIG is being administered (2–5 days).[4]

CONCLUSION

IVIG is currently being used to treat several autoimmune diseases. Cancer and autoimmunity diseases share several characteristics. RPL could occur from an autoimmune disease or from an unknown cause. Generally, in RPL there are few autoimmune factors. Therefore, both cancer and RPL represent potent target diseases for IVIG therapy. Beneficial effects have been observed in a variety of autoimmune diseases, cancerous diseases, and RPL conditions (TABLES 1–3). The mechanisms of action of IVIG are diverse and not fully elucidated. IVIG clearly has the ability to neutralize pathogenic autoantibodies, modulate the immune system, and inhibit metastatic spread. IVIG is a safe product if given properly and to selected patients.

The only disadvantage of IVIG is its high cost. Therefore, clinicians should balance the cost of IVIG therapy against symptom amelioration and quality of life, minus costs of conventional therapy, decreased complications, fewer hospital admissions, and time off from work.[1] IVIG can affect every component of the immune system. It should be considered in immune-mediated diseases as a treatment for patients whose disease is refractory to conventional therapies.

Important steps for the future include: (1) the generation of specific-IVIG (sIVIG), an immunoglobulin preparation consisting of anti-idiotypic antibodies against specific antibodies, purified from an IVIG preparation by affinity chromatography[39]; and (2) the production of less expensive alternatives for IVIG, such as a synthetic preparation.

REFERENCES

1. Mydlarski, P.R., N. Mittmann & N.H. Shear. 2004. Intravenous immunoglobulin: use in dermatology. Skin Ther. Lett. **9:** 1–6.
2. Rauova, L., J. Rovensky & Y. Shoenfeld. 2000. High dose intravenous immunoglobulins: a new step in the treatment of systemic lupus erythematosus. Isr. Med. Assoc. J. **2:** 388–392.
3. Kazatchkine, M.D. & S.V. Kaveri. 2001. Immunomodulation of autoimmune and inflammatory diseases with intravenous immune globulin. N. Engl. J. Med. **345:** 747–755.
4. Dalakas, M.C. 1997. Intravenous immune globulin therapy for neurologic diseases. Ann. Intern. Med. **126:** 721–730.
5. Sherer, Y., Y. Levy & Y. Shoenfeld. 2002. IVIG in autoimmunity and cancer—efficacy versus safety. Expert Opin. Drug Saf. **1:** 153–158.
6. Krause, I., M. Blank & Y. Shoenfeld. 1998. Anti-DNA and antiphospholipid antibodies in IVIG preparations: *in vivo* study in naive mice. J. Clin. Immunol. **18:** 52–60.
7. Terryberry, J.F., Y. Shoenfeld, Y. Sherer, *et al.* 2000. Detection of antibodies to gangliosides and glycolipids in various intravenous immunoglobulin (IVIg) preparations. Immunol. Invest. **29:** 337–347.
8. Blasczyk, R., U. Westhoff & H. Grosse-Wilde. 1993. Soluble CD4, CD8, and HLA molecules in commercial immunoglobulin preparations. Lancet **341:** 789–790.
9. Kekow, J., D. Reinhold, T. Pap & S. Ansorge. 1998. Intravenous immunoglobulins and transforming growth factor beta. Lancet **351:** 184–185.
10. Altznauer, F., S. von Gunten, P. Spath & H.U. Simon. 2003. Concurrent presence of agonistic and antagonistic anti-CD95 autoantibodies in intravenous Ig preparations. J. Allergy Clin. Immunol. **112:** 1185–1190.
11. Sherer, Y., R. Wu, I. Krause, *et al.* 2001. Cytokine levels in various intravenous immunoglobulin (IVIg) preparations. Hum. Antibodies **10:** 51–53.
12. Omwandho, C.O., S.E. Gruessner, T.K. Roberts & H.R. Tinneberg. 2004. Intravenous immunoglobulin (IVIG): modes of action in the clinical management of recurrent pregnancy loss (RPL) and selected autoimmune disorders. Clin. Chem. Lab. Med. **42:** 359–370.
13. Finland, M. 1930. The serum treatment of lobar pneumonia. N. Engl. J. Med. **202:** 1244–1247.
14. Cohn, E.J. 1948. The history of plasma fractionation. *In* Company in Advances in Military Medicine, Vol. 1. E.C. Andrus, D.W. Bronk, G.A. Carden, Jr., *et al.*, Eds.: 364–443. Little, Brown. Boston.
15. Oncley, J.L., M. Melin, D.A. Richert, *et al.* 1949. The separation of the antibodies, isoagglutinins, prothrombin, plasminogen and 1-lipoprotein into subfractions of human plasma. J. Am. Chem. Soc. **71:** 541–550.
16. Berger, M. 2002. A history of immune globulin therapy, from the Harvard crash program to monoclonal antibodies. Curr. Allergy Asthma Rep. **2:** 368–378.

17. JANEWAY, C.A. 1970. The development of clinical uses of immunoglobulins: a review. *In* Immunoglobulins. E. Merler, Ed.: 3–14. National Academy of Sciences. Washington, DC.
18. MARTIN, N.H. 1971. Recognition of the hypogammaglobulinaemia syndrome. *In* Hypogammaglobulinaemia in the United Kingdom. MRC Working Party on Hypogammaglobulinaemia: 1–3. Her Majesty's Stationery Office. London.
19. IMBACH, P., V. D'APUZZO, A. HIRT, *et al.* 1981. High-dose intravenous gammaglobulin for idiopathic thrombocytopenic purpura in childhood. Lancet **1:** 1228–1231.
20. SHOENFELD, Y. & I. KRAUSE. 2004. IVIG for autoimmune, fibrosis, and malignant conditions: our experience with 200 patients. J. Clin. Immunol. **24:** 107–114.
21. MRC WORKING PARTY ON HYPOGAMMAGLOBULINAEMIA. 1971. Hypogammaglobulinaemia in the United Kingdom. Her Majesty's Stationery Office. London.
22. MARINOS, C., M.C. DALAKAS & P.J. SPATH. 2004. *In* Intravenous Immunoglobulins in the Third Millennium. C. Marinos, M.C. Dalakas & P.J. Spath, Eds. The Parthenon Publishing Group. New York/London.
23. SEGAL, E. & Y. SHOENFELD. 2001. IVIG therapy in sepsis. Harefuah **140:** 955–958.
24. KRAUSE, I., R. WU, Y. SHERER, *et al.* 2002. In vitro antiviral and antibacterial activity of commercial intravenous immunoglobulin preparations—a potential role for adjuvant intravenous immunoglobulin therapy in infectious diseases. Transfus. Med. **12:** 133–139.
25. NATIONAL INSTITUTES OF HEALTH. 1990. Intravenous immunoglobulin: prevention and treatment of disease. NIH Consensus Statement Online **8:** 1–23. Http://consensus.nih.gov/cons/080/080_intro.htm. Accessed March 18, 2002.
26. FURUSHO, K., T. KAMIYA, H. NAKANO, *et al.* 1984. High-dose intravenous gammaglobulin for Kawasaki disease. Lancet **ii:** 1055–1058.
27. SULTAN, Y., M.D. KAZATCHKINE, P. MAISONNEUVE & U.E. NYDEGGER. 1984. Anti-idiotypic suppression of autoantibodies to factor VIII (antihaemophilic factor) by high-dose intravenous gammaglobulin. Lancet **ii:** 765–768.
28. GAJDOS, P.H., H. OUTIN, D. ELKHARRAT, *et al.* 1984. High-dose intravenous gammaglobulin for myasthenia gravis. Lancet **1:** 406–407.
29. ARSURA, E.L., A. BICK, N.G. BRUNNER, *et al.* 1986. High-dose intravenous immunoglobulin in the management of myasthenia gravis. Arch. Intern. Med. **146:** 1365–1368.
30. KLEYWEG, R.P., F.G. VAN DER MECHE & J. MEULSTEE. 1988. Treatment of Guillain-Barré syndrome with high-dose gamma globulin. Neurology **38:** 1639–1641.
31. VERMUELEN, M., F.G.A. VAN DER MECHE, J.D. SPEELMAN, *et al.* 1985. Plasma and gamma-globulin infusion in chronic inflammatory polyneuropathy. J. Neurol. Sci. **70:** 317–326.
32. LATOV, N., V. CHAUDHRY, C.L. KOSKI, *et al.* 2001. Use of intravenous gamma globulins in neuroimmunologic diseases. J. Allergy Clin. Immunol. **108:** S126–S132.
33. DALAKAS, M.C. 1998. Mechanism of action of intravenous immunoglobulin and therapeutic considerations in the treatment of autoimmune neurologic diseases. Neurology **51:** S2–S8.
34. DALAKAS, M.C., M. FUJII, M. LI, *et al.* 2001. High-dose intravenous immune globulin for stiff-person syndrome. N. Engl. J. Med. **345:** 1870–1876.
35. SHERER, Y., Y. LEVY, F. FABBRIZZI & Y. SHOENFELD. 2000. Treatment of hematologic disorders other than immune thrombocytopenic purpura with intravenous immunoglobulin (IVIg)—report of seven cases and review of the literature. Eur. J. Intern. Med. **11:** 85–88.
36. CARP, H., R.A. ASHERSON & Y. SHOENFELD. 2001. Intravenous immunoglobulin in pregnancies complicated by the antiphospholipid syndrome: what is its role? J. Clin. Rheumatol. **7:** 291–294.
37. KONOVA, E., H. ANDREEVA, P. PETROVA, *et al.* 2001. Intravenous immunoglobulin in the treatment of antiphospholipid-associated miscarriages—our experience. Clin. Appl. Immunol. Invest. **1:** 75–79.
38. SHOENFELD, Y., R. KENNEDY & S. FERRANO. 1997. *In* Idiotypes in Autoimmunity, Infectious Diseases and Cancer. Y. Shoenfeld, R. Kennedy & S. Ferrano, Eds. Elsevier. Amsterdam.

39. SHOENFELD, Y., L. RAUOVA, B. GILBURD, *et al.* 2002. Efficacy of IVIG affinity-purified anti-double-stranded DNA anti-idiotypic antibodies in the treatment of an experimental murine model of systemic lupus erythematosus. Int. Immunol. **14:** 1303–1311.
40. IBANEZ, C. & J.B. MONTORO-RONSANO. 2003. Intravenous immunoglobulin preparations and autoimmune disorders: mechanisms of action. Curr. Pharm. Biotechnol. **4:** 239–247.
41. KIMBERLY, R.P., J.E. SALMON, J.B. BUSSEL, *et al.* 1984. Modulation of mononuclear phagocyte function by intravenous gamma-globulin. J. Immunol. **132:** 745–750.
42. FEHR, J., V. HOFMANN & U. KAPPELER. 1982. Transient reversal of thrombocytopenia in idiopathic thrombocytopenic purpura by high-dose intravenous gamma globulin. N. Engl. J. Med. **306:** 1254–1258.
43. SAMUELSSON, A., T.L. TOWERS & J.V. RAVETCH. 2001. Anti-inflammatory activity of IVIG mediated through the inhibitory Fc receptor. Science **291:** 484–486.
44. LEUNG, D.Y., R.S. COTRAN, E. KURT-JONES, *et al.* 1989. Endothelial cell activation and high interleukin-1 secretion in the pathogenesis of acute Kawasaki disease. Lancet **ii:** 1298–1302.
45. AUKRUST, P., S.S. FROLAND, N.B. LIABAKK, *et al.* 1994. Release of cytokines, soluble cytokine receptors, and interleukin-1 receptor antagonist after intravenous immunoglobulin administration in vivo. Blood **84:** 2136–2143.
46. BAUDET, V., V. HUREZ, C. LAPEYRE, *et al.* 1996. Intravenous immunoglobulin (IVIg) modulates the expansion of V beta 3+ and V beta 17+ T cells induced by staphylococcal enterotoxin B superantigen in vitro. Scand. J. Immunol. **43:** 277–282.
47. LEUNG, D.Y. 1996. Kawasaki syndrome: immunomodulatory benefit and potential toxin neutralization by intravenous immune globulin. Clin. Exp. Immunol. **104** (Suppl 1): 49–54.
48. BASTA, M. & M.C. DALAKAS. 1994. High-dose intravenous immunoglobulin exerts its beneficial effect in patients with dermatomyositis by blocking endomysial deposition of activated complement fragments. J. Clin. Invest. **94:** 1729–1735.
49. SHARIEF, M.K., D.A. INGRAM, M. SWASH & E.J. THOMPSON. 1999. I.V. immunoglobulin reduces circulating proinflammatory cytokines in Guillain-Barré syndrome. Neurology **52:** 1833–1838.
50. ASHKENAZI, S., T.G. CLEARY, E. LOPEZ & L.K. PICKERING. 1988. Anticytotoxin-neutralizing antibodies in immune globulin preparations: potential use in hemolytic-uremic syndrome. J. Pediatr. **113:** 1008–1014.
51. ROSSI, F., Y. SULTAN & M.D. KAZATCHKINE. 1988. Anti-idiotypes against autoantibodies and alloantibodies to VIII:C (anti-haemophilic factor) are present in therapeutic polyspecific normal immunoglobulins. Clin. Exp. Immunol. **74:** 311–316.
52. ROSSI, F., D.R. JAYNE, C.M. LOCKWOOD & M.D. KAZATCHKINE. 1991. Anti-idiotypes against anti-neutrophil cytoplasmic antigen autoantibodies in normal human polyspecific IgG for therapeutic use and in the remission sera of patients with systemic vasculitis. Clin. Exp. Immunol. **83:** 298–303.
53. KRAUSE, I., M. BLANK, J. KOPOLOVIC, *et al.* 1995. Abrogation of experimental systemic lupus erythematosus and primary antiphospholipid syndrome with intravenous gamma globulin. J. Rheumatol. **22:** 1068–1074.
54. LEVY, Y., Y. SHERER, A. AHMED, *et al.* 1998. Autoantibody level modification in adult patients with idiopathic thrombocytopenic purpura following intravenous immunoglobulin treatment. Nat. Immun. **16:** 207–214.
55. KRAUSE, I., M. BLANK, Y. SHERER, *et al.* 2002. Induction of oral tolerance in experimental antiphospholipid syndrome by feeding with polyclonal immunoglobulins. Eur. J. Immunol. **32:** 3414–3424.
56. MACIAS, A., S. ARCE, J. LEON, *et al.* 1999. Novel cross-reactive anti-idiotype antibodies with properties close to the human intravenous immunoglobulin (IVIg). Hybridoma **18:** 263–272.
57. TOMER, Y. & Y. SHOENFELD. 2000. Autoantibodies, autoimmunity and cancer. *In* Cancer and Autoimmunity. Y. Shoenfeld & E.M. Gershwin, Eds.: 141–150. Elsevier. Amsterdam.
58. TISHLER, M. & Y. SHOENFELD. 2000. Paraneoplastic syndromes. *In* Cancer and Autoimmunity. Y. Shoenfeld & E.M. Gershwin, Eds.: 121–132. Elsevier. Amsterdam.

59. Sherer, Y. & Y. Shoenfeld. 2000. Thymoma and autoimmune diseases. *In* Cancer and Autoimmunity. Y. Shoenfeld & E.M. Gershwin, Eds.: 249–252. Elsevier. Amsterdam.
60. Huminer, D., Y. Tomer, S. Pitlick & Y. Shoenfeld. 1991. Autoantibodies in cancer patients. Are they tumor related or age related? Autoimmunity **5:** 232–233.
61. Swissa, M., Y. Cohen & Y. Shoenfeld. 1990. Autoantibodies in neoplasia: unresolved enigma. Cancer **65:** 2554–2558.
62. Shoenfeld, Y. & D.A. Isenberg. 1989. The mosaic of autoimmunity. Immunol Today **10:** 123–126.
63. Fishman, P., S. Bar-Yehuda & Y. Shoenfeld. 2002. IVIg to prevent tumor metastases [Review]. Int. J. Oncol. **21:** 875–880.
64. Shoenfeld, Y. & P. Fishman. 1999. Gamma-globulin inhibits tumor spread in mice. Int. Immunol. **11:** 1247–1252.
65. Shapiro, S., Y. Shoenfeld, B. Gilburd, *et al.* 2002. Intravenous gamma globulin inhibits the production of matrix metalloproteinase-9 in macrophages. Cancer **95:** 2032–2037.
66. United States Patents no. 5,562,902. Immunotherapeutic method of treating cancerous diseases by administration of intravenous immunoglobulin. 1996.
67. United States Patents no. 5,965,130. Immunotherapeutic method of treating cancerous diseases by administration of intravenous immunoglobulin. 1999.
68. Bar-Dayan, T., I. Barshack, M. Blank, *et al.* 1999. Antibodies to the cytoplasm, cell membrane and nuclear membrane of malignant neoplasms in pooled normal human polyspecific immunoglobulin G. Int. J. Oncol. **15:** 1091–1096.
69. Girardi, G., P. Redecha & J.E. Salmon. 2004. Heparin prevents antiphospholipid antibody-induced fetal loss by inhibiting complement activation. Nat. Med. **10:** 1222–1226.
70. Sherer, Y., Y. Levy & Y. Shoenfeld. 2000. Intravenous immunoglobulin therapy of antiphospholipid syndrome. Rheumatology (Oxford) **39:** 421–426.
71. Matalon, S.T., M. Blank, Y. Levy, *et al.* 2003. The pathogenic role of anti-thyroglobulin antibody on pregnancy: evidence from an active immunization model in mice. Hum. Reprod. **18:** 1094–1099.
72. Practice Committee of the American Society for Reproductive Medicine. 2004. Intravenous immunoglobulin (IVIG) and recurrent spontaneous pregnancy loss. Fertil. Steril. **82** (Suppl 1): S199–S200.
73. Kwak, J.Y., F.M. Kwak, S.W. Ainbinder, *et al.* 1996. Elevated peripheral blood natural killer cells are effectively downregulated by immunoglobulin G infusion in women with recurrent spontaneous abortions. Am. J. Reprod. Immunol. **35:** 363–369.
74. Graphou, O., A. Chioti, A. Pantazi, *et al.* 2003. Effect of intravenous immunoglobulin treatment on the Th1/Th2 balance in women with recurrent spontaneous abortions. Am. J. Reprod. Immunol. **49:** 21–29.
75. Simon, H.U. & P.J. Spath. 2003. IVIG—mechanisms of action. Allergy **58:** 543–552.
76. Erduran, E., Y. Aslan, Y. Gedik & F. Orhan. 2003. A randomized and comparative study of intravenous immunoglobulin and mega dose methylprednisolone treatments in children with acute idiopathic thrombocytopenic purpura. Turk. J. Pediatr. **45:** 295–300.
77. Song, S., A.R. Crow, J. Freedman & A.H. Lazarus. 2003. Monoclonal IgG can ameliorate immune thrombocytopenia in a murine model of ITP: an alternative to IVIG. Blood **101:** 3708–3713.
78. Orbach, H., M. Tishler & Y. Shoenfeld. 2004. Intravenous immunoglobulin and the kidney—a two-edged sword. Semin. Arthritis Rheum. **34:** 593–601.
79. Rauova, L., J. Lukac, Y. Levy, *et al.* 2001. High dose intravenous immunoglobulins for lupus nephritis—a salvage immunomodulation. Lupus **10:** 209–213.
80. Benesch, M., R. Kerbl, H. Lackner, *et al.* 2003. Low-dose versus high-dose immunoglobulin for primary treatment of acute immune thrombocytopenic purpura in children: results of a prospective, randomized single-center trial. J. Pediatr. Hematol. Oncol. **25:** 797–800.
81. Nuchprayoon, I., P. Seksarn, P. Vanichsetakul & R. O-Chareon. 2001. Low dose intravenous immunoglobulin for acute immune thrombocytopenic purpura in children. Asian Pac. J. Allergy Immunol. **19:** 11–16.

82. SHAHAR, E. & M. LEIDERMAN. 2003. Outcome of severe Guillain-Barré syndrome in children: comparison between untreated cases versus gamma-globulin therapy. Clin. Neuropharmacol. **26:** 84–87.
83. REUBEN, S., M.G. SUMI, A. MATHAI, *et al.* 2003. Intravenous immunoglobulin reduces serum tumor necrosis factor alpha in patients with Guillain-Barré syndrome. Neurol. India **51:** 487–489.
84. ECHANIZ-LAGUNA, A., F. BATTAGLIA, B. ELLERO, *et al.* 2004. Chronic inflammatory demyelinating polyradiculoneuropathy in patients with liver transplantation. Muscle Nerve **30:** 501–504.
85. MENDELL, J.R., R.J. BAROHN, M.L. FREIMER, *et al.*, for the Working Group on Peripheral Neuropathy. 2001. Randomized controlled trial of IVIg in untreated chronic inflammatory demyelinating polyradiculoneuropathy. Neurology **56:** 445–449.
86. HAHN, A.F., C.F. BOLTON, D. ZOCHODNE & T.E. FEASBY. 1996. Intravenous immunoglobulin treatment in chronic inflammatory demyelinating polyneuropathy. A double-blind, placebo-controlled, cross-over study. Brain **119:** 1067–1077.
87. VERMEULEN, M., P.A. VAN DOORN, A. BRAND, *et al.* 1993. Intravenous immunoglobulin treatment in patients with chronic inflammatory demyelinating polyneuropathy: a double blind, placebo controlled study. J. Neurol. Neurosurg. Psychiatry **56:** 36–39.
88. VAN DOORN, P.A., A. BRAND, P.F. STRENGERS, *et al.* 1990. High-dose intravenous immunoglobulin treatment in chronic inflammatory demyelinating polyneuropathy: a double-blind, placebo-controlled, crossover study. Neurology **40:** 209–212.
89. COSI, V., M. LOMBARDI, G. PICCOLO & A. ERBETTA. 1991. Treatment of myasthenia gravis with high-dose intravenous immunoglobulin. Acta Neurol. Scand. **84:** 81–84.
90. WEGNER, B. & I. AHMED. 2002. Intravenous immunoglobulin monotherapy in long-term treatment of myasthenia gravis. Clin. Neurol. Neurosurg. **105:** 3–8.
91. ACHIRON, A., Y. BARAK, S. MIRON & I. SAROVA-PINHAS. 2000. Immunoglobulin treatment in refractory myasthenia gravis. Muscle Nerve **23:** 551–555.
92. TERENGHI, F., A. CAPPELLARI, A. BERSANO, *et al.* 2004. How long is IVIg effective in multifocal motor neuropathy? Neurology **62:** 666–668.
93. AZULAY, J.P., P. RIHET, J. POUGET, *et al.* 1997. Long term follow up of multifocal motor neuropathy with conduction block under treatment. J. Neurol. Neurosurg. Psychiatry **62:** 391–394.
94. VAN DEN BERG, L.H., H. KERKHOFF, P.L. OEY, *et al.* 1995. Treatment of multifocal motor neuropathy with high dose intravenous immunoglobulins: a double blind, placebo controlled study. J. Neurol. Neurosurg. Psychiatry **59:** 248–252.
95. DALAKAS, M.C., I. ILLA, J.M. DAMBROSIA, *et al.* 1993. A controlled trial of high-dose intravenous immune globulin infusions as treatment for dermatomyositis. N. Engl. J. Med. **329:** 1993–2000.
96. GOTTFRIED, I., A. SEEBER, B. ANEGG, *et al.* 2000. High dose intravenous immunoglobulin (IVIG) in dermatomyositis: clinical responses and effect on sIL-2R levels. Eur. J. Dermatol. **10:** 29–35.
97. SANGTAWESIN, C., T. KIRAWITAYA, T. LAYANGKOOL, *et al.* 2003. Treatment of Kawasaki disease using locally product intravenous immunoglobulin. J. Med. Assoc. Thai. **6** (Suppl 3): S656–S660.
98. KHOWSATHIT, P., C. HONG-HGAM, A. KHOSITSETH & S. WANITKUN. 2002. Treatment of Kawasaki disease with a moderate dose (1 g/kg) of intravenous immunoglobulin. J. Med. Assoc. Thai. **85** (Suppl 4): S1121–S1126.
99. JAYNE, D.R. & C.M. LOCKWOOD. 1996. Intravenous immunoglobulin as sole therapy for systemic vasculitis. Br. J. Rheumatol. **35:** 1150–1153.
100. LEVY, Y., Y. SHERER, J. GEORGE, *et al.* 1999. Serologic and clinical response to treatment of systemic vasculitis and associated autoimmune disease with intravenous immunoglobulin. Int. Arch. Allergy Immunol. **119:** 231–238.
101. JAYNE, D.R., V.L. ESNAULT & C.M. LOCKWOOD. 1993. ANCA anti-idiotype antibodies and the treatment of systemic vasculitis with intravenous immunoglobulin. J. Autoimmun. **6**: 207–219.
102. LEVY, Y., J. GEORGE, F. FABBRIZZI, *et al.* 1999. Marked improvement of Churg–Strauss vasculitis with intravenous gammaglobulins. South Med. J. **92:** 412–414.

103. SULLIVAN, K.M., J. STOREK, K.J. KOPECKY, *et al.* 1996. A controlled trial of long-term administration of intravenous immunoglobulin to prevent late infection and chronic graft-vs.-host disease after marrow transplantation: clinical outcome and effect on subsequent immune recovery. Biol. Blood Marrow Transpl. **2:** 44–53.
104. ACHIRON, A., I. KISHNER, I. SAROVA-PINHAS, *et al.* 2004. Intravenous immunoglobulin treatment following the first demyelinating event suggestive of multiple sclerosis: a randomized, double-blind, placebo-controlled trial. Arch. Neurol. **61:** 1515–1520.
105. HOMMES, O.R., P.S. SORENSEN, F. FAZEKAS, *et al.* 2004. Intravenous immunoglobulin in secondary progressive multiple sclerosis: randomised placebo-controlled trial. Lancet **364:** 1149–1156.
106. LEBRUN, C., G. GHETAU, V. BOURG, *et al.* 2003. Intravenous immunoglobulins for relapsing-remitting multiple sclerosis after failure of treatment with other immunomodulators. Rev. Neurol. (Paris) **159:** 648–651.
107. STANGEL, M., F. BOEGNER, C.H. KLATT, *et al.* 2000. Placebo controlled pilot trial to study the remyelinating potential of intravenous immunoglobulins in multiple sclerosis. J. Neurol. Neurosurg. Psychiatry **68:** 89–92.
108. ROSENBAUM, J.T., R.K. GEORGE & C. GORDON. 1999. The treatment of refractory uveitis with intravenous immunoglobulin. Am. J. Ophthalmol. **127:** 545–549.
109. SUNAKAWA, M. 1989. High-dose intravenous gammaglobulin therapy for uveitis. Metab. Pediatr. Syst. Ophthalmol. **12:** 93–95.
110. FLORES, G., C. CUNNINGHAM-RUNDLES, A.C. NEWLAND & J.B. BUSSEL. 1993. Efficacy of intravenous immunoglobulin in the treatment of autoimmune hemolytic anemia: results in 73 patients. Am. J. Hematol. **44:** 237–242.
111. HILGARTNER, M.W. & J. BUSSEL. 1987. Use of intravenous gamma globulin for the treatment of autoimmune neutropenia of childhood and autoimmune hemolytic anemia. Am. J. Med. **83:** 25–29.
112. ALLIOT, C., M. BARRIOS, S. TABUTEAU & B. DESABLENS. 2000. Autoimmune cytopenias associated with malignancies and successfully treated with intravenous immune globulins: about two cases. Therapie **55:** 371–374.
113. SCHWARTZ, R.S., D.A. GABRIEL, L.M. ALEDORT, *et al.* 1995. A prospective study of treatment of acquired (autoimmune) factor VIII inhibitors with high-dose intravenous gammaglobulin. Blood **86:** 797–804.
114. CHERIN, P., S. PELLETIER, A. TEIXEIRA, *et al.* 2002. Results and long-term followup of intravenous immunoglobulin infusions in chronic, refractory polymyositis: an open study with thirty-five adult patients. Arthritis Rheum. **46:** 467–474.
115. JANN, S., S. BERETTA, M. MOGGIO, *et al.* 1992. High-dose intravenous human immunoglobulin in polymyositis resistant to treatment. J. Neurol. Neurosurg. Psychiatry **55:** 60–62.
116. CLARK, A.L., D.W. BRANCH, R.M. SILVER, *et al.* 1999. Pregnancy complicated by the antiphospholipid syndrome: outcomes with intravenous immunoglobulin therapy. Obstet. Gynecol. **93:** 437–441.
117. SPINNATO, J.A., A.L. CLARK, S.S. PIERANGELI & E.N. HARRIS. 1995. Intravenous immunoglobulin therapy for the antiphospholipid syndrome in pregnancy. Am. J. Obstet. Gynecol. **172:** 690–694.
118. KAAJA, R., H. JULKUNEN, P. AMMALA, *et al.* 1993. Intravenous immunoglobulin treatment of pregnant patients with recurrent pregnancy losses associated with antiphospholipid antibodies. Acta Obstet. Gynecol. Scand. **72:** 63–66.
119. VALENSISE, H., E. VAQUERO, C. DE CAROLIS, *et al.* 1995. Normal fetal growth in women with antiphospholipid syndrome treated with high-dose intravenous immunoglobulin (IVIG). Prenat. Diagn. **15:** 509–517.
120. MARZUSCH, K., J. DIETL, R. KLEIN, *et al.* 1996. Recurrent first trimester spontaneous abortion associated with antiphospholipid antibodies: a pilot study of treatment with intravenous immunoglobulin. Acta Obstet. Gynecol. Scand. **75:** 922–926.
121. MAKSYMOWYCH, W.P., A. AVINA-ZUBIETA, M. LUONG & A.S. RUSSELL. 1996. High dose intravenous immunoglobulin (IVIg) in severe refractory rheumatoid arthritis: no evidence for efficacy. Clin. Exp. Rheumatol. **14:** 657–660.
122. TUMIATI, B., P. CASOLI, M. VENEZIANI & G. RINALDI. 1992. High-dose immunoglobulin therapy as an immunomodulatory treatment of rheumatoid arthritis. Arthritis Rheum. **35:** 1126–1133.

123. SILVERMAN, E.D., G.D. CAWKWELL, D.J. LOVELL, *et al.* 1994. Intravenous immunoglobulin in the treatment of systemic juvenile rheumatoid arthritis: a randomized placebo controlled trial. Pediatric Rheumatology Collaborative Study Group. J. Rheumatol. **21:** 2353–2358.
124. UZIEL, Y., R.M. LAXER, R. SCHNEIDER & E.D. SILVERMAN. 1996. Intravenous immunoglobulin therapy in systemic onset juvenile rheumatoid arthritis: a followup study. J. Rheumatol. **23:** 910–918.
125. LEVY, Y., Y. SHERER, A. AHMED, *et al.* 1999. A study of 20 SLE patients with intravenous immunoglobulin—clinical and serologic response. Lupus **8:** 705–712.
126. FRANCIONI, C., M. GALEAZZI, A. FIORAVANTI, et al. 1994. Long-term i.v. Ig treatment in systemic lupus erythematosus. Clin. Exp. Rheumatol. **12:** 163–168.
127. WINDER, A., Y. MOLAD, I. OSTFELD, *et al.* 1993. Treatment of systemic lupus erythematosus by prolonged administration of high dose intravenous immunoglobulin: report of 2 cases. J. Rheumatol. **20:** 495–498.
128. AKASHI, K., K. NAGASAWA, T. MAYUMI, *et al.* 1990. Successful treatment of refractory systemic lupus erythematosus with intravenous immunoglobulins. J. Rheumatol. **17:** 375–379.
129. SCHROEDER, J.O., R.A. ZEUNER, H.H. EULER & H. LOFFLER. 1996. High dose intravenous immunoglobulins in systemic lupus erythematosus: clinical and serological results of a pilot study. J. Rheumatol. **23:** 71–75.
130. AMITAL, H., E. REWALD, Y. LEVY, *et al.* 2003. Fibrosis regression induced by intravenous gammaglobulin treatment. Ann. Rheum. Dis. **62:** 175–177.
131. LEVY, Y., H. AMITAL, P. LANGEVITZ, *et al.* 2004. Intravenous immunoglobulin modulates cutaneous involvement and reduces skin fibrosis in systemic sclerosis: an open-label study. Arthritis Rheum. **50:** 1005–1007.
132. LEVY, Y., Y. SHERER, P. LANGEVITZ, *et al.* 2000. Skin score decrease in systemic sclerosis patients treated with intravenous immunoglobulin—a preliminary report. Clin. Rheumatol. **19:** 207–211.
133. KAHALY, G., S. PITZ, W. MULLER-FORELL & G. HOMMEL. 1996. Randomized trial of intravenous immunoglobulins versus prednisolone in Graves' ophthalmopathy. Clin. Exp. Immunol. **106:** 197–202.
134. BASCHIERI, L., A. ANTONELLI, S. NARDI, *et al.* 1997. Intravenous immunoglobulin versus corticosteroid in treatment of Graves' ophthalmopathy. Thyroid **7:** 579–585.
135. LEIBE, A., Y. LEVY & Y. SHOENFELD. 2001. Intravenous immunoglobulins treatment of patients with Graves' ophthalmopathy. Harefuah **140:** 392–394, 454, 455.
136. LEHOANG, P., N. CASSOUX, F. GEORGE, *et al.* 2000. Intravenous immunoglobulin (IVIg) for the treatment of birdshot retinochoroidopathy. Ocul. Immunol. Inflamm. **8:** 49–57.
137. ROMANELLO, C., F. GROSSI, L. RADILLO, *et al.* 1991. Comparison of high-dose immunoglobulin and cyclosporine in newly diagnosed diabetic children. Pediatr. Med. Chir. **13:** 355–358.
138. AHMED, A.R. 2001. Intravenous immunoglobulin therapy in the treatment of patients with pemphigus vulgaris unresponsive to conventional immunosuppressive treatment. J. Am. Acad. Dermatol. **45:** 679–690.
139. HERZOG, S., E. SCHMIDT, M. GOEBELER, *et al.* 2004. Serum levels of autoantibodies to desmoglein 3 in patients with therapy-resistant pemphigus vulgaris successfully treated with adjuvant intravenous immunoglobulins. Acta Derm. Venereol. **84:** 48–52.
140. SAMI, N., A. QURESHI, E. RUOCCO & A.R. AHMED. 2002. Corticosteroid-sparing effect of intravenous immunoglobulin therapy in patients with pemphigus vulgaris. Arch. Dermatol. **138:** 1158–1162.
141. SAMI, N., A. QURESHI & A.R. AHMED. 2002. Steroid sparing effect of intravenous immunoglobulin therapy in patients with pemphigus foliaceus. Eur. J. Dermatol. **12:** 174–178.
142. AHMED, A.R. & N. SAMI. 2002. Intravenous immunoglobulin therapy for patients with pemphigus foliaceus unresponsive to conventional therapy. J. Am. Acad. Dermatol. **46:** 42–49.

143. KLOS, K. & J. KRUSZEWSKI. 2001. Preliminary estimation of results of high-dose intravenous immunoglobulin in severe steroid-dependent adult asthma. Pol. Merkuriusz. Lek. **11:** 379–383.
144. HAQUE, S., N. BOYCE, F.C. THIEN, *et al.* 2003. Role of intravenous immunoglobulin in severe steroid-dependent asthma. Intern. Med. J. **33:** 341–344.
145. LANDWEHR, L.P., J.D. JEPPSON, M.G. KATLAN, *et al.* 1998. Benefits of high-dose i.v. immunoglobulin in patients with severe steroid-dependent asthma. Chest **114:** 1349–1356.
146. SHORTT, R., M. GOMEZ, N. MITTMAN & R. CARTOTTO. 2004. Intravenous immunoglobulin does not improve outcome in toxic epidermal necrolysis. J. Burn. Care. Rehabil. **25:** 246–255.
147. VIARD, I., P. WEHRLI, R. BULLANI, *et al.* 1998. Inhibition of toxic epidermal necrolysis by blockade of CD95 with human intravenous immunoglobulin. Science **282:** 490–493.
148. DALAKAS, M.C., B. SONIES, J. DAMBROSIA, *et al.* 1997. Treatment of inclusion-body myositis with IVIg: a double-blind, placebo-controlled study. Neurology **48:** 712–716.
149. DALAKAS, M.C., B. KOFFMAN, M. FUJII, *et al.* 2001. A controlled study of intravenous immunoglobulin combined with prednisone in the treatment of IBM. Neurology **56:** 323–327.
150. WINDER, A., Y. SHOENFELD, R. HOCHMAN, *et al.* 1998. High-dose intravenous gammaglobulins for heparin-induced thrombocytopenia: a prompt response. J. Clin. Immunol. **18:** 330–334.
151. PRULL, A., R. NECHWATAL, H. RIEDEL & W. MAURER. 1992. The therapy of the heparin-induced thrombosis-thrombocytopenia syndrome with immunoglobulins. Dtsch. Med. Wochenschr. **117:** 1838–1842.
152. BUSSEL, J., P. LALEZARI, M. HILGARTNER, *et al.* 1983. Reversal of neutropenia with intravenous gammaglobulin in autoimmune neutropenia of infancy. Blood **62:** 398–400.
153. KODURI, P.R., R. KUMAPLEY, J. VALLADARES & C. TETER. 1999. Chronic pure red cell aplasia caused by parvovirus B19 in AIDS: use of intravenous immunoglobulin—a report of eight patients. Am. J. Hematol. **61:** 16–20.
154. MOUDGIL, A., H. SHIDBAN, C.C. NAST, *et al.* 1997. Parvovirus B19 infection-related complications in renal transplant recipients: treatment with intravenous immunoglobulin. Transplantation **64:** 1847–1850.
155. WICKI, J., K. SAMII, P. CASSINOTTI, *et al.* 1997. Parvovirus [correction of Parovirus] B19-induced red cell aplasia in solid-organ transplant recipients. Two case reports and review of the literature. Hematol. Cell Ther. **39:** 199–204.
156. HUANG, Y.W. & P. SAIDI. 2004. Acquired von Willebrand disease in a patient with monoclonal gammopathy of undetermined significance. Am. J. Med. Sci. **327:** 98–101.
157. MACIK, B.G., D.A. GABRIEL, G.C. WHITE II, *et al.* 1988. The use of high-dose intravenous gamma-globulin in acquired von Willebrand syndrome. Arch. Pathol. Lab. Med. **112:** 143–146.
158. VIALLARD, J.F., J.L. PELLEGRIN, C. VERGNES, *et al.* 1999. Three cases of acquired von Willebrand disease associated with systemic lupus erythematosus. Br. J. Haematol. **105:** 532–537.
159. SAMPSON, B., D.R. ANDERSON, M. DUGAL, *et al.* 1997. Acquired type 2a von Willebrand's disease: response to immunoglobulin infusion. Haemostasis **27:** 286–289.
160. BREEDVELD, F.C., A. BRAND & W.G. VAN AKEN. 1985. High dose intravenous gamma globulin for Felty's syndrome. J. Rheumatol. **12:** 700–702.
161. JOLLES, S., J. HUGHES & M. RUSTIN. 2000. The treatment of atopic dermatitis with adjunctive high-dose intravenous immunoglobulin: a report of three patients and review of the literature. Br. J. Dermatol. **142:** 551–554.
162. JOLLES, S., C. SEWELL, D. WEBSTER, *et al.* 2003. Adjunctive high-dose intravenous immunoglobulin treatment for resistant atopic dermatitis: efficacy and effects on intracellular cytokine levels and CD4 counts. Acta Derm. Venereol. **83:** 433–437.
163. JOLLES, S. 2002. A review of high-dose intravenous immunoglobulin treatment for atopic dermatitis. Clin. Exp. Dermatol. **27:** 3–7.

164. KORBER, J., E. KOTTGEN & H. RENZ. 1998. A case of Crohn's disease with increased CD8 T-cell activation and remission during therapy with intravenous immunoglobulins. Scand. J. Gastroenterol. **33:** 1113–1117.
165. WOLF, A., G. GAEDICKE, D. LEUPOLD & E. KOHNE. 1988. Treatment of Crohn disease with intravenous immunoglobulin. Monatsschr. Kinderheilkd. **136:** 101–103.
166. LEVINE, D.S., S.H. FISCHER, D.L. CHRISTIE, *et al.* 1992. Intravenous immunoglobulin therapy for active, extensive, and medically refractory idiopathic ulcerative or Crohn's colitis. Am. J. Gastroenterol. **87:** 91–100.
167. BANERJEE, D., W. KUPIN & D. ROTH. 2003. Hemolytic uremic syndrome after multivisceral transplantation treated with intravenous immunoglobulin. J. Nephrol. **16:** 733–735.
168. GATTI, S., M. ARRU, P. REGGIANI, *et al.* 2003. Successful treatment of hemolytic uremic syndrome after liver-kidney transplantation. J. Nephrol. **16:** 586–590.
169. ROBSON, W.L., G.H. FICK, T. JADAVJI & A.K. LEUNG. 1991. The use of intravenous gammaglobulin in the treatment of typical hemolytic uremic syndrome. Pediatr. Nephrol. **5:** 289–292.
170. SEIDER, N., I. BEIRAN, J. SCHARF & B. MILLER. 2001. Intravenous immunoglobulin therapy for resistant ocular Behcet's disease. Br. J. Ophthalmol. **85:** 1287–1288.
171. SHOENFELD, Y., Y. LEVY & P. FISHMAN. 2001. Shrinkage of melanoma metastases following high dose intravenous immunoglobulin treatment. Isr. Med. Assoc. J. **3:** 698–699.
172. MERIMSKY, O., I. MELLER, M. INBAR, *et al.* 2002. A possible role for IVIg in the treatment of soft tissue sarcoma: a clinical case and an experimental model. Int. J. Oncol. **20:** 839–843.
173. CARMELI, Y., D. MEVORACH, N. KAMINSKI & E. RAZ. 1994. Regression of Kaposi's sarcoma after intravenous immunoglobulin treatment for polymyositis. Cancer **73:** 2859–2861.
174. BESA, E.C. 1984. Use of intravenous immunoglobulin in chronic lymphocytic leukemia. Am. J. Med. **76:** 209–218.
175. MAEDA, H., O. FURONAKA, K. MATSUSHIMA, *et al.* 2001. Successful treatment of "malignant rheumatoid arthritis" in Japan with pooled intravenous immunoglobulin. Rheumatology (Oxford) **40:** 955–956.
176. STERIO, M., E. GEBAUER, G. VUCICEVIC, *et al.* 1990. Intravenous immunoglobulin in the treatment of malignant epilepsy in children. Wien Klin. Wochenschr. **102:** 230–233.
177. SIPAK-SZMIGIEL, O., E. RONIN-WALKNOWSKA & A. MIKLASZWICZ. 2003. Application of intravenous immunoglobulin therapy (IVIG) in pregnant patients with recurrent spontaneous abortions. Ginekol. Pol. **74:** 350–355.
178. CHRISTIANSEN, O.B., B. PEDERSEN, A. ROSGAARD & M. HUSTH. 2002. A randomized, double-blind, placebo-controlled trial of intravenous immunoglobulin in the prevention of recurrent miscarriage: evidence for a therapeutic effect in women with secondary recurrent miscarriage. Hum. Reprod. **17:** 809–816.
179. COULAM, C.B., L. KRYSA, J.J. STERN & M. BUSTILLO. 1995. Intravenous immunoglobulin for treatment of recurrent pregnancy loss. Am. J. Reprod. Immunol. **34:** 333–337.
180. CARP, H.J., V. TODER, E. GAZIT, *et al.* 2001. Further experience with intravenous immunoglobulin in women with recurrent miscarriage and a poor prognosis. Am. J. Reprod. Immunol. **46:** 268–273.
181. CARP, H.J., R. AHIRON, S. MASHIACH, *et al.* 1996. Intravenous immunoglobulin in women with five or more abortions. Am. J. Reprod. Immunol. **35:** 360–362.

Response of Vasculitic Peripheral Neuropathy to Intravenous Immunoglobulin

YAIR LEVY,[a] YOSEF UZIEL,[b] GIESELE ZANDMAN,[c,d] PNINA ROTMAN,[a] HAWARED AMITAL,[c] YANIV SHERER,[c] PNINA LANGEVITZ,[d] BOLECK GOLDMAN,[e] AND YEHUDA SHOENFELD[c,f]

[a]*Department of Medicine E, Meir Medical Center, Sackler Faculty of Medicine, Tel Aviv University, Tel Aviv, Israel*

[b]*Pediatric Rheumatology Unit, Meir Medical Centre, Kfar Saba, Sackler Faculty of Medicine, Tel Aviv University, Tel Aviv, Israel*

[c]*Department of Medicine B and Centre for Autoimmune Diseases, Sheba Medical Centre Tel Hashomer, Sackler Faculty of Medicine, Tel Aviv University, Tel Aviv, Israel*

[d]*Rheumatic Diseases Unit, Sheba Medical Centre Tel Hashomer, Sackler Faculty of Medicine, Tel Aviv University, Tel Aviv, Israel*

[e]*Institute of Genetics, Sheba Medical Centre Tel Hashomer, Sackler Faculty of Medicine, Tel Aviv University, Tel Aviv, Israel*

ABSTRACT: Peripheral neuropathy is a prominent feature of the systemic and secondary vasculitides. Usually, it responds to corticosteroids therapy, but in certain cases it may resist corticosteroid or immunosuppressive treatment, or both. The objective of this study is to present case reports of patients who exhibited various inflammatory diseases, accompanied with vasculitic peripheral neuropathies, for which intravenous immunoglobulin (IVIg) was used for treatment. The study included 10 patients with the following: Sjögren's syndrome (1), systemic lupus erythematosus (2), vaccination-induced vasculitis (1), Churg-Strauss vasculitis (1), mixed cryoglobulinemia (2), polyarteritis nodosa (1), sarcoidosis (1), and scleroderma (1). All developed vasculitic peripheral neuropathy and were treated with 1–13 cycles of high-dose IVIg (2 g/kg body weight). The patients were followed up for 1–5 years after this treatment. Results showed that in all but two patients (mixed cryoglobulinemia associated with hepatitis C and sarcoidosis), neuropathy improved or completely resolved after IVIg treatment. In conclusion, IVIg may be beneficial in cases of resistant vasculitic peripheral neuropathy. IVIg should probably be considered as a sole or adjuvant treatment in patients for whom conventional treatment is contraindicated, or for patients in whom conventional treatment has failed.

KEYWORDS: peripheral neuropathy; vasculitis; immunoglobulin; corticosteroids

Address for correspondence: Prof. Y. Shoenfeld, Department of Medicine B, Sheba Medical Centre, Tel Aviv University, Tel Aviv, Israel. Voice: +972-3-5302652; fax: +972-3-5352855.
shoenfel@post.tau.ac.il

[f]Incumbent of the Laura Schwartz-Kipp Chair for Research of Autoimmunity Diseases, Tel Aviv University, Tel Aviv, Israel.

Ann. N.Y. Acad. Sci. 1051: 779–786 (2005).
doi: 10.1196/annals.1361.121

INTRODUCTION

Peripheral neuropathy is a prominent feature of diverse systemic and secondary vasculitides. In patients with mononeuritis multiplex, vasculitis of the vasa nervorum results in neuronal deficits. Patients with vasculitis restricted to the peripheral nervous system usually respond to combined treatment with high-dose corticosteroids, plasmapheresis, and cyclophosphamide.[1–2]

Increasingly, intravenous immunoglobulin (IVIg) has been used in neurological manifestations of autoimmune diseases.[3] However, only a few case reports have discussed the administration of IVIg in patients with vasculitis and peripheral neuropathy who were unresponsive to conventional treatment.[4–6] Previously, we described six patients with vasculitic peripheral neuropathy, to whom IVIg was administered, eliciting a good response in four patients.[7] Herein, we describe our experience with IVIg treatment in ten patients with peripheral neuropathy associated with vasculitis that was, in most cases, unresponsive to conventional immunosuppressive treatment. Six of the patients who had been described previously had longer follow-ups, and four new patients were added to our series.

CASE REPORTS

Systemic Lupus Erythematosus

A 12-year-old girl was admitted after a convulsive episode. Two weeks earlier, she had developed fever, arthralgias, facial rash, hair loss, abdominal pain, and pain and burning sensations in her legs. On examination, pathological neurological findings were noted: anxiety, agitation, confusion with memory impairment, and a fine tremor. Her muscular strength was impaired, and increased sensitivity to touch was apparent. Fundus examination of the eye was compatible with retinal vasculitis.

The serological analysis disclosed a high positive antinuclear antibody titer, anti-double-stranded DNA (anti-dsDNA), anti-Sm, and anti-Ro antibodies. Lumbar puncture, brain single-photon emission computed tomography (SPECT), brain computed tomography (CT), and magnetic resonance imaging (MRI) were compatible with central nervous system involvement. Nerve conduction velocity was compatible with peripheral neuropathy.

Diagnosis for this patient was systemic lupus erythematosus (SLE) with active central and peripheral nervous system involvement, together with hematologic and dermatologic manifestations. A 3-day course of intravenous methylprednisolone was started, 1 g every day, followed by 20 mg i.v. methylprednisolone three times a day for a week, followed by prednisone 20 mg three times a day. Two weeks later, she remained in agony, with unbearably painful legs that did not respond to narcotic drugs.

At this point, we decided to institute high-dose IVIg in the form of Omr-IgG-am (Omrix Biopharmaceuticals, Tel Aviv, Israel) at a dose of 2 g/kg body weight given for 2 days. The day after, a drastic response was noticed, with a significant decrease in her excruciating pain. Gradually her depression, agitation, and confusion improved as well. Two months later, she went back to school and continued treatment with low-dose prednisone, hydroxychloroquine, and cyclophosphamide. Later on, the cyclophosphamide and prednisone were stopped, and for 3 years since the IVIg therapy, the patient has been in good health receiving hydroxychloroquine therapy.

Systemic Lupus Erythematosus

A 55-year-old woman received a diagnosis of SLE 20 years ago. The criteria for diagnosis were arthritis, butterfly rash, high titer of anti-dsDNA, and positive antinuclear factor (ANF). The patient was treated with hydroxychloroquine and low-dose steroids. Six months before the IVIg treatment, the patient started to complain of pain in both her legs. Electromyography (EMG) revealed severe sensory polyneuropathy without motor deficit. Her steroid dose was increased, and azathioprine was started without any improvement. Six months later, IVIg (Omr-IgG-am) was added at a dose of 2 g/kg, and rapid improvement of her pain followed. Repeated EMG tests also demonstrated significant improvement.

Mixed Cryoglobulinemia Type II Associated with Hepatitis C Infection

A 67-year-old man with type II mixed cryoglobulinemia associated with hepatitis C infection was referred for evaluation. He suffered from severe symmetrical sensorimotor polyneuropathy. For six years, the patient had experienced distal motor and sensory deficits. On examination, symmetrical hyperesthesia and hyperalgasia were found, along with bilateral loss of vibration and position sense and loss of ankle jerks. Nerve conduction studies were consistent with severe sensorimotor polyneuropathy. Treatment with prednisone, interferon-alpha, cyclosporine, and pulse cyclophosphamide did not help. IVIg treatment with Pentaglobin (Biotest Pharma, Dreieich, Germany) comprising 38 g/L IgG, 6 g/L IgM, and 6 g/L IgA was instituted at a dosage of 400 mL/day for 3 days. Although the patient was treated with two monthly courses, no clinical benefit was seen.

Mixed Cryoglobulinemia Type II Associated with CMV Infection

A 44-year-old woman was diagnosed with mixed cryoglobulinemia based on purpuric rash on her legs and positive cryoglobulins in her blood. Positive IgM cytomegalovirus (CMV) serology was found at that time. Later on, the patient developed proteinuria (3–4 grams per 24 hours), and her creatinine increased from 0.7 to 1.2 mg/dL with nephritic urine sediment. She also reported severe abdominal cramps, although an investigation that included gastroscopy, colonoscopy, and CT scanning of the abdomen appeared normal. The patient was treated with high-dose prednisone and pulse therapy of cyclophosphamide and showed some improvement. At that time, severe pain appeared in her right hand with a decline in the function of her hand. EMG revealed mononeuritis multiplex of the right hand. Because the patient was already taking steroids and cyclophosphamide, high-dose IVIg therapy was initiated. Her severe pain immediately disappeared, and, after six IVIg courses, there remained only minor disturbance in her hand functioning. Repeated EMG tests demonstrated significant improvement.

Scleroderma

A 65-year-old man who had scleroderma diagnosed 3 years previously was referred to us because of severe pain in his legs and, to a lesser extent, in his hands. The patient also suffered from dyspnea due to restrictive lung disease, a manifestation of scleroderma lung disease. EMG/nerve conduction study (NCS) testing demonstrated asymmetrical sensorimotor polyneuropathy with mixed axonal and demyelinating features. The patient was treated with prednisone (1 mg/kg), which did not achieve a beneficial response, and developed steroid-induced diabetes mellitus. The steroid therapy was thereafter tapered down to 5 mg/day of prednisone. Treatment with high-dose IVIg (2 g/kg/cycle Omr-IgG-am) was initiated. After 12 cycles of treatment, the patient's symptoms significantly improved, and an EMG study revealed partial improvement of his polyneuropathy.

Polyarteritis Nodosa

A 77-year-old woman presented with pain and cyanosis of the fingers and toes in all four extremities. Two months later, drop foot appeared first in the left and later in the right foot. EMG demonstrated motor neuropathy of both legs. A sural nerve biopsy showed necrotizing vasculitis of the polyarteritis nodosa type with subacute axonopathy. Treatment with pulse cyclophosphamide and methylprednisolone was initiated, with 30 mg prednisone given daily between the pulses. The patient received four cycles of therapy; afterward, oral cyclophosphamide was given in a dose of 100 mg per day. While on this treatment regimen, weakness appeared in the patient's left hand, and EMG disclosed severe neuropathy of the ulnar and median nerves. Four months after initiating the immunosuppressive therapy, IVIg (Omr-IgG-am) was given at a dose of 400 mg/kg/day for 5 days per month with oral cyclophosphamide and prednisone (15 mg/day) over a course of 13 months. After 13 months, impressive improvement was seen in the right foot and the left hand, as confirmed in an EMG study.

Sjögren's Syndrome

A 41-year-old man was admitted with Sjögren's syndrome (SS) associated with severe distal hand and leg pains. Neurophysiological studies showed a distal, chronic, axonal, demyelinating, and mainly sensory neuropathy. Right-leg sural nerve biopsy demonstrated mononuclear infiltrates around the vasa nervorum, with ischemic nerve injury consistent with vasculitis. Treatment with corticosteroids and methotrexate was started, but the distal hyperesthesia and cramps were aggravated. Upon referral, hypertension and diabetes mellitus were noticed, and therefore the corticosteroid dose was tapered down, and IVIg treatment (Pentaglobin) was initiated. His symptoms improved gradually. The clinical improvement lasted for 3 months. Four additional cycles of IVIg treatments were instituted (two with Pentaglobin; two with Omr-IgG-am) every 4–6 months. His ongoing clinical improvement has been accompanied by the normalization of neurophysiological studies.

Peripheral Localized Neuropathy after Influenza Vaccination

A 64-year-old man developed peripheral neuropathy 1 month after an influenza vaccination. EMG demonstrated axonal and motor neuropathy of the right ulnar nerve. Treatment with nonsteroidal anti-inflammatory drugs, corticosteroids, and azathioprine did not help. One course of high-dose IVIg treatment (2 g/kg body weight of Omr-IgG-am) was given. A week later, a dramatic improvement in right-hand functioning was noticed. His symptoms resolved completely. A repeated EMG test was normal.

Sarcoidosis

A 41-year-old female patient had a diagnosis of sarcoidosis affecting her lungs and liver 12 years before the referral. The patient was treated with prednisolone and methotrexate.

For 10 months before admission, she had reported severe numbness and cramps in both legs. Neurophysiological studies confirmed a distal, chronic, axonal, demyelinating, and mainly sensory neuropathy. Right-leg sural nerve biopsy demonstrated mononuclear infiltrates around the vasa nervorum and an ischemic nerve injury consistent with vasculitis. Two courses of IVIg in the form of Pentaglobin (400 mL/day for 3 days) were given, but no change in the results of clinical or neurophysiological studies was seen after a few months of follow-up.

Churg-Strauss Vasculitis

A 47-year-old man with Churg-Strauss vasculitis was admitted with subacute onset of distal paresthesias and progressive weakness in the arms and legs. On examination, the following were noted: discrete proximal muscle weakness in the arms and legs along with severe distal muscle wasting of the arms, hyporeflexia, and touch-temperature-pain hypoesthesia in a stocking-and-glove pattern. The results of neurophysiological studies were consistent with a symmetrical sensorimotor polyneuropathy. Histological investigations of a skin lesion demonstrated cutaneous necrotizing vasculitis with eosinophilic infiltrates.

High-dose prednisolone (1 mg/kg body weight) was given for 6 months with no apparent response, and then gradually tapered to a maintenance dose of 12.5 mg/day. Two months after administering steroids, cyclophosphamide was added (2 mg/kg every day). During the next 9 months, the patient did not show any adequate response. Six cycles of high-dose IVIg treatment (2 g/kg body weight; in the form of Isiven; Instituto Sierovaccinogeno, Italiano ISI SpA, Pisa, Italy) were given. The patient gradually regained his normal weight, and progressive neurological improvement was seen. The paresthesias, hypoesthesia, and muscle weakness markedly improved. Laboratory tests and nerve-conduction velocity measures returned to normal.

DISCUSSION

In this study, we describe 10 patients with peripheral neuropathy associated with vasculitis. All the patients had severe disease with vasculitic peripheral neuropathy that did not respond to corticosteroids and/or cytotoxic drugs, and therefore IVIg was initiated. IVIg was administered in the regular high IV dose: 2 g/kg body weight per cycle of treatment, or as Pentaglobin, dosed at 5 mL per day (38 g/L IgG, 6 g/L IgM, and 6 g/L IgA) for 3 consecutive days. Follow-up of these patients included subjective clinical parameters, serological and laboratory investigations, and EMG studies.

Eight of the patients responded to this treatment, but the patients with sarcoidosis and one of the patients with mixed cryoglobulinemia did not show any clinical benefit.

IVIg use has become increasingly prevalent in patients with autoimmune and systemic inflammatory diseases.[7–10] In this article, we have reported our extended experience with IVIg treatment in patients with vasculitic peripheral neuropathy.

Systemic vascular injury is common in SLE. Although peripheral neuropathies occur in 6–28% of patients with SLE, vasculitis is present histologically in just a small proportion of those neuropathies.[11] Our SLE patient was treated with IVIg because of her central nervous system involvement.[12] Interestingly, a drastic improvement was noticed in her peripheral neuropathy. The girl with SLE was treated for 2 weeks with high-dose steroids with no improvement in her neuropathic pain, yet she showed a immediate and drastic response only 1 day after IVIg treatment was started. Cyclophosphamide was initiated a week after the IVIg therapy while the patient was already in a remission. Therefore, it seems that the IVIg led to the change in her neuropathy.

In SS, peripheral neuropathies are prominent, and their prevalence ranges from 10% to 50%.[13,14] There are two case reports of such patients in which IVIg was of benefit. In contrast with our patient, whose improvement was gradual, the reported patients responded promptly to IVIg.[5,15] Two other patients in this series had severe peripheral neuropathy due to mixed cryoglobulinemia. This disease is strongly associated with peripheral neuropathy.[16] Both patients were treated with immunosuppressive therapy: the first patient with interferon, cyclosporine, and cyclophosphamide without showing any improvement, and the second patient with prednisone and cyclophosphamide, also without showing any improvement. In the first patient, two monthly courses of IVIg did not lead to a remission, but the other patient showed remarkable improvement.

The patient who developed localized mononeuritis after influenza vaccination emphasizes the association between vaccination and autoimmunity.[17] This patient's symptoms resolved completely after one course of IVIg treatment. This was not the case with the patient who had long-standing sarcoidosis with a rare involvement of a peripheral distal neuropathy.[18]

The last patient, with Churg-Strauss vasculitis, was treated with high-dose IVIg after 11 months of treatment with steroids and cyclophosphamide. At that point, no improvement had been noted in his agonizing pain due to the peripheral neuropathy. About two months after initiating IVIg treatment, the peripheral neuropathy improved. Improvement continued alongside the IVIg treatment. Although a contribution by the previous treatment cannot be ruled out, it is plausible that the IVIg played a pivotal role in the improvement. Peripheral neuropathy is one of the American College of Rheumatology classification criteria for Churg-Strauss vasculitis[19]; 60–71% of these patients have mononeuritis multiplex, 5–29% display asymmetrical polyneuropathy, and 0–35% show signs of symmetric polyneuropathy.[6,19–21]

The benefits of IVIg in our four patients are most probably multifactorial—acting through complement deactivation, receptor blockade, anti-idiotypes, and modulation of cytokine production. In our study, patients were more likely to have their disease remit if they were treated during an acute or subacute phase, in contrast with those who were treated after long-standing disease. In all the patients, IVIg was found to be safe and did not cause any adverse effects.

In conclusion, in this report we show that IVIg may be beneficial in vasculitic peripheral neuropathy, especially in acute multisystem diseases such as SLE and SS. IVIg may be considered as either a sole or an adjuvant treatment, particularly in patients for whom other immunosuppressive treatment has failed or is contraindicated.

REFERENCES

1. GRIFFIN, J.W. Vasculitic neuropathies. 2001. Rheum. Dis. Clin. North Am. **27:** 751–760.
2. PAGNOUX, C. & L. GUILLEVIN. 2005. Peripheral neuropathy in systemic vasculitides. Curr. Opin. Rheumatol. **17:** 41–48.
3. WILES, C.M., P. BROWN, H. CHAPEL, *et al.* 2002. Intravenous immunoglobulin in neurological disease: a specialist review. J. Neurol. Neurosurg. Psychiatry **72:** 440–448.
4. LESPRIT, P., F. MOULOUD, P. BIERLING, *et al.* 1996. Prolonged remission of SLE-associated polyradiculoneuropathy after a single course of intravenous immunoglobulin. Scand. J. Rheumatol. **25:** 177–179.
5. PASCUAL, J., C. CID & J. BERCIANO. 1998. High-dose i.v. immunoglobulin for peripheral neuropathy associated with Sjögren's syndrome. Neurology **51:** 650–651.
6. TSURIKISAWA, N., M. TANIGUCHI, H. SAITO, *et al.* 2004. Treatment of Churg-Strauss syndrome with high-dose intravenous immunoglobulin. Ann. Allergy Asthma Immunol. **92:** 80–87.
7. LEVY, Y., Y. UZIEL, G.G. ZANDMAN, *et al.* 2003. Intravenous immunoglobulins in peripheral neuropathy associated with vasculitis. Ann. Rheum. Dis. **62:** 1221–1223.
8. LEVY, Y., Y. SHERER, A. AHMED, *et al.* 1999. A study of 20 SLE patients with intravenous immunoglobulin—clinical and serologic response. Lupus **8:** 705–712.
9. LEVY, Y., Y. SHERER, J. GEORGE, *et al.* 2000. Intravenous immunoglobulin treatment of lupus nephritis. Semin. Arthritis Rheum. **29:** 321–327.
10. AMITAL, H., E. REWALD, Y. LEVY, *et al.* 2003. Fibrosis regression induced by intravenous gammaglobulin treatment. Ann. Rheum. Dis. **62:** 175–177.
11. OMDAL, R., O.A. HENRIKSEN, S.I. MELLGREN & G. HUSBY. 1991. Peripheral neuropathy in systemic lupus erythematosus. Neurology **41:** 808–811.
12. SHERER, Y., Y. LEVY, P. LANGEVITZ, *et al.* 1999. Successful treatment of systemic lupus erythematosus cerebritis with intravenous immunoglobulin. Clin. Rheumatol. **18:** 170–173.
13. LAFITTE, C., Z. AMOURA, P. CACOUB, *et al.* 2001. Neurological complications of primary Sjögren's syndrome. J. Neurol. **248:** 577–584.
14. BARENDREGT, P.J., M.J. VAN DEN BENT, V.J. VAN RAAIJ-VAN DEN AARSSEN, *et al.* 2001. Involvement of the peripheral nervous system in primary Sjögren's syndrome. Ann. Rheum. Dis. **60:** 876–881.
15. MOLINA, J.A., J. BENITO-LEON, F. BERMEJO, *et al.* 1996. Intravenous immunoglobulin therapy in sensory neuropathy associated with Sjögren's syndrome. J. Neurol. Neurosurg. Psychiatry **60:** 699.
16. FERRI, C., L. LA CIVITA, C. CIRAFISI, *et al.* 1992. Peripheral neuropathy in mixed cryoglobulinemia: clinical and electrophysiologic investigations. J. Rheumatol. **19:** 889–895.
17. SHOENFELD, Y., A. AHARON-MAOR & Y. SHERER. 2000. Vaccination as an additional player in the mosaic of autoimmunity. Clin. Exp. Rheumatol. **18:** 181–184.
18. SCOTT, T.S., J. BRILLMAN & J.A. GROSS. 1993. Sarcoidosis of the peripheral nervous system. Neurol. Res. **15:** 389–390.
19. MASI, A.T., G.G. HUNDER, J.T. LIE, *et al.* 1990. The American College of Rheumatology 1990 criteria for the classification of Churg-Strauss syndrome (allergic granulomatosis and angiitis). Arthritis Rheum. **33:** 1094–1100.

20. Hattori, N., K. Mori, K. Misu, *et al.* 2002. Mortality and morbidity in peripheral neuropathy associated Churg-Strauss syndrome and microscopic polyangiitis. J. Rheumatol. **29:** 1408–1414.
21. Sehgal, M., J.W. Swanson, R.A. DeRemee & T.V. Colby. 1995. Neurologic manifestations of Churg-Strauss syndrome. Mayo Clin. Proc. **70:** 337–341.

Involvement of Innate Immunity in the Development of Inflammatory and Autoimmune Diseases

HELENA TLASKALOVÁ-HOGENOVÁ,[a] LUDMILA TUCKOVÁ,[a] RENATA STEPÁNKOVÁ,[a] TOMÁS HUDCOVIC,[a] LENKA PALOVÁ-JELÍNKOVÁ,[a] HANA KOZÁKOVÁ,[a] PAVEL ROSSMANN,[a] DANIEL SANCHEZ,[a] JANA CINOVÁ,[a] TOMÁS HRNČÍŘ,[a] MILOSLAV KVERKA,[a] LENKA FROLOVÁ,[a] HOLM UHLIG,[b] FIONA POWRIE,[b] AND PAUL BLAND[c]

[a]*Department of Immunology and Gnotobiology, Institute of Microbiology, Academy of Sciences of the Czech Republic, 1st Faculty of Medicine, Charles University, Prague, Czech Republic*

[b]*University of Oxford, Oxford, United Kingdom*

[c]*University of Goteborg, Goteborg, Sweden*

ABSTRACT: **Initial events and effector mechanisms of most inflammatory and autoimmune diseases remain largely unknown. Dysfunction of the innate and adaptive immune systems associated with mucosae (the major interface between the organism and its environment, e.g., microbiota, food) can conceivably cause impairment of mucosal barrier function and development of localized or systemic inflammatory and autoimmune processes. Animal models help in elucidating the etiology and pathogenetic mechanisms of human diseases, such as the inflammatory bowel diseases, Crohn's disease and ulcerative colitis, severe chronic diseases affecting the gut. To study the role of innate immunity and gut microbiota in intestinal inflammation, colitis was induced by dextran sulfate sodium (DSS) in mice with severe combined immunodeficiency (SCID). Conventionally reared (microflora-colonized) SCID mice displayed severe inflammation like that seen in immunocompetent Balb/c mice, whereas only minor changes appeared in the intestinal mucosa of DSS-fed gnotobiotic germ-free SCID mice. The presence of microflora facilitates the inflammation in DSS-induced colitis that develops in immunodeficient SCID mice, that is, in the absence of T and B lymphocytes. Celiac disease, a chronic autoimmune small bowel disorder, afflicts genetically susceptible individuals with wheat gluten intolerance. We showed that, in contrast with any other food proteins, wheat gliadin and its peptic fragments activate mouse macrophages and human monocytes to produce proinflammatory cytokines through the nuclear factor–κB signaling pathway. Activation of innate immunity cells by food proteins or components from gut microbiota thus could participate in the impairment of intestinal mucosa and the development of intestinal and/or systemic inflammation.**

Address for correspondence: Prof. Helena Tlaskalová-Hogenová, M.D., Ph.D., Institute of Microbiology, Academy of Sciences of the Czech Republic, Department of Immunology and Gnotobiology, Víde-ská 1083, Prague 4, Czech Republic. Voice: +420-2-4106-2363; fax: +420-2-4172-1143.
tlaskalo@biomed.cas.cz

Ann. N.Y. Acad. Sci. 1051: 787–798 (2005).
doi: 10.1196/annals.1361.122

KEYWORDS: **innate immunity; mucosal immunity; mucosal barrier; inflammation; autoimmunity; animal models; germ-free animals; commensal bacteria; gut microbiota; inflammatory bowel diseases; celiac disease; gluten; gliadin**

INTRODUCTION

Body surfaces covered by epithelial cells come into contact with a number of microoganisms and foreign substances immediately after birth. Although the surface of the skin (~2 m^2) is protected mechanically by several epithelial layers, the surfaces of the gastrointestinal, respiratory, and urogenital tracts (~300 m^2) are mostly covered with a single-layered epithelium. To resist the invasion of microorganisms, they require extensive protection, as represented by a complex of mechanical and chemical mechanisms responsible for the degradation and removal of heterogeneous substances, and by highly effective innate and highly specific adaptive immune systems. However, the interface between the organism and the outside world is also the site of the exchange of nutrients, and the export of products and waste components. Mucosae must, therefore, be selectively permeable; at the same time, they must constitute a barrier equipped with local defense mechanisms against environmental threats (e.g., invading pathogens). The mucosal immune system has evolved mechanisms for discriminating between harmless antigens from food and microflora and dangerous antigens. Characteristic features of mucosal immunity distinguishing it from systemic immunity are (1) strongly developed mechanisms of innate defense; (2) the existence of characteristic populations of unique types of lymphocytes and their products; (3) colonization of the mucosal and exocrine glands by cells originating from the mucosal-organized tissues ("common mucosal system"); (4) transport of polymeric immunoglobulins through epithelial cells into secretions (sIgA); and (5) preferential induction of inhibitory mechanisms directed against mucosal nondangerous antigens ("oral/mucosal tolerance"). The innate mucosal immune system is represented by cells (epithelial cells, macrophages, dendritic cells, mast cells, and other cells) and their humoral products (e.g., antimicrobial proteins and peptides). Basic functions of the mucosal immune system are protection against pathogenic microorganisms and prevention of penetration of immunogenic components from mucosal surfaces into the internal environment of the organism (barrier and anti-infectious functions). Another important function is the induction of unresponsiveness of systemic immunity to antigens present on mucosal surfaces (oral/mucosal tolerance) and the maintenance of homeostasis on mucosal surfaces (immunoregulatory function).[1–4]

INNATE IMMUNE MECHANISMS IN INFLAMMATORY AND AUTOIMMUNE PROCESSES: THE ROLE OF MUCOSAL BARRIER

The basic mechanism of mucosal immunity is innate, natural immunity, as represented by processes that protect the host immediately, within the first minutes and hours of exposure to infection. It is of interest that these defense mechanisms of vertebrates are implemented by structurally related effector molecules present in plants and insects, which do not possess higher, specialized forms of adaptive immunity. A characteristic, although not yet clearly defined, feature of innate immunity is an ability to distinguish between potentially pathogenic microbial components and harmless antigens by pattern recognition receptors (PRRs). Examples of these molecules are the so-called Toll-like receptors (TLRs) that enable mammalian cells to recognize conserved characteristic molecules present on microorganisms that represent so-called pathogen-associated molecular patterns (PAMPs).[5–7] Because these molecules (e.g., lipopolysaccharides, peptidoglycans) also are present on commensal bacteria, it seems more precise to call them microbe-associated molecular patterns (MAMPs). Toll receptors were originally described in *Drosophila*; their extracellular domain contains leucine-rich repeats, whereas the cytoplasmic domain is homologous to the IL-1 receptor (IL-1R). In insects, they were found to play an essential role in the immune response to fungal infection. In mammals, PRRs are present on macrophages, neutrophils, dendritic cells, epithelial cells, and other cells belonging to the innate immune system. It was demonstrated that recognition of microbes activates the NF-κB signaling pathway, triggering cytokine production and upregulation of costimulatory molecules on antigen-presenting cells that leads to activation of T cells. We have shown that human intestinal epithelial cells express an important lipopolysaccharide-binding molecule, CD14, which, together with Toll-like receptors, can participate in maintaining the intricate balance between self and the outer environment in the gut. Western blotting and reverse transcriptase polymerase chain reaction (RT-PCR) confirmed CD14 positivity. Furthermore, we found that these cells release a soluble form of CD14 that may have important implications in shaping the interaction between the mucosal immune system and gut bacteria.[8] Innate immunity is closely linked to adaptive, acquired immunity; the link is represented by dendritic cells.

In addition to well-known humoral components of innate immunity (humoral forms of PRRs) present on mucosal surfaces such as complement, lysozyme, lactoferrin, and mannan-binding protein, recently described factors have been the subject of intensive study. Important components of nonspecific mechanisms are antimicrobial peptides widely distributed throughout the plant and animal kingdoms. Various antibiotic peptides, defensins, were found in epithelial cells (e.g., in apical granules of Paneth epithelial cells). In addition to their wide antimicrobial activity, defensins display chemotactic activity toward T cells; in other words, they represent components of innate immunity interacting with adaptive immunity.[4,9]

The intestine harbors an enormously complex microflora of a large variety of indigenous bacteria. These bacteria are in close proximity to a large population of rapidly renewing epithelial cells and other components of the mucosal innate immune system. Components of normal microflora maintain a balanced, "physiological" inflammatory response that is missing in animals reared under germ-free conditions.[10,11] Starting from the first hours after delivery from the sterile uterine environment, microorganisms colonize most of the mucosal surfaces and skin. The number of autochthonous bacteria (~1×10^{14}) exceeds the number of cells forming the human body. The highest numbers of commensal bacteria, exhibiting enormous diversity, are found in distal parts of the gut; their identification and characterization is, however, hampered by the fact that many intestinal bacteria are not cultivable. Molecular biological methods help in analyzing the complexity of the microflora and in identifying its components.[12] The highly protective colonization of the mucosal surfaces by commensals has an important stimulatory effect on innate and adaptive immunity, metabolic processes (e.g., nutrition), and other host activities.[13–15] Using gnotobiotic animal models (animals reared in germ-free conditions), we and others demonstrated that components of intestinal microflora play a crucial role during early postnatal development of the immune system.[10] However, unlimited immune activation in response to signals from commensal bacteria could pose the risk of pathological inflammation. The mucosal immune system has developed specialized regulatory, anti-inflammatory mechanisms for eliminating or tolerating non-dangerous commensal microorganisms and food antigens (oral/mucosal tolerance).[16,17] Still, under specific conditions, commensal bacteria could participate in the development of intestinal or systemic inflammation.[11,18]

The epithelium of most mucosal surfaces consists of a layer of interconnected, polarized epithelial cells separated by a basal membrane from the connective and supporting tissue surrounding various types of cells present in the lamina propria. The epithelial layer is reinforced by tight junctions present in paracellular spaces of epithelial cells and forming an interconnected network. In addition to laterally situated tight junctions present in zonula occludens, there are intermediary junctions and desmosomes in the so-called zonula adherens. Tight junctions were found to act as a dynamic and strictly regulated port of entry that opens and closes in response to various signals (e.g., cytokines) originating in the lumen, the lamina propria, and the epithelium. Tight junctions participate in preserving cellular polarity and are regarded as key elements in intestinal diffusion mechanisms. Occludin, members of claudin family, and junctional adhesion molecule (JAM) were identified as the molecules forming transmembrane tight junction strands. The cytoplasmic plaque of tight junctions includes many proteins (e.g., zonula occludens–1 [ZO-1], ZO-2, ZO-3) that interact with each other and with cytoskeletal proteins. Tight junction proteins also appear to be direct targets and effectors of different signaling pathways. Although our knowledge of the ultrastructure of tight junctions has progressed during the last several years, the pathogenic mechanism of diseases where tight junctions are affected remained poorly understood, because of limited knowledge about their regulation.[19–21]

The intestinal epithelium represents the primary site for active transport of fluid and electrolytes from the gut lumen through the transcellular pathway; however, the predominant route for passive transepithelial solute flow is the paracellular pathway. Gut mucosa serves as the main barrier to the passage of macromolecules, that is, foreign antigens entering the host via the oral route, components of commensal flora such as toxins. The majority of luminal proteins cross the intestinal barrier through the transcellular pathway, followed by lysosomal degradation. Lysosomal degradation changes proteins into nonimmunogenic peptides. Small but immunologically significant amounts of antigens cross the barrier in intact form through the paracellular pathway. The paracellular pathway involves a subtle regulation of intercellular tight junctions that leads to antigen (mucosal) tolerance. When the integrity of tight junctions is compromised, for example, as a consequence of prematurity, exposure to toxins, drugs, or radiation, aberrant immune reactions to environmental antigens occur and could lead to inflammatory and autoimmune diseases.[19–21] Various types of epithelial cells participate in the mucosal barrier function; the main and most common cells are conventional enterocytes (colonocytes in colon). Also of importance are goblet cells producing both mucus and trefoil peptides required for epithelial growth and repair, enteroendocrine cells producing neuroendocrine molecules having a paracrine effect, and Paneth's cells secreting antibiotic peptides-defensins. Epithelial cells are maintained on a network of interconnected myofibroblasts, which produce molecules necessary for the basal membrane, in addition to factors required for epithelial growth. Mucosal barrier function is greatly influenced by the products of the nervous system (neurotransmitters), increasing, for instance, the passage of macromolecules through tight junctions.[4]

Initial events leading to the development of chronic inflammatory and autoimmune diseases have not yet been elucidated. We propose that dysfunction of the immune system associated with the gut and other mucosal surfaces is a prerequisite for impairment of physiologically developing regulatory mechanisms. The balance in intestinal mucosa may be disturbed by pathogenic microorganisms and toxins attacking the mucosae by qualitative or quantitative changes in the composition of mucosal microbiota, or by inadequately functioning components of the innate or adaptive immune system occurring in cases of dysregulated mechanisms of mucosal immunity, or in immunodeficiencies. An expression of pathologically increased immunological activity may induce inflammatory processes of a different character, depending on the type and mediators of inflammation. Thus, numerous chronic diseases may occur as a result of disturbances of mucosal barrier function or of changes in mechanisms regulating mucosal immunity.[2,11,14] The main characteristics of chronic, "idiopathic," inflammatory, and autoimmune diseases are tissue destruction and functional impairment as a consequence of immunologically mediated mechanisms that are principally the same as those functioning against dangerous (pathogenic) infections. One of the most attractive explanations for inflammatory and autoimmune phenomena has centered on various infections as natural events capable of initiating the process in genetically predisposed individuals.[2,11,22–25] We propose that not only pathogenic microorganisms but also components of normal microflora could participate in the triggering and development of inflammatory and autoimmune processes.

THE ROLE OF COMMENSAL BACTERIA AND INNATE IMMUNE MECHANISMS IN INFLAMMATORY BOWEL DISEASES: STUDY IN EXPERIMENTAL MODELS

Both forms of inflammatory bowel disease (IBD), that is, Crohn's disease (CD) and ulcerative colitis (UC), are severe chronic disorders that affect approximately 0.2% of the human population. They represent an important medical problem because they have a devastating impact on quality of life and require long-standing medical care. Despite the long-lasting efforts, the etiology and pathogenesis of IBD remain unclear. The inflammatory bowel diseases seem to involve interactions among immune, environmental, and genetic factors; the combination of these factors results in induction of inflammation, subsequent mucosal lesions, and then repair.[26] Environmental factors seem to be responsible for the remarkably growing incidence of IBD, Crohn's disease, in particular, observed during the last half-century. It has been shown that northern geographic location and high social and economic status increase the risk of IBD. This finding is in agreement with "the hygiene hypothesis" for allergic and autoimmune diseases.

Recently, experimental models of intestinal inflammation, induced chemically or developing spontaneously, have been described that make it possible to examine early events during the induction of disease, to control all steps in disease progression, and to develop new preventive and therapeutic strategies.[27–29] Chemically induced intestinal inflammation is used to study the participation of immunological mechanisms in the pathogenesis of the diseases. Several murine and rat models with spontaneously developing colitis suggest that disruption of T lymphocyte regulatory functions or mucosal barrier defects could lead to intestinal inflammation. Mice with a null mutation in the interleukin-2 (IL-2), interleukin-10 (IL-10), transforming growth factor β1 (TGF-β1), MHC class II, T cell receptor (TCR)-α chain, and TCR-β chain, and mice lacking signaling protein G protein subunit Gαi2 chain were shown to develop chronic intestinal inflammation spontaneously. Interestingly, when some of these mice were reared in germ-free conditions, disease did not appear.[27,30]

Dysregulation of the intestinal immune response to bacterial flora was suggested to play a crucial role. Loss of physiologically normal regulatory mechanisms of the local immune system, perhaps a breakdown of oral tolerance to environmental antigens/commensal gut bacteria, could be involved in the pathogenic mechanism. Findings from experimental models of IBD indicate that T cells are responsible for the regulation of the intestinal immunological response to luminal antigens.[16] The finding that there is an abnormal T cell responsiveness against indigenous microflora in human inflammatory bowel disease, and its experimental model, awakened interest in the possibility that commensals may initiate and/or maintain IBD lesions.[30,31] Breakdown of oral tolerance to microfloral antigens was suggested to play a role in the development of intestinal inflammat ion. Under conditions of an immunoregulatory or mucosal barrier defect, the common intestinal flora obviously is capable of evoking stimulation leading to a chronic intestinal or systemic inflammation.[29,31] The solutions to the questions of which and how gut bacteria, and which cells, are involved in the induction and maintenance of chronic intestinal inflammation are of great importance because they could bring about new approaches to the therapy and/or prevention of this severe disease.

We used colitis induced by dextran sulfate sodium (DSS) feeding of mice to study the immunological factors involved in the pathogenetic mechanisms of chemically triggered intestinal inflammation. The role of adhesion molecules in intestinal inflammation was studied in our laboratory using mice with deletion of the gene for ICAM-1, in comparison with genetically corresponding wild-type controls.[32] Acute and chronic colitis was induced by oral administration of DSS in drinking water. Only minor changes were found in ICAM-1 knockout (KO) mice; in contrast, wild-type controls exhibited severe intestinal changes with ulcerations, suggesting direct involvement of ICAM-1 molecules in the development of the inflammatory response. The chronic colitis was accompanied by an increased level of anti-epithelial IgA autoantibodies detected in wild-type control mice.[32]

These experimental models were used also to analyze the role of commensal bacteria and innate immunity in the development of intestinal inflammation. Using the DSS-induced model of intestinal inflammation, we have shown that, as in conventionally reared, immunocompetent Balb/c mice, mice with severe combined immunodeficiency (SCID) developed profound inflammatory changes in colonic mucosa. Immunocompetent Balb/c and immunodeficient SCID mice were transferred into isolators for germ-free rearing by special gnotobiological techniques. Balb/c and

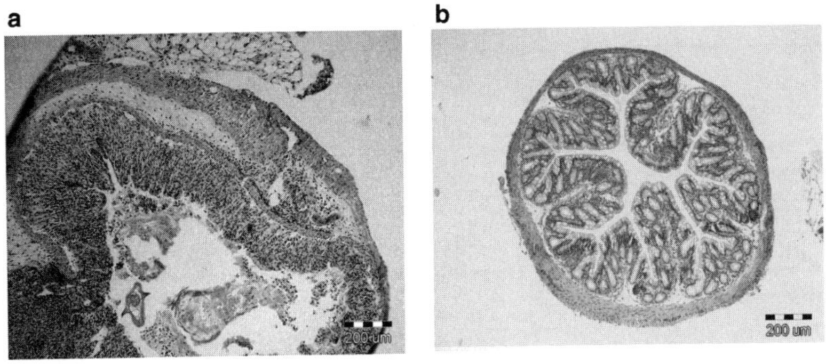

FIGURE 1. The colon after 1 week of ingestion of dextran sodium sulfate in (**a**) conventional SCID mice, showing ulcerative colitis with severe infiltration of inflammatory cells (grade 4 inflammation); and (**b**) germ-free SCID mice, in which no inflammation is observed.

SCID mice reared in germ-free conditions developed only minor signs of mucosal inflammation.[33] Interestingly, conventionally reared SCID mice, lacking T and B cells, developed intestinal inflammation similar to the inflammation that developed in immunocompetent Balb/c mice (FIG. 1). This finding suggests that under physiological conditions, innate immunity components are able to regulate (keep in balance) the interaction of the macroorganism with commensal bacteria, and, after chemically induced breakdown of mucosal barrier, commensal bacteria could induce severe forms of intestinal inflammation in the absence of components of adaptive immunity (T and B cells).

Another model of intestinal inflammation, developing spontaneously in the colons of conventional SCID mice restored with the CD45 RB^{high} subset of $CD4^+$ T cells isolated from the spleens of normal Balb/c mice, was used in further studies.[16,17] The $CD4^+$ $CD45RB^{high}$ subpopulation of T cells was purified from the spleens of conventional Balb/c mice and transferred to SCID mice. As recipients, germ-free SCID mice, conventional SCID mice, or SCID mice monoassociated with defined bacterial strains or colonized with bacterial mixtures were used. The clinical picture as well as morphological results revealed that severe colitis was present only in conventional SCID mice and in mice colonized with the cocktail of specific pathogen–free (SPF) microflora plus segmented filamentous bacteria (SFB). A monoassociation of SCID mice with SFB or colonization with the cocktail of SPF bacteria did not lead to intestinal inflammation.[34] Signs of impairment of tight junctions of the intestinal barrier in the terminal ileum of colitic mice was documented by anti–ZO-1 antibody (FIG. 2). Our studies performed in the model of reconstituted SCID mice suggest that noncultivable segmented filamentous bacteria, together with a defined mixture of cultivable bacteria from SPF mice, were effective in triggering intestinal inflammation.[34]

Experiments performed in gnotobiotic models suggest that the composition of gut microbiota plays a decisive role in the pathogenetic mechanism of intestinal inflammation. Exogenous application of commensal organisms (probiotics) exerting beneficial effects on host health has recently been shown to have protective and

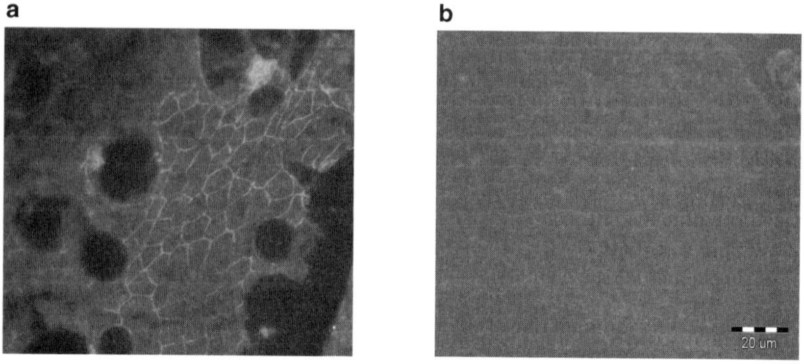

FIGURE 2. Tight junctions in terminal ileum of SCID mice colonized 12 weeks after transfer of $CD4^{+}CD45RB^{high}$ T cells with (**a**) specific pathogen–free (SPF) microflora, showing preserved integrity of tight junctions; and (**b**) mixture of SPF microflora and segmented filamentous bacteria, showing altered structure of tight junctions (staining for zonula occludens–1).

therapeutic effects on diarrheal diseases, including IBD, and to reduce the risk of infections and allergies.[35–38] Oral introduction of probiotic bacteria is associated with an alleviation of intestinal inflammation and normalization of increased intestinal permeability, together with promotion of intestinal barrier functions. Orally ingested probiotic microorganisms do not exert health effects entirely in the intestine. Investigations in germ-free mice have shown that after oral monoassociation of the mice with a *Bifidobacterium longum* strain, bifidobacteria translocated and were found in the mesenteric lymph nodes, liver, and kidneys 1 week later. Translocation of probiotic bacteria had no harmful effects but increased the barrier function of the intestinal mucosa and inhibited translocation of other bacteria. Recently, we showed that monoassociation with *B. bifidum* speeds up the biochemical maturation of enterocytes, resulting in a shift of specific activities of brush-border enzymes between the values found for germ-free and conventionally reared mice.[39] Regulation of microflora composition (e.g., by probiotics and prebiotics) offers the potential to influence the development of mucosal and systemic immunity but also can play a role in the prevention and treatment of human IBD.[30,31,40]

INNATE IMMUNITY MECHANISMS IN PATHOGENESIS OF CELIAC DISEASE

Celiac disease is a disorder characterized by gluten-dependent enteropathy. Small intestinal mucosal villous atrophy with hyperplasia of the crypts, abnormal surface epithelium, and increased inflammatory cell infiltration are regularly found in biopsy specimens taken from the jejunum or duodenum of patients with active disease. The features of the mucosal lesions suggest that gliadin and related prolamins of other cereals lead to an aberrant, pathologically increased immune response in genetically predisposed individuals. The pathogenetic concept of celiac disease is based on

TABLE 1. Effects of gliadin, soy protein, ovalbumin, and their proteolytic fragments on IL-8 and TNF-α secretion by THP-1 (monocytic cell line) cells, measured after 24 h of cell cultivation

	Food proteins only			+IFN-γ 150 U	
	0 μg	100 μg	500 μg	100 μg	500 μg
IL-8					
Gliadin crude	81.2 (10.9)	14.1 (6.0)	77.5 (25.6)	191.3 (17.5)	245.0 (68.6)
Soy crude	81.2 (10.9)	19.1 (8.7)	24.2 (2.3)	86.3 (11.3)	114.2 (12.8)
OVA crude	81.2 (10.9)	21.7 (2.3)	21.7 (3.1)	67.2 (8.4)	127.0 (25.1)
Gliadin digest	81.2 (10.9)	71.7 (15.2)[a]	216.5 (13.6)[b]	166.3 (30.2)[a]	481.3 (30.0)[b]
Soy digest	81.2 (10.9)	12.0 (1.2)	24.3 (5.8)	90.6 (10.4)	133.5 (19.6)
OVA digest	81.2 (10.9)	27.3 (2.2)	21.3 (3.1)	82.3 (12.6)	162.2 (14.4)
TNF-α					
Gliadin crude	21.6 (6.5)	20.6 (2.5)	29.8 (10.1)	24.3 (7.2)	32.4 (6.0)
Soy crude	21.6 (6.5)	4.7 (3.6)	9.2 (1.2)	17.9 (4.4)	24.1 (7.2)
OVA crude	21.6 (6.5)	2.5 (2.1)	8.5 (2.2)	23.5 (4.2)	23.9 (2.0)
Gliadin digest	21.6 (6.5)	27.2 (4.4)[b]	66.4 (8.4)[b]	52.9 (7.5)[a]	107.6 (12.0)[b]
Soy digest	21.6 (6.5)	0.0 (0.0)	12.8 (7.1)	25.3 (5.9)	27.7 (4.0)
OVA digest	21.6 (6.5)	8.0 (5.1)	16.1 (3.5)	31.5 (3.5)	34.5 (5.6)

Right: Synergistic effect of IFN-γ applied together with food proteins. Data are expressed as mean (± SEM).

[a]$P < .05$, [b]$P < .01$.[50]

OVA, ovalbumin.

the interaction of toxic gliadin peptides with HLA-DQ2 antigens, which occurs in antigen-presenting dendritic cells of the lamina propria. Intolerance to gluten seems to be caused by increased activity of gliadin-specific lamina propria $CD4^+$ T cells producing Th0/Th1 cytokines, and cytotoxic intraepithelial $CD8^+$ T cells expressing NK receptors.[41–44] The increased level of antibodies to gliadin in sera of patients is regularly accompanied by the presence of autoantibodies. The molecular target of antiendomysial autoantibodies recently was identified as tissue transglutaminase. We identified common epitopes on gliadin and another autoantigen, calreticulin, recognized by antibodies present in sera of patients with celiac disease.[45] Also, other features of the disease suggest that celiac disease fulfills the criteria for autoimmune diseases.[22,46]

Based on our previous findings, it seems that the unique structure of gliadin and its fragments could be responsible for the involvement of innate immunity mechanisms in the pathogenetic mechanism of this disease.[47] The question of how gliadin affects innate immunity was answered by experiments in which mouse macrophages were used. We have shown that in contrast with other dietary proteins tested, gliadin stimulated IFN-γ–treated mouse macrophages to produce nitric oxide and secrete cytokines (TNF-α, IL-10, RANTES).[48] Moreover, the active gliadin peptide was separated and identified.[49] Using the human monocytic cell line THP-1, we tried to see whether human monocytes could be activated similarly by a peptic digest of gliadin.

Cultivation of THP-1 cells with a digest of gliadin was found to lead to the production of IL-8 and TNF-α; the production was augmented by pretreatment of cells with IFN-γ or its addition to the culture. Ovalbumin and soy protein or their peptic digests had no effect on IL-8 and TNF-α production when applied alone or in combination with IFN-γ (TABLE 1). The participation of nuclear factor–κB (NF-κB) in the stimulatory effect of the gliadin digest on monocytes was documented by a marked increase of the DNA-binding activities of NF-κB subunits p50 and p65. Moreover, the inhibition of p65 and p50 subunit binding was detected using NF-κB inhibitors sulfasalazine, PDTC, and TPCK.[50] Because NF-κB activation involves phosphorylation and subsequent degradation of Iκ-Bα, the phosphorylation of Iκ-Bα was determined by immunoblotting. We found that stimulation of THP cells with gliadin and/or with IFN-γ leads to an increase of phosphorylation of Iκ-Bα, suggesting that NF-κB is involved in the activation pathway triggered by gliadin fragments. Similar findings were recently described by other authors.[43,44,51,52]

ACKNOWLEDGMENTS

This work was supported by grants A 5020205, A 5020210, B 5020407 (Grant Agency of the Academy of Sciences of the Czech Republic), 310/05/2245, 310/03/H147, 303/05/2249, 310/04/P242(Grant Agency of the Czech Republic), S 5020203 (Academy of Sciences of the Czech Republic), NR/8356-3 (Internal Grant Agency of Ministry of Health of the Czech Republic), and AVOZ 50200510 (Institute of Microbiology).

REFERENCES

1. MESTECKY, J., M.W. RUSSEL, S. JACKSON, *et al.* 1995. Advances in Mucosal Immunology. Plenum Press. New York, London.
2. TLASKALOVÁ-HOGENOVÁ, H., L. TUCKOVÁ, R. LODINOVÁ-ZÁDNÍKOVÁ, *et al.* 2002. Mucosal immunity: its role in defense and allergy. Int. Arch. Allergy Immunol. **128:** 77–89.
3. BRANDTZAEG, P. & R. PABST. 2004. Let's go mucosal: communication on slippery ground. Trends Immunol. **25:** 570–577.
4. MESTECKY, J., M.E. LAMM, W. STROBER, *et al.* 2005. Mucosal Immunology, 3rd ed. Elsevier Academic Press. Amsterdam.
5. MEDZHITOV, R. & C. JANEWAY, JR. 2000. Innate immune recognition: mechanisms and pathways. Immunol. Rev. **173:** 89–97.
6. ADEREM, A. & R.J. ULEVITCH. 2000. Toll-like receptors in the induction of the innate immune response. Nature **406:** 782–787.
7. AKIRA, S. & K. TAKEDA. 2004. Toll-like receptor signalling. Nat. Rev. Immunol. **4:** 499–511.
8. FUNDA, D.P., L. TUCKOVÁ, M. FARRÉ, *et al.* 2001. CD14 is expressed and released as soluble CD14 by human intestinal epithelial cells in vitro: lipopolysaccharide activation of epithelial cells revisited. Inf. Immun. **69:** 3772–3781.
9. BEVINS, C.L. 2004. The Paneth cell and the innate immune response. Curr. Opin. Gastroenterol. **20:** 572–580.
10. TLASKALOVÁ-HOGENOVÁ, H., J. STERZL, R. STEPÁNKOVÁ, *et al.* 1983. Development of immunological capacity under germfree and conventional conditions. Ann. N.Y. Acad. Sci. **409:** 96–113.
11. TLASKALOVÁ-HOGENOVÁ, H. 1997. Gnotobiology as a tool—an introduction. *In* Immunology Methods Manual. I. Lefkovits, Ed.: 1524–1559. Academic Press. London.

12. HARMSEN, H.J., G.C. RAANGS, T. HE, *et al.* 2002. Extensive set of 16S rRNA-bases probes for detection of bacteria in human feces. Appl. Environ. Microbiol. **68:** 2982–2990.
13. HOOPER, L.V., M.H. WONG, A. THELIN, *et al.* 2001. Molecular analysis of commensal host-microbial relationships in the intestine. Science **291:** 881–884.
14. TLASKALOVÁ-HOGENOVÁ, H., R. STEPÁNKOVÁ, T. HUDCOVIC, *et al.* 2004. Commensal bacteria (normal microflora), mucosal immunity and chronic inflammatory and autoimmune diseases. Immun. Lett. **93:** 97–108.
15. CEBRA, J.J., H.Q. JIANG, N. BOIKO & H. TLASKALOVÁ-HOGENOVÁ. 2005. The role of mucosal microbiota in the development, maintenance, and pathologies of the mucosal immune system. *In* Mucosal Immunology, 3rd ed. J. Mestecky, M.E. Lamm, W. Strober, *et al.*, Eds.: 335–368. Elsevier Academic Press. Amsterdam.
16. SINGH, B., S. READ, C. ASSEMAN, *et al.* 2001. Control of intestinal inflammation by regulatory T cells. Immunol. Rev. **182:** 190–200.
17. POWRIE, F. & H. UHLIG. 2004. Animal models of intestinal inflammation: clues to the pathogenesis of inflammatory bowel disease. Novartis Found. Symp. **263:** 164–174.
18. RAKOFF-NAHOUM, S., J. PAGLINO, F. ESLAMI-VARZANEH, *et al.* 2004. Recognition of commensal microflora by toll-like receptors is required for intestinal homeostasis. Cell **118:** 229–241.
19. FASANO, A., T. NOT, W. WANG, *et al.* 2000. Zonulin, a newly discovered modulator of intestinal permeability, and its expression in coeliac disease. Lancet **355:** 1518–1519.
20. FASANO, A. 2001. Intestinal zonulin: open sesame! Gut **49:** 159–162.
21. NEUTRA M.P. & J.P. KRAEHENBUHL. 2005. Cellular and molecular basis for antigen transport across epithelial barriers. *In* Mucosal Immunology, 3rd ed. J. Mestecky, M.E. Lamm, W. Strober, *et al.*, Eds.: 111–130. Elsevier Academic Press. Amsterdam.
22. SHOENFELD, Y. & N.R. ROSE. 2004. Infection and Autoimmunity. Elsevier. Amsterdam.
23. BACH, J.F. 2002. The effect of infections on susceptibility to autoimmune and allergic diseases. N. Engl. J. Med. **347:** 930–931.
24. KITA, H., X.S. HE & M.E. GERSHWIN. 2004. Autoimmunity and environmental factors in the pathogenesis of primary biliary cirrhosis. Ann. Med. **36:** 72–80.
25. TOUBI, E. & Y. SHOENFELD. 2004. Toll-like receptors and their role in the development of autoimmune diseases. Autoimmunity **73:** 183–188.
26. MACDONALD, T.T., G. MONTELEONE & S.L. PENDER. 2000. Recent developments in the immunology of inflammatory bowel disease. Scand. J. Immunol. **52:** 2–9.
27. STROBER, W. & R.O. EHRHARDT. 1993. Chronic intestinal inflammation: an unexpected outcome in cytokine or T cell receptor mutant mice. Cell **78:** 203–295.
28. STROBER, W., I.J. FUSS & R.S. BLUMBERG. 2002. The immunology of mucosal models of inflammation. Annu. Rev. Immunol. **20:** 495–549.
29. ELSON, C.O., A. KONRAD, Y. CONGH, *et al.* 2004. Gene disruption and immunity in experimental colitis. Inflamm. Bowel Dis. **10:** S25–S28.
30. SARTOR, R.B. 2005. Therapeutic manipulation of the enteric microflora in inflammatory bowel diseases: antibiotics, probiotics, and prebiotics. Gastroenterology **126:** 1620–1633.
31. SARTOR, R.B. 2003. Innate immunity in the pathogenesis and therapy of IBD. J. Gastroenterol. **38** (Suppl. 15)**:** 43–47.
32. BENDJELLOUL, F., P. MALY, V. MANDYS, *et al.* 2000. Intercellular adhesion molecule-1 (ICAM-1) deficiency protects mice against severe forms of experimentally induced colitis. Clin. Exp. Immunol. **119:** 57–63.
33. HUDCOVIC, T., R. STEPÁNKOVÁ, J. CEBRA, *et al.* 2001. The role of microflora in the development of intestinal inflammation: acute and chronic colitis induced by dextran sulfate in germ-free and conventionally reared immunocompetent and immunodeficient mice. Folia Microbiol. (Praha) **46:** 565–572.
34. STEPÁNKOVÁ, R., H. TLASKALOVÁ, F. POWRIE, *et al.* 2004. The role of segmented filamentous bacteria (SFB) in experimental colitis induced in SCID mice reconstituted with CD4+CD45RB/hight T cells [abstract]. Gut **36** (Suppl. 1): A305.
35. CUKROWSKA, B., R. LODINOVÁ-ZÁDNÍKOVÁ, C. ENDERS, *et al.* 2002. Specific proliferative and antibody responses of premature infants to intestinal colonization with nonpathogenic probiotic *E. coli* strain Nissle 1917. Scand. J. Immunol. **55:** 204–209.

36. Lodinová-Zádníková, R., B. Cukrowska & H. Tlaskalová-Hogenová. 2003. Oral administration of probiotic *Escherichia coli* after birth reduces frequency of allergies and repeated infections later in life. Int. Arch. Allergy Immunol. **131:** 209–211.
37. Kalliomaki, M.A. & E. Isolauri. 2004. Probiotics and down-regulation of the allergic response. Immunol. Allergy Clin. North Am. **24:** 739–752.
38. Cumming, J.H., J.M. Antoine, E. Azpiroz, *et al.* 2004. PASSCLAIM—gut health and immunity. Eur. J. Nutr. **43** (Suppl. 2)**:** II118–II173.
39. Kozáková, H., Z. Reháková & J. Kolínská. 2001. Bifidobacterium bifidum monoassociation of gnotobiotic mice: effect on enterocyte brush-border enzymes. Folia Microbiol. (Praha) **46:** 573–576.
40. Danese, S., M. Sans & C. Fiocchi. 2004. Inflammatory bowel disease: the role of environmental factors. Autoimmun. Rev. **3:** 394–400.
41. Stepánková, R., H. Tlaskalová, J. Sinkora, *et al.* 1996. Changes in jejunal mucosa after long-term feeding of germfree rats with gluten. Scand. J. Gastroenterol. **31:** 551–557.
42. Sollid, L.M. 2002. Coeliac disease: dissecting a complex inflammatory disorder. Nat. Rev. Immunol. **2:** 647–655.
43. Schuppan, D., B. Esslinger & W. Dietrich. 2003. Innate immunity and coeliac disease. Lancet **362:** 3–5.
44. Cerf-Bensussan, N., N. Brousse, C. Caillat-Zucman, *et al.* 2003. Coeliac Disease. John Libbey Eurotext. Esber, UK.
45. Krupicková, S., L. Tucková, Z. Flegelová, *et al.* 1999. Identification of common epitopes on gliadin, enterocytes, and calreticulin recognised by antigliadin antibodies of patients with celiac disease. Gut **44:** 168–173.
46. Rose, N.R. 2002. Mechanisms of autoimmunity. Semin. Liver Dis. **22:** 387–394.
47. Novák, P., P. Man, L. Tucková, *et al.* 2002. Monitoring of in vitro deamidation of gliadin peptic fragments by mass spectrometry may reflect one of the molecular mechanisms taking place in celiac disease development. J. Mass Spectrom. **37:** 507–511.
48. Tucková, L., H. Tlaskalová-Hogenová, Z. Flegelová, *et al.* 2000. Activation of macrophages by food antigens: enhancing effect of gluten on nitric oxide and cytokine production. J. Leukoc. Biol. **67:** 312–318.
49. Tucková, L., J. Novotná, P. Novák, *et al.* 2002. Activation of macrophages by gliadin fragments: isolation and characterization of active peptide. J. Leukoc. Biol. **71:** 625–631.
50. Jelínková, L., L. Tucková, J. Cinová, *et al.* 2004. Gliadin stimulates human monocytes to production of IL-8 and TNF-γ through a mechanism involving NF-κB. FEBS Letters **571:** 81–85.
51. Maiuri, M.C., D. De Stefano, G. Mele, *et al.* 2003. Nuclear factor -B is activated in small intestinal mucosa of celiac patients. J. Mol. Med. **81:** 373–379.
52. Nikulina, M., C. Habich, S.B. Flohe, *et al.* 2004. Wheat gluten causes dendritic cell maturation and chemokine secretion. J. Immunol. **173:** 1925–1933.

Do We Need New Treatment That Goes beyond Tumor Necrosis Factor Blockers for Rheumatoid Arthritis?

REINHARD E. VOLL[a,b] AND JOACHIM R. KALDEN[a]

[a]*Department of Internal Medicine III, Friedrich-Alexander University of Erlangen–Nuremberg, 91054 Erlangen, Germany*

[b]*IZKF-N2 Research Group, Nikolaus-Fiebiger Center for Molecular Medicine, Friedrich-Alexander University of Erlangen–Nuremberg, 91054 Erlangen, Germany*

ABSTRACT: Rheumatoid arthritis (RA) has a prevalence of approximately 1%, making it the most common inflammatory rheumatic disease. The outcome for RA patients has significantly improved during recent years. Factors include the introduction of new therapies such as tumor necrosis factor (TNF)–blocking agents and new treatment strategies, especially early and aggressive therapy, including combinations of several disease-modifying antirheumatic drugs (DMARDs). However, only 60–70% of RA patients respond to treatment with a TNF-blocking agent. In addition, most of these patients show only a partial response according to ACR20 criteria. Therefore, to ameliorate painful joint inflammation and prevent disability in RA patients, new treatment principles and more intelligent combination therapies are urgently needed. Interestingly, the strategy of switching patients who no longer respond to one of the TNF blockers to another has often turned out to be effective. Areas of ongoing research include combining TNF-blocking agents with DMARDs other than methotrexate. Also, several new biologics are being tested in clinical trials that promise to soon enhance the therapeutic armamentarium to fight RA. These biologics' mechanisms of action feature blockade of T cell costimulation by a CTLA4Ig fusion protein (abatacept); blockade of interleukin (IL)–6 signaling with an antibody to the IL-6 receptor (MRA); neutralizing IL-15 by a monoclonal antibody; and targeting B cells with an anti-CD20 antibody (rituximab). Other therapeutic approaches, such as blockade of chemokine receptors, adhesion molecules, complement components, and transcription factors regulating the inflammatory response, appear promising; however, they still need careful evaluation in placebo-controlled clinical studies.

KEYWORDS: rheumatoid arthritis; TNF blockade; disease-modifying antirheumatic drugs; DMARDs; interleukin signaling blockade; methotrexate; monoclonal antibodies

Address for correspondence: Prof. Dr. Med. Dr. H.C. Joachim R. Kalden, Department of Internal Medicine III, University of Erlangen-Nuremberg, Krankenhausstrasse 12, 91054 Erlangen, Germany. Voice: +49-9131-853-3363; +fax: 49-9131-853-4770.
joachim.kalden@med3.imed.uni-erlangen.de

**Ann. N.Y. Acad. Sci. 1051: 799–810 (2005). © 2005 New York Academy of Sciences.
doi: 10.1196/annals.1361.123**

INTRODUCTION

Rheumatoid arthritis (RA) has a prevalence of approximately 1%, making it the most common inflammatory rheumatic disease. It features extra-articular manifestations such as nodules in the subcutaneous tissue and involvement of internal organs. However, the primary site of pathogenesis is within the synovial tissue. The perpetuating relapsing inflammatory process results in destruction of the joint structures, and eventually, even in ankylosis. Hence, if not adequately controlled, RA often leads to permanent disability, with high social and economic costs.

The long-term prognosis for RA patients is generally serious with respect to joint function and mobility. Radiographic evidence of bony erosions was detected in 30% of patients at the time of diagnosis, and in 60% 2 years later, in spite of treatment with conventional DMARDs.[1] More importantly, nearly half of RA patients become severely disabled after 5 years with the disease. Less than 3% of patients achieve a complete remission lasting more than 3 years. The mortality rate of patients with RA is increased mainly because of comorbidities. Most of the excess mortality can be attributed to cardiovascular diseases, which presumably are directly fostered by chronic, systemic inflammation in general. In addition, evidence is accumulating that some antirheumatic drugs, including higher dose glucocorticoids, promote atherosclerosis.[2]

The treatment of RA has recently been revolutionized by the introduction of tumor necrosis factor (TNF)–blocking agents. Although monotherapy with TNF inhibitors may not be significantly more efficacious than methotrexate (MTX) alone, the combination of a TNF inhibitor with MTX has proved to be a clearly superior and highly efficient medication for RA, as shown in several randomized, placebo-controlled multicenter trials.[3–5] However, 30–40% of patients with established RA do not respond clinically to TNF-blocking therapy. In addition, the majority of anti-TNF responders experience only a partial clinical improvement of their disease, as evaluated by the American College of Rheumatology (ACR) response criteria or by the Disease Activity Score (DAS28) and the Health Assessment Questionnaire (HAQ).[3–5]

Nevertheless, in the majority of patients, combinations of TNF inhibitors and MTX are the first treatment regimens that can virtually stop radiographic progression (indicating structural joint damage) over at least 1 or 2 years. Importantly, even patients who do not fulfill clinical response criteria showed significant delays in radiographic progression.[5] More efficacious combination therapies and new drugs are still needed to control pain and inflammation in the approximately 30–40% of clinical nonresponders to TNF blockade, and to achieve a higher proportion of complete remissions, allowing patients with RA to participate in nearly normal occupational and social activities.

The etiopathogenesis of RA remains largely elusive. Even so, our knowledge of important factors and mechanisms that contribute to pathogenesis has greatly improved during recent years. Data from RA patients and animal models of RA have helped to identify new potential therapeutic targets, which can then be specifically addressed using biologics or conventional small-molecule drugs. However, even after sophisticated animal experiments, the final burden of proof for the relevance of certain factors in the pathogenesis of RA rests with placebo-controlled clinical that specifically target these suspected pathogens. In this article, we provide an overview of promising novel treatment principles and therapeutics that are undergoing clinical

TABLE 1. New principles for the treatment of rheumatoid arthritis

Clinical studies necessary for the optimization of combination therapy	• Optimal step-down regimens after inducing remission • Combination therapy of anti-TNF agents with one or more conventional DMARDs (apart from MTX) • Combinations of TNF antagonists with other biologics, with and without conventional DMARDs
New therapeutics currently in clinical trials	• IL-6 receptor blockade (MRA) • Neutralization of IL-15 • CTLA4Ig (abatacept) for blockade of costimulation • LFA-3-IgG1 (alefacept) fusion protein for blockade of T cell activation • Anti-LFA-1 (efalizumab) for blockade of T cell activation • B cell depletion by anti-CD20 monoclonal antibodies (rituximab) • Blockade of chemokine receptors such as CCR1 • Anti-complement component C5a (pexelizumab)
Novel therapeutic strategies/targets	• Selective IκB kinase β inhibitors • Inhibitors of the p38 MAP kinase • Induction of regulatory T cells • Induction of a Th1-to-Th2 shift • Modulation of Toll-like receptors/signal transduction pathways • Immune modulation by galectins • Neutralization of proinflammatory factors such as HMGB-1 and heat-shock proteins • Tailor-made therapies based on genetic and acquired factors

ABBREVIATIONS: DMARD, disease-modifying antirheumatic drug; HMGB, high-mobility group box; LFA, lymphocyte function–associated antigen; MTX, methotrexate; Th1, T-helper cell type 1; TNF, tumor necrosis factor.

trials, and briefly discuss some new potential treatment strategies/targets that are in preclinical investigation (see overview in TABLE 1).

EMERGING THERAPIES

TNF Inhibitors

TNF plays a crucial role in the pathobiology of RA, because it appears to be upstream of other proinflammatory cytokines such as interleukin (IL)–1, IL-6, and IL-8. In addition, TNF induces the expression of adhesion molecules on endothelial cells, stimulates the secretion of tissue-degrading matrix metalloproteinases by macrophages and fibroblasts, and contributes to pannus formation.[6]

Currently, three TNF inhibitors are approved for clinical use in RA:

(1) Etanercept represents a fusion protein consisting of the extracellular domain of the human p75 TNF receptor and the Fc region of human immunoglobulin G1 (IgG1). In addition to TNF, this molecule also neutralizes

lymphotoxin β but does not induce cell death in membrane TNF-bearing cells, although binding is observed.

(2) Infliximab is a chimeric (mouse/human) monoclonal antibody with a TNF-binding Fab region of mouse origin, whereas the rest of the antibody molecule is derived from a human IgG1 antibody.

(3) Adalimumab is a fully human anti-TNF antibody of the IgG1 isotype.

Infliximab and adalimumab each can induce the death of cells expressing the membrane-bound form of TNF. A polyethylene glycol–conjugated (pegylated) p55 TNF receptor and other TNF antagonists are still in clinical trials but may have similar efficacy and side effects as the currently available TNF blockers.[6] No ongoing studies are directly comparing the efficacies and toxicities of TNF-blocking agents. Small-molecule TNF blockers, which might be administered orally and be less expensive to produce, are in development.

Similar to conventional DMARDs, TNF antagonists rarely induce complete remission of the disease, and only 60–70% of patients respond to TNF-blocking therapies, even with the use of modest criteria such as the ACR20. However, evidence is growing that at least some patients who fail to respond to one TNF antagonist may respond to another one.[7] These observations might be explained by differences in structure, pharmacokinetics, binding specificity (TNF only vs. TNF and lymphotoxin β), or the presence of neutralizing antibodies against a particular TNF blocker. Well-designed studies investigating switching from one TNF antagonist to another are needed to provide a rationale for this clinical practice.

Combination Therapy

The goal of combining RA therapies is to enhance efficacy without increasing toxicity. This goal is best achieved by combining medications with different mechanisms of action and side-effect profiles but without relevant pharmacokinetic interactions. The COBRA trial (Combinatietherapie Bij Reumatoide Artritis) showed much higher response rates among patients, without increased side effects, for a combination of MTX, sulfasalazine, and hydroxychloroquine compared with either MTX alone or sulfasalazine plus hydroxychloroquine.[8] Up to now, TNF antagonists have been used mainly in combination with MTX. This pairing has been shown to significantly improve response rates as well as lower the risk of developing an antibody response toward the TNF antagonist—especially against the chimeric antibody infliximab.

An important goal of research is to identify optimal, alternative, or additional DMARDs to combine with TNF-blocking agents. Theoretically, or considering only animal data, combining TNF antagonists with leflunomide, sulfasalazine, hydroxychloroquine, cyclosporin A, or various combinations of these may display synergistic effects; however, placebo-controlled, multicenter studies are still missing. In a small prospective study, the combination of leflunomide with infliximab led to a high percentage of patients responding to the treatment (ACR20 >80%), although all patients experienced adverse events.[9] In a German multicenter, open-label trial, infliximab was added to a stable regimen of leflunomide in patients who did not respond satisfactorily to leflunomide. In this add-on setting, almost 50% of patients achieved an ACR20 response. The overall adverse event rate (76%) was no higher than in previous trials with either monotherapy, and the combination showed a similar safety profile.[10]

Also, combining different biologics could result in favorable response rates and safety profiles. For instance, in animal experiments, TNF blockade and anti-CD4 treatment have displayed a synergistic effect in collagen-induced arthritis but have not yet been tested in RA.[11] Even with a theoretical rationale and encouraging animal data, combined treatment with the IL-1 receptor antagonist anakinra (Amgen's Kineret) and TNF antagonists did not show synergistic effects in RA, although it did result in an unacceptably increased risk of serious infections (Amgen Inc.: Kineret Prescribing Information; available at: www.kineretrx.com).

Anti–Interleukin-6 Receptor (MRA)

IL-6 is a pleiotropic cytokine that regulates the immune response, hematopoiesis, and bone metabolism while inducing the production of acute-phase reactants, such as C-reactive protein, in the liver. Elevated levels of IL-6 (which is produced mainly by RA fibroblasts and macrophages) have been found in the synovial fluid and serum of patients with RA.[12] Remarkably, serum IL-6 levels correlated with disease activity and joint damage.[13]

Recently, the humanized anti–IL-6 receptor antibody MRA, which blocks the binding of IL-6 to its receptor complex, was evaluated for safety and efficacy in treatment-refractory RA patients. In this multicenter double-blind, placebo-controlled clinical trial, 164 patients with active RA who had not responded to previous DMARD therapy (median: five to six DMARDs per patient) were randomized into 3 treatment arms: (1) MRA dosed at 4 mg/kg body weight, (2) MRA dosed at 8 mg/kg body weight, or (3) placebo. The study medication was administered intravenously every 4 weeks for 3 months. After 3 months of treatment, an encouraging reduction in disease activity according to ACR criteria was noted: 78% of patients in the 8 mg/kg body-weight group, 57% in the 4 mg/kg body-weight group, and 11% in the placebo group achieved an ACR20 response. Moreover, 40% of patients in the 8 mg/kg body-weight group, but only 1.9% in the placebo group, achieved an ACR50 response.[14]

Generally, the treatment was well tolerated and did not significantly increase the risk of infections. Most adverse events were mild, and they included transient liver function disorders and a decrease in leukocyte counts. Although serum cholesterol levels increased in 44% of patients receiving MRA, the clinical relevance of the latter finding remains unclear.[14] Considering the difficult-to-treat patient group in this study, the results appear very promising. However, additional trials investigating long-term safety and efficacy, influence on radiographic progression, and potential combination partners are needed.

Anti–Interleukin-15

IL-15 is produced by several cell types, including activated monocytes/macrophages, dendritic cells, osteoclasts, and fibroblasts. The IL-15 receptor is formed by the β chain of the IL-2 receptor, the common γ chain, and the IL-15 receptor–specific α chain. IL-15 receptor signaling uses the JAK1/3 and STAT3/5 pathways. IL-15–deficient mice display marked lymphopenia and severe impairment of mature $CD8^+$ lymphocytes' proliferation and homing.

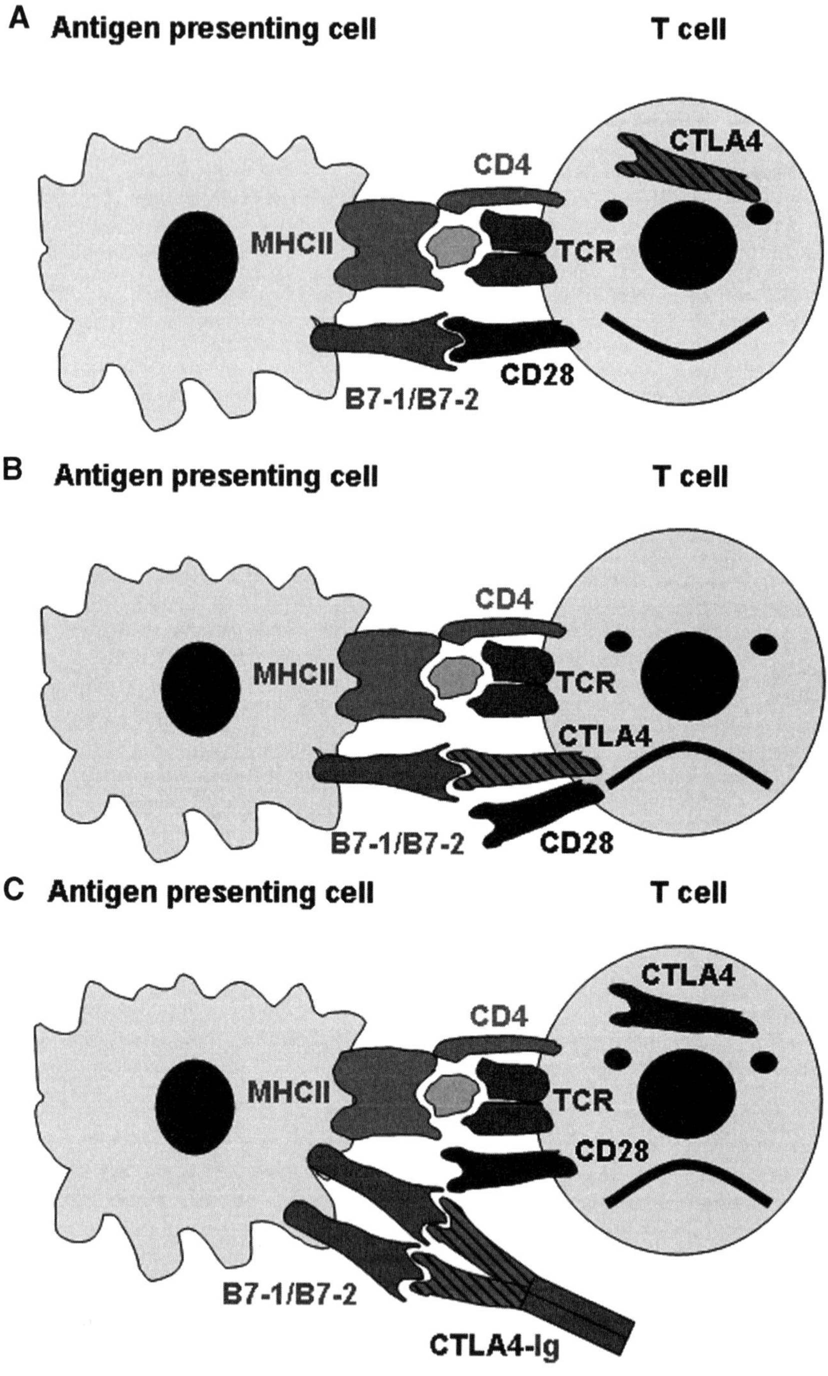

FIGURE 1. *See following page for legend.*

Within inflamed RA joints, IL-15 is produced predominantly by the macrophages of the synovial lining layer. In addition, activated RA fibroblasts and endothelial cells produce IL-15. From animal experiments, further evidence has emerged that IL-15 contributes markedly to the pathogenesis of arthritis and therefore should be a useful target for the treatment of RA.[15] Successful phase I trials and ongoing phase II clinical trials investigating a humanized neutralizing IL-15 antibody reportedly indicate a favorable response; however, the final results of the studies have not been published.

Costimulation Blockade with CTLA4Ig (Abatacept)

To fully activate T cells, two signals are required. Signal 1 originates from the T cell receptor engaging its antigen presented by major histocompatibility complex (MHC) molecules. Signal 2 is delivered by costimulatory molecules (such as CD28) on the surface of T cells. CD28 signaling is initiated by the interaction with members of the B7 family, which are expressed on activated antigen-presenting cells (FIG. 1A). If a T cell receives only signal 1 by T cell receptor stimulation, in the absence of costimulation, the T cell becomes anergic or even undergoes apoptotic cell death. CTLA4, which has a higher affinity for B7 family members than CD28, is expressed by activated T cells, competes for B7 binding, and thereby limits T cell responses (FIG. 1B). A soluble CTLA4Ig fusion protein was developed to specifically block the interaction of CD28 on T cells with its costimulatory ligands of the B7 family on antigen-presenting cells, thereby interfering with T cell activation (FIG. 1C).

In a recently published placebo-controlled, randomized, multicenter study, a total of 339 patients with active RA despite treatment with methotrexate were included and randomized to receive either CTLA4Ig 2 mg/kg body weight, CTLA4Ig 10 mg/kg body weight, or placebo for 6 months in addition to MTX, which was continued throughout the study. The dose-dependent application of CTLA4Ig improved the level of disease activity, as evaluated by the ACR criteria. In the CTLA4Ig 10 mg/kg body-weight group, 60% of patients achieved an ACR20 response, in contrast to 35% of patients in the placebo group. Approximately 23% of patients in the CTLA4Ig 2 mg/kg body-weight group and 36% of patients in the CTLA4Ig 10 mg/kg body-weight group met the ACR50 criteria, in contrast with only 12% of patients in the placebo group.

CTLA4Ig was well tolerated and displayed an overall safety profile similar to placebo.[16] In summary, in RA patients whose disease remains active despite receiving

---

FIGURE 1. Costimulation blockade by CTLA4Ig. **(A)** For their activation, T cells require two signals: Signal 1 originates from the T cell receptor (TCR) engaging its antigen presented by MHC molecules. Signal 2 is delivered by costimulatory molecules such as CD28 on the surface of T cells. CD28 signaling is initiated by the interaction with members of the B7 family, which are expressed on activated antigen-presenting cells such as dendritic cells and macrophages. **(B)** CTLA4, which has a higher affinity for B7 family members than CD28, is expressed by activated T cells, competes for B7 binding, and thereby limits T cell responses. **(C)** A soluble CTLA4Ig fusion protein was developed to specifically block the interaction of CD28 on T cells with its costimulatory ligands of the B7 family on antigen-presenting cells, thereby interfering with T cell activation.

MTX, the addition of the costimulation blocker CTLA4Ig significantly improved signs and symptoms of RA as well as health-related quality of life.

Inhibition of T Cell Activation by Blocking CD2 or CD11a

CD2 is an important stimulatory/costimulatory surface molecule on T cells that binds specifically to CD58 (lymphocyte activation–associated antigen-3 [LFA-3]). Depending on the mode of CD2 ligation, inhibitory or stimulatory signals are delivered to the T cell, or CD2 can just function as an adhesion molecule. A soluble fusion protein consisting of the extracellular domain of CD58 (LFA-3) and the Fc part of human IgG1, named alefacept (Biogen Idec's Amevive), has been shown to efficiently inhibit T cell activation. In psoriasis vulgaris, alefacept treatment resulted in marked clinical improvement associated with a strong reduction in lesional $CD8^+$ lymphocytes and reduced expression of interferon γ, inducible nitric oxide synthase, and IL-8.[17] Alefacept is already approved for the treatment of psoriasis.

CD11a comprises the α subunit of LFA-1 and represents another surface molecule involved in the adhesion and activation of T lymphocytes. CD11a is expressed on T and B lymphocytes, natural killer cells, monocytes/macrophages, and polymorphonuclear cells. Efalizumab is a humanized recombinant antibody against CD11a that interferes with T cell activation.[18] This anti-CD11a antibody was recently licensed for the treatment of psoriasis vulgaris. Alefacept and efalizumab may also be efficacious for the treatment of RA, because T cell activation plays a crucial role in the pathogenesis of RA as well.

Anti-CD20 (Rituximab)

The exact roles of B cells in the pathogenesis of RA remain to be fully elucidated. Most obviously, B cells and plasma cells may play a role as producers of pathogenic autoantibodies, especially rheumatoid factors (RFs), which can form immunocomplexes with IgGs. These immunocomplexes can trigger Fc receptors on macrophages along with the consecutive release of TNF and other proinflammatory cytokines. In addition, B cells may play an even more important role as atypical antigen presenters, thereby contributing to the loss of self-tolerance. In the RA synovial membrane, significant numbers of B cells are present that produce cytokines and contribute to the formation of ectopic lymphoid follicles within the inflamed tissue. The first strong evidence for a role for B cells in RA came from a small open-label study that used the anti-CD20 antibody rituximab in combination with glucocorticoids and cyclophosphamide for the treatment of RA.[19]

The CD20 antigen is expressed on all mature B cells but is absent from B cell precursors and plasma cells. Rituximab is a chimeric anti-CD20 antibody that causes B cell depletion; it does so most likely via antibody-dependent cytotoxicity and, perhaps, additional complement-mediated mechanisms. Rituximab has been approved for the treatment of B cell non-Hodgkin's lymphomas since 1997.

In a recent placebo-controlled, multicenter trial, 161 RA patients whose disease remained active despite MTX treatment were randomly assigned to four treatment arms: (1) oral MTX (as control); (2) rituximab (1000 mg on days 1 and 15); (3) rituximab plus cyclophosphamide (750 mg on days 3 and 17); or (4) rituximab plus MTX. In addition, all groups received glucocorticoids for 17 days. Responses were evaluated at weeks 24 and 48 according to ACR and European League Against Rheumatism (EULAR) criteria. At week 24, 43% of patients treated with rituximab plus MTX and 41% of patients treated with rituximab plus cyclophosphamide had achieved an ACR50 response, compared with 13% of the MTX-only group. At week 48, the rituximab plus MTX group still showed significant improvements according to the ACR20, ACR50, and ACR70 criteria.[20]

Adverse events were observed mainly during the first rituximab infusion and were similar, but generally less severe, than in lymphoma patients. Although the treatment induced a long-lasting depletion of B cells, no major decrease in total immunoglobulin levels and no significant increase in infectious complications were observed during the study period.[20] This trial demonstrated that B cells play a crucial role in the pathogenesis of RA, and that B cell depletion by rituximab represents an efficacious new therapeutic strategy, especially in combination with MTX.

Further Novel Therapeutics in Clinical Investigation for RA

Animal experiments and immunohistochemical studies in RA suggest that complement activation makes an important contribution to the inflammatory process of arthritis. C5a, a 74–amino acid peptide, is released after complement activation and represents a potent chemoattractant for leukocytes, including neutrophils and monocytes/macrophages. A monoclonal antibody against C5 (pexelizumab) is in clinical trials in patients undergoing coronary bypass surgery and angioplasty. Complement inhibition may also prove useful for the treatment of inflammatory diseases such as RA and systemic lupus erythematosus. Recently, peptide and nonpeptide C5a antagonists that are administered orally have been developed.[21]

Chemokines and their receptors are involved in the recruitment of leukocytes to inflamed joints. Therefore, the blockade of certain chemokine receptors such as CCR-1 may also yield a new treatment approach for RA, as suggested by *in vitro* and animal experiments and an initial phase I clinical trial.[22–25]

NEW THERAPEUTIC STRATEGIES FOR IMMUNE SYSTEM INTERVENTION

Mainly based on data from animal experiments, multiple therapeutic approaches are emerging, some of which might be tested in the future for their applicability and efficacy in the treatment of RA. Certain components of the innate immune system appear to be potential drug targets. Promising strategies include blocking toll-like receptors, which mediate a proinflammatory response via nuclear factor kappa beta (NF-κb) activation; neutralizing the proinflammatory activity of extracellular heat-shock proteins and high-mobility group box–1; and interfering with complement activation.[26–28]

Modulating the immune system by inducing antigen-specific regulatory T cells or a shift in T-helper cells (from Th1 to Th2) may profoundly modify the disease course of RA.[29] However, more research will be necessary to enable us to modulate T cell differentiation *in vivo*.

Small molecules that specifically interfere with intracellular signal transduction pathways, such as the MAP-kinase pathway or transcriptional activation of proinflammatory genes, should provide an efficient and cost-effective treatment.[30] However, such drugs may also have more side effects in terms of general immunosuppression compared with the highly specific biologics, which selectively block one effector molecule. The transcription factor NF-κB is critically involved in the expression of many proinflammatory factors and represents a "master switch" for the inflammatory and immune response. Therefore, NF-κB inhibitors have potent anti-inflammatory effects. Specific inhibitors of the IκB kinase β, a key enzyme for NF-κB activation, are now available and have resulted in very efficient amelioration of established arthritis in animal models.[30] Similarly, the transcription factor hypoxia-inducible factor 1α (HIF1α) is activated within inflamed RA synovial tissue. HIF1α appears to play an important role in angiogenesis and the inflammatory response and, hence, represents a potential drug target.[31]

CONCLUSION

Despite considerable progress in the treatment of RA because of the new TNF-blocking biologics (and the presumably somewhat less efficacious IL-1 receptor antagonist), more efficient drugs are urgently needed, especially in nonresponders to anti-TNF therapies. We hope that several new and efficacious biologics now in advanced clinical trials will soon improve our therapeutic armamentarium to fight RA. In addition, a large number of promising novel strategies are in preclinical development. Another important goal of RA research is to identify genetic and other factors that would help predict disease course and the most appropriated drugs for individual patients, enabling tailor-made treatment with increased efficacy and fewer side effects.

REFERENCES

1. van der Heijde, D.M. 1995. Joint erosions and patients with early rheumatoid arthritis. Br. J. Rheumatol. **34** (Suppl 2): 74–78.
2. del Rincon, I. & A. Escalante. 2003. Atherosclerotic cardiovascular disease in rheumatoid arthritis. Curr. Rheumatol. Rep. **5:** 278–286.
3. Weinblatt, M.E., E.C. Keystone, D.E. Furst, *et al.* 2003. Adalimumab, a fully human anti-tumor necrosis factor alpha monoclonal antibody, for the treatment of rheumatoid arthritis in patients taking concomitant methotrexate: the ARMADA trial. Arthritis Rheum. **48:** 35–45.
4. Weinblatt, M.E., J.M. Kremer, A.D. Bankhurst, *et al.* 1999. A trial of etanercept, a recombinant tumor necrosis factor receptor:Fc fusion protein, in patients with rheumatoid arthritis receiving methotrexate. N. Engl. J. Med. **340:** 253–259.
5. Lipsky, P.E., D.M. van der Heijde, E.W. St. Clair, *et al.* 2000. Infliximab and methotrexate in the treatment of rheumatoid arthritis. Anti-Tumor Necrosis Factor Trial in Rheumatoid Arthritis with Concomitant Therapy Study Group. N. Engl. J. Med. **343:** 1594–1602.
6. Mikuls, T.R. & A.L. Weaver. 2003. Lessons learned in the use of tumor necrosis factor-alpha inhibitors in the treatment of rheumatoid arthritis. Curr. Rheumatol. Rep. **5:** 270–277.
7. Hansen, K.E., J.J. Cush, S. Patel, *et al.* 2002. The efficacy of switching from etanercept to infliximab in patients with rheumatoid arthritis. Arthritis Rheum. **46** (Suppl): S538.
8. O'Dell, J.R., C.E. Haire, N. Erikson, *et al.* 1996. Treatment of rheumatoid arthritis with methotrexate alone, sulfasalazine and hydroxychloroquine, or a combination of all three medications. N. Engl. J. Med. **334:** 1287–1291.

9. KIELY, P.D. & D.M. JOHNSON. 2002. Infliximab and leflunomide combination therapy in rheumatoid arthritis: an open-label study. Rheumatology (Oxford). **41:** 631–637.
10. ANTONI, C.E., H.G. NUESSLEIN, J. WOLLENHAUPT, G.R. BURMESTER, *et al.* 2004. Combination treatment with infliximab and leflunomide in patients with active rheumatoid arthritis: safety and efficacy in an open label clinical trial. Ann. Rheum. Dis. **63** (Suppl. I): 276.
11. WILLIAMS, R.O., L.J. MASON, M. FELDMANN & R.N. MAINI. 1994. Synergy between anti-CD4 and anti-tumor necrosis factor in the amelioration of established collagen-induced arthritis. Proc. Natl. Acad. Sci. USA **91:** 2762–2766.
12. HOUSSIAU, F.A., J.P. DEVOGELAER, J. VAN DAMME, *et al.* 1988. Interleukin-6 in synovial fluid and serum of patients with rheumatoid arthritis and other inflammatory arthritides. Arthritis Rheum. **31:** 784–788.
13. MADHOK, R., A. CRILLY, J. WATSON & H.A. CAPELL. 1993. Serum interleukin 6 levels in rheumatoid arthritis: correlations with clinical and laboratory indices of disease activity. Ann. Rheum. Dis. **52:** 232–234.
14. NISHIMOTO, N., K. Yoshizaki, N. Miyasaka, *et al.* 2004. Treatment of rheumatoid arthritis with humanized anti-interleukin-6 receptor antibody: a multicenter, double-blind, placebo-controlled trial. Arthritis Rheum. **50:** 1761–1769.
15. MCINNES, I.B. & J.A. GRACIE. 2004. Interleukin-15: a new cytokine target for the treatment of inflammatory diseases. Curr. Opin. Pharmacol. **4:** 392–397.
16. KREMER, J.M., R. WESTHOVENS, M. LEON, *et al.* 2003. Treatment of rheumatoid arthritis by selective inhibition of T-cell activation with fusion protein CTLA4Ig. N. Engl. J. Med. **349:** 1907–1915.
17. CHAMIAN, F., M.A. LOWES, S.L. LIN, *et al.* 2005. Alefacept reduces infiltrating T cells, activated dendritic cells, and inflammatory genes in psoriasis vulgaris. Proc. Natl. Acad. Sci. USA **102:** 2075–2080.
18. MENTER, A., K. GORDON, W. CAREY, *et al.* 2005. Efficacy and safety observed during 24 weeks of efalizumab therapy in patients with moderate to severe plaque psoriasis. Arch. Dermatol. **141:** 31–38.
19. EDWARDS, J.C. & G. CAMBRIDGE. 2001. Sustained improvement in rheumatoid arthritis following a protocol designed to deplete B lymphocytes. Rheumatology (Oxford). **40:** 205–211.
20. EDWARDS, J.C., L. SZCZEPANSKI, J. SZECHINSKI, *et al.* 2004. Efficacy of B-cell-targeted therapy with rituximab in patients with rheumatoid arthritis. N. Engl. J. Med. **350:** 2572–2581.
21. ALLEGRETTI, M., A. MORICONI, A.R. BECCARI, *et al.* 2005. Targeting C5a: recent advances in drug discovery. Curr. Med. Chem. **12:** 217–236.
22. BERTINI, R., M. ALLEGRETTI, C. BIZZARRI, *et al.* 2004. Noncompetitive allosteric inhibitors of the inflammatory chemokine receptors CXCR1 and CXCR2: prevention of reperfusion injury. Proc. Natl. Acad. Sci. USA. **101:** 11791–11796.
23. SOUZA, D.G., R. BERTINI, A.T. VIEIRA, *et al.* 2004. Repertaxin, a novel inhibitor of rat CXCR2 function, inhibits inflammatory responses that follow intestinal ischaemia and reperfusion injury. Br. J. Pharmacol. **143:** 132–142.
24. HARINGMAN, J.J., M.C. KRAAN, T.J. SMEETS, *et al.* 2003. Chemokine blockade and chronic inflammatory disease: proof of concept in patients with rheumatoid arthritis. Ann. Rheum. Dis. **62:** 715–721.
25. GLADUE, R.P., S.H. ZWILLICH, A.T. CLUCAS & M.F. BROWN. 2004. CCR1 antagonists for the treatment of autoimmune diseases. Curr. Opin. Investig. Drugs. **5:** 499–504.
26. ANDREAKOS, E., B. FOXWELL & M. FELDMANN. 2004. Is targeting Toll-like receptors and their signaling pathway a useful therapeutic approach to modulating cytokine-driven inflammation? Immunol. Rev. **202:** 250–265.
27. TANIGUCHI, N., K. KAWAHARA, K. YONE, *et al.* 2003. High mobility group box chromosomal protein 1 plays a role in the pathogenesis of rheumatoid arthritis as a novel cytokine. Arthritis Rheum. **48:** 971–981.
28. KOKKOLA, R., J. LI, E. SUNDBERG, *et al.* 2003. Successful treatment of collagen-induced arthritis in mice and rats by targeting extracellular high mobility group box chromosomal protein 1 activity. Arthritis Rheum. **48:** 2052–2058.

29. SCHULZE-KOOPS, H. & J.R. KALDEN. 2001. The balance of Th1/Th2 cytokines in rheumatoid arthritis. Best Pract. Res. Clin. Rheumatol. **15:** 677–691.
30. MOREL, J. & F. BERENBAUM. 2004. Signal transduction pathways: new targets for treating rheumatoid arthritis. Joint Bone Spine. **71:** 503–510.
31. GIATROMANOLAKI, A., E. SIVRIDIS, E. MALTEZOS, *et al.* 2003. Upregulated hypoxia inducible factor-1alpha and -2alpha pathway in rheumatoid arthritis and osteoarthritis. Arthritis Res. Ther. **5:** R193–R201.

Index of Contributors